Essential Atlas of
Cardiovascular Disease

Peter Libby, MD

Mallinckrodt Professor of Medicine
Harvard Medical School
Chief
Cardiovascular Division
Brigham and Women's Hospital
Boston, Massachusetts

With 31 Contributors
Developed by Current Medicine Group LLC

Springer

CURRENT MEDICINE GROUP LLC, PART OF SPRINGER SCIENCE+BUSINESS MEDIA LLC

400 Market Street, Suite 700 • Philadelphia, PA 19106

Senior Developmental Editor . . . . Lee Klein
Editorial Assistant . . . . Juleen Deaner
Design and Layout . . . . Daniel Britt and William Whitman Jr
Illustrators . . . . Kim Broadbent, Marie Dean, Heather Hoch, Sara Krause, Wieslawa Langenfeld,
Jacqueline Leonard, Maureen Looney, Andrea Penko
Creative Director . . . . Wendy Vetter
Production Coordinator . . . . Carolyn Naylor
Indexer . . . . Holly Lukens

Library of Congress Cataloging-in-Publication Data

Essential atlas of cardiovascular disease / editor, Peter Libby ; with 31 contributors. -- 1st ed.
  p. ; cm.
 Includes bibliographical references and index.
 ISBN-13: 978-1-57340-309-2 (alk. paper)
 ISBN-10: 1-57340-309-1 (alk. paper)
 1. Cardiovascular system--Diseases--Atlases. I. Libby, Peter. II. Title.
 [DNLM: 1. Cardiovascular Diseases--Atlases. WG 17 E778 2009]

RC669.9.E87 2009
616.1--dc22

2009000297

ISBN 978-1-57340-309-2
ISBN 1-57340-309-1

www.springer.com

For more information, please call 1 (800) 777-4643
or email us at orders-ny@springer.com

www.currentmedicinegroup.com

10 9 8 7 6 5 4 3 2 1

Printed in China by L. Rex Printing Company Limited

This book was printed on acid-free paper

Preface

No medical specialty depends more on images and graphics than cardiovascular diseases. No medical specialty moves faster than contemporary cardiovascular medicine. How can the busy practitioner keep apace to learn and apply the rapid advances and ever-increasing palette of diagnostic and management strategies available for our patients?

Visual imagery and concise "take home" bullets provide a very effective teaching and learning tool. The *Atlas of Heart Diseases* series, founded by Dr. Eugene Braunwald, recognized this need and offered a solution, and also provided a strong foundation for this atlas. The *Essential Atlas of Cardiovascular Disease* has the ambitious goal of providing a condensed and palatable yet comprehensive update of major principles and recent advances in cardiovascular medicine of practical importance to cardiovascular specialists, internists, primary care physicians, and practitioners of non-medical specialties in their daily clinical work. For this purpose, we have assembled an expert team of leading authorities in their areas to contribute a series of chapters that embrace the most important areas in cardiovascular medicine. By focusing on images, graphical representations of essential data, and highly distilled textual material, this compendium aims to provide a convenient and practical tool to help practitioners master key aspects of cardiovascular medicine. We focus on the most important and common clinical problems that confront physicians on a regular basis. We highlight the availability of new diagnostic and management tools without neglecting the tried-and-true, while striving to acquaint the reader with the strengths and weaknesses of these modalities in a balanced fashion. The contributors and editor have designed this volume to serve as a ready reference for a specific problem confronted by the physician in practice, as well as a background source for easy perusal during spare moments. We offer this update to the previous compilation atlas edited by Dr. Eugene Braunwald with the hope that we meet our goal of providing a convenient and palatable source for reference and continued learning.

Dedication

I take great pride in dedicating this book to my career-long mentor, Dr. Eugene Braunwald, the founder and editor of the series on which this atlas is based. I met Dr. Braunwald on my first day of medical school, and over the past four decades he has provided an unending and generous source of inspiration and learning. In medical school, Dr. Braunwald whetted my appetite for what has been a lifelong quest for understanding pathophysiology in the service of clinical medicine. As a research fellow in his laboratory he guided my fledgling steps as a cardiovascular investigator. When I was a house officer in the program that Dr. Braunwald directed he spurred me to apply the same rigor and reasoning to clinical problems that we applied in the research laboratory, while never neglecting the human aspects of medicine. As a fellow and faculty member, his example of indefatigable devotion and unrelenting quest for excellence served as a north star for me, among hundreds of others whose careers he shaped. When entrusted with a leadership position later in my career, I continued to learn from Dr. Braunwald, both by example and by patient mentorship, how to navigate the challenges without losing sight of fundamental values and guiding principles. Over the last decade, I have had the privilege of learning the art of medical editing from the Master. I learn still from him at every encounter, and therefore dedicate this edition of the *Essential Atlas of Cardiovascular Disease* to Eugene Braunwald.

Acknowledgment

I thank Ms. Joan Perry for her skillful and dedicated editorial assistance, Ms. Patricia Yee and Mr. David Lynn for their daily help, and my wife Beryl Benacerraf, MD, for her continuous loving and infinitely patient support and forbearance during the preparation of this volume and so many other projects over the last third of a century.

Peter Libby, MD

Contributors

Elliott Antman, MD
Professor of Medicine
Cardiovascular Division
Brigham and Women's Hospital
Senior Investigator, TIMI Study Group
Boston, Massachusetts

Kenneth L. Baughman, MD
Professor
Department of Medicine
Harvard Medical School
Director
Advanced Heart Disease Section
Brigham and Women's Hospital
Boston, Massachusetts

Matthew J. Budoff, MD
Associate Professor of Medicine-UCLA
  School of Medicine
Director of Cardiac CT
Los Angeles Biomedical Research Institute
Harbor-UCLA Medical Center
Los Angeles, California

Wilson S. Colucci, MD, FACC, FAHA
Thomas J. Ryan Professor of Medicine
Boston University School of Medicine
Chief, Cardiovascular Medicine
Department of Medicine
Boston University Medical Center
Boston, Massachusetts

Mark A. Creager, MD
Professor of Medicine
Harvard Medical School
Director, Vascular Center
Simon C. Fireman Scholar in
  Cardiovascular Medicine
Department of Medicine
Brigham and Women's Hospital
Boston, Massachusetts

Marcelo F. Di Carli, MD
Chief of Nuclear Medicine
Brigham and Women's Hospital
Assistant Professor of Radiology and Medicine
Harvard Medical School
Boston, Massachusetts

Vasken Dilsizian, MD
Professor
Department of Medicine and Radiology
University of Maryland School of Medicine
Chief
Division of Nuclear Medicine
Director
Cardiovascular Nuclear Medicine and
  PET Imaging
University of Maryland School of Medicine
Baltimore, Maryland

Jean-Francois Dorval, MD
Advanced Interventional Cardiovascular
  Medicine Fellow
Department of Cardiovascular Medicine
Harvard Medical School
Brigham and Women's Hospital
Boston, Massachusetts

Laurence M. Epstein, MD
Associate Professor of Medicine
Department of Medicine
Harvard Medical School
Chief
Arrhythmia Service
Cardiovascular Division
Brigham and Women's Hospital
Boston, Massachusetts

J. Michael Gaziano, MD
Associate Professor of Medicine
Harvard Medical School
Chief
Division of Aging
Department of Medicine
Brigham and Women's Hospital
Director, MAVERIC
VA Boston Healthcare System
Boston, Massachusetts

Michael M. Givertz, MD
Associate Professor of Medicine
Harvard Medical School
Brigham and Women's Hospital
Boston, Massachusetts

Samuel Z. Goldhaber, MD
Professor of Medicine
Harvard Medical School
Senior Physician
Director, Cardiovascular Division
Co-Director, Venous Thromboembolism
Research Group,
  Anticoagulation Management Service
Boston, Massachusetts

Norman K. Hollenberg, MD, PhD
Professor
Department of Medicine
Harvard Medical School
Director
Radiology/Physiologic Research Division
Brigham and Women's Hospital
Boston, Massachusetts

Marc Z. Krichavsky, MD
Advanced Interventional Cardiovascular
  Medicine Fellow
Department of Medicine
Harvard Medical School
Department of Internal
  Medicine/Cardiovascular Medicine
Brigham and Women's Hospital
Boston, Massachusetts

Raymond Y. Kwong, MD, MPH, FACC
Assistant Professor
Cardiovascular Division
Department of Medicine
Harvard Medical School
Boston, Massachusetts

Michael J. Landzberg, MD
Assistant Professor
Department of Medicine
Harvard Medical School
BACH (Boston Adult Congenital Heart) and
  Pulmonary Hypertension Group
Departments of Cardiology and Medicine
Children's Hospital and Brigham and
  Women's Hospital
Boston, Massachusetts

Judy Mangion, MD
Assistant Professor
Department of Cardiovascular Medicine
Harvard Medical School
Associate Director
Noninvasive Cardiac Laboratory
Brigham and Women's Hospital
Boston, Massachusetts

David A. Morrow, MD, MPH
Associate Professor of Medicine
Harvard Medical School
Attending Physician
Cardiovascular Division
Brigham and Women's Hospital
Boston, Massachusetts

Jagat Narula, MD, PhD
Professor of Medicine
Chief
Division of Cardiology
Associate Dean for Research
University of California Irvine Medical Center
Orange, California

Patrick T. O'Gara, MD
Associate Professor of Medicine
Harvard Medical School
Director
Clinical Cardiology
Cardiovascular Division
Brigham and Women's Hospital
Boston, Massachusetts

Gregory Piazza, MD
Clinical Instructor in Medicine
Harvard Medical School
Fellow in Vascular Medicine
Brigham and Women's Hospital
Boston, Massachusetts

Andrew J. Powell, MD
Assistant Professor
Department of Pediatrics
Harvard Medical School
Associate in Cardiology
Department of Cardiology
Children's Hospital Boston
Affiliate Staff
Department of Newborn Medicine
Brigham and Women's Hospital
Boston, Massachusetts

Frederic S. Resnic, MD, MSc
Assistant Professor
Department of Medicine
Harvard Medical School
Director
Cardiac Catheterization Laboratory
Cardiovascular Division
Brigham and Women's Hospital
Boston, Massachusetts

Kurt C. Roberts-Thomson, MBBS
Research Fellow
Department of Medicine
Harvard Medical School
Cardiovascular Division
Brigham and Women's Hospital
Boston, Massachusetts

Vincent Y. See, MD
Fellow
Cardiac Arrhythmia Service
Cardiovascular Division
Brigham and Women's Hospital
Fellow
Department of Genetics
Harvard Medical School
Boston, Massachusetts

Jens Seiler, MD
Research Fellow in Medicine
Department of Medicine/Cardiology
Harvard Medical School
Brigham and Women's Hospital
Boston, Massachusetts

Pinak B. Shah, MD
Assistant Professor of Medicine
Harvard Medical School
Director
Interventional Cardiology Fellowship
Cardiovascular Division
Brigham and Women's Hospital
Boston, Massachusetts

Scott D. Solomon, MD
Associate Professor
Department of Medicine
Harvard Medical School
Director
Noninvasive Cardiac Laboratory
Cardiovascular Division
Brigham and Women's Hospital
Boston, Massachusetts

Daniel Steven, MD
Research Fellow
Harvard Medical School
Cardiac Arrhythmia Service
Brigham and Women's Hospital
Boston, Massachusetts

William G. Stevenson, MD
Professor of Medicine
Department of Internal Medicine
Cardiovascular Division
Harvard Medical School
Brigham and Women's Hospital
Boston, Massachusetts

Anne Marie Valente, MD
Instructor
Department of Pediatrics
Harvard Medical School
Assistant in Cardiology
Division of Cardiology
Brigham and Women's Hospital
Assistant in Cardiology
Department of Cardiology
Children's Hospital Boston
Boston, Massachusetts

Contents

Atherosclerosis Risk Factors

J. Michael Gaziano and Peter Libby

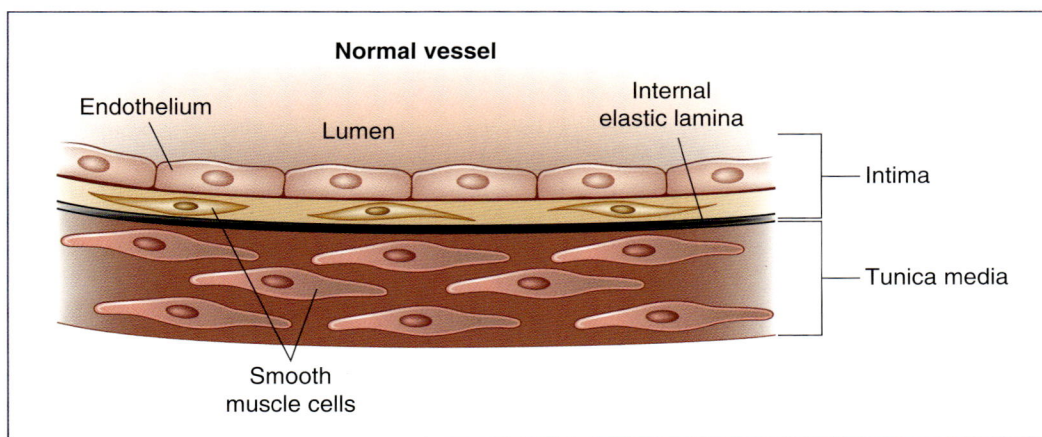

Figure 1-1. The normal artery consists of a monolayer of endothelial cells that overlie the innermost layer or the tunica intima of the artery. The intima of human arteries most often contains resident smooth muscle cells. The normal endothelial cell displays an array of homeostatic properties including tonic vasodilatation due to nitric oxide production. The normal endothelial monolayer also resists prolonged contact with inflammatory cells, maintains blood in a liquid state, and exerts a number of other atheroprotective functions. The internal elastic lamina divides the intima from the underlying tunica media. This middle layer of human arteries normally consists of vascular smooth muscle cells arrayed in a complex but well-ordered extracellular matrix made of interstitial collagen and elastin, among other constituents. This figure does not depict the outermost layer, the adventitia.

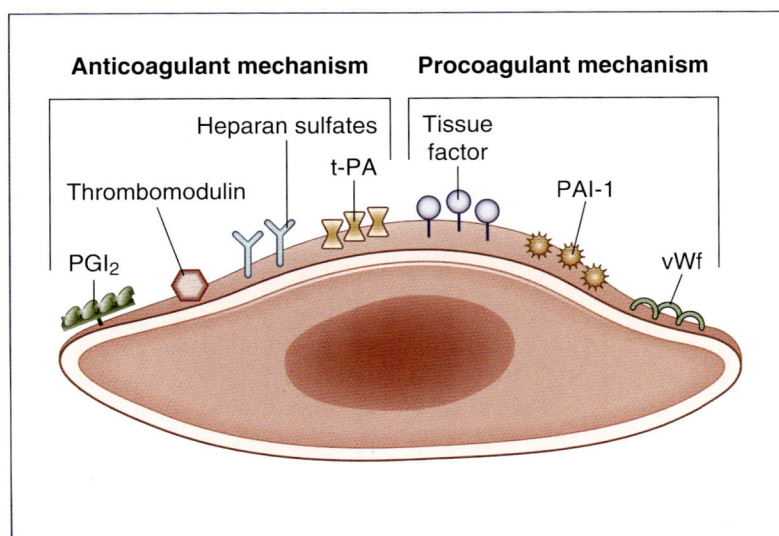

Figure 1-2. The normal endothelial monolayer resists blood coagulation by production of surface-linked thrombomodulin, an activator of the anticoagulant protein C pathway, as well as the elaboration of endogenous heparin-like molecules. The normal endothelium also promotes fibrinolysis due to the expression of endogenous plasminogen activators of the tissue (t-PA) and urokinase type. Under normal conditions, endothelial cells make relatively little plasminogen activator inhibitor-1 (PAI-1). When stimulated, for example by exposure to proinflammatory cytokines, or disturbed flow, the endothelium changes this normal homeostatic balance toward one that favors coagulation of blood and resists fibrinolysis, in part by heightened expression of PAI-1 [1]. PGI_2—prostacyclin; vWf—von Willebrand factor.

Figure 1-3. When the artery wall encounters stimuli—such as those associated with risk factors, including dyslipidemia, hypertension, and insulin resistance—the normal homeostatic panel of endothelial functions becomes dysregulated. The endothelial cells can express adhesion molecules that cause the attachment of blood leukocytes. Vascular cell adhesion molecule-1 (VCAM-1), an adhesion molecule from monocytes not expressed by normal endothelial cells, increases rapidly after initiation of an atherogenic diet in several animal species. Chemokines, such as monocyte chemoattractant protein-1 (MCP-1) that interact with receptors such as chemokine receptor 2 (CCR2) on the surface of the leukocyte, cause the cell to penetrate into the tunica media. Blood monocytes, the most numerous inflammatory cells that enter atherosclerotic lesions, change into macrophage-derived foam cells after recruitment to the intima. The expression of scavenger receptors allows these macrophages to capture modified lipoproteins and engulf the lipid, creating the characteristic foamy appearance. Among the mediators that cause monocyte differentiation into macrophages and promote the division of macrophages, macrophage-colony stimulating factor (M-CSF) plays a prominent role. Once resident in the artery wall, the activated macrophage can secrete many mediators, including matrix metalloproteinases (MMPs), cytokines (proinflammatory proteins), reactive oxygen species (ROS), and the procoagulant protein tissue factor. These mediators can spur the progression and complication of the atherosclerotic lesions. Ultimately, many macrophages can die, often due to programmed cell death or apoptosis. Tissue factor–rich apoptotic bodies spun off by dying macrophages may provide an important procoagulant stimulus if they enter the circulation. (*Adapted from* Libby [2]; with permission).

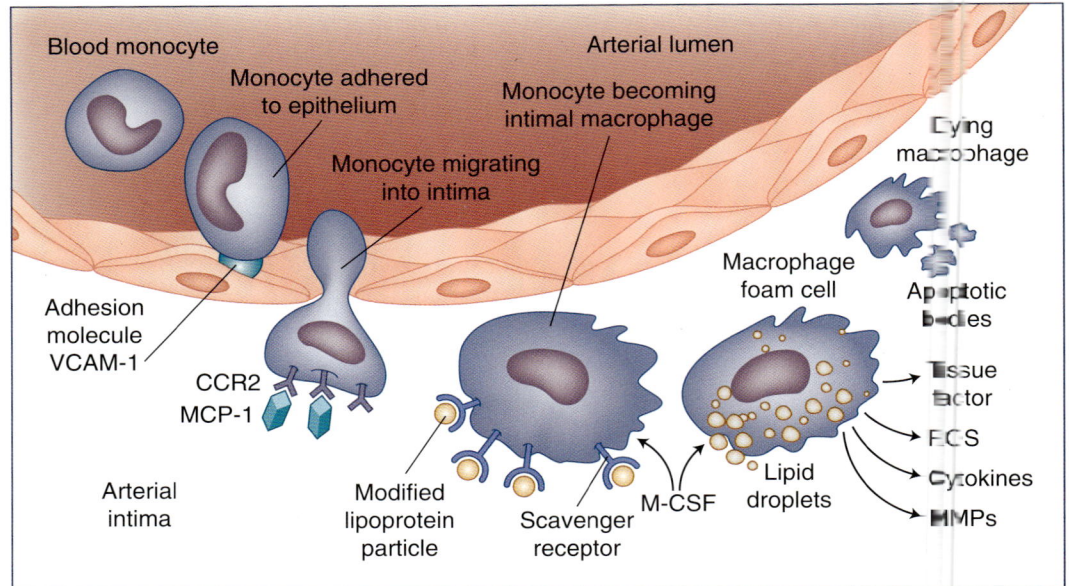

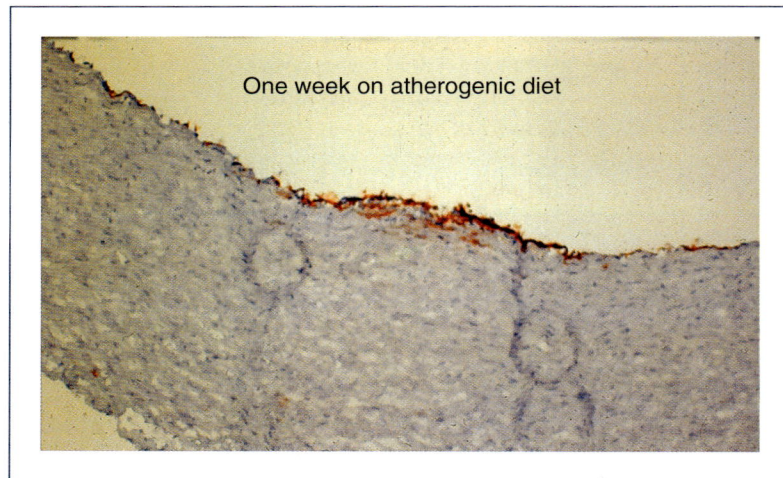

Figure 1-4. Vascular cell adhesion molecule-1 (VCAM-1) expression in rabbit aorta. This figure shows a cross-section of the aorta of a rabbit that has consumed an atherogenic diet enriched in cholesterol and saturated fat for one week. The red-stained patch of endothelial cells indicates the presence of VCAM-1 stained with a monoclonal antibody. Genetic studies in mice have proven a role for VCAM-1 in lesion initiation during experimental atherosclerosis. Other adhesion molecules also contribute to leukocyte recruitment during early atherogenesis, including P-selectin, for example. (*Adapted from* Li et al. [3]; with permission.)

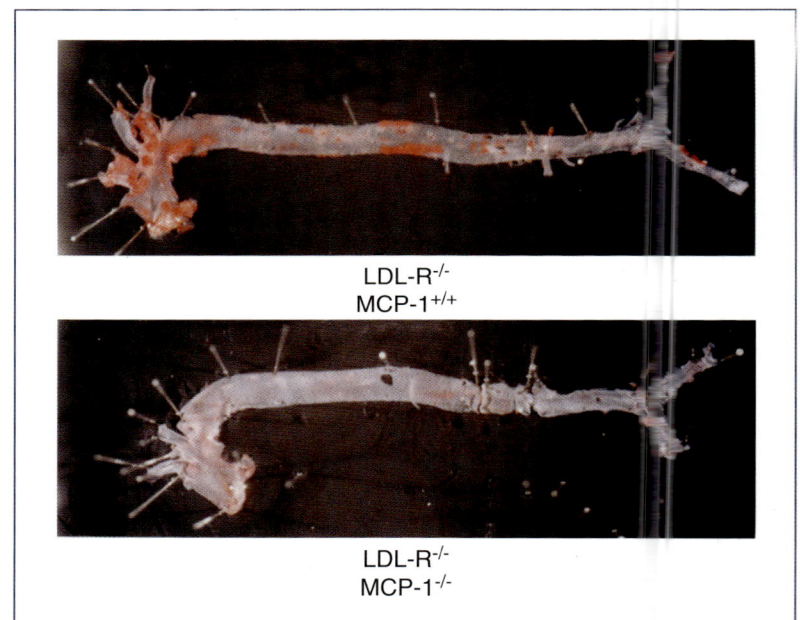

Figure 1-5. Reduced lipid deposition in monocyte chemoattractant protein-1 (MCP-1)–deficient atherosclerotic mice. This figure depicts aortas from mice that have undergone genetic alterations and consumed an atherogenic diet. The red staining indicates accumulation of lipid. In the upper panel the mouse has been rendered susceptible to diet-induced atherosclerosis by inactivation of both alleles that encode the low-density lipoprotein (LDL) receptor, yielding a mouse that resembles humans with homozygous familial hypercholesterolemia. Note the considerable lipid accumulation in the aortic arch and descending aorta. The representative figure shown in the lower panel depicts the lipid-stained aorta from a mouse that lacks LDL receptors and has also undergone genetic inactivation of both alleles that encode MCP-1. Note the marked reduction in atherosclerosis. Such experiments in compound-mutant mice have allowed researchers to unravel various steps in the pathogenesis of atherosclerosis and the mediators that cause these changes in arterial biology. (*Adapted from* Gu et al. [4]; with permission.)

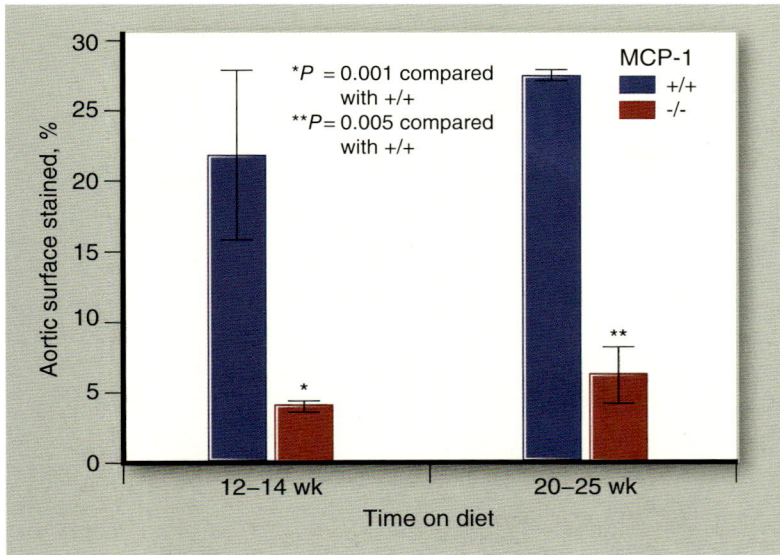

Figure 1-6. This figure depicts quantitative data from experiments exemplified in Figure 1-5. The lipid staining in aortas removed at two timepoints shows the marked reduction in atherosclerotic lesion formation in the animals that lack monocyte chemoattractant protein-1 (*red bars*). MCP-1—monocyte chemoattractant protein-1. (*Adapted from* Gu *et al.* [4]; with permission.)

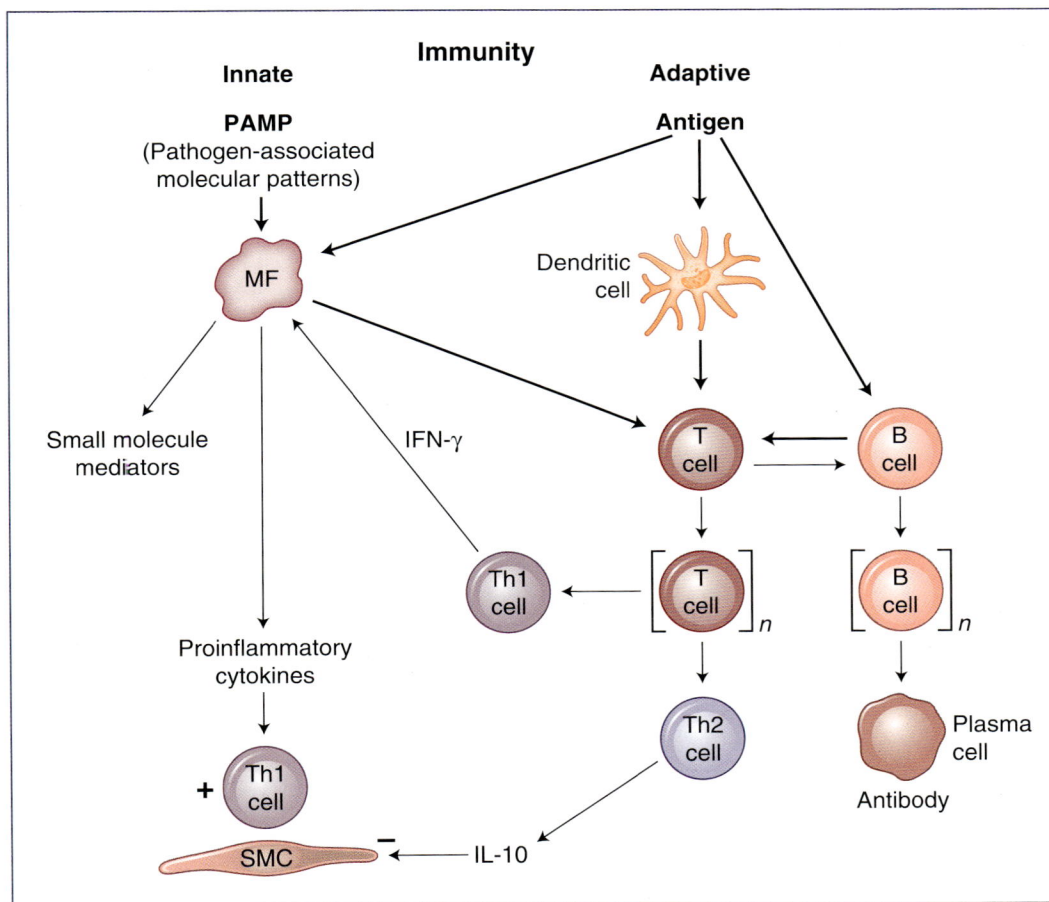

Figure 1-7. In addition to macrophages (MF), an entire spectrum of leukocytes involved in both innate and adaptive immunity operate in atherosclerotic lesions. Innate immunity involves activation of macrophages that produce small molecule proinflammatory mediators and proinflammatory cytokines invoked in atherogenesis and lesion complication. Dendritic cells present in the artery wall can survey the environment for potential antigens and present them to T cells. When T cells encounter their cognate antigen including candidates such as oxidatively modified low-density lipoprotein, the T cells can proliferate and differentiate either into Th1 or Th2 helper T cells. The Th1 cells secrete interferon gamma (IFN-γ) that can augment innate immunity by stimulating macrophages. The activated macrophage can elaborate many mediators that amplify and sustain the inflammatory process in the artery wall (*see* Fig. 1-3). Th2 cells may limit inflammation by secreting anti-inflammatory cytokines, such as interleukin-10 (IL-10), that can dampen the inflammatory response. The Th2 response also involves elaboration of antibodies by B cells. The humoral limb of the innate immune response may also regulate aspects of atherogenesis. (*Adapted from* Hansson *et al.* [5]; with permission.)

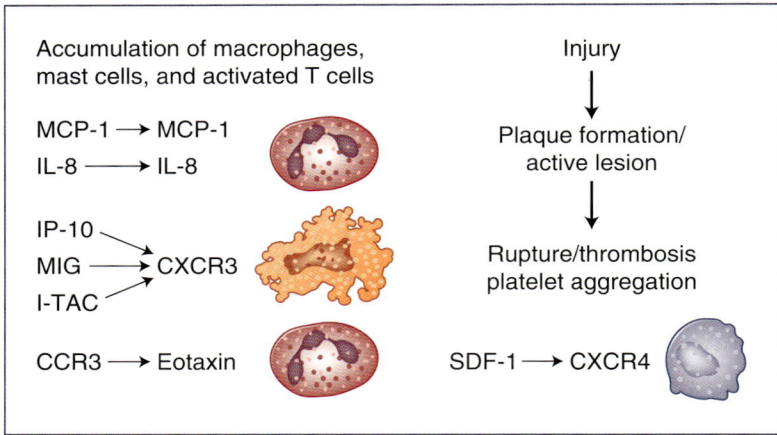

Figure 1-8. Chemokines and atherosclerosis. Many chemokines in addition to monocyte chemoattractant protein-1 (MCP-1) may contribute to cellular recruitment and activation during atherogenesis. Many of these chemoattractant cytokines and their cognate receptors recruit or activate different cell types. MCP-1 and interleukin-8 (IL-8) tend to recruit primarily monocytes. A trio of chemokines that are induced by interferon gamma (IFN-γ), known as inducible protein 10 (IP-10), monokine induced by gamma–interferon (MIG), and interferon-inducible T cell alpha-chemoattractant (I-TAC), can recruit T lymphocytes to plaques by engaging the receptor CXCR3. The chemokine Eotaxin may recruit mast cells to plaques. The chemokine stromal cell derived factor-1 (SDF-1) can activate platelets, causing their aggregation. Thus, inflammation involving not only leukocytes but also platelets can participate in atherogenesis.

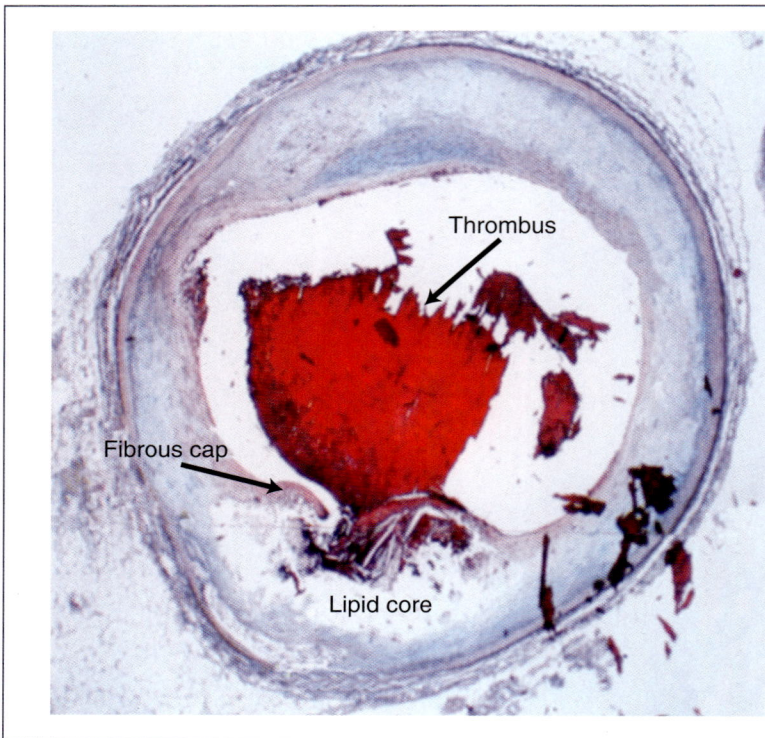

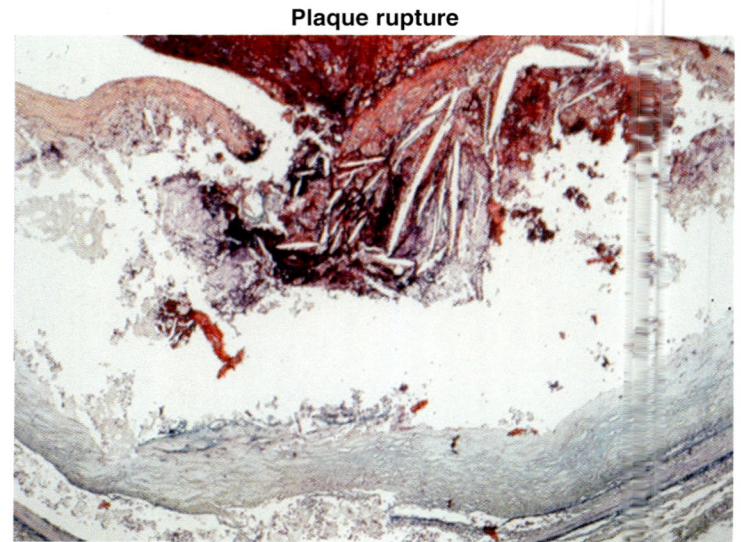

Figure 1-9. Most fatal coronary thromboses result from a rupture of the atherosclerotic plaque. This figure shows a cross-section through a coronary artery from a patient who succumbed due to the thrombus shown in red. Note that this fatal thrombus occurred despite the lack of a critical stenosis in this artery. The thrombus arose because of a fracture of the plaque's fibrous cap that allowed the blood with its coagulation proteins contact with the tissue-factor rich lipid core. Thus, the plaque disruption, shown at higher power in the inset, precipitated the thrombus that killed this patient. (*Courtesy of* Dr. M.L. Higuchi.)

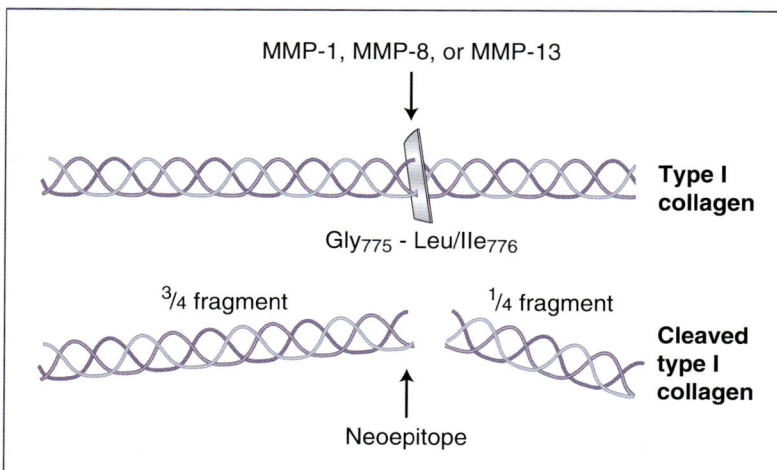

Figure 1-10. Interstitial collagenases. The integrity of the plaque's protective fibrous cap depends on interstitial collagens (*triple helix*). Ordinarily very stable, interstitial collagenases produced by activated macrophages in the plaque can attack the intact collagen fibril and initiate its breakdown. The interstitial collagenases matrix metalloproteinase (MMP)-1, -8, and -13 abound in atheromatous plaques. Excessive catabolism of collagen can weaken the fibrous cap, rendering it thin and susceptible to rupture and hence thrombosis (*see* Fig. 1-9).

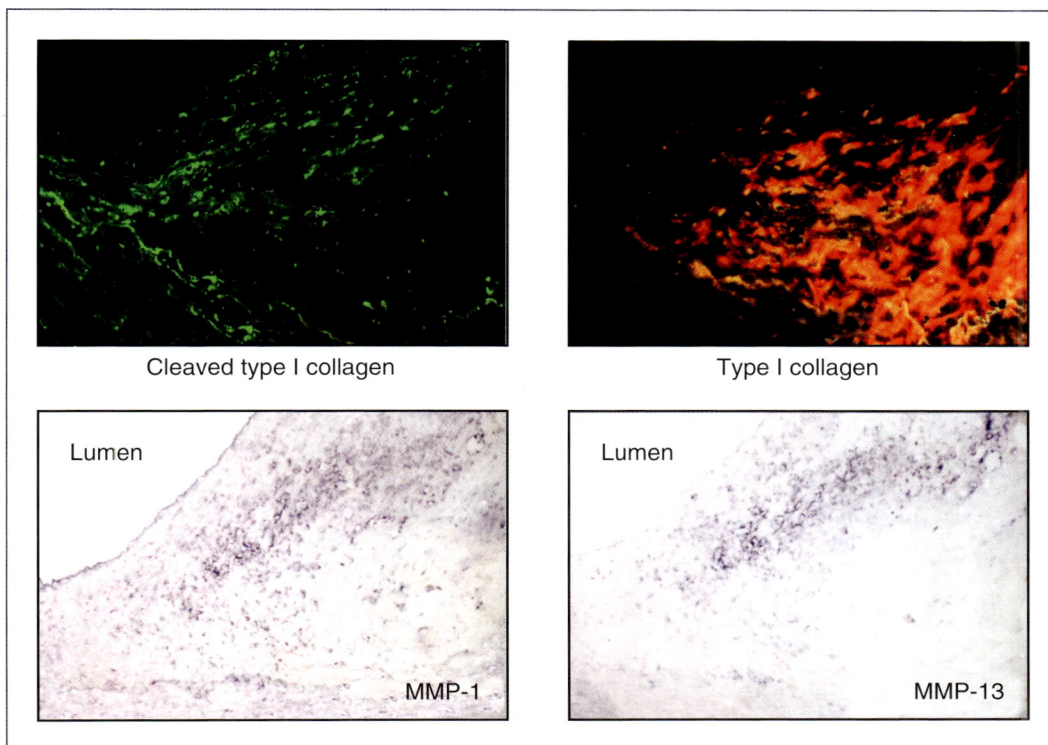

Figure 1-11. Cleaved collagen colocalizes with matrix metalloproteinase (MMP)-1 and MMP-13 in human atheroma. Regions of overexpression of the interstitial collagenases MMP-1 and MMP-13 (*bottom panels*) correlate with regions of collagen cleavage (*fluorescent green in upper left panel*) signal due to binding of an antibody that selectively recognizes partially degraded collagen. The area of MMP overexpression and collagen cleavage surrounds a region of intact type 1 collagen in the plaque's cap (*orange in upper right panel*). (*Adapted from* Sukhova *et al.* [6]; with permission.)

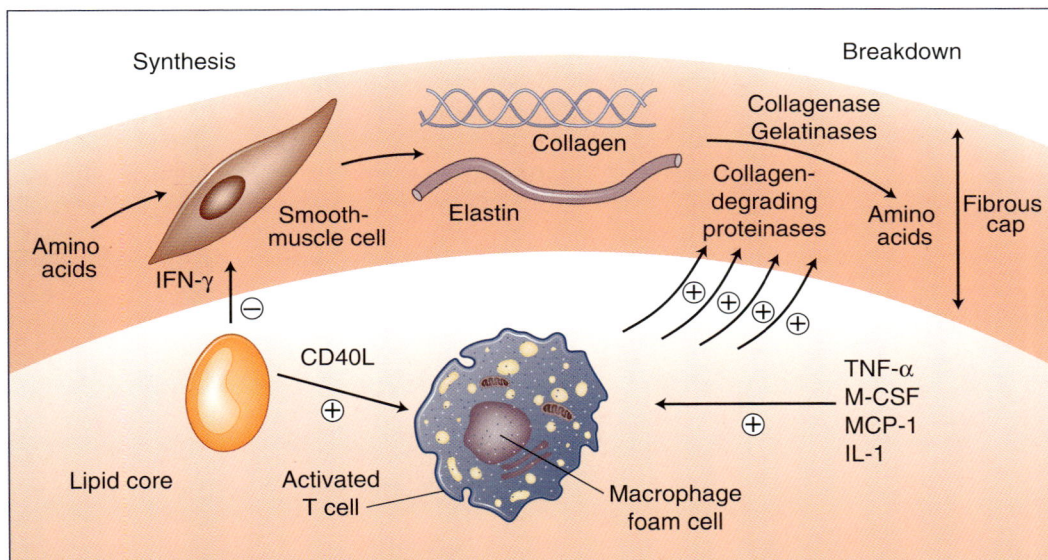

Figure 1-12. Molecular biology of the high-risk plaque. We now understand in considerable detail the molecular and cellular pathogenesis of plaque rupture in the acute coronary syndromes. According to this scheme, the activated T cell in blue can elaborate an inhibitor of collagen synthesis by smooth muscle cells (*red*). The T lymphocyte can also elicit the overproduction of collagen-degrading proteinases from the macrophage foam cell in the center due to the action of the cytokine CD-40 ligand (CD40L), a product of activated T cells. CD40L can also induce overexpression of tissue factor procoagulant by human mononuclear phagocytes. Proinflammatory cytokines present in the atherosclerotic plaque—such as interleukin-1 (IL-1), tumor necrosis factor alpha (TNF-α), the chemokine monocyte chemoattractant protein-1 (MCP-1), and macrophage colony stimulating factor (M-CSF)—can all amplify macrophage activation. Thus, inflammation regulates both the stability of the plaque's protective fibrous cap and the thrombogenicity of the lipid core. This schema, supported by substantial experimental data and many observations on human specimens, points to the pivotal role of inflammation in precipitation of the acute coronary syndromes. (*Adapted from* Libby [7]; with permission.)

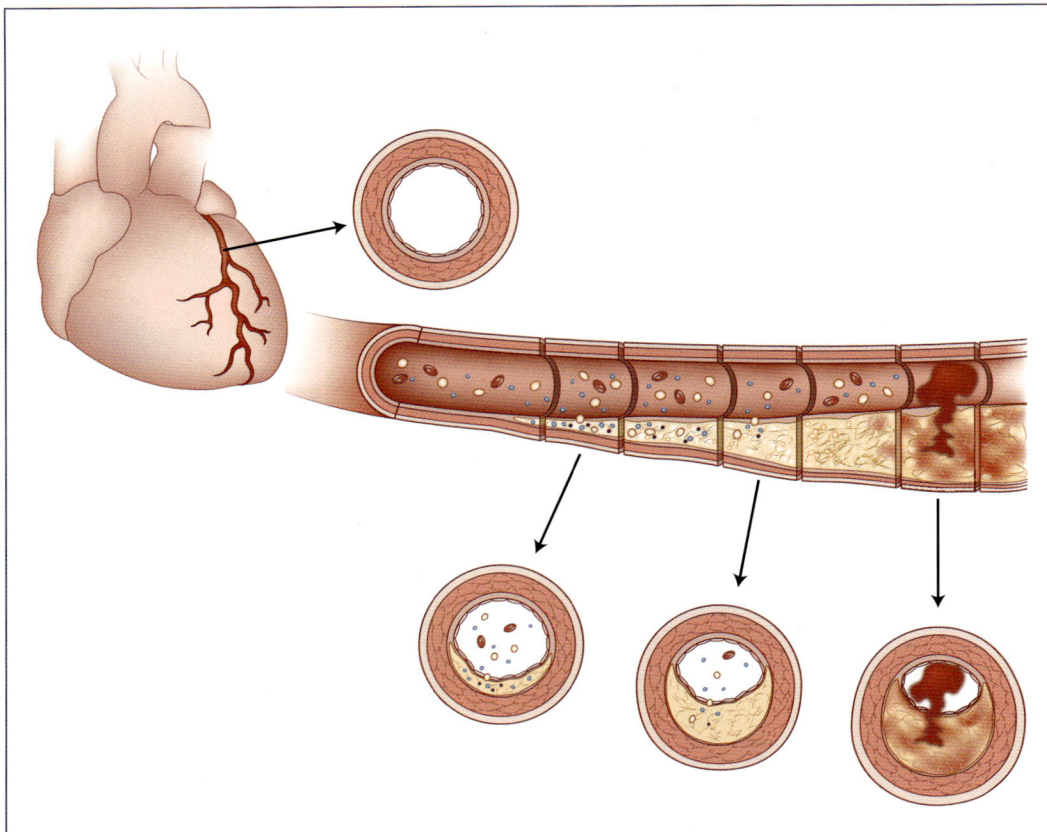

Figure 1-13. All stages of atherosclerosis from initiation (*left inset*), progression (*middle*), and thrombotic complications (*right side*) involve inflammation [8].

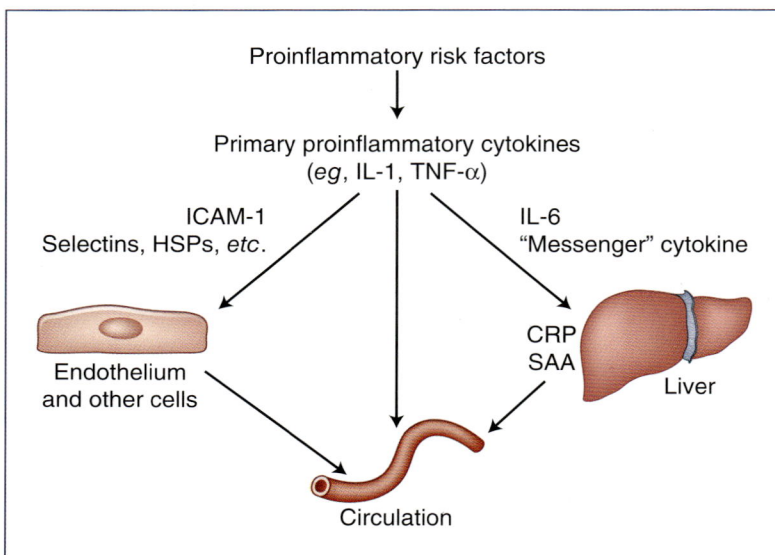

Proinflammatory risk factors

↓

Primary proinflammatory cytokines
(*eg*, IL-1, TNF-α)

ICAM-1
Selectins, HSPs, *etc*.

IL-6
"Messenger" cytokine

Endothelium
and other cells

CRP
SAA

Liver

Circulation

Figure 1-14. Proinflammatory pathways. Biomarkers provide a window on the inflammatory process in individuals at risk for cardiovascular events. Various proximal proinflammatory risk factors (*eg*, dyslipidemia, hypertension, obesity, cigarette smoking) can elicit the production of a first wave of primary proinflammatory cytokines, including interleukin-1 (IL-1) and tumor necrosis factor alpha (TNF-α). These primary cytokines can in turn beget the production of many molecules of interleukin-6 (IL-6), a soluble cytokine that can transfer messages to the liver from various remote sites of inflammation ranging from adipose tissue to the atherosclerotic plaque itself. IL-6 modulates the pattern of protein synthesis in the liver and augments the production of the proteins of the acute phase reaction including C-reactive protein (CRP) and serum amyloid A (SAA). These acute phase reactants, sampled from the peripheral circulation, reflect the level and activity of the proinflammatory risk factors. The proinflammatory cytokines can also induce the expression of adhesion molecules on the endothelial cell (*see* Fig. 1-3 and Fig. 1-4). Shed forms of adhesion molecules such as intercellular adhesion molecule 1 (ICAM-1) or the selectins, also released into the peripheral blood, provide additional biomarkers of inflammation. Endothelial cells subjected to inflammatory activation can also overproduce mediators, such as the heat shock proteins (HSPs) invoked as candidate antigens in the adaptive immune response during atherogenesis. (*Adapted from* Libby et al. [9]; *with permission.*)

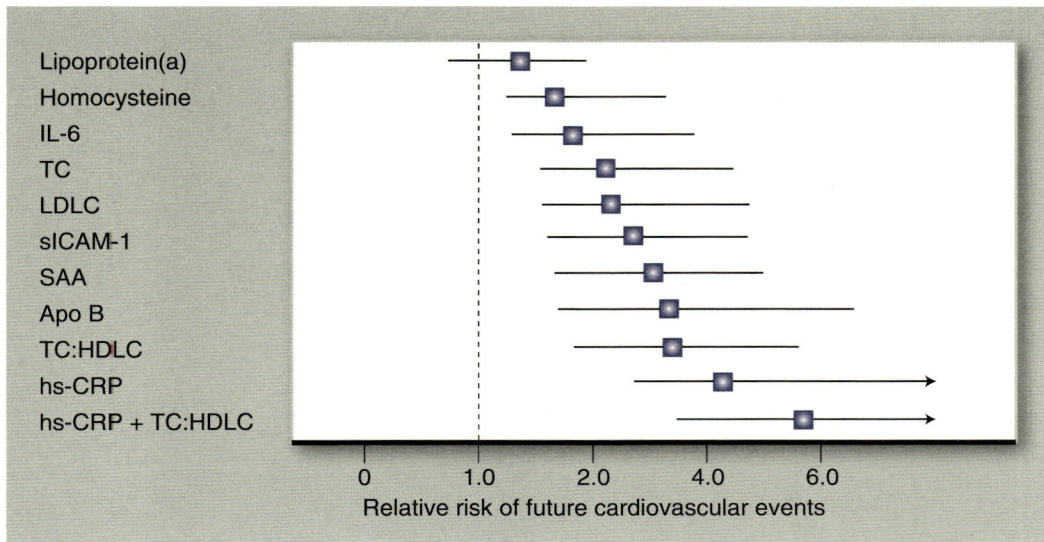

Figure 1-15. Risk factors for future cardiovascular events. Biomarkers of atherosclerotic risk in the Women's Health Study (WHS). Ridker *et al.* [10] have extensively studied the value of various biomarkers of cardiovascular risk in large patient populations. This example shows the relative risk of future cardiovascular events with confidence intervals for a variety of biomarkers. Although perhaps important in individuals, lipoprotein(a) and homocysteine appear to be relatively weak risk markers in populations. The total cholesterol to high-density lipoprotein cholesterol ratio (TC:HDLC) predicts first ever cardiovascular events quite well in the WHS. Those women with higher levels of C-reactive protein, measured by a highly sensitive assay (hs-CRP), also have greater cardiovascular risk. Combination of the classical lipid parameter, TC:HDLC and hs-CRP predicts future cardiovascular events best of all. As many as 24 large prospective trials concordantly show a correlation of higher levels of C-reactive protein with increased cardiovascular risk in broad categories of individuals, men and women, and those with or without prior cardiovascular events [10]. Apo B—apolipoprotein B; IL-6—interleukin 6; LDLC—low-density lipoprotein cholesterol; SAA—serum amyloid A; sICAM-1—soluble intercellular adhesion molecule-1.

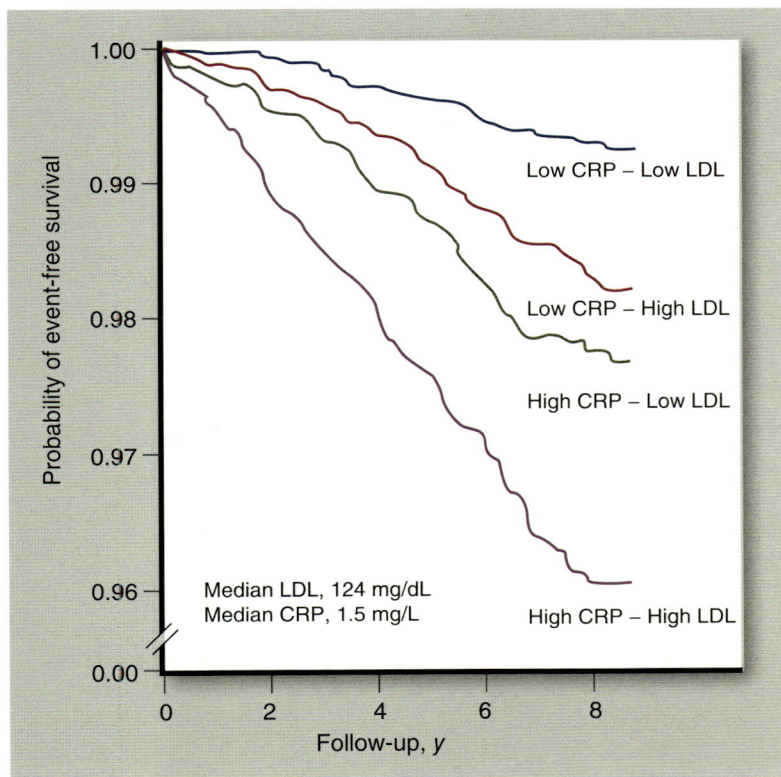

Figure 1-16. Cardiovascular event-free survival using combined high-sensitivity C-reactive protein (CRP) assay and low-density lipoprotein (LDL) cholesterol measurements. The inflammatory biomarker CRP and the lipid biomarker LDL appear to independently correlate with cardiovascular risk. In this example, those with higher levels of inflammation and LDL (*purple line*) have the lowest event-free survival. Those who have low levels of inflammation, indicated by low CRP levels, and low levels of LDL, have the best prognosis (*blue line*). (*Adapted from* Ridker *et al.* [11]; with permission.)

Figure 1-17. Lipoprotein disorders rank among the best studied and best understood risk factors for atherosclerosis. Lipids, which are water insoluble, require coating with proteins or other more polar moieties, such as phospholipids, for transport through the blood and interstitium. The lipoprotein particles consist of a lipid core coated with phospholipids, occasional cholesterol molecules, and various apolipoproteins. The apolipoproteins serve as "addresses" on the surface of various fractions of lipoprotein particles that help guide their transport, uptake by cells, and metabolic fate. Lipids can enter the blood compartment by intestinal absorption, forming large lipoprotein particles known as chylomicrons. The enzyme lipoprotein lipase (LPL) can trim fatty acids from the triglycerides in chylomicrons forming chylomicron, remnants and generating free fatty acids (FFA) that, when bound to albumin for transport through the aqueous medium of blood, can provide nutrition for aerobic tissues, such as the heart muscle. Chylomicron remnants can enter the liver, where they furnish an extrinsic source of cholesterol and triglyc-

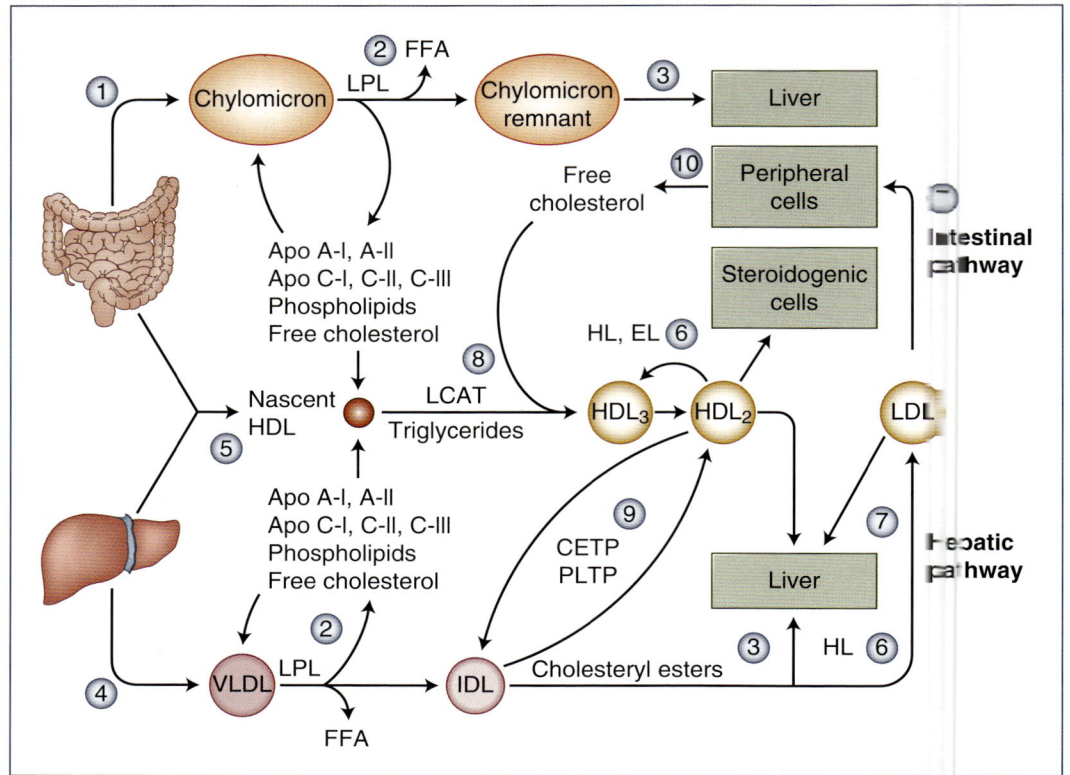

erides for hepatic metabolism. Most of the body's cholesterol arises from synthesis within the liver. Hepatocytes package cholesterol in lipoprotein particles known as very low-density lipoprotein particles (VLDL). Removal of FFAs due to hydrolysis of triglycerides in VLDL by the action of lipoprotein lipase can give rise to intermediate density lipoproteins (IDL). IDL can in turn become LDL particles that can deliver cholesterol to peripheral cells for membrane biogenesis and other metabolic uses. High-density lipoprotein (HDL) particles initially arise as phospholipid-rich discs with phospholipids and the signature apolipoprotein, apo A-I. These nascent HDL particles can arise from the intestine or from the liver. Esterification of free cholesterol taken up from tissues by HDL leads to the formation of more mature HDL3 and HDL2 particles The enzyme lecithin cholesterol acyltransferase (LCAT) catalyzes the formation of cholesteryl ester from free cholesterol within HDL particles. Hepatic lipase (HL) and endothelial lipase (EL) can interconvert various forms of HDL particles. HDL can participate in reverse cholesterol transport by unloading cholesterol from peripheral cells. HDL particles can also deliver cholesterol to steroidogenic cells such as the adrenal gland and the gonads for steroid hormone synthesis. Cholesteryl ester transfer protein (CETP) and phospholipid transfer protein (PLTP) shuttle cholesteryl or phospholipids between the apo A-I–containing HDL particle family and the apo B–containing family that includes LDL, IDL, and VLDL [12].

Figure 1-18. Dyslipidemia of insulin resistance. Insulin-resistant states, including diabetes mellitus and the metabolic syndrome, typically involve a dyslipidemia characterized by high levels of triglycerides, low levels of high-density lipoprotein (HDL), and accumulation of a population of particularly small and dense low-density lipoprotein particles. This dyslipidemia arises in part because of increased delivery of fatty acids due to excessive lipolysis and from decreased utilization of fatty acids by insulin-resistant skeletal and cardiac muscle. The liver faced with a surfeit of fatty acids augments its production of very low-density lipoprotein (VLDL), a triglyceride-rich lipoprotein particle. VLDL particles contain much of the excessive triglyceride associated with diabetic dyslipidemia. The increased VLDL also provides a sink for accumulating cholesteryl ester derived from HDL particles due to the action of cholesteryl ester transfer protein (CETP). Thus triglyceride levels (reflecting VLDL content) and HDL levels tend to vary reciprocally. The small, dense LDL particles that accumulate in insulin-resistant states appear particularly atherogenic, as they have an increased dwell time in the artery wall and may thus undergo modification and uptake by macrophages at accelerated rates [13]. FFA—free fatty acid.

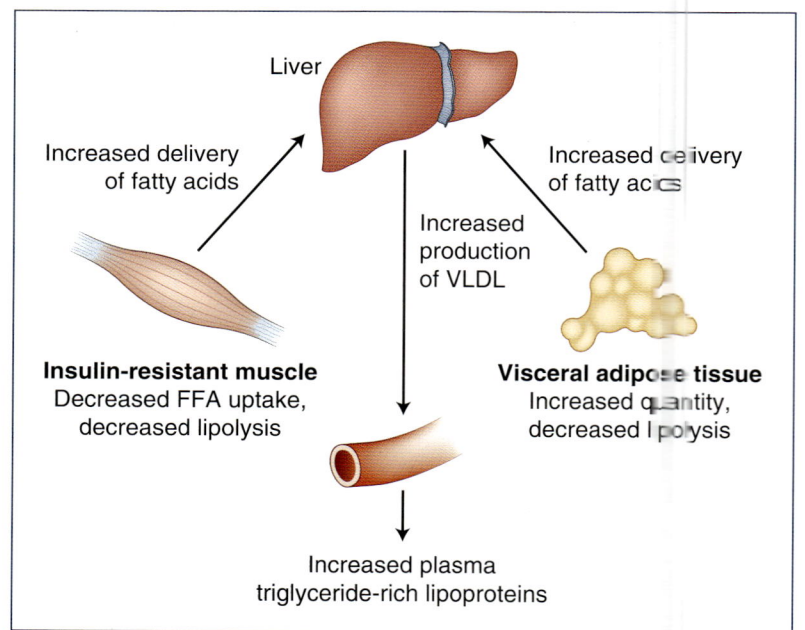

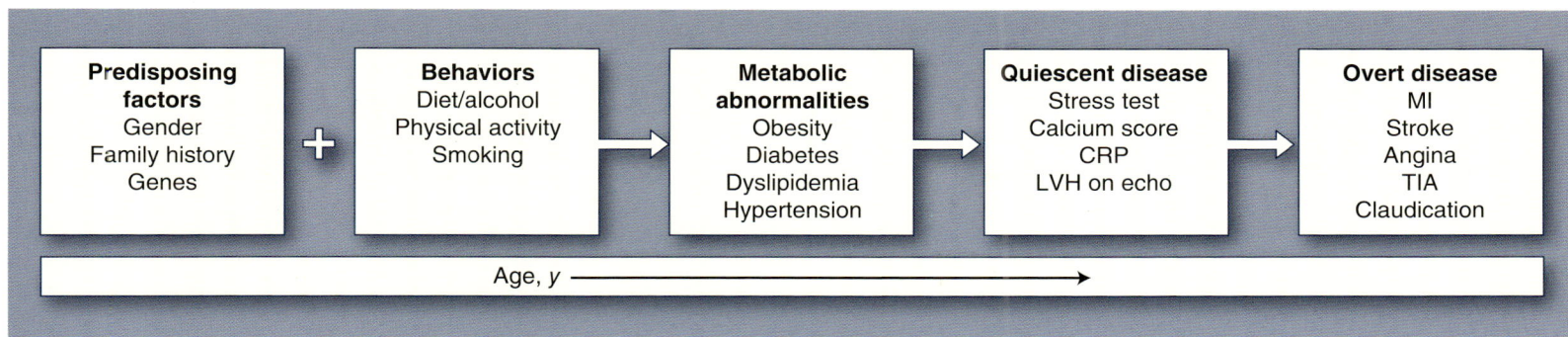

Predisposing factors		Behaviors		Metabolic abnormalities		Quiescent disease		Overt disease
Gender		Diet/alcohol		Obesity		Stress test		MI
Family history	+	Physical activity	→	Diabetes	→	Calcium score	→	Stroke
Genes		Smoking		Dyslipidemia		CRP		Angina
				Hypertension		LVH on echo		TIA
								Claudication

Age, y →

Figure 1-19. Progression of atherosclerosis. As discussed above, our knowledge of the biologic process of atherosclerosis has led to a working model for the progression of this disease. A convergence of risk factors often causes atherosclerosis. Most people with cardiovascular disease have small, concurrent adverse changes in multiple risk factors rather than extreme deviations in any single risk factor. Left unchecked, atherosclerosis will progress. Predisposing factors such as genes interact with behavioral factors (eg, type of diet and amount of regular exercise). This combination of predisposing factors and behaviors can lead to metabolic abnormalities—such as dyslipidemia, hypertension, obesity, and diabetes—that may eventually result in atherosclerosis. Atherosclerosis first develops silently, often beginning early in life. Various imaging modalities, including carotid ultrasound or calcium scores, can detect subclinical disease (see also Chapter 15). Symptoms or an exercise stress test can disclose stenoses that cause ischemia. Biomarkers, such as lipid parameters or C-reactive protein (CRP) measurement, can assess the underlying risk of cardiovascular events (see Fig. 1-15). Over time, atherosclerosis may become overt in the form of a transient ischemic attack (TIA), a myocardial infarction (MI), or another cardiovascular event. A risk factor can operate at any point along this continuum. The remainder of this chapter discusses risk factors with interventions that can delay or even reverse the progression of disease and/or prevent events.

Figure 1-20. Factors in cardiovascular disease prevention. Risk factors can be divided into two broad categories based on their use in clinical practice: risk predictors and potential risk "reducers," or causal risk factors. Certain factors, such as cigarette smoking and blood pressure, fall into both categories. Further, just because a given risk factor has predictive value, it does not necessarily follow that modification of that factor will lead to reduced risk. The benefit of any intervention must clearly exceed the risks and be worth the cost.

Useful factors that predict risk are readily and reproducibly measured and have sufficient prevalence in the population to warrant screening. Risk assessment should include nonmodifiable factors, such as age, gender, and family history of premature coronary disease, as well as modifiable factors, such as smoking, hypertension, dyslipidemia, excess weight, and physical inactivity. Because many of these factors coexist, when building a prediction model, such as the Framingham Risk Score, once we have a dozen or so factors, our model will not be greatly enhanced by including more factors. ACE—angiotensin-converting enzyme; ARB—angiotensin-receptor blocker; ASA—acetylsalicylic acid; CABG—coronary artery bypass graft; CEA—carotid endarterectomy; CRP—C-reactive protein; EBT—electron-beam tomography; ECHO—echocardiogram; ETT—exercise tolerance test; PCI—percutaneous coronary intervention.

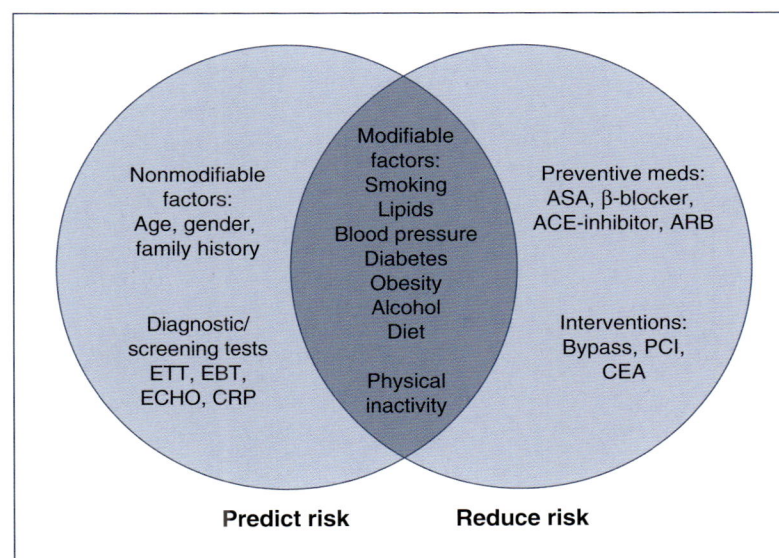

Figure 1-21. Determining which preventive strategies will be most beneficial to individuals involves assessing the risk of developing a clinically relevant outcome because the cost efficacy of any intervention varies according to global risk in an individual or population. Many risk factors are correlated, making it possible to predict an individual's risk with data on just a few of these factors. Even though it is possible to assess many factors, in most cases, when a clinician conducts an initial screening, a handful of easily measured risk factors suffice to determine an individual's overall risk of coronary heart disease.

Risk Assessment Tool for Estimating 10-Year Risk of Developing Hard CHD (Myocardial Infarction and Coronary Death)

The risk assessment tool below uses recent data from the Framingham Heart Study to predict a person's chance of having a heart attack in the next 10 years. This tool is designed for adults aged 20 and older who do not have heart disease or diabetes. To find your risk score, enter your information in the calculator below.

Age: ⬚ Years
Gender: ○ Female ○ Male
Total cholesterol: ⬚ mg/dL
HDL cholesterol: ⬚ mg/dL
Smoker: ○ No ○ Yes
Systolic blood pressure: ⬚ mm Hg
Are you currently on any medication to treat high blood pressure ○ No ○ Yes

As testament to the importance of individual risk assessment, the National Cholesterol Education Program (NCEP) Adult Treatment Panel (ATP) III developed a risk-assessment tool, illustrated in the figure, that is widely used to estimate the future risk of a coronary heart disease (CHD) event and can be accessed online or downloaded [14]. HDL—high-density lipoprotein.

Figure 1-22. Many risk-prediction engines exist, proposed for applicability to particular populations or geographic locales. One recently developed tool, denoted the Reynolds Risk Score, emerged from an unbiased statistical analysis of nearly 40 biomarkers in a generation subset of the Women's Health Study ($n = 16,400$). Using procedures that drove the model to parsimony (the Bayesian Information Coefficient) the model that emerged included the key "Framingham" risk factors (see Fig. 1-21), and two elements not captured by the Framingham model: family history of a cardiovascular event before age 60 and the high-sensitivity C-reactive protein measurement (hsCRP). Validation on a randomly reserved portion of the same cohort ($n = 8158$) showed that the Reynolds Risk Score raised or lowered the risk level in about 40% of those at intermediate risk according to the Framingham instrument by the addition of hsCRP and family history. Comparison of predicted to observed event rates showed that this reclassification was correct in more than 98% of cases. This depiction of the Reynolds Risk Score site illustrates its use for a hypothetical woman [15]. The Reynolds Risk Score for men and women is now available (www.reynoldsriskscore.org).

Reynolds Risk Score
Calculating Heart and Stroke Risk for Women

For healthy women without diabetes, the Reynolds Risk score predicts the risk of having a heart attack, stroke, or other major heart disease in the next 10 years.

Beyond age, blood pressure, cholesterol levels, and current smoking status, the Reynolds Risk Score uses information from two other risk factors: a blood test called hsCRP (a measure of inflammation) and whether one of your parents had a heart attack before age 60 (a measure of genetic risk). To calculate your risk, fill in the information below with your most recent values.

Age | 62 | Years
Do you currently smoke? | ● Yes ○ No
Systolic blood pressure | 140 | mm Hg
Total cholesterol | 235 | mg/dL
HDL or "good" cholesterol | 45 | mg/dL
High sensitivity C-reactive protein (hsCRP) | 4 | mg/L
Did your mother or father have a heart attack before age 60? | ● Yes ○ No

Calculate 10-year risk

As shown below, at age 72, your chance of having a heart attack, stroke, or other heart disease event in the next 10 years is 37%.

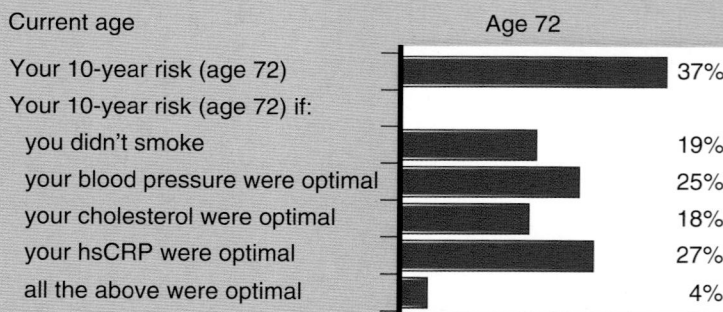

Current age | Age 72
Your 10-year risk (age 72) | 37%
Your 10-year risk (age 72) if:
you didn't smoke | 19%
your blood pressure were optimal | 25%
your cholesterol were optimal | 18%
your hsCRP were optimal | 27%
all the above were optimal | 4%

The graph above also compares your risk to that of a 72-year-old woman who has optimal levels for all modifiable risk factors, and shows what your risk would be if you improved your individual risk factors. For young women, risk may appear to be low over the next 10 years, yet can be very high over a lifetime.

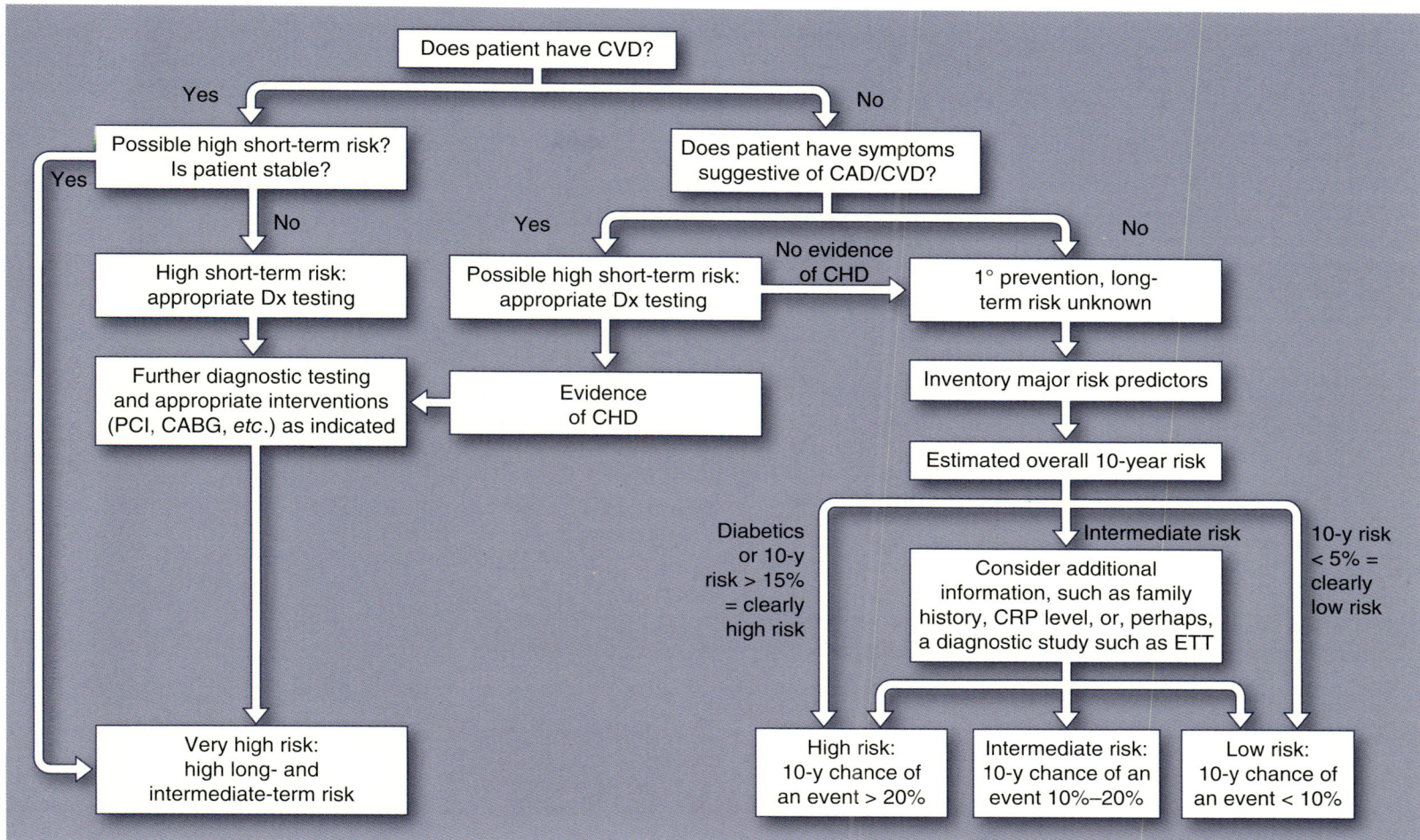

Figure 1-23. Algorithm for risk assessment of cardiovascular disease (CVD). Using this algorithm, clinicians can classify a patient's long-term risk of a coronary heart disease (CHD) event using a few simple questions and measurements, such as blood pressure. The first branch point is "Does the patient have known CVD?" and, if so, "Is it stable?" If the patient is stable, no further classification is necessary. This person is already at very high long-term risk. If there is an indication of instability, the patient needs to be referred for further diagnostic testing and intervention as appropriate. For patients without known CVD, it is important to determine if they have symptoms suggestive of CVD, such as new chest pain when walking up stairs. If so, they also need referral for short-term risk assessment and intervention. For individuals without CVD or symptoms, the first step is taking inventory of major risk predictors. Men and women with diabetes automatically enter the high-risk category because long-term risk is clearly high. In those without diabetes, determination of a risk score is useful. For individuals who have intermediate risk after initial screening, particularly if they are on the cusp between high and intermediate risk, consider a secondary screen such as measuring C-reactive protein (CRP) [16]. CAD—coronary artery disease; Dx—diagnostic; ETT—exercise tolerance test.

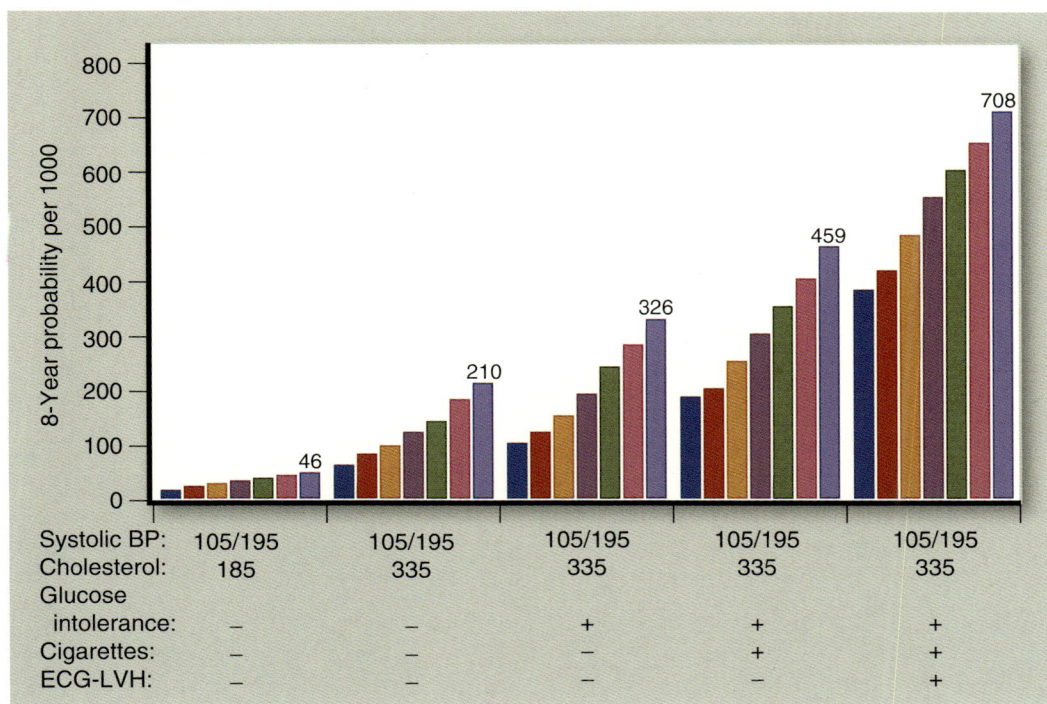

Figure 1-24. Risk of cardiovascular disease according to a number of risk factors. Many adults have multiple cardiac risk factors working together to increase risk. This image from the Framingham Heart Study shows that having multiple risk factors can dramatically increase the 8-year probability of developing coronary heart disease. In 1976, Kannel [17] wrote, "Most cases of angina pectoris or myocardial infarction represent medical failures; the conditions should have been detected years earlier for preventive management." (*Adapted from* Kannel [17]; with permission.) BP—blood pressure; ECG-LVH—electrocardiographic left ventricular hypertrophy.

Figure 1-25. Association between myocardial infarction and risk factors. The INTERHEART study further illustrates how risk factors can work together. This case-control study investigated the strength of the association between acute myocardial infarction (MI) and nine risk factors in 15,152 cases and 14,820 control subjects recruited from 52 countries [18]. The study found that abnormal lipids, smoking, hypertension, diabetes, abdominal obesity, psychosocial factors, low consumption of fruits and vegetables, no alcohol intake, and irregular physical activity account for most MI risk, regardless of gender, age, or region. Conversely, a healthy lifestyle that includes daily consumption of fruits and vegetables and regular exercise was associated with reduced risk of acute MI, conferring an OR of 0.60. The risk was further reduced (OR, 0.21) if in addition to eating a healthy diet and exercising, an individual also avoided smoking. Although the relative importance of every risk factor varied, raised lipids, smoking, and psychosocial factors were the most important risk factors in all regions of the world. (*Adapted from Yusuf et al.* [18]; with permission.)

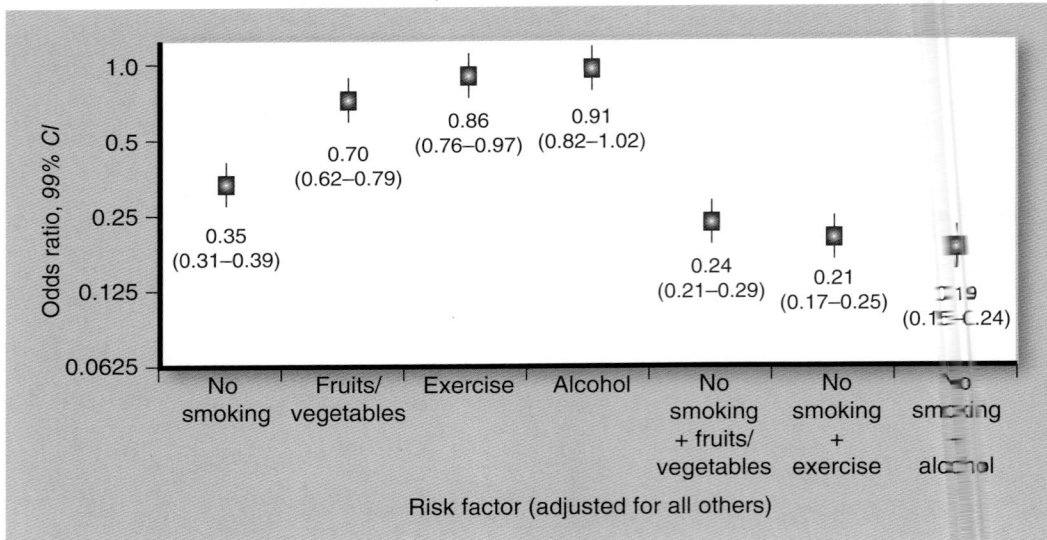

Interventions to Lower Cardiovascular Disease Risk

Class I	Class II	Class III
Cigarette smoking	Diabetes/pre-diabetes	Postmenopausal estrogen
Dyslipidemia	Physical inactivity	Dietary supplements
Hypertension	Obesity	Psychological factors
Prophylactic medications	Diet and alcohol intake	Novel biochemical and genetic markers
Aspirin		Multiple risk factor intervention programs
β-Blockers		
ACE-I, ARB		

Figure 1-26. Interventions to lower risk should be prioritized according to the likelihood of achieving success. Interventions can be classified into three categories based on the quality of the evidence that a particular intervention will reduce risk. Class I risk factors have a clear causal relationship with heart disease. Data have demonstrated the magnitude of an associated intervention's benefit, as well as its risks and cost. Hypertension and dyslipidemia are causally related to coronary heart disease, and the corresponding interventions—blood pressure management and lipid profile management—are cost-effective in both primary and secondary prevention. For Class II risk factors, the available data strongly indicate a causal relationship and suggest that intervention will probably reduce the incidence of events but for which data on the benefits, risks, and costs of intervention are limited. Diabetes/prediabetes is in Class II, as are obesity, physical inactivity, and various dietary factors. For risk factors that fall into Class III, which include menopause and use of micronutrients, an independent causal relationship with cardiovascular disease has not been established and interventions to lower risk have not yet been proven. ACE-I—angiotensin-converting enzyme inhibiitor; ARB—angiotensin-receptor blocker.

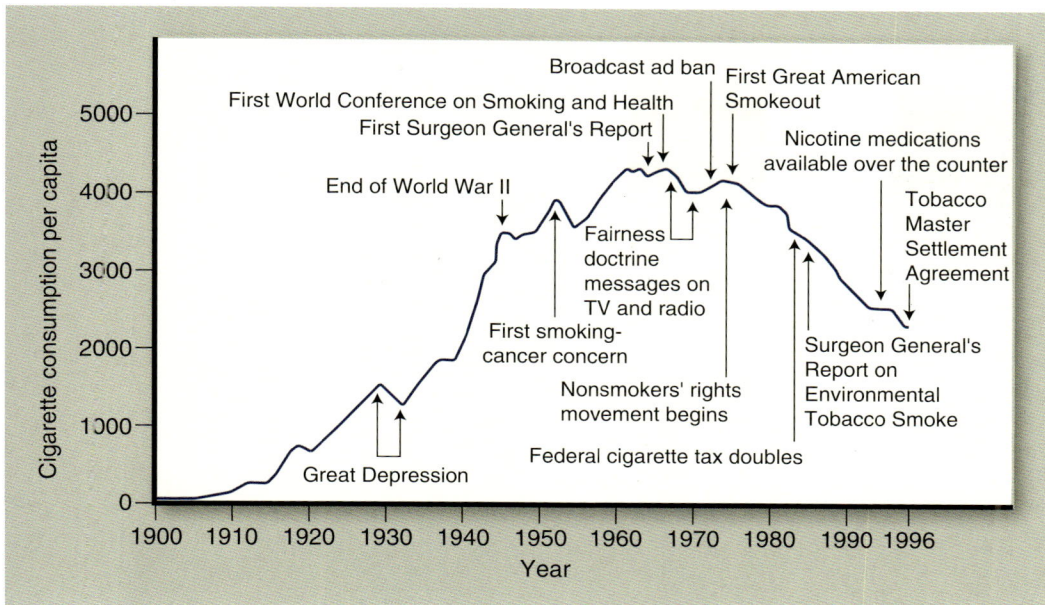

Figure 1-27. Yearly adult cigarette consumption per capita and major smoking and health events. More than 65% of men born between 1911 and 1920 were smoking by 1945. In the 20th century, rates of cigarette smoking increased, with few pauses, until the 1960s. The health warnings issued at that time by the US Surgeon General and the beginning of antitobacco efforts resulted in a steady decline over the next 40 years. Education about health risks, improved therapies for cessation, taxes on tobacco, litigation, and legislation to create smoke-free public places have all contributed to this trend. [19].

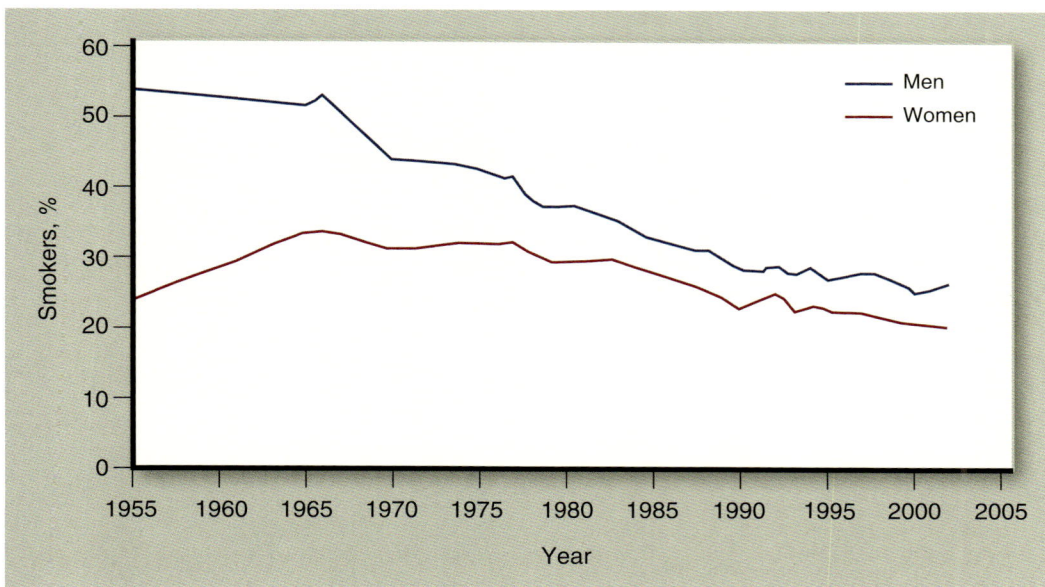

Figure 1-28. Cigarette smoking trends from 1955 to 1997 among men and women older than 18 years. Since the 1960s, smoking rates have continued to decline, and by 2002 there were more former smokers than current smokers in the United States. Persistent gender differences in smoking rates have narrowed over time. In 2002, the rate among men (25.2%) remained higher than among women (20.0%) [20,21].

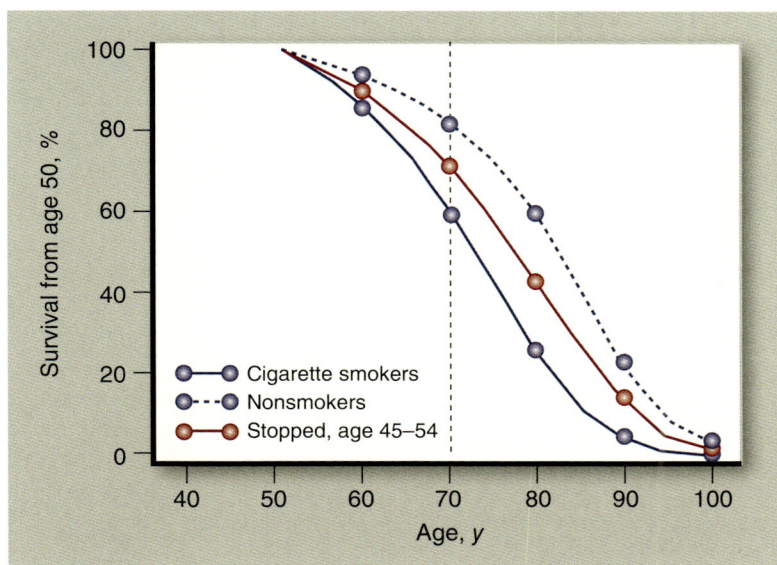

Figure 1-29. Reduction in mortality with smoking cessation after myocardial infarction, age 45 to 54 years. In a meta-analysis, smoking cessation was associated with a lower mortality rate after a myocardial infarction in 12 cohorts over a mean of 4.8 years. OR ranged from 0.29 to 0.84, with a combined OR of 0.54 (95% CI, 0.46–0.62), a magnitude comparable with other therapeutic interventions. A benefit to smoking cessation was observed in every group, with results consistent across study location, patient gender, year of study, and length of follow-up. (*Adapted from* Wilson *et al.* [22].)

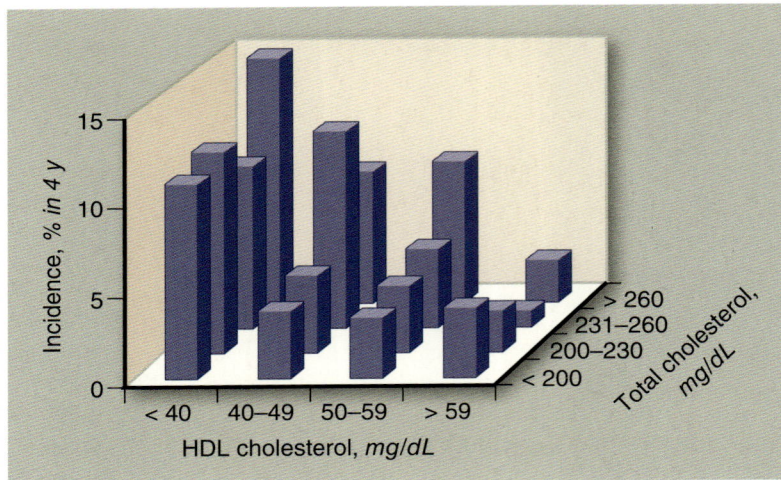

Figure 1-30. Total and high-density lipoprotein (HDL) cholesterol value: men and women without coronary heart disease (CHD) history. The Framingham Heart Study and other cohort studies identified a number of risk factors for CHD. In the 1960s and 1970s, smoking and high blood pressure were clearly established as risk factors for CHD. In addition, blood-based markers appeared as important predictors of disease, with the emergence of cholesterol levels as clear risk factors. This image illustrates the independent relationship of total cholesterol and HDL cholesterol with incident CHD in men and women. In addition to the Framingham Heart Study, a number of other large-scale cohort studies, as well as smaller case-control studies, have clearly established factors, such as smoking, high blood pressure, and lipids, as causative agents in the development of CHD. (*Adapted from* Castelli *et al.* [23].)

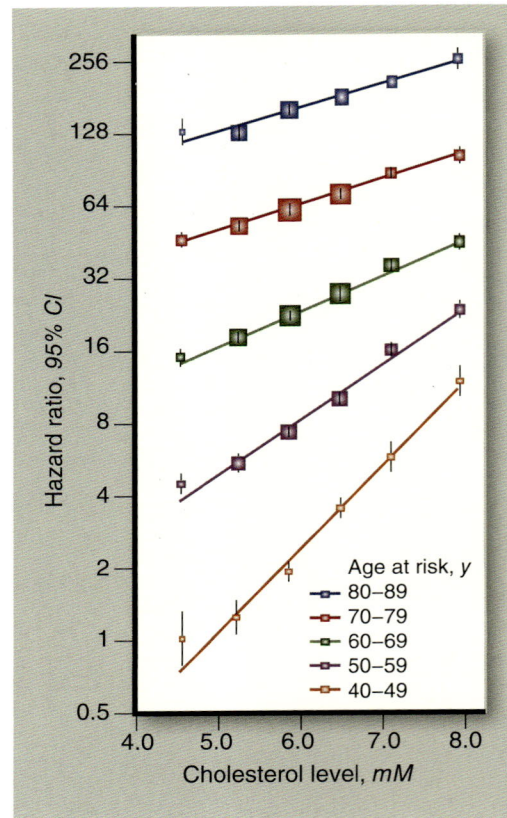

Figure 1-31. A recent meta-analysis clearly demonstrates the largely log linear relationship of total cholesterol levels and level of risk of death from ischemic heart disease. (*Adapted from* Prospective Studies Collaboration *et al.* [24]; with permission.)

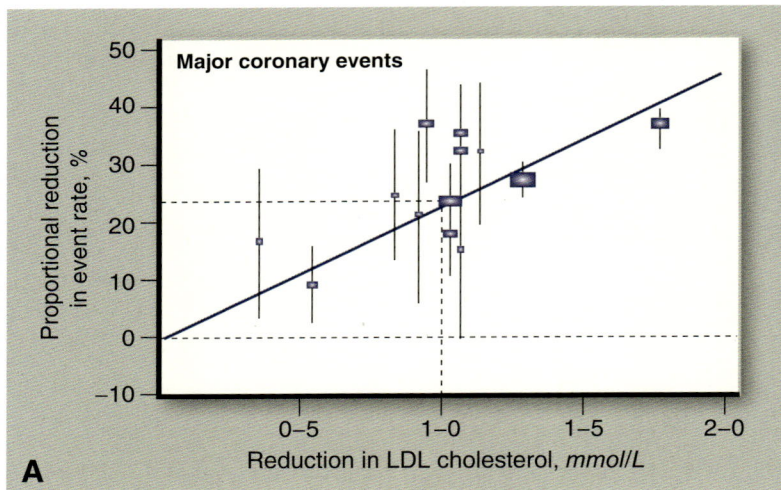

A

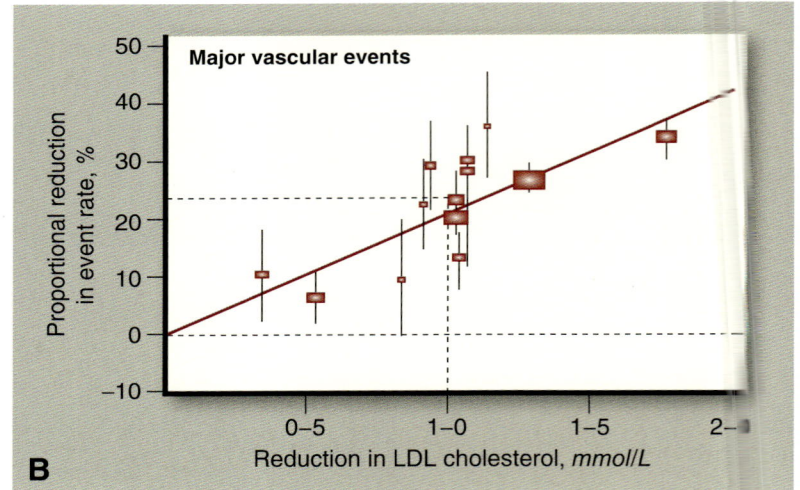

B

Figure 1-32. Relationship of reduction in low-density lipoprotein (LDL) cholesterol to reduction in risk of cardiovascular disease events. While lifestyle modification remains important in modifying lipids, the discovery of 3-hydroxy-3-methylglutaryl coenzyme A reductase inhibitors, the "statins," and their ability to reduce LDL levels by 30% to 60% has resulted in significant clinical benefits. Emerging evidence suggests that statins may have direct anti-inflammatory effects that contribute to clinical benefit beyond their LDL-lowering action. Several large-scale primary and secondary prevention trials of these drugs have demonstrated significant reductions in coronary heart disease and stroke in a variety of populations. **A** and **B**, For example, a

2005 meta-analysis of 14 randomized trials with 90,056 participants showed that statin therapy can reduce the 5-year incidence of major coronary events by about one fifth per mmol/L reduction in LDL level, regardless of the pretreatment cholesterol level, age, sex, or preexisting disease and without any increases in cancer. This reduction in risk is linear, resulting in comparable risk reductions across the spectrum of lipid levels. Pharmacologic intervention is clearly cost-effective under certain conditions, and available data permit tailoring recommendations to the level of baseline coronary heart disease risk. (*Adapted from* Cholesterol Treatment Trialists' Collaborators *et al.* [25]; with permission.)

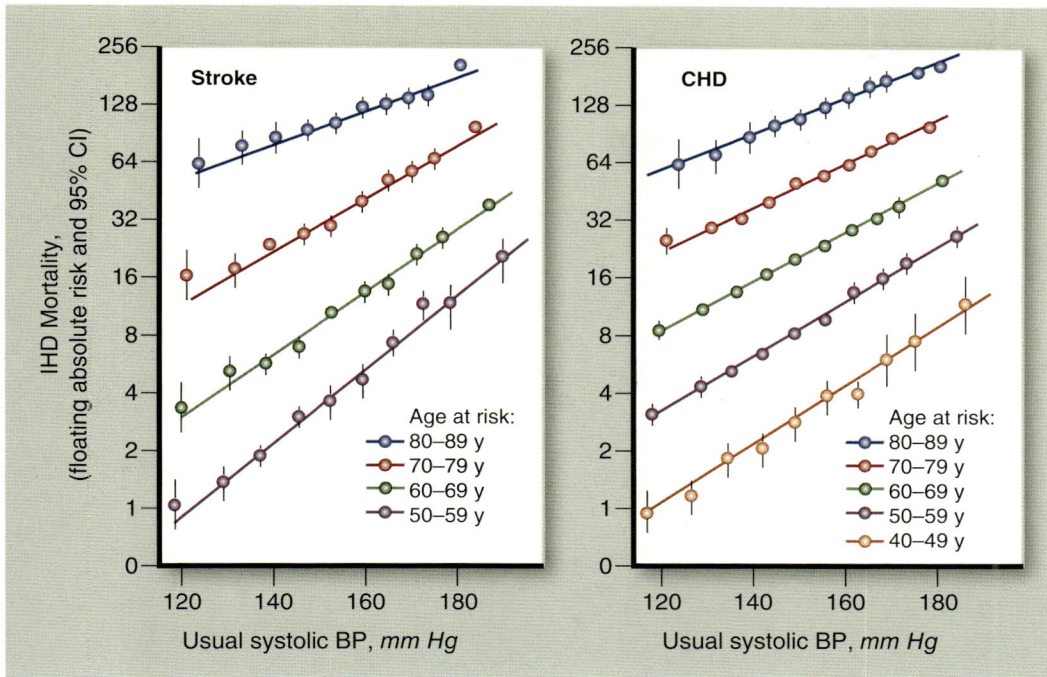

Figure 1-33. Ischemic heart disease (IHD) rates by systolic blood pressure (BP), diastolic BP, and age. Studies have demonstrated a significant linear correlation between the degree of hypertension and the risk of cardiovascular disease or stroke. Even small increases in the level of hypertension can influence cardiovascular morbidity and mortality (*see* Ch. 8). (*Adapted from* Lewington *et al.* [26]; with permission.) CHD—coronary heart disease.

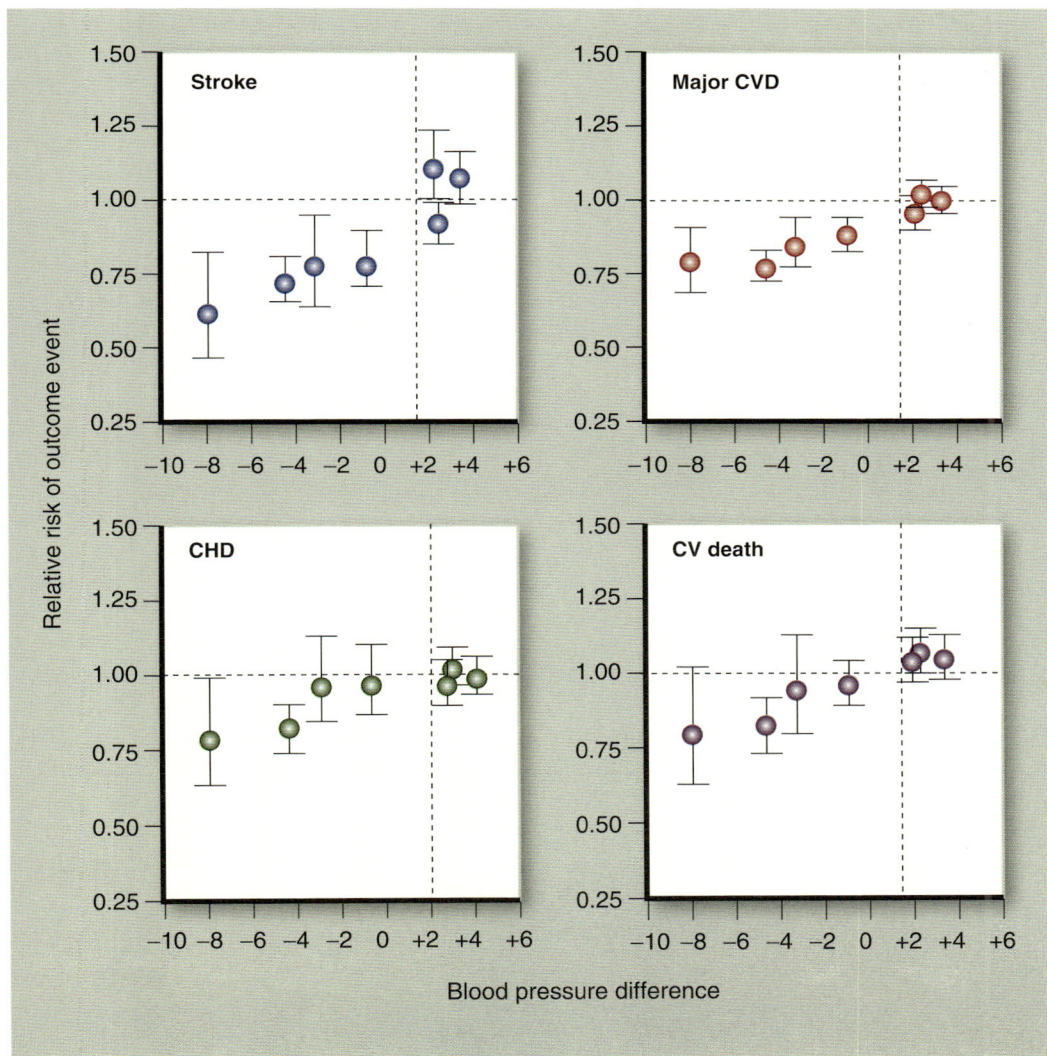

Figure 1-34. Meta-analysis: blood pressure differences and risk of major vascular outcomes. Over the past 40 years, a number of randomized trials have confirmed the protective effect of treating mild to moderate hypertension. As with lipid reduction, the shape of the relationship is linear. This meta-analysis of randomized trials demonstrated a linear relationship between levels of blood pressure lowering achieved and lowered risk of stroke, major cardiovascular disease (CVD) events, coronary heart disease (CHD), and CV death (*see* Ch. 8).

Detection and management of hypertension have proven highly cost-effective in both primary and secondary prevention. However, those at high risk based on the existence of cardiovascular disease or diabetes warranted more aggressive management based on greater cost efficacy. (*Adapted from* Blood Pressure Lowering Treatment Trialists' Collaboration *et al.* [27]; with permission.)

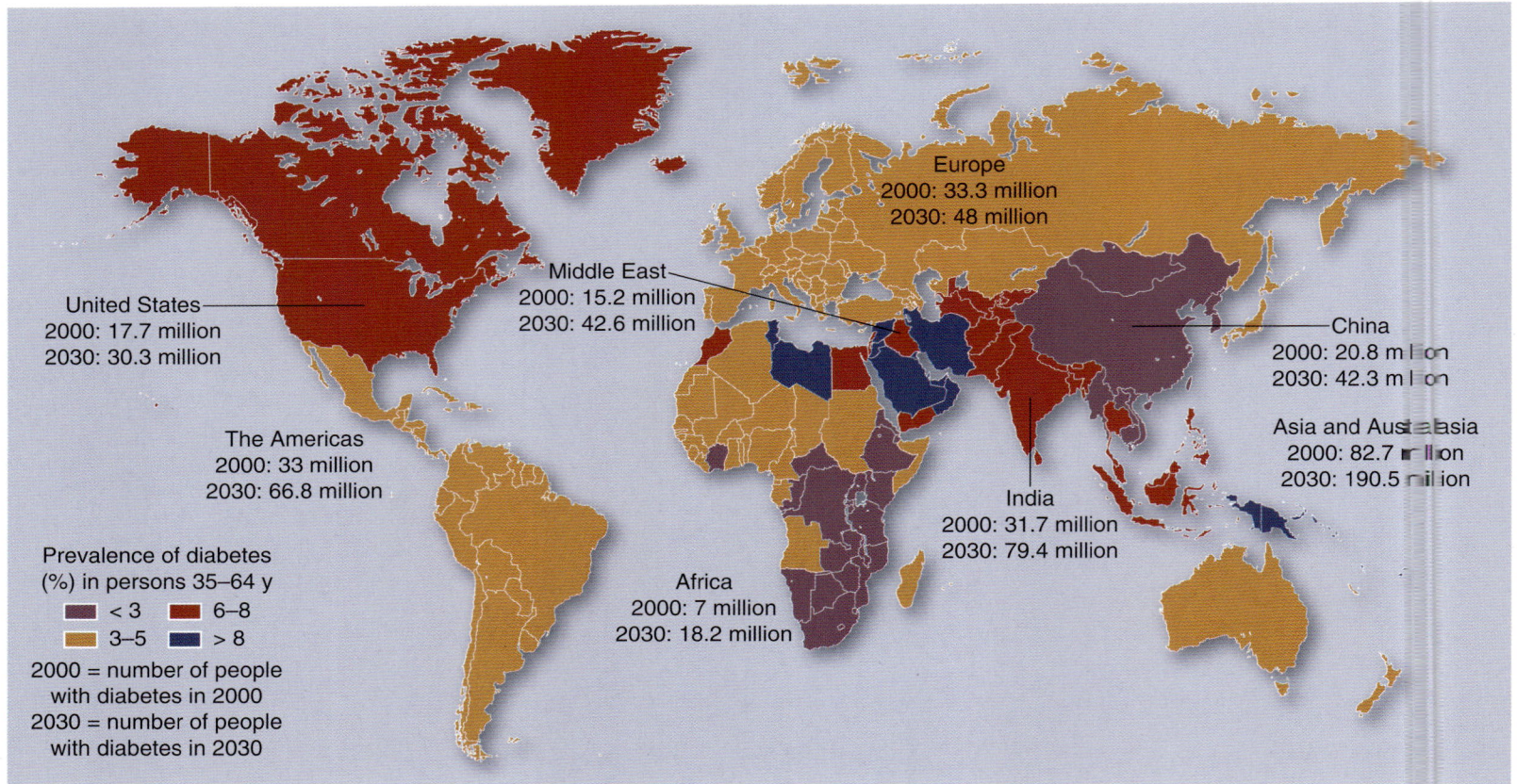

Figure 1-35. Prevalence of diabetes. Nearly 21 million Americans—7% of the population—have diabetes mellitus. Type 2 diabetes accounts for approximately 90% of cases. Fully one third of people with diabetes are not aware that they have this increasingly common disease [28].

This figure illustrates the prevalence of diabetes worldwide. Diabetes is a powerful risk factor for atherosclerotic disease, its complications, and cardiovascular-related mortality. By age 40, coronary heart disease (CHD) is the leading cause of death in men and women with diabetes, with surveys showing heart disease listed on 69% of death certificates in a representative national cohort of adults with diabetes. However, data demonstrating reduced risk of CHD with tight glycemic control are scant, and currently controversial. Those with type 2 diabetes more often have multiple coronary risk factors than the general population. Thus, aggressive modification of associated risk factors—including treatment of hypertension, aggressive reduction of serum cholesterol, reduction of weight, and increased physical activity—assumes paramount importance in reducing the risk of CHD among people with diabetes. Diet and physical activity are integral components of the treatment strategy for patients with diabetes.

Diagnosing metabolic syndrome
Three of these five criteria must be met:

Fasting glucose:	Triglycerides:	Blood pressure:
At least 100 mg/dL	At least 150 mg/dL	At least 130/85 mm Hg

High-density lipoprotein cholesterol:
Below 50 mg/dL in women; below 40 mg/dL in men

Central obesity:
Abdominal waist circumference > 35 inches in women
Abdominal waist circumference > 40 inches in men

Figure 1-36. Adult Treatment Panel (ATP) III metabolic syndrome criteria. The metabolic syndrome is a cluster of metabolic abnormalities that includes insulin resistance, dyslipidemia, hypertension, a proinflammatory state, and excess weight, particularly abdominal adiposity. While debate persists over whether this cluster confers risk greater than the individual components, it provides a useful operating concept in clinical practice. This constellation of risk factors is quite common: approximately 27% of US adults and 10% of adolescents between age 12 and 19 meet the criteria for metabolic syndrome [29,30].

Both the ATP III and the Joint National Committee for Prevention, Detection, Evaluation, and Treatment of Hypertension (JNC-7) guidelines address the metabolic syndrome. Patients are classified as having it if they have three or more of the following: waist circumference greater than 40 inches for men or 35 inches for women; blood pressure more than 130/85 mm Hg; high-density lipoprotein lower than 40 mg/dL for men or 50 mg/dL for women; triglycerides more than 150 mg/dL; and fasting blood sugar more than 100 mg/dL [31,32].

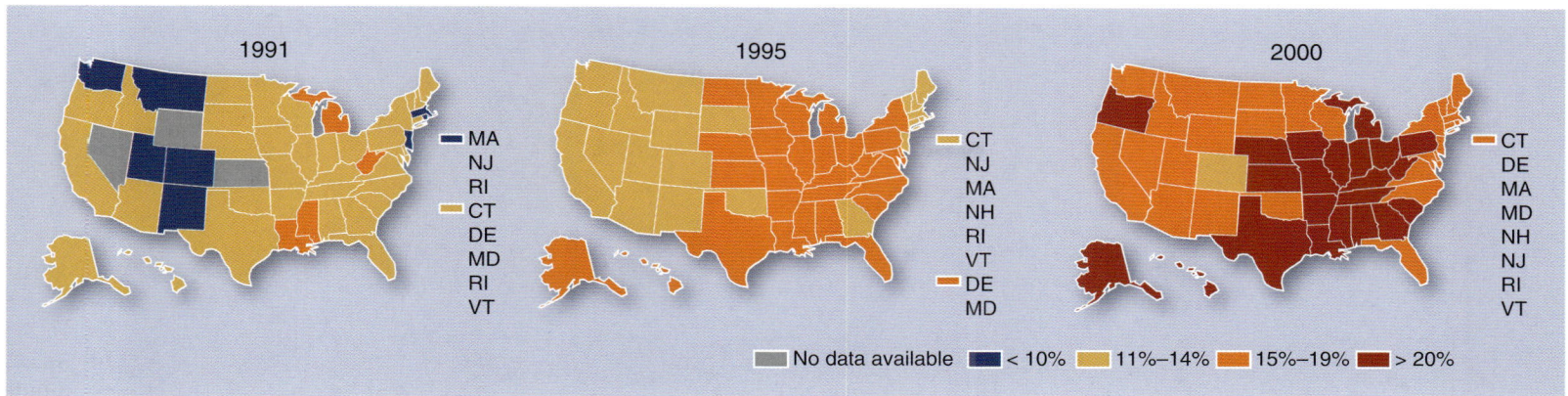

1991   **1995**   **2000**

| No data available | < 10% | 11%–14% | 15%–19% | > 20% |

Figure 1-37. Obesity trends among US adults. Over the past four decades, the proportion of the US population considered to be overweight (body mass index [BMI] > 25) has risen dramatically. The prevalence of overweight and obesity in children and adolescents is rising in parallel with that in adults. Obesity is defined as BMI of 30 or greater or approximately 30 pounds overweight for a 5'4" individual. These data are based on self-reported weight and height [33].

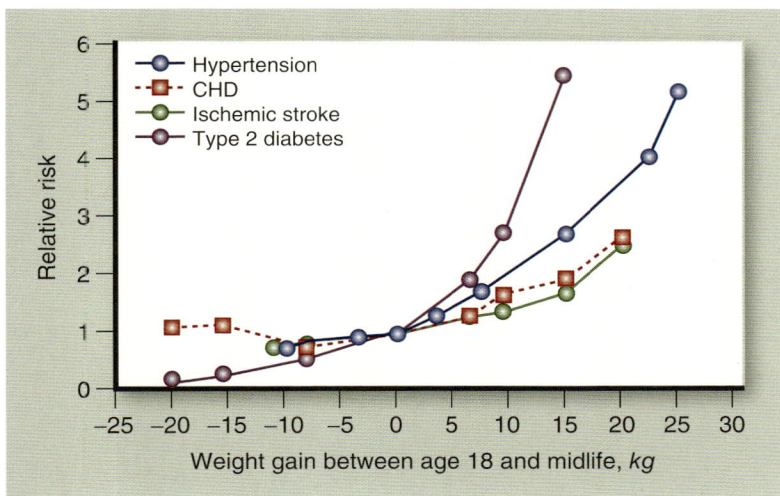

Figure 1-38. Weight change and risk of cardiovascular heart disease, hypertension, stroke, and diabetes. Obesity and overweight strongly associate with risks of coronary heart disease (CHD) and stroke. This figure demonstrates the exponential increase in diabetes, hypertension, CHD, and stroke risks with weight gain in adulthood. No large-scale randomized trials of weight reduction as an isolated intervention are available on which to estimate the benefits of weight loss in lowering risk of CHD. However, sufficient information is available from numerous observational studies and small or short-term randomized clinical trials to conclude that weight loss offers substantial health benefits. (*Data from* Willet *et al.* [34], Huang *et al.* [35], Rexrode *et al.* [36], Goldhaber *et al.* [37], and Colditz *et al.* [38].)

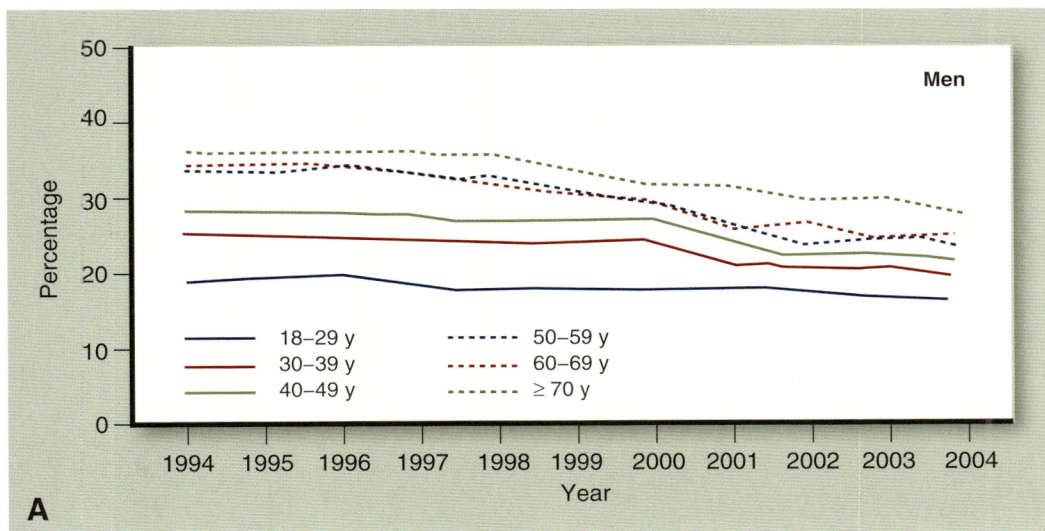

A

Figure 1-39. Prevalence of leisure-time physical inactivity among men (**A**) and women (**B**) by age group and survey year. Physical inactivity is one of the most common modifiable risk factors for coronary heart disease (CHD). Nearly one quarter do not engage in any leisure-time physical activity at all, with women being more sedentary than men, and older individuals being the most inactive.

Continued on the next page

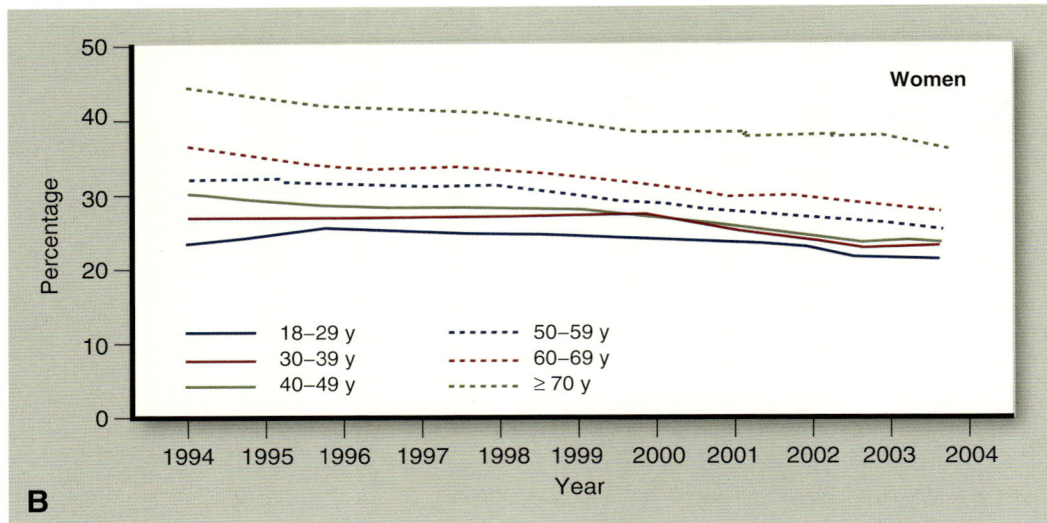

B

Figure 1-39. (Continued) Data from more than 40 observational studies demonstrate clear evidence of an inverse linear dose-response relation between physical activity and all-cause mortality rates in younger and older men and women. While cessation of activity appears to result in increased risk of CHD, the lack of large-scale, randomized, primary prevention trials on the benefits of physical activity makes it difficult to determine the precise magnitude of benefit of exercise in terms of CHD reduction. Physical activity does, however, have clearly demonstrated benefits on cardiovascular risk factors [39].

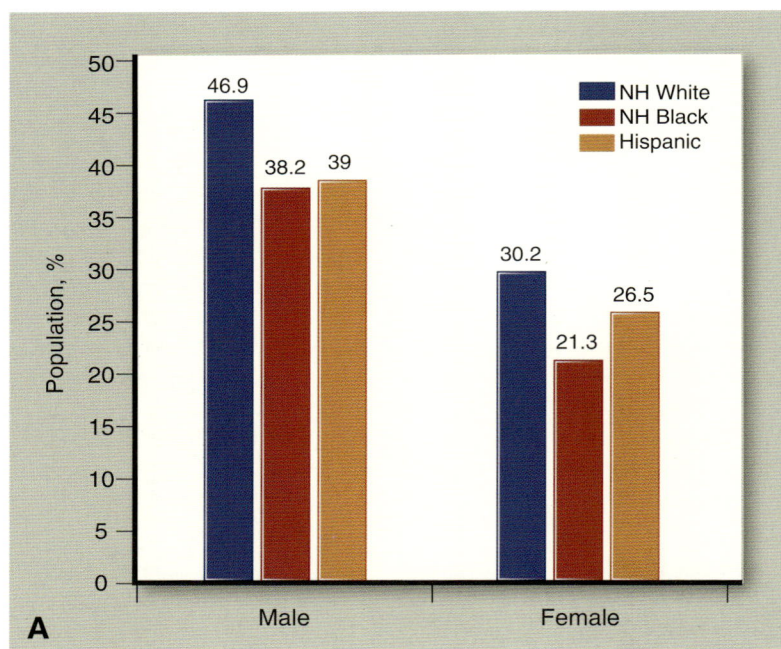

A

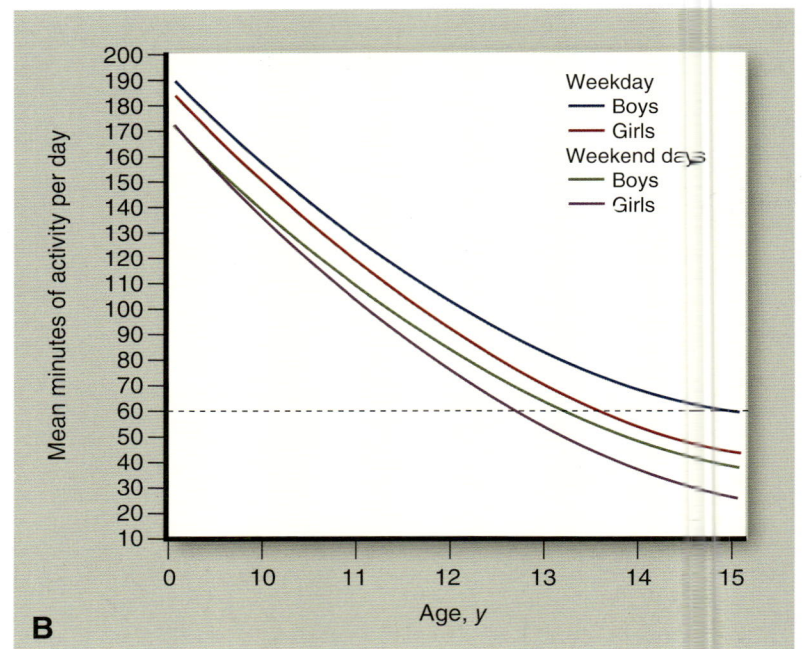

B

Figure 1-40. A, Prevalence of students in grades 9 through 12 who in 2005 met recommended levels of physical activity during the past seven days, by race/ethnicity and sex. Most adolescents do not achieve currently recommended levels of physical activity, which was defined as activity that often increased heart rates and hard breathing for a total of at least 60 minutes per day, five days per week [40]. NH—non-Hispanic.

B, Moderate to vigorous physical activity (MVPA) declines precipitously with age in US adolescents. This graph shows average weekday and weekend minutes of MVPA by sex [41].

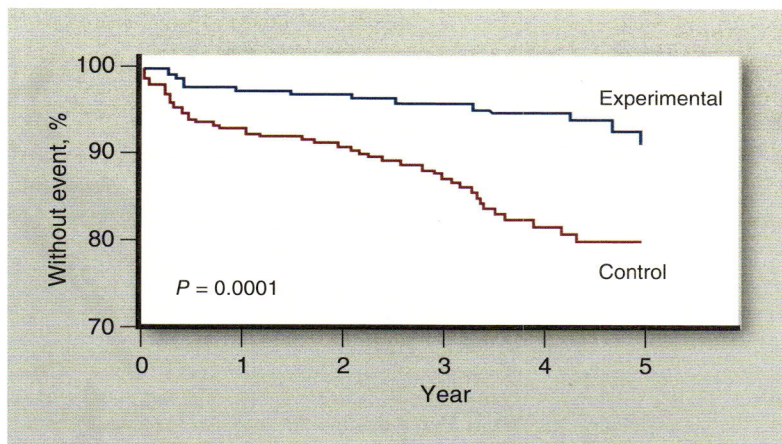

Figure 1-41. Diet has an important impact on coronary heart disease (CHD) risk. Cross-cultural studies suggest that diet plays a role in CHD as well as other chronic diseases. Observational studies suggest a number of dietary factors that may influence the risk of CHD. A key feature of the Western lifestyle is an excess of caloric intake relative to caloric expenditure. Trial data exploring the impact of dietary changes alone on CHD events are very limited. The Lyon Diet Heart Study randomized 605 survivors of a first myocardial infarction to a Mediterranean-type diet (*eg*, canola oil–based margarine, fiber, low cholesterol, low saturated fat, fruits, vegetables) or a "prudent Western-type diet." After a mean follow-up of 46 months, the risk of cardiac death or acute myocardial infarction was 65% lower for those consuming the Mediterranean diet [42].

Summary: AIM

Assess risk using simple tools

Inventory modifiable factors with established beneficial interventions

Modify risk with a multifactorial, comprehensive program: risk-reduction prescription

Figure 1-42. The "AIM" mnemonic aids application of prevention in clinical practice. The process of risk reduction begins with an assessment (A) of an individual's risk. The next step is to inventory (I) the major modifiable risk factors and prioritize interventions to modify (M) risk. These interventions must be implemented, and finally, the risk factors must be reassessed and the information fed back to the patient. Best results are achieved when the patient is fully empowered to actively participate in this process.

References

1. Libby P: The Vascular Biology of Atherosclerosis. In *Braunwald's Heart Disease: A Textbook of Cardiovascular Medicine*, edn 8. Edited by Libby P, Bonow RO, Mann DL, Zipes DP, Braunwald E. Philadelphia: WB Saunders;2007:987.

2. Libby P: Inflammation in atherosclerosis. *Nature* 2002, 420:868–874.

3. Li HM, Cybulsky MI, Gimbrone MA Jr, Libby P: An atherogenic diet rapidly induces VCAM-1, a cytokine-regulatable mononuclear adhesion molecule, in rabbit aortic endothelium. *Arterioscler Thromb* 1993, 15:197–204.

4. Gu L, Okada Y, Clinton SK, *et al.*: Absence of monocyte chemoattractant protein-1 reduces atherosclerosis in low density lipoprotein receptor-deficient mice. *Molecular Cell* 1998, 2:275–281.

5. Hansson G, Libby P, Schoenbeck U, Yan Z-Q: Innate and adaptive immunity in the pathogenesis of atherosclerosis. Review. *Circ Res* 2002, 91:281–291.

6. Sukhova GK, Schoenbeck U, Rabkin E, *et al.*: Evidence for increased collagenolysis by interstitial collagenases-1 and -3 in vulnerable human atheromatous plaques. *Circulation* 1999, 99:2503–2509.

7. Libby P: Molecular bases of the acute coronary syndromes. From bench to bedside. *Circulation* 1995, 91:2844–2850.

8. Libby P: Atherosclerosis: the new view. *Sci Am* 2002, 286:46–55.

9. Libby P, Ridker P: Novel inflammatory markers of coronary risk: theory versus practice. Editorial. *Circulation* 1999, 100:1148–1150.

10. Ridker PM, Hennekens CH, Buring JE, Rifai N: C-reactive protein and other markers of inflammation in the prediction of cardiovascular disease in women. *N Engl J Med* 2000, 342:836–843.

11. Ridker PM, Rifai N, Rose L, *et al.*: Comparison of C-reactive protein and low-density lipoprotein cholesterol levels in the prediction of first cardiovascular events. *N Engl J Med* 2002, 347:1557–1565.

12. Genest J, Libby P: Lipoprotein disorders in cardiovascular disease. In Libby P, Bonow RO, Mann DL, Zipes DP, Braunwald E, eds. *Braunwald's Heart Disease: A Textbook of Cardiovascular Medicine*, edn. 8. Philadelphia: WB Saunders; 2007:1073.

13. Beckman JA, Libby P, Creager MA: Diabetes mellitus, the metabolic syndrome, and atherosclerotic vascular disease. In Libby P, Bonow RO, Mann DL, Zipes DP, Braunwald E, eds. *Braunwald's Heart Disease: A Textbook of Cardiovascular Medicine*, edn 8. Philadelphia: WB Saunders; 2007:1093–1106.

14. Third Report of the National Cholesterol Education Program (NCEP) Expert Panel on Detection, Evaluation, and Treatment of High Blood Cholesterol in Adults (Adult Treatment Panel III) final report. *Circulation* 2002, 106:3143–3421.

15. Ridker PM, Buring JE, Rifai N, Cook NR: Development and validation of improved algorithms for the assessment of global cardiovascular risk in women: the Reynolds Risk Score. *JAMA* 2007, 297:611–619.

16. Gaziano JM, Manson JE, Ridker PM: Primary and secondary prevention of coronary heart disease. In Libby P, Bonow RO, Mann DL, Zipes DP, Braunwald E, eds. *Braunwald's Heart Disease: A Textbook of Cardiovascular Medicine*, edn 8. Philadelphia: WB Saunders, 2007:1119–1148.

17. Kannel WB: High-density lipoproteins: epidemiologic profile and risks of coronary artery disease. *Am J Cardiol* 1983, 4:B9–B12.

18. Yusuf S, Hawken S, Ounpuu S, on behalf of the INTERHEART Study Investigators. Effect of potentially modifiable risk factors associated with myocardial infarction in 52 countries (the INTERHEART study): case-control study. *Lancet* 2004, 364:937–952.

19. US Department of Health and Human Services. *The Health Consequences of Involuntary Smoking: A Report of the Surgeon General*. Washington, DC: Department of Health and Human Services; 1986.

20. Schoenborn CA, Adams PF, Barnes PM, *et al.*: Health behaviors of adults: United States 1999–2001. *Vital Health Stat 10* 2004, 219:1–79.

21. Centers for Disease Control and Prevention: Cigarette smoking among adults: United States, 2002. *MMWR* 2004, 53:427–431.

22. Wilson K, Gibson N, Willan A, Cook D: Effect of smoking cessation on mortality after myocardial infarction: meta-analysis of cohort studies. *Arch Intern Med* 2000, 160:939–944.

23. Castelli WP, Garrison RJ, Wilson PW, *et al.*: Incidence of coronary heart disease and lipoprotein cholesterol levels. The Framingham Study. *JAMA* 1986, 256, 2:835–838.

24. Prospective Studies Collaboration, Lewington S, Whitlock G, *et al.*: Blood cholesterol and vascular mortality by age, sex, and blood pressure: a meta-analysis of individual data from 61 prospective studies with 55,000 vascular deaths. *Lancet* 2007, 370:1829–1839.

25. Cholesterol Treatment Trialists' Collaborators, Kearney PM, Blackwell L, *et al.*: Efficacy and safety of cholesterol-lowering treatment: prospective meta-analysis of data from 90,056 participants in 14 randomised trials of statins. *Lancet* 2005, 366:1267–1278.

26. Lewington S, Clarke R, Qizilbash N, *et al.*: Age-specific relevance of usual blood pressure to vascular mortality: a meta-analysis of individual data for one million adults in 61 prospective studies. *Lancet* 2002, 360:1903–1913.

27. Blood Pressure Lowering Treatment Trialists' Collaboration, Turnbull F, Neal B, *et al.*: Effects of different blood-pressure-lowering regimens on major cardio-vascular events: results of prospectively-designed overviews of randomized trials. *Lancet* 2003, 362:1527–1535.

28. National Diabetes Fact Sheet: *General Information and National Estimates on Diabetes in the United States, 2005.* Atlanta: US Department of Health and Human Services, Centers for Disease Control and Prevention, 2005.

29. Ford ES, Giles WH, Mokdad AH: Increasing prevalence of the metabolic syndrome among U.S. Adults. *Diabetes Care* 2004, 27:2444–2449.

30. de Ferranti SD, Gauvreau K, Ludwig DS, *et al.*: Prevalence of the metabolic syndrome in American adolescents: findings from the Third National Health and Nutrition Examination Survey. *Circulation* 2004, 110:2494–2497.

31. Third Report of the National Cholesterol Education Program (NCEP) Expert Panel on Detection, Evaluation, and Treatment of High Blood Cholesterol in Adults (Adult Treatment Panel III) final report. *Circulation* 2002, 106:3143–3421.

32. Chobanian AV, Bakris GL, Black HR, *et al.*: The Seventh Report of the Joint National Committee on Prevention, Detection, Evaluation, and Treatment of High Blood Pressure: the JNC 7 report. *JAMA* 2003, 289:2560–2572.

33. Centers for Disease Control and Prevention, Department of Health and Human Services: Preventing chronic diseases: investing wisely in health. Preventing obesity and chronic diseases through good nutrition and physical activity. Available at http://www.cdc.gov/nccdphp/pe_factsheets/pe_pa.htm.

34. Willett WC, Manson JE, Stampfer MJ, *et al.*: Weight, weight change, and coronary heart disease in women. Risk within the "normal" weight range. *JAMA* 1995, 273:461–465.

35. Huang Z, Willett WC, Manson JE, *et al.*: Body weight, weight change, and risk for hypertension in women. *Ann Intern Med* 1998, 128:81–88.

36. Rexrode KM, Hennekens CH, Willett WC, *et al.*: A prospective study of body mass index, weight change, and risk of stroke in women. *JAMA* 1997, 277:1539–1545.

37. Goldhaber SZ, Grodstein F, Stampfer MJ, *et al.*: A prospective study of risk factors for pulmonary embolism in women. *JAMA* 1997, 277:642–645.

38. Colditz GA, Willett WC, Rotnitzky A, Manson JE: Weight gain as a risk factor for clinical diabetes mellitus in women. *Ann Intern Med* 1995, 122:481–486.

39. Kruger J; Division of Nutrition and Physical Activity; National Center for Chronic Disease Prevention and Health Promotion; Centers for Disease Control. Trends in leisure-time physical inactivity by age, sex, and race/ethnicity—United States, 1994–2004. *MMWR* 2005, 54(39):991–994.

40. Eaton DK, Kann L, Kinchen S, *et al.*: Division of Adolescent and School Health; Division of Adult and Community Health; National Center for Chronic Disease Prevention and Health Promotion; Centers for Disease Control. Youth risk behavior surveillance—United States, 2005. *MMWR* 2006, 55(SS05):1–108.

41. Nader PR, Bradley RH, Houts RM, *et al.*: Moderate-to-vigorous physical activity from ages 9 to 15 years. *JAMA* 2008, 300:295–305.

42. de Lorgeril M, Salen P, Martin J-L, *et al.*: Mediterranean diet, traditional risk factors, and the rate of cardiovascular complications after myocardial infarction. *Circulation* 1999, 99:779–785.

Acute Coronary Syndromes

Elliott Antman

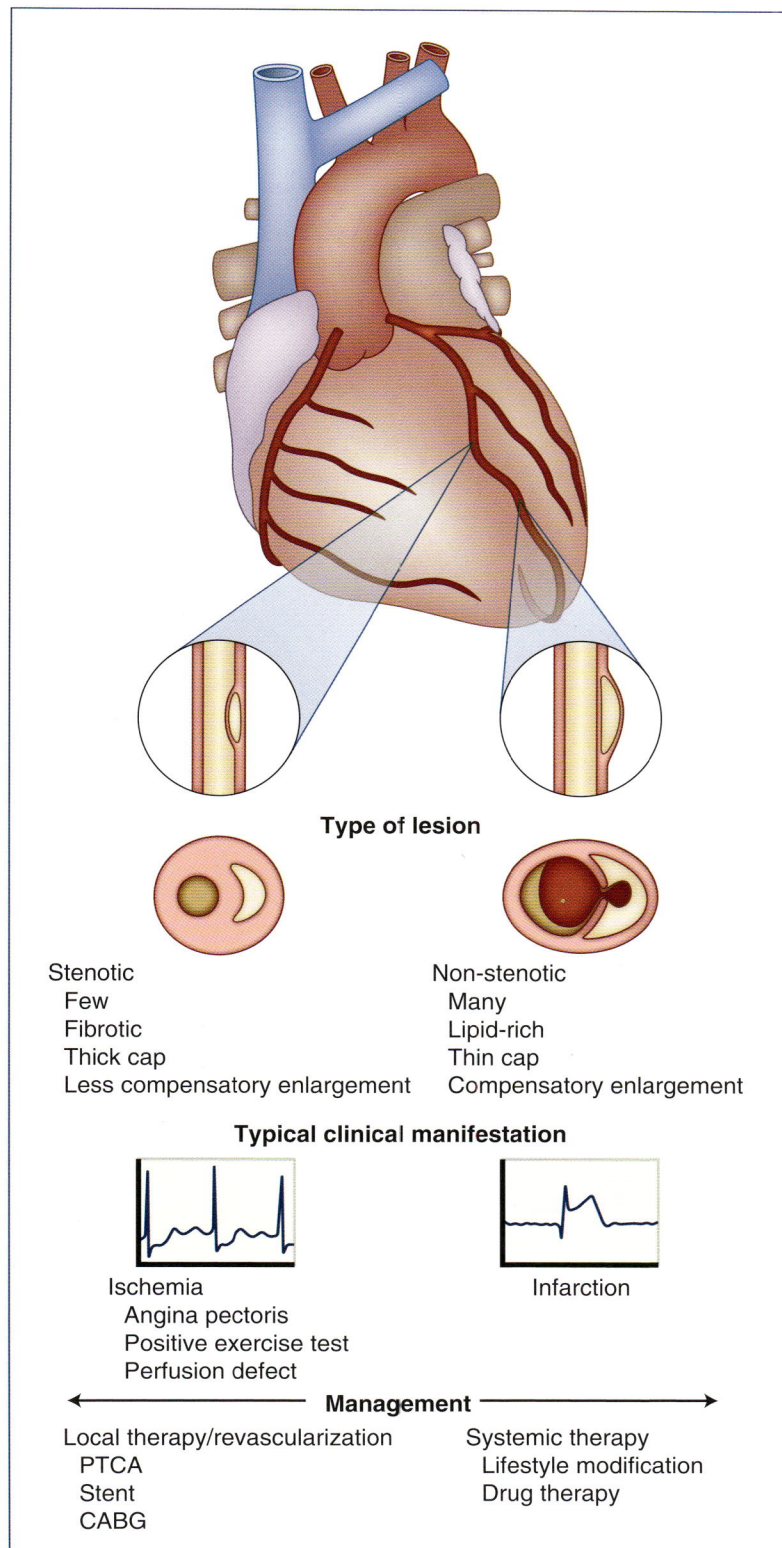

Type of lesion

Stenotic
Few
Fibrotic
Thick cap
Less compensatory enlargement

Non-stenotic
Many
Lipid-rich
Thin cap
Compensatory enlargement

Typical clinical manifestation

Ischemia
  Angina pectoris
  Positive exercise test
  Perfusion defect

Infarction

← **Management** →

Local therapy/revascularization
  PTCA
  Stent
  CABG

Systemic therapy
  Lifestyle modification
  Drug therapy

Figure 2-1. Simplified schema of lesion diversity in human coronary atherosclerosis. This schematic depicts two morphologic extremes of coronary atherosclerotic plaques. Stenotic lesions (*top*) tend to have smaller lipid cores, more fibrosis and calcification, thick fibrous caps, and less compensatory enlargement (positive remodeling). They typically produce ischemia that can be managed by a combination of medications from different drug classes and, in selected patients, revascularization for symptom relief. Nonstenotic lesions (*bottom*) generally outnumber stenotic plaques and tend to have large lipid cores and thin, fibrous caps susceptible to rupture and thrombosis. They often undergo substantial compensatory enlargement that leads to underestimation of lesion size by angiography. Nonstenotic plaques may cause no symptoms for many years but when disrupted can provoke an acute coronary syndrome. Management of nonstenotic lesions should include lifestyle modification (and pharmacotherapy in high-risk individuals). Enlarged segments of the schematic show longitudinal section (*left*) and cross-section (*right*). Many coronary atherosclerotic lesions may lie between these two extremes, produce mixed clinical manifestations and require multipronged management. Because both types of lesions usually coexist in a given high-risk individual, optimum management often requires revascularization and systemic medical therapy. CABG—coronary artery bypass graft; PTCA—percutaneous transluminal coronary angioplasty. (*Adapted from* Libby and Théroux [1].)

Figure 2-2. Chronology of atherosclerotic process. Longitudinal section of artery depicting the timeline of human atherogenesis from normal artery to atheroma that caused clinical manifestations by thrombosis or stenosis (*top*). Cross-sections of artery during various stages of atheroma evolution (*bottom*). From left to right: 1) Normal artery. 2) Lesion initiation occurs when endothelial cells, activated by risk factors such as hyperlipoproteinemia, express adhesion and chemoattractant molecules that recruit inflammatory leukocytes, such as monocytes and T lymphocytes. Extracellular lipid begins to accumulate in intima at this stage. 3) Evolution to fibrofatty stage. 4) As lesion progresses, inflammatory mediators cause expression of tissue factor, a potent procoagulant, and of matrix-degrading proteinases that weaken fibrous cap of plaque. 5) If fibrous cap ruptures at the point of weakening, coagulation factors in blood can gain access to a thrombogenic, tissue factor–containing lipid core, causing thrombosis on a nonocclusive atherosclerotic plaque, and an acute coronary syndrome may occur, depending on the balance of prothrombotic and fibrinolytic mechanisms. 6) When thrombus resorbs, products associated with thrombosis, such as thrombin and mediators released from degranulating platelets, including platelet-derived growth factor and transforming growth factor-β, can cause a healing response, leading to increased collagen accumulation and smooth muscle cell growth. In this manner,

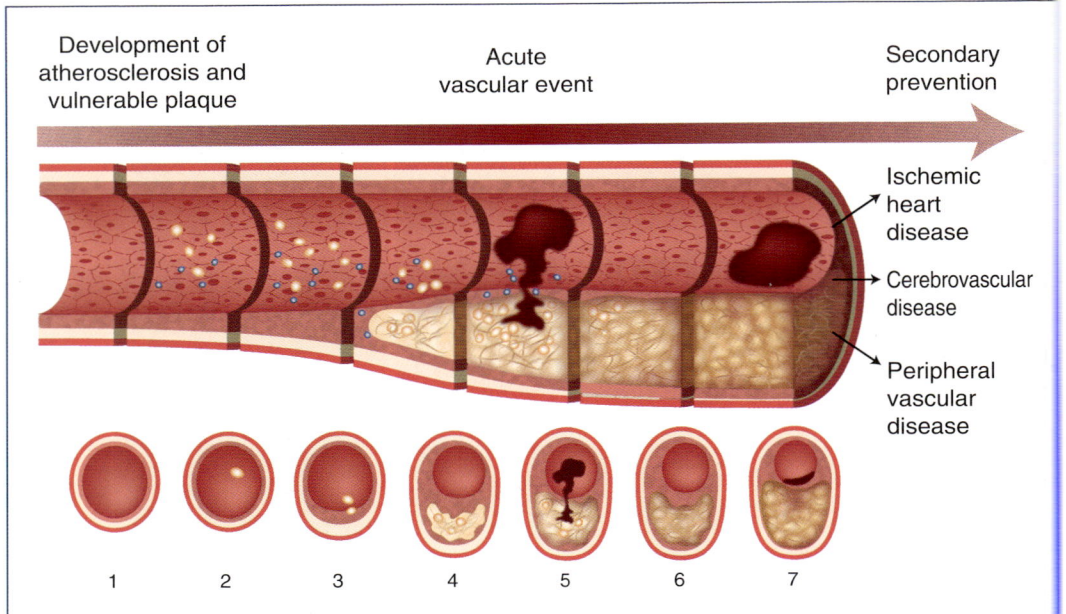

the fibrofatty lesion can evolve into advanced fibrous and often calcified plaque, one that may cause significant stenosis and produce symptoms of stable angina pectoris. 7) In some cases, occlusive thrombi arise not from fracture of fibrous cap but from superficial erosion of the endothelial layer. As noted along the right side of the figure, atherosclerosis is a generalized vascular process, emphasizing that clinicians should evaluate patients with clinically evident ischemic heart disease for coexisting atherosclerosis in cerebral and peripheral arterial beds. (*Adapted from* Libby [2].)

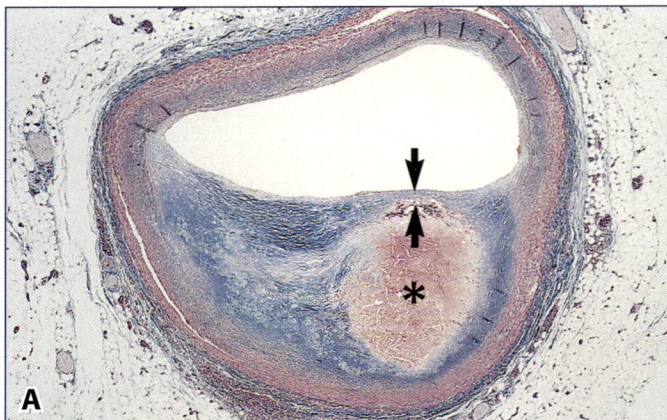

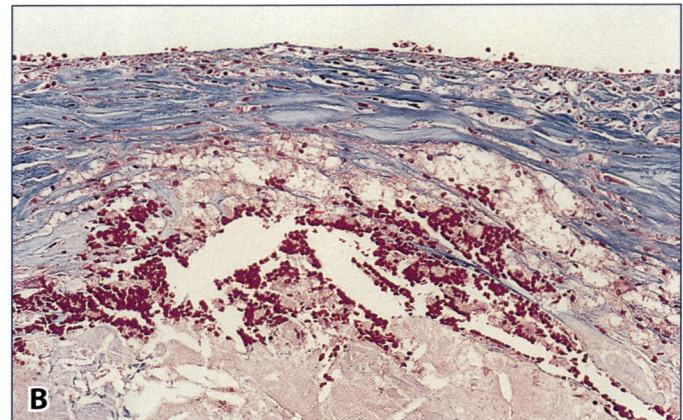

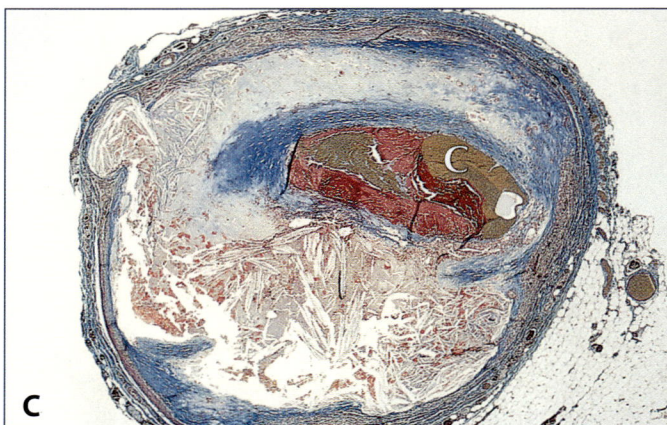

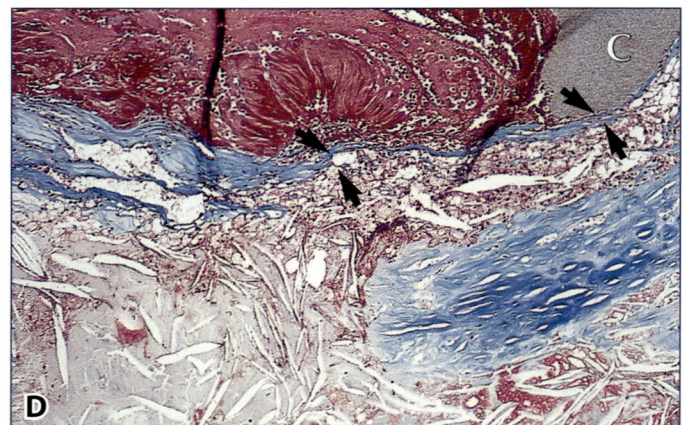

Figure 2-3. The consistency of coronary plaques and their vulnerability to rupture differ. The collagen-rich sclerotic plaque component is hard and stable, whereas the lipid-rich atheromatous component is soft and unstable. **A,** A thin cap of fibrous tissue (*between arrows*) separates the soft, lipid-rich pool (*asterisk*) from the lumen [3]. Such a thin fibrous cap, infiltrated with macrophage foam cells (clearly seen in **B**), overlying an extracellular lipid pool is mechanically weak and vulnerable to rupture. **C** and **D,** In this case, the thin foam cell-infiltrated cap (*between arrows in* **D**) has ruptured nearby, and a mural thrombus has evolved at the rupture site where thrombogenic material has been exposed (trichrome stain, showing collagen as *blue* and thrombus as *red*) [4]. The presence of erythrocytes just beneath the cap indicates that the cap is ruptured nearby. C—contrast medium in residual lumen.

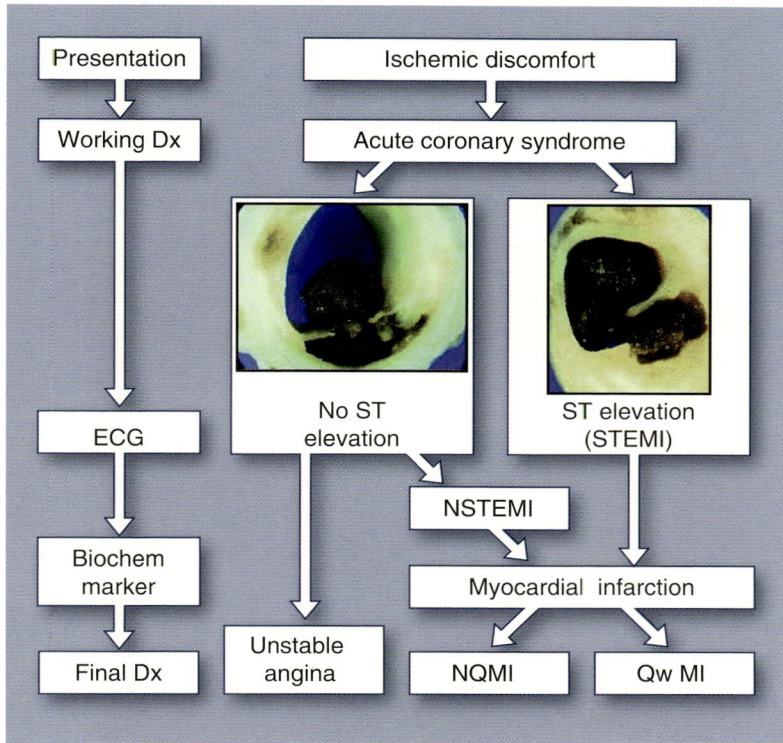

Figure 2-4. Acute coronary syndromes. Following disruption of a vulnerable plaque, patients may experience an acute coronary syndrome, characterized by ischemic discomfort resulting from a reduction of flow through the affected epicardial coronary artery. The flow reduction may be caused by a completely occlusive thrombus (*right side*) or subtotally occlusive thrombus (*left side*). Patients with ischemic discomfort may present with or without ST-segment elevation on the electrocardiogram (ECG). Of patients with ST-segment elevation myocardial infarction (STEMI), most ultimately develop a Q-wave MI (QwMI), while a few develop a non–Q-wave MI (NQMI). Patients who present without ST-segment elevation are suffering from either unstable angina or a non–ST-segment elevation MI (NSTEMI), a distinction that is ultimately made on the presence or absence of a serum cardiac marker such as the MB isoenzyme of creatine kinase or preferably a cardiac troponin detected in the blood. Most patients presenting with NSTEMI ultimately develop an NQMI on the ECG; a few may develop a QwMI. The spectrum of clinical presentations ranging from unstable angina through NSTEMI and STEMI are referred to as the acute coronary syndromes. Dx—diagnosis. (*Adapted from* Libby [2], Libby *et al.* [5], Hamm *et al.* [6], Davies [7], *and* Antman *et al.* [8].)

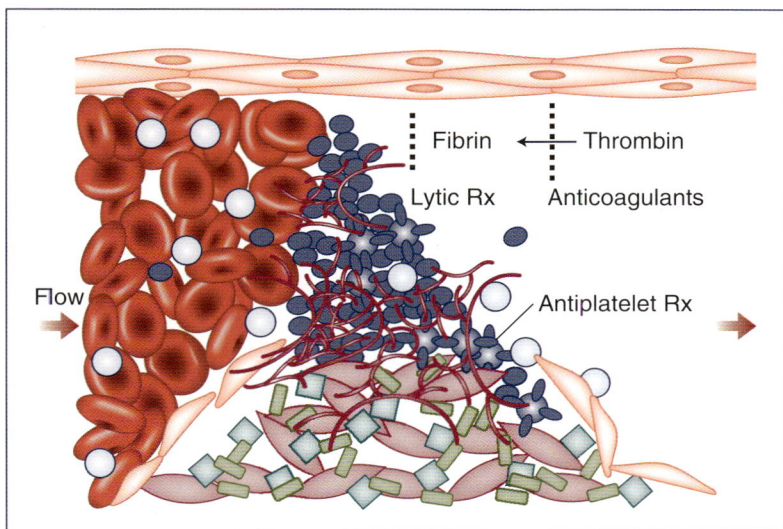

Figure 2-5. Thrombus in infarct-related artery. This figure shows a schematic view of a longitudinal section of an infarct-related artery at the level of the obstructive thrombus. Rupture of a vulnerable plaque (*bottom center*) activates the coagulation cascade, ultimately leading to the deposition of fibrin strands (*red curvilinear arcs*); platelets are activated and begin to aggregate (transition from flat blue discs representing inactive platelets to blue spiked ball elements representing activated and aggregating platelets). The mesh of fibrin strands and platelet aggregates obstructs flow (normally moving from left to right) in the infarct-related artery; this would correspond to thrombolysis in myocardial infarction (TIMI) grade 0 on angiography. Pharmacologic reperfusion is a multipronged approach consisting of fibrinolytic agents that digest fibrin, antithrombins that prevent the formation of thrombin and inhibit the activity of thrombin that is formed, and antiplatelet therapy (Rx) [5].

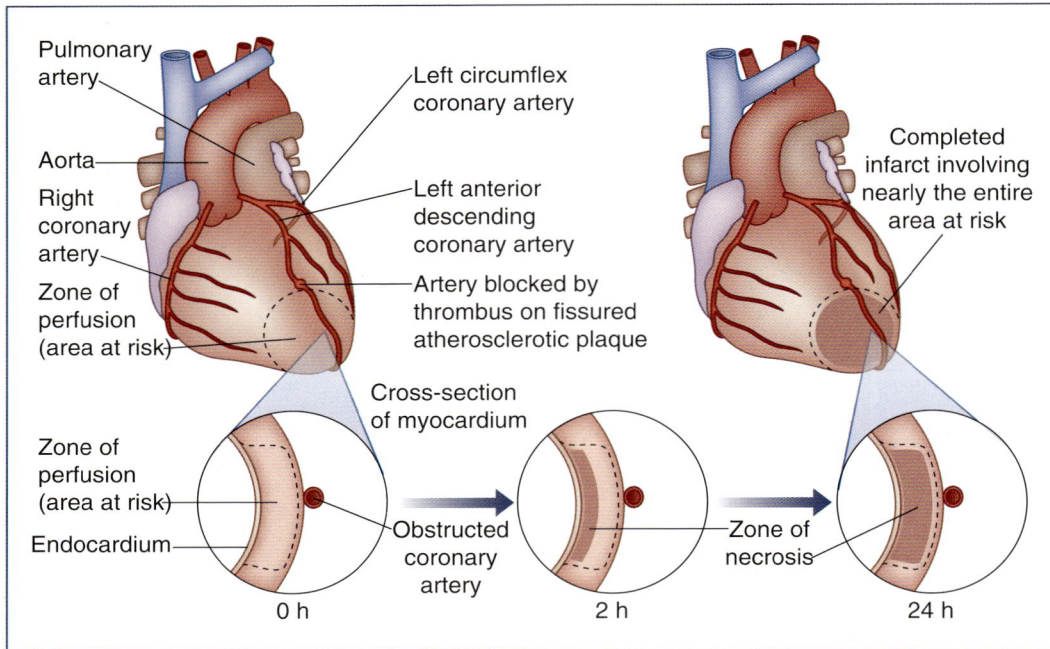

Pulmonary artery
Left circumflex coronary artery
Aorta
Left anterior descending coronary artery
Right coronary artery
Artery blocked by thrombus on fissured atherosclerotic plaque
Zone of perfusion (area at risk)
Completed infarct involving nearly the entire area at risk

Cross-section of myocardium

Zone of perfusion (area at risk)
Endocardium
Obstructed coronary artery
Zone of necrosis

0 h   2 h   24 h

Figure 2-6. Schematic representation of the progression of myocardial necrosis after coronary artery occlusion. Necrosis begins in a small zone of the myocardium beneath the endocardial surface in the center of the ischemic zone. This entire region of myocardium (*dashed outline*) depends on the occluded vessel for perfusion and is the area at risk. Note that a very narrow zone of myocardium immediately beneath the endocardium is spared from necrosis because it can be oxygenated by diffusion from the ventricle [5,9].

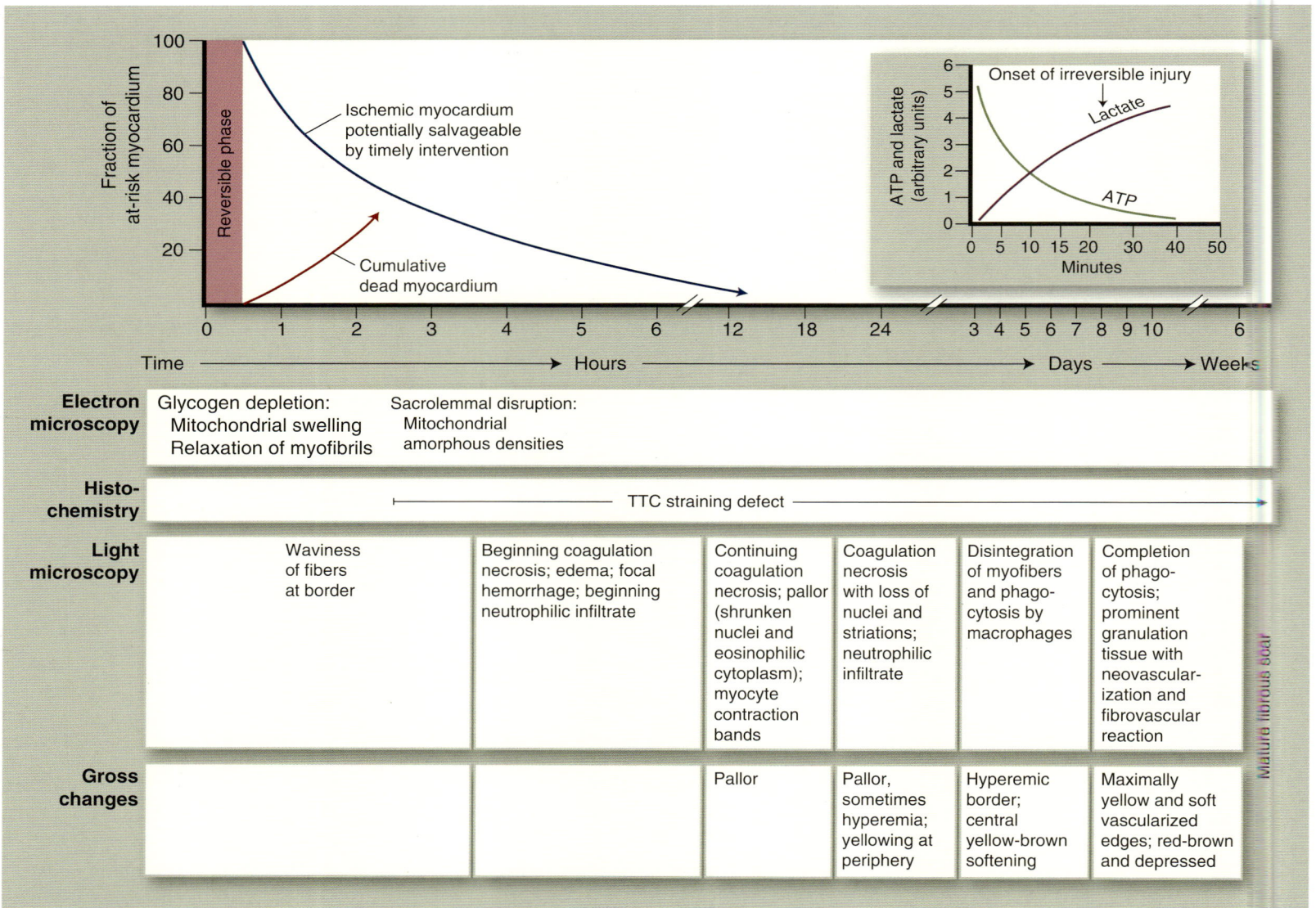

Inset graph: Onset of irreversible injury — Lactate, ATP; ATP and lactate (arbitrary units) vs Minutes (0 5 10 15 20 30 40 50)

Fraction of at-risk myocardium — Reversible phase; Ischemic myocardium potentially salvageable by timely intervention; Cumulative dead myocardium

Time — Hours — Days — Weeks

Electron microscopy	Glycogen depletion: Mitochondrial swelling Relaxation of myofibrils	Sacrolemmal disruption: Mitochondrial amorphous densities				
Histo-chemistry		TTC straining defect				
Light microscopy	Waviness of fibers at border	Beginning coagulation necrosis; edema; focal hemorrhage; beginning neutrophilic infiltrate	Continuing coagulation necrosis; pallor (shrunken nuclei and eosinophilic cytoplasm); myocyte contraction bands	Coagulation necrosis with loss of nuclei and striations; neutrophilic infiltrate	Disintegration of myofibers and phago-cytosis by macrophages	Completion of phago-cytosis; prominent granulation tissue with neovascular-ization and fibrovascular reaction
Gross changes			Pallor	Pallor, sometimes hyperemia; yellowing at periphery	Hyperemic border; central yellow-brown softening	Maximally yellow and soft vascularized edges; red-brown and depressed

Mature fibrous scar

Figure 2-7. Temporal sequence of early biochemical, ultrastructural, histochemical, and histologic findings after myocardial infarction onset. Time frames (*top*) are shown for early and late reperfusion of the myocardium supplied by an occluded coronary artery. For about 30 minutes after onset of even the most severe ischemia, myocardial injury may be reversed, although progressive loss of viability is complete by 6 to 12 hours. Reperfusion benefits are greatest when achieved early, with progressively smaller benefits occurring with delay. Pathologic findings after reperfusion vary depending on reperfusion timing, prior infarction, and collateral flow [5,10]. ATP—adenosine triphosphate; TTC—triphenyltetrazolium chloride.

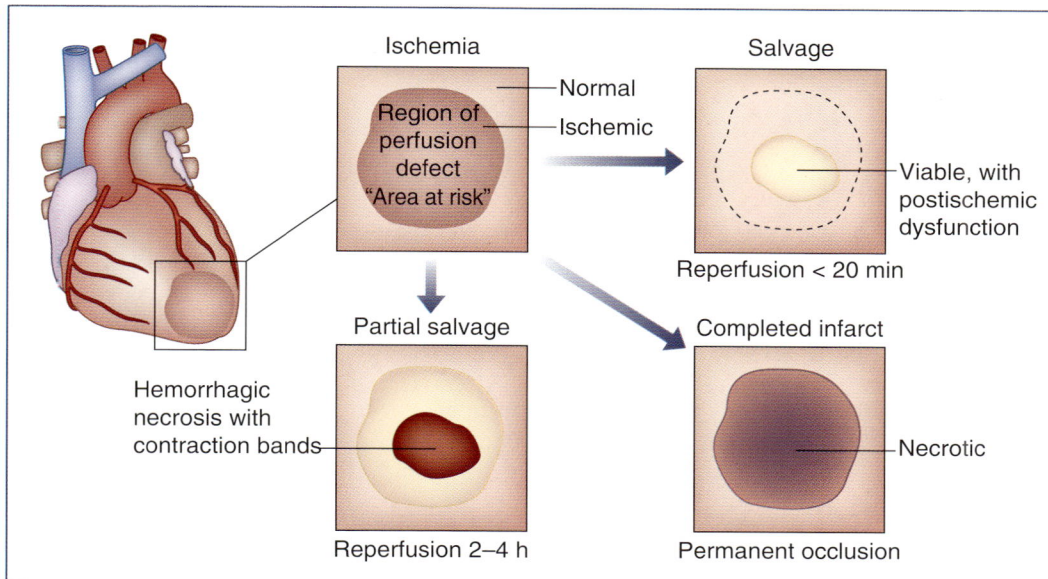

Figure 2-8. Consequences of reperfusion at various times after coronary adhesion. In this example, the midportion of the left anterior descending coronary artery is occluded and a large zone of anterior and apical ischemic myocardium develops—the "area at risk." Reperfusion in less than 20 minutes does not result in permanent tissue loss, but there may be a period of contractile dysfunction of the reperfused myocardium—a condition referred to as "stunning." Later reperfusion results in hemorrhagic necrosis with contraction bands. Permanent occlusion results in necrosis of myocardium [5,11].

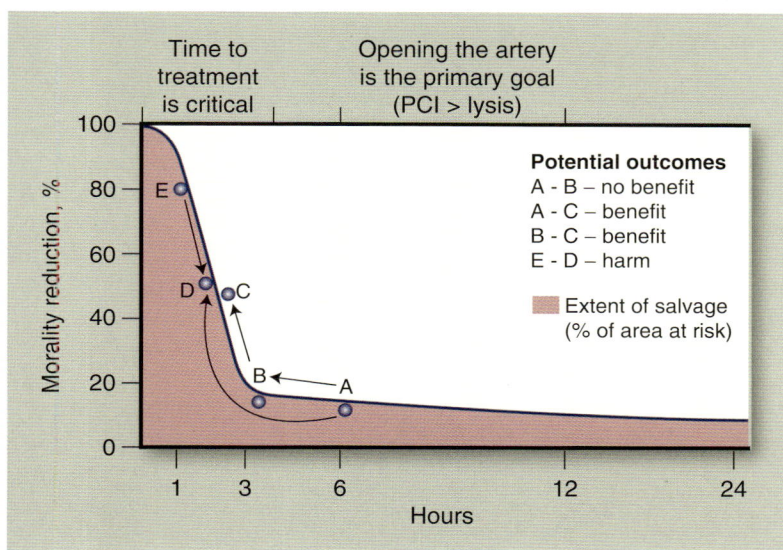

Figure 2-9. Time and myocardial salvage. Mortality reduction as a benefit of reperfusion therapy is greatest in the first 2 to 3 hours after the onset of symptoms of acute myocardial infarction, most likely a consequence of myocardial salvage. The exact duration of this critical early period depends on several factors, including the presence of functioning collateral coronary arteries, ischemic preconditioning, myocardial oxygen demands, and duration of sustained ischemia. After this early period, the magnitude of the mortality benefit is much reduced, and as the mortality-reduction curve flattens, time to reperfusion therapy is less critical. The magnitude of benefit depends on how far up the curve the patient can be shifted. The benefit of a shift from points *A* or *B* to point *C* would be substantial, but the benefit of a shift from point A to point B would be small. A treatment strategy that delays therapy during the early critical period, such as patient transfer for percutaneous coronary intervention (PCI), would be harmful (*eg*, shift from point D to point B) [5,12].

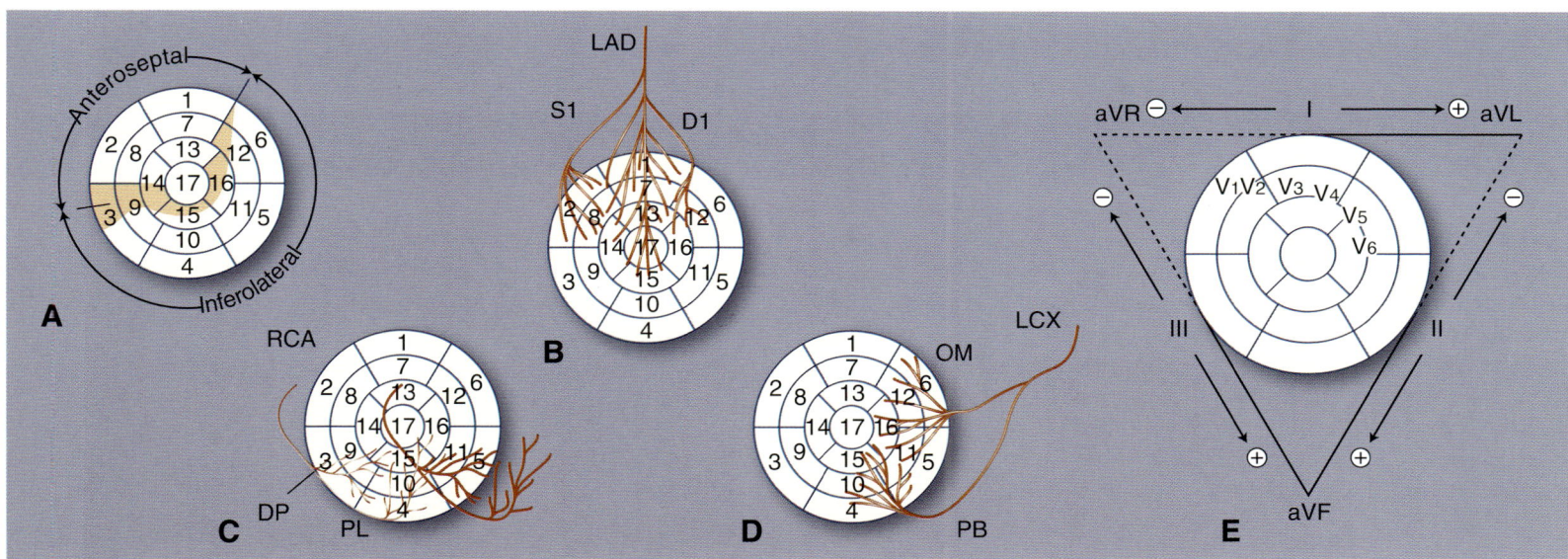

Figure 2-10. Identification of infarct artery from 12-lead electrocardiogram (ECG). This figure shows the 17 myocardial segments in a polar map format (**A**) with superimposition of the arterial supply provided by the left anterior descending (LAD) (**B**), right coronary artery (RCA) (**C**), and left circumflex (LCX) (**D**). The position of the standard ECG leads relative to the polar map is shown (**E**). The infarct artery can be deduced by identifying the leads that show ST elevation and referencing that information to **A–D**. For example, ST elevation seen most prominently in the leads overlying segments 1, 2, 7, 8, 13, 14, and 17 indicates that the LAD is the infarct artery [5,13]. D1—first diagonal; DP—posterior descending; OM—obtuse marginal; PB—posterobasal; PL—posterolateral; S1—first septal.

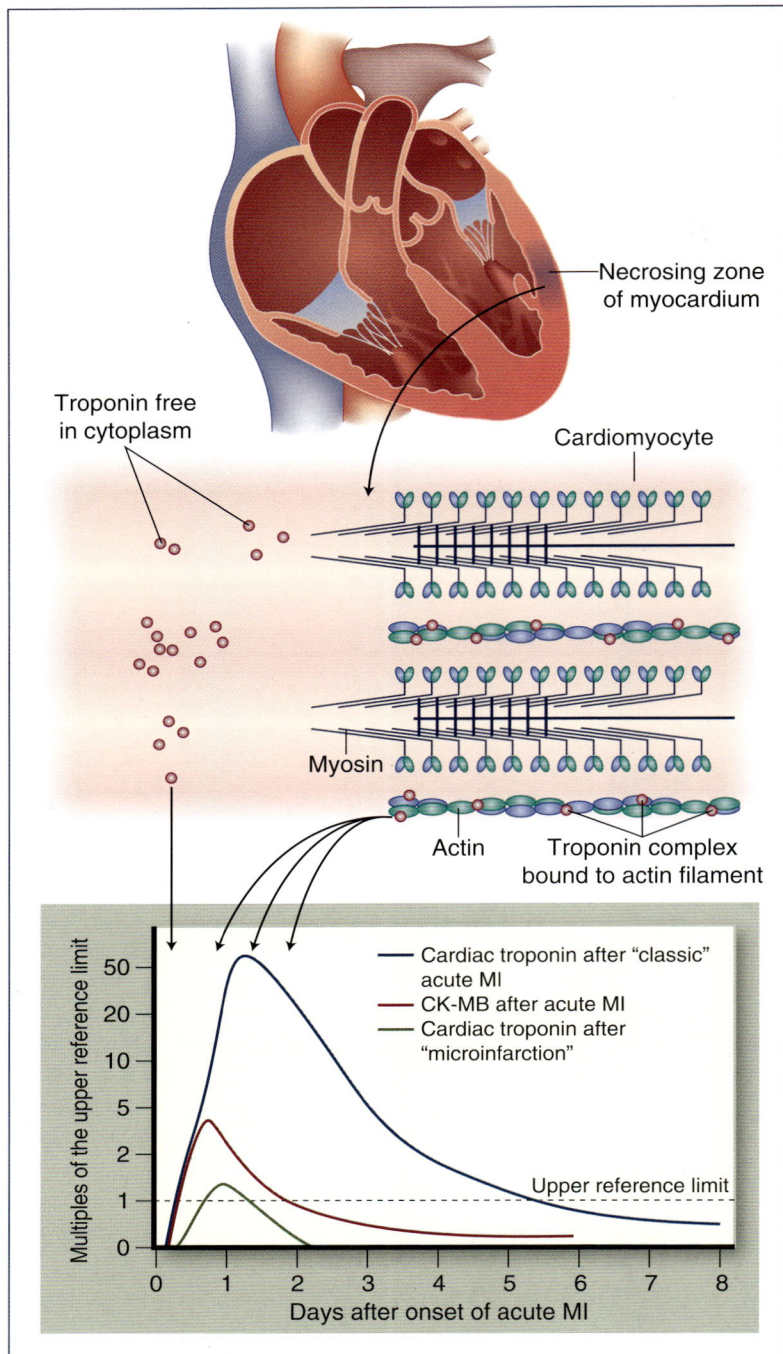

Figure 2-11. The zone of necrosing myocardium (*top*), followed by a cardiomyocyte (*middle*) that is in the process of releasing biomarkers. After disruption of the sarcolemmal membrane of the cardiomyocyte, the cytoplasmic pool of biomarkers is released first (*leftmost arrow in bottom portion*). Markers such as myoglobin and creatine kinase (CK) isoforms are rapidly released and blood levels rise quickly above the cutoff limit. This is then followed by a more protracted release of biomarkers from the disintegrating myofilaments that may continue for several days (*three-headed arrow*). Cardiac troponin levels rise to about 20 to 50 times the upper reference limit (the 99th percentile of values in a reference control group) in patients who have a "classic" acute myocardial infarction (MI) and sustain sufficient myocardial necrosis to result in abnormally elevated levels of the MB fraction of creatine kinase (CK-MB). Clinicians can now diagnose episodes of microinfarction by sensitive assays that detect cardiac troponin elevations above the upper reference limit, even though CK-MB levels may still be in the normal reference range (*not shown*) [5,14,15].

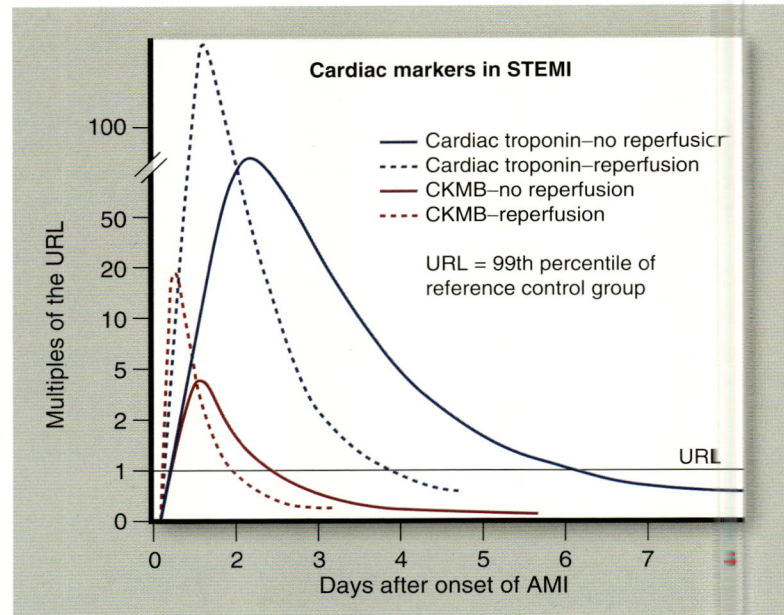

Figure 2-12. The kinetics of release of MB fraction of creatine kinase (CK-MB) and cardiac troponin in patients who do not undergo reperfusion (*solid green and red curves*) shown as multiples of the upper reference limit (URL). Note that when patients with ST-segment elevation myocardial infarction (STEMI) undergo reperfusion (*dashed green and red curves*), the cardiac biomarkers are detected sooner, rise to a higher peak value, but decline more rapidly, resulting in a smaller area under the curve and limitation of infarct size [5,8,16]. AMI—acute myocardial infarction.

Revised Definition of Myocardial Infarction

Critieria for Acute, Evolving, or Recent MI

Either of the following criteria satisfies the diagnosis for acute, evolving, or recent MI:

1. Typical rise and/or fall of biochemical markers of myocardial necrosis with at least one of the following:

   Ischemic symptoms

   Development of pathological Q waves in the ECG

   ECG changes indicative of ischemia (ST segment elevation or depression)

   Imaging evidence of new loss of viable myocardium or new regional wall motion abnormality

2. Pathological findings of an acute myocardial infarction

Criteria for Healing or Healed Myocardial Infarction

Any of the following criteria satisfies the diagnosis for healing or healed myocardial infarction:

   Development of new pathological Q waves in serial ECGs. Patients may or may not remember previous symptoms. Biochemical markers of myocardial necrosis may have normalized depending on the time since the infarction developed

   Pathological findings of a healed or healing infarction

Figure 2-13. Revised definition of myocardial infarction. ECG—electrocardiogram. (*Adapted from* Bayes de Luna *et al.* [13].)

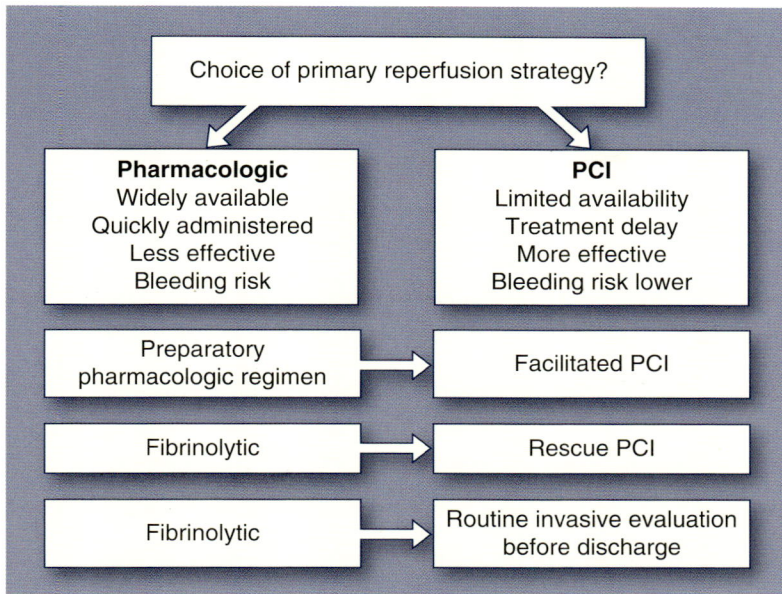

Figure 2-14. Interface of pharmacologic and catheter-based reperfusion strategies for ST-segment elevation myocardial infarction (STEMI). The *top row* illustrates the choice between pharmacologic and mechanical reperfusion for STEMI and outlines the advantages and disadvantages of each approach. If the percutaneous coronary intervention (PCI) is routinely performed very shortly after a preparatory pharmacologic regimen, it is referred to as facilitated PCI. Rescue PCI refers to PCI performed when there is clinical suspicion of failure of an initial attempt at pharmacologic reperfusion. Some clinicians elect to perform diagnostic angiography and PCI as indicated even if pharmacologic reperfusion was successful [5,17].

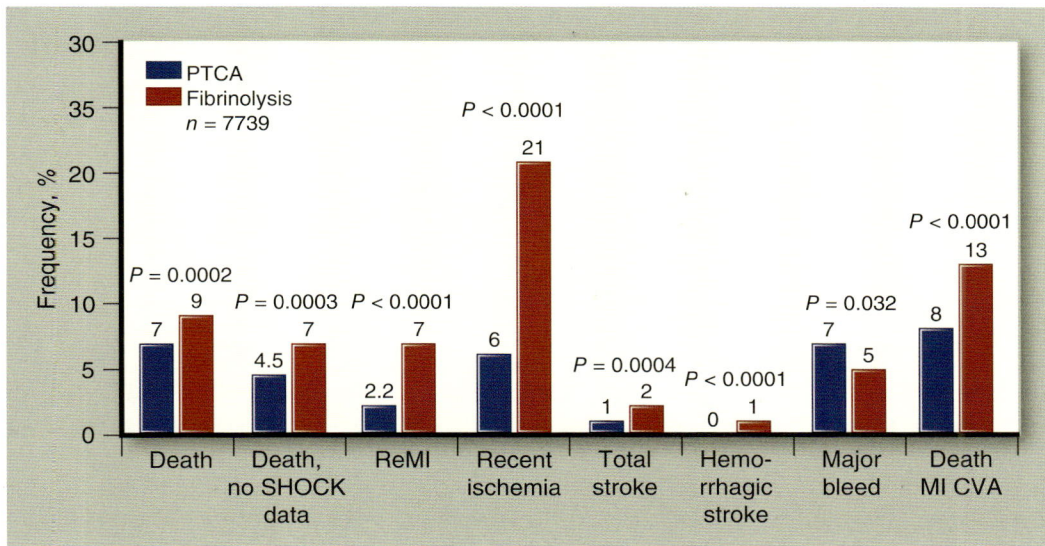

Figure 2-15. Short-term clinical outcomes in patients with ST-segment elevation myocardial infarction (STEMI) treated either with fibrinolysis or percutaneous coronary intervention (PCI) [18]. CVA—cerebrovascular accident.

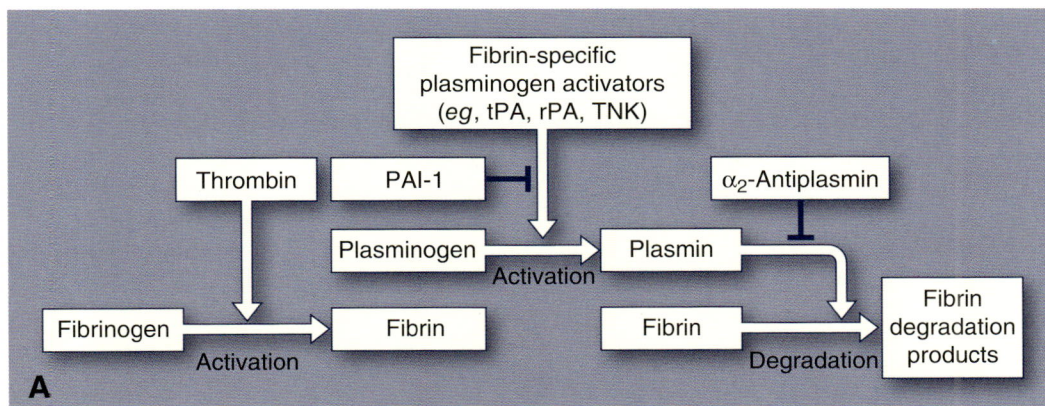

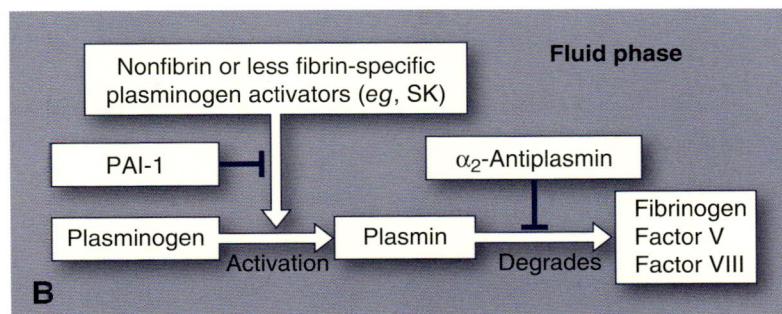

Figure 2-16. Overview of fibrinolytic agents. **A,** Plasminogen is converted by either intrinsic or extrinsic activators to plasmin, which in turn degrades fibrin. **B,** More fibrin-specific activators preferentially activate plasminogen at the fibrin surface, whereas nonfibrin or less-specific plasminogen activators induce extensive systemic plasminogen activation, with degradation of several plasma proteins including fibrinogen, factor V, and factor VIII. Plasminogen activator inhibitor (PAI) 1 and α_2-antiplasmin are serine protease inhibitors (members of the serpin superfamily) that are the main inhibitors of plasminogen activators and plasmin, respectively, in human plasma [19].

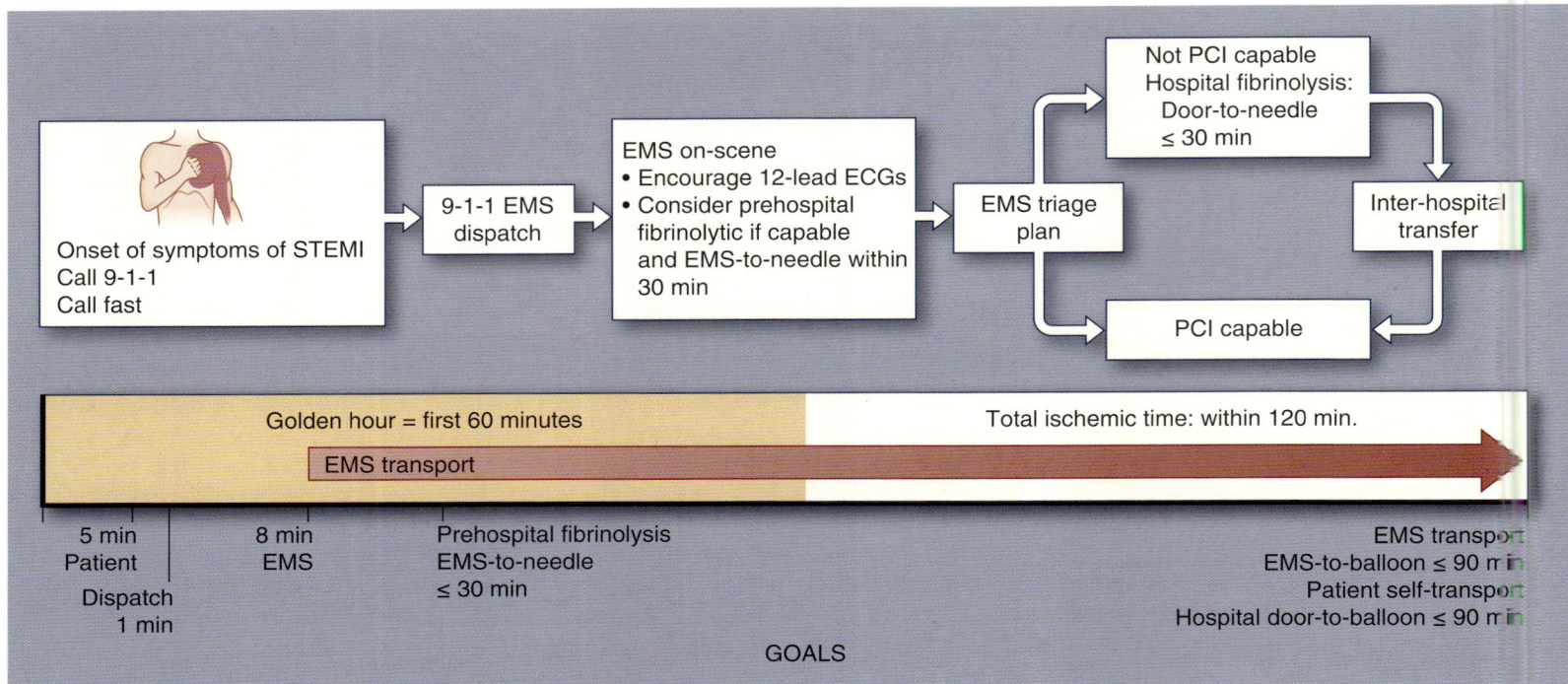

Figure 2-17. Options for transportation of ST-segment elevation myocardial infarction (STEMI) patients and initial reperfusion treatment. Reperfusion in patients with STEMI can be accomplished by the pharmacologic (fibrinolysis) or catheter-based (primary percutaneous coronary intervention [PCI]) approaches. Implementation of these strategies varies based on the mode of transportation of the patient and capabilities at the receiving hospital. Patients are transported by emergency medical services (EMS) after calling 911. Transport time to the hospital varies from case to case, but the goal is to limit total ischemic time to less than 120 minutes. There are three possibilities: 1) If EMS has fibrinolytic capability and the patient qualifies for therapy, prehospital fibrinolysis should be started within 30 minutes of EMS arrival. 2) If EMS cannot administer prehospital fibrinolysis and the patient is transported to a non–PCI-capable hospital, the hospital-to-needle time should be less than or equal to 30 minutes for patients in whom fibrinolysis is indicated. 3) If EMS is not capable of administering prehospital fibrinolysis and the patient is transported to a PCI-capable hospital, the hospital door-to-balloon time should be less than or equal to 90 minutes.

It is also appropriate to consider emergency interhospital transfer to a PCI-capable hospital for mechanical revascularization if 1) there is a con-

traindication to fibrinolysis; 2) PCI can be initiated promptly ($\leq$ 90 min after the patient presented to the initial receiving hospital or $\leq$ 60 min compared with when fibrinolysis could be initiated at the initial receiving hospital); 3) fibrinolysis is administered and is unsuccessful (ie, "rescue PCI"). Secondary nonemergency interhospital transfer can be considered for recurrent ischemia.

Patient self-transportation is discouraged. If the patient arrives at a non–PCI-capable hospital, the door-to-needle time should be 30 minutes or less. If the patient arrives at a PCI-capable hospital, the door-to-balloon time should be 90 minutes or less. The treatment options and time recommendations after first hospital arrival are the same.

The medical system goal is to facilitate rapid recognition and treatment of patients with STEMI such that door-to-needle (or EMS-to-needle for initiation of fibrinolytic therapy can be achieved within 30 minutes or that door-to-balloon (or EMS-to-balloon) or PCI can be achieved within 90 minutes. These goals should not be understood as ideal times, but rather the longest times that should be considered acceptable for a given system. Systems that are able to achieve even more rapid times for treatment of patients with STEMI should be encouraged [5,8,20].

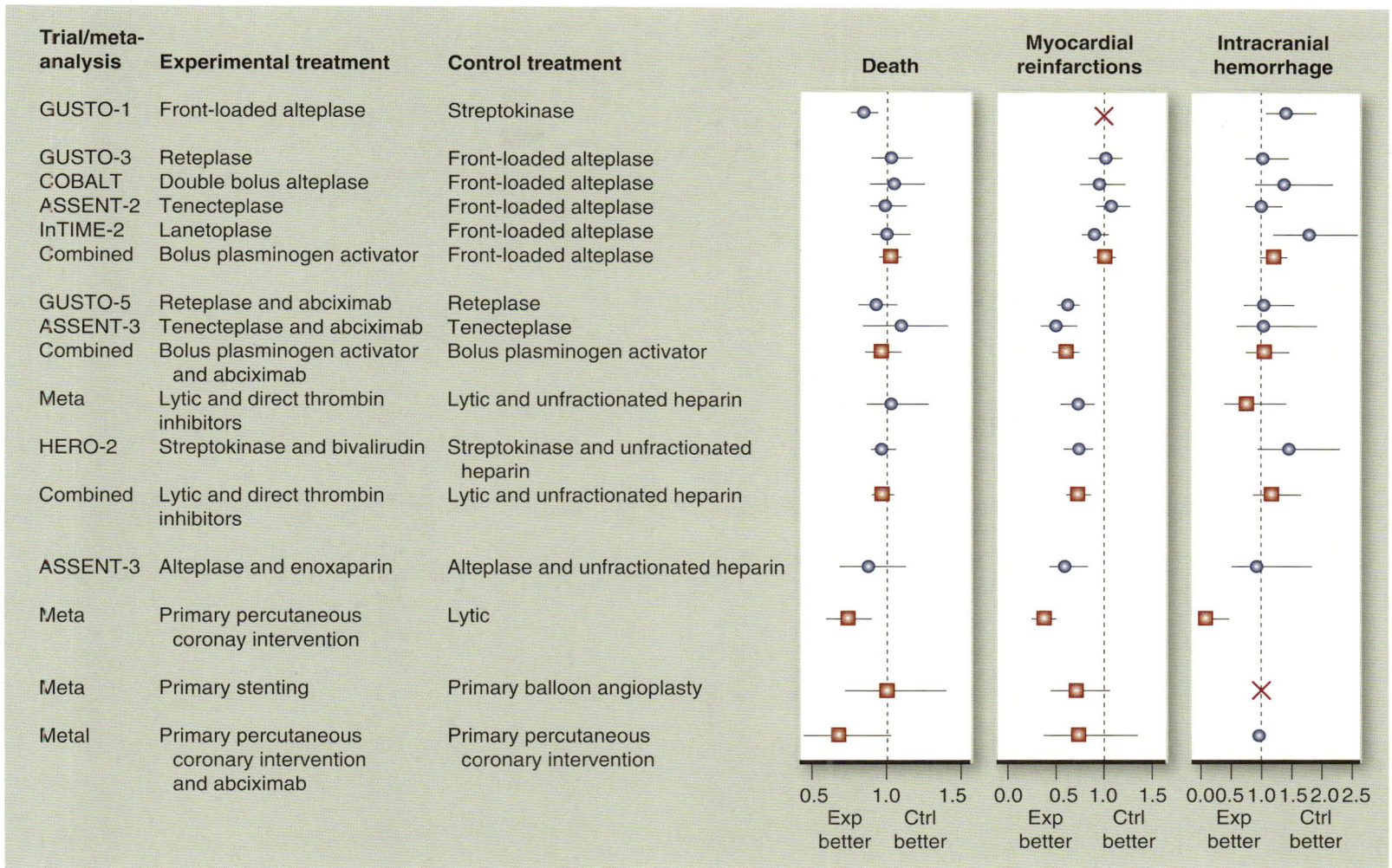

Figure 2-18. Relative treatment effect associated with several acute reperfusion modalities in patients presenting with ST-segment elevation myocardial infarction (STEMI). Data are OR and 95% CI [5,21]. Ctrl—control treatment; Exp—experimental treatment.

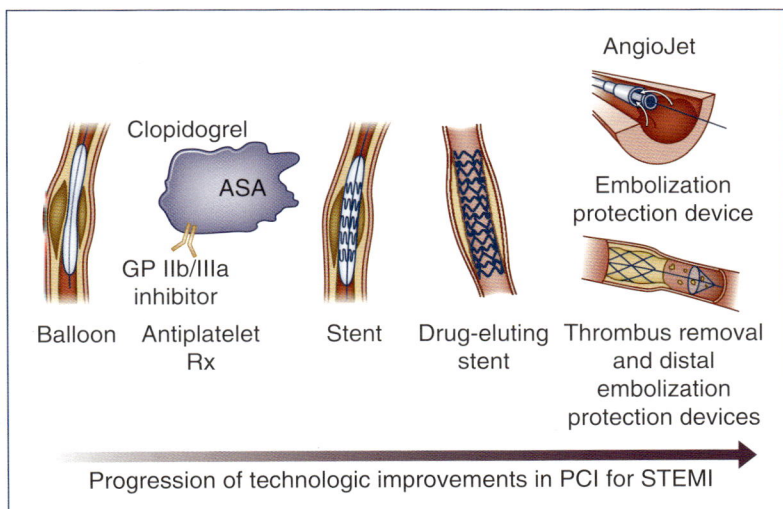

Figure 2-19. Progression of technologic improvements in percutaneous coronary intervention (PCI) for ST-segment elevation myocardial infarction (STEMI). Initial attempts at PCI used balloon angioplasty. Progressive improvements include antiplatelet therapy, bare metal followed by drug-eluting stents, and, more recently, thrombus removal and distal embolization protection devices [22]. ASA—aspirin; Rx—therapy.

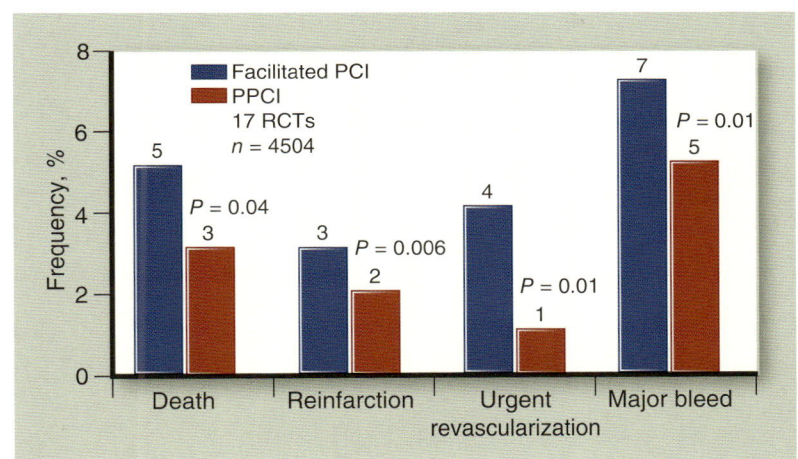

Figure 2-20. Short-term clinical outcomes in patients with ST-segment elevation myocardial infarction treated with facilitated percutaneous coronary intervention (PCI) or primary percutaneous coronary intervention (PPCI) [23].

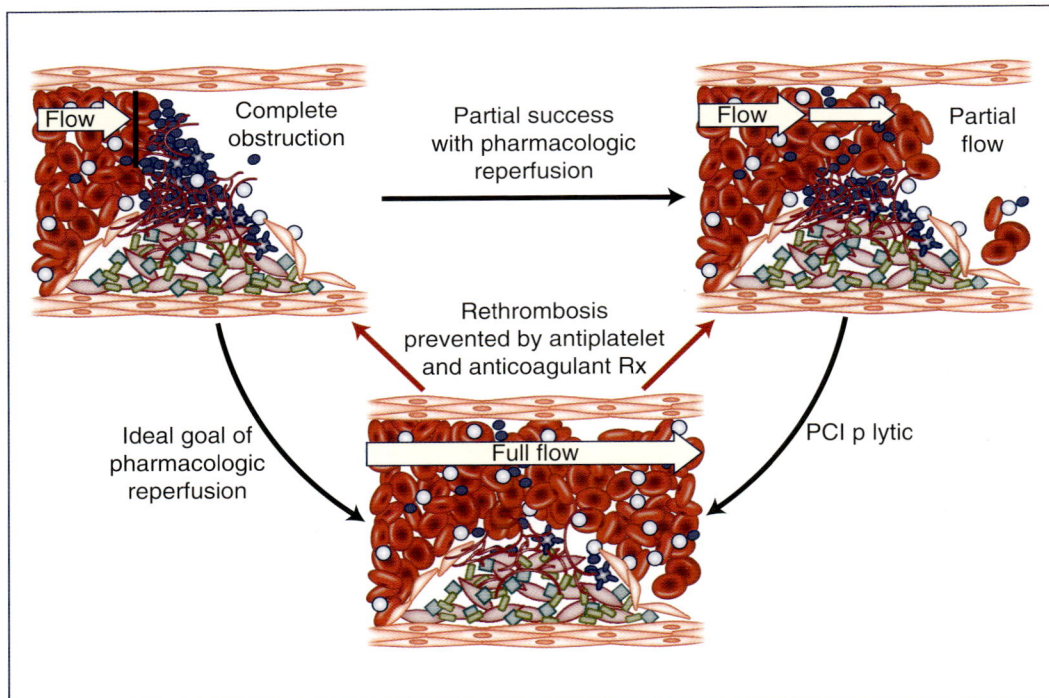

Figure 2-21. Overview of reperfusion for ST-segment elevation myocardial infarction (STEMI). A longitudinal view of an infarct artery in a patient with STEMI (top left). A vulnerable plaque has ruptured, resulting in the formation of a completely occlusive thrombus (see Fig. 2-5) that causes total cessation of antegrade flow (occurring from left to right). The ideal goal of pharmacologic reperfusion is to achieve full antegrade flow (bottom center). Partial success with pharmacologic reperfusion is apparent (top right) where some fibrin strands have broken up and there is partial antegrade flow. Percutaneous coronary intervention (PCI) is performed after administration of a lytic if there is judged to be either total failure to restore antegrade flow (remaining at top left) or only partial success (top right). A catheter-based intervention in such circumstances is referred to as rescue PCI (arrows at bottom right) (see Fig. 2-14). Antiplatelet and anticoagulant therapies are typically administered to prevent rethrombosis (red arrows), an occurrence that causes a relapse to either no flow (top left) or only partial flow (top right). Rx—therapy.

Figure 2-22. Summary of recommendations for the use of β-blockers in patients with an acute coronary syndrome [24,25]. HF—heart failure; HR—heart rate; SBP—systolic blood pressure.

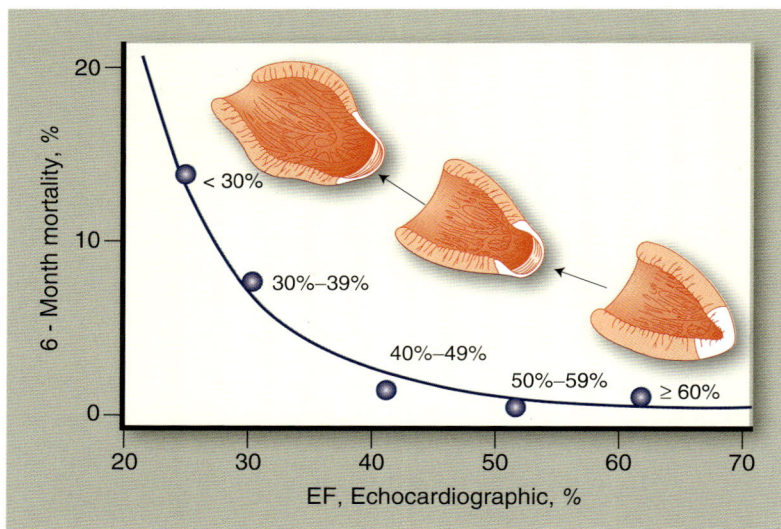

Figure 2-23. Remodeling of the left ventricle after ST-segment elevation myocardial infarction (STEMI). Above the curve on the right side of the figure is an apical STEMI (white zone of left ventricle). Over time, the infarct zone elongates and thins. Progressive remodeling of the left ventricle occurs (center and left images), ultimately converting the left ventricle from an oval shape to a spherical shape. Pharmacologic and catheter-based reperfusion strategies for STEMI have a favorable impact on this process by minimizing the extent of myocardial necrosis (left) through prompt restoration of flow in the epicardial infarct vessel [26]. This figure also demonstrates the impact of left ventricular function on survival following myocardial infarction. The curvilinear relationship between left ventricular ejection fraction (LVEF) for patients treated in the fibrinolytic era is shown. Among patients with an LVEF below 40%, the mortality rate is markedly increased at 6 months. Thus, interventions such as thrombolysis, aspirin, and angiotensin-converting enzyme inhibitors should be of considerable benefit in patients with acute myocardial infarction to minimize the amount of left ventricular damage and interrupt the neurohumoral activation seen with congestive heart failure [5,27].

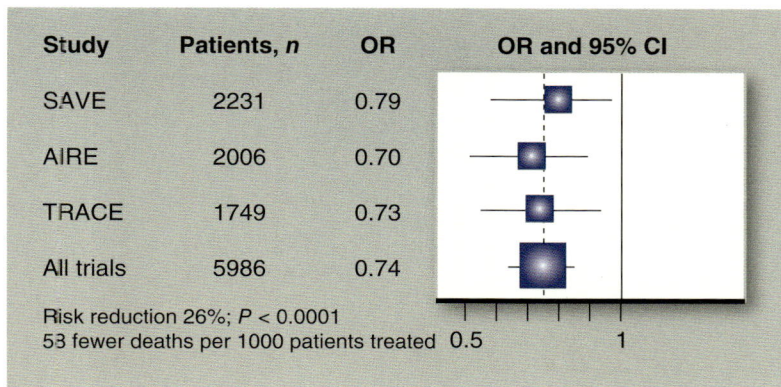

Study	Patients, n	OR	OR and 95% CI
SAVE	2231	0.79	
AIRE	2006	0.70	
TRACE	1749	0.73	
All trials	5986	0.74	

Risk reduction 26%; P < 0.0001
53 fewer deaths per 1000 patients treated   0.5   1

Figure 2-24. Effect of angiotensin-converting enzyme inhibitors (ACEIs) on mortality after myocardial infarction. Results from long-term trials show a consistent benefit of ACEIs [5,28]. AIRE—Acute Infarction Ramipril Efficacy Study; SAVE—Survival and Ventricular Enlargement Study; TRACE—Trandolapril Cardiac Evaluation Study.

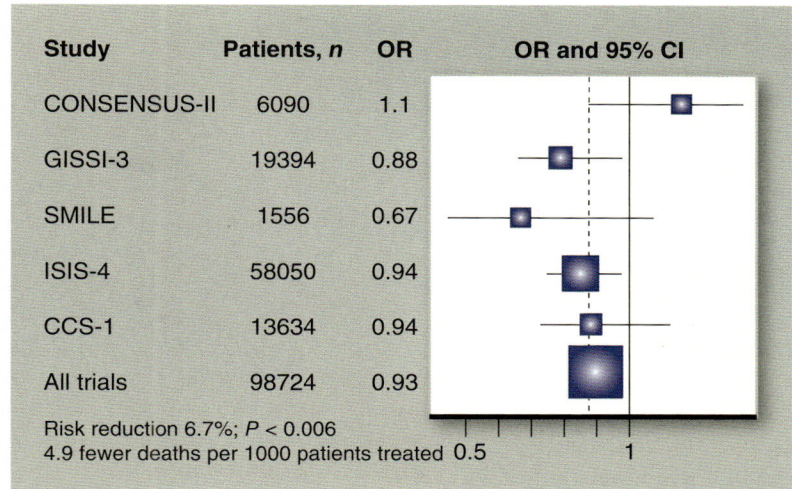

Study	Patients, n	OR	OR and 95% CI
CONSENSUS-II	6090	1.1	
GISSI-3	19394	0.88	
SMILE	1556	0.67	
ISIS-4	58050	0.94	
CCS-1	13634	0.94	
All trials	98724	0.93	

Risk reduction 6.7%; P < 0.006
4.9 fewer deaths per 1000 patients treated   0.5   1

Figure 2-25. Effects of angiotensin-converting enzyme inhibitors on mortality after myocardial infarction. Results from short-term trials show a consistent benefit, except for the Cooperative New Scandinavian Enalapril Survival Study (CONSENSUS II), which used an intravenous preparation early in the course of myocardial infarction treatment [5,28]. CCS-1—Chinese Cardiac Study; GISSI-3—Gruppo Italiano per lo Studio Della Sopravvivenza; ISIS-4—Fourth International Study of Infarct Survival; SMILE—Survival of Myocardial Infarction Long-term Evaluation.

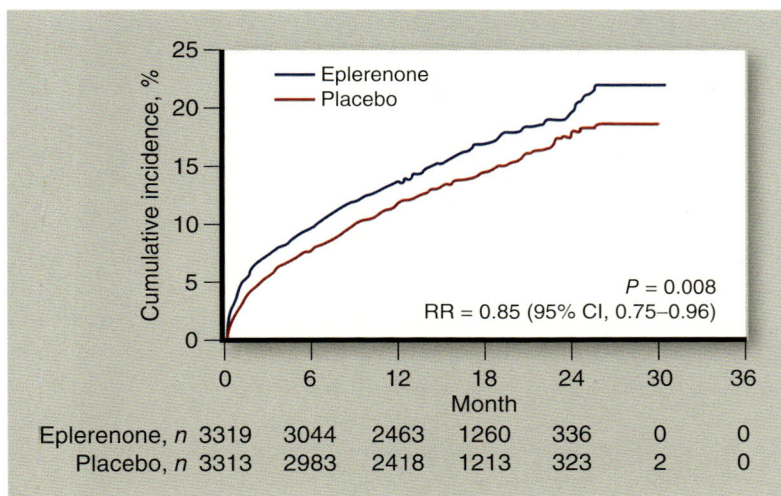

	0	6	12	18	24	30	36
Eplerenone, n	3319	3044	2463	1260	336	0	0
Placebo, n	3313	2983	2418	1213	323	2	0

P = 0.008
RR = 0.85 (95% CI, 0.75–0.96)

Figure 2-26. Effect of an aldosterone antagonist after myocardial infarction. Kaplan–Meier estimates of the rate of death from any cause, the rate of death from cardiovascular causes or hospitalization for cardiovascular events, and the rate of sudden death from cardiac causes [29].

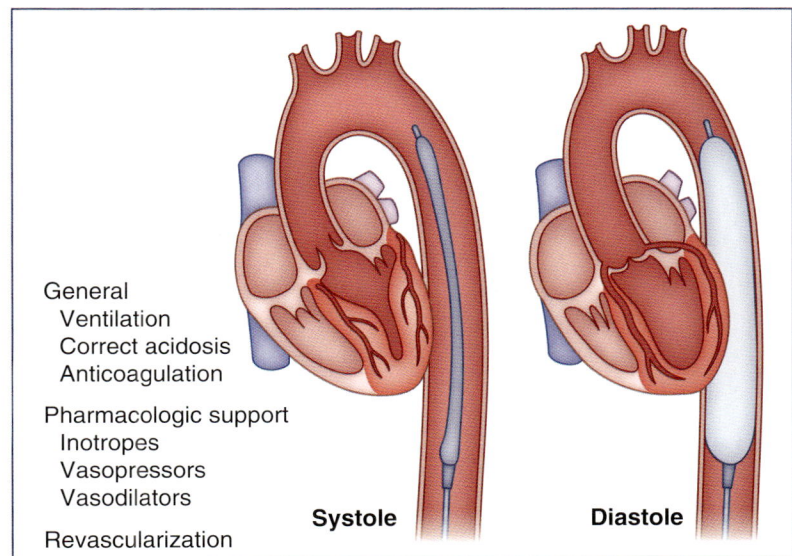

General
Ventilation
Correct acidosis
Anticoagulation

Pharmacologic support
Inotropes
Vasopressors
Vasodilators

Revascularization

Systole   **Diastole**

Figure 2-27. Overview of the management of left ventricular dysfunction after myocardial infarction. In addition to the general, pharmacologic, and revascularization aspects of care, clinicians should consider temporary mechanical support of the circulation with an intra-aortic balloon pump as shown in the systolic and diastolic diagrams.

Right ventricular infarction

Proximal occlusion of right coronary artery		ST-segment elevation ≥ 1 mm and positive T wave
Distal occlusion of right coronary artery		No ST-segment elevation and positive T wave
Occlusion of circumflex coronary artery		ST-segment depression ≥ 1 mm and negative T wave

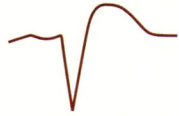

Clinical findings:
  Shock with clear lungs, elevated JVP
  Kussmaul sign
Hemodynamics:
  Increased RA pressure (y descent)
  Square root sign in RV tracing
ECG:
  ST elev in R sided leads (lead V₄R)
Echo:
  Depressed RV function
Rx:
  Maintain RV preload
  Lower RV afterload (PA–PCW)
  Inotropic support
  Reperfusion

Figure 2-28. The clinical features and management of right ventricular infarction. Patients with hemodynamically significant right ventricular infarction present with shock but clear lungs and elevated (elev) jugular venous pressure (JVP). ST elevation exists in right-sided electrocardiogram (ECG) leads with variation in the repolarization pattern depending on the infarct artery and the location of the occlusion. Management recommendations (*bottom right*) [8,30]. PA—pulmonary artery; PCW—pulmonary capillary wedge; RA—right atrial; RV—right ventricular; Rx—therapy.

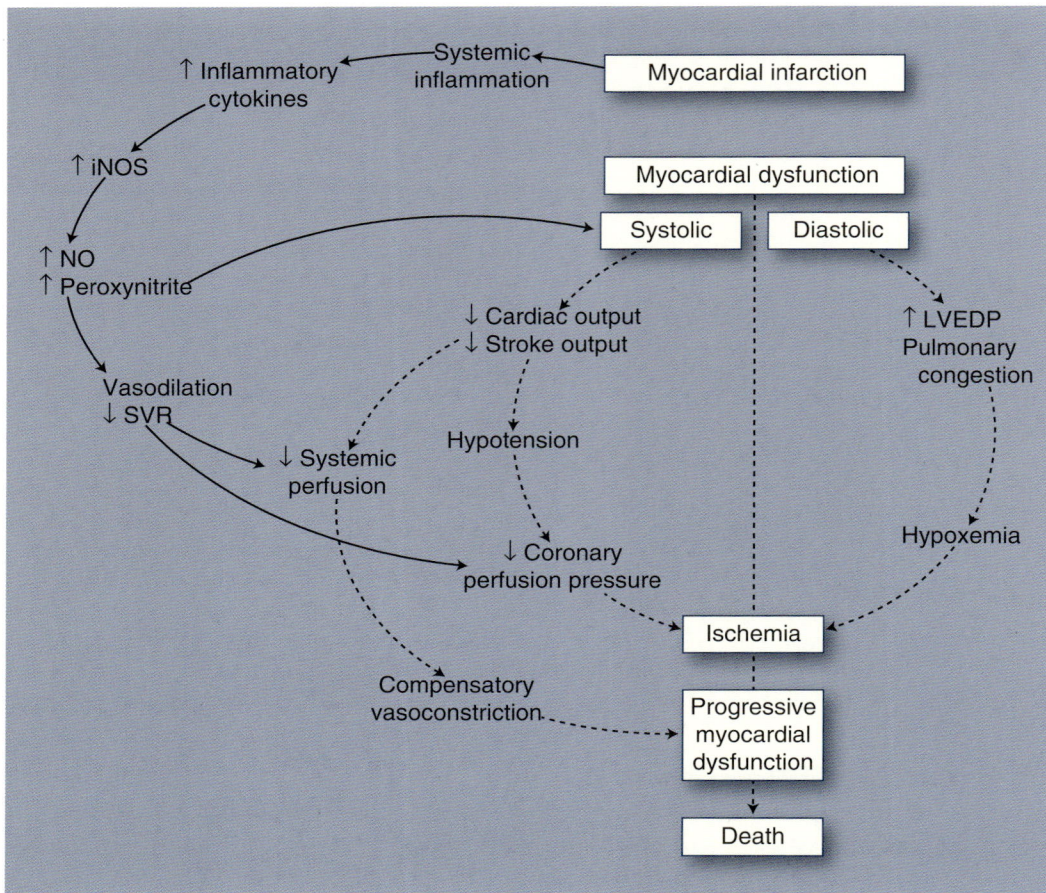

Figure 2-29. Classic shock paradigm (*solid line*) and the influence of the inflammatory response syndrome initiated by a large myocardial infarction (*dotted line*) [5,31]. iNOS—inducible nitric oxide synthase; LVEDP—left ventricular end-diastolic pressure; NO—nitric oxide; SVR—systemic vascular resistance.

	Ventricular septal rupture	Free wall rupture	Mitral regurgitation (Pap M dysfunction)
Incidence	1–2%	1–6%	1–2%
Timing	3–5 d p MI	3–6 d p MI	3–5 d p MI
Phy exam	Murmur 90%	JVD, PEA	Murmur 50%
Thrill	Common	No	Rare
Echo	Shunt	Pericardial effusion	Regurg jet
PA cath	O_2 step up	Diast press equal	C-V wave in PCW

Figure 2-30. Mechanical complications of myocardial infarction (MI) [32,33]. Diast press—diastolic pressure; Echo—echocardgiogram; JVD—jugular venous distention; PA cath—pulmonary artery catheter; Pap M—papillary muscle; p—post; PCW—pulmonary capillary wedge; PEA—pulseless electrical activity; Phy exam—physical examination; Regurg—regurgitation.

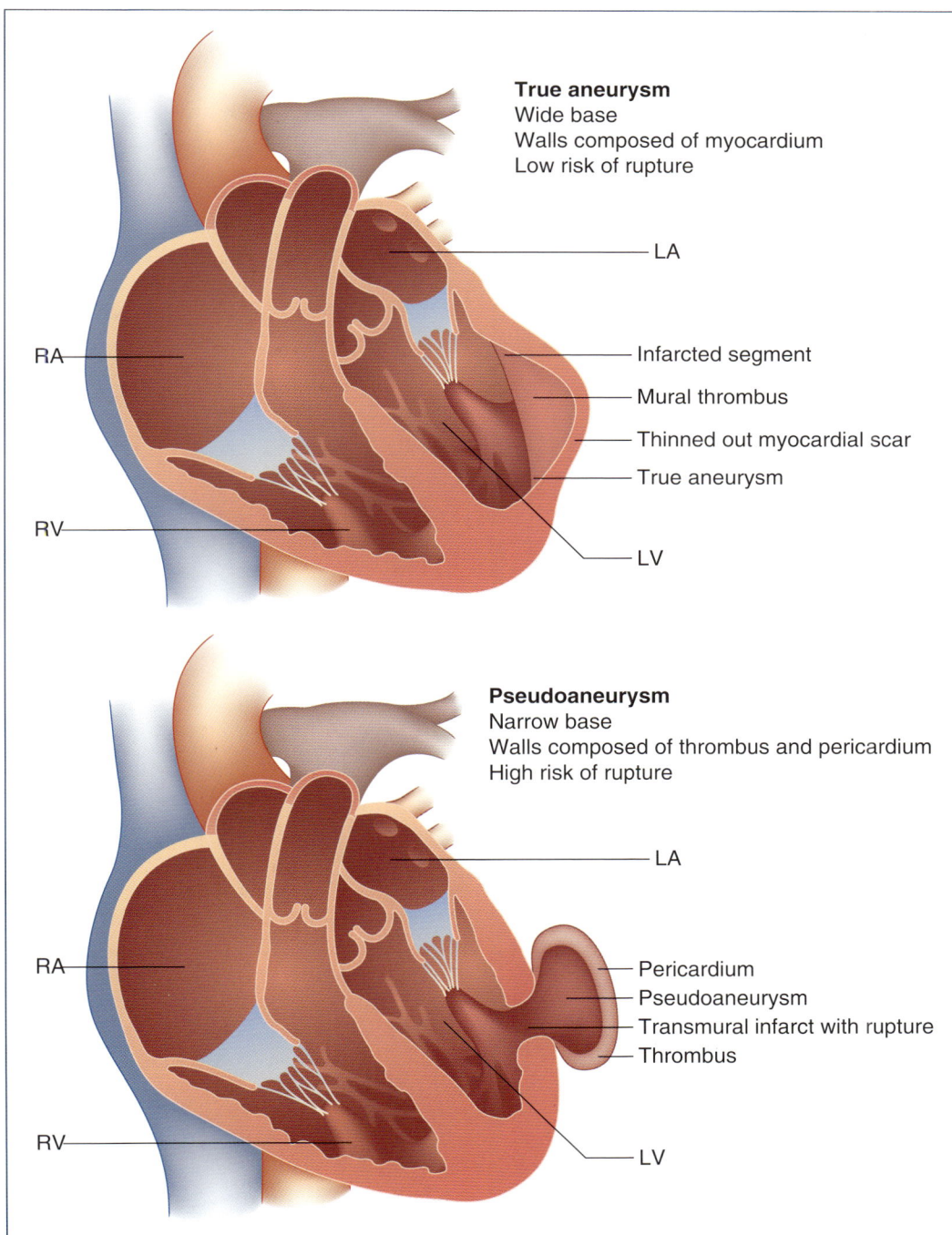

True aneurysm
Wide base
Walls composed of myocardium
Low risk of rupture

LA
RA
Infarcted segment
Mural thrombus
Thinned out myocardial scar
True aneurysm
RV
LV

Pseudoaneurysm
Narrow base
Walls composed of thrombus and pericardium
High risk of rupture

LA
RA
Pericardium
Pseudoaneurysm
Transmural infarct with rupture
Thrombus
RV
LV

Figure 2-31. Comparison of true and false (pseudo) aneurysms after ST-segment elevation myocardial infarction [34]. LA—left atrium; LV—left ventricle; RA—right atrium; RV—right ventricle.

Figure 2-32. Algorithm for implantation of an implantable cardioverter-defibrillator (ICD) in ST-segment elevation myocardial infarction (STEMI) patients without ventricular fibrillation or sustained ventricular tachycardia more than 48 hours after STEMI. The appropriate management path is based on measurement of left ventricular ejection fraction (LVEF). LVEF measurements obtained 3 or fewer days after STEMI should be repeated before proceeding with the algorithm. Patients with an LVEF less than 30% to 40% at least 40 days after STEMI are referred for insertion of an ICD if in New York Heart Association (NYHA) Class II-III. Patients with a more depressed LVEF of less than 30% to 35% are referred for ICD implantation even if they are NYHA Class I because of their increased risk of sudden cardiac death (SCD). Patients with preserved LV function (LVEF > 40%) do not receive an ICD and are treated with medical therapy after STEMI [5,35].

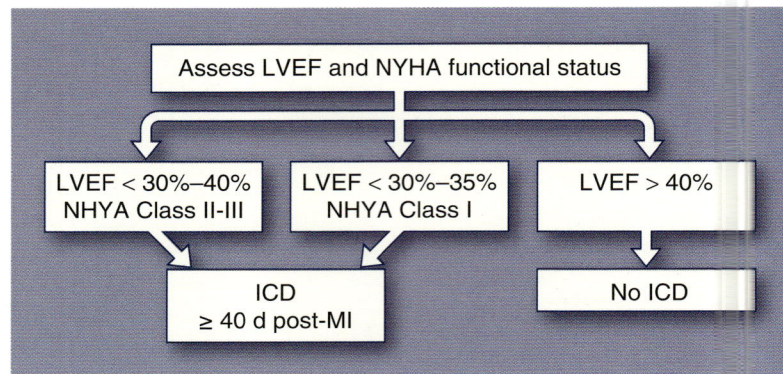

Figure 2-33. Networking of coagulation cascade and aggregation of platelets (Plt). The extrinsic limb triggers activation of the coagulation cascade when tissue factor (TF) is exposed in a disrupted plaque. Coagulation factor VII is activated (VIIa) and can activate factor X to Xa and promote perpetuation of the coagulation process via the intrinsic limb that results in formation of IXa and VIIIa. The prothrombinase complex of Xa, Va, Ca^{++} forms on a phospholipid surface (eg, membrane of a platelet) and converts prothrombin to thrombin. The thrombin that is formed binds to the thrombin receptor on platelets promoting activation and aggregation of platelets, as well as amplifying the coagulation cascade by promoting formation of VIIIa and Va. This diagram depicts the amplification nature of the coagulation process because one molecule of Xa leads to the downstream production of a large number of thrombin molecules (stoichiometric relationship not completely depicted to prevent obscuring the diagram with thrombin molecules). Activated platelets express numerous copies of the active form of the fibrinogen receptor GP IIb/IIIa on their surface. GP IIb/IIIa recognizes specific amino acid sequences on circulating ligands. One such ligand is fibrinogen (FGN), which has multiple copies of the RGD amino acid sequence and serves to bridge platelets together, promoting formation of aggregates. The more aggregates formed, the greater the surface area for the prothrombinase complex and amplification of the reactions of the coagulation cascade.

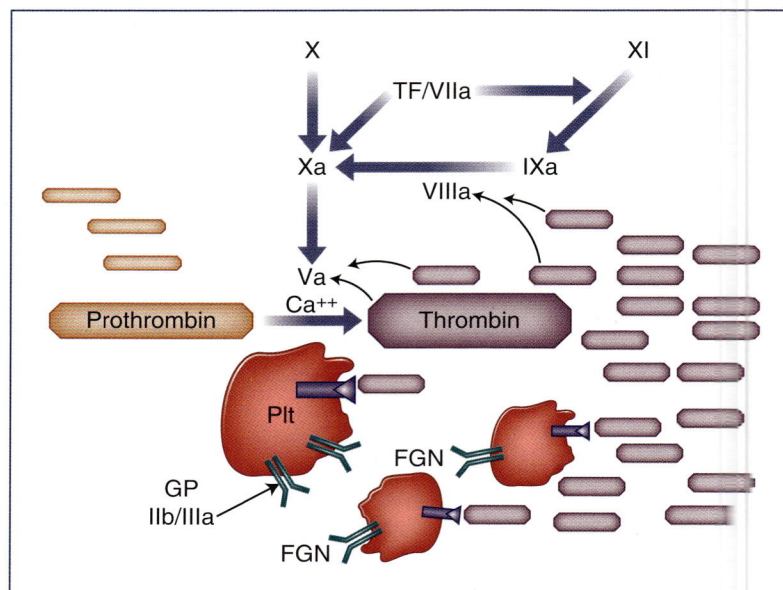

Figure 2-34. Overview of anticoagulant and antiplatelet therapies. These processes may be inhibited by various agents acting at different points. Anticoagulants inhibit the coagulation cascade either in a single position (proximally as in the case of the critical pentasaccharide or distally as in the case of direct thrombin inhibitors [DTIs]) or multiple positions (as shown for unfractionated heparin [UFH] or low molecular weight heparin [LMWH]). Font size depicts the relative inhibitory activity of the anticoagulants. For example, LMWHs have an anti-Xa:IIa ratio greater than or equal to 1, whereas the ratio is 1:1 for UFH. Platelets can be inhibited by cyclooxygenase inhibitors, such as aspirin (ASA), GP IIb/IIIa inhibitors (abciximab, tirofiban, eptifibatide), and thienopyridines such as clopidogrel, which blocks the P2Y12 receptor that is activated by adenosine diphosphate (see Fig. 2-35).

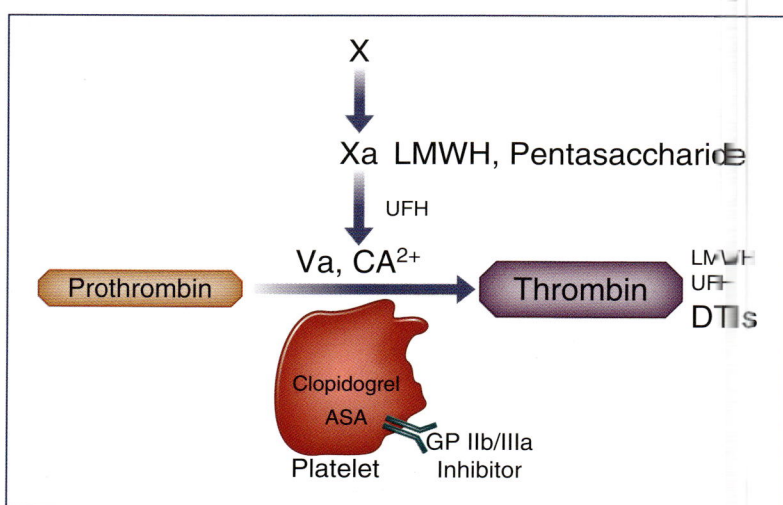

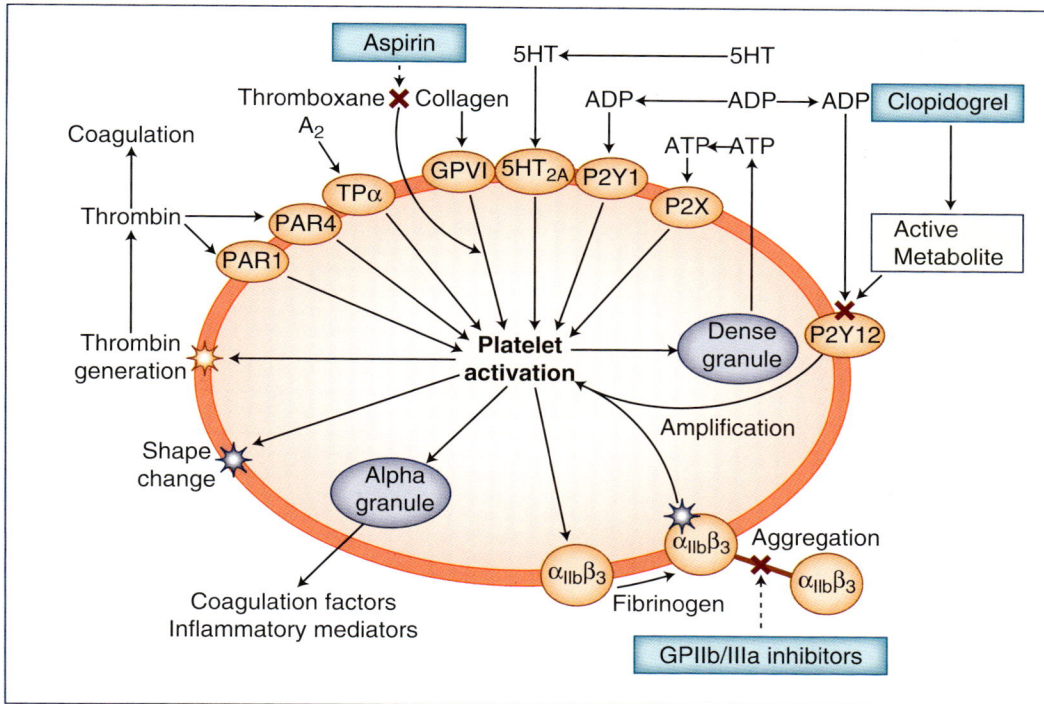

Figure 2-35. Pathways involved in platelet activation and aggregation. This diagram depicts some of the many platelet targets. Aspirin, a cyclo-oxygenase inhibitor, reduces the formation of thromboxane A_2. Thienopyridines, such as clopidogrel, block P2Y12, an ADP receptor, and thus inhibit platelet activation and aggregation. GP IIb/IIIa inhibitors block GP IIb/IIIa (also referred to as $\alpha_{IIb}\beta_3$) and thereby prevent the formation of fibrinogen bridges between platelets [36].

Antiplatelet Scorecard for Acute Coronary Syndromes

	Aspirin	Clopidogrel	GP IIb/IIIa Inhibitor
Route	PO	PO	IV
Monitor	No (?)	No (?)	No
UA/NSTEMI STEMI	Yes (Indefinitely)	Yes (1 year)	Yes
Bleeding	Yes	Yes	Yes
PCI	Dual antiplatelet Rx prolonged therapy for at least 1 year important after DES		Yes
CABG	Yes	Stop before CABG	
Antidote	None	None	None
Issues		Variable response	Need with clopidogrel? Timing pre-PCI?
	Avoid MD > 325 mg	Optimum timing and magnitude of LD uncertain	
Adjustment for renal dysfunction	None	None	Decrease MD by 50% if: Eptifibatide: CrCl < 50 mL/min
			Tirofiban: CrCl < 30 mL/min

Figure 2-36. Antiplatelet scorecard for acute coronary syndromes. CABG—coronary artery bypass graft; CrCl—creatinine clearance; DES—drug-eluting stents; IV—intravenous; GP—glycoprotein; MD—maintenance dose; PCI—percutaneous coronary intervention; PO—by mouth; LD—loading dose; UA/NSTEMI—unstable angina non–ST-segment elevation myocardial infarction.

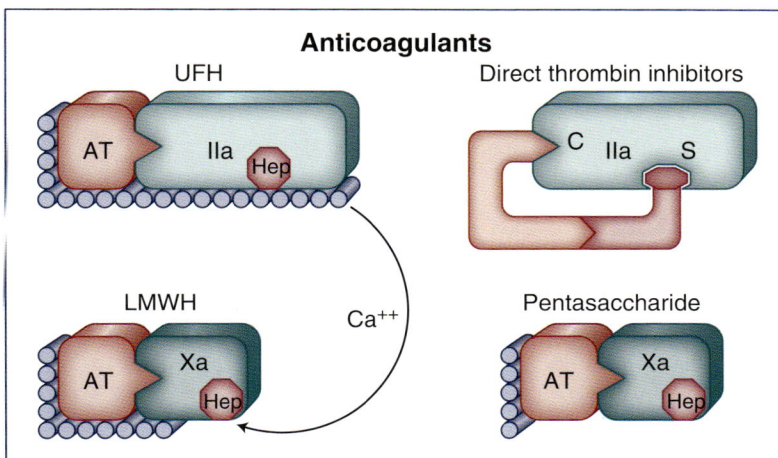

Figure 2-37. The mechanism of action of anticoagulants, showing thrombin (coagulation factor IIa; *top*) and factor Xa (*bottom*). Unfractionated heparin (UFH), a glycosaminoglycan polymer, depicted by the *blue cylinders*, serves as a bridge to bring antithrombin (AT) closer to the catalytic center of thrombin. UFH accomplishes this through a critical pentasaccharide sequence that binds to AT (causing a conformational change in AT, allowing it to fit into the catalytic center of thrombin) and at least an additional 13 sugar residues that attach at the heparin-binding domain (Hep) on thrombin. In contrast, direct thrombin inhibitors (*eg*, bivalirudin, argatroban, hirudin) do not require AT, but block the catalytic center (C) directly, with or without simultaneous attachment at the substrate-recognition domain (S) of thrombin. Factor Xa is inhibited when AT undergoes a conformational change after binding of the pentasaccharide sequence of a LMWH or by the synthetic pentasaccharide fondaparinux. In the presence of Ca^{++}, a heparin-binding domain is exposed on Xa and longer chains of UFH may participate in Xa inhibition via bridging (*see* Fig. 2-34, Fig. 2-35, and Fig. 2-39).

Anticoagulant Scorecard for Acute Coronary Syndromes

	UFH	ENOX	FONDA	BIVAL
Route	IV (SC)	IV, SC	SC (IV)	IV
Monitor	aPTT, ACT	No	No	aPTT, ACT
UA/NSTEMI STEMI	Yes	Yes	Yes	To support PCI
Bleeding	Yes	Yes	Less	Less
HIT	Yes	Less	None	None
PCI	Yes	Yes	Need anti-IIa Rx	Yes
CABG	Yes	No	No	Possible
Antidote	Protamine	Protamine	None	None
Adjustment for renal dysfunction	None	Extend SC dosing to every 24 h for CrCl < 30 mL/min	Avoid in patients with CrCl < 30 mL/min	Reduce maintenance infusion from 1.75 to 1.0 mg/kg/h for CrCl < 30 mL/min

Figure 2-38. Anticoagulant scorecard for acute coronary syndromes. ACT—activated clotting tissue; aPTT—activated partial thromboplastin time; BIVAL—bivalirudin; CABG—coronary artery bypass graft; CrCl—creatinine clearance; ENOX—enoxaparin; FONDA—fondaparinux; HIT—heparin-induced thrombocytopenia; IV—intravenous; PCI—percutaneous coronary intervention; SC—subcutaneous UA/NSTEMI—unstable angina non–ST-segment elevation myocardial infarction; UFH—unfractionated heparin.

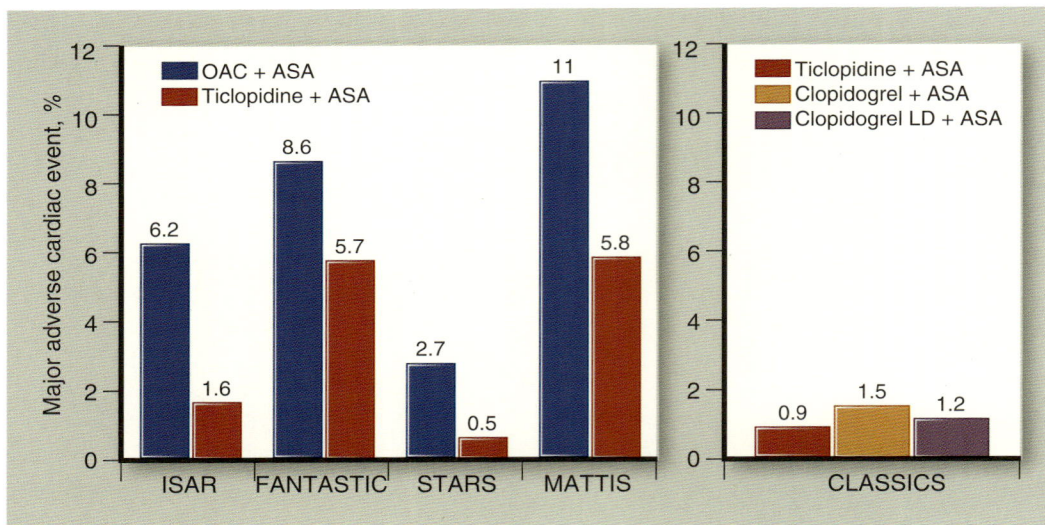

Figure 2-39. Comparison of major adverse cardiac event (MACE) rates (%) in CLASSICS with ISAR [6], FANTASTIC [7], STARS [8], and MATTIS [9,37]. ASA—aspirin; CLASSICS—Clopidogrel Aspirin Stent International Cooperation Study; FANTASTIC—Full Anticoagulation Versus Aspirin and Ticlopidine; ISAR—Intracoronary Stenting and Antithrombotic Regimen; LD—loading dose; MATTIS—Multicenter Aspirin and Ticlopidine Trial after Intracoronary Stenting; OAC—oral anticoagulants; STARS—Stent Antithrombotic Regimen Study.

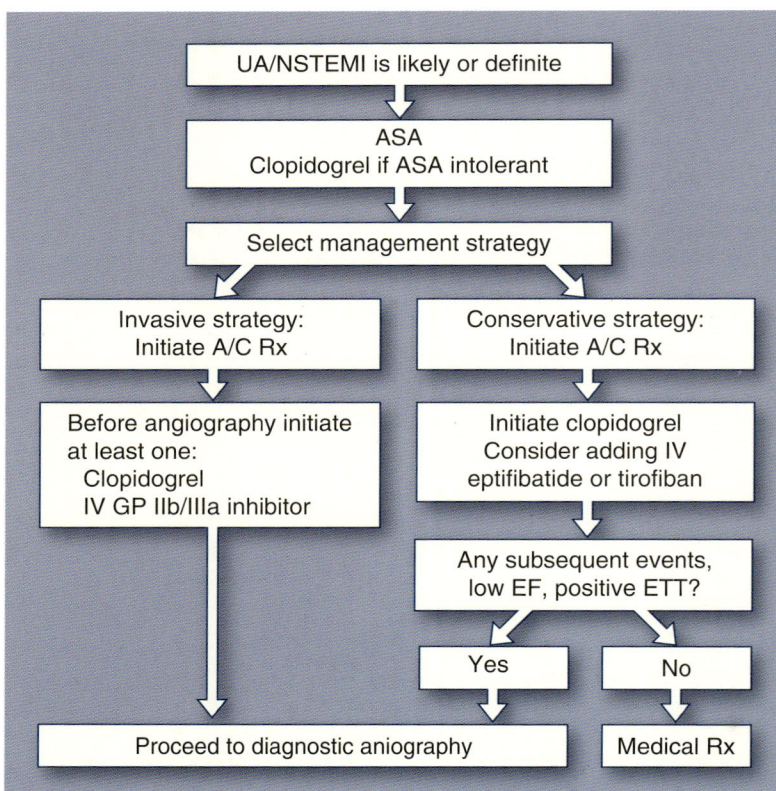

Figure 2-40. Algorithm for management of patients in whom unstable angina (UA) or non–ST-elevation myocardial infarction (NSTEMI) is likely or definite. Anticoagulant therapy (A/C Rx) is given and the patient is managed either by an early invasive strategy or an initial conservative strategy [25]. ASA—aspirin; EF—ejection fraction; ETT—exercise tolerance test; IV—intravenous.

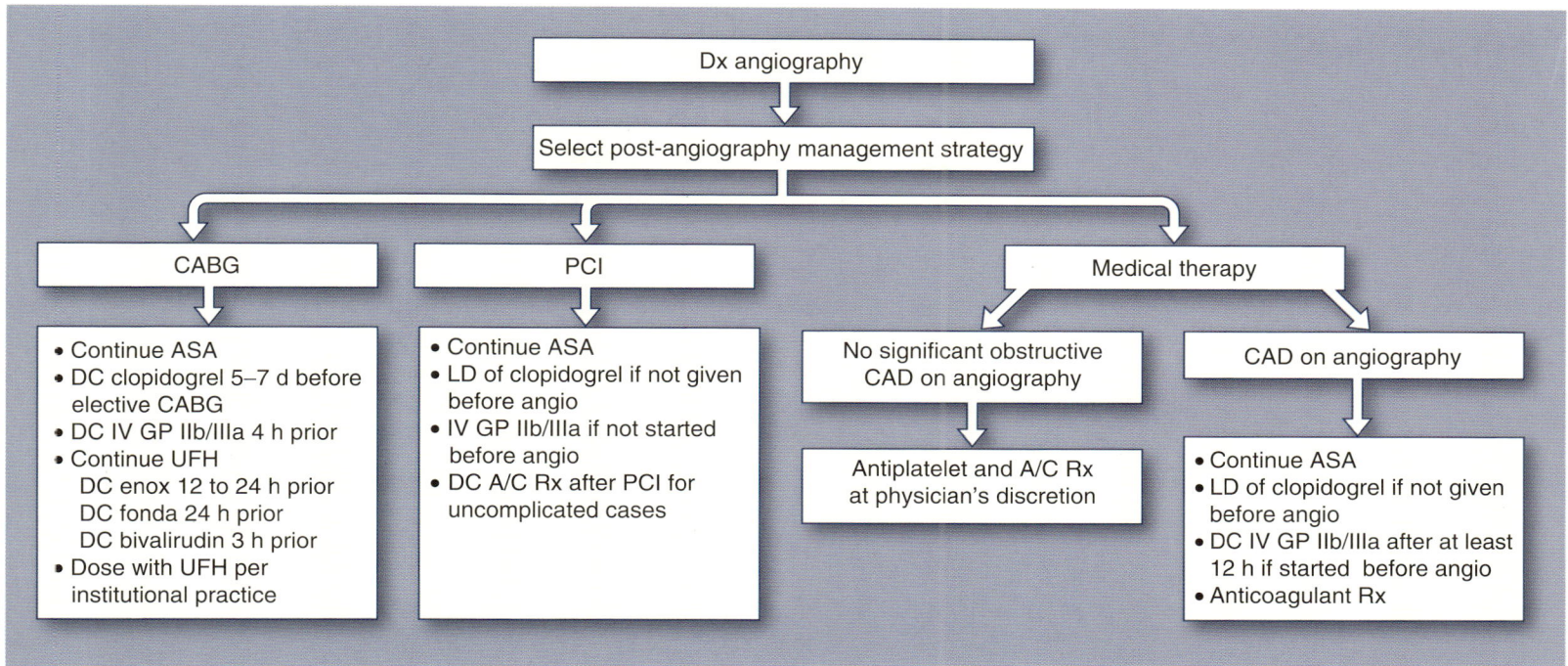

Figure 2-41. Management of patients with unstable angina (UA) or non–ST-elevation myocardial infarction (NSTEMI) following diagnostic (Dx) angiography. Patients are treated either with coronary artery bypass graft (CABG) surgery, percutaneous coronary intervention (PCI), or medically as shown [25]. A/C—anticoagulant; ASA—aspirin; CAD—coronary artery disease; DC—discontinue; enox—enoxaparin; fonda—fondaparinux; LD—loading dose; UFH—unfractionated heparin; Rx—therapy.

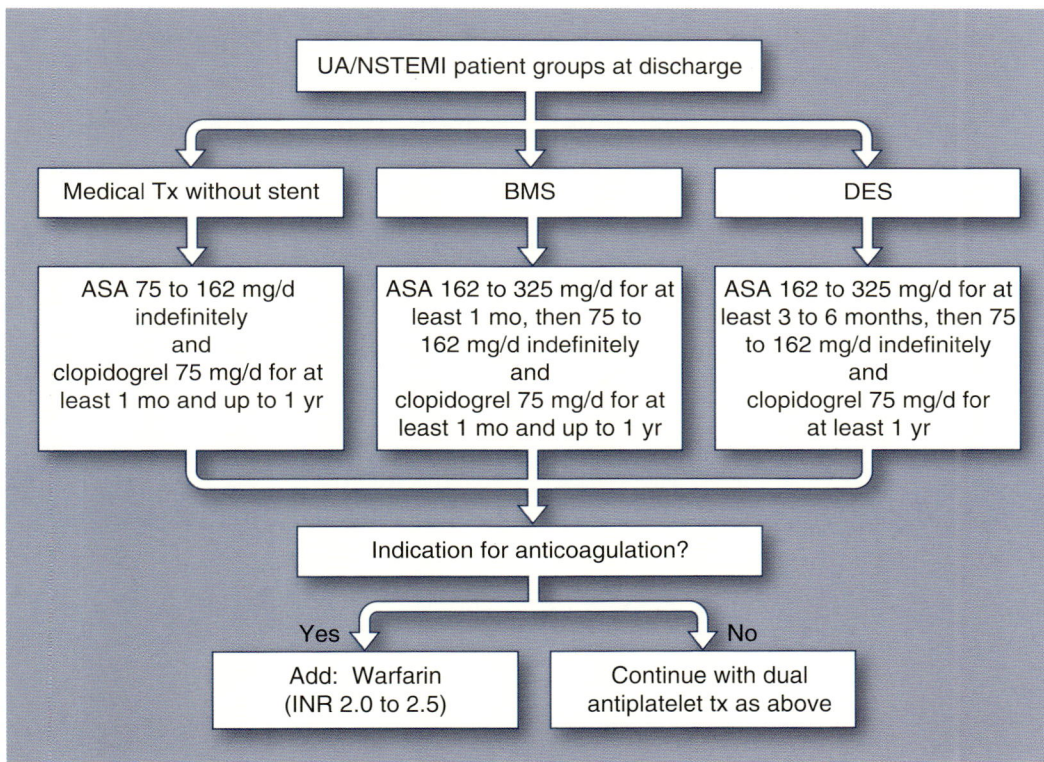

Figure 2-42. Long-term antithrombotic therapy at hospital discharge after unstable angina (UA) or non–ST-elevation myocardial infarction (NSTEMI). Dual antiplatelet therapy with aspirin (ASA) and clopidogrel is given at different doses and for different durations depending on whether a patient receives medical treatment (Tx), a bare metal stent (BMS), or a drug-eluting stent (DES) [25]. INR—international normalized ratio.

Secondary Prevention and Long-Term Management

Smoking goal: complete cessation

Blood-pressure control goal: < 140/90 mm Hg or < 130/80 mm Hg if chronic kidney disease or diabetes

Physical activity minimum goal: 30 min 3–4 d per wk; daily is optimal

Diabetes management goal: hemoglobin A1c < 7%

Weight management goal: BMI 18.5 to 24.9 kg/m²; waist circumference < 35 in (women) and < 40 in (men)

Figure 2-43. Secondary prevention and long-term management. BMI—body mass index. (*Adapted from* Anderson *et al.* [25].)

References

1. Libby P, Théroux P: Pathophysiology of coronary artery disease. *Circulation* 2005, 111:3481–3488.

2. Libby P: Current concepts of the pathogenesis of the acute coronary syndromes. *Circulation* 2001, 104:365–372.

3. Falk E, Andersen HR: Pathology of atherosclerotic plaque: stable, unstable, and infarctional. In *Interventional Cardiovascular Medicine: Principles and Practice.* Edited by Roubin GS, Califf RM, O'Neill WW, et al. New York: Churchill Livingstone; 1994:57–68.

4. Falk E: Why do plaques rupture? *Circulation* 1992, 86(Suppl 3):30–42.

5. Libby P, Bonow RO, Zipes DP, Mann DL, eds: *Braunwald's Heart Disease*, edn 8. Philadelphia: WB Saunders; 2008.

6. Hamm CW, Bertrand M, Braunwald E: Acute coronary syndrome without ST elevation: implementation of new guidelines. *Lancet* 2001, 358:1533–1548.

7. Davies MJ: The pathophysiology of acute coronary syndromes. *Heart* 2000, 83:361–366.

8. Antman EM, Anbe DT, Armstrong PW, et al.: ACC/AHA Guidelines for the Management of Patients with ST-Elevation Myocardial Infarction: a report of the American College of Cardiology/American Heart Association Task Force on Practice Guidelines (Committee to Revise the 1999 Guidelines for the Management of Patients with Acute Myocardial Infarction). *J Am Coll Cardiol* 2004, 44:671–719.

9. Schoen FJ: The heart. In *Robbins & Cotran Pathologic Basis of Disease*, edn 7. Edited by Kumar V, Abbas AK, Fausto N, et al. Philadelphia: WB Saunders; 2005:678.

10. Schoen FJ: The heart. In *Robbins & Cotran Pathologic Basis of Disease*, edn 7. Edited by Kumar V, Abbas AK, Fausto N, et al. Philadelphia: WB Saunders; 2005:581.

11. Schoen FJ: The heart. In *Robbins & Cotran Pathologic Basis of Disease*, edn 7. Edited by Kumar V, Abbas AK, Fausto N, et al. Philadelphia: WB Saunders; 2005:682.

12. Gersh BJ, Stone GW, White HD, Homes DR Jr: Pharmacological facilitation of primary percutaneous coronary intervention for acute myocardial infarction: is the slope of the curve the shape of the future? *JAMA* 2005, 293:979–986.

13. Bayes de Luna A, Wagner G, Birnbaum Y, et al.: A new terminology for left ventricular walls and location of myocardial infarcts that present Q wave based on the standard of cardiac magnetic resonance imaging: a statement for healthcare professionals from a committee appointed by the International Society for Holter and Noninvasive Electrocardiography. *Circulation* 2006, 114:1755–1760.

14. Antman EM: Decision making with cardiac troponin tests. *N Engl J Med* 2002, 346:2079–2082.

15. Jaffe AS, Babiun L, Apple FS: Biomarkers in acute cardiac disease: the present and the future. *J Am Coll Cardiol* 2006, 48:1–11.

16. Antman EM, Braunwald E: ST-Elevation myocardial infarction: pathology, pathophysiology, and clinical features. In *Braunwald's Heart Disease*, edn 8. Edited by Libby P, Bonow RO, Zipes DP, Mann DL. Philadelphia: WB Saunders; 2008:1208.

17. Bates ER, Kushner FG: ST-elevation myocardial infarction. In *Cardiovascular Therapeutics: A Companion to Braunwald's Heart Disease*, edn 3. Edited by Antman EM. Philadelphia: WB Saunders; 2007:253.

18. Keeley EC, Boura JA, Grines CL: Primary angioplasty versus intravenous thrombolytic therapy for acute myocardial infarction: a quantitative review of 23 randomised trials. *Lancet* 2003, 361:13–20.

19. Llevadot J, Giugliano RP, Antman EM: Bolus fibrinolytic therapy in acute myocardial infarction. *JAMA* 2001, 286:442–449:443.

20. Armstrong PW, Collen D, Antman E: Fibrinolysis for acute myocardial infarction: the future is here and now. *Circulation* 2003, 107:2533–2537.

21. Boersma E, Mercado N, Poldermans D, et al.: Acute myocardial infarction. *Lancet* 2003, 361:851–858.

22. Antman EM, Van de Werf F: Pharmacoinvasive therapy: the future of treatment for ST-elevation myocardial infarction. *Circulation* 2004, 109:2480–2486.

23. Keeley EC, Boura JA, Grines CL: Comparison of primary and facilitated percutaneous coronary interventions for ST-elevation myocardial infarction: quantitative review of randomised trials. *Lancet* 2006, 367:579–588.

24. Antman EM, Hand M, Armstrong PW, et al.: 2007 focused update of the ACC/AHA 2004 Guidelines for the Management of Patients With ST-Elevation Myocardial Infarction. *Circulation* 2008, 117:296–329.

25. Anderson JL, Adams CD, Antman EM, et al.: ACC/AHA 2007 guidelines for the management of patients with unstable angina/non ST-elevation myocardial infarction: a report of the American College of Cardiology/American Heart Association Task Force on Practice Guidelines (Writing Committee to Revise the 2002 Guidelines for the Management of Patients With Unstable Angina/Non ST Elevation Myocardial Infarction). *Circulation* 2007, 116:e148–e304.

26. McMurray JJV, Pfeffer MA, eds: *Heart Failure Updates*. London: Martin Dunitz 2003.

27. Volpi A, De VC, Franzosi MG, et al.: Determinants of 6-month mortality in survivors of myocardial infarction after thrombolysis. Results of the GISSI-2 data base. The Ad Hoc Working Group of the Gruppo Italiano per lo Studio della Sopravvivenza nell'Infarto Miocardico (GISSI)-2 Data Base. *Circulation* 1993, 88:416–429.

28. Gornik H, O'Gara PT: Adjunctive medical therapy. In *Clinical Trials in Heart Disease: A Companion to Braunwald's Heart Disease*. Edited by Manson JE, Buring JE, Ridker PM, Gaziano JM. Philadelphia: WB Saunders; 2004:114.

29. Pitt B, Remme W, Zannad F, et al.: Eplerenone, a selective aldosterone blocker, in patients with left ventricular dysfunction after myocardial infarction. *N Engl J Med* 2003, 348:1309–1321.

30. Wellens HJ: The value of the right precordial leads of the electrocardiogram. *N Engl J Med* 1999, 340:381–383.

31. Hochman J: Cardiogenic shock complicating acute myocardial infarction: expanding the paradigm. *Circulation* 2003, 107:2998–3002.

32. Wilansky S, Moreno CA, Lester SJ: Complications of myocardial infarction. *Crit Care Med* 2007, 35(Suppl 8):S348–S354.

33. Birnbaum Y, Fishbein MC, Blanche C, Siegel RJ: Ventricular septal rupture after acute myocardial infarction. *N Engl J Med* 2002, 347:1426–1432.

34. Shah PK: Complications of acute MI in cardiology. In *Cardiology*. Edited by Parmley WW, Chatterjee K. Philadelphia: JB Lippincott; 1987.

35. Zipes DP, Camm AJ, Borggrefe M, et al.: ACC/AHA/ESC 2006 guidelines for management of patients with ventricular arrhythmias and the prevention of sudden cardiac death: a report of the American College of Cardiology/American Heart Association Task Force and the European Society of Cardiology Committee for Practice Guidelines (Writing Committee to Develop Guidelines for Management of Patients with Ventricular Arrhythmias and the Prevention of Sudden Cardiac Death). Developed in collaboration with the European Rhythm Association and the Heart Rhythm Society. *Circulation* 2006, 114:e385–e484.

36. Storey RF: Biology and pharmacology of the platelet P2Y12 receptor. *Curr Pharm Des* 2006, 12:1255–1259.

37. Bertrand ME, Rupprecht H, Urban P, et al.: Double-blind study of the safety of clopidogrel with and without a loading dose in combination with aspirin compared with ticlopidine in combination with aspirin after coronary stenting. *Circulation* 2000, 102:624–629.

Chronic Ischemic Heart Disease 3

David A. Morrow

The importance of ischemic heart disease in the practice of clinical medicine relates to both its pervasiveness in contemporary society and its morbid complications. Some 16 million Americans have coronary artery disease, 9.1 million of whom have angina pectoris and 8.1 million have had prior myocardial infarction. Ischemic heart disease causes one of every five deaths in the United States. Importantly, advances over the past several decades have reduced death rates due to ischemic heart disease. These advances in management include more aggressive risk factor modification, with lifestyle and behavioral interventions, and effective disease-modifying pharmacotherapy, along with improvements in technology for revascularization. This chapter reviews the pathophysiology, clinical presentation, diagnosis, natural history, risk stratification, and the pharmacologic and invasive management of ischemic heart disease, with particular attention to the appropriate use of noninvasive and invasive testing, and guideposts for therapeutic decision making.

Pathophysiology of Coronary Artery Disease and Angina

Figure 3-1. Endothelial dysfunction leads to atherogenesis and progression.

Injury causing endothelial dysfunction is an inciting event in the onset of atherogenesis. The vascular endothelium is a complex organ capable of many functions, including regulation of vasomotor tone, modification of lipoproteins, and mediation of cellular traffic stimulated by the release of intercellular messengers. The endothelium may be injured by a variety of insults, including oxidative stress, hemodynamic forces, and modified lipoproteins. Advanced glycosylation end products may also injure the endothelium. Classic atherosclerotic risk factors, such as diabetes, dyslipidemia, smoking, and hypertension adversely affect endothelial function and contribute to the development and progression of coronary atherosclerosis. Genetic and environmental factors modulate the susceptibility of the endothelium to damage and subsequent dysfunction, which lead to impaired vasomotor tone, a prothrombotic state, a proinflammatory state, and smooth muscle proliferation or intima expansion in the arterial wall. These processes contribute to plaque rupture, intravascular thrombosis, vasospasm, and progression of the atherosclerotic process, culminating in clinical syndromes, such as angina, myocardial infarction, peripheral vascular disease, and stroke. Many of the pharmacologic therapies for patients with chronic ischemic heart disease improve endothelial function as one mechanism of reducing the risk of future cardiac events. (*Adapted from* Widlansky *et al.* [1].)

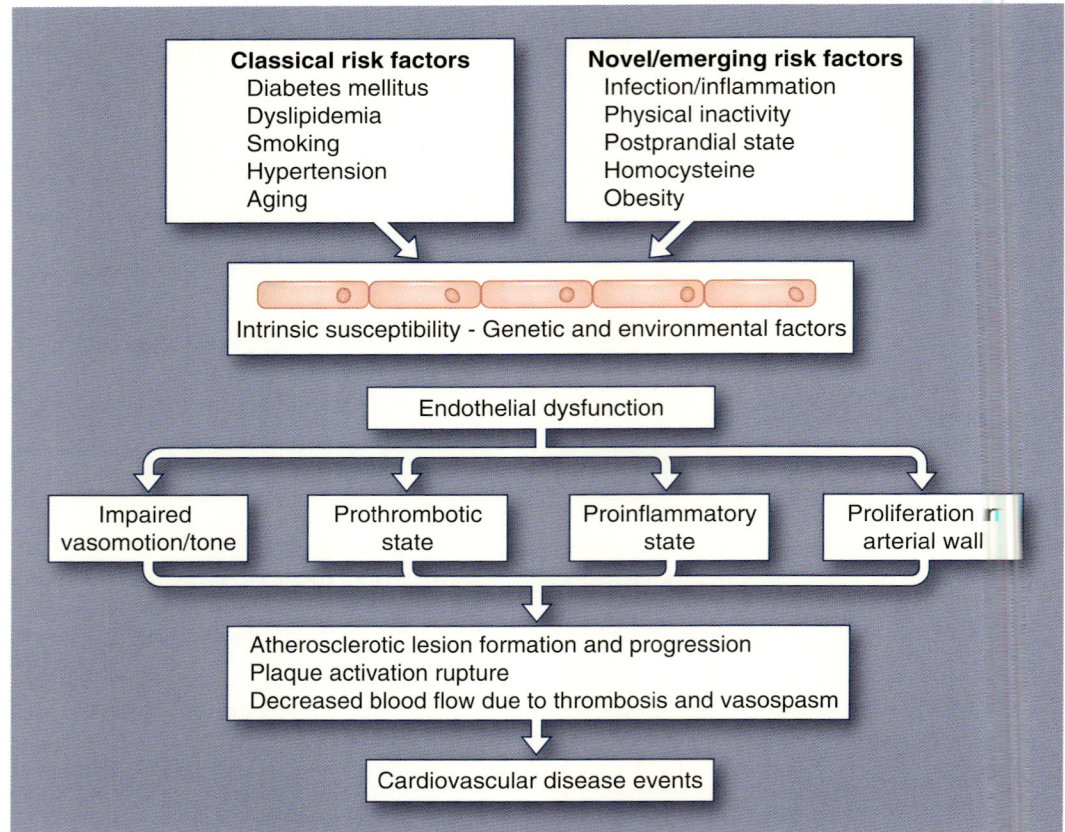

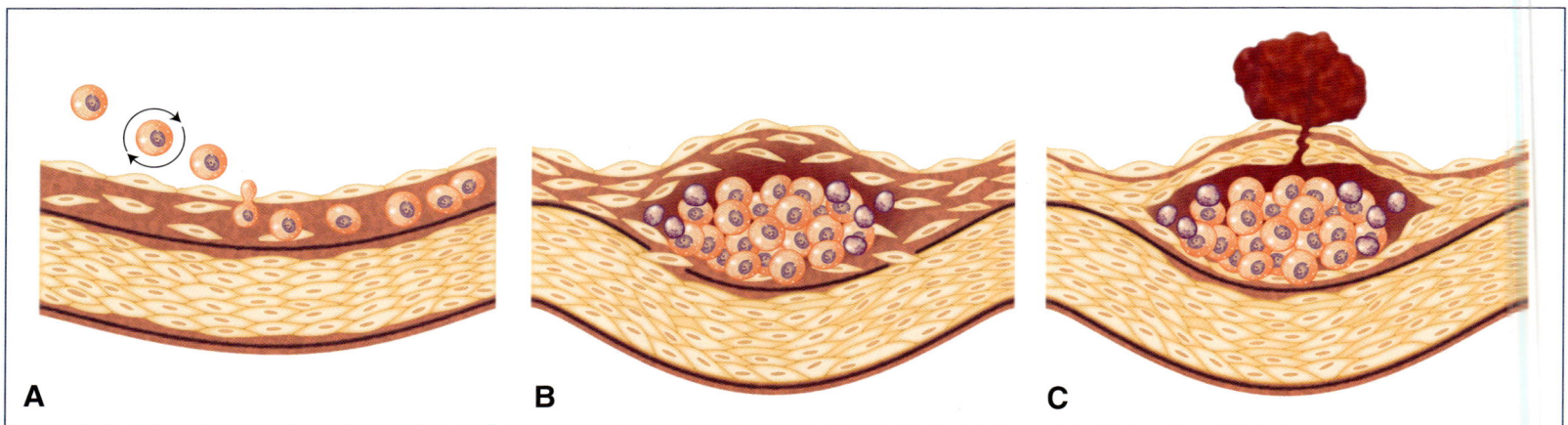

Figure 3-2. Atherosclerosis is an inflammatory disease. Inflammatory processes participate at every stage of atherothrombosis, from initiation of the earliest progenitor of an atheroma (**A**), to maturation and progression of atherosclerotic plaque (**B**), as well as plaque destabilization (**C**). The activation of endothelial cells leads to upregulation of intercellular adhesion molecules and the elaboration of chemokines that stimulate increased adhesion and migration of inflammatory cells into the subendothelial space. Uptake of low-density lipoproteins (LDL) by macrophages changes them into lipid-laden foam cells. The continued generation of inflammatory cytokines by arriving monocytes promotes additional expression of adhesion molecules, cellular recruitment, the oxidation and uptake of LDL, and the production of reactive oxygen species that exacerbate the endothelial injury. Simultaneously, released mitogens trigger the proliferation of smooth muscle cells that foster maturation of plaque into an intermediate atheroma. Both macrophages and T lymphocytes appear to produce inflammatory cytokines and mitogens that promote this progression of the atheroma. Concurrently, a resilient fibrous cap forms over the mixture of inflammatory and smooth muscle cells, intra- and extracellular lipids, and the necrotic cellular debris that form the core of the advanced atherosclerotic lesion. Ultimately, plaque rupture and thrombosis can provoke acute coronary syndromes or through a healing response promote lesion progression. (*Adapted from* Libby *et al.* [2].)

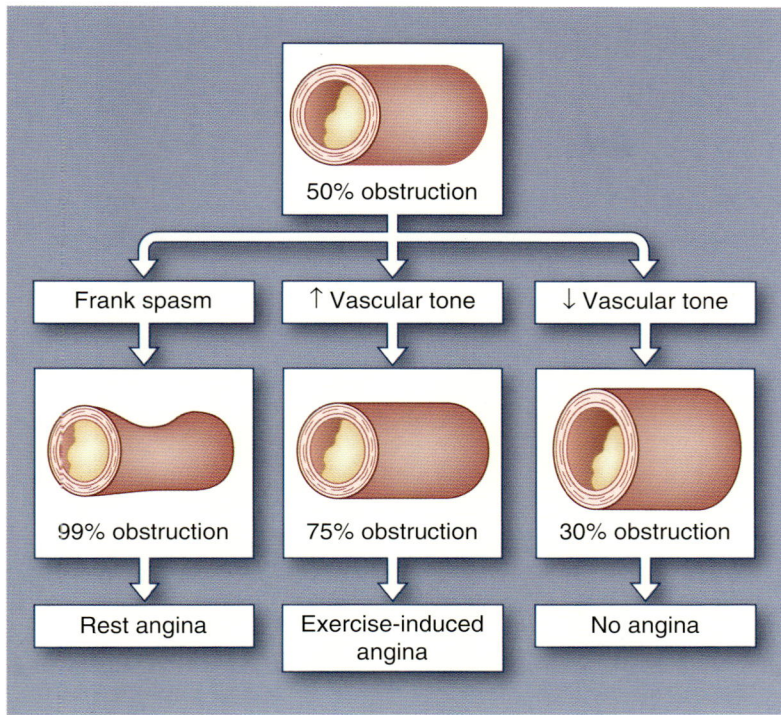

Figure 3-3. Coronary obstruction is a dynamic phenomenon. Chronic angina is most commonly caused by obstruction of the coronary arteries by atheromatous plaque. However, it is now recognized that coronary artery obstructions are capable of changing caliber, and that constriction of a preexisting lesion can be a factor in precipitating angina. If the coronary segment has sufficient smooth muscle (media) that is not involved in the atherosclerotic process, the vessel can dilate or constrict at the site of the stenosis. In general, vasoconstriction is most likely to occur in association with asymmetric atherosclerotic lesions, which consist of coronary atherosclerotic plaque in a segment of the wall with some arterial media intact. It is believed that at least 25% of an arc or rim of media in the coronary artery must be preserved to allow for stenosis due to vasomotion. This figure shows how the caliber of eccentric coronary artery stenoses may change, with considerable variation in the degree of stenosis and the propensity to produce angina. Both increased vascular tone and decreased vascular tone are depicted. This phenomenon has been called dynamic stenosis with resulting variable-threshold angina, emphasizing the variability of the actual obstruction. (*Adapted from* Epstein and Talbot [3].)

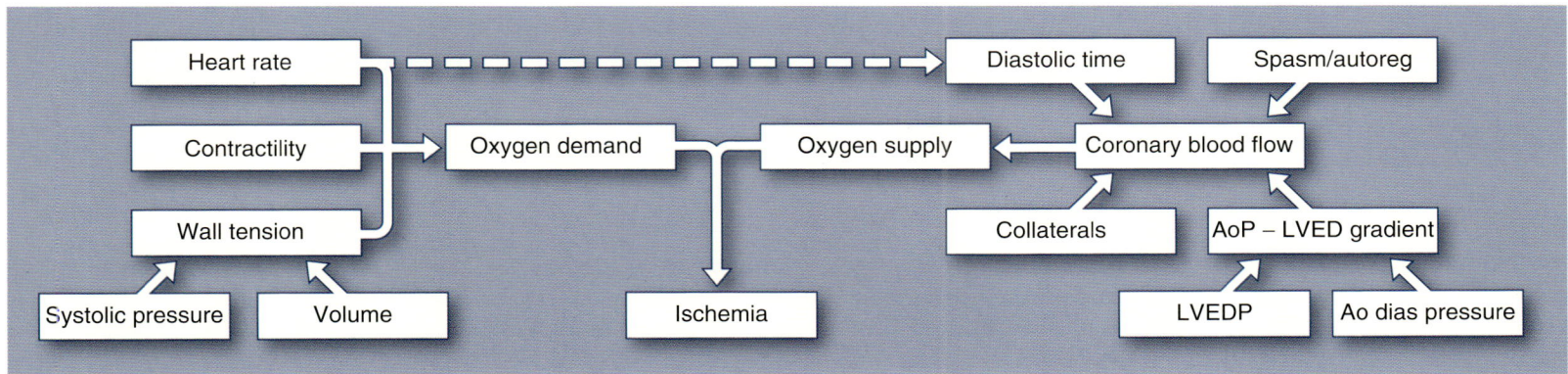

Figure 3-4. Factors influencing the balance between myocardial oxygen requirement and supply. Angina results from myocardial ischemia, which is caused by an imbalance between myocardial oxygen requirements and myocardial oxygen supply. The principle determinants of myocardial oxygen demand are heart rate, myocardial contractility, and left ventricular wall stress. Pharmacologic therapy for angina targets these determinants directly (heart rate) or indirectly by modulating systolic afterload and preload. Myocardial oxygen supply is determined by coronary blood flow and coronary arterial oxygen content. Percutaneous and surgical coronary revascularization directly improve coronary blood flow by reducing or bypassing epicardial coronary obstructions. In addition, pharmacologic agents also can improve myocardial oxygen supply by reducing vasoconstriction, increasing the time for diastolic (dias) coronary flow, and decreasing left ventricular end diastolic pressure (LVEDP), favorably influencing the gradient established with aortic pressure (AoP). autoreg—autoregulation. (*Adapted from* Morrow and Gersh [4].)

Natural History and Characteristics of Angina

Figure 3-5. Characteristics of angina and differentiation from other causes of chest pain. Differentiation of angina pectoris from other causes of chest pain relies on a thorough clinical history in conjunction with a physical examination and the results of noninvasive testing. Angina is usually brought on by exertion and often described as "strangling," "constricting," "crushing," "heavy," or "squeezing." However, in some patients, the quality of the sensation is more vague. **A,** The location of the discomfort is usually retrosternal, but radiation is common. Epigastric discomfort may also occur. Discomfort above the mandible or below the epigastrium is unusual for angina. **B,** The quality, duration, and aggravating factors may be used to help distinguish chest symptoms due to angina. Angina typically begins gradually over a period of minutes. Patients with angina usually prefer to rest during episodes. Chest discomfort while walking in the cold or after a meal is suggestive of angina. Symptoms unusual for angina include pain localized to a small area, pain reproduced by motion of the arms or palpation of the chest, and constant pain lasting many hours or only seconds. (*Adapted from* Braunwald [5].)

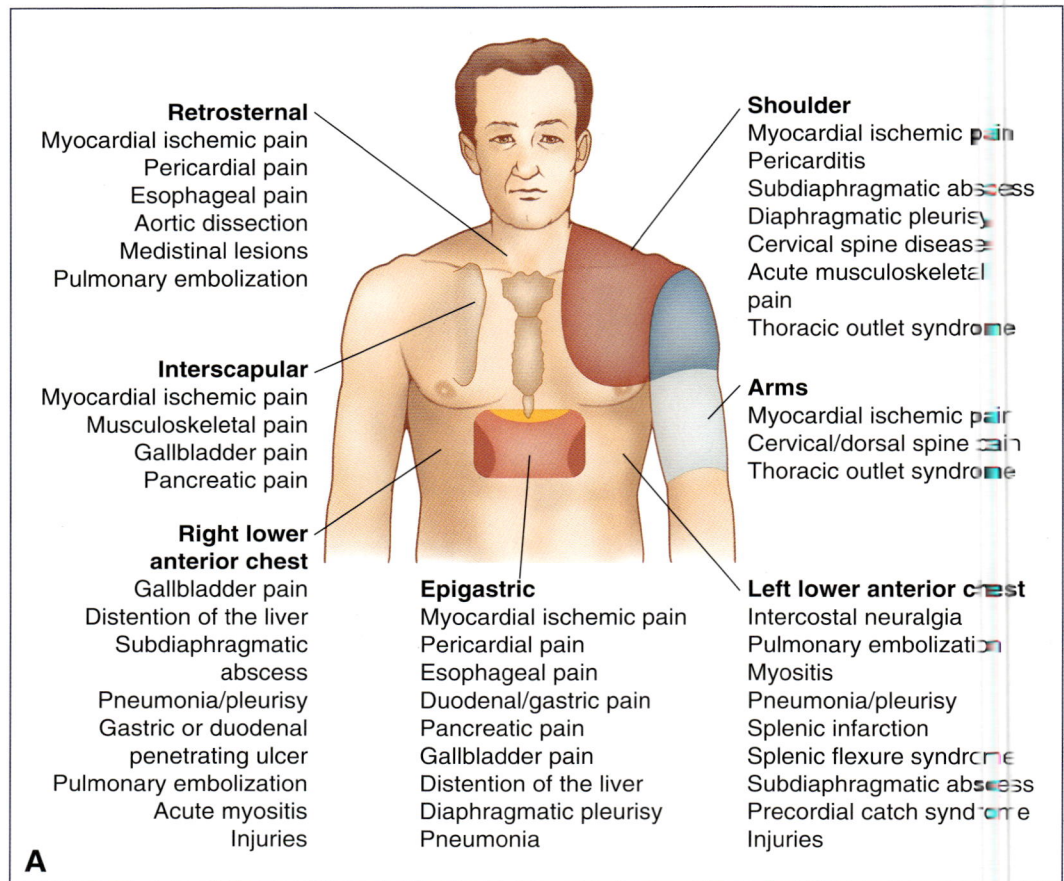

Retrosternal
Myocardial ischemic pain
Pericardial pain
Esophageal pain
Aortic dissection
Medistinal lesions
Pulmonary embolization

Shoulder
Myocardial ischemic pain
Pericarditis
Subdiaphragmatic abscess
Diaphragmatic pleurisy
Cervical spine disease
Acute musculoskeletal pain
Thoracic outlet syndrome

Interscapular
Myocardial ischemic pain
Musculoskeletal pain
Gallbladder pain
Pancreatic pain

Arms
Myocardial ischemic pain
Cervical/dorsal spine pain
Thoracic outlet syndrome

Right lower anterior chest
Gallbladder pain
Distention of the liver
Subdiaphragmatic abscess
Pneumonia/pleurisy
Gastric or duodenal penetrating ulcer
Pulmonary embolization
Acute myositis
Injuries

Epigastric
Myocardial ischemic pain
Pericardial pain
Esophageal pain
Duodenal/gastric pain
Pancreatic pain
Gallbladder pain
Distention of the liver
Diaphragmatic pleurisy
Pneumonia

Left lower anterior chest
Intercostal neuralgia
Pulmonary embolization
Myositis
Pneumonia/pleurisy
Splenic infarction
Splenic flexure syndrome
Subdiaphragmatic abscess
Precordial catch syndrome
Injuries

A

Cardiovascular Causes of Chest Pain

Condition	Location	Quality	Duration	Aggravating or relieving factors	Associated symptoms or signs
Angina	Retrosternal region: radiates to or occasionally isolated to neck, jaw, epigastrium, shoulder, or arms (left common)	Pressure, burning, squeezing, heaviness, indigestion	< 2–10 min	Precipitated by exercise, cold weather, or stress; relieved by rest or nitroglycerin	S_4, or murmur of papillary muscle dysfunction during pain
Myocardial infarction	Same as angina	Same as angina	Sudden onset, 30 min or longer, but variable	Unrelieved by rest or nitroglycerin	Same as angina, plus shortness of breath, sweating, nausea, vomiting
Pericarditis	Usually begins over sternum or toward cardiac apex and can radiate to neck or left shoulder; often more localized than the pain of myocardial ischemia	Sharp, stabbing, knifelike	Lasts many hours to days; many wax and wane	Aggravated by deep breathing, rotating chest, or supine position; relieved by sitting up and leaning forward	Pericardial friction rub
Aortic dissection	Anterior chest; can radiate to back	Excruciating, tearing, knifelike	Sudden onset, unrelenting	Usually occurs in setting of hypertension or predisposition such as Marfan Syndrome	Murmur of aortic insufficiency, pulse or blood pressure asymmetry; neurological deficit
Pulmonary embolism (chest pain often not present)	Substernal or over region of pulmonary infarction	Pleuritic (with pulmonary infarction) or angina-like	Sudden onset; minutes to hours	Can be aggravated by breathing	Dyspnea, tachypnea, tachycardia; signs of acute right-sided heart failure and pulmonary hypertension with large emboli; rales, pleural rub, hemoptysis with pulmonary infarction
Pulmonary hypertension	Substernal	Pressure, oppressive		Aggravated by effort	Pain usually associated with dyspnea; signs of pulmonary hypertension

B

Grading of Angina: Canadian Cardiovascular Society Classification

I	Ordinary physical activity does not cause angina
	Angina occurs with strenuous, rapid, or prolonged exertion at work or recreation but not with ordinary activity such as walking, climbing stairs
II	Slight limitation of ordinary activity
	Angina occurs on walking or climbing stairs rapidly, walking uphill, walking or climbing stairs after meals, or in cold, or in wind, or under emotional stress, or only during the few hours after wakening; or occurs on walking more than two city blocks (150 meters) on the level and climbing more than one flight of stairs at a normal pace and in normal conditions
III	Marked limitation of ordinary physical activity
	Angina occurs on walking one or two blocks on the level or on climbing one flight of stairs in normal conditions and at normal pace
IV	Inability to carry out any physical activity without discomfort
	Angina may be present at rest

Figure 3-6. The Canadian Cardiovascular Society proposed a simple system for grading the severity of angina that is a modification of the New York Heart Association (NYHA) functional classification.

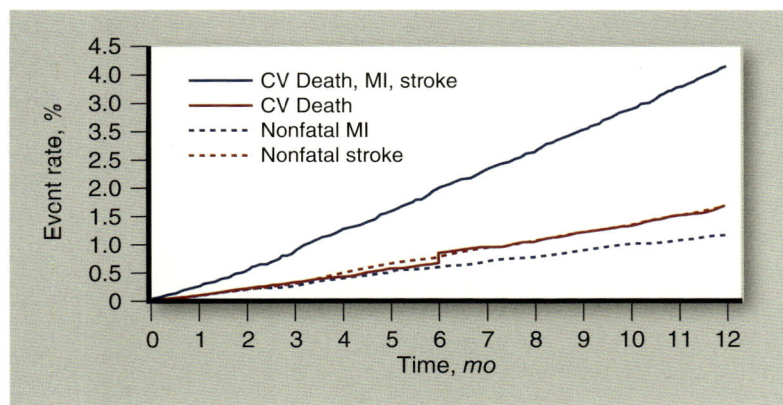

Figure 3-7. Natural history. Coronary heart disease (CHD) is the cause of more than half of all cardiovascular (CV) events in men and women younger than age 75. The lifetime risk of developing CHD after age 40 is 49% for men and 32% for women. The incidence of CHD in women lags behind men by 10 years for total CHD and 20 years for myocardial infarction (MI) and sudden death. In 2004, CHD caused one of every five (20%) deaths in the United States [6]. It has been estimated that by 2020, CV disease will be the leading cause of death worldwide. Data from long-term follow-up of individuals with prevalent CHD indicate an annual mortality rate of 1% to 3% and an annual rate of major ischemic events of 1% to 2%. For example, among 38,602 patients with stable coronary artery disease followed in an outpatient registry, the 1-year rate of CV death was 1.9% (95% CI; 1.7–2.1), all-cause mortality was 2.9% (95% CI; 2.6–3.2), and CV death, myocardial infarction, or stroke was 4.5% (95% CI; 4.2–4.8). (*Adapted from* Steg *et al.* [7].)

Noninvasive Testing

Selection of Noninvasive Testing for Ischemia

Likelihood of Coronary Artery Disease in Symptomatic Patients According to Age and Sex*

Age, y	Nonanginal chest pain		Atypical angina		Typical angina	
	Men	Women	Men	Women	Men	Women
30–39	4	2	34	12	76	26
40–49	13	3	51	22	87	55
50–59	20	7	65	31	93	73
60–69	27	14	72	51	94	86

*Each value represents the percentage with significant coronary artery disease at coronary angiography.

Figure 3-8. Pretest likelihood of coronary artery disease (CAD) in symptomatic patients. Noninvasive stress testing is valuable to establish the diagnosis of CAD and estimate the prognosis in patients with chronic stable angina. However, the indiscriminate use of such tests may generate misleading results. Appropriate application of noninvasive tests requires consideration of Bayesian principles, which state that the predictive value of a test depends not only on the sensitivity and specificity, but also on the prevalence of disease (or pretest probability) in the population of interest.

The value of noninvasive stress testing is greatest when the pretest likelihood is intermediate because the test result is likely to have the greatest effect on the posttest probability of CAD and, hence, on clinical decision making. A clinical assessment using the patient's age, sex, and a careful history of symptoms can provide an initial estimate of the probability of underlying CAD. The incremental diagnostic value of exercise testing is limited in patients in whom the estimated prevalence of CAD is either high or low. (*Adapted from* Gibbons *et al.* [8].)

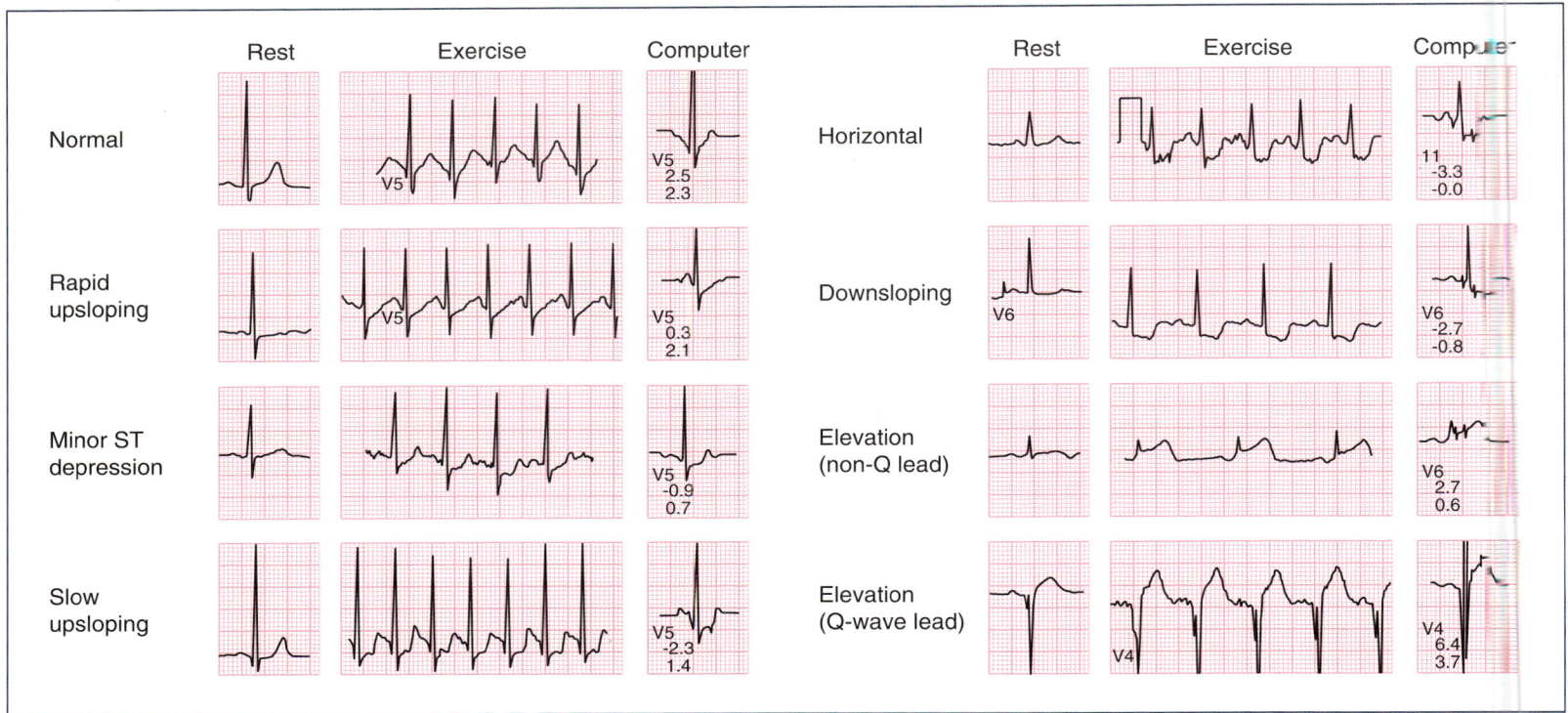

Figure 3-9. Exercise electrocardiography (ECG). Illustration of typical exercise electrocardiographic patterns at rest and at peak exertion. The computer-processed incrementally averaged beat corresponds with the raw data taken at the same time during exercise. The patterns represent a gradient of worsening ECG response to myocardial ischemia. In the column of computer-averaged beats, ST-80 displacement (*top number*) indicates the magnitude of ST-segment displacement 80 ms after the J-point. ST-segment slope measurement (*bottom number*) indicates the ST-segment slope at a fixed time after the J-point to the ST-80 measure-ment. The first two tracings illustrate normal and rapid upsloping ST-segments; both are normal responses to exercise. Slight ST depression can occur occasionally at submaximal workloads in patients with coronary disease. A slow upsloping ST-segment pattern often demonstrates an ischemic response in patients with known coronary disease. Classic criteria for myocardial ischemia include horizontal and/or downsloping ST-segment depression. ST-segment elevation in an infarct territory (Q-wave lead) indicates a severe wall motion abnormality and is usually not an ischemic response.

Approach to Stress Testing

Modality	Patients, *n*	Sensitivity, %*	Specificity, %†
Exercise ECG	24,047	68	77
Exercise SPECT	5272	88	72
Adenosine SPECT	2137	90	82
Exercise echocardiography	2788	85	81
Dobutamine echocardio graphy	2582	81	79

*Without correction for referral bias.
†Weighted average pooled across individual trials.

A

Figure 3-10. Selection of approach to stress testing. The exercise electrocardiography (ECG) is the most reasonable initial diagnostic test in patients with chest pain syndromes who have a moderate pretest probability of coronary artery disease (CAD), have a normal resting ECG and are likely to be able to achieve an adequate workload. **A,** Exercise imaging using either nuclear perfusion imaging or echocardiography with simultaneous ECG is superior to exercise ECG alone in detecting CAD, and in identifying multivessel disease.

Continued on the next page

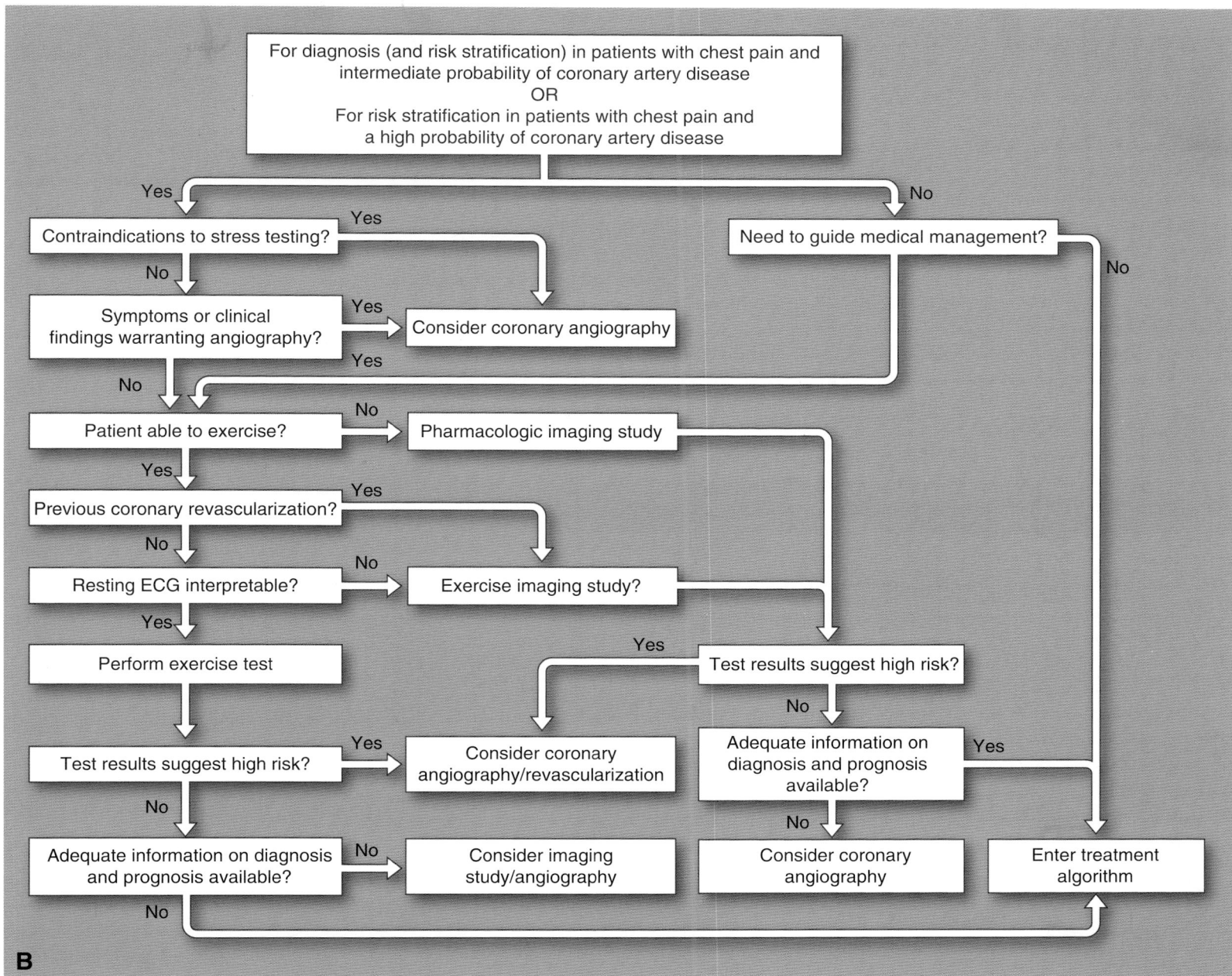

For diagnosis (and risk stratification) in patients with chest pain and intermediate probability of coronary artery disease
OR
For risk stratification in patients with chest pain and a high probability of coronary artery disease

Figure 3-10. *(Continued)* **B,** A stress-imaging technique should be considered for patients with ST-segment abnormalities at rest, left bundle-branch block, ventricular paced rhythm, or ventricular preexcitation, and those taking digoxin. Patients unable to exercise because of physical limitations (*eg,* arthritis, severe claudication, or severe lung dysfunction) should undergo pharmacologically induced stress imaging. SPECT—single-photon emission computed tomography. (**A,** *adapted from* Morrow and Gersh [4]; **B,** *adapted from* Gibbons *et al.* [8].)

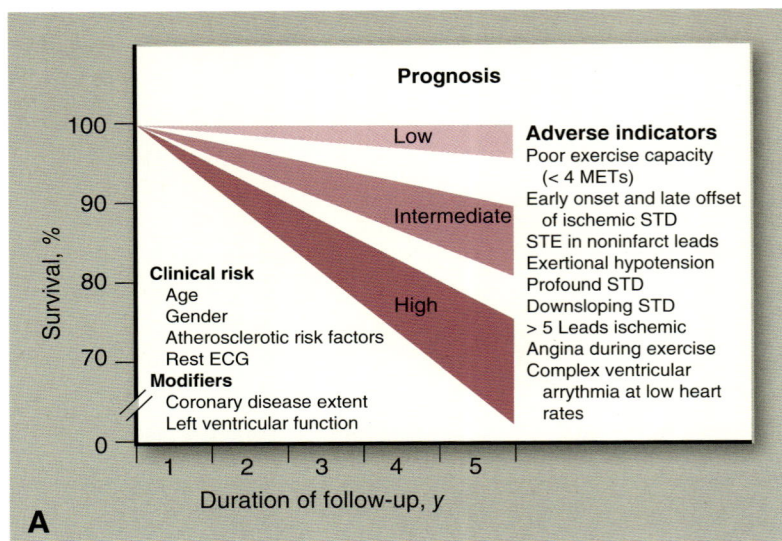

A

Prognosis

Low

Intermediate

High

Clinical risk
Age
Gender
Atherosclerotic risk factors
Rest ECG
Modifiers
Coronary disease extent
Left ventricular function

Adverse indicators
Poor exercise capacity
　(< 4 METs)
Early onset and late offset
　of ischemic STD
STE in noninfarct leads
Exertional hypotension
Profound STD
Downsloping STD
> 5 Leads ischemic
Angina during exercise
Complex ventricular
　arrythmia at low heart
　rates

Survival, %

Duration of follow-up, y

Risk Stratification on the Basis of Noninvasive Testing

High risk (> 3% annual mortality rate)

1. Severe resting LV dysfunction (LVEF < 35%)

2. High-risk treadmill score (score ≤ -11)

3. Severe exercise LV dysfunction (exercise LVEF < 35%)

4. Stress-induced large perfusion defect (particularly if anterior)

5. Stress-induced multiple perfusion defects of moderate size

6. Large, fixed perfusion defect with LV dilation or increased lung uptake (thallium-201)

7. Stress-induced moderate perfusion defect with LV dilation or increased lung uptake (thallium-201)

8. Echocardiographic wall motion abnormality (involving > 2 segments) developing at low dose of dobutamine (≤ 10mg/kg/min) or at a low heart rate (< 120 beats/min)

9. Stress echocardiographic evidence of extensive ischemia

Intermediate risk (1%–3% annual mortality rate)

1. Mild/moderate resting LV dysfunction (LVEF, 0.35–0.49)

2. Intermediate-risk treadmill score (-11 < score < 5)

3. Stress-induced moderate perfusion defect without LV dilation or increased lung intake (thallium-201)

4. Limited stress echocardiographic ischemia with a wall motion abnormality only at higher doses of dobutamine involving ≤ 2 segments

Low risk (<1% annual mortality rate)

1. Low-risk treadmill score (score ≥ 5)

2. Normal or small myocardial perfusion defect at rest or with stress*

3. Normal stress echocardiographic wall motion or no change of limited resting wall motion abnormalities during stress*

*Although the published data are limited, patients with these findings will probably not be at low risk in the presence of either a high-risk treadmill score or severe resting LV dysfunction (LVEF < 0.35).
LV—left ventricular; LVEF—LV ejection fraction.

B

Figure 3-11. Risk stratification on the basis of exercise testing. **A,** Actuarial survival curves of patients with normal or mildly impaired left ventricular function who have prognostic low-, intermediate-, and high-risk mortality estimates based on exercise test results. Patients able to exercise to at least seven metabolic equivalent of task units (METs) with a normal exercise electrocardiography (ECG) have an excellent 5-year prognosis for survival, even in the presence of obstructive coronary disease. The presence of several adverse indicators, such as poor exercise capacity and early onset and late resolution of myocardial ischemia on the exercise ECG, and slow recovery of heart rate, places the patient into a prognostic high-risk group. Patients in the intermediate category, who have fewer marked adverse indicators than individuals in the higher-risk group, fall into a subgroup for which myocardial perfusion imaging would significantly enhance the prognostic information used to guide the decision for coronary angiography and revascularization. **B,** Information regarding left ventricular function during exercise, and the extent of ischemia provides additional data regarding prognosis. STD—ST-segment depression; STE—ST-segment elevation. (**A,** *adapted from* Chaitman [9]; **B,** *adapted rom* Gibbons *et al.* [8].)

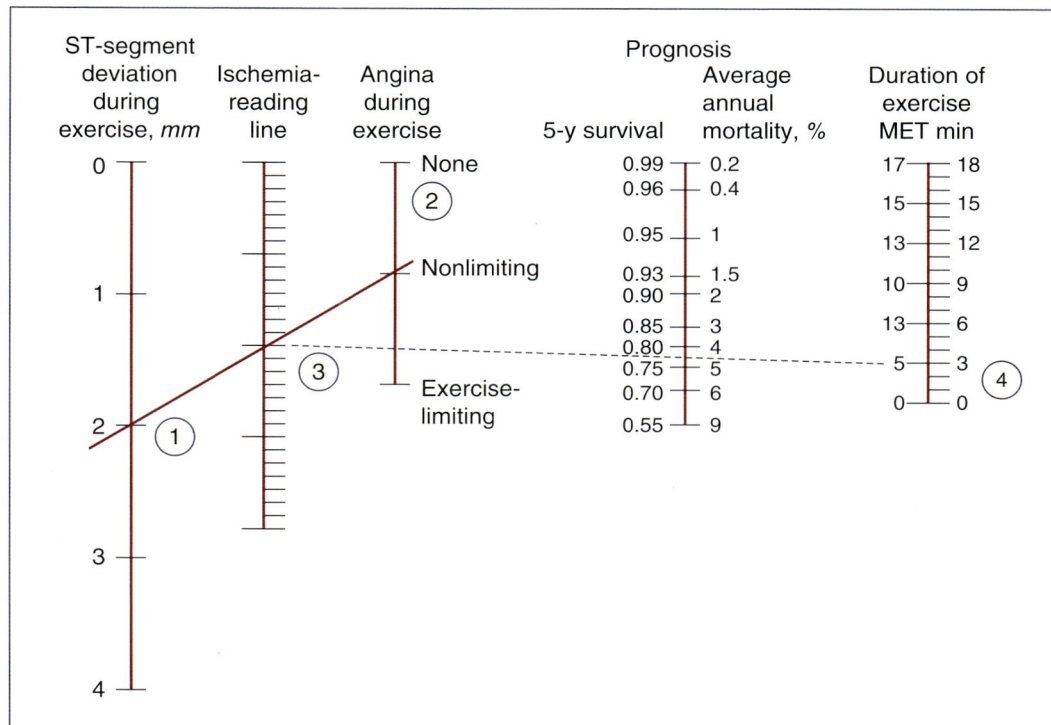

Figure 3-12. Prognostic nomogram using the Duke outpatient treadmill score. The score incorporates duration of exercise (in minutes) – (5 × maximal ST-segment deviation during/after exercise) – (4 × treadmill angina index). Treadmill angina index is 0 for no angina, 1 for nonlimiting angina, and 2 for exercise-limiting angina. The observed amount of exercise-induced ST-segment deviation (minus resting changes) is marked on the line for ST-segment deviation during exercise (*1*). Next, the degree of angina during exercise is plotted (*2*), and the two points are connected with a straightedge. The point of intersection on the ischemia reading line is noted (*3*). Next, the number of metabolic equivalent of task units (METs; or minutes of exercise if the Bruce method is used) is marked on the exercise duration line (*4*). The mark on the ischemia reading line and duration of exercise line are connected (*dashed line*), and the point of intersection on the prognosis line determines the 5-year survival rate and average annual mortality for patients with the selected specific variables. The 5-year prognosis is estimated at 78% for an example of exercise-induced 2 mm ST-depression, nonlimiting exercise-induced angina, and workload of 5 METs [10].

Echocardiography

Figure 3-13. Evaluation of left ventricular function in ischemic heart disease. Echocardiography is useful in the evaluation of patients with chronic ischemic heart disease because it can assess global and regional left ventricular function, as well as detect associated valve disease. Echocardiography is not necessary for all patients with angina, such as those with a normal echocardiogram (ECG) and no history of myocardial infarction. However, among patients with a history of myocardial infarction, ST-T wave changes, conduction defects, or Q waves on the ECG, or suspicion of significant associated valvular heart disease, echocardiography is likely to be valuable. A wall motion abnormality is the hallmark of coronary artery disease on echocardiography. This abnormality is one of the earliest signs of myocardial

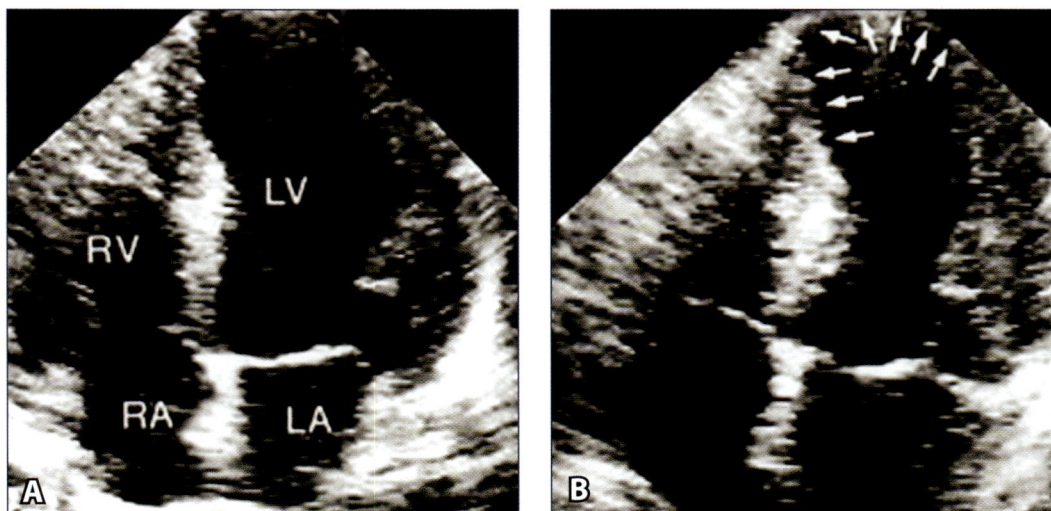

ischemia or infarction. **A,** Two-dimensional echocardiographic apical four-chamber view at end-diastole. **B,** Two-dimensional echocardiographic apical four-chamber view at end-systole. The right ventricle (RV) and the septal and lateral walls at the base of the left ventricle (LV) demonstrate normal inward motion from diastole through systole; however, the distal septum and apex demonstrate akinesis (*arrows*). The wall motion abnormality demonstrated in this frame was caused by ischemia from a lesion in the mid-left anterior descending artery. LA—left atrium; RA—right atrium.

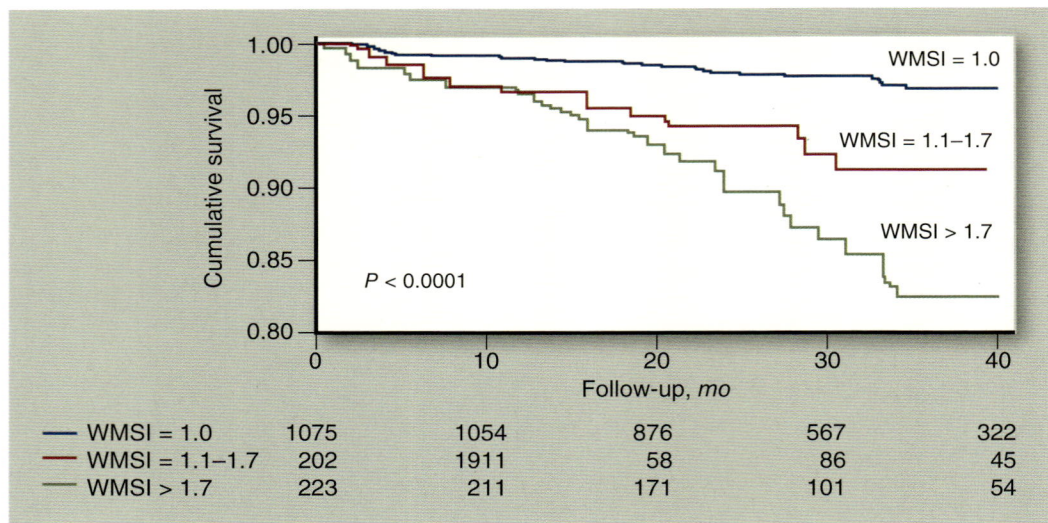

Figure 3-14. Prognostic information provided by stress echocardiography.

Stress echocardiography may be performed with either exercise-induced or pharmacologic stress and allows the detection of regional ischemia by identifying areas of wall motion abnormality. Pharmacologic stress using dobutamine should be employed in patients unable to exercise, or unable to achieve an adequate increase in heart rate with exercise. Exercise echocardiography can be used for the diagnosis of coronary artery disease with an accuracy that is similar to that of stress myocardial perfusion imaging and superior to exercise echocardiography alone.

— WMSI = 1.0	1075	1054	876	567	322
— WMSI = 1.1–1.7	202	1911	58	86	45
— WMSI > 1.7	223	211	171	101	54

Stress echocardiography also provides important prognostic information in patients with known or suspected ischemic heart disease. When stratified by a wall motion score index (WMSI), which is a measure of regional function at peak stress, patients with a normal WMSI (*upper curve*) have an excellent prognosis, whereas patients with a WMSI greater than 1.7 have a significantly worse event-free survival. (*Adapted from* Yao et al. [11].)

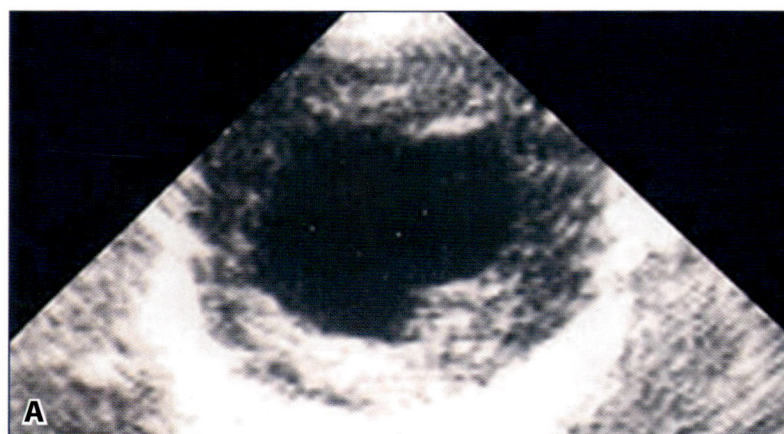
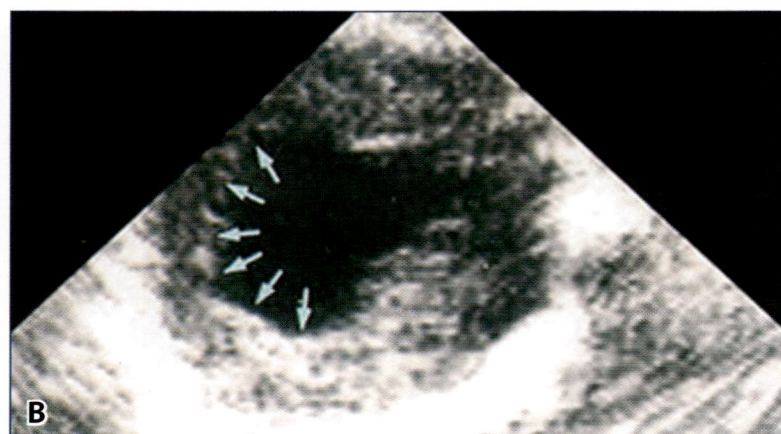
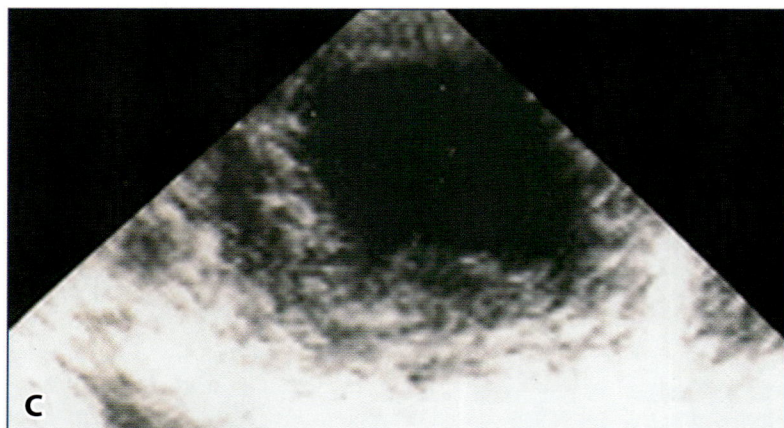
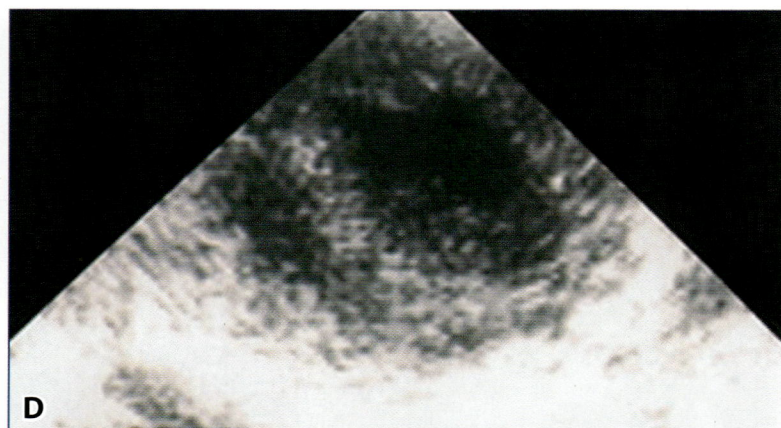

Figure 3-15. Assessment of myocardial viability using dobutamine stress echocardiography. Studies with dobutamine echocardiography (as well as nuclear techniques; *see* Fig. 3-19) have demonstrated that patients with left ventricular dysfunction and evidence of viable myocardium have improved outcomes with revascularization. Patients selected for revascularization on the basis of an imaging study demonstrating myocardial viability also have lower operative and long-term mortality rates than do those who have no evidence of important myocardial viability. This figure provides an example of the detection of viable myocardium by low-dose dobutamine echocardiography in an experimental model of ischemic but viable myocardium. **A,** Short-axis end-diastolic image of the left ventricular apex at rest. **B,** Accompanying end-systolic image. A wall motion abnormality is present (*arrows*) involving 50% of the circumference and results from reduction of flow in the mid-left anterior descending artery. **C** and **D,** With a 3-minute infusion of 10 μg/kg/min of dobutamine, an improvement in wall motion is noted in the segments that formerly exhibited abnormal wall motion. **C** is of the apex at end-diastole, and **D** is at end-systole. Following restoration of normal flow in the left anterior descending artery, wall motion in the apex returned to normal.

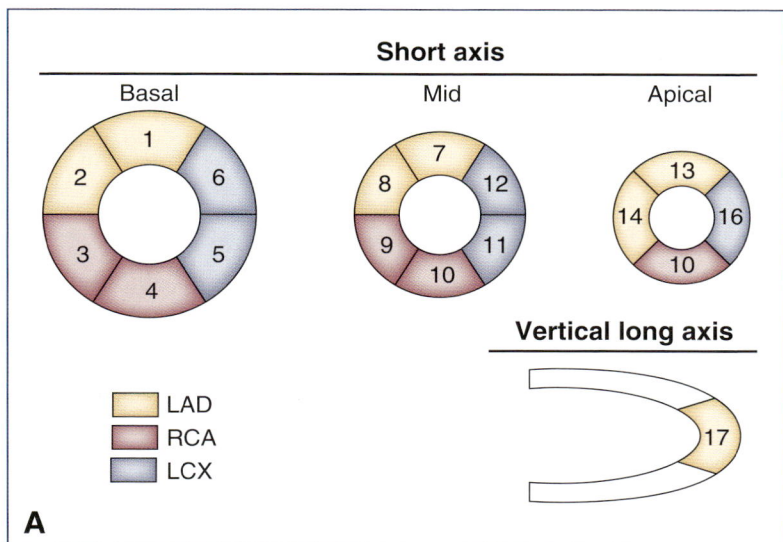

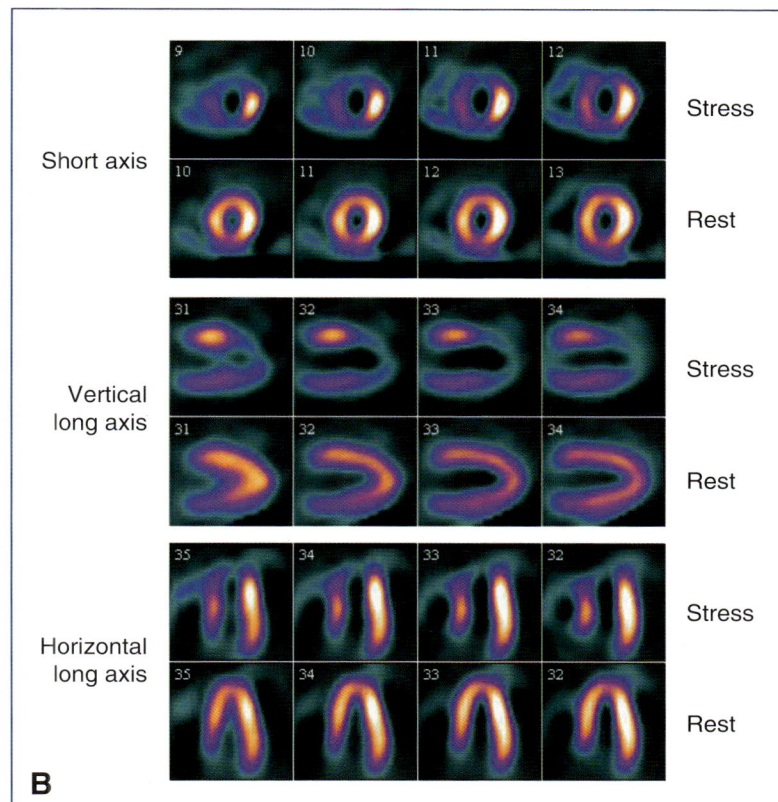

Figure 3-16. Single-photon emission computed tomography (SPECT; *see also* Chapter 14). Exercise perfusion imaging with simultaneous electrocardiography (ECG) is superior to exercise ECG alone in detecting coronary artery disease (CAD), in identifying multivessel disease, in localizing diseased vessels, and in determining the magnitude of ischemic and infarcted myocardium. Stress myocardial scintigraphy is particularly helpful in the diagnosis of CAD in patients with abnormal resting ECGs and those in whom ST segment responses cannot be interpreted accurately, such as patients with repolarization abnormalities due to left ventricular hypertrophy, those with left bundle branch block, and those receiving digitalis. Because stress myocardial perfusion imaging is a relatively expensive test (three to four times the cost of an exercise ECG), stress myocardial perfusion scintigraphy should not be used as a screening test in patients in whom the prevalence of CAD is low because the majority of abnormal tests will yield false-positive results, and a regular exercise ECG should always be considered first in patients with chest pain and a normal resting ECG for screening and detection of CAD. **A,** Anatomic correlation of the images. **B,** A stress SPECT study showing a marked anteroapical and inferior perfusion defect, present with stress but not at rest, consistent with ischemia in the absence of infarction. LAD—left anterior descending; LCX—left circumflex; RCA—right coronary artery.

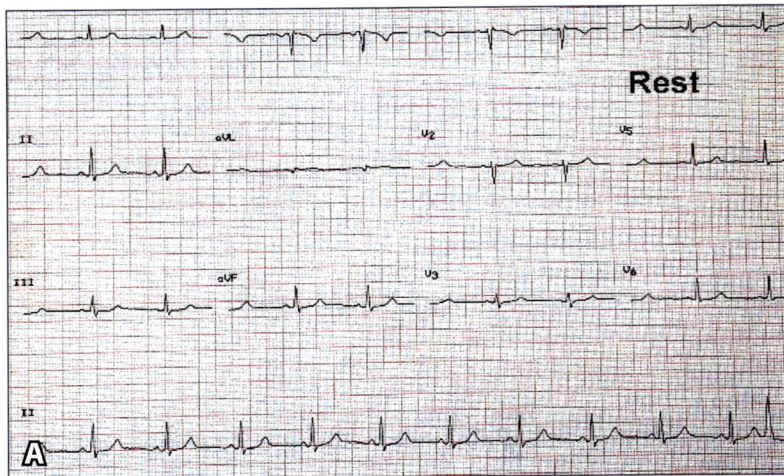

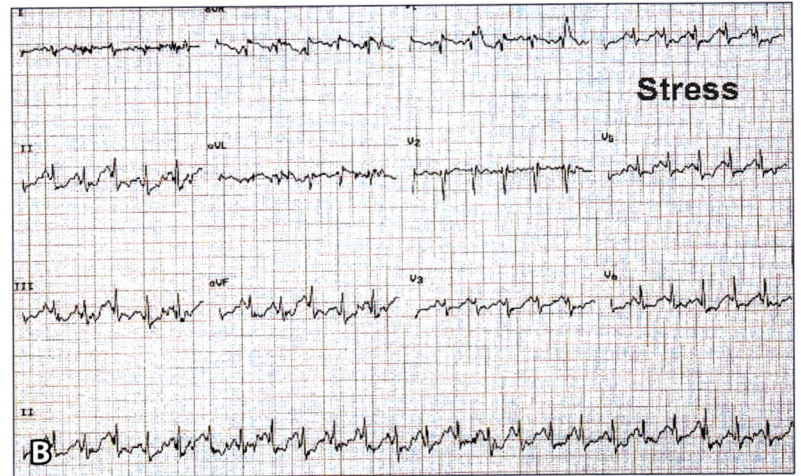

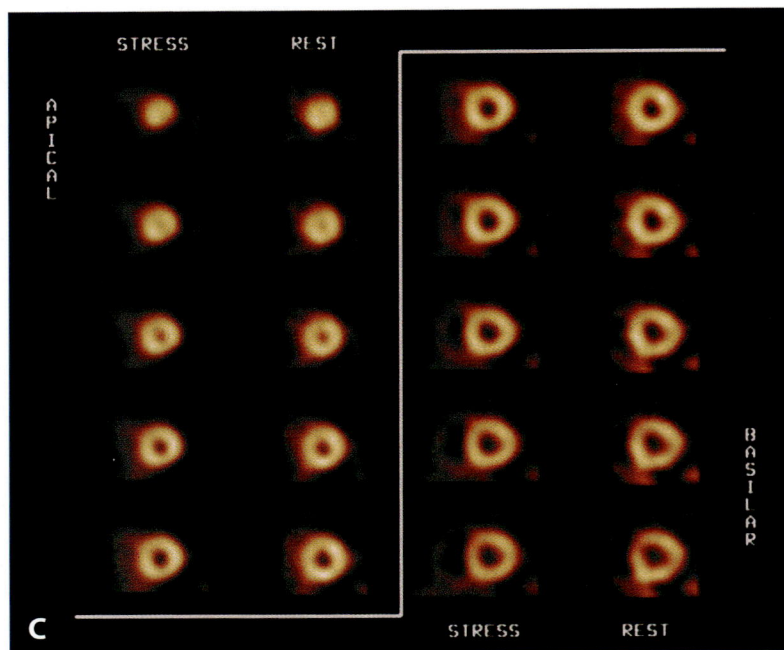

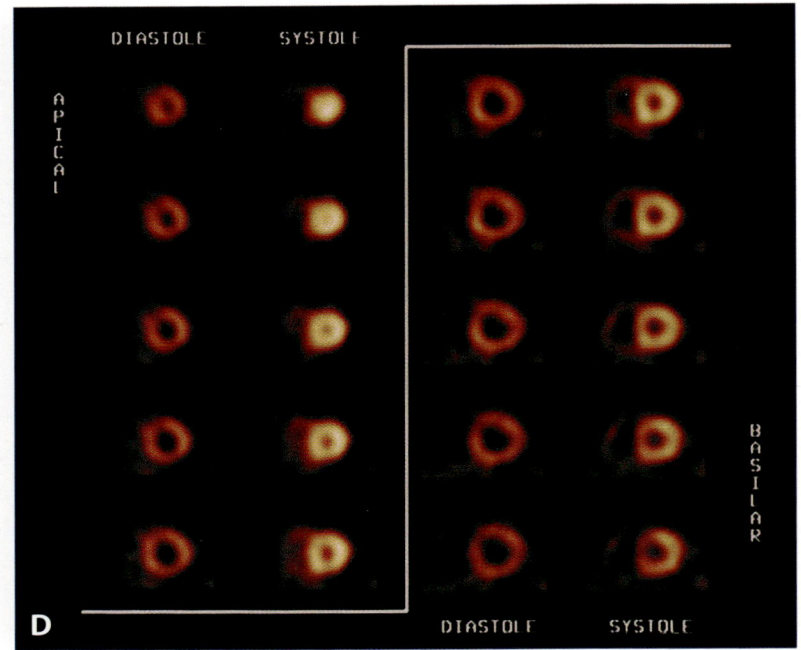

Figure 3-17. Use of myocardial perfusion imaging when a false-positive stress electrocardiography (ECG) is suspected (*see also* Chapter 14). Stress perfusion imaging is useful in differentiating true- from false-positive ST-segment responses on exercise treadmill testing. This is an example of a patient with a false-positive exercise ECG response, who had a normal gated single-photon emission computed tomography (SPECT) perfusion scan. **A,** Resting ECG showing no abnormalities. **B,** The exercise ECG at peak stress showing ST-segment depression in multiple leads and most prominent in leads V_4–V_6. For most complexes, the ST depression is approximately 1 mm. **C,** Stress and rest short-axis tomographic images showing uniform technetium-99m–sestamibi uptake in all myocardial segments. The resting study is also within normal limits. **D,** End-diastolic and end-systolic short-axis images showing uniform systolic thickening of all myocardial segments. This patient was told that the ST-segment response was false-positive for ischemia and that there was a very low likelihood of functionally important coronary artery disease.

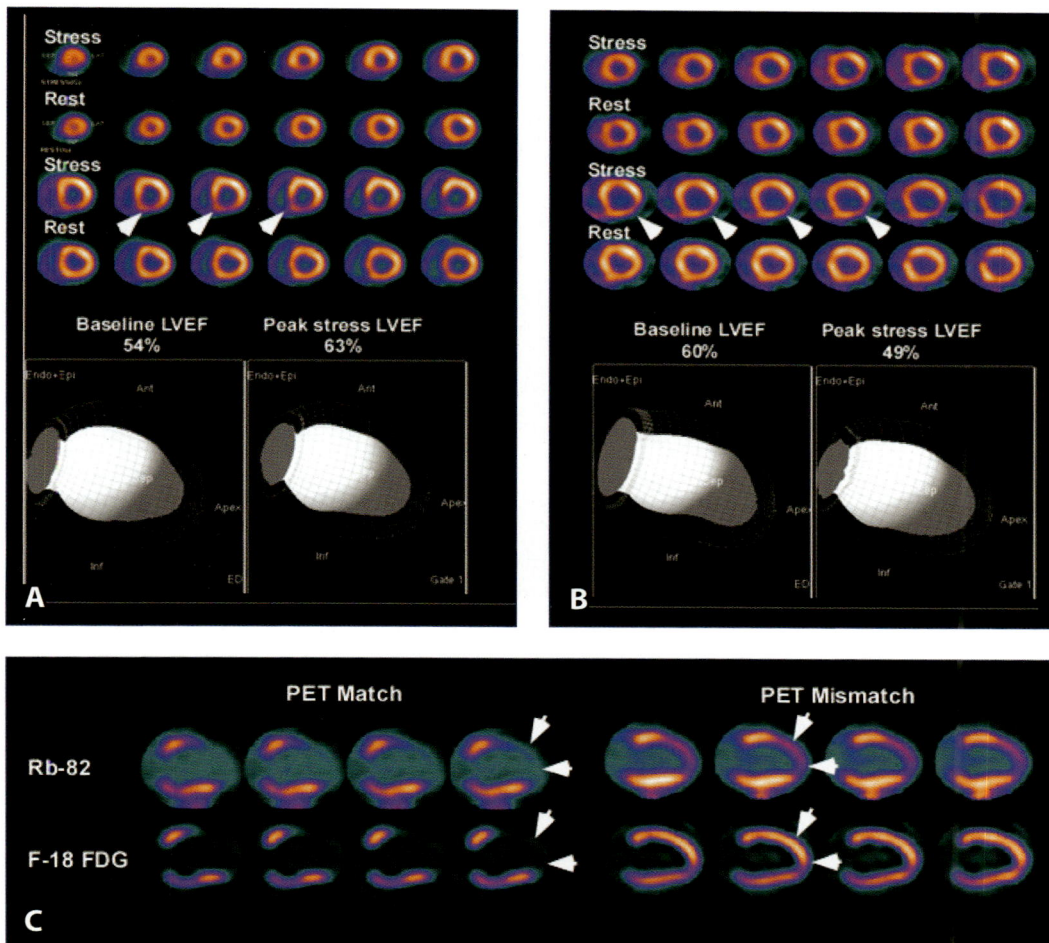

Figure 3-18. Advantages of positron emission tomography (PET; *see also* Chapter 14). PET employs positron emitting radionuclides to obtain images of myocardial perfusion and metabolism. Because carbon, oxygen, and nitrogen have radionuclide species that decay by positron emission, important biological processes may be quantified (*eg*, glucose and fatty acid metabolism). Several technical advantages provide for an improved quality of the images and associated superior diagnostic ability of PET compared with single-photon emission computed tomography (SPECT), particularly in patients with suboptimal SPECT images, such as those with obesity. The use of short-lived radiopharmaceuticals also enables rapid staging of rest/stress images, facilitating throughput. PET allows assessment of left ventricle (LV) function at rest and peak stress (as opposed to only post-stress with SPECT), facilitating the detection of balanced perfusion defects due to global ischemia [12].

A, Gated rest-stress myocardial perfusion PET images illustrating a normal rise in left ventricle ejection fraction (LVEF) from rest to peak stress (*bottom*) in a patient with angiographic single-vessel coronary artery disease (CAD), showing a single perfusion defect in the inferior wall on the PET images (*arrowheads*).

B, Abnormal drop in LVEF from rest to peak stress (*bottom*) in a patient with angiographic multivessel CAD, also showing only a single perfusion defect in the inferolateral wall on the PET images (*arrowheads*). (*From* Di Carli and Hachamovitch [12].)

C, The use of metabolic imaging with fluorodeoxyglucose (FDG) for evaluating myocardial viability has been well validated. Contractile dysfunction is predicted to be reversible in regions with increased FDG uptake or a perfusion-FDG mismatch. PET patterns of myocardial viability. Concordant reductions in myocardial perfusion (Rb-82), and glucose metabolism (FDG), reflecting myocardial infarction (*left*). Preserved glucose metabolism (FDG) in a territory with decreased myocardial perfusion (Rb-82), reflecting complete tissue viability (*right*). (*From* Di Carli and Hachamovitch [12].)

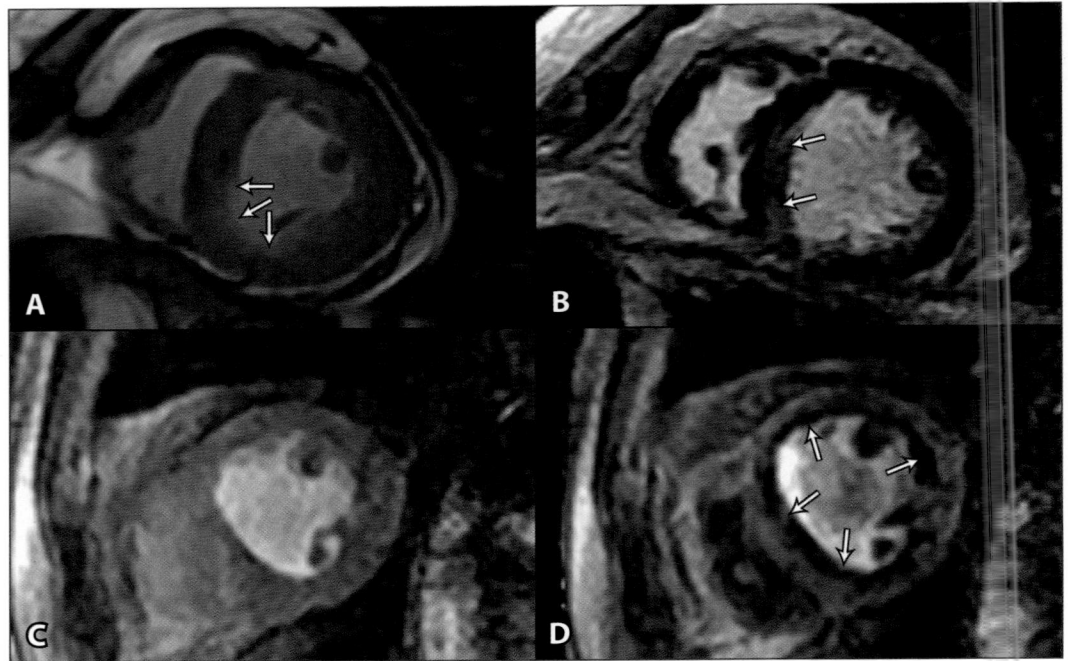

Figure 3-19. Uses of cardiac magnetic resonance imaging (MRI) in ischemic heart disease (*see also* Chapter 16). Cardiac MRI is emerging as a valuable approach to noninvasive cardiac imaging with ischemic heart disease. Similarly to nuclear perfusion imaging, cardiac MRI has been shown to identify myocardial viability that is associated with functional recovery after revascularization. Pharmacologic stress perfusion imaging may also be performed with MRI, and compares favorably to other methods. Cardiac MRI also provides accurate characterization of left ventricular (LV) function and may be used to differentiate ischemic from nonischemic causes of regional myocardial dysfunction. By virtue of its ability to visualize arteries in three dimensions and differentiate tissue constituents, MRI angiography has received intense interest as a potential, but as yet not established, modality to characterize arterial atheroma and assess vulnerability to rupture on the basis of compositional analysis [13].

A, Systolic frame of the LV cine shows inferior and inferoseptal hypokinesis. **B,** Late enhancement of the myocardium in these segments indicates a subendocardial infarction. **C,** A resting first-pass perfusion does not show any significant perfusion abnormality. **D,** However, upon adenosine stress infusion, circumferential subendocardial perfusion abnormality indicates multivessel flow-limiting coronary disease, which was confirmed upon coronary angiography.

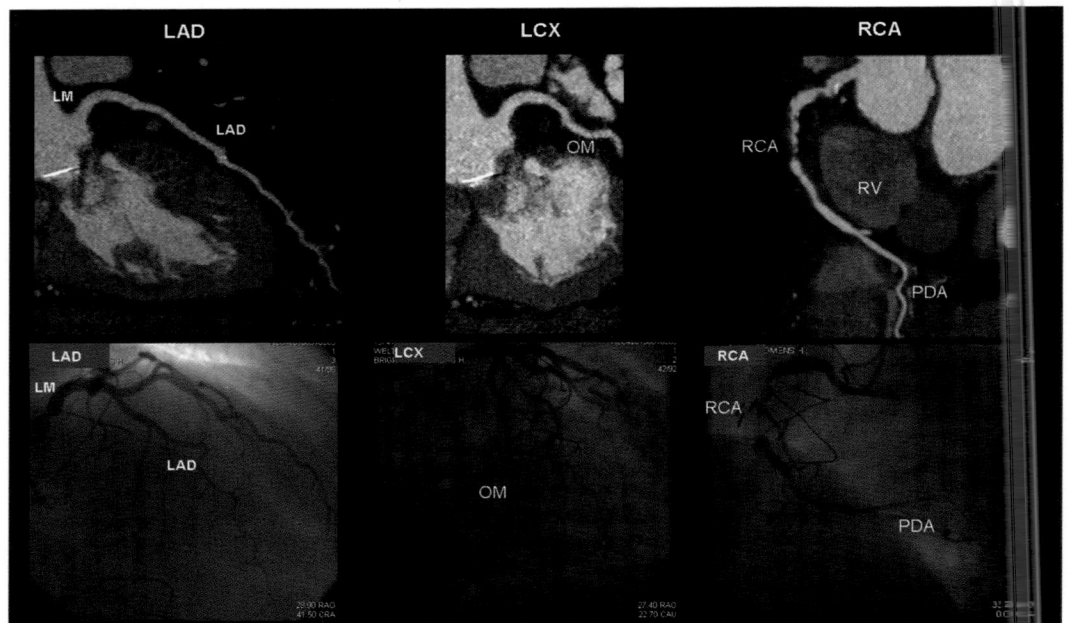

Figure 3-20. Cardiac computed tomography (CT) in ischemic heart disease. Electron-beam, and now multislice cardiac, CT is recognized as a highly sensitive method for detecting coronary calcification and may be used as a screening technique for coronary artery disease (CAD; *see also* Chapter 15). The calcium score, a quantitative index of total coronary artery calcium detected by CT, is a good marker of the total coronary atherosclerotic burden. In addition to application for detection of coronary calcification, CT technology continues to evolve toward providing reliable noninvasive coronary angiography. Newer multislice spiral CT technology in conjunction with aggressive β-blockade to reduce heart rate during imaging has shown promise for detection of obstructive CAD in the major epicardial arteries, but at present has not yet overcome limitations related to false-positive and nonevaluable results. Delayed-enhancement multislice CT is under investigation as a method for detection and quantification of myocardial infarction [12]. This CT angiogram (*top*) reveals serial critical stenosis of the proximal right coronary artery (RCA). Severe right CAD was confirmed at invasive coronary arteriography. LAD—left anterior descending; LCX—left circumflex; LM—left main; OM—obtuse marginal; PDA—patent ductus arteriosus; RV—right ventricle.

Medical Therapy

Prevention of Death and Ischemic Events

American Heart Association/American College of Cardiology Recommendations for Secondary Prevention in Patients With Coronary Disease *(Continued on the next page)*

Goal	Intervention Recommendations With Class of Recommendation and Level of Evidence
Smoking	
Complete cessation; no exposure to environmental tobacco smoke	Ask about tobacco use status at every visit. I (B)
	Advise every tobacco user to quit. I (B)
	Assist by counseling and developing a plan for quitting. I (B)
	Arrange follow-up, referral to special programs, or pharmacotherapy. I (B)
	Urge avoidance of exposure to environmental tobacco smoke at work and home. I (B)
Blood pressure control	*For all patients:*
≤ 140/90 mm Hg	Initiate or maintain lifestyle modification, including weight control; increased physical activity; alcohol moderation; sodium reduction; and emphasis on increased consumption of fresh fruits, vegetables, and low-fat dairy products. I (B)
or ≤130/80 mm Hg if patient has diabetes or chronic kidney disease	*For patients with* blood pressure > 140/90 mm Hg (or > 130/80 mm Hg for individuals with chronic kidney disease or diabetes):
	As tolerated, add blood pressure medication, treating initially with β-blockers and/or ACE inhibitors, with addition of other drugs such as thiazides as needed to achieve goal blood pressure. I (A)
Lipid management	*For all patients (see* Fig. 3-23 for pharmacotherapy):
LDL-C < 100 mg/dL; if triglycerides are ≥ 200 mg/dL, non-HDL-C should be < 130 mg/dL*	Start dietary therapy. Reduce intake of saturated fats (to < 7% of total calories), trans-fatty acids, and cholesterol (to < 200 mg/d). I (B)
	Adding plant stanol/sterols (2 g/d) and viscous fiber (> 10 g/d) will further lower LDL-C.
	Promote daily physical activity and weight management. I (B)
	Encourage increased consumption of omega-3 fatty acids in the form of fish[†] or in capsule form (1 g/d) for risk reduction. For treatment of elevated triglycerides, higher doses are usually necessary for risk reduction. IIb (B)
Physical activity	*For all patients,* assess risk with a physical activity history and/or an exercise test, to guide prescription. I (B)
	For all patients, encourage 30–60 minutes of moderate-intensity aerobic activity, such as brisk walking, on most, preferably all, days of the week, supplemented by an increase in daily lifestyle activities (*eg*, walking breaks at work, gardening, household work). I (B)
	Encourage resistance training 2 days per week. IIb (C)
	Advise medically supervised programs for high-risk patients (*eg*, recent acute coronary syndrome or revascularization, heart failure). I (B)
Weight management	
Body mass index: 18.5 to 24.9 kg/m²; waist circumference: men < 40 in, women < 35 in	Assess body mass index and/or waist circumference on each visit and consistently encourage weight maintenance/reduction through an appropriate balance of physical activity, caloric intake, and formal behavioral programs when indicated to maintain/achieve a body mass index between 18.5 and 24.9 kg/m². I (B)
	If waist circumference (measured horizontally at the iliac crest) is ≥ 35 inches in women and ≥ 40 inches in men, initiate lifestyle changes and consider treatment strategies for metabolic syndrome as indicated. I (B)
	The initial goal of weight loss therapy should be to reduce body weight by approximately 10% from baseline.
	With success, further weight loss can be attempted if indicated through further assessment. I (B)

*Non–high density lipoprotein cholesterol (HDL-C)—total cholesterol minus HDL-C.
[†]Pregnant and lactating women should limit their intake of fish to minimize exposure to methylmercury.
LDL-C—low-density lipoprotein cholesterol.

Figure 3-21. American College of Cardiology/American Heart Association recommendations for secondary prevention in patients with coronary disease. The management of patients with chronic angina includes both interventions to reduce the risk of disease progression and treatments to alleviate angina. Risk factors should be modified aggressively with lifestyle changes, behavior modification, or pharmacologic therapy. Recommendations are shown for interventions to prevent myocardial infarction and death in patients with established atherosclerotic vascular disease. In separate figures, recommendations are discussed for lipid-lowering pharmacotherapy, antiplatelet therapy, and angiotensin-converting enzyme (ACE) inhibitors. (*Adapted from* Smith *et al.* [14].)

Continued on the next page

American Heart Association/American College of Cardiology Recommendations for Secondary Prevention in Patients With Coronary Disease *(Continued)*

Diabetes management	Initiate lifestyle and pharmacotherapy to achieve near-normal HbA1c. I (B)
	Begin vigorous modification of other risk factors (*eg*, physical activity, weight management, blood pressure control, and cholesterol management as recommended above). I (B)
	Coordinate diabetic care with patient's primary care physician or endocrinologist. I (C)
β-Blockers	Start and continue indefinitely in all patients who have had myocardial infarction, acute coronary syndrome, or left ventricular dysfunction with or without heart failure symptoms, unless contraindicated. I (A)
	Consider chronic therapy for all other patients with coronary or other vascular disease or diabetes unless contraindicated. IIa (C)
Influenza vaccination	Patients with cardiovascular disease should have an influenza vaccination. I (B)

Non–high density lipoprotein cholesterol (HDL-C)—total cholesterol minus HDL-C.
†*Pregnant and lactating women should limit their intake of fish to minimize exposure to methylmercury.*
LDL-C—low-density lipoprotein cholesterol.

Figure 3-21. *(Continued)*

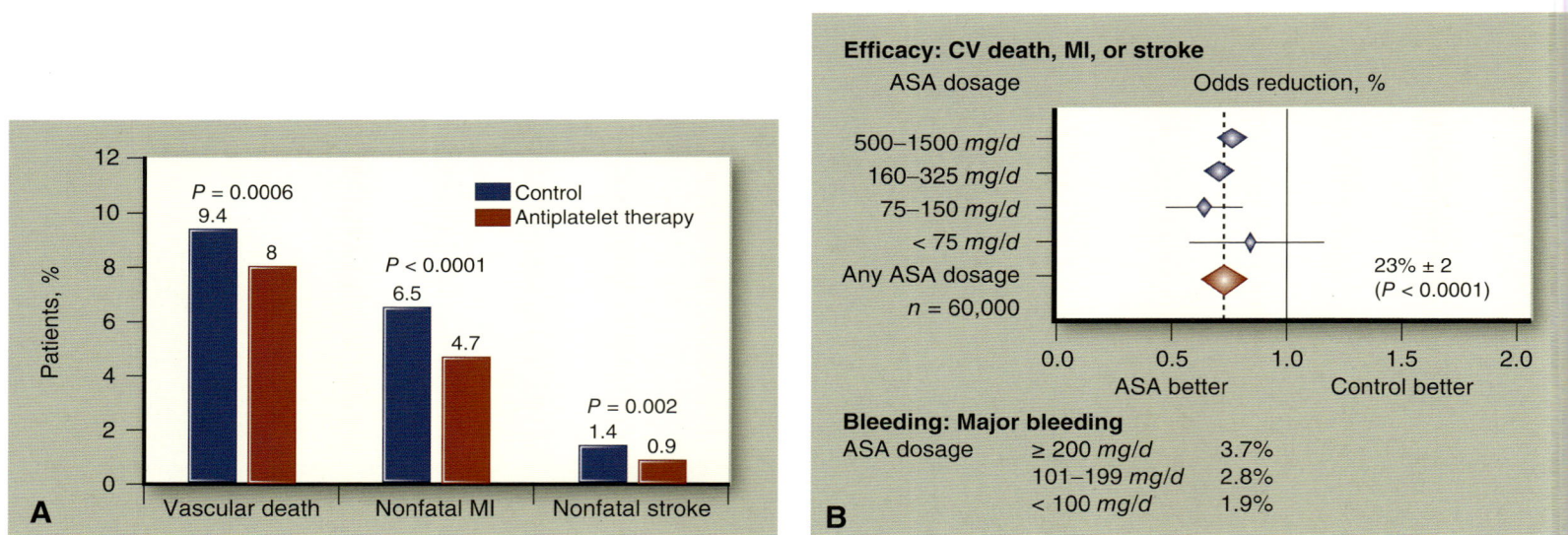

Antiplatelet Agents

Start aspirin 75–162 mg/d and continue indefinitely in all patients unless contraindicated. I (A)

For patients undergoing coronary artery bypass grafting, aspirin should be started within 48 hours after surgery to reduce saphenous vein graft closure. Dosing regimens ranging from 100–325 mg/d appear to be efficacious. Dosages higher than 162 mg/d can be continued for up to 1 year. I (B)

Start and continue clopidogrel 75 mg/d in combination with aspirin for up to 12 months in patients after acute coronary syndrome or percutaneous coronary intervention with stent placement (≥ 1 month for bare metal stent, ≥ 3 months for sirolimus-eluting stent, and ≥ 6 months for paclitaxel-eluting stent). I (B)

Patients who have undergone percutaneous coronary intervention with stent placement should initially receive higher-dose aspirin at 325 mg/d for 1 month for bare metal stent, 3 months for sirolimus-eluting stent, and 6 months for paclitaxel-eluting stent. I (B)

C

Figure 3-22. Antiplatelet therapy in chronic ischemic heart disease. The benefits of antiplatelet therapy in patients with ischemic heart disease is established. A meta-analysis of 140,000 patients in 300 studies confirmed the prophylactic benefit of aspirin in both men and women with angina pectoris, previous myocardial infarction, or previous stroke and after bypass surgery.

A, The benefit of acetylsalicylic acid (ASA) in approximately 20,000 patients with prior myocardial infarction is shown. **B,** Dosing at 75 to 162 mg/d appears to have comparable effects for secondary prevention to dosing at 160 to 325 mg/d and appears to be associated with lower bleeding risk [15,16]. **C,** Therefore, administration of aspirin is recommended by the American College of Cardiology and American Heart Association in patients with chronic stable angina but without contraindications to this drug. Aspirin, 75 to 162 mg/d, is preferred for secondary prevention in the absence of recent revascularization procedures [14]. CV—cardiovascular; MI—myocardial infarction.

Figure 3-23. Lipid-lowering therapy in chronic ischemic heart disease. Clinical trials in patients with atherosclerotic vascular disease have demonstrated improved outcomes in patients treated with 3-hydroxy-3-methylglutaryl coenzyme A (HMG-CoA) reductase inhibitors (statins). The benefits are apparent in patients with a wide range of cholesterol levels.

A, Among patients with coronary heart disease (CHD) with a total cholesterol > 135 mg/dL enrolled in the Heart Protection Study, 40 mg/d of simvastatin reduced the risk of major vascular events (cardiovascular death, myocardial infarction [MI], stroke, or arterial revascularization) by 24% compared with placebo. (*Adapted from* Heart Protection Study Collaborative group [17].)

B, Moreover, in a pooled evaluation of intensive versus standard (Std) dosing of statin therapy for patients with established CHD in four randomized trials, intensive therapy was associated with significantly lower achieved levels of low-density lipoprotein cholesterol (75 mg/dL vs 101 mg/dL) and a 16% lowering of the risk of death or MI. (*Adapted from* Cannon et al. [18].)

C, These and other trials have supported the American College of Cardiology/American Heart Association recommendations for the management of lipid-lowering therapy in patients with established atherosclerotic vascular disease [14].

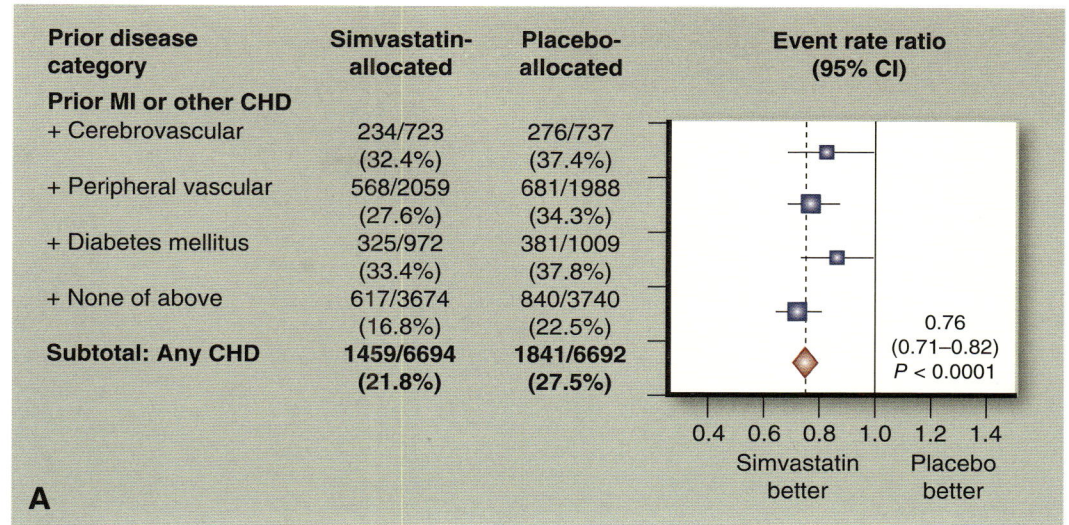

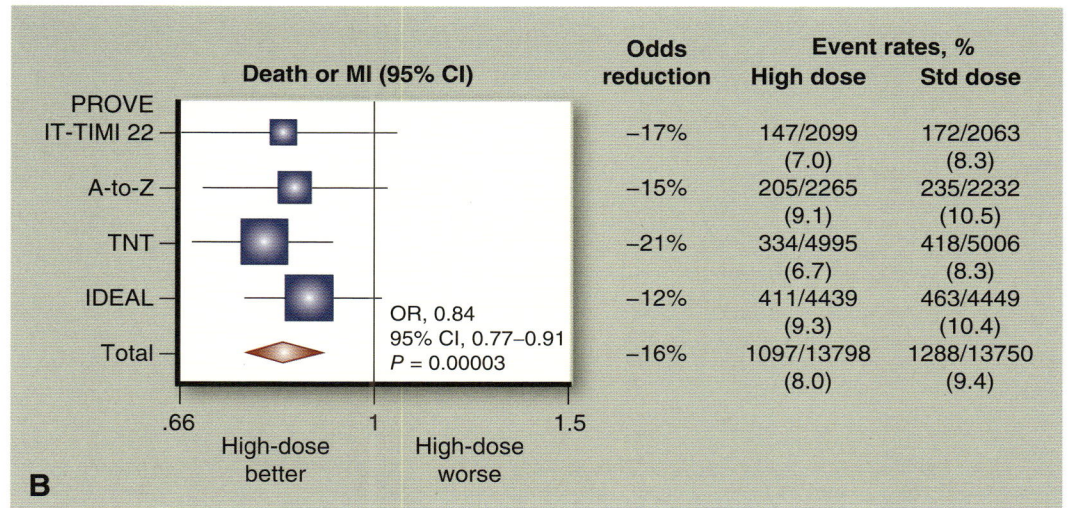

Prior disease category	Simvastatin-allocated	Placebo-allocated	Event rate ratio (95% CI)
Prior MI or other CHD			
+ Cerebrovascular	234/723 (32.4%)	276/737 (37.4%)	
+ Peripheral vascular	568/2059 (27.6%)	681/1988 (34.3%)	
+ Diabetes mellitus	325/972 (33.4%)	381/1009 (37.8%)	
+ None of above	617/3674 (16.8%)	840/3740 (22.5%)	
Subtotal: Any CHD	**1459/6694 (21.8%)**	**1841/6692 (27.5%)**	0.76 (0.71–0.82) $P < 0.0001$

	Death or MI (95% CI)	Odds reduction	Event rates, % High dose	Event rates, % Std dose
PROVE IT-TIMI 22		−17%	147/2099 (7.0)	172/2063 (8.3)
A-to-Z		−15%	205/2265 (9.1)	235/2232 (10.5)
TNT		−21%	334/4995 (6.7)	418/5006 (8.3)
IDEAL		−12%	411/4439 (9.3)	463/4449 (10.4)
Total	OR, 0.84 95% CI, 0.77–0.91 $P = 0.00003$	−16%	1097/13798 (8.0)	1288/13750 (9.4)

Lipid-Lowering Therapy in Chronic Ischemic Heart Disease

Lipid management: LDL-C < 100 mg/dL; if triglycerides are ≥ 200 mg/dL, non–HDL-C should be < 130 mg/dL*	In addition to measures described in Fig. 3-23:
	Assess fasting lipid profile in all patients, and within 24 h of hospitalization for those with an acute cardiovascular or coronary event. For hospitalized patients, initiate lipid-lowering medication as recommended below before discharge according to the following schedule:
	LDL-C should be < 100 mg/dl I (A), and:
	Further reduction of LDL-C to < 70 mg/dL is reasonable. IIa (A)
	If baseline LDL-C is ≥ 100 mg/dL, initiate LDL-lowering drug therapy.† I (A)
	If on-treatment LDL-C is > 100 mg/dL, intensify LDL-lowering drug therapy (may require LDL-lowering drug combination). I (A)
	If baseline LDL-C is 70 to 100 mg/dL, it is reasonable to treat to LDL-C < 70 mg/dL. IIa (B)
	If triglycerides are 200–499 mg/dL, non–HDL-C should be < 130 mg/dL. I (B), and
	Further reduction of non–HDL-C to ≤ 100 mg/dL is reasonable. IIa (B)
	Therapeutic options to reduce non–HDL-C are:
	More intense LDL-C–lowering therapy I (B), or
	Niacin† (after LDL-C–lowering therapy) IIa (B), or
	Fibrate therapy§ (after LDL-C–lowering therapy) IIa (B)
	If triglycerides are ≥ 500 mg/dL§, therapeutic options to prevent pancreatitis are fibrate† or niacin† before LDL-lowering therapy; and treat LDL-C to goal after triglyceride-lowering therapy. Achieve non–HDL-C < 130 mg/dL if possible. I (C)

*Non–high density lipoprotein cholesterol (HDL-C)—total cholesterol minus HDL-C.
†When low-density lipoprotein (LDL)-lowering medications are used, obtain at least a 30%–40% reduction in LDL-cholesterol (C) levels. If LDL-C ≤ 70 mg/dL is the chosen target, consider drug titration to achieve this level to minimize side effects and cost. When LDL-C ≤ 70 mg/dL is not achievable because of high baseline LDL-C levels, it generally is possible to achieve reductions of ≥ 50% in LDL-C levels by either statins or LDL-C–lowering drug combinations.
‡The combination of high-dose statin-fibrate can increase risk for severe myopathy. Statin doses should be kept relatively low with this combination. Dietary supplement niacin must not be used as a substitute for prescription niacin.
§Patients with very high triglycerides should not consume alcohol. The use of bile acid sequestrant is relatively contraindicated when triglycerides are ≥ 200 mg/dL.

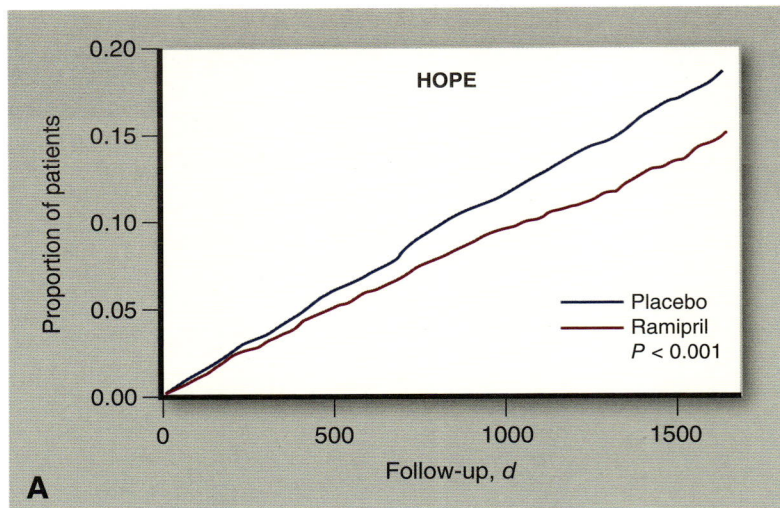

A

Renin–Angiotensin–Aldosterone System Blockers

ACE inhibitors

Start and continue indefinitely in all patients with left ventricular ejection fraction ≤ 40% and in those with hypertension, diabetes, or chronic kidney disease, unless contraindicated. I (A)

Consider for all other patients. I (B)

Among lower-risk patients with normal left ventricular ejection fraction in whom cardiovascular risk factors are well controlled and revascularization has been performed, use of ACE inhibitors may be considered optional. IIa (B)

Angiotensin receptor blockers

Use in patients who are intolerant of ACE inhibitors and have heart failure or have had a myocardial infarction with left ventricular ejection fraction ≤ 40%. I (A)

Consider in other patients who are ACE inhibitor intolerant. I (B)

Consider use in combination with ACE inhibitors in systolic-dysfunction heart failure. IIb (B)

Aldosterone blockade

Use in post–myocardial infarction patients, without significant renal dysfunction* or hyperkalemia†, who are already receiving therapeutic doses of an ACE inhibitor and β-blocker, have a left ventricular ejection fraction ≤ 40%, and have either diabetes or heart failure. I (A)

*Creatinine should be < 2.5 mg/dL in men and < 2.0 mg/dL in women.
†Potassium should be < 5.0 mEq/L.

B

Figure 3-24. Use of renin-angiotensin-aldosterone blockers in chronic ischemic heart disease. Inhibitors of the renin-angiotensin-aldosterone system appear to have important benefits in reducing the risk of ischemic events in some patients with cardiovascular disease. Angiotensin-converting enzyme (ACE) inhibitors, in particular, may have favorable effects on inflammation and endothelial function. Two trials have provided strong evidence supporting the benefit of ACE inhibitors in patients with atherosclerotic vascular disease, normal ejection fraction, and absence of heart failure. **A,** In the Heart Outcomes Protection Evaluation (HOPE) study, ramipril decreased the risk of cardiovascular death, myocardial infarction (MI), and stroke by 22%. In the European Trial on Reduction of Cardiac Events with Perindopril in stable CAD

(EUROPA), another ACE inhibitor reduced the risk of cardiovascular death, MI, or cardiac arrest by 20%. In contrast, trandolapril showed no effect on the risk of cardiovascular death, MI, or coronary revascularization in 8290 patients with stable coronary artery disease (CAD) at low risk after receiving intensive preventive therapy, usually including revascularization and lipid-lowering agents (PEACE). The absence of an additional reduction with trandolapril in this trial is plausibly related to the lower risk of the population in the setting of other advances in preventive therapy. (*Adapted from* Morrow and Gersh [4].)

B, ACE inhibitors are recommended for all patients with CAD with left ventricular dysfunction, and in those with hypertension, diabetes, or chronic kidney disease. (*Adapted from* Smith *et al.* [14].)

Treatment of Angina

Anti-ischemic Mechanisms of Medical Therapy in Stable Angina

	Drug Class		
Action	Nitroglycerin or nitrates	β-Blockers	Calcium antagonists
Decreased myocardial demand	++	+++	+ to ++
Increased coronary blood supply	+++	0 to +	++ to +++
Prevent coronary spasm or vasoconstriction	++	0 to +	++ to +++
Coronary stenosis enlargement	++	0 to +	+ to ++
Left ventricular function	Improves	− to 0	− to 0
Other	Reverse disordered endothelial function; antiplatelet action	Electrical stabilization; antiarrhythmic; antihypertensive	Antihypertensive

0—no effects; −—negative effects or may worsen; +—minor effects; ++—moderate effects; +++—major effects

Figure 3-25. Anti-ischemic mechanisms of traditional antianginal agents. Most classes of antianginals act predominantly through lowering myocardial oxygen consumption, thereby lessening cardiac energy demands. The β-adrenergic blocking agents (β-blockers) are the most potent in this regard. However, the nitrates and calcium antagonists increase coronary blood flow and thus are used in the presence of coronary artery vasoconstriction. Coronary atherosclerotic stenosis constriction may be an important cause of angina in some patients. Data are limited regarding drugs other than the nitrates in preventing or reversing stenosis constriction. Nitrates are the favored drugs for patients with angina and left ventricular dysfunction or congestive heart failure. β-Blockers and calcium antagonists are ideal for angina occurring in the presence of hypertension.

Physiologic Activities of β-Adrenergic Receptors

Organ	Receptor type	Response to stimulus
Heart		
SA node	β1	Increased heart rate
Atria	β1	Increased contractility and conduction velocity
AV node	β1	Increased contractility and conduction velocity
His-Purkinje system	β1	Increased contractility and conduction velocity
Ventricles	β1	Increased automaticity, contractility, and conduction velocity
Arteries		
Peripheral	β2	Dilation
Coronary	β2	Dilation
Carotid	β2	Dilation
Other	β1	Increased insulin release
		Increased liver and muscle glycogenolysis
Lungs	β2	Dilation of bronchi
Uterus	β2	Smooth muscle relaxation

AV—atrioventricular; SA—sinoatrial.

A

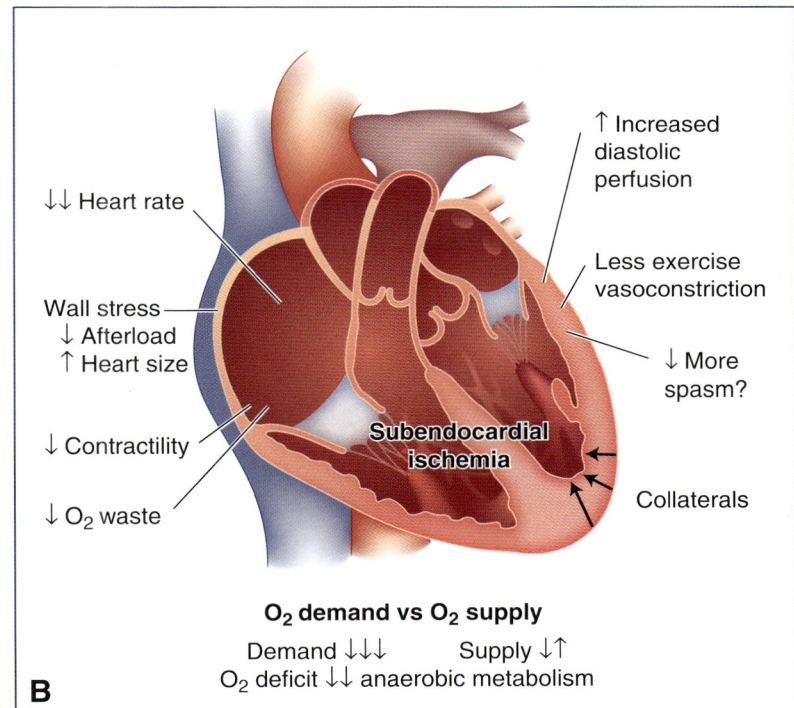

↑ Increased diastolic perfusion

↓↓ Heart rate

Less exercise vasoconstriction

Wall stress
↓ Afterload
↑ Heart size

↓ More spasm?

↓ Contractility

Subendocardial ischemia

Collaterals

↓ O₂ waste

O₂ demand vs O₂ supply
Demand ↓↓↓   Supply ↓↑
O₂ deficit ↓↓ anaerobic metabolism

B

Figure 3-26. Actions of β-blockers. β-Blockers have a number of important effects in patients with chronic ischemic heart disease. β-Blockers are effective antianginals, antihypertensives, and antiarrhythmics, and they reduce mortality in patients after myocardial infarction and in patients with heart failure.

A, β-Blockers competitively inhibit the effects of neuronally released and circulating catecholamines on β-adrenergic receptors. By this mechanism, β-blockers reduce myocardial oxygen requirements, primarily by slowing the heart rate. In addition, these drugs reduce blood pressure and limit exercise-induced increases in contractility. Thus, β-blockers reduce myocardial oxygen demand primarily during activity or excitement, when surges of increased sympathetic activity occur. (*Adapted from* Beller [19].)

B, β-Blocker administration has a beneficial effect on ischemic myocardium unless 1) the preload rises substantially as in left-sided heart failure or 2) vasospastic angina is present, in which case spasm may be promoted in some patients. (*Adapted from* Morrow and Gersh [4].)

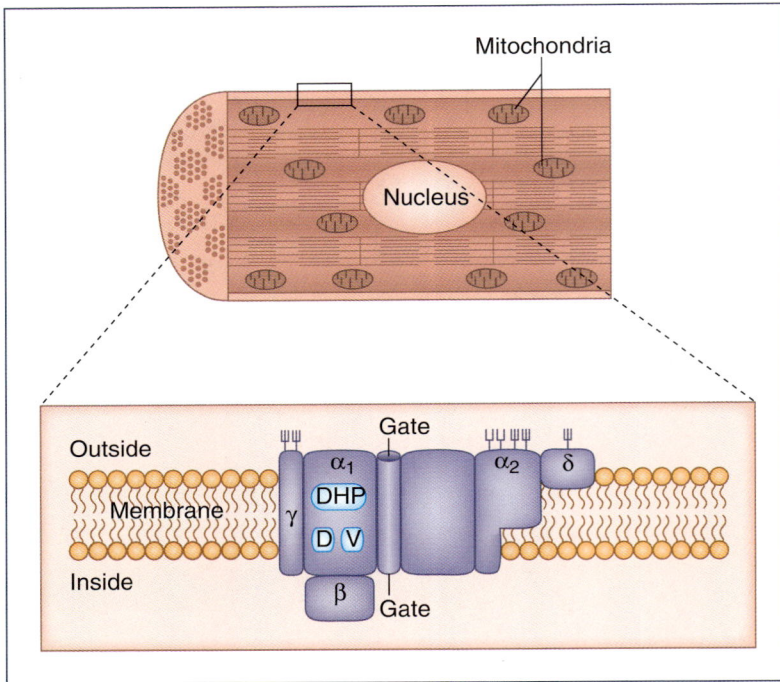

Figure 3-27. Mechanism of action of calcium channel blockers. Calcium antagonists inhibit calcium ion movement by noncompetitive blockade of voltage-sensitive L-type calcium channels in cardiac and smooth muscle membranes. The three major classes of calcium antagonists have different binding sites within the calcium channel. These classes include the dihydropyridines (nifedipine is the prototype), the phenylalkylamines (verapamil is the prototype), and the modified benzothiazepines (diltiazem is the prototype). Phenylalkylamines slow recovery of the calcium channel and thereby exert depressant effects on cardiac pacemakers and conduction, whereas dihydropyridines, which do not impair channel recovery, have little effect on the conduction system. Each relaxes vascular smooth muscle in both the systemic arterial and coronary arterial beds. The efficacy of calcium antagonists for treating angina is related to the reduction in myocardial oxygen demand and the increase in oxygen supply that they induce. The blockade of the entry of calcium into myocytes results in a negative inotropic effect, which must be taken into consideration in patients with significant left ventricular dysfunction. D—diltiazem; DHP—dihydropyridine; V—verapamil.

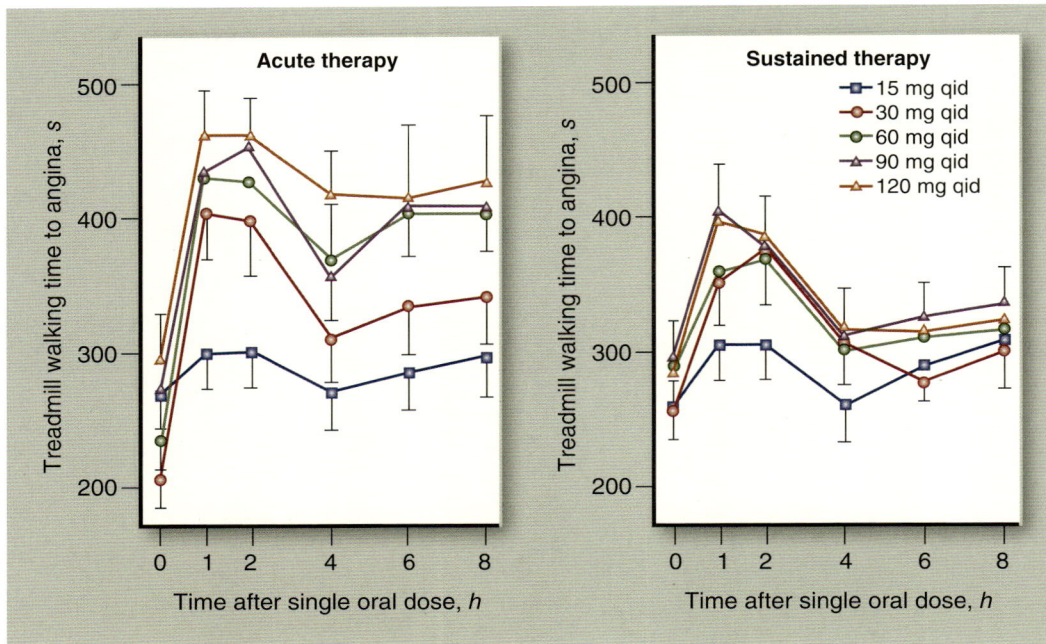

Figure 3-28. Nitrate tolerance. This study of nitrate tolerance in patients with angina is typical of numerous clinical trials in the literature. This study was a pivotal investigation documenting the appearance of tolerance with various doses of oral isosorbide dinitrate. In this placebo-controlled, double-blind study, dosing with 15 mg or more of isosorbide four times daily (qid) for 1 to 2 weeks resulted in decreased duration of nitrate efficacy as well as a loss of the dose-response relationship. There is now evidence that the mechanism of tolerance may relate to inhibition of mitochondrial aldehyde dehydrogenase, an enzyme that contributes to the biotransformation of nitroglycerin. To minimize nitrate tolerance, a dosage schedule that allows a 10- to 12-hour nitrate-free interval should be adopted [20].

Newer Antianginal Pharmacotherapy

Agent	Effect on heart rate or blood pressure	Proposed mechanism of action
Fasudil	Reduces afterload	Relaxes smooth muscle cells via inhibition of Rho-kinase
Ivabradine	Reduces heart rate	Reduces sinoatrial node activity via inhibition of I_f ion channel
Nicorandil	Reduces afterload and preload	Promotes peripheral and coronary vasodilation via nitrate-like effects and interaction with ATP-sensitive potassium channel
Ranolazine	No meaningful effect	Decreases intracellular sodium and calcium overload by inhibiting the late sodium current
Trimetazidine	No meaningful effect	Improved myocardial metabolism via partial inhibition of fatty acid oxidase

ATP—adenosine triphosphate.

A

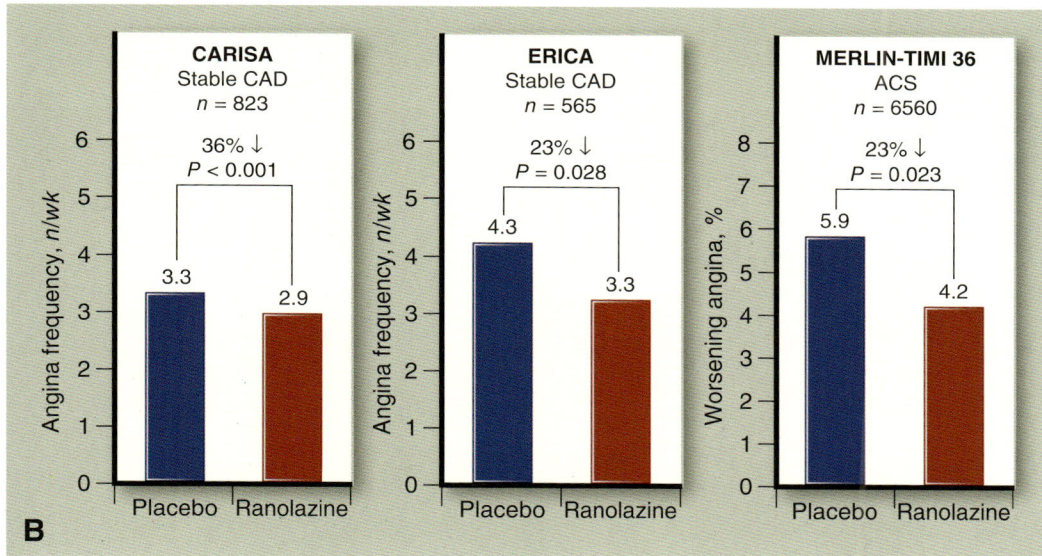

B

Figure 3-29. A, Newer anti-anginal pharmacotherapy. Several newer antianginal agents have either been approved, or remain under active investigation for the treatment of chronic angina. Among these agents, some share mechanisms of action with traditional antianginals, such as decreasing myocardial demand via reducing heart rate, contractility, or afterload. However, they do so by mechanisms that differ from those for traditional agents. Of the listed agents, at the time of this writing, only ranolazine is available for clinical use in the United States. Each has been shown to have antianginal effects. For example, in 939 patients with chronic angina, ivabradine proved comparable to atenolol, 100 mg, with respect to exercise performance on treadmill testing, and both agents equally reduced ischemic episodes and sublingual nitroglycerin consumption. Similarly, nicorandil was evaluated in a trial of 5126 patients with stable angina and found to reduce cardiovascular death, myocardial infarction, and hospitalization for angina (13.1% vs 15.5%; $P = 0.014$). **B,** Ranolazine has been studied in randomized trials of patients with established coronary artery disease (CAD) and found to reduce angina and ischemia. Ranolazine achieves these antianginal effects without a clinically important effect on heart rate or blood pressure. ACS—acute coronary syndrome.

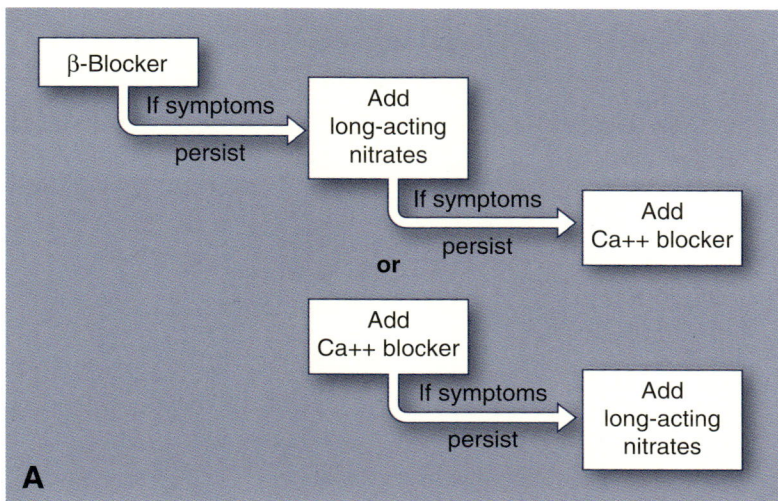

A

Figure 3-30. Selection of antianginal pharmacotherapy. β-Blockers, calcium antagonists, nitrates, and ranolazine can ameliorate angina. Because β-blockers improve survival after acute myocardial infarction, it is reasonable to consider a β-blocker as the initial agent in most patients. **A,** The majority of patients will require more than one antianginal agent, which may be added in a staged approach [21].

Continued on the next page

Selection of Antianginal Pharmacotherapy

Agent	Favors use	Relative or absolute contraindications to use
β-Blockers	Post–myocardial infarction	Severe bradycardia
	Chronic heart failure	Significant AV block
	Sinus tachycardia	Severe depression
	Tachyarrhythmia	Raynaud's phenomenon
	Systemic hypertension	Poorly controlled diabetes
	Hyperthyroidism	Symptomatic peripheral artery disease
	Pre-existing headaches	Severe reactive airway disease
		Decompensated heart failure
		Low blood pressure
Calcium antagonist (dihydropyridine)	Systemic hypertension	Low blood pressure
	Raynaud's phenomenon	
	Prinzmetal's angina	
	Severe bradycardia or atrioventricular block	
Calcium antagonist (verapamil or diltiazem)	Systemic hypertension	Severe bradycardia
	Supraventricular tachycardia	Significant AV block
		Left ventricular dysfunction or heart failure
		Low blood pressure
Nitrates	Left ventricular dysfunction or heart failure	Severe aortic stenosis
		Relative hypotension
		Phosphodiesterase type 5 inhibitor use
Ranolazine	Bradycardia or atrioventricular block	End-stage renal disease
	Low blood pressure	QT prolongation or treatment with QT-prolonging agents
	Left ventricular dysfunction limiting other antianginal therapy	Moderate or severe hepatic dysfunction
	Diabetes mellitus*	
	Tachyarrhythmia*	

*Emerging evidence.

B

Figure 3-30. *(Continued)* **B,** In some cases, clinical factors may influence the selection of agents other than a β-blocker as initial therapy. For example, a dihydropyridine calcium antagonist may be the agent of choice in patients with significant atrioventricular conduction disturbances. Calcium channel blockers are also preferred in patients with angina due to coronary vasospasm, and may be better tolerated in patients with symptomatic peripheral arterial disease. Other relative contraindications to the use of β-blockers include significant depression, sexual dysfunction, or sleep disturbance. The clinical experience with ranolazine is more limited than with the traditional antianginal agents. However, because it does not lower blood pressure or heart rate, ranolazine is an alternative for patients with conduction disease or blood pressure that limits use of traditional antianginals. Moreover, emerging evidence suggests potential antiarrhythmic properties and a favorable influence on hemoglobin A1c. AV—atrioventricular.

Nonpharmacologic Options

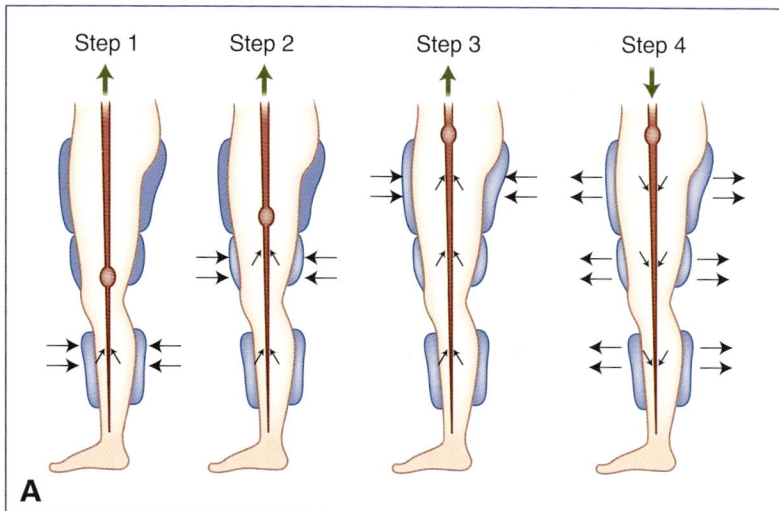

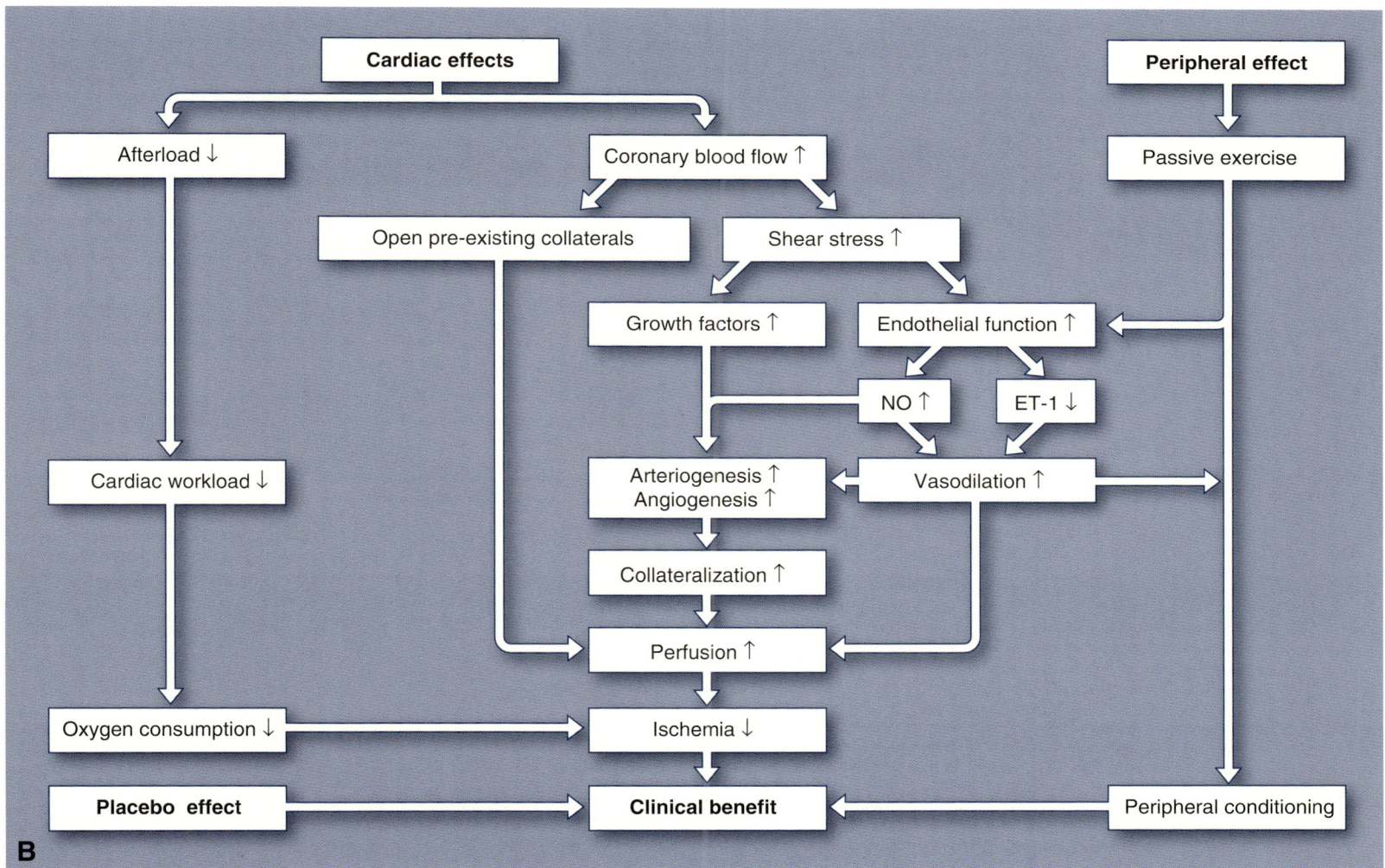

Figure 3-31. Enhanced external counterpulsation (EECP) is an effective treatment for patients with coronary artery disease and angina refractory to conventional medical therapy when revascularization is not an option. **A,** EECP involves the use of three paired inflatable cuffs wrapped around the patient's lower extremities. The cuffs are sequentially inflated during diastole: the calves followed by lower thighs and followed by upper thighs and buttocks. The pressure is released at the onset of systole. The sequential cuff compression enhances venous return and significantly augments diastolic pressure. **B,** Acute afterload reduction decreases myocardial demand. By increasing coronary blood flow, EECP may promote myocardial collateralization. Increased blood flow and shear stress also may improve coronary endothelial function. In addition to a peripheral training effect, a minor placebo effect has been suggested to contribute to the symptomatic benefit of EECP. Data from observational studies and clinical trials suggest that 70% to 80% of patients will experience a sustained improvement in angina with EECP. ET-1—endothelin-1; NO—nitric oxide. (*Adapted from* Manchanda and Soran [22].)

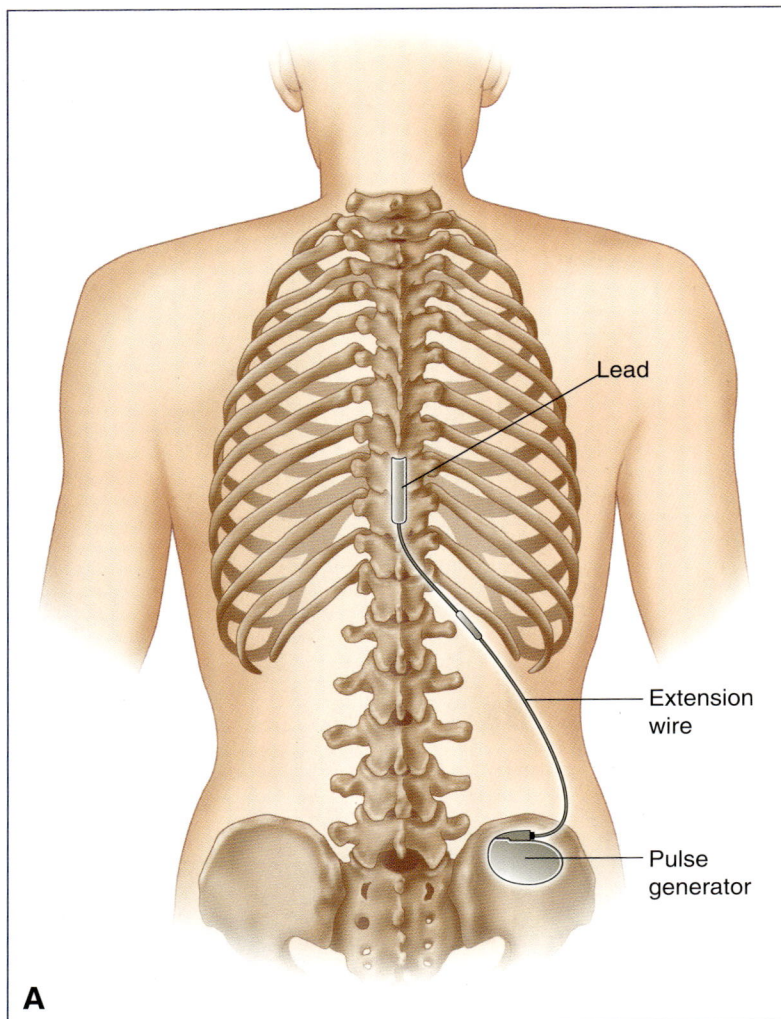

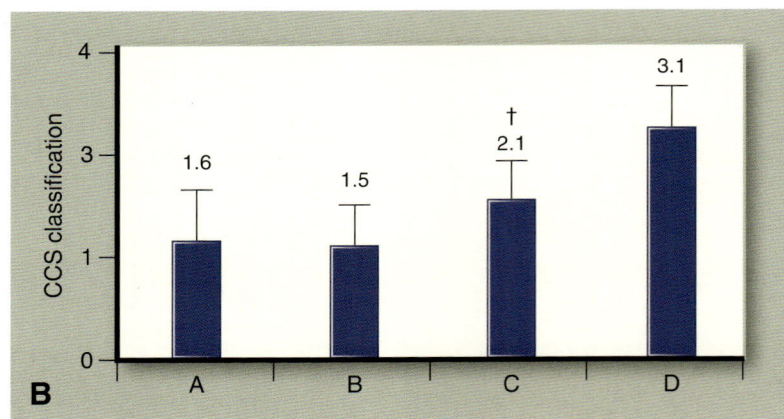

Figure 3-32. Spinal cord stimulation. Spinal cord stimulation is an option for patients with refractory angina who are not candidates for coronary revascularization. **A,** A specially designed electrode is inserted into the epidural space. Stimulation of axons in the spinal cord that do not transmit pain to the brain can reduce input to the brain from pain-transmitting axons (gate theory). Several observational studies have reported that up to 80% of patients experience a reduction in the frequency and severity of angina. **B,** In a small randomized study of differing stimulation patterns (*A*—conventional periodic; *B*—conventional continuous; *C*—reduced periodic; *D*—low output "placebo") among 12 patients with spinal cord stimulators, angina graded using the Canadian Cardiovascular Society (CCS) classification (*see* Fig. 3-6) was significantly reduced with active compared with "placebo" stimulation [23]. In a randomized trial of spinal cord simulation compared with coronary artery bypass grafting in patients with angina and coronary artery disease not amenable to percutaneous coronary intervention, spinal cord stimulation was associated with similar symptom relief and long-term quality of life compared with surgery. Large, randomized, placebo-controlled trials have not been conducted. This approach should be reserved for patients in whom other treatment options have been exhausted.

Coronary Revascularization

American College of Cardiology/American Heart Association Recommendations for Coronary Angiography in Patients With Suspected Stable Angina

For diagnosis

Class I

Patients with known or possible angina pectoris who have survived sudden cardiac death. (Level of Evidence: B)

Class II

1. Patients with an uncertain diagnosis after noninvasive testing in whom the benefit of a more certain diagnosis outweighs the risk and cost of coronary angiography. (Level of Evidence: C)

2. Patients who cannot undergo noninvasive testing because of disability, illness, or morbid obesity. (Level of Evidence: C)

3. Patients with an occupational requirement for a definitive diagnosis. (Level of Evidence: C)

4. Patients who by virtue of young age at onset of symptoms, noninvasive imaging, or other clinical parameters are suspected of having a nonatherosclerotic cause for myocardial ischemia. (Level of Evidence: C)

5. Patients in whom coronary artery spasm is suspected and provocative testing may be necessary. (Level of Evidence: C)

6. Patients with a high pretest probability of left main or three-vessel coronary artery disease (CAD). (Level of Evidence: C)

Class IIb

1. Patients with recurrent hospitalization for chest pain in whom a definite diagnosis is judged necessary. (Level of Evidence: C)

2. Patients with an overriding desire for a definitive diagnosis and a greater-than-low probability of CAD. (Level of Evidence: C)

Class III

1. Patients with significant comorbidity in whom the risk of coronary arteriography outweighs the benefit of the procedure. (Level of Evidence: C)

2. Patients with an overriding personal desire for a definitive diagnosis and a low probability of CAD. (Level of Evidence: C)

For risk stratification and guiding revascularization

Class I

1. Patients with disabling (Canadian Cardiovascular Society [CCS] classes III and IV) chronic stable angina despite medical therapy. (Level of Evidence: B)

2. Patients with high-risk criteria on noninvasive testing regardless of anginal severity. (Level of Evidence: B)

3. Patients with angina who have survived sudden cardiac death or serious ventricular arrhythmia. (Level of Evidence: B)

4. Patients with angina and symptoms and signs of congestive heart failure. (Level of Evidence: C)

5. Patients with clinical characteristics that indicate a high likelihood of severe CAD. (Level of Evidence: C)

Class IIa

1. Patients with significant left ventricular (LV) dysfunction (ejection fraction less than 45%), CCS class I or II angina, and demonstrable ischemia but less than high-risk criteria on noninvasive testing. (Level of Evidence: C)

2. Patients with inadequate prognostic information after noninvasive testing. (Level of Evidence: C)

Class IIb

1. Patients with CCS class I or II angina, preserved LV function (ejection fraction greater than 45%), and less than high-risk criteria on noninvasive testing. (Level of Evidence: C)

2. Patients with CCS class III or IV angina, which with medical therapy improves to class I or II. (Level of Evidence: C)

3. Patients with CCS class I or II angina but intolerance (unacceptable side effects) to adequate medical therapy. (Level of Evidence: C)

Class III

1. Patients with CCS class I or II angina who respond to medical therapy and who have no evidence of ischemia on noninvasive testing. (Level of Evidence: C)

2. Patients who prefer to avoid revascularization. (Level of Evidence: C)

Figure 3-33. Selection of patients for coronary angiography. Selection of coronary angiography as the initial diagnostic test for stable angina is rarely indicated. Coronary angiography, with a view toward coronary revascularization, is indicated in patients with refractory symptoms or ischemia despite optimal medical therapy, in patients with "high-risk" noninvasive test results who may derive a survival benefit from revascularization, and in those with occupations or lifestyles that require a more aggressive approach [21].

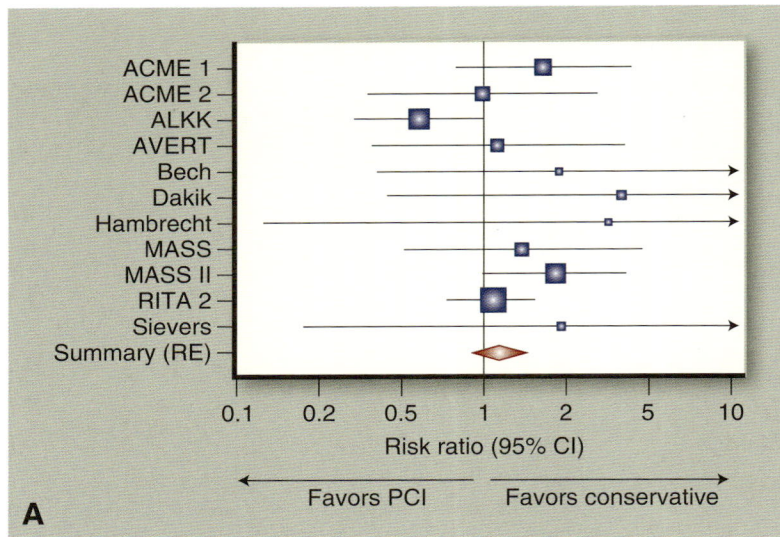

A

Favors PCI ← → Favors conservative

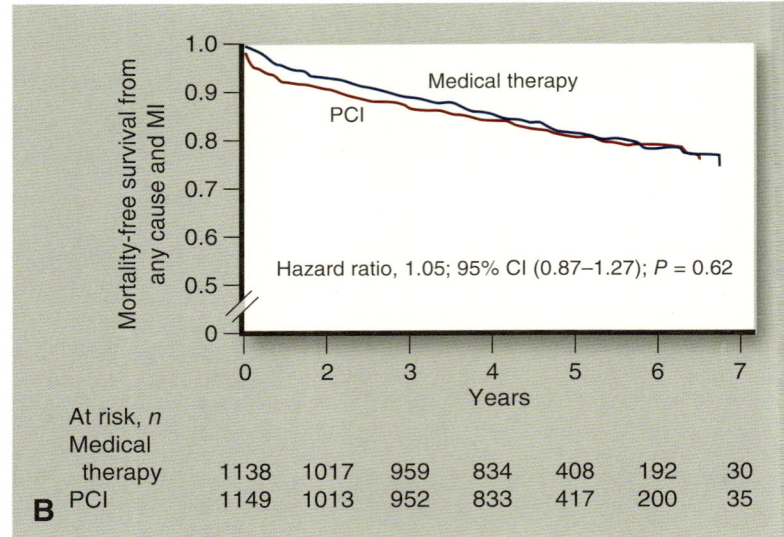

Hazard ratio, 1.05; 95% CI (0.87–1.27); P = 0.62

At risk, n							
Medical therapy	1138	1017	959	834	408	192	30
B PCI	1149	1013	952	833	417	200	35

Figure 3-34. Randomized trials of percutaneous coronary intervention (PCI) versus medical therapy. Randomized clinical trials comparing PCI to medical therapy in patients with stable angina are few in number and have involved fewer than 5000 patients (total). The majority of these trials were completed before routine use of coronary stenting and contemporary preventive medical therapy, and recruited patients predominantly with single-vessel disease.

A, In aggregate, the results of trials completed before 2005 indicated superior control of angina, improved exercise capacity, and improved quality of life, but showed no reduction of death or myocardial infarction

(MI) with PCI compared with medical therapy. (*Adapted from* Katritsis and Laonnidis [24].)

B, The Clinical Outcomes Utilizing Revascularization and Aggressive drug Evaluation (COURAGE) trial tested whether PCI (predominantly with stenting) coupled with optimal medical therapy reduced the risk of death or MI in patients with stable coronary artery disease (CAD) compared with medical therapy alone. The main study finding in 2287 patients with evidence of myocardial ischemia and significant CAD was that, as an initial strategy in patients with stable CAD, PCI did not reduce death, MI, or other major cardiovascular events when added to optimal medical therapy (*From* Boden *et al.* [25].)

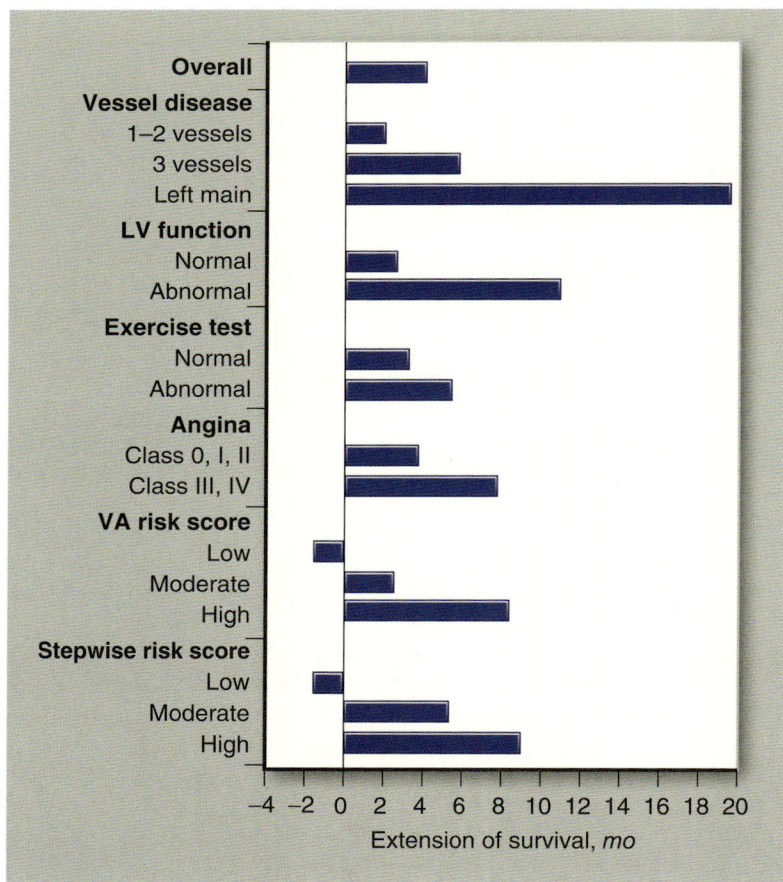

Figure 3-35. Studies of medical therapy versus coronary artery bypass grafting (CABG). Although now outdated, several randomized trials started in the 1970s and 1980s comparing CABG versus medical therapy remain informative with respect to the potential for revascularization to prolong survival in some groups of patients. A meta-analysis of these trials involving about 2500 patients showed a 25% reduction in mortality at 7 years with CABG as initial therapy, with particular benefit in those patients with left main disease (66% relative risk reduction) and those with three-vessel disease and left ventricular (LV) dysfunction, and a moderate benefit in those with one- or two-vessel disease and proximal left anterior descending coronary artery (LAD) stenosis [8]. VA—Veterans affairs.

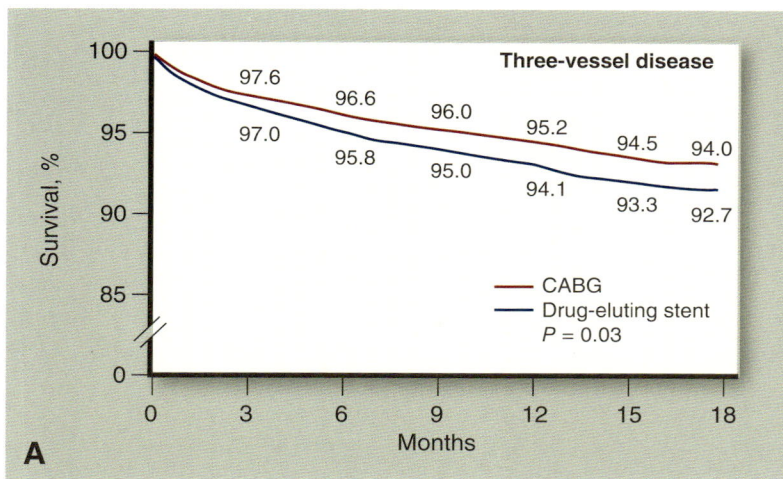

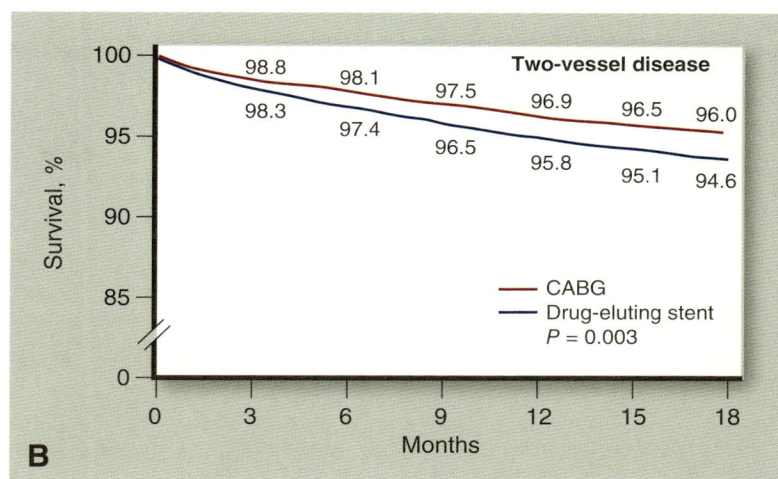

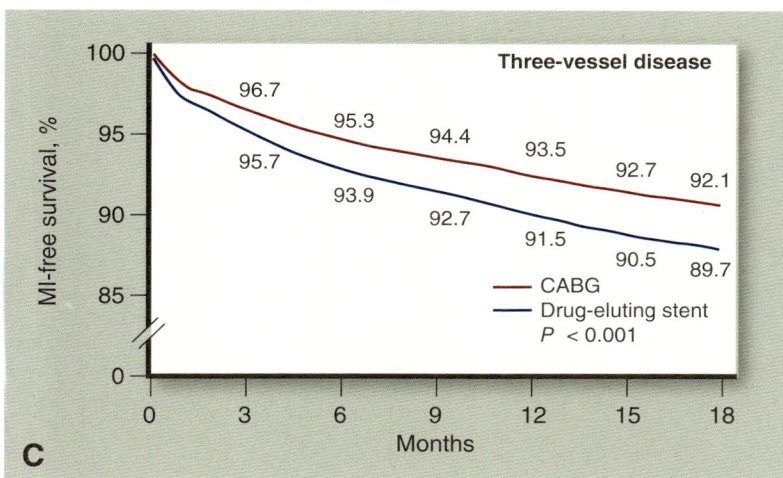

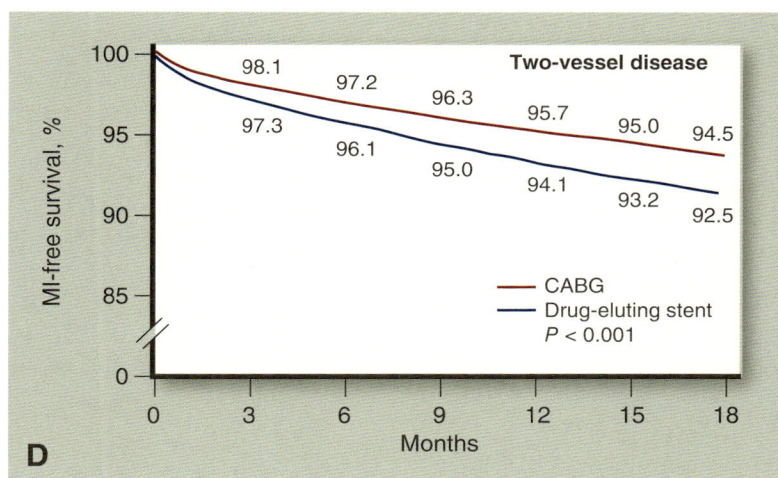

Figure 3-36. Studies of percutaneous coronary intervention (PCI) versus coronary artery bypass grafting (CABG). The results of randomized trials have provided a generally consistent perspective of CABG and PCI in selected patients with multivessel disease. These trials excluded patients with significant left main coronary artery disease and those with impaired left ventricular systolic function. Among patients with preserved ventricular function and multivessel disease amenable to PCI, overall survival rates and rates of myocardial infarction (MI) in individual studies did not differ between PCI and CABG. However, CABG was associated with a greater initial improvement in angina and with a diminished frequency of repeat revascularization procedures compared with PCI. An observational study from the New York State Registry suggested that CABG confers a mortality benefit compared with PCI with drug-eluting stents. **A** through **D** show survival curves adjusted for age; sex; ejection fraction; hemodynamic state; history or no history of MI before the procedure; the presence or absence of cerebrovascular disease, peripheral arterial disease, congestive heart failure, chronic obstructive pulmonary disease, diabetes, and renal failure; and involvement of the proximal left anterior descending artery. (*From* Hannan *et al.* [26].)

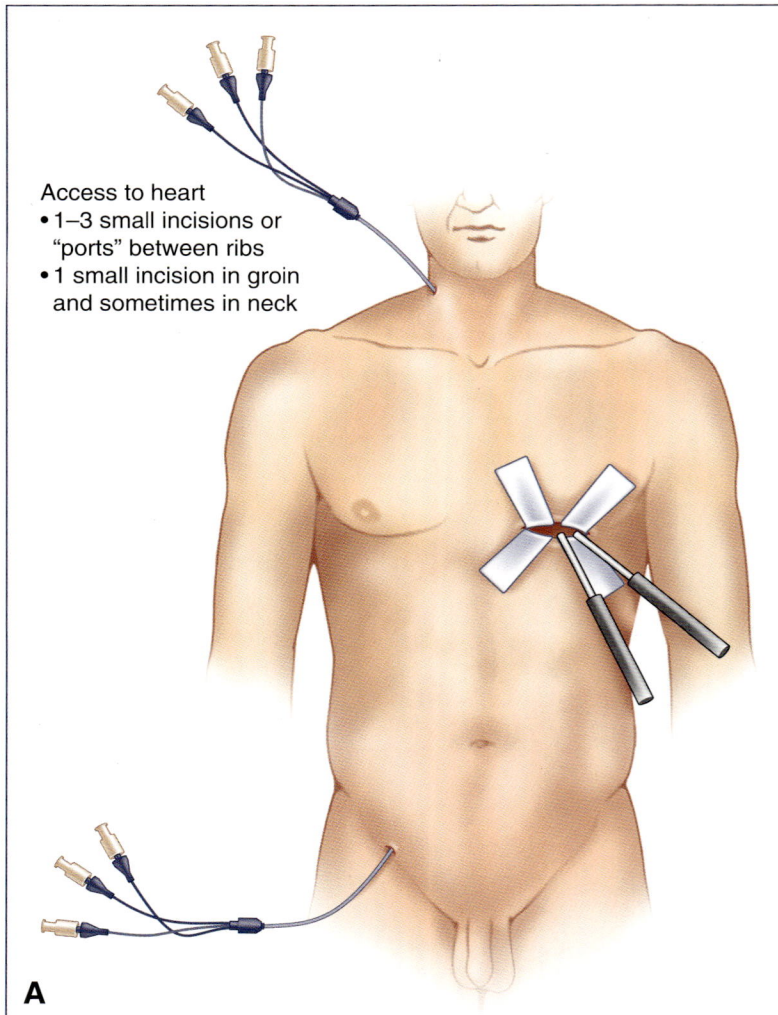

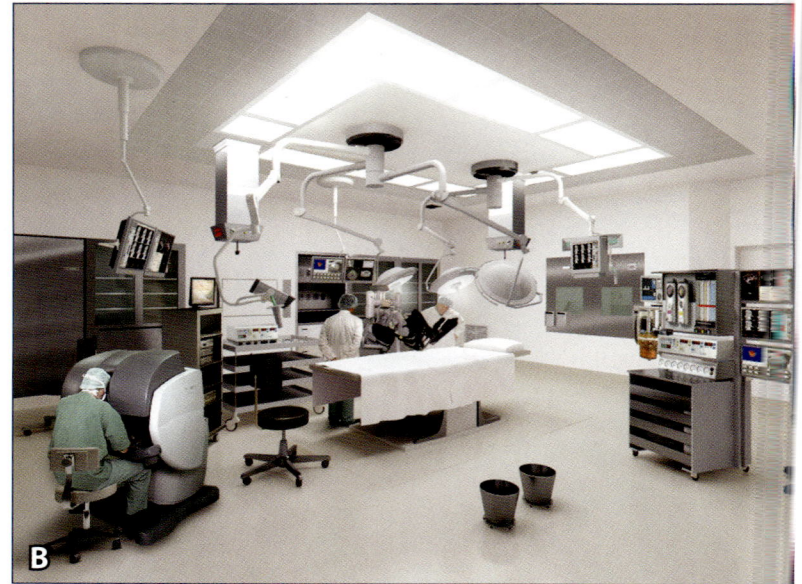

Figure 3-37. Less invasive approaches to coronary artery bypass grafting. Minimally invasive approaches may be divided into four major categories on the basis of the approach and use of cardiopulmonary bypass (CPB). **A,** Port-access coronary artery bypass grafting (CABG) is performed using limited incisions with femoral–femoral CPB and cardioplegic arrest. **B,** Totally endoscopic robotically assisted CABG may be performed on the arrested heart using port-access technology. (*Courtesy of* Dr. Tomislav Mihaljevic, Cleveland, OH.)

Continued on the next page

In illustration A:

Access to heart
- 1–3 small incisions or "ports" between ribs
- 1 small incision in groin and sometimes in neck

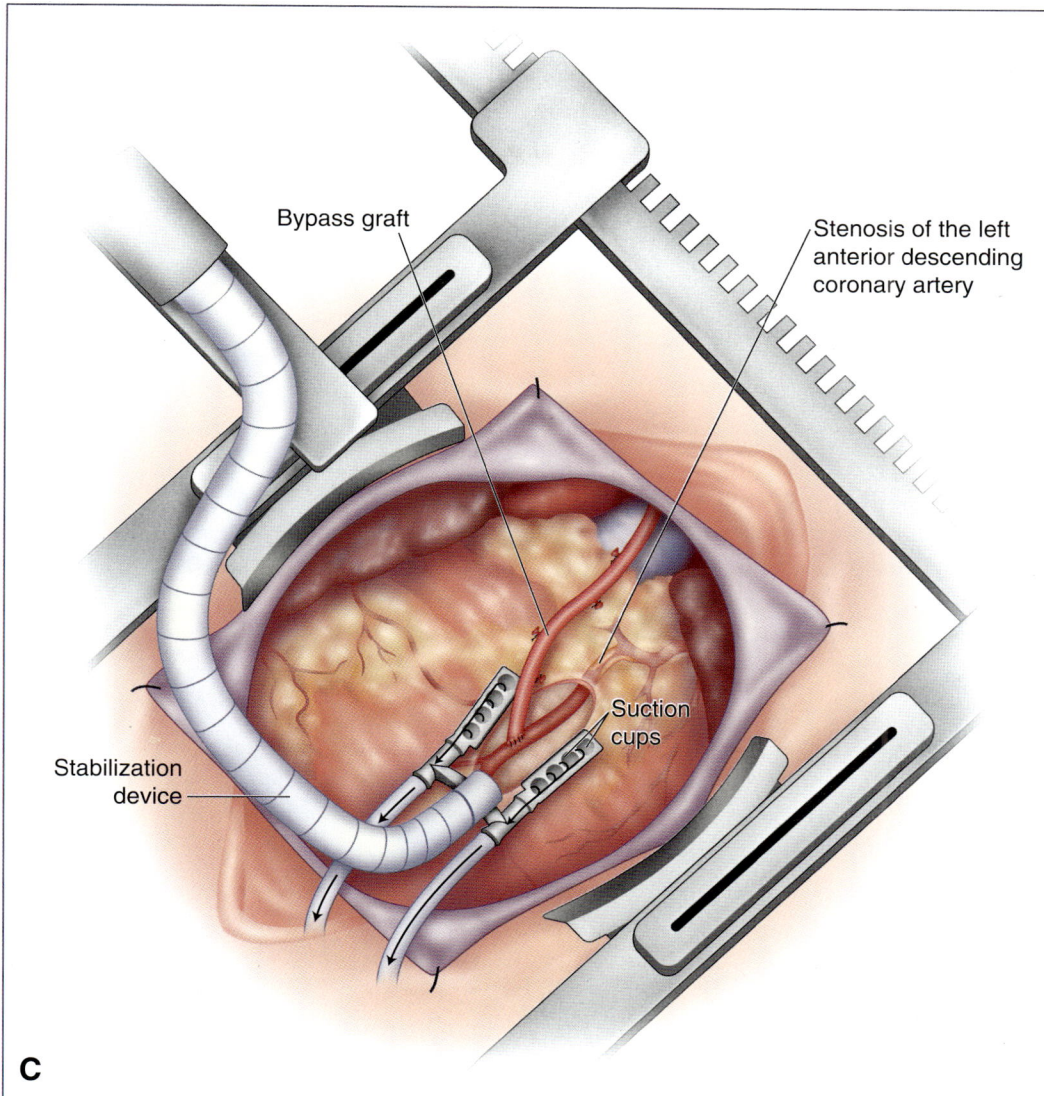

C

Bypass graft

Stenosis of the left
anterior descending
coronary artery

Suction
cups

Stabilization
device

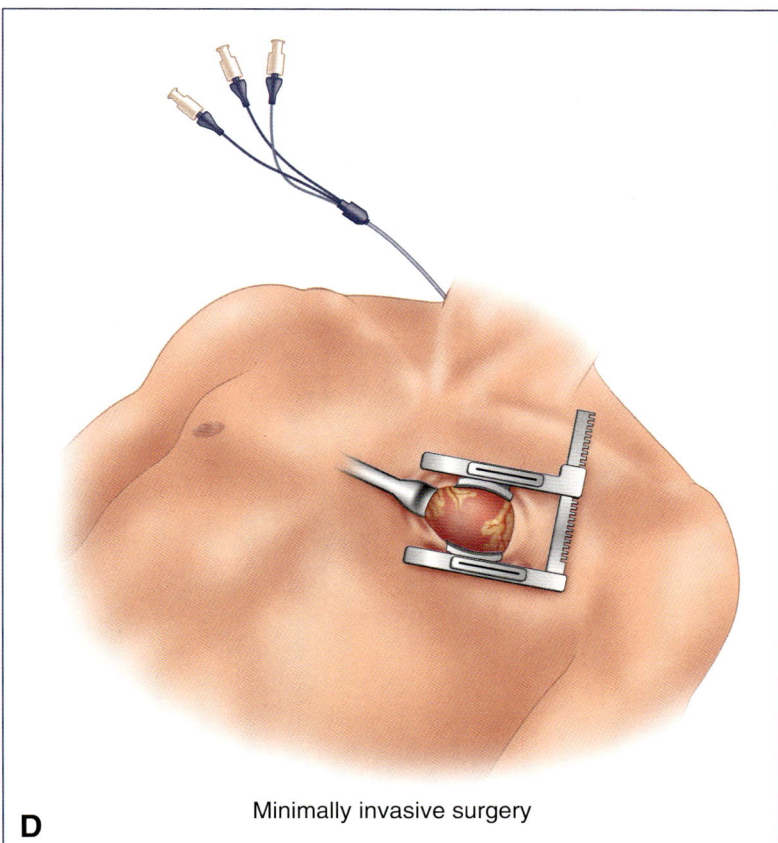

D

Minimally invasive surgery

Figure 3-37. *(Continued)* **C,** Off-pump CABG is performed using a standard sternotomy with stabilization devices to reduce motion of the target vessels, whereas anastomoses are performed without CPB. **D,** Finally, minimally invasive direct coronary artery bypass is performed through a left anterior thoracotomy using smaller incisions without CPB. The potential advantages of these minimally invasive approaches include less postoperative patient discomfort, lower risk of wound infection, and shorter recovery times. The avoidance of CPB may reduce the risk of bleeding, thromboembolism, renal insufficiency, and damaging neurological effects of bypass, particularly in patients with heavy aortic calcification. Newer "hybrid" approaches to coronary revascularization may also include CABG with percutaneous coronary intervention (PCI) by combining a minimally invasive CABG on the left anterior descending artery with PCI on the remaining vessels.

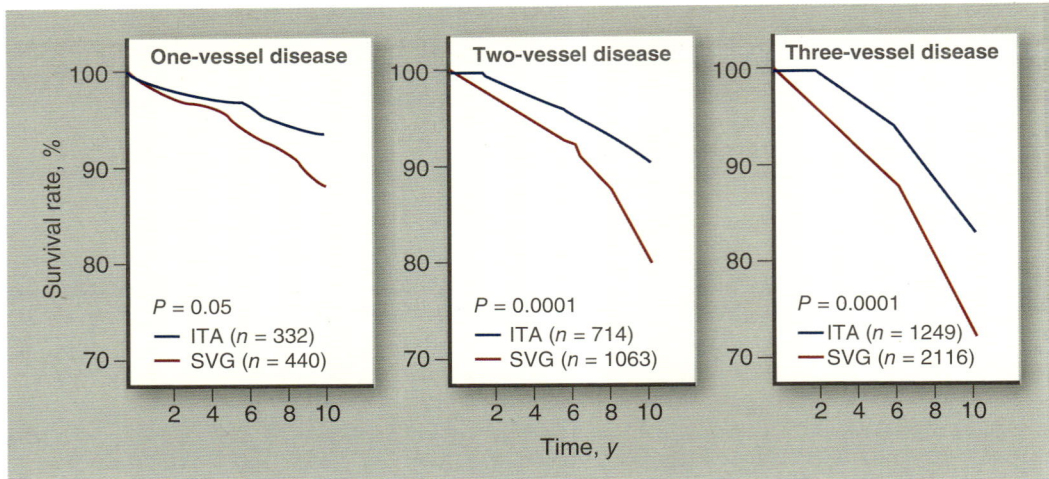

Figure 3-38. Importance of grafting with the internal mammary artery. The relative importance of the type of conduit, regardless of the extent of disease, is apparent through study of disease affecting one, two, or three vessels. All groups demonstrated statistically significant improved survival when an internal thoracic artery (ITA) as opposed to a saphenous vein graft (SVG) was used. (*Adapted from Loop et al.* [27].)

Indications for Revascularization in Patients With Stable Angina

Symptom relief	Persistence of unacceptable angina despite medical therapy
	Unacceptable side effects of medical therapy or patient's desire for fewer medications
Potential for survival benefit	Significant left-main coronary artery disease
	Three-vessel coronary artery disease, particularly with left ventricular dysfunction
	Two-vessel coronary artery disease with left ventricular dysfunction or demonstrable ischemia on noninvasive testing, particularly when there is involvement of the proximal left anterior descending (LAD) coronary artery
	High-risk criteria on noninvasive testing regardless of anginal severity, particularly with large territory of viable myocardium
	Patients with angina who have survived sudden cardiac death or serious ventricular arrhythmia
Other considerations	Restenosis at site of prior percutaneous coronary intervention either associated with a large territory of viable myocardium or high-risk criteria on noninvasive testing.
	Prior coronary artery bypass graft with graft stenosis, particularly if significant stenosis of a graft to the LAD

Figure 3-39. Selection of patients for revascularization. Medical management of chronic ischemic heart disease involves aggressive management of risk factors, treatment of conditions that intensify angina, pharmacologic management of ischemia, and administration of agents shown to be effective for secondary prevention. When an unaccept-able level of angina persists despite appropriate medical management, or when treatment is limited by side effects, and/or when the patient manifests high-risk features on clinical evaluation, the coronary anatomy should be defined to enable consideration of revascularization. (*Adapted from Gibbons et al.* [8].)

Figure 3-40. Selection of the approach to revascularization (percutaneous coronary intervention [PCI] versus coronary artery bypass grafting [CABG]). Both PCI and CABG offer effective approaches to coronary revascularization. The selection of the approach to revascularization should be made on the basis of integrated consideration of the 1) technical feasibility of each approach, including the achievable completeness of revascularization; 2) specific coronary anatomy and/or associated structural heart disease for which a survival benefit may be present with CABG; 3) history of diabetes mellitus; 4) patient-specific risks associated with each approach; and 5) patient preferences. The survival benefits of CABG are established in patients with left ventricular dysfunction and multivessel disease, and with significant left main coronary artery disease. Patients with chronic stable angina and two-vessel coronary artery disease with significant proxi-

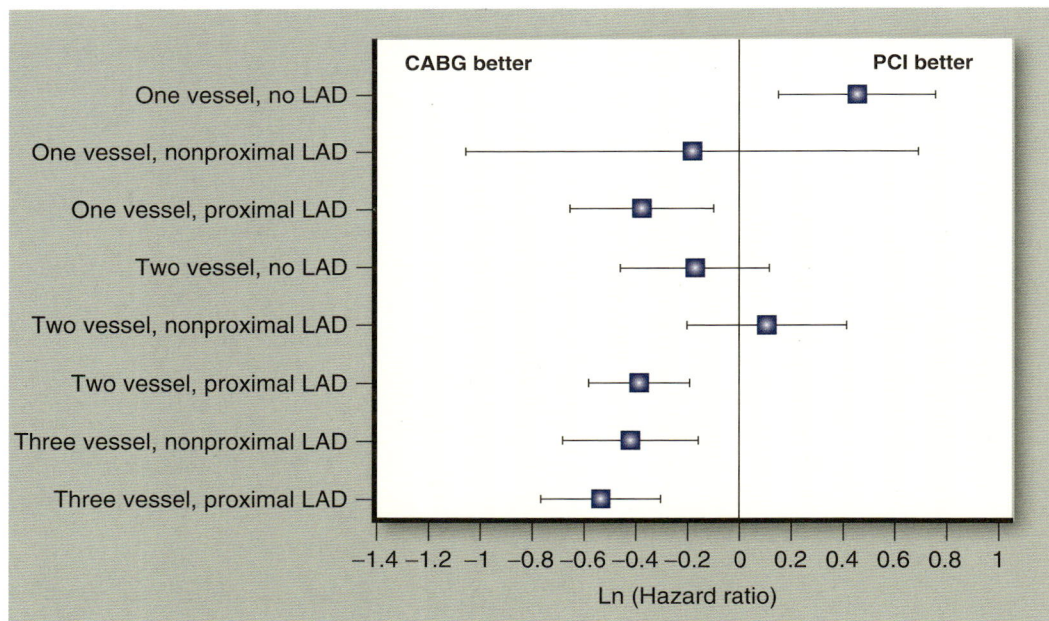

mal disease of the left anterior descending artery and either left ventricular dysfunction, high-risk findings on noninvasive testing, or diabetes mellitus should also be considered for CABG. In patients with single-vessel disease, the primary objective is relief of significant symptoms and PCI is usually the preferred approach to revascularization when indicated and techni-cally feasible. These anatomic considerations are supported by an analysis of approximately 60,000 patients in the New York State registry treated with CABG or angioplasty. Ln—natural log. (*Adapted from Hannan et al.* [28].)

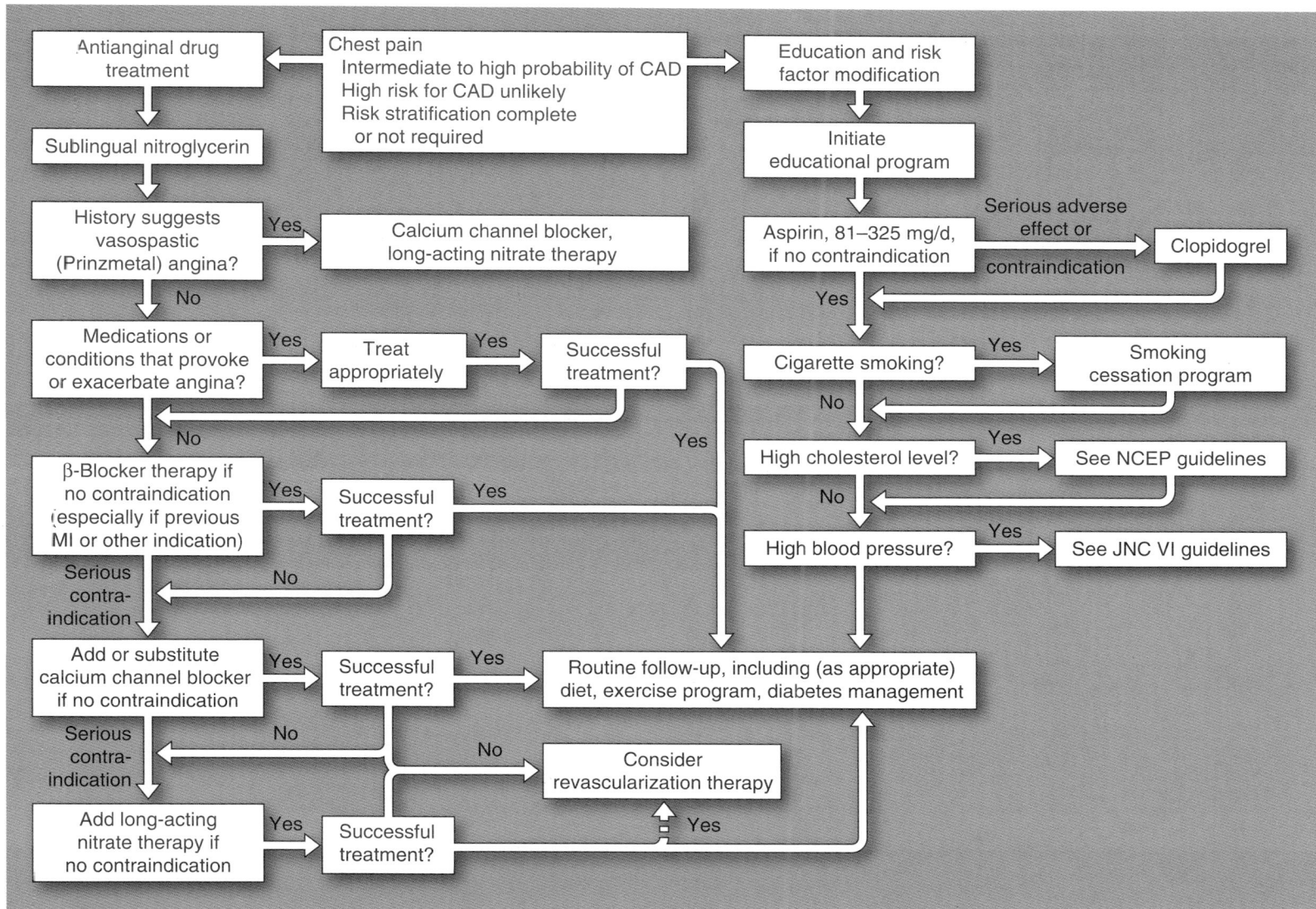

Figure 3-41. American College of Cardiology/American Heart Association guidelines for management of chronic coronary disease. Guidelines for the management of patients with chronic stable coronary artery disease (CAD) are shown in this diagram. The essentials of antianginal pharmacologic therapy include β-blockers, calcium antagonists, and nitrates. β-Blockers are particularly indicated in patients with previous myocardial infarction (MI). Contraindications to β-blockers are severe bradycardia, advanced atrial ventricular block, sick sinus syndrome with bradyarrhythmias, severe bronchospasm, and perhaps severe depression or severe peripheral vascular disease. Patients intolerant of β-blockers can be treated with a heart rate–lowering calcium channel blocker. Long-acting nitrates are also effective in reducing episodes of angina. Antianginal agents should be used in conjunction with risk factor–modifying pharmacotherapy and lifestyle interventions. Invasive evaluation with a view toward revascularization is recommended for patients with refractory symptoms, those with high-risk noninvasive findings consistent with extensive ischemia, and those patients with noninvasive or invasive findings indicating left main disease or proximal three-vessel disease or two-vessel disease, including a high-grade stenosis of the proximal left anterior descending coronary artery. JNC—Joint National Committee on Prevention, Detection, Evaluation, and Treatment of High Blood Pressure; NCEP—National Cholesterol Education Program. (*Adapted* from Gibbons *et al.* [8].)

References

1. Widlansky ME, Gokce N, Keaney JF Jr, Vita JA: The clinical implications of endothelial dysfunction. *J Am Coll Cardiol* 2003, 42:1149–1160.

2. Libby P, Ridker PM, Maseri A: Inflammation and atherosclerosis. *Circulation* 2002, 105:1135–1143.

3. Epstein SE, Talbot TL: Dynamic coronary tone in precipitation, exacerbation and relief of angina pectoris. *Am J Cardiol* 1981, 48:797–803.

4. Morrow DA, Gersh BJ: Chronic coronary artery disease. In *Braunwald's Heart Disease*, edn 8. Edited by Libby P, Bonow RO, Mann DL, Zipes D. Philadelphia: WB Saunders; 2008.

5. Braunwald E: The history. In *Braunwald's Heart Disease*, edn 7. Edited by Zipes D, Libby P, Bonow RO, Braunwald E. Philadelphia: WB Saunders; 2005.

6. American Heart Association: Heart Disease and Stroke Statistics—2008 Update. Dallas: American Heart Association; 2008.

7. Steg PG, Bhatt DL, Wilson PW, *et al.*: One-year cardiovascular event rates in outpatients with atherothrombosis. *JAMA* 2007, 297:1197–1206.

8. Gibbons RJ, Balady GJ, Bricker JT, *et al.*: ACC/AHA 2002 guideline update for exercise testing: summary article: a report of the American College of Cardiology/American Heart Association Task Force on Practice Guidelines (Committee to Update the 1997 Exercise Testing Guidelines). *Circulation* 2002, 106:1883–1892.

9. Chaitman B: Exercise stress testing. In *Braunwald's Heart Disease*, edn 8. Edited by Libby P, Bonow RO, Mann DL, Zipes D. Philadelphia: WB Saunders; 2008.

10. Kligfield P, Lauer MS: Exercise electrocardiogram testing: beyond the ST segment. *Circulation* 2006, 114:2070–2082.

11. Yao SS, Qureshi E, Sherrid MV, Chaudhry FA: Practical applications in stress echocardiography: risk stratification and prognosis in patients with known or suspected ischemic heart disease. *J Am Coll Cardiol* 2003, 42:1084–1090.

12. Di Carli MF, Hachamovitch R: New technology for noninvasive evaluation of coronary artery disease. *Circulation* 2007, 115:1464–1480.

13. Wu HD, Kwong RY: Cardiac magnetic resonance imaging in patients with coronary disease. *Curr Treat Options Cardiovasc Med* 2008, 10:83–92.

14. Smith SC Jr, Allen J, Blair SN, *et al.*: AHA/ACC guidelines for secondary prevention for patients with coronary and other atherosclerotic vascular disease: 2006 update: endorsed by the National Heart, Lung, and Blood Institute. *Circulation* 2006, 113:2363–2372.

15. Antithrombotic Trialists' Collaboration: Collaborative meta-analysis of randomised trials of antiplatelet therapy for prevention of death, myocardial infarction, and stroke in high risk patients. *BMJ* 2002, 324:71–86.

16. Peters RJ, Mehta SR, Fox KA, *et al.*: Effects of aspirin dose when used alone or in combination with clopidogrel in patients with acute coronary syndromes: observations from the Clopidogrel in Unstable angina to prevent Recurrent Events (CURE) study. *Circulation* 2003, 108:1682–1687.

17. Heart Protection Study Collaborative Group: MRC/BHF Heart Protection Study of cholesterol lowering with simvastatin in 20,536 high-risk individuals: a randomised placebo-controlled trial. *Lancet* 2002, 360:7–22.

18. Cannon CP, Steinberg BA, Murphy SA, *et al.*: Meta-analysis of cardiovascular outcomes trials comparing intensive versus moderate statin therapy. *J Am Coll Cardiol* 2006, 48:438–445.

19. Beller: *Atlas of Heart Disease*, vol 5. Philadelphia: WB Saunders; 1995:7.

20. Gori T, Parker JD: Long-term therapy with organic nitrates: the pros and cons of nitric oxide replacement therapy. *J Am Coll Cardiol* 2004, 44:632–634.

21. Gibbons RJ, Abrams J, Chatterjee K, *et al.*: ACC/AHA 2002 guideline update for the management of patients with chronic stable angina—summary article: a report of the American College of Cardiology/American Heart Association Task Force on practice guidelines (Committee on the Management of Patients With Chronic Stable Angina). *J Am Coll Cardiol* 2003, 41:159–168.

22. Manchanda A, Soran O: Enhanced external counterpulsation and future directions: step beyond medical management for patients with angina and heart failure. *J Am Coll Cardiol* 2007, 50:1523–1531.

23. Eddicks S, Maier-Hauff K, Schenk M, *et al.*: Thoracic spinal cord stimulation improves functional status and relieves symptoms in patients with refractory angina pectoris: the first placebo-controlled randomised study. *Heart* 2007 93:585–590.

24. Katritsis DG, Ioannidis JP: Percutaneous coronary intervention versus conservative therapy in nonacute coronary artery disease: a meta-analysis. *Circulation* 2005, 111:2906–2912.

25. Boden WE, O'Rourke RA, Teo KK, *et al.*: Optimal medical therapy with or without PCI for stable coronary disease. *N Engl J Med* 2007, 356:1503–1516.

26. Hannan EL, Wu C, Walford G, *et al.*: Drug-eluting stents vs. coronary-artery bypass grafting in multivessel coronary disease. *N Engl J Med* 2008, 358:331–341.

27. Loop FD, Lytle BW, Cosgrove DM, *et al.*: Influence of the internal-mammary-artery graft on 10-year survival and other cardiac events. *N Engl J Med* 1986, 314:1–6.

28. Hannan EL, Racz MJ, McCallister BD, *et al.*: A comparison of three-year survival after coronary artery bypass graft surgery and percutaneous transluminal coronary angioplasty. *J Am Coll Cardiol* 1999, 33:63–72.

Vascular Disease

4

Mark A. Creager

Vascular diseases are among the most frequent problems encountered by the cardiovascular specialist. Atherosclerotic vascular disease is a systemic disorder with regional manifestations in the heart, brain, limbs, and kidneys. Diseases of the aorta, including aortic dissection and aortic aneurysms, have life-threatening consequences unless recognized and properly treated. Advances in vascular imaging, therapeutics, and intervention have provided cardiovascular physicians with important tools to diagnose and treat patients with vascular diseases. The images in this chapter highlight the clinical evaluation, medical treatment, and interventional strategies that are used to manage peripheral atherosclerotic vascular diseases, including peripheral artery disease of the lower extremity, renal artery disease, and carotid artery disease, and diseases of the aorta, including aortic dissection and aortic aneurysms. Most of these images have been reproduced from *The Atlas of Vascular Disease*, to which the reader is referred for more extensive review [1]. The authors of the chapters from which these images are derived are gratefully acknowledged.

Peripheral Artery Disease

Peripheral artery disease (PAD) is defined as the presence of a stenosis or occlusion in the aorta or the arteries of the limbs. It is usually caused by atherosclerosis and is associated with an increased risk of death, myocardial infarction, and stroke. Symptoms of PAD include functional limitations characterized by impaired walking ability, intermittent claudication, and rest pain. Necrosis and gangrene may occur in patients with critical limb ischemia. Patients with critical limb ischemia are at risk of limb loss if viability cannot be restored by a revascularization procedure.

The diagnosis of PAD is made by a vascular history and examination. The examination includes palpation of peripheral pulses, auscultation for bruits, and careful inspection of the legs and feet. Noninvasive vascular tests that provide hemodynamic information include the ankle-brachial index (ABI), segmental pressure measurements, and pulse volume recordings. Duplex ultrasonography may localize and quantify arterial stenoses. Magnetic resonance angiography and computed tomographic angiography are useful methods to evaluate the vascular anatomy of patients with PAD. Catheter-based angiographic procedures also provide important diagnostic data, but are usually performed in anticipation of percutaneous or surgical revascularization procedures.

Risk factor modification and antiplatelet therapy should be prescribed to decrease the risk of fatal and non-fatal myocardial infarction, stroke, amputation, and death. Exercise rehabilitation and pharmacotherapy are indicated to improve symptoms of claudication and quality of life. Catheter-based and surgical revascularization procedures are used to improve symptoms in patients with disabling claudication and to relieve rest pain and prevent limb loss in patients with critical limb ischemia. Evidenced-based care of patients with PAD is reviewed in recent guideline and consensus documents [2,3].

Most of the following figures and legends were originally published in the *Atlas of Vascular Disease* in the chapter by Hirsch and Creager entitled, "Peripheral Arterial Disease" [1].

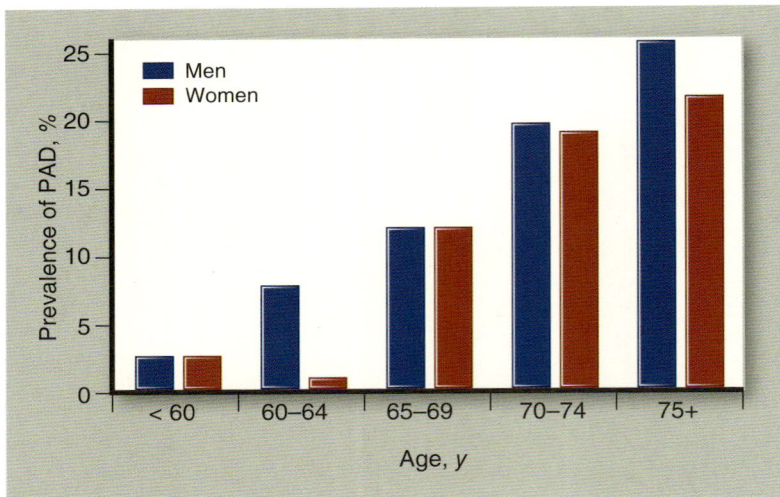

Figure 4-1. Age-dependent prevalence of peripheral arterial disease (PAD). The prevalence of PAD, as defined by an abnormal ankle-brachial index, increases with age. At 60 years of age, it is approximately 2% to 3%, and increases to 20% to 25% of the population older than 70 years of age. The prevalence of PAD rises in both men and women with increasing age, but it is more common in women after menopause. (*Adapted from* Criqui *et al.* [4].)

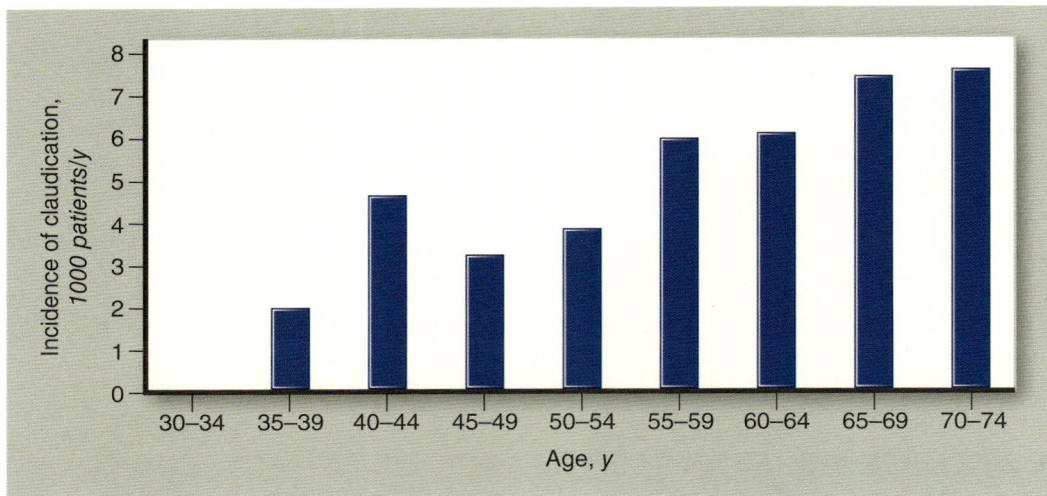

Figure 4-2. Age-dependent incidence of claudication. The incidence of intermittent claudication increases with advancing age, rising from 2% to 7% of adults between the third and seventh decades of life. Classic symptoms of claudication include fatigue, aching, heaviness, or pain in the muscles of the calves, thighs, and buttocks that occurs reproducibly with walking and resolves with rest. Claudication can be differentiated from pain due to other causes by the reproducible stop-start nature of the symptoms in relation to exercise. Sedentary individuals with moderate to severe peripheral arterial disease (PAD) may not experience claudication. (*Adapted* from Norgren *et al.* [3].)

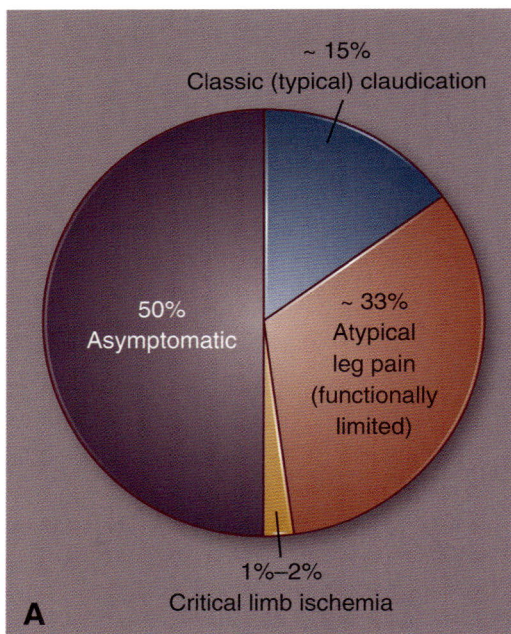

Clinical Presentation of Claudication

Exertional pain, cramping, tightness, fatigue

Occurs in muscle groups, not joints

Reproducible from day to day (consistent level of walking ability)

Resolves completely in 3–4 min

Occurs at same distance once activity resumes

Figure 4-3. A, Clinical presentations of peripheral arterial disease (PAD). Approximately half of individuals with PAD are asymptomatic, 15% experience classic claudication, and at least one third experience leg symptoms that are not typical for claudication. A small fraction of individuals with PAD (1%–2%) have signs or symptoms of critical limb ischemia. (*Modified from* Hirsch *et al.* [2].) **B,** Clinical presentation of claudication. Claudication is often described as an ache, cramp, fatigue, or frank pain provoked by walking and relieved by rest (usually within 10 min). It may occur in the buttocks, thigh, calf, or foot, and the location of discomfort often correlates with a more proximal flow-limiting stenosis. In contrast to the leg discomfort caused by spinal stenosis ("pseudoclaudication"), vascular claudication does not occur with standing or bending. Ischemic rest pain typically occurs in the foot of the affected leg and is an ominous sign that limb blood flow is critically diminished. It is worse when the leg is horizontal or elevated, and may interfere with sleep.

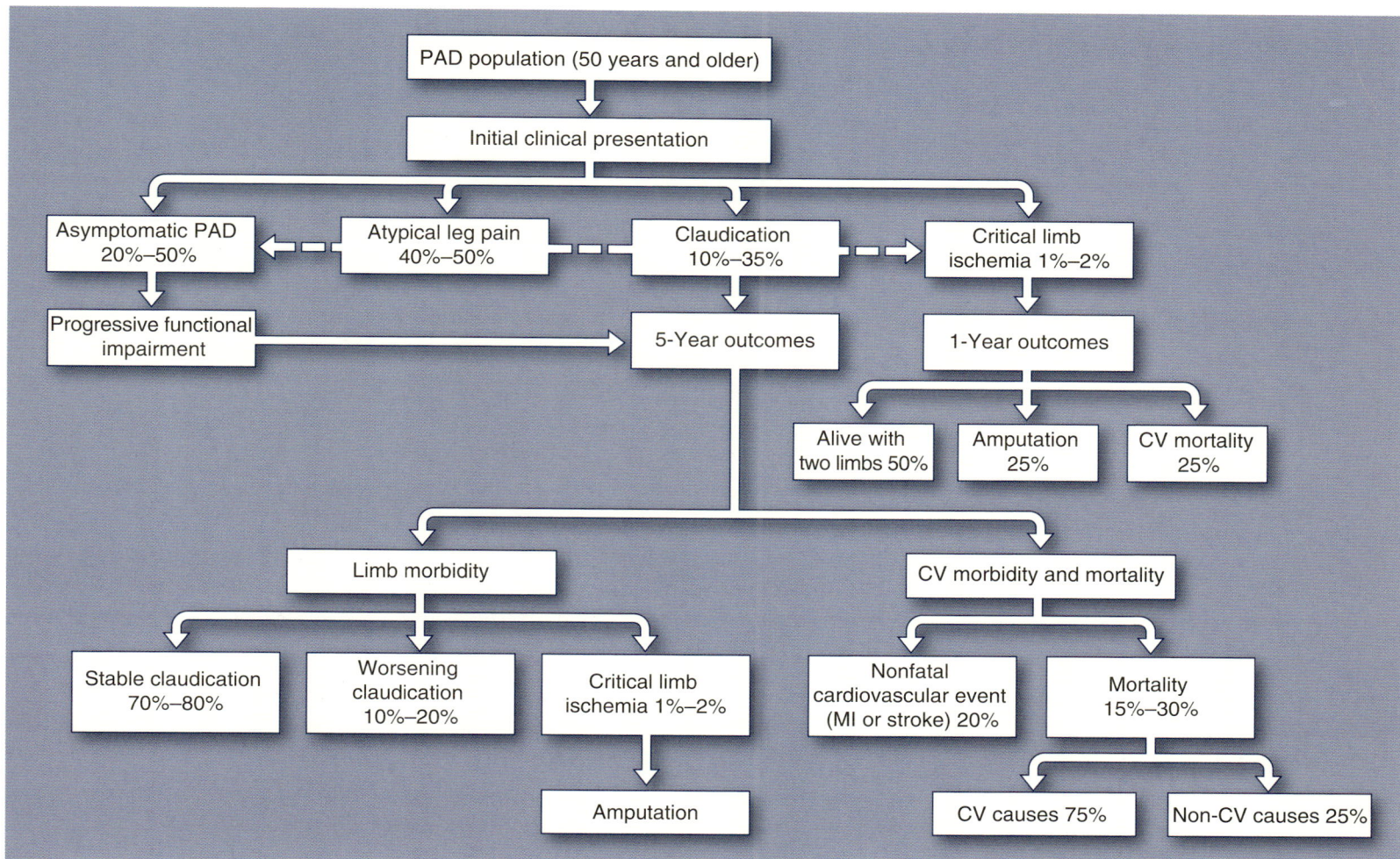

Figure 4-4. Natural history of peripheral arterial disease (PAD). Patients with PAD are at increased risk of adverse cardiovascular events, including fatal and nonfatal myocardial infarction (MI) and stroke. Death may occur in 15% to 30% of patients with PAD over the next 5 years. The major-

ity of patients with intermittent claudication do not experience worsening of symptoms, but claudication severity may increase in 10% to 20% and critical limb ischemia develops in 1% to 2% of patients over 5 years [2,5]. CV—cardiovascular. (*Adapted from* Hirsch *et al.* [2].)

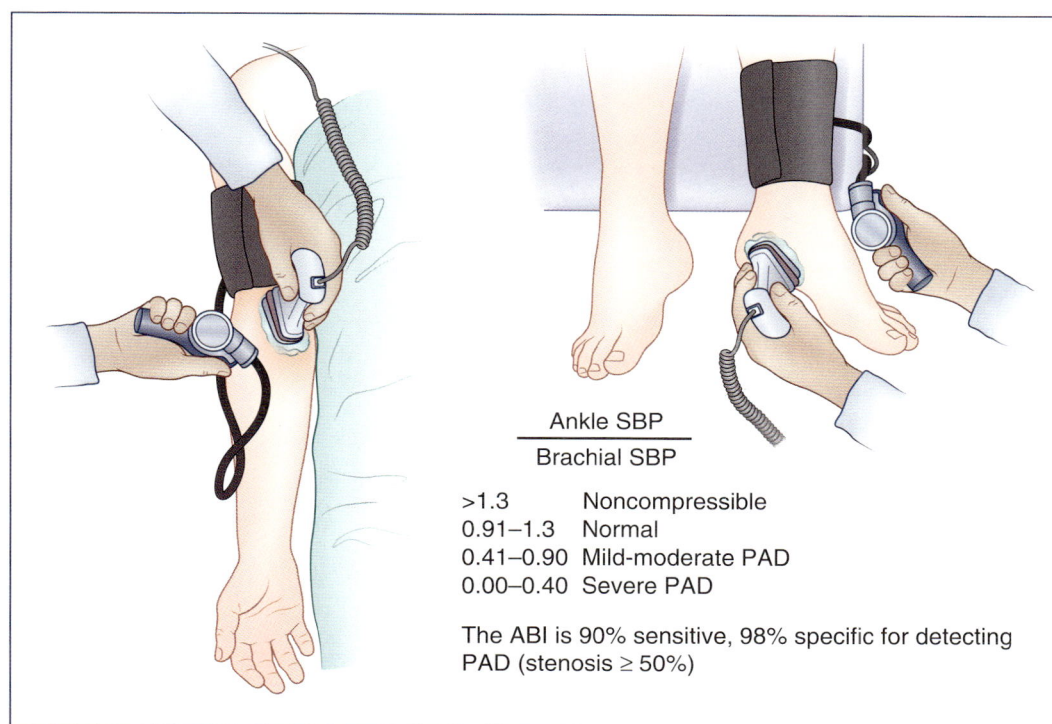

$$\frac{\text{Ankle SBP}}{\text{Brachial SBP}}$$

>1.3   Noncompressible
0.91–1.3   Normal
0.41–0.90 Mild-moderate PAD
0.00–0.40 Severe PAD

The ABI is 90% sensitive, 98% specific for detecting PAD (stenosis ≥ 50%)

Figure 4-5. The Ankle-Brachial Index (ABI) is the ratio of the systolic pressure measured at the ankle using the posterior tibial or dorsalis pedis artery and the systolic pressure measured in the arm over the brachial artery. A sphygmomanometric cuff is placed above the elbow of each arm and above the ankle of each leg and inflated to suprasystolic pressure. The onset of systole is detected with a hand-held Doppler device during cuff deflation. The higher of the ankle pressures in each leg is used in the numerator and the higher of the two brachial systolic pressures is used for the denominator. The normal ABI ranges from 0.91 to 1.30. An ABI < 0.90 is considered diagnostic of peripheral artery disease. An ABI greater than 1.3 is an indication of calcified, noncompressible arteries at the ankle.

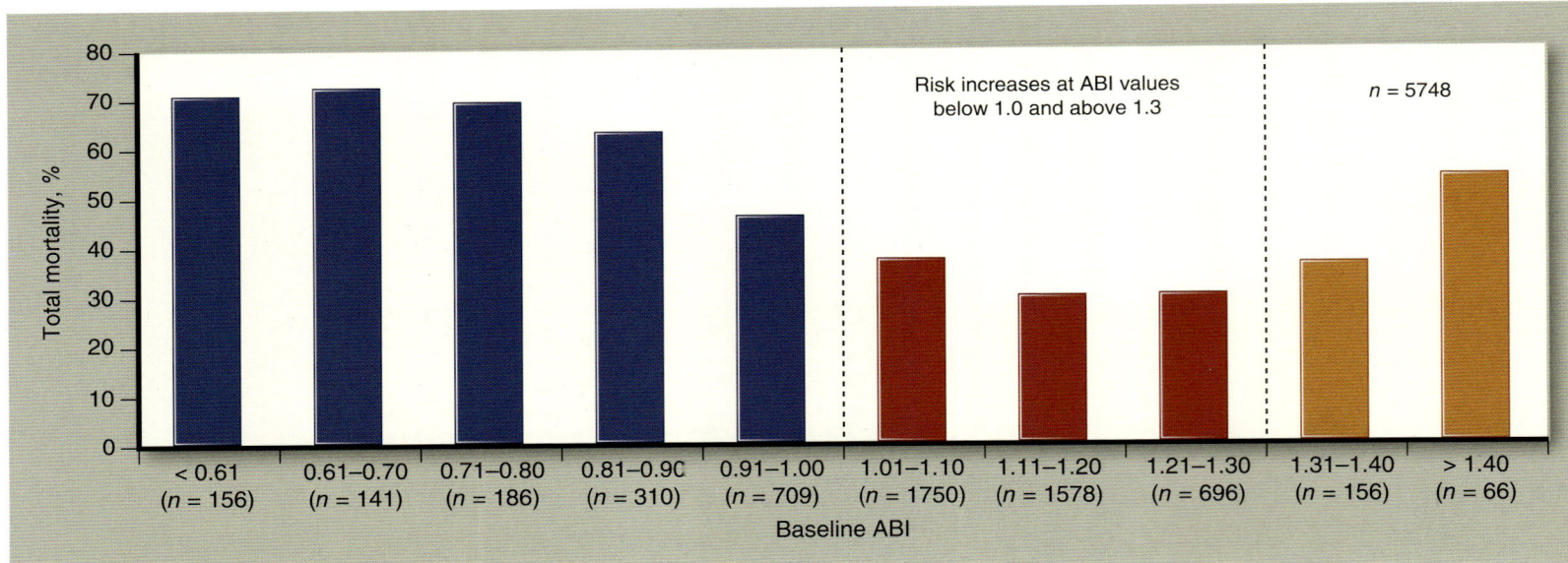

Figure 4-6. Ankle-brachial index (ABI) and mortality. The mortality rate of patients with peripheral arterial disease (PAD) is high. Epidemiologic studies have confirmed the inverse relationship between the ABI and subsequent patient survival [6]. O'Hare et al. [6] examined total and cardiovascular mortality and cardiovascular events across the ABI spectrum among 5748 participants in the Cardiovascular Health Study. The mean age of the sample population was 73 years. The median duration of follow-up was 11.1 years. Higher mortality rates occurred in patients with low ABI compared with the reference group (ABI 1.1 to 1.2). Mortality rates were also increased among patients with elevated ABIs, which are indicative of vascular calcification. (*From* O'Hare et al. [6].)

Noninvasive Vascular Testing for PAD

Test	Disease localization	Quantitation of disease severity	Relative cost	Benefits (limitations)
ABI	–	++	+	Ideal office screening tool; predicts limb and patient survival
Segmental pressure analysis	++	++	+	Excellent arterial localization
Pulse volume recordings	+	+	+	Objective qualitative data
Transcutaneous oximetry	+	+++	++	Assess small vessel disease; predicts wound healing
Exercise ABI testing	–	+++	++	Objective functional assessment; assesses exercise pain etiology; coronary ischemia assessment
Doppler waveform analysis	+++	++	++	Accurate in all populations
Arterial duplex ultrasound	+++	++	+++	Excellent anatomic localization
Gadolinium-enhanced MRA	+++	+++	+++	Contraindicated in individuals with implanted devices and with renal disease
CTA	+++	+++	+++	Contraindicated in individuals with renal disease

Figure 4-7. Noninvasive testing. Noninvasive vascular examinations of the lower extremity are performed to establish the presence of peripheral arterial disease (PAD); assess the severity of disease; localize lesions to specific arterial segments of the limb; and to determine the temporal progression of disease or its response to therapy. Hemodynamic tests include the ankle-brachial index (ABI) at rest and with exercise, segmental pressure measurements, Doppler waveform analysis, and pulse volume recordings. Duplex ultrasonography is used to determine the location and significance of stenotic and occlusive lesions. Both magnetic resonance angiography (MRA) and CT angiography (CTA) provide high-resolution arterial imaging.

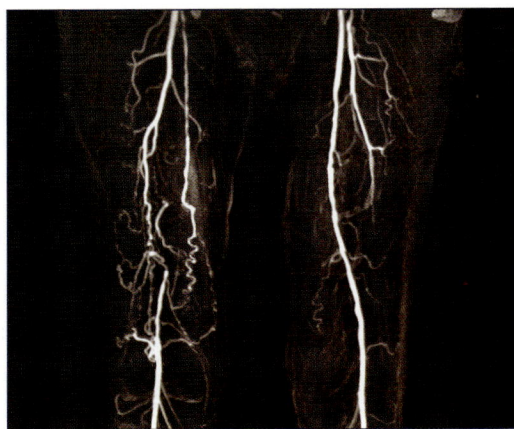

Figure 4-8. Magnetic resonance angiography (MRA), performed with gadolinium enhancement, is useful to assess vascular anatomy and select patients who are candidates for endovascular or surgical revascularization. MRA tends to overestimate the anatomic stenosis, is contraindicated in individuals with significant renal impairment, and is limited in individuals with implanted metallic devices. This MRA image displays a total occlusion of the right mid-superficial femoral artery, with bridging collaterals from the deep femoral artery. There is diffuse atherosclerosis of the left superficial femoral artery.

Management of PAD

Risk factor modification	Antiplatelet therapies
Smoking cessation	Aspirin, clopidogrel
Goal: complete cessation	Goal: reduction in risk of MI, stroke
Lipid management	**Symptom-directed therapies**
Goal: LDL < 100 mg/dL	Supervised exercise rehabilitation
Blood pressure control	Cilostazol, pentoxifylline
Goal: < 140/90 mm Hg	Selective use of revascularization (PTA, bypass)
Blood sugar control in patients with diabetes	**General supportive care**
Goal: HBA1c < 7%	Foot care
	Psychosocial support

Figure 4-9. Management of peripheral arterial disease (PAD). Risk factor modification reduces the risk of adverse cardiovascular events. Smoking cessation, effective lipid management (low-density lipoprotein [LDL] cholesterol < 100 mg/dL), normalization of blood pressure (< 140/90 mm Hg and <130/80 in patients with diabetes or renal insufficiency), and normalization of blood sugar (HbA1c < 7.0%) should be achieved in all patients with PAD [2]. Antiplatelet medications should be prescribed unless otherwise contraindicated [2,3]. For patients with limb symptoms, supervised exercise training (rehabilitation), use of pharmacotherapies, or selective use of revascularization may improve symptoms [2,3]. Attention to foot care will diminish the incidence of ischemic wounds and amputation. PTA—percutaneous transluminal angioplasty.

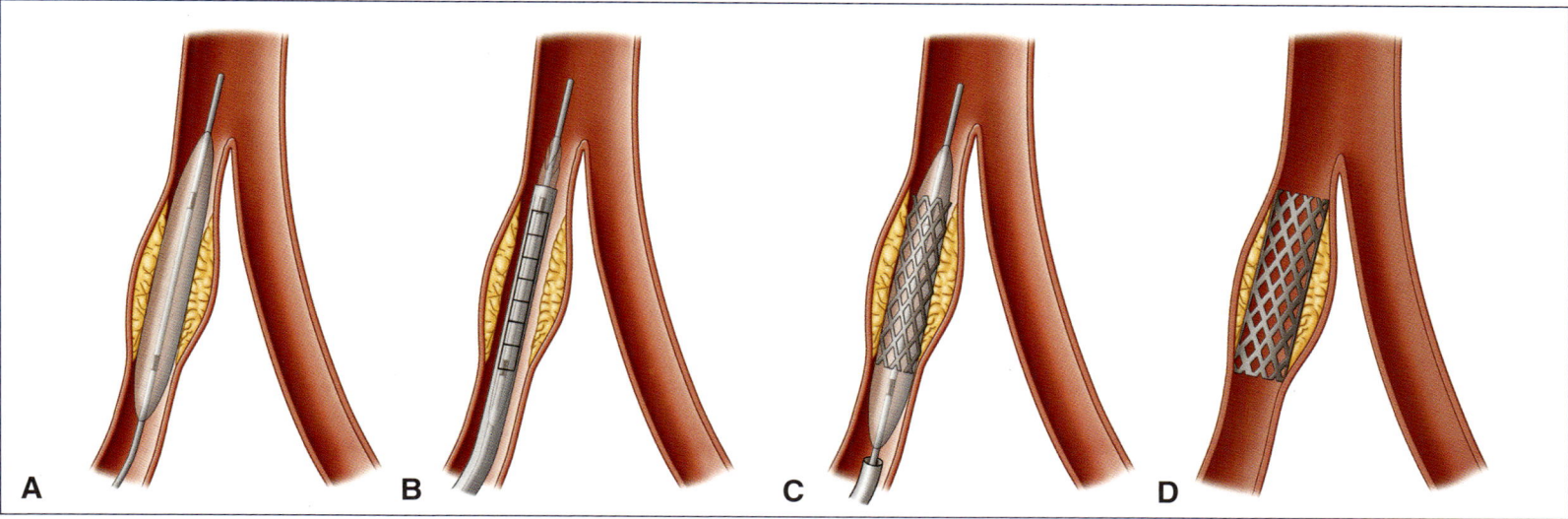

Figure 4-10. Placement of iliac stent for the treatment of iliac artery stenosis. **A,** Standard balloon angioplasty is used initially to decrease the diameter of the iliac stenosis. **B,** The stent is then loaded onto a balloon catheter and guided to the diseased arterial segment. **C,** Balloon inflation permits the stent to enlarge to its maximal diameter. **D,** After removal of the catheter, the stent retains its position and intima will eventually grow to encompass the metallic mesh.

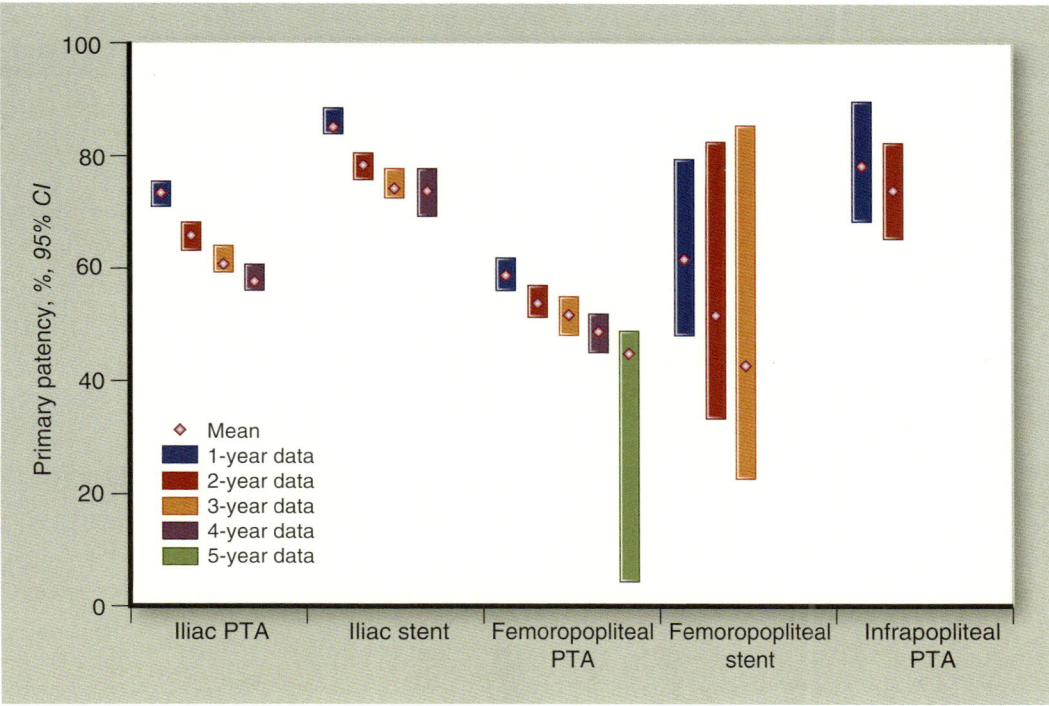

Figure 4-11. Durability of endovascular procedures. While revascularization can often be achieved with endovascular procedures, patency rates are dependent on many patient-derived and anatomic factors [7]. Iliac percutaneous transluminal angioplasty (PTA) without stenting is associated with approximate 75% 1-year patency rates and 60% 4-year patency rates. Iliac artery stenting is associated with 1- and 4-year patency rates of approximately 85% and 75%, respectively. Femoropopliteal PTA is associated with 1-year patency rates of 55%–60% and 4-year patency rates of 50%. Patency is better with shorter, discrete lesions than long segment occlusions. In most studies, stenting of the femoral artery does not improve patency rates, but in one study patency rate after placement of a nitinol stent was better than with PTA alone [8]. (*Adapted from* Hirsch et al. [2].)

Renal Artery Disease

Atherosclerotic renal artery disease usually occurs in older individuals with other manifestations of atherosclerosis. It may cause hypertension, renal failure (ischemic nephropathy), or congestive heart failure. Tests to screen for the presence of renal artery disease include duplex ultrasound, magnetic resonance angiography, and CT angiography. Catheter-based arteriography is occasionally required for diagnostic purposes.

Medical management includes risk factor modification, as occurs with other clinical manifestations of atherosclerosis, and particularly antihypertensive therapy. Indications for revascularization include a significant stenosis of one or both renal arteries and inability to adequately control blood pressure despite a good antihypertensive regimen, or renal insufficiency attributed to bilateral renal artery stenoses or stenosis to a solitary functioning kidney. Other indications for revascularization include recurrent congestive heart failure

or flash pulmonary edema not attributed directly to heart disease. Renal artery stenting has replaced surgical revascularization for most patients with atherosclerotic disease who require an intervention. There is considerable controversy regarding the efficacy of renal artery stenting in patients with renal artery disease. The National Institutes of Health–sponsored Cardiovascular Outcomes in Renal Atherosclerotic Lesions (CORAL) trial is a randomized clinical trial comparing optimum medical therapy alone to stenting with optimal medical therapy. The primary endpoint is a composite of cardiovascular and renal events (cardiovascular or renal death, myocardial infarction, hospitalization for congestive heart failure, stroke, doubling of serum creatinine, and need for renal replacement therapy) [9].

The following figures and legends were originally published in the *Atlas of Vascular Disease* in the chapter by Olin entitled, "Renal Artery Disease" [1].

Clinical Clues to the Diagnosis of Renovascular Disease

Onset of hypertension after age 55 or before age 30 years

Exacerbation of previously well-controlled hypertension

Malignant hypertension

Resistant hypertension

Epigastric bruit (systolic and diastolic)

Unexplained azotemia

Azotemia while receiving ACE inhibitors or AII receptor blocking agents

Atrophic kidney or discrepancy in size between the kidneys

Atherosclerosis elsewhere

Flash pulmonary edema or recurrent congestive heart failure

Figure 4-12. Clinical clues to the diagnosis of renal artery disease. The onset of diastolic hypertension after age 55 years is a strong clue for atherosclerotic renal artery disease, because most patients with primary (essential) hypertension have onset of hypertension between ages 30 and 55 years. Resistant hypertension, malignant hypertension, unexplained azotemia, azotemia while receiving angiotensin-converting enzyme (ACE) inhibitor or angiotensin receptor blocker (ARB) therapy, and atherosclerosis elsewhere are additional findings that should increase suspicion for renal artery disease.

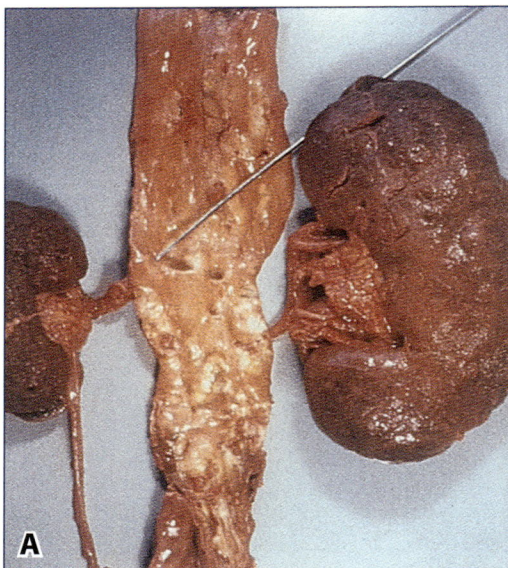

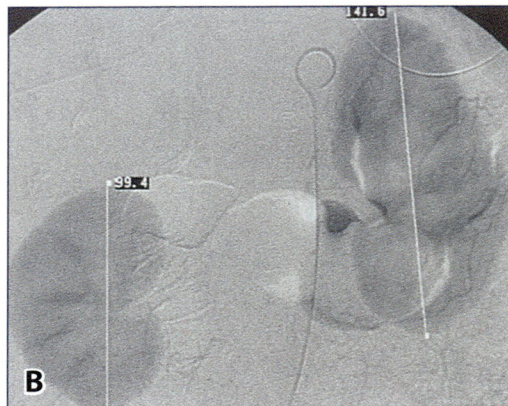

Figure 4-13. Atrophic kidney. **A**, If a kidney is atrophic or there is a difference in kidney size, the smaller kidney usually has a severe stenosis or occlusion of the renal artery supplying that kidney. **B**, The contralateral renal artery also is stenotic approximately 60% of the time. Therefore, discovery of a small kidney should prompt investigation for renal artery disease.

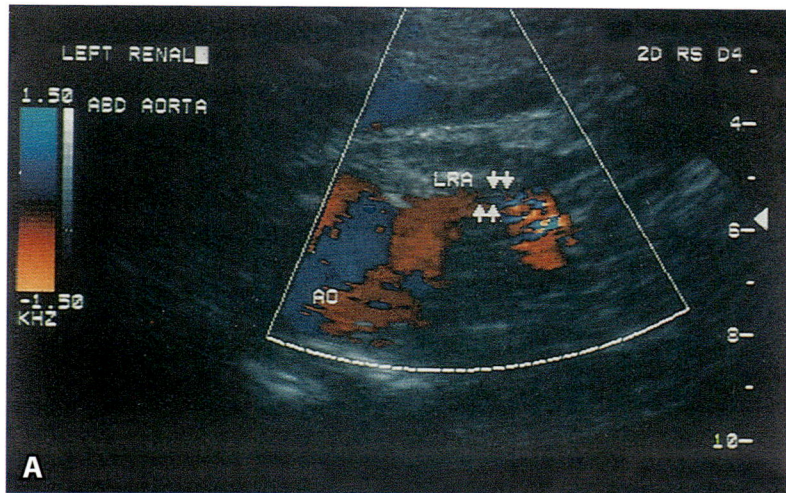

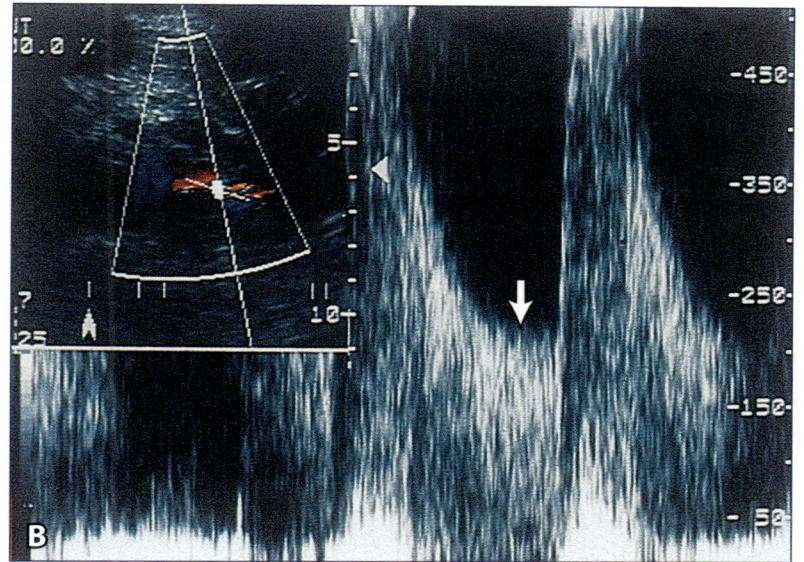

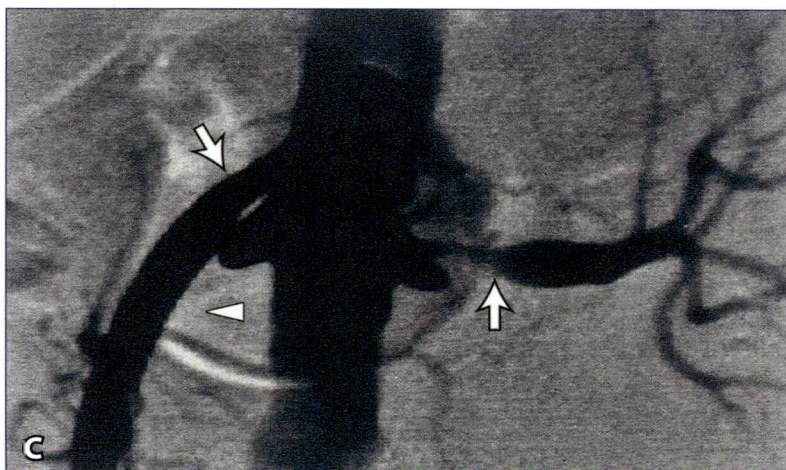

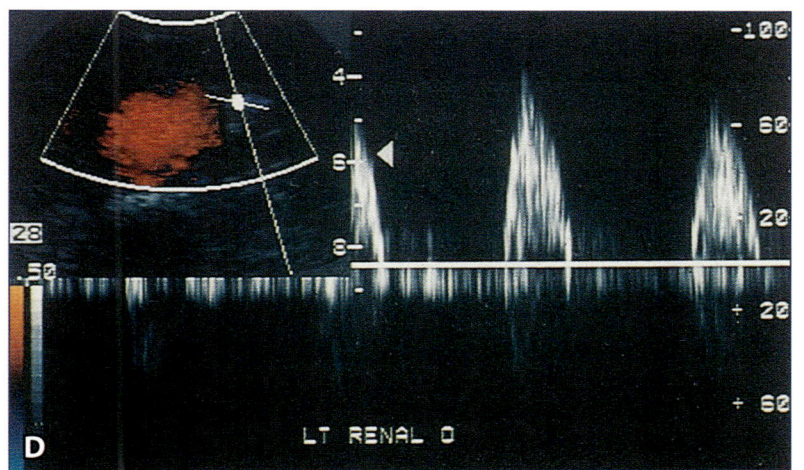

Figure 4-14. Renal artery duplex scanning. **A,** Renal artery duplex scan demonstrating excellent visualization of the left renal artery from the origin in the anterior approach. Note the mosaic color pattern just distal to the *arrows*, indicating turbulence of flow. This area should be carefully insonated with the Doppler.

B, The Doppler was placed in the proximal left renal artery at the correct angle of 60°. The peak systolic velocity was more than 450 cm/sec and the end diastolic velocity (*arrow*) is 220 cm/sec, indicating a stenosis of over 80% of the left renal artery. The right renal artery could not be found and the right kidney was atrophic.

C, Aortogram showing a total occlusion of the right renal artery (*arrowhead*) and a severe eccentric stenosis of the left renal artery (*right arrow*) with post-stenotic dilatation. The superior mesenteric artery is also visualized (*upper-left arrow*).

D, Duplex ultrasound of the left renal artery after a renal artery stent was placed. Note normal velocities (peak systolic velocity 70 cm/sec) compared with the markedly elevated velocities before the placement of the renal artery stent. (*From* Olin and Begelman [10]; with permission.)

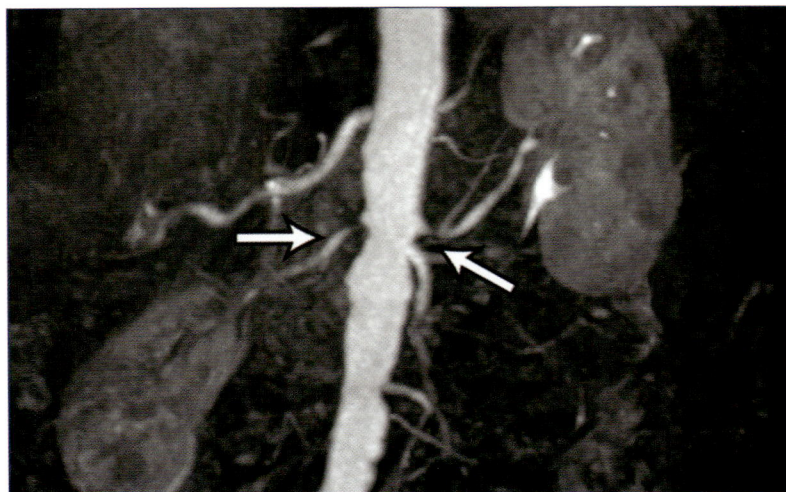

Figure 4-15. Magnetic resonance angiography (MRA) demonstrating severe bilateral renal artery stenoses (*arrows*). MRA is a useful screening test for renal artery stenosis. The sensitivity and specificity for detecting stenosis greater than 60% ranges from 73% to 100% and 76% to 100%, respectively. Patients with metal clips or staples, pacemakers, or other metallic devices may not be candidates for MRA.

Medical Treatment of Renal Artery Disease

Control blood pressure

Follow recommendations of JNC 7

ACE inhibitor ± diuretic for initial therapy for unilateral disease

Preserve renal function

Follow serum creatinine

Follow renal size (ultrasound)

Follow progression of renal artery stenosis with serial duplex ultrasound

Modify all cardiovascular risk factors

Figure 4-16. Medical treatment of renal artery disease. Patients should receive risk factor modification and antiplatelet therapy, even those undergoing a revascularization procedure. This includes smoking cessation, treatment of hypertension, hypercholesterolemia, and diabetes, as recommended for other atherosclerotic conditions. JNC7—The Seventh Report of the Joint National Committee on Prevention, Detection, Evaluation, and Treatment of High Blood Pressure.

Indications for Revascularization for Atherosclerotic Renal Artery Stenosis

Inability to control blood pressure

Preservation of renal function

Control of congestive heart failure

Figure 4-17. Indications for revascularization for atherosclerotic renal artery disease. Despite advances in the technical aspects of angioplasty and stent implantation, there are few controlled clinical trials assessing the role of renal artery angioplasty and stenting to control hypertension or preserve renal function. Despite the lack of randomized controlled trials, the consensus of experts supports the use of angioplasty and stenting for most patients with atherosclerotic renal artery stenosis who meet the criteria for intervention.

Figure 4-18. Renal artery stenting for atherosclerotic renal artery stenosis. Due to the high restenosis rate with percutaneous transluminal angioplasty (PTA) alone, stents offer a significant advantage in patients with atherosclerotic disease, especially those with ostial stenosis. The degree of stenosis post-stenting approaches zero, and most dissection flaps caused by PTA alone are successfully sealed with stents.

A, Angiogram showing marked atherosclerosis in the abdominal aorta. Note the severe stenosis (*arrow*) at the ostium and in the proximal portion of the left renal artery with post-stenotic dilatation. The guiding catheter comes from above in this case due to the angle of the takeoff of the left renal artery. **B,** Excellent angiographic result after renal artery stenting (*arrow*). Note that the stent extends 1 to 2 mm into the aorta, which is perfect position in patients with ostial renal artery stenosis. (*Courtesy of* J. Michael Bacharach, MD, MPH.)

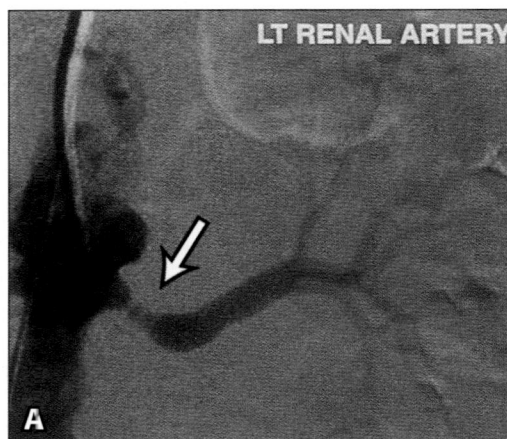

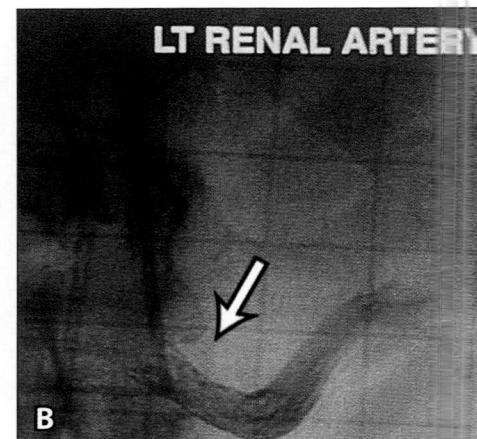

Carotid Artery Disease

There are approximately 700,000 new or recurrent stroke cases each year in the United States, of which approximately 75% are ischemic and 20% are hemorrhagic [11–13]. Carotid artery disease accounts for approximately 15% to 20% of ischemic strokes. Carotid artery disease occurs commonly in patients with other manifestations of atherosclerosis. Patients with carotid artery disease may be asymptomatic or present with transient hemispheric ischemia, amaurosis fugax, or stroke. Tests to diagnose carotid artery disease include duplex ultrasonography, CT, magnetic resonance angiography, and catheter angiography. Strategies for secondary prevention include platelet inhibitors, risk factor modification, carotid endarterectomy, and carotid stenting.

The following figures and legends were originally published in the *Atlas of Vascular Disease* in the chapter by Feske, Jensen, and Creager entitled, "Carotid Artery Disease" [1].

Carotid Artery Disease: TIA

Transient hemispheric ischemia

Duration < 24 h, usually 30 min

Symptoms: motor and/or sensory dysfunction of contralateral limbs (face and arm > leg); aphasia (left hemisphere); neglect (right hemisphere)

Transient monocular blindness

Duration usually briefer

Symptoms: monocular visual loss or obscuration, typically with vertical progression and recovery (like a shade descending and rising)

Figure 4-19. Carotid artery disease: transient ischemic attack (TIA). TIAs affecting the cerebral territory in the distribution of the carotid artery must, by definition, last less than 24 hours. The great majority of TIAs last for less than 30 minutes. The clinical presentation may include motor and/or sensory deficits affecting the contralateral side of the face and limbs. Cognitive deficits, such as aphasia (left hemisphere), apraxia, or neglect (usually right hemisphere), may also develop with cerebral cortical ischemia. Transient monocular blindness may be caused by retinal ischemia.

Carotid Artery Disease: Stroke

Territory

Anterior cerebral artery

Middle cerebral artery

Mechanisms

Proximal stenosis or occulsion

Artery-to-artery embolism

Clinical presentation

Contralateral weakness

Contralateral sensory loss

Aphasia, apraxia, neglect

Visual loss

Figure 4-20. Carotid artery disease: stroke. Stroke caused by carotid artery disease affects the middle cerebral artery (MCA) and/or anterior cerebral artery (ACA) territories. In about 15% of patients, the posterior cerebral artery (PCA) receives its major supply from the anterior circulation via a large posterior communicating artery; in such patients, the PCA territory may be affected by carotid disease. The major mechanisms of ischemic injury in the carotid territory are artery-to-artery embolism and reduced flow distal to severe stenosis. Regardless of the cause, transient ischemic attacks (TIAs) often precede stroke. The most common symptoms are contralateral weakness and/or sensory deficits. With MCA territory ischemia, the face and arm symptoms and signs are usually greater than those in the leg; with ACA territory symptoms, the leg symptoms may be most prominent. Patients may also have visual field deficits from involvement of the visual fibers in the temporal and parietal lobes, or the occipital lobes in cases involving the PCA. Cognitive deficits from left hemisphere ischemia typically include language dysfunction, aphasia. Lesions of either hemisphere may cause apraxia. Right or left hemisphere lesions may cause a contralateral neglect syndrome, but this is typically much more marked with right hemisphere lesions. Ocular infarction from central retinal artery occlusion is uncommon. Such patients present with monocular blindness or scotomas.

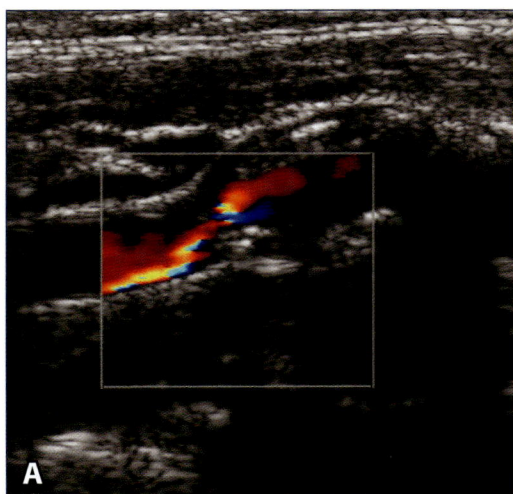

Figure 4-21. Color-assisted duplex ultrasound of a stenotic internal carotid artery. **A,** Color-assisted duplex ultrasound examination of a stenotic right internal carotid artery (RT ICA). Flow becomes turbulent at the site of the stenosis, which is depicted by the color examination showing both dropout of color at the site of the plaque as well as turbulence of flow (*red, yellow, and blue colors*).

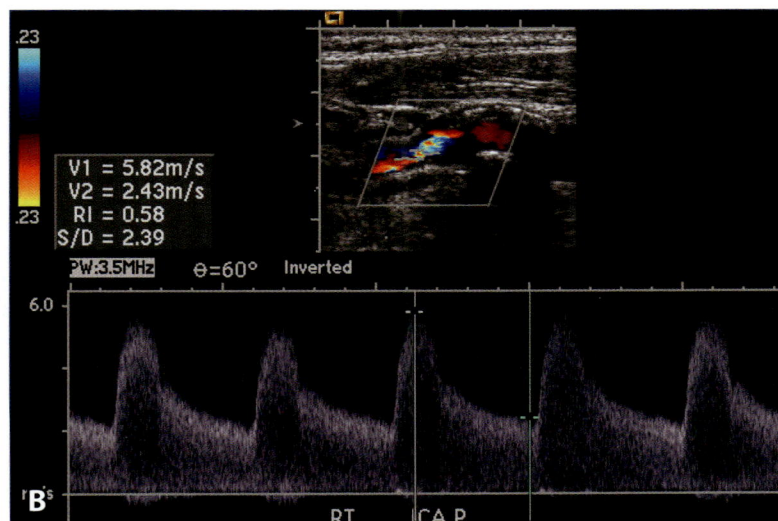

B, The pulsed-wave Doppler component of the carotid ultrasound examination enables interrogation of the blood flow velocity within the lumen of the vessel. In the presence of a significant stenosis, the velocity accelerates through the stenotic lesion. In this example, the peak systolic velocity is increased (582 cm/sec), indicative of more than 80% stenosis. Furthermore, cells are not moving at the same rate of speed, accounting for broadening of the Doppler display.

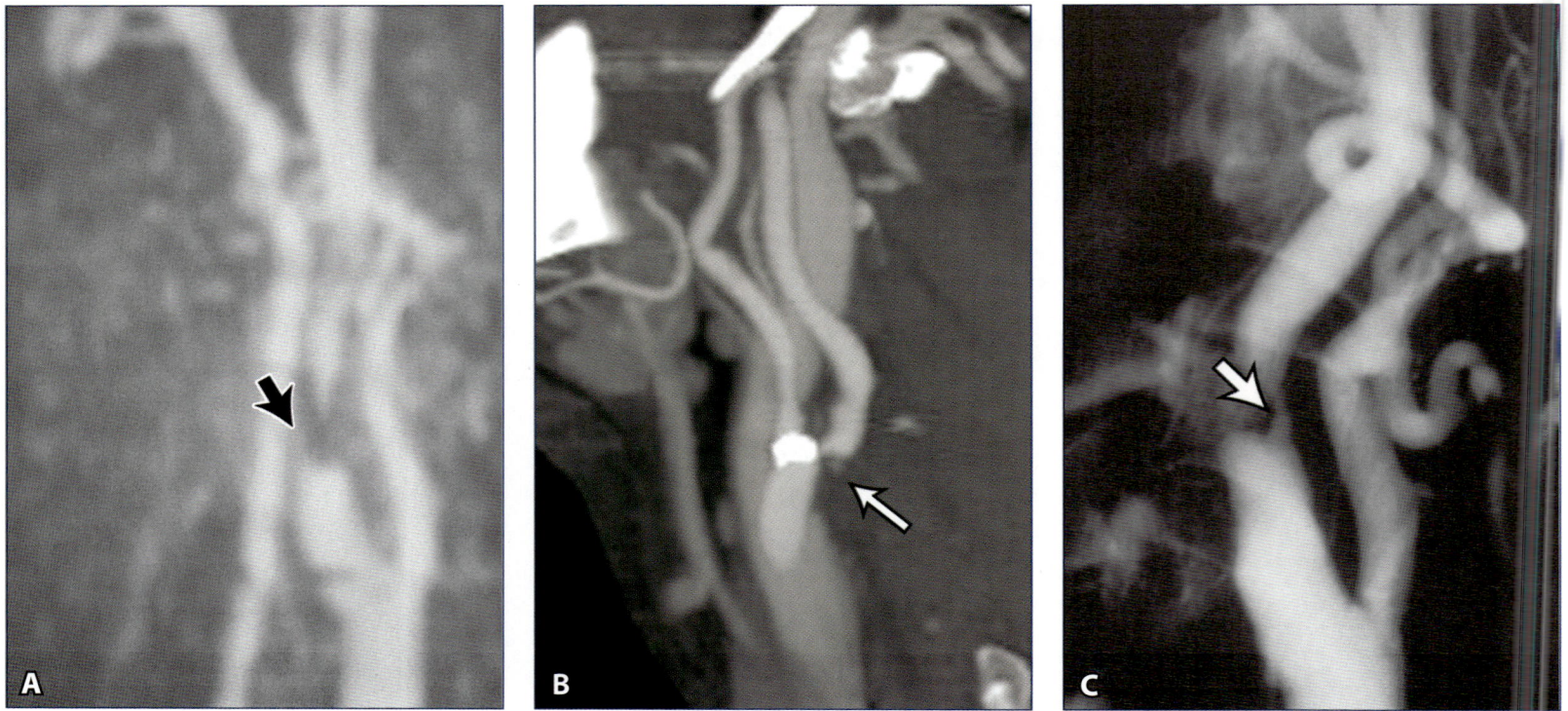

Figure 4-22. Magnetic resonance (MR), CT, and conventional angiograms of the extracranial carotid arteries of the same patient, showing high-grade stenosis at the origin of the left internal carotid artery.

A, MR angiogram demonstrating a short segment of narrowing and drop-out of the flow signal (*arrow*) of the left internal carotid artery. MR angiography is a reliably sensitive technique; however, it cannot differentiate among different degrees of severe stenosis.

B, CT angiogram of the left cervical carotid arteries showing a short segment of severe carotid stenosis at the origin of the left internal carotid

artery (*arrow*). Calcification in the carotid bulb is seen adjacent to the short segment of stenosis. In many cases, CT angiography is adequate to replace conventional angiography; however, resolution is variable, and local calcification may obscure interpretation in some cases.

C, Conventional contrast angiogram of the carotid arteries demonstrating high-grade stenosis in the proximal internal carotid artery (*arrow*). Conventional angiography is still the most accurate test for carotid stenosis, and it is used when duplex ultrasonography and MR or CT angiography have yielded ambiguous results.

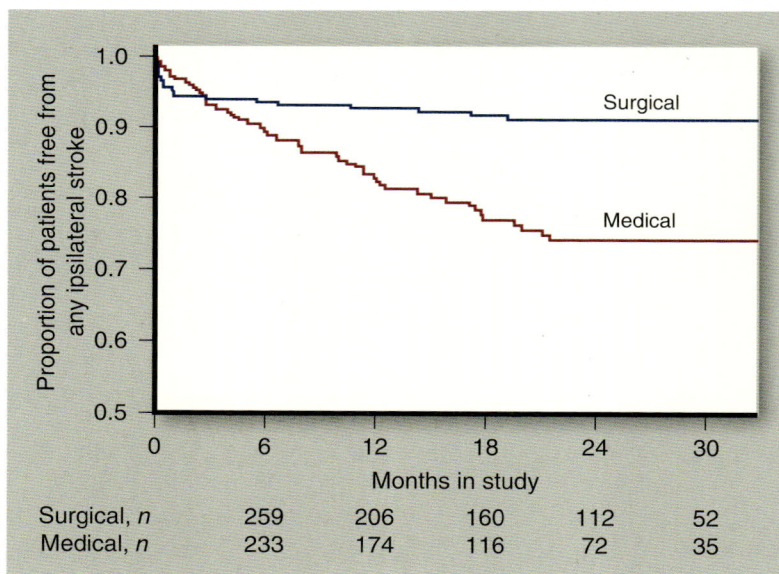

Surgical, *n*	259	206	160	112	52
Medical, *n*	233	174	116	72	35

Figure 4-23. Carotid endarterectomy for patients with symptomatic high-grade carotid artery stenosis: North American Symptomatic Carotid Endarterectomy Trial (NASCET) [14]. In this trial, patients with carotid artery stenosis of 70% to 90% who had transient hemispheric symptoms, amaurosis fugax, or a nondisabling stroke were randomized to carotid endarterectomy or optimal medical care, including antiplatelet therapy. The cumulative risk of any ipsilateral stroke at 2 years was 26% in the medical care group and 9% in the surgical group, resulting in an absolute risk reduction of 17%. Carotid endarterectomy was also found to be beneficial when all strokes and deaths were included in the analysis. (*Adapted from* North American Symptomatic Carotid Endarterectomy Trial Collaborators [14].)

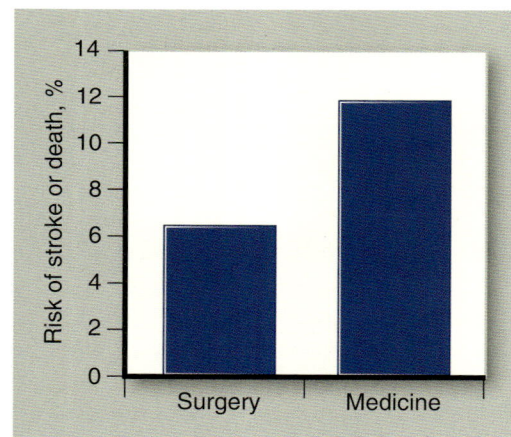

Figure 4-24. Carotid endarterectomy for asymptomatic carotid artery stenosis. The Asymptomatic Carotid Surgery Trial (ACST) [15] was a multicenter randomized controlled clinical trial that examined the effect of carotid endarterectomy versus nonsurgical therapy in patients with asymptomatic carotid artery stenosis of greater than 60%. Of the 3120 eligible patients who participated in the ACST trial, 1560 were randomized to each group. Results were reported for 5 years of follow-up. The risk of any stroke or perioperative death was 6.42% in the surgical group and 11.78% in the medical group. The relative risk reduction conferred by surgery was 46% ($P < 0.0001$).

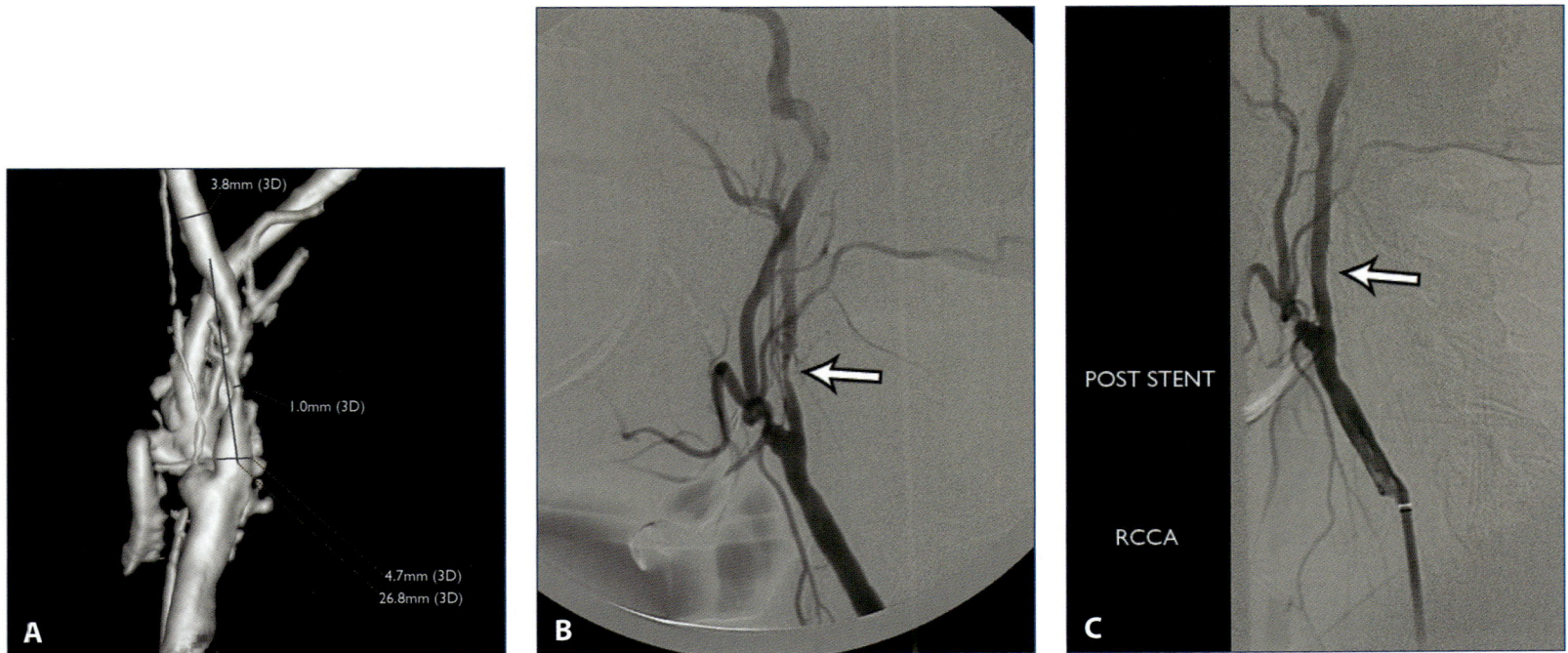

Figure 4-25. A 71-year-old man developed recurrent stenosis at the origin of the right internal carotid artery 1.5 years after stenting of this artery. Three-dimensional reconstruction of angiographic data (**A**) shows the residual lumen to be narrowed to 1 mm with approximately 75% stenosis. The next two panels show the angiogram with the arrow indicating the site of stenosis before (**B**) and after (**C**) repeat stenting.

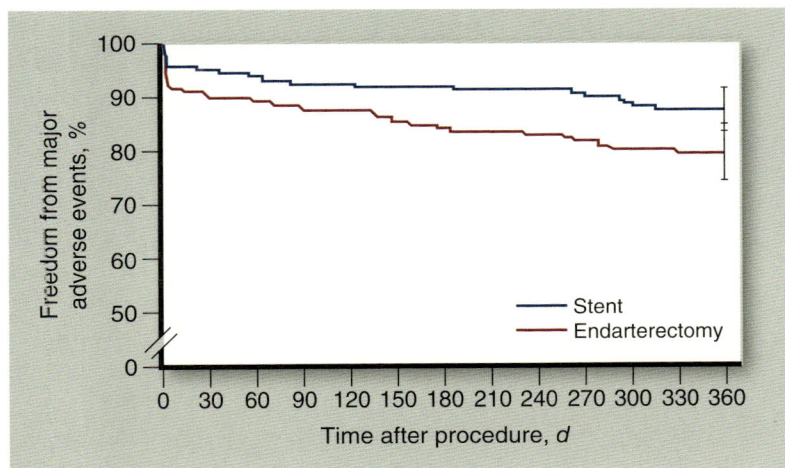

Figure 4-26. Carotid endarterectomy (CEA) versus carotid artery stenting in high-risk patients. The Stenting and Angioplasty with Protection in Patients at High Risk for Endarterectomy (SAPPHIRE) study compared carotid stenting with an embolic protection device against carotid endarterectomy in patients considered to be at high risk [16]. Symptomatic patients with greater than 50% stenosis and asymptomatic patients with greater than 80% stenosis were enrolled. Of 334 patients enrolled, 167 were randomly assigned to each group. Patients were followed for myocardial infarction within the first 30 days, and stroke or death within the first year. In a non-inferiority analysis, 20 patients undergoing stenting and 32 patients undergoing CEA reached the study endpoint, demonstrating non-inferiority of carotid artery stenting ($P = 0.004$ for non-inferiority) (*Modified from* Yadav et al. [16].)

Aortic Dissection

Aortic dissection is a life-threatening disorder requiring prompt diagnosis and treatment. It is the most common of the acute aortic syndromes, the others being aortic intramural hematoma and penetrating aortic ulcer. Aortic dissection affects approximately 3 to 3.5 per 100,000 people each year. It usually occurs in the setting of preexisting aortic disease, but may develop in a patient with no history of aortic disease. Coexisting conditions associated with aortic dissection include aortic aneurysm, hypertension, bicuspid aortic valve, and inherited disorders of connective tissue, such as Marfan syndrome and pregnancy. The most common symptom is chest or back pain, occurring in over 90% of patients; abdominal pain occurs less frequently. Most patients are hypertensive, though hypotension may occur in patients with dissection of the ascending aorta complicated by cardiac tamponade, acute myocardial infarction, or aortic regurgitation. Clinical clues on the examination include asymmetric blood pressure, pulse deficits, neurologic deficits, and limb ischemia. Diagnostic testing, including transesophageal echocardiography, computed tomography, or magnetic resonance imaging, should occur urgently in patients who present with symptoms and findings suggestive of acute aortic dissection. Up to 20% of patients die before presentation to a medical facility and mortality rates within the first 48 hours of presentation to hospital approximate 1% per hour. Prompt medical therapy, including α-adrenergic blockers and other drugs to lower blood pressure and dP/dT, as well as emergent surgery in appropriate circumstances, reduces mortality rate. Endovascular interventions, including fenestration procedures and stent grafts, are emerging as additional options in selected patients.

The following figures and legends were originally published in the *Atlas of Vascular Disease* in the chapter by Spooner and Isselbacher entitled, "Aortic Dissection" [1].

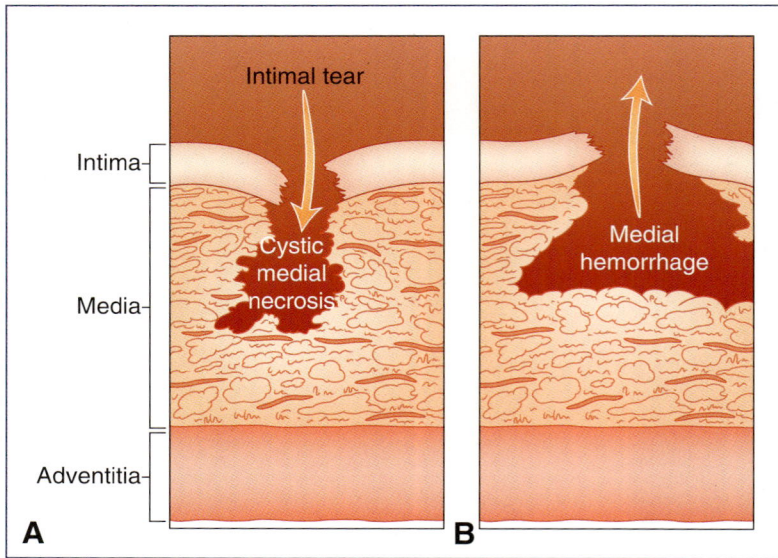

Figure 4-27. The mechanism of intimal tearing in aortic dissection. This illustration shows the two possible mechanisms for the pathogenesis of aortic dissection. **A,** In this mechanism of intimal tear, which is believed to be the more likely one, there is a primary intimal tear followed by dissection of blood from the aorta into the media. Propagation usually occurs antegrade, driven by the natural forward pressure of blood flow in the aorta, but retrograde propagation may occur as well. The presence of an intimal tear allows the transmission of aortic pressure into the disrupted media, causing progressive separation of the tissue planes and propagation of the dissection. **B,** In this mechanism, the primary event is rupture of the vasa vasorum with hemorrhage in the aortic media and then through the intima into the aortic lumen. When such medial hemorrhage occurs without intimal rupture, it produces a variant of aortic dissection called intramural hematoma. (*Adapted from* Eagle *et al.* [17].)

Etiology of Aortic Dissection: Predisposing Factors

Advanced age (mean age, 63 years)
Male gender (65%)
History of hypertension (72%)
Known aortic aneurysm (16%)
Marfan syndrome (5%)
Bicuspid aortic valve (5%)
Peripartum period of pregnancy (1%)
Cardiac catheterization (2%)
Prior cardiac surgery (18%)

Figure 4-28. Etiology of aortic dissection in 464 patients in the International Registry of Acute Aortic Dissection. Other uncommon but important predisposing factors include cocaine abuse and blunt trauma. Any disease process or other condition that undermines the integrity of the aortic media (either its elastic or muscular component) may predispose to aortic dissection. Cystic medial degeneration is the common denominator in nontraumatic cases. Elderly patients with a history of hypertension are the most typical population presenting with aortic dissection. Patients with Marfan syndrome are at particularly high risk for aortic dissection—as well as for recurrent dissection—and therefore often require a more aggressive diagnostic and therapeutic approach. Younger patients (age < 40 years at presentation) are more likely to have underlying Marfan syndrome or a bicuspid aortic valve and tend to have larger aortic diameters at presentation [18].

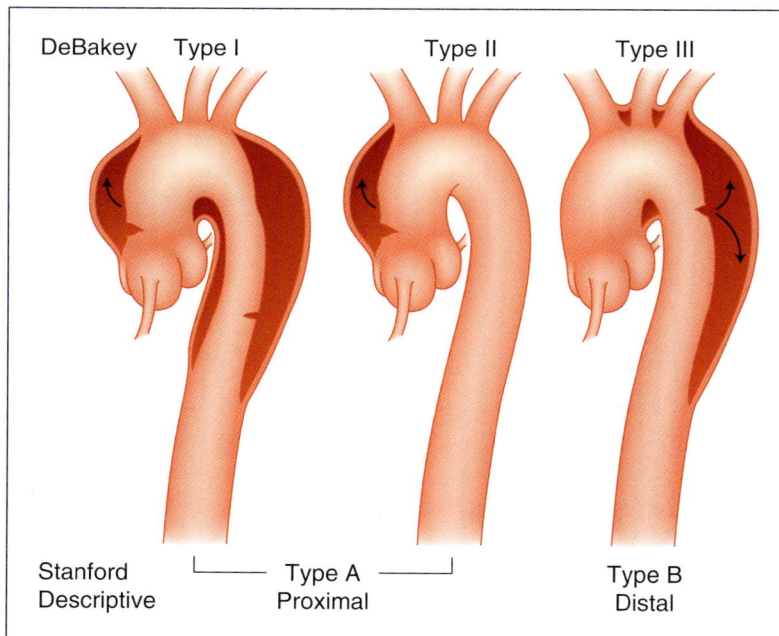

Figure 4-29. Classification of aortic dissection by the extent of aortic involvement. This diagrammatic representation of aortic dissection shows the anatomy of the three most common types. The intimal tear is represented by the arrows, which cross from the true lumen out into the false lumen (*darker red*). Three classification systems are commonly used to describe aortic dissections. These three systems share the same basic principle of distinguishing dissections that involve the ascending aorta from those that do not, because involvement of the ascending aorta has important prognostic and therapeutic implications. Most would consider involvement of the ascending aorta an indication for surgery, whereas a lack of involvement would favor medical therapy. Because management of DeBakey types I and II is usually similar, the other classification systems have combined these two types into a single group called type A, or proximal. Type A aortic dissections outnumber type B aortic dissections by approximately 2 to 1. (*Adapted from* Eagle *et al.* [17].)

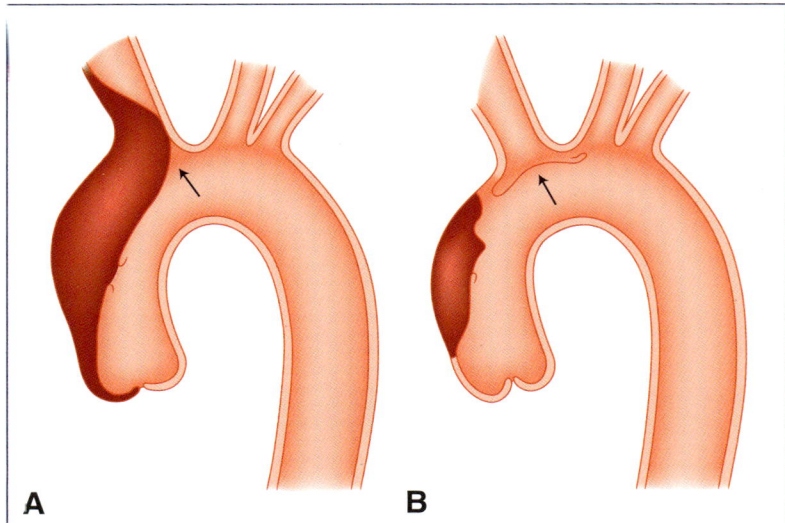

Figure 4-30. The mechanisms by which aortic dissection may cause loss of pulses. **A,** The intimal flap and false lumen extend into the right innominate artery to narrow or occlude the lumen. **B,** A mobile portion of the intimal flap has folded over the orifice of the right innominate artery, obstructing blood flow. (*Adapted from* Eagle *et al.* [17].)

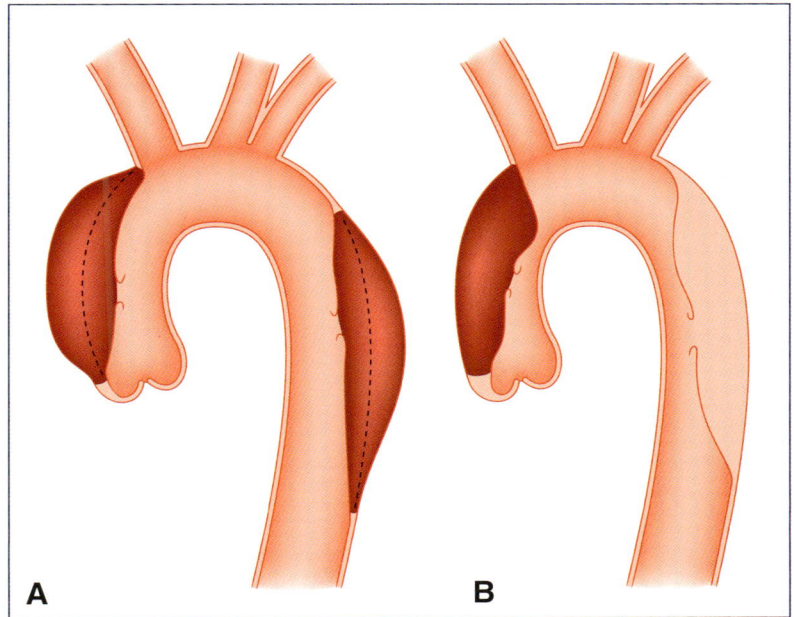

Figure 4-31. A dissecting hematoma may variably affect aortic size and contour on a chest radiograph or aortogram. **A,** The proximal and distal false lumina have expanded outward, producing an enlarged aortic silhouette with an abnormal bulging contour, whereas the diameter of the true lumen is narrowed minimally. **B,** The false lumen has expanded inward, causing marked narrowing of the true lumen, but this results in little or no change in the silhouette of the ascending or descending aorta. An unremarkable chest radiograph might be seen in this case. (*Adapted from* O'Gara and DeSanctis [19].)

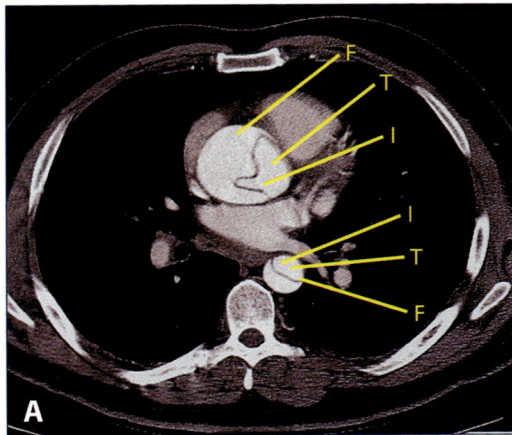

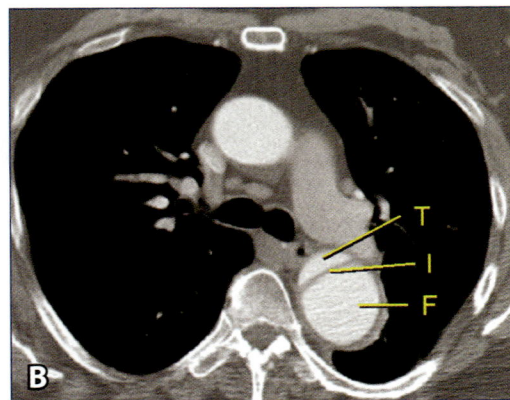

Figure 4-32. Computed tomography (CT) for diagnosing aortic dissection. **A,** A contrast-enhanced spiral CT scan of the chest at the level of the pulmonary artery showing an intimal flap (I) in both the ascending thoracic aorta (*above*) and descending thoracic aorta (*below*) separating the true (T) and false (F) lumina in a type A aortic dissection. **B,** A contrast-enhanced spiral CT scan of the chest at the level of the pulmonary artery showing an intimal flap (I) in the descending thoracic aorta separating the larger false (F) and the true (T) lumina in a type B aortic dissection.

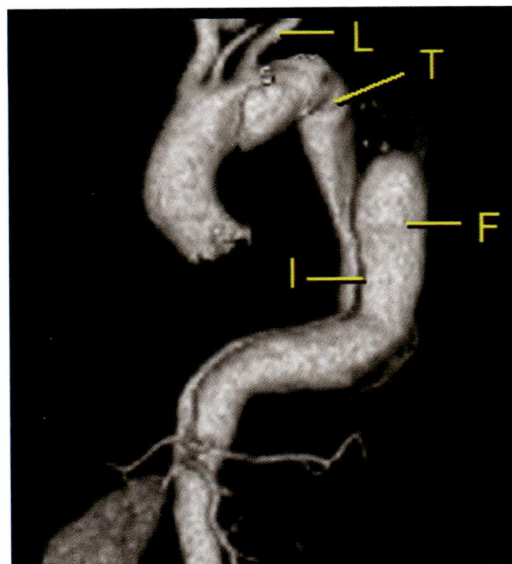

Figure 4-33. Advanced computed tomography (CT) scan of aortic dissection. Three-dimensional reconstruction technique, as shown in this example of a type B dissection in the left anterior oblique projection with surface shaded display, provides superior resolution and anatomic detail compared with standard axial CT imaging. This technique is particularly useful in defining the extent of dissection and the complexity of aortic anatomy. The intimal flap (I) arises just distal to the left subclavian artery (L) and extends distally beyond the aortic bifurcation and into the common iliac arteries. The true lumen (T) is smaller than the false lumen (F), which is typical. The most proximal segment of the false lumen is thrombosed. Also evident is the fact that the patient's status is postsurgical left nephrectomy.

Figure 4-34. Steps in the early medical management of a patient presenting with suspected aortic dissection. The risk of complications from aortic dissection is highest within the first hours after onset, with a mortality rate for those untreated as high as 1% per hour. It is therefore essential to institute appropriate therapy as soon as the diagnosis of dissection is reasonably suspected, rather than waiting for the diagnosis to be confirmed. Specific management goals include 1) comprehensively examining the patient for evidence of aortic dissection and the associated complications; 2) stabilizing the patient as necessary and treating the patient pharmacologically to minimize the risk of progression or rupture of the dissection by reducing the slope of increasing pressure (dP/dT); and 3) selecting and obtaining a diagnostic imaging study as promptly as possible, and deciding between medical and surgical therapy if the diagnosis of dissection is confirmed. ECG—electrocardiogram.

Figure 4-35. Indications for definitive surgery in aortic dissection. As a general rule, aortic repair is indicated for the management of acute type A aortic dissection, because survival in this group is improved when compared with medical management [20,21]. Overall in-hospital mortality remains high (approximately 25%), but with greater risk in those presenting with shock, tamponade, hypotension, limb ischemia, migrating chest pain, or history of aortic valve replacement [22]. For acute and uncomplicated type B aortic dissection, however, aortic repair does not provide a survival advantage over medical therapy [23]; in such cases, medical therapy is preferred. Nevertheless, if an acute distal dissection leads to complications, surgery may well be indicated. In-hospital mortality for the surgical management of type B dissection was 29% in a recent analysis, with greater risk associated with age greater than 70 years and preoperative shock, as well as univariate factors of perioperative altered mental status, partial thrombosis of the false lumen, periaortic hematoma, descending aortic diameter greater than 6 cm, right ventricular dysfunction, or early surgery [24]. In the setting of chronic aortic dissection, surgery is indicated when there is evidence of significant degenerative aortic aneurysm formation. The role of endovascular stent-grafting to repair degenerative thoracic aneurysm, as well as thoracic aortic pseudoaneurysm, penetrating ulcer, traumatic tear, and acute dissection, is currently being compared with open surgical repair, with promising early results with respect to operative morbidity and mortality [25]. (*Adapted from* Isselbacher [26].)

Figure 4-36. Options for intervention in type B aortic dissection. In-hospital management of acute type B aortic dissection and its effect on survival were recently evaluated among patients enrolled in the International Registry of Acute Aortic Dissection. Although all were subject to initial medical management, 11% subsequently underwent surgery and 11% subsequently underwent endovascular therapy (stenting and/or fenestration), primarily as the result of limb and visceral ischemia, extension of dissection, refractory hypertension, or recurrent pain. One-year and 3-year survival rates for those treated medically, surgically, or with an endovascular approach alive at discharge were 90% and 78%, 96% and 83%, and 89% and 76%, respectively (median, 2.3 years; log-rank $P = 0.61$). These results suggest that management technique itself does not significantly alter future mortality, so determining the optimal treatment strategy for these patients requires further study [27].

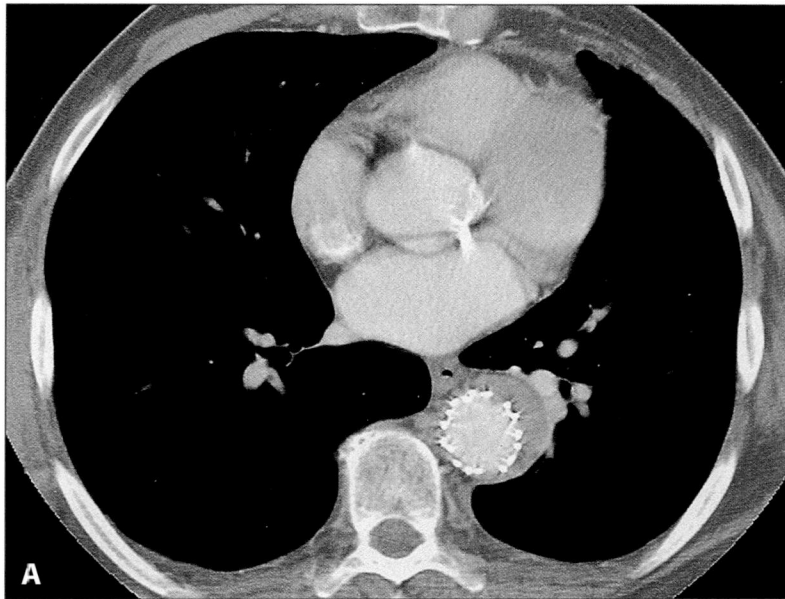

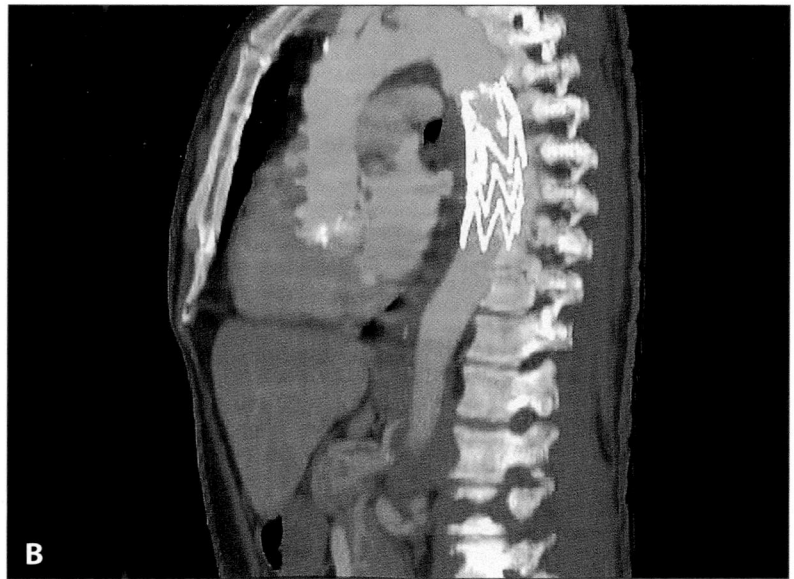

Figure 4-37. Endovascular aortic stent-grafts for nonsurgical management of type B dissection. Stent-grafts can be placed percutaneously via the transfemoral catheter technique. The purpose of the stent-graft is to close off the site of entry into the false lumen (*ie*, the intimal tear), thus decompressing the distended false lumen and promoting its thrombosis. For those with acute vascular complications, this should in turn relieve any obstruction of branch arteries. Such stent-grafts can be placed only in the descending aorta (*ie*, to treat distal dissections) because they cannot be passed through the aortic arch to reach the ascending aorta. In a study by Dake *et al.* [28] of 19 patients with acute dissection and a patent false lumen, this technique produced complete thrombosis of false lumen in 79%, partial thrombosis in 21%, and restoration of flow to ischemic arteries with relief of corresponding symptoms in 76%. Larger studies with more patients and longer follow-up are needed before stent-graft therapy becomes a standard therapy for distal aortic dissection.

A, A contrast-enhanced CT scan of the chest demonstrating a stent-graft in the descending aorta of a patient who presented with a type B aortic dissection. Note that there is flow in the true lumen (within the stent) but the false lumen (outside the stent) has thrombosed.

B, A three-dimensional reconstruction in the left anterior oblique view of the contrast-enhanced CT scan of the same patient demonstrating the position of the stent-graft within the descending thoracic aorta.

Aortic Aneurysms

Aortic aneurysm refers to enlargement of the aorta when its maximal diameter is greater than 1.5 times that of the adjacent proximal normal segment. The normal diameter of the thoracic aorta is approximately 2.5 cm at the aortic annulus, 3 cm at the tubular ascending portion, 2.5 cm at the descending thoracic aorta, and 2 cm in the infrarenal abdominal aorta. Abdominal aortic aneurysm is also defined when the diameter of the abdominal aorta exceeds 3 cm. Aneurysms are classified according to the segment of aorta affected and include thoracic, thoracoabdominal, and abdominal aortic aneurysms. Aneurysms of the thoracic aorta are associated with advanced age, hypertension, bicuspid aortic valve, and inherited disorders, such as familial thoracic aortic aneurysm syndrome, Marfan syndrome, and Ehlers-Danlos type IV syndrome. These are often characterized by elastic fiber degeneration, necrosis of muscle cells, and cystic spaces filled with mucoid material, particularly in Marfan syndrome. Other etiologies of thoracic aortic aneurysms include infections (such as tuberculosis and syphilis), vasculitis (such as Takayasu and giant cell arteritis), aortic dissection, trauma, and congenital defects. Aneurysms of the descending thoracic aorta and abdominal aorta are usually degenerative and often associated with atherosclerosis and some of its risk factors, particularly cigarette smoking. The pathobiology is characterized by an inflammatory process including production of matrix metalloproteinases, which leads to degradation of the extracellular matrix of the aortic wall with subsequent aortic remodeling and dilatation.

Tests used to diagnose aortic aneurysms include ultrasonography, and computed tomographic and magnetic resonance angiography. Catheter-based aortography is used in some circumstances to determine the relationship of the aneurysm to adjacent vascular structures in patients with concomitant arterial occlusive disease and to guide endovascular repair. The risk of aortic aneurysms rupture correlates with diameter. Thoracic aortic aneurysm are generally repaired using standard surgical techniques. The use of endovascular techniques to repair thoracic and thoracoabdominal aortic aneurysms is an ongoing area of clinical research. Open surgical repair is used commonly to treat large abdominal aortic aneurysms. Endovascular repair of abdominal aortic aneurysms is an attractive alternative and has become the procedure of choice for eligible patients in experienced centers. Several controlled trials have found no survival advantage of early elective repair of small abdominal aortic aneurysms compared with careful surveillance when surgical repair is deferred until aneurysm size exceeds 5.5 cm or expands at a rate of 1 cm or more per year. A successful outcome depends upon close serial evaluation by means of appropriate noninvasive imaging methodology and timely, judicious intervention. The long-term survival of patients with abdominal aortic aneurysm is also affected by concomitant coronary and cerebrovascular disease. Cardiovascular risk factor modification is indicated for patients with abdominal aortic aneurysm.

The following figures and legends were originally published in the *Atlas of Vascular Disease* in the chapter by Gornik *et al.* entitled, "Aortic and Arterial Aneurysms" [1].

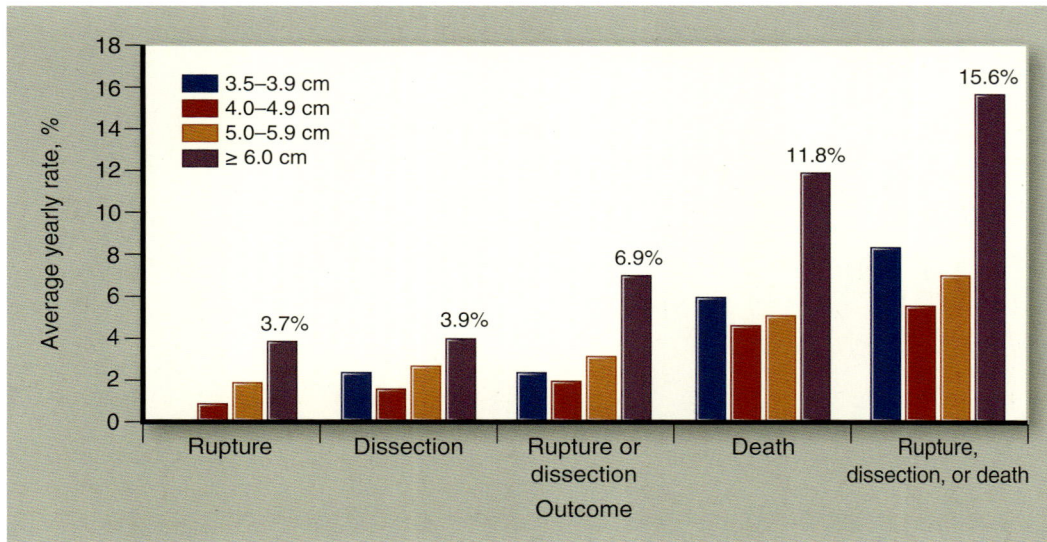

Figure 4-38. Natural history of thoracic aortic aneurysm. The likelihood of an adverse outcome, namely rupture, dissection, or death, increases with aneurysm size. At or above a maximal aortic dimension of 6 cm, the annual rate of a catastrophic event exceeds the risk of surgical repair in most cases. Ascending aortic aneurysms have a slower growth rate (average 0.07 cm/y) compared with descending or thoracoabdominal aortic aneurysms (0.19 cm/y) [29]. (*Adapted from* Davies *et al.* [29], with permission.)

Timing of Surgical Repair of Thoracic Aortic Aneurysm

Ascending aorta
≥ 5.5 cm for most patients
≥ 6.0 cm with comorbidities
≥ 4.5–5.0 cm Marfan syndrome, bicuspid aortic valve, family history of aortic dissection, rapid aneurysm expansion
Descending TAA
≥ 6.5–7.0 cm for most patients
≥ 6.0 Marfan syndrome for prior aortic dissection

Figure 4-39. Timing of surgical repair of thoracic aortic aneurysms (TAA). The operative risk for each patient must be weighed against the risk of rupture or dissection. A lower threshold for repair is generally applied to patients with high-risk features for dissection, such as the Marfan syndrome or the familial aortic aneurysm syndromes. For high-risk patients of advanced age with multiple comorbidities, or for high-risk surgical procedures, such as descending thoracic aneurysm repair, a higher threshold for repair is applied.

Prevalence of Abdominal Aortic Aneurysm, by Size

Diameter, *cm*	Prevalence, %
≥ 3.0	4.2
≥ 4.0	1.3
≥ 5.0	0.5
≥ 6.0	0.2
≥ 7.0	0.1
≥ 8.0	0.03

Figure 4-40. Prevalence of abdominal aortic aneurysm (AAA). Prevalence of AAA by diameter in the Veterans Administration Cooperative Study of 126,196 men between 50 and 79 years of age with no history of documented AAA who underwent ultrasound screening [30].

Variables Associated With Aneurysm Rupture

Baseline Variable*	Hazard Ratio (95% CI)	P
Age, *y*	1.02 (0.93–1.13)	0.067
Female sex	4.50 (1.98–10.2)	0
AAA diameter, *cm*	2.51 (1.08–5.80)	0.032
Current smoker†	2.11 (0.95–4.67)	0.066
Mean BP, *mm Hg*	1.04 (1.02–1.07)	0.002

*Cox regression analysis; all baseline variables adjusted for one another.
†People who never smoked and ex-smokers were combined and compared with current smokers.

Figure 4-41. Variables associated with abdominal aortic aneurysm (AAA) rupture. In addition to initial AAA diameter in the United Kingdom Small Aneurysm Trial of 2257 patients, estimated hazard ratios identified female sex, higher mean arterial blood pressure (BP), and current smoking as factors associated with increased risk of aneurysm rupture. The cohort included patients whose AAA diameter never exceeded 4.0 cm or who were unfit for or refused surgery. When the analysis was limited to a more homogenous group of 1090 otherwise healthy patients with AAAs 4.0 to 5.5 cm in diameter (with 25 that ruptured), current smoking had borderline significance, whereas initial AAA diameter, female sex, and higher mean BP were independently and significantly associated with rupture [31].

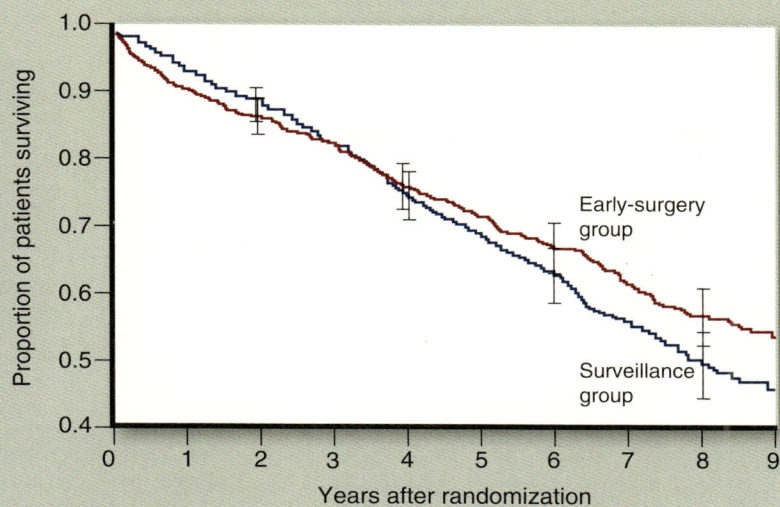

Figure 4-42. Surveillance versus early repair of small abdominal aortic aneurysms (AAAs). The risk of rupture is low for AAAs smaller than 5 cm in diameter. The UK Small Aneurysm Trial [32] and a Veterans Administration Cooperative Study [33] addressed whether early elective surgery would reduce mortality. In the UK study, 1090 patients 60 to 76 years of age with asymptomatic AAAs 4.0 to 5.5 cm in diameter were randomized to early elective open surgery (*n* = 563) or ultrasonographic surveillance (*n* = 527) and were followed for a mean of 8 years, with surgical repair recommended if the diameter of aneurysms in the surveillance group exceeded 5.5 cm. There was a survival disadvantage for patients in the elective surgery group early in the follow-up period, balanced by a higher rate of aneurysm rupture in the surveillance group. Mortality did not differ significantly between groups at 8 years, though women had a higher risk of aneurysm rupture than men. Ultrasonographic surveillance for small AAAs was a safe initial strategy [32]. Findings in the Veterans Administration Cooperative Trial were similar [33].

Indications for Repair of Abdominal Aortic Aneurysm

≥ 5.5 cm for most patients

> 5 cm an option for good surgical and/or endovascular candidates

Consider referral for repair for female patients at 5 cm

Expansion > 1 cm per year

Symptomatic compression of surrounding structures

Aortic wall tenderness

Distal atheroembolism

Figure 4-43. Indications for repair of abdominal aortic aneurysms.

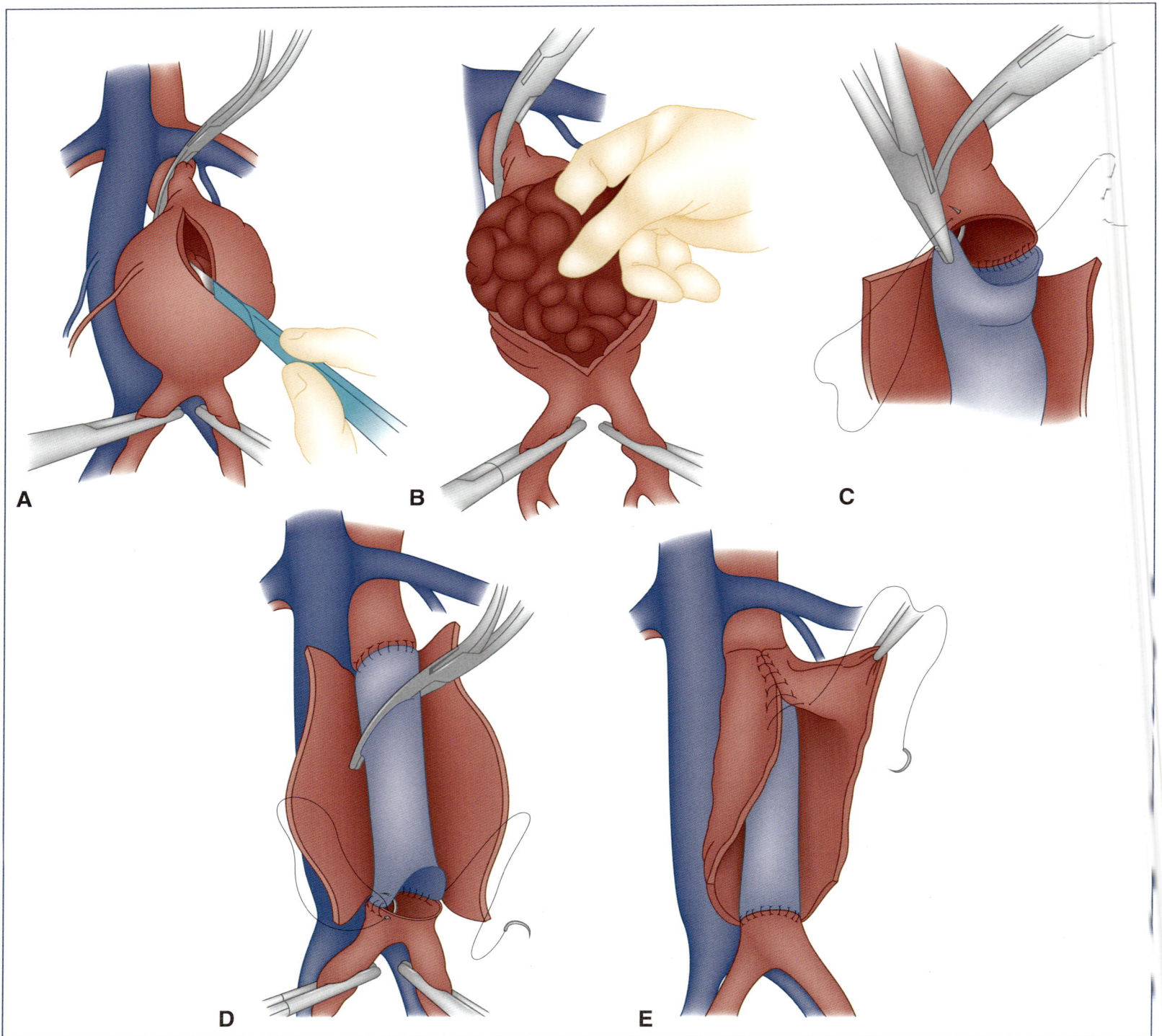

Figure 4-44. Surgical technique for repair of infrarenal abdominal aortic aneurysm. **A,** Following retroperitoneal exposure, the aneurysm is isolated between occluding cross-clamps and the sac is incised longitudinally. **B,** Intraluminal thrombus is evacuated and backbleeding lumbar vessels are oversewn. **C,** The proximal anastomosis is formed by continuously suturing the graft end-to-end to the neck of the aneurysm. **D,** The distal anastomosis is completed at the aortic bifurcation, also using monofilament suture. **E,** After flow is restored, the wall of the aneurysm is reapproximated over the graft to protect adjacent viscera. Open surgical repair of nonruptured abdominal aortic aneurysm is associated with a mortality rate of approximately 5% [34,35]. (*Adapted from* Greenhalgh [36].)

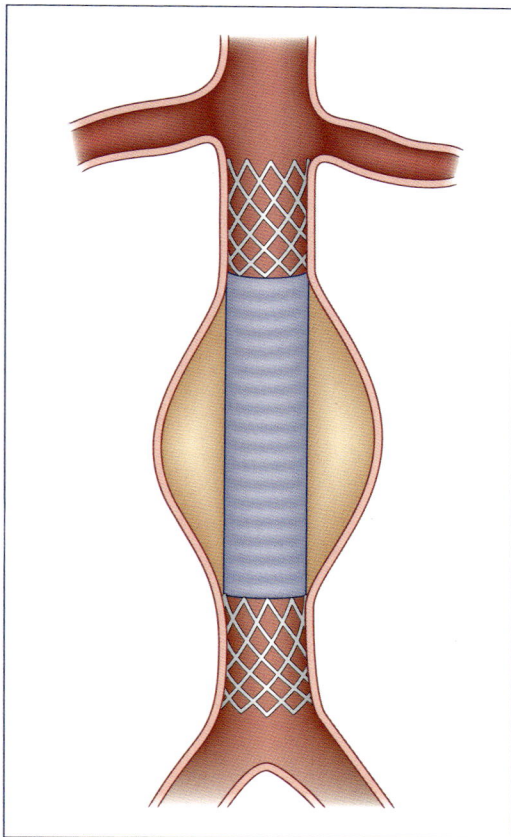

Figure 4-45. Diagram showing an endovascular stent graft in an infrarenal abdominal aortic aneurysm. (*Adapted from* Parodi *et al.* [37].)

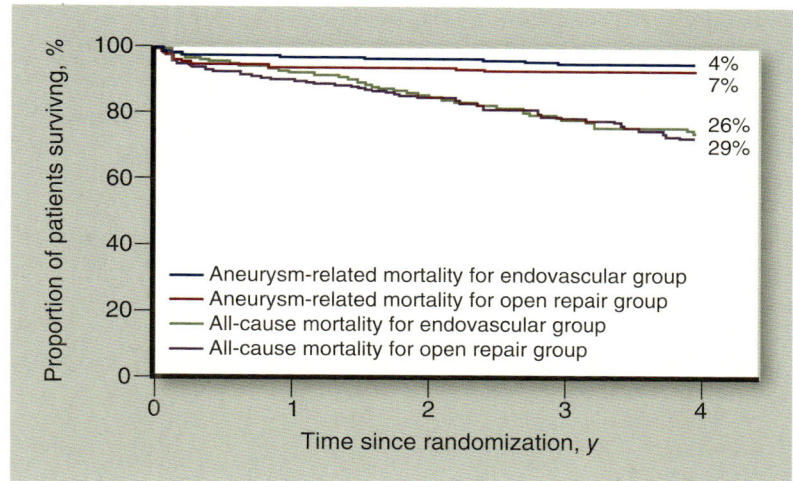

Figure 4-46. Open versus endovascular repair of abdominal aortic aneurysms: mid-term outcomes from the Endovascular Aneurysm Repair (EVAR)-1 trial. Two large randomized clinical trials randomly allocated patients with abdominal aortic aneurysm to undergo open or endovascular repair [38,39]. In the EVAR-1 trial, although there was decreased 30-day mortality in the endovascular aneurysm repair group, there were no differences in overall survival during a 4-year follow-up period. Endovascular aneurysm repair was associated with improved aneurysm-related survival, which was largely due to a reduction in perioperative events compared with open repair. Endovascular repair was associated with a much higher rate of reintervention during the follow-up period, 41% versus 20% in the open repair group. The general findings of the DREAM (Diabetes REduction Assessment with ramipril and rosiglitazone Medication) study were similar during a 2-year follow-up period. (*Adapted from* EVAR Trial [39].)

References

1. *Atlas of Vascular Disease*, edn 3. Edited by Creager MA. Philadelphia: Current Medicine Group; 2008.

2. Hirsch AT, Haskal ZJ, Hertzer NR, *et al.*: ACC/AHA 2005 guidelines for the management of patients with peripheral arterial disease (lower extremity, renal, mesenteric, and abdominal aortic): executive summary a collaborative report from the American Association for Vascular Surgery/Society for Vascular Surgery, Society for Cardiovascular Angiography and Interventions, Society for Vascular Medicine and Biology, Society of Interventional Radiology, and the ACC/AHA Task Force on Practice Guidelines (Writing Committee to Develop Guidelines for the Management of Patients With Peripheral Arterial Disease) endorsed by the American Association of Cardiovascular and Pulmonary Rehabilitation; National Heart, Lung, and Blood Institute; Society for Vascular Nursing; TransAtlantic Inter-Society Consensus; and Vascular Disease Foundation. *J Am Coll Cardiol* 2006, 47:1239–1312.

3. Norgren L, Hiatt WR, Dormandy JA, *et al.*: Inter-Society Consensus for the Management of Peripheral Arterial Disease (TASC II). *J Vasc Surg* 2007, 45:S5–S67.

4. Criqui MH, Fronek A, Barrett-Connor E, *et al.*: The prevalence of peripheral arterial disease in a defined population. *Circulation* 1985, 71:510–515.

5. McDaniel MD, Cronenwett JL: Basic data related to the natural history of intermittent claudication. *Ann Vasc Surg* 1989, 3:273–277.

6. O'Hare AM, Katz R, Shlipak MG, *et al.*: Mortality and cardiovascular risk across the ankle-arm index spectrum: results from the Cardiovascular Health Study. *Circulation* 2006, 113:388–393.

7. Hirsch AT, Rooke TW: Peripheral vascular diseases. In *Cardiovascular Medicine*, edn 2. Edited by Cohn JN, Willerson JT. New York: Churchill-Livingstone; 2000:1398–1416.

8. Hiatt WR, Regensteiner JG, Hargarten ME, *et al.*: Benefit of exercise conditioning for patients with peripheral arterial disease. *Circulation* 1990, 81:602–609.

9. Cooper CJ, Murphy TP, Matsumoto A, *et al.*: Stent revascularization for the prevention of cardiovascular and renal events among patients with renal artery stenosis and systolic hypertension: rationale and design of the CORAL trial. *Am Heart J* 2006, 152:59–66.

10. Olin JW, Begelman SM: Renal artery disease. In *Textbook of Cardiovascular Medicine*. Edited by Topol EJ. Philadelphia: Lippincott-Raven; 2002:2139–2159.

11. Rosamond W, Flegal K, Friday G, *et al.*: Heart disease and stroke statistics–2007 update: a report from the American Heart Association Statistics Committee and Stroke Statistics Subcommittee. *Circulation* 2007, 115:e69–e171.

12. Thrift AG, Dewey HM, Macdonell RA, *et al.*: Incidence of the major stroke subtypes: initial findings from the North East MElbourne Stroke Incidence Study (NEMESIS). *Stroke* 2001, 32:1732–1738.

13. Petty GW, Brown RD Jr, Whisnant JP, *et al.*: Ischemic stroke subtypes: a population-based study of incidence and risk factors. *Stroke* 1999, 30:2513–2516.

14. North American Symptomatic Carotid Endarterectomy Trial Collaborators. Beneficial effect of carotid endarterectomy in symptomatic patients with high-grade carotid stenosis. *N Engl J Med* 1991, 325:445–453.

15. Halliday A, Mansfield A, Marro J, *et al.*: Prevention of disabling and fatal strokes by successful carotid endarterectomy in patients without recent neurological symptoms: randomised controlled trial. *Lancet* 2004, 363:1491–1502.

16. Yadav JS, Wholey MH, Kuntz RE, *et al.*: Protected carotid-artery stenting versus endarterectomy in high-risk patients. *N Engl J Med* 2004, 351:1493–1501.

17. Eagle KA, Doroghazi RM, DeSanctis RW, Austen WG: Aortic dissection. In *The Practice of Cardiology*, edn 2. Edited by Eagle KA, *et al.* Boston: Little Brown; 1989:1369-1392.

18. Januzzi JL, Isselbacher EM, Fattori R, *et al.*: Characterizing the young patient with aortic dissection: results from the International Registry of Aortic Dissection (IRAD). *J Am Coll Cardiol* 2004, 43:665–669.

19. O'Gara PT, DeSanctis RW: Aortic dissection. In *Vascular Medicine*. Edited by Loscalzo J, Creager MA, Dzau VJ. Boston: Little Brown; 1992:931–956.

20. Debakey ME, Henly WS, Cooley DA, *et al.*: Surgical management of dissecting aneurysms of the aorta. *J Thorac Cardiovasc Surg* 1965, 49:130–149.

21. Miller DC, Mitchell RS, Oyer PE, *et al.*: Independent determinants of operative mortality for patients with aortic dissections. *Circulation* 1984, 70:I153–I164.

22. Trimarchi S, Nienaber CA, Rampoldi V, *et al.*: Contemporary results of surgery in acute type A aortic dissection: the International Registry of Acute Aortic Dissection experience. *J Thorac Cardiovasc Surg* 2005, 129:112–122.

23. Glower DD, Fann JI, Speier RH, *et al.*: Comparison of medical and surgical therapy for uncomplicated descending aortic dissection. *Circulation* 1990, 82:IV39–IV46.

24. Trimarchi S, Nienaber CA, Rampoldi V, *et al.*: Role and results of surgery in acute type B aortic dissection: insights from the International Registry of Acute Aortic Dissection (IRAD). *Circulation* 2006, 114:I357–I364.

25. Stone DH, Brewster DC, Kwolek CJ, *et al.*: Stent-graft versus open-surgical repair of the thoracic aorta: mid-term results. *J Vasc Surg* 2006, 44:1188–1897.

26. Isselbacher EM: Disease of the aorta. In *Heart Disease: A Textbook of Cardiovascular Medicine*, edn 6. Edited by Braunwald E, Zipes DP, Libby P. Philadelphia: WB Saunders; 2001:422–456.

27. Tsai TT, Fattori R, Trimarchi S, *et al.*: Long-term survival in patients presenting with type B acute aortic dissection: insights from the International Registry of Acute Aortic Dissection. *Circulation* 2006, 114:2226–2231.

28. Dake MD, Kato N, Mitchell RS, *et al.*: Endovascular stent-graft placement for the treatment of acute aortic dissection. *N Engl J Med* 1999, 340:1546–1552.

29. Davies RR, Goldstein LJ, Coady MA, *et al.*: Yearly rupture or dissection rates for thoracic aortic aneurysms: simple prediction based on size. *Ann Thorac Surg* 2002, 73:17–27; discussion 27–28.

30. Lederle FA, Johnson GR, Wilson SE, *et al.*: The aneurysm detection and management study screening program: validation cohort and final results. Aneurysm Detection and Management Veterans Affairs Cooperative Study Investigators. *Arch Intern Med* 2000, 160:1425–1430.

31. Brown LC, Powell JT: Risk factors for aneurysm rupture in patients kept under ultrasound surveillance. UK Small Aneurysm Trial Participants. *Ann Surg* 1999, 230:289–296; discussion 96–97.

32. United Kingdom Small Aneurysm Trial Participants: Long-term outcomes of immediate repair compared with surveillance of small abdominal aortic aneurysms. *N Engl J Med* 2002, 346:1445–1452.

33. Lederle FA, Wilson SE, Johnson GR, *et al.*: Immediate repair compared with surveillance of small abdominal aortic aneurysms. *N Engl J Med* 2002, 346:1437–1444.

34. Prinssen M, Verhoeven EL, Buth J, *et al.*: A randomized trial comparing conventional and endovascular repair of abdominal aortic aneurysms. *N Engl J Med* 2004, 351:1607–1618.

35. Greenhalgh RM, Brown LC, Kwong GP, *et al.*: Comparison of endovascular aneurysm repair with open repair in patients with abdominal aortic aneurysm (EVAR trial 1), 30-day operative mortality results: randomised controlled trial. *Lancet* 2004, 364:843–848.

36. Greenhalgh RM: *Vascular Surgical Techniques: An Atlas*. Philadelphia: WB Saunders; 1989.

37. Parodi JC, Palmaz JC, Barone HD: Transfemoral intraluminal graft implantation for abdominal aortic aneurysms. *Ann Vasc Surg* 1991, 5:491–499.

38. Blankensteijn JD, de Jong SE, Prinssen M, *et al.*: Two-year outcomes after conventional or endovascular repair of abdominal aortic aneurysms. *N Engl J Med* 2005, 352:2398–2405.

39. Endovascular aneurysm repair versus open repair in patients with abdominal aortic aneurysm (EVAR trial 1): randomised controlled trial. *Lancet* 2005, 365:2179–2186.

Heart Failure

5

Michael M. Givertz and Wilson S. Colucci

Epidemiology

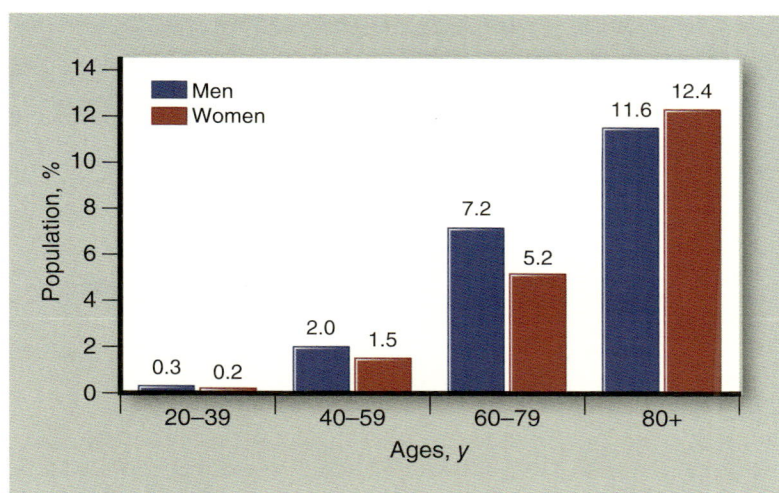

Figure 5-1. Prevalence of heart failure. In the United States, 5.2 million adults are affected by heart failure. Heart failure is more commonly a disease of the elderly and this is reflected in age-specific prevalence rates. Less than 1% of men and women experience heart failure between the ages of 20 and 39 years, compared with approximately 12% of men and women 80 years old or older. (*Adapted from* American Heart Association [1].)

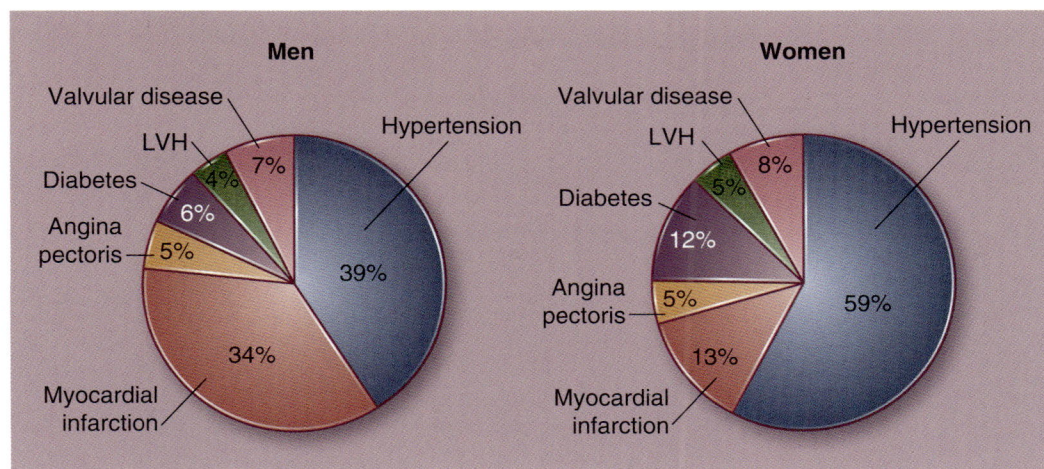

Figure 5-2. Population attributable risk (PAR) for heart failure incidence. Based on longitudinal data from the Framingham Heart Study, the risk factors contributing most significantly to the PAR of heart failure in men were previous myocardial infarction and hypertension (in men both represented equal contributions to heart failure PAR). In contrast, hypertension was the risk factor accounting for the majority of total PAR in women. In women, previous myocardial infarction accounted for only 13% of the PAR of heart failure compared with 34% in men. LVH—left ventricular hypertrophy. (*Adapted from* Levy et al. [2].)

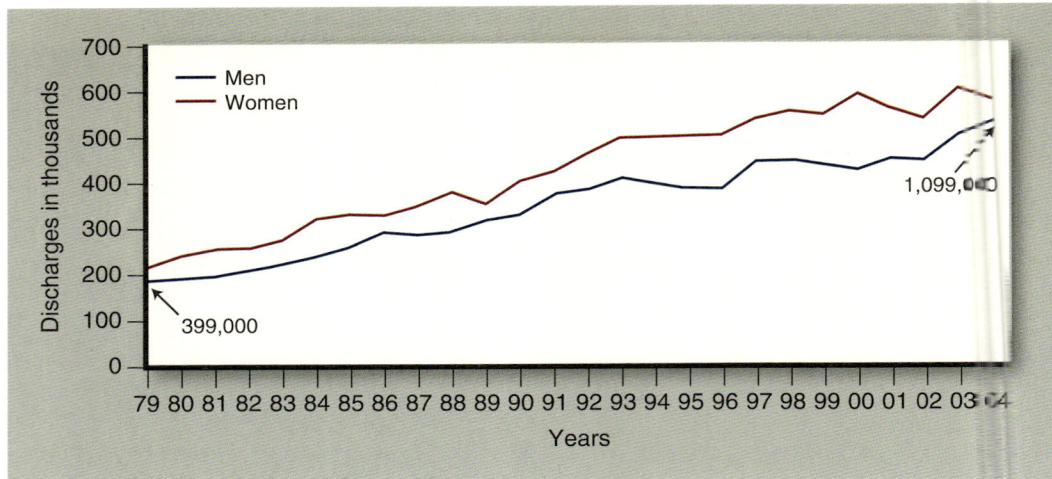

Figure 5-3. Hospital discharges for heart failure from 1979 to 2005. Rates of hospital discharges among men and women increased 175% from 399,000 visits in 1979 to over 1 million visits in 2005. From 1999 to 2000, the number of ambulatory medical visits for heart failure was 3.4 million. (*Adapted from* Rosamond *et al.* [3].)

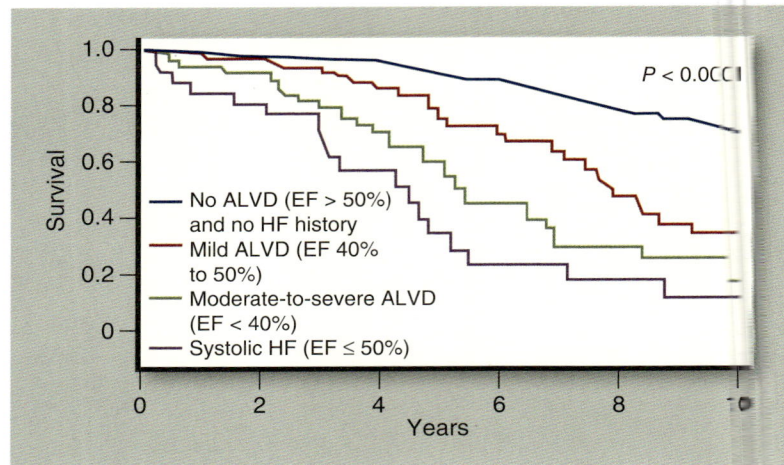

Figure 5-4. Natural history of patients with asymptomatic left ventricular dysfunction (ALVD) in the Framingham Heart Study. The referent group consists of subjects with normal left ventricular systolic function (ejection fraction [EF] > 50%) and no history of heart failure (HF). Mild ALVD indicates mild asymptomatic left ventricular systolic dysfunction (EF 40%–50%). Moderate-to-severe ALVD indicates moderate-to-severe asymptomatic left ventricular systolic dysfunction (EF < 40%). Systolic HF indicates HF with EF ≤ 50%. The median survival for subjects was 7.9 years for those with mild ALVD, 5.4 years for those with moderate-to-severe ALVD, and 4.6 years for those with a history of overt HF and left ventricular (LV) systolic dysfunction. The age- and sex-adjusted hazard ratios for mortality associated with mild ALVD, moderate-to-severe ALVD, and overt systolic HF were 1.9 (CI, 1.3–2.8), 3.1 (CI, 2.0–4.7), and 5.0 (CI, 3.1–8.0), respectively (with no ALVD as the referent). The findings indicate that mild ALVD is prognostically important, with rates of HF and death that are two- to fourfold higher than those of individuals with normal LV systolic function. Importantly, the median survival free of HF was almost 10 years in those with mild ALVD, suggesting a window of opportunity during which these individuals could be identified and treated, provided optimal therapy could be determined. (*Adapted from* Wang *et al.* [4].)

Ventricular Function and Remodeling

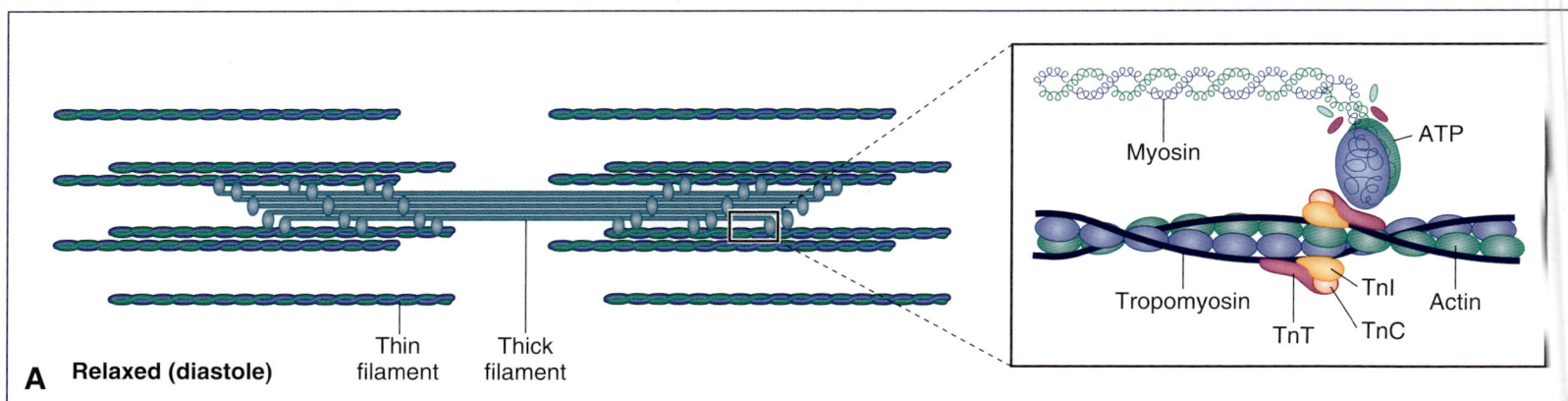

A **Relaxed (diastole)**

Figure 5-5. Cardiac contraction is brought about by interactions between actin in the thin filament and myosin cross-bridges that project from the thick filament. **A,** In relaxed muscle, where troponin C (TnC) is not bound to calcium, the "relaxed" conformation of the troponin complexes and tropomyosin prevents actin in the thin filament from interacting with the myosin cross-bridges. As a result, actin is unable to convert the chemical energy of the adenosine triphosphatase (ATP) bound to the myosin cross-bridges into mechanical work.

Continued on the next page

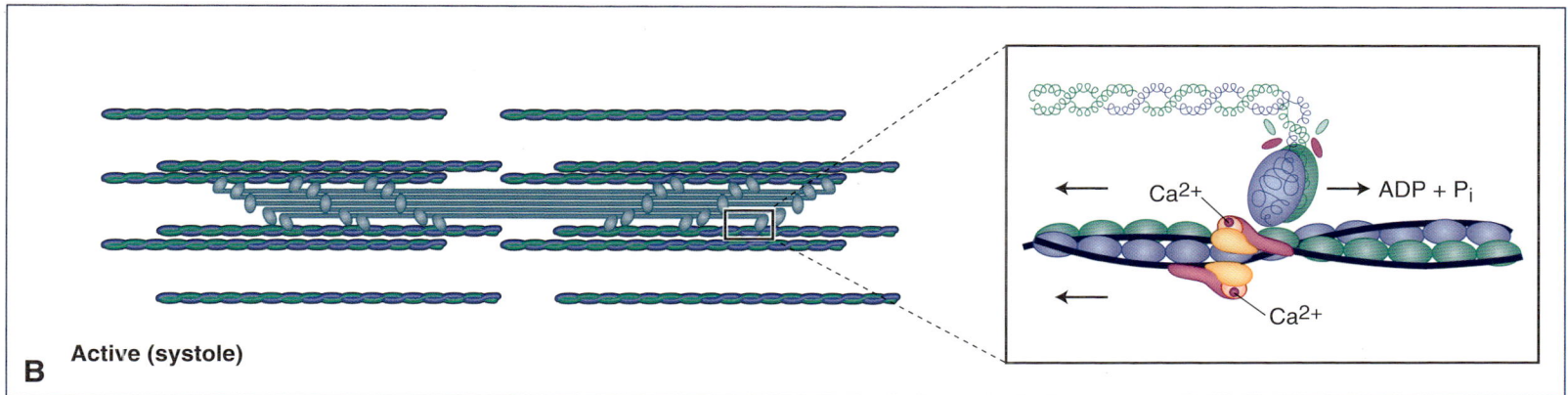

B Active (systole)

Figure 5-5. *(Continued)* **B,** In active muscle, Ca^{2+} bound to TnC has shifted the troponin complexes and tropomyosin to an "active" conformation that enables actin to interact with the myosin cross-bridges. Release of chemical energy when actin stimulates hydrolysis of myosin-bound ATP enables the cross-bridges to "row" the thin filaments toward the center of the sarcomere. ADP—adenosine diphosphate; TnI—troponin I; TnT—troponin T.

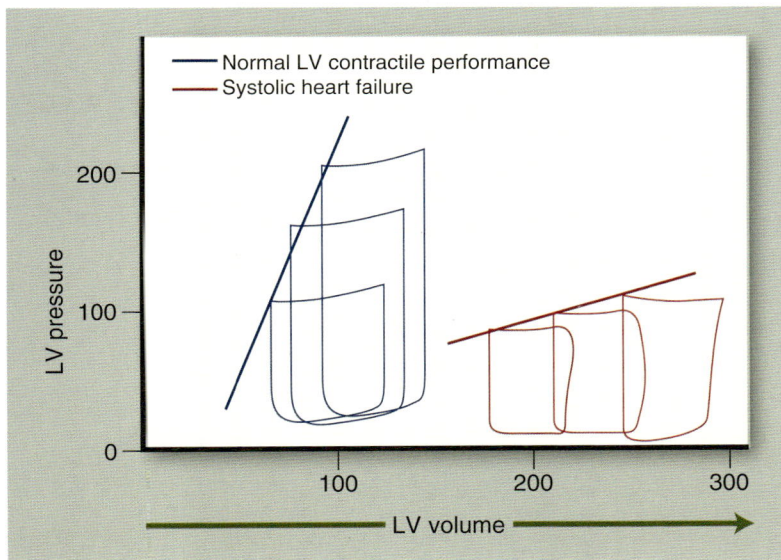

Figure 5-6. Series of left ventricular (LV) pressure–volume loops for a heart with normal myocardial contractility and a heart with contractile dysfunction. The principal problem with systolic heart failure because of myocardial injury is LV remodeling through dilatation, altered arterial characteristics and, thereby, afterload, and assumption of a spherical geometric shape. All of these adaptations result in a reduction in systolic performance. As seen in these pressure–volume loops, the normal heart has a steep slope indicating that little change occurs in end-systolic volume over a wide range of LV pressures. In contrast, the heart with systolic heart failure demonstrates little change in these pressures over a wide range of LV end-systolic volumes. If the slope of this relationship, end-systole elastance, is less than 1 mm Hg/mL, this reflects depressed myocardial contractility as in patients with systolic heart failure [5].

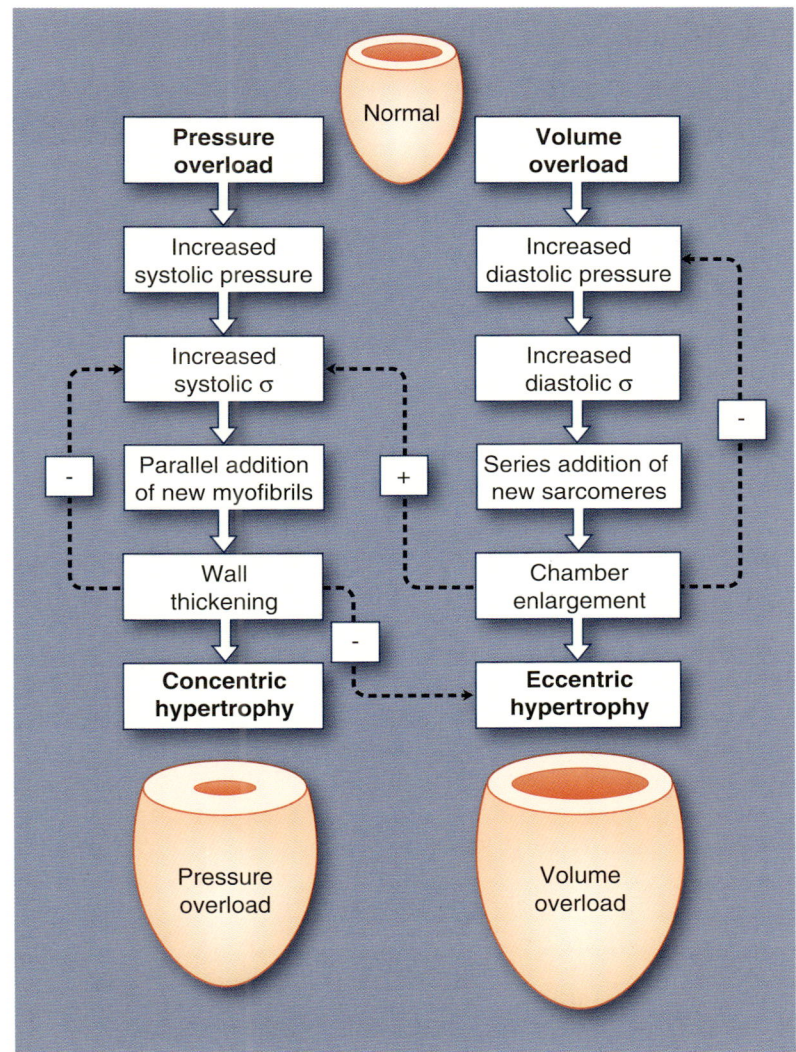

Figure 5-7. Patterns of ventricular hypertrophy. Specific patterns of ventricular remodeling occur in response to the imposed augmentation in workload. A pattern of hypertrophic growth characterized as concentric, in which increased mass is out of proportion to chamber volume, is particularly effective in reducing systolic wall stress(es) under conditions of heightened pressure load. In contrast, in volume overload conditions in which the major stimulus is diastolic loading, a predominant finding is a great increase in the cavity size or volume. Although there can be extensive increases in mass, the relationship between mass and volume is preserved or, in severe cases, reduced. The fundamental response is generated by cellular hypertrophy. However, the configuration of the new contractile tissue is specific and offsets the major mechanical stimulus. (*Adapted from* Grossman and Carabello [6].)

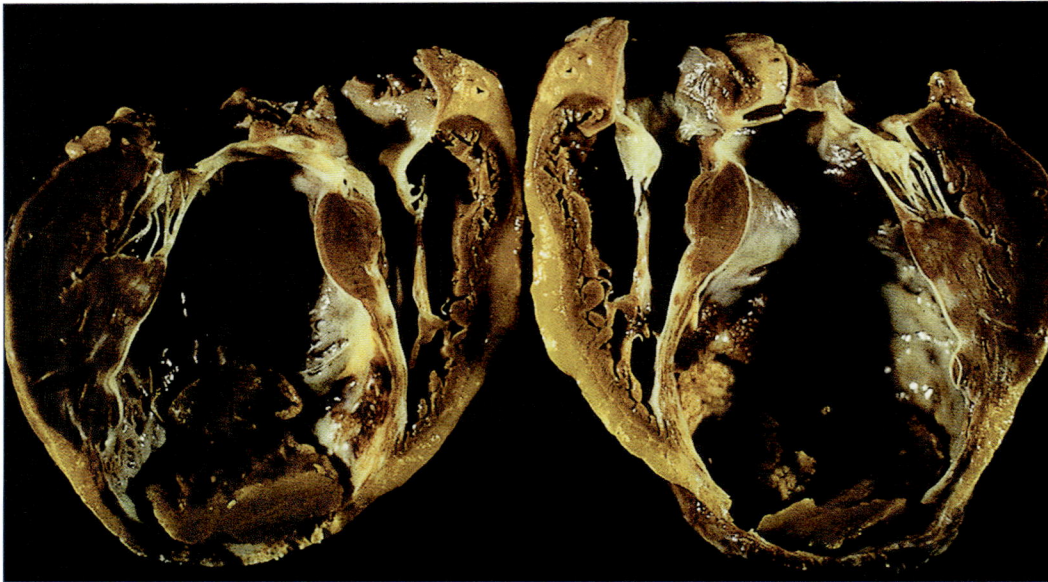

Figure 5-8. A heart removed from a cardiac transplant recipient. This specimen, from a survivor of a large anterior, septal, and apical infarction, demonstrates the thinning and elongation of the infarcted region, the cavity enlargement, and hypertrophy of the remaining segment, as well as a large apical thrombus. (*Courtesy of* Dr. Lynda Biedrzycki, Boston, MA.)

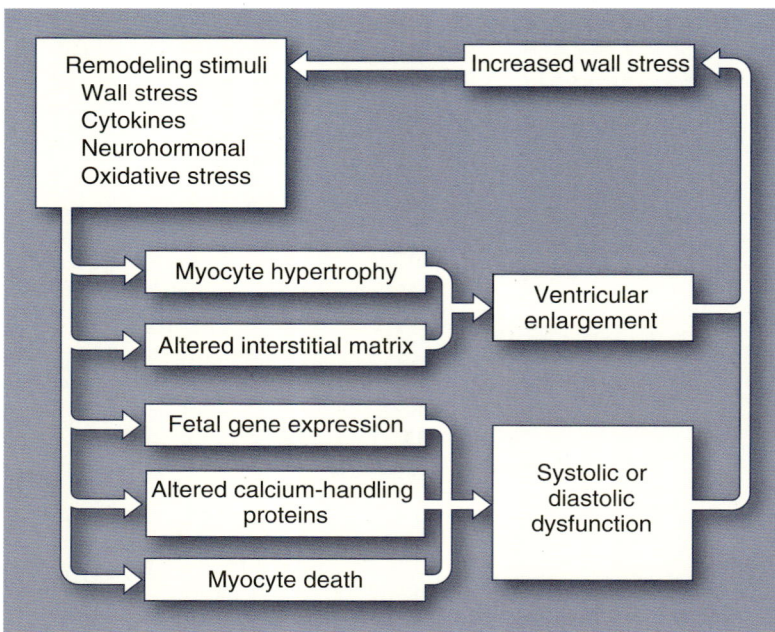

Figure 5-9. Remodeling stimuli. Chronic hemodynamic stimuli such as pressure and volume overload lead to ventricular remodeling through increases in myocardial wall stress, cytokines, signaling peptides, neuroendocrine signals, and perhaps, oxidative stress. The myocardium responds with adaptive as well as maladaptive changes. Re-expression of fetal contractile proteins and calcium handling proteins may contribute to impaired contraction and relaxation. Myocytes unable to adapt might be triggered to undergo programmed cell death (apoptosis). The net result of these changes is further impairment in pump function and increased wall stress, thus completing a vicious cycle that leads to further progression of myocardial dysfunction.

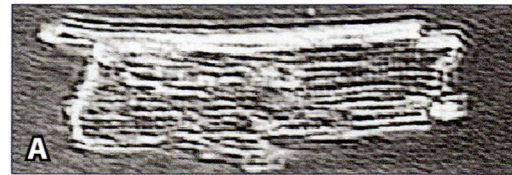

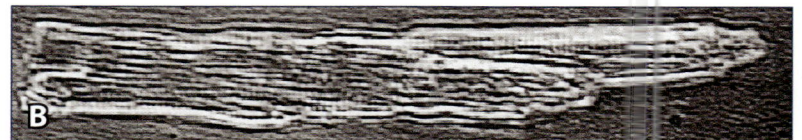

Figure 5-10. Isolated cardiac myocytes obtained from mice showing cellular hypertrophy. **A,** Myocyte from the left ventricle of the normal mouse heart. **B,** Hypertrophied myocyte from the left ventricle of a mouse 6 months after myocardial infarction, viewed at the same magnification as in *A.* In the myocyte from the failing heart, there has been a series of sarcomeres added, which are otherwise organized into a normal pattern. The resulting myocyte elongation, a form of hypertrophy, likely contributes to ventricular dilatation that occurs during myocardial remodeling.

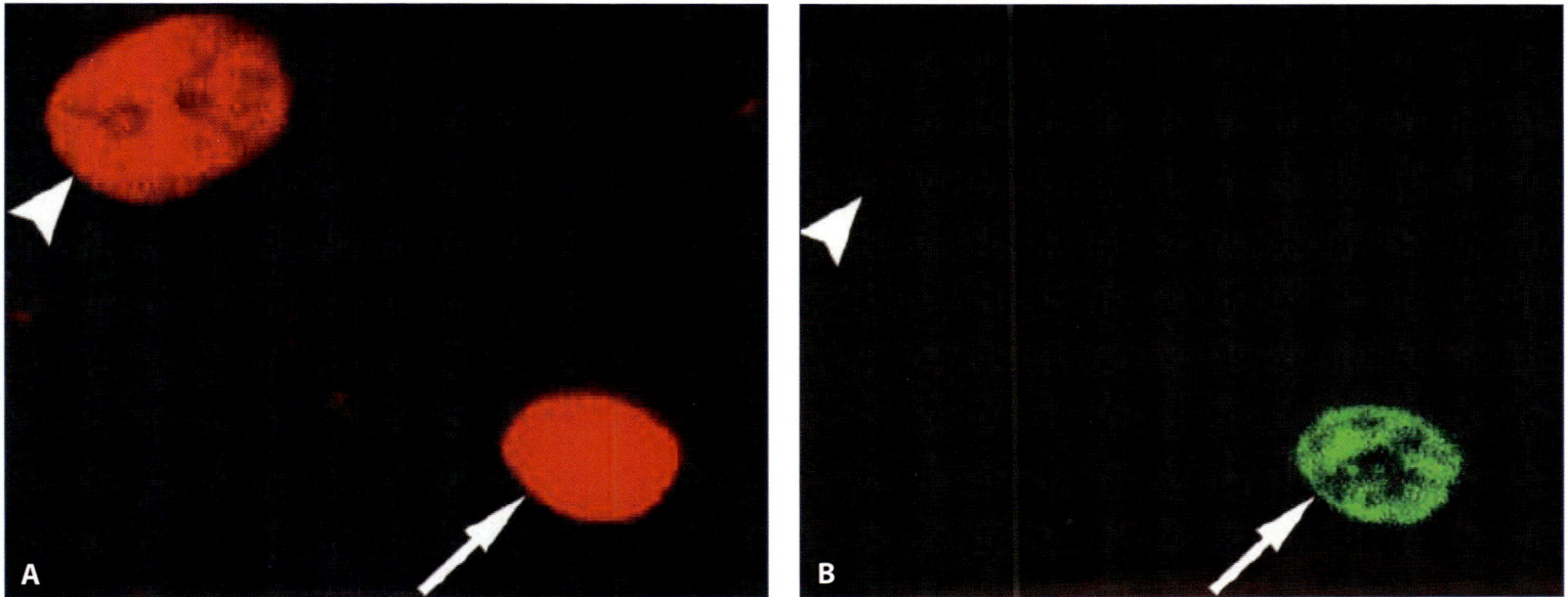

Figure 5-11. Loss of myocytes in heart failure. The slow loss of myocytes may contribute to the progressive decline in systolic function in heart failure. All cells have the ability to undergo programmed cell death, or apoptosis, in the presence of stimuli that activate the necessary signaling cascades. Cardiac apoptosis appears to play an important role in embryonic life as the heart "remodels" during development. Thus, apoptosis may be part of a fetal gene program. Apoptosis also occurs as a defense mechanism to rid an organ of infected or damaged cells without activation of inflammatory systems as would occur with necrosis. Olivetti *et al.* [7] demonstrated that apoptosis occurs in myocardium obtained from patients with heart failure by staining for fragmented DNA, a hallmark of the apoptotic process. **A,** Confocal microscopy of myocardial nuclei stained with propidium iodide. **B,** DNA fragments labeled with deoxyuridine triphosphate (Tunel) in apoptotic nucleus (*arrow*) but not normal nucleus (*arrowhead*). (*Adapted from* Olivetti *et al.* [7].)

Neurohormonal, Renal, and Vascular Adjustments

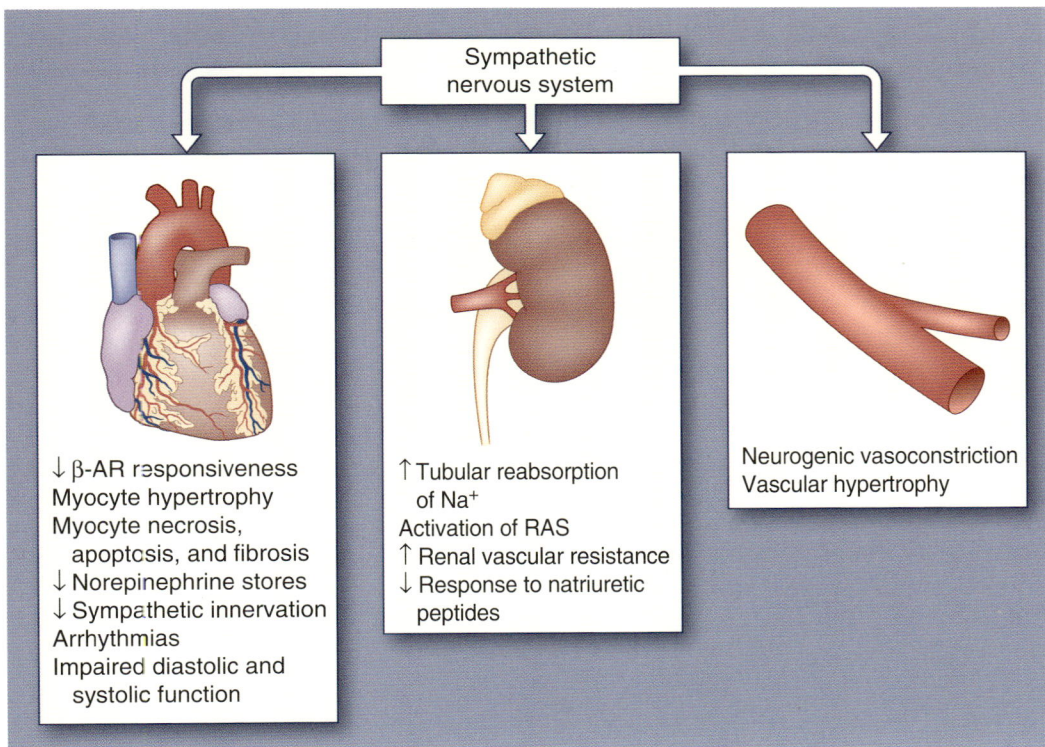

Figure 5-12. Increased sympathetic nervous system activity may contribute to the pathophysiology of heart failure by multiple mechanisms involving cardiac, renal, and vascular function. In the heart, increased sympathetic nervous system outflow may lead to desensitization of postsynaptic β-adrenergic receptors (β-AR), nonuniform depletion of norepinephrine stores, nonuniform destruction of sympathetic innervation, arrhythmias, and impairment of diastolic and systolic function, and act directly on myocardial cells, causing myocyte hypertrophy, necrosis, apoptosis, and fibrosis. In the kidneys, increased sympathetic activation induces arterial and venous vasoconstriction, activation of the renin-angiotensin system (RAS), increase in salt and water retention, and an attenuated response to natriuretic peptides. In the peripheral vessels, neurogenic vasoconstriction and vascular hypertrophy are induced by increased sympathetic activity. (*Adapted from* Floras [8].)

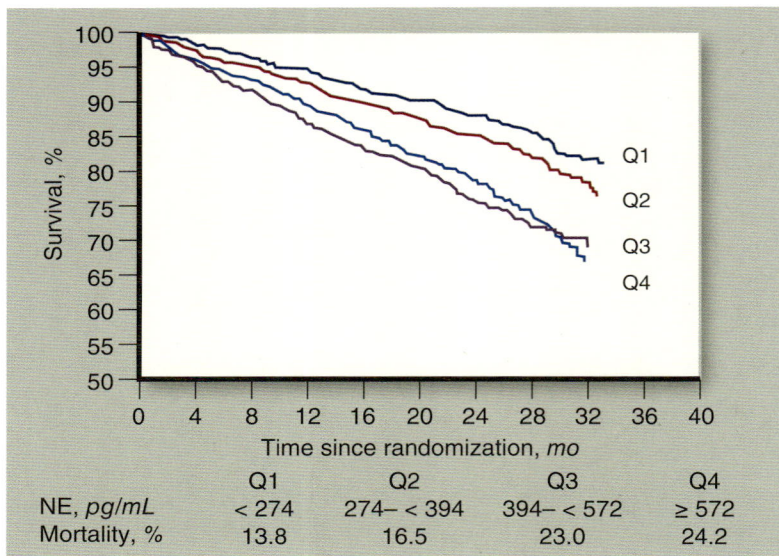

Figure 5-13. The level of activation of the sympathetic nervous system predicts survival in patients with chronic heart failure (HF).

Anand *et al.* [9] measured plasma norepinephrine (NE) levels in approximately 4300 patients with stable symptomatic HF and a left ventricular ejection fraction less than 40% enrolled in the Valsartan Heart Failure Trial (Val-HeFT). After randomization, patients were observed prospectively for all-cause mortality or first morbid event (defined as death, sudden death with resuscitation, hospitalization for HF, or intravenous inotropic or vasodilator therapy for at least 4 hours). The mean ± SD for plasma NE was 464 ± 323 pg/mL (median, 394 pg/mL). As shown by the Kaplan-Meier curves, baseline NE in quartiles showed a significant quartile-dependent increase in mortality and first morbid event. (*Adapted from* Anand *et al.* [9].)

	Q1	Q2	Q3	Q4
NE, *pg/mL*	< 274	274– < 394	394– < 572	≥ 572
Mortality, %	13.8	16.5	23.0	24.2

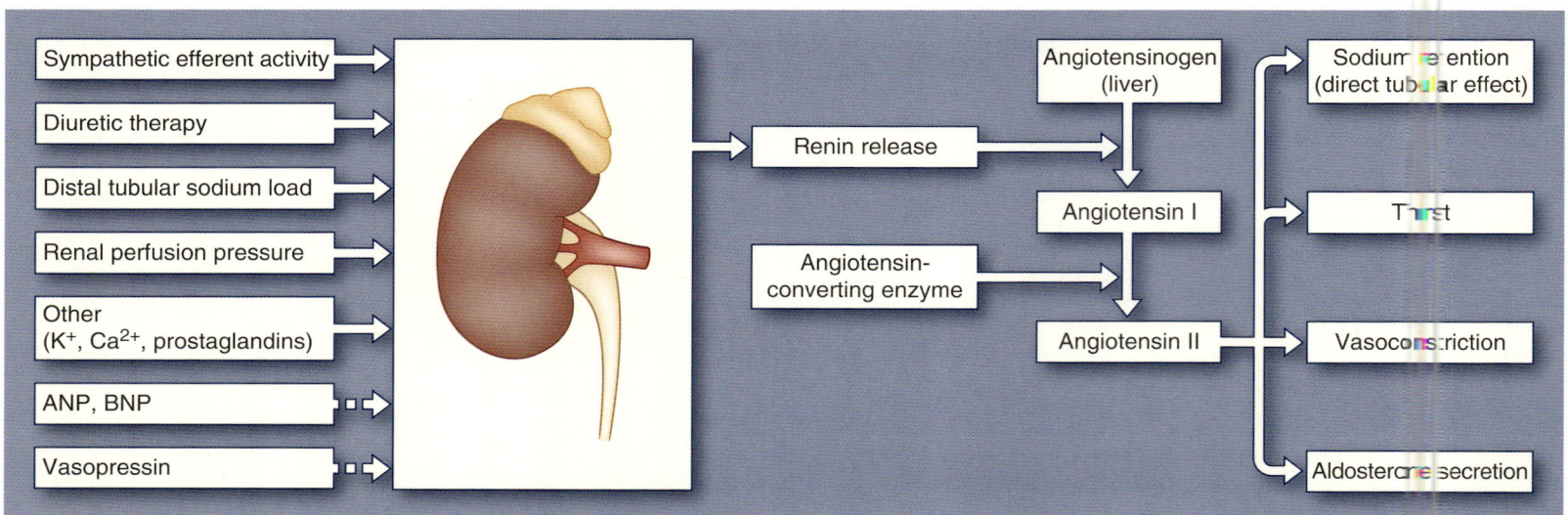

Figure 5-14. The renin-angiotensin system is activated in patients with heart failure. The major site of release of circulating renin is the juxtaglomerular apparatus of the kidney, where multiple stimuli may contribute to renal release of renin into the systemic circulation, including increased renal sympathetic efferent activity, decreased distal tubular sodium delivery, reduced renal perfusion pressure, and diuretic therapy. Natriuretic peptides (ANP, BNP), and vasopressin (*dashed arrows*) may inhibit the release of renin. Renin enzymatically cleaves angiotensinogen, a tetrapeptide produced in the liver, to form the inactive decapeptide angiotensin I. Angiotensin I is converted to the octapeptide angiotensin II by angiotensin-converting enzyme. Angiotensin II is a potent vasoconstrictor; it promotes sodium reabsorption by increasing aldosterone secretion and by a direct effect on the tubules, and it stimulates water intake by acting on the thirst center. Angiotensin II causes vasoconstriction directly and may also facilitate the release of norepinephrine by acting on sympathetic nerve endings. (*Adapted from* Paganelli *et al.* [10].)

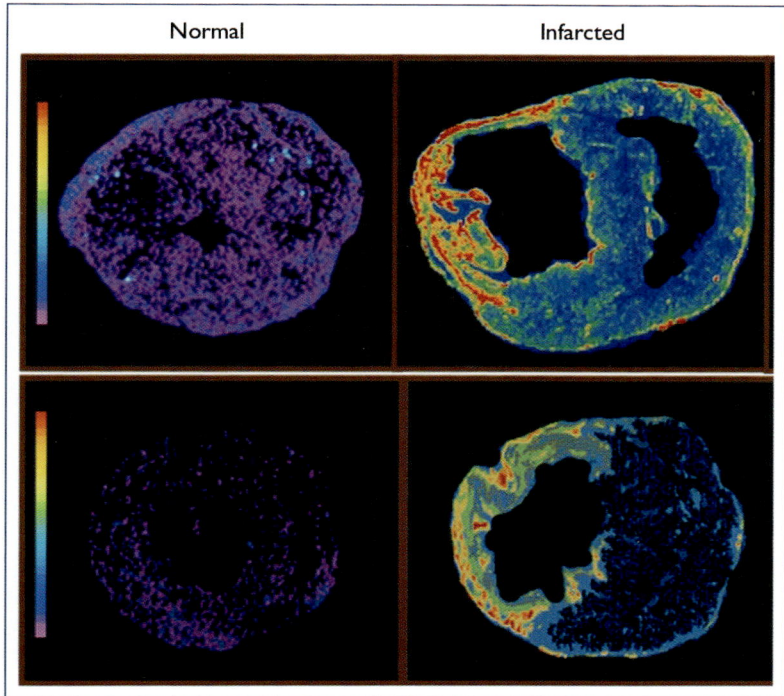

Figure 5-15. Autoradiograph showing angiotensin-converting enzyme (ACE) binding (*upper panel*) in the normal (*left*) and infarcted (*right*) rat heart. The lower panel shows angiotensin II receptor binding in the normal (*left*) and infarcted (*right*) rat heart. These data demonstrate upregulation of binding of ACE and the angiotensin receptor after infarction. (*Adapted from* Sun and Weber [11,12].)

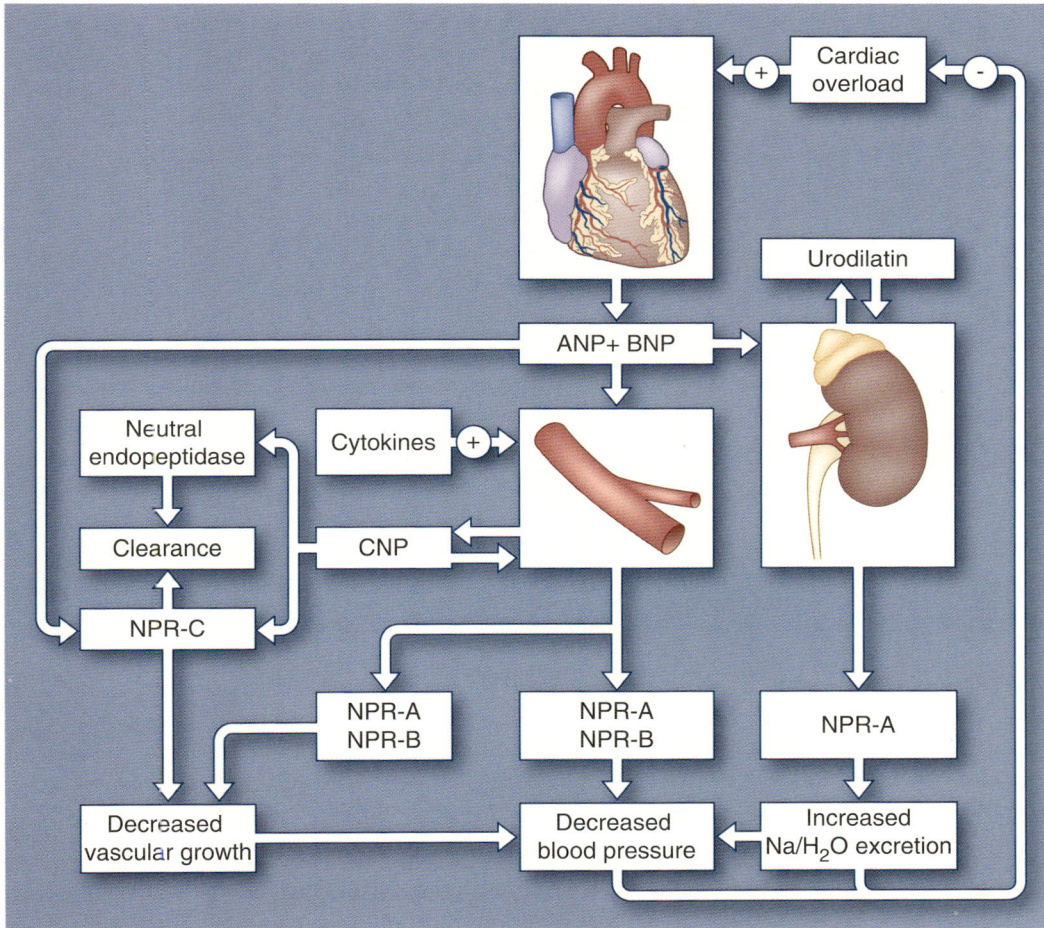

Figure 5-16. The natriuretic peptide family. The natriuretic peptides include atrial natriuretic peptide (ANP), B-type natriuretic peptide (BNP), C-type natriuretic peptide (CNP), and urodilatin. ANP is derived from a prohormone composed of 126 amino acids, and it is secreted primarily from cardiac atria. The prohormone is cleaved to an N-terminal fragment (ANP1-98) and a C-terminal fragment (ANP99-126). BNP, identified initially in brain, is secreted from atria and ventricles, particularly the latter. CNP has been identified primarily in brain but is also present in vascular endothelial cells. Urodilatin, or ANP95-126, is found in urine. Stretch receptors in the atria and ventricles detect changes in cardiac chamber volume related to increased cardiac filling pressures, resulting in release of ANP and BNP, but not CNP. The natriuretic peptides are inactivated by neutral endopeptidases. The actions of the natriuretic peptides are mediated by natriuretic peptide receptors (NPRs), designated NPR-A, NPR-B, and NPR-C. NPR-A and NPR-B are particulate guanylate cyclases, activation of which increases levels of cGMP. Natriuretic peptide receptors have been localized in vascular smooth muscle, endothelium, platelets, the adrenal glomerulosa, and the kidney. ANP and BNP increase urine volume and sodium (Na) excretion, decrease vascular resistance, and inhibit release of renin and secretion of aldosterone and vasopressin. CNP reduces vascular resistance but, despite its name, does not have natriuretic properties. (*Adapted from* Wilkins *et al.* [13].)

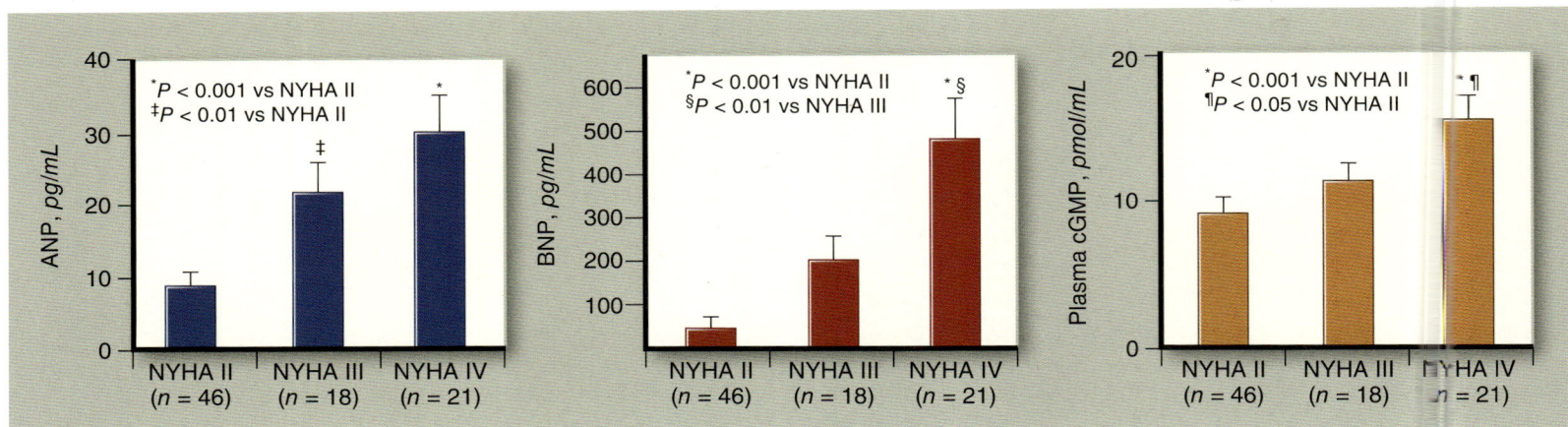

Figure 5-17. Measurement of natriuretic peptides in patients with heart failure. The prognostic information derived from measurement of natriuretic peptides in patients with heart failure was assessed by Tsutamoto et al. [14]. Plasma levels of atrial natriuretic peptide (ANP), B-type natriuretic peptide (BNP), and cGMP were measured in 85 patients with chronic heart failure who were observed for 2 years. The concentrations of ANP, BNP, and cGMP increased proportionally with the functional severity of heart failure. In a Kaplan-Meier analysis of the cumulative rates of survival in patients with heart failure stratified into two groups on the basis of the median plasma concentration of BNP (73 pg/mL), it was shown that survival was significantly worse in the group with the higher plasma BNP levels. A stepwise multivariate analysis, which included ANP, BNP, norepinephrine, New York Heart Association (NYHA) functional class, selected hemodynamic indices, and demographic features found that only a high concentration of plasma BNP ($P < 0.0001$) and pulmonary capillary wedge pressure ($P = 0.003$) were significant independent predictors of mortality. (Adapted from Tsutamoto et al. [14].)

Clinical Features

Framingham Criteria for Diagnosis of Heart Failure

Major criteria	Minor criteria
Paroxysmal nocturnal dyspnea	Extremity edema
Neck vein distention	Dyspnea on exertion
Rales	Hepatomegaly
Cardiomegaly	Pleural effusion
Acute pulmonary edema	Vital capacity reduced by one third from normal
S_3 gallop	Tachycardia ($\geq$ 120 bpm)
Increased venous pressure (> 16 cm H_2O)	
Positive hepatojugular reflux	**Major or minor**
	Weight loss $\geq$ 4.5 kg over 5 days' treatment

Figure 5-18. A constellation of symptoms and abnormal physical findings may be used in making the diagnosis of heart failure. The Framingham Study, for example, suggested that several specific clinical criteria be combined and weighted. To establish a clinical diagnosis of heart failure by this method, at least one major and two minor criteria are required [15]. bpm—beats per minute.

Figure 5-19. Complementary classification schemes of the heart failure syndrome. The approach most commonly used to quantify the degree of functional limitation imposed by heart failure is the New York Heart Association (NYHA) classification system, whereby patients are assigned a score based on the degree of effort needed to elicit symptoms. However, the NYHA classification is a subjective assessment that may change over short periods of time, and there is a poor relation between functional capacity and measured cardiac performance. This has led to a new approach to the classification of heart failure that emphasizes the development and progression of disease, allowing objective classification of patients and initiation of preventive therapies. Stage A includes patients at risk for heart failure, including those with hypertension, atherosclerotic heart disease, diabetes, obesity, the metabolic syndrome, or those using cardiotoxins or with a family history of cardiomyopathy. Stage B denotes patients with structural heart disease but no heart failure symptoms, including those with previous myocardial infarction, left ventricular hypertrophy, reduced ejection fraction, or asymptomatic valvular heart disease. Stage C describes patients with known structural heart disease and heart failure symptoms, while stage D is reserved for patients with severe, refractory heart failure requiring frequent hospitalizations and consideration of advanced therapies such as transplant. The staging and functional classification systems are complementary, since patients with stage B heart failure have no symptoms. Patients with stage C heart failure move between NYHA class I, II, III, and IV, and stage D heart failure includes those patients with NYHA class IV symptoms. ACC—American College of Cardiology; AHA—American Heart Association. (*Adapted from* Farrell *et al.* [16].)

Classification of Heart Failure

ACC-AHA Stage	NYHA Functional classification
A At high risk for heart failure but without structural heart disease or symptoms	None
B Structural heart disease but without symptoms of heart failure	**I** Asymptomatic
C Structural heart disease with prior or current symptoms of heart failure	**II** Symptoms with moderate exertion
	III Symptoms with minimal exertion
D Severe, refractory heart failure requiring specialized interventions	**IV** Symptoms at rest

Figure 5-20. Initial assessment of patients presenting with heart failure. The American College of Cardiology/American Heart Association guidelines on chronic heart failure provide recommendations for the initial evaluation of patients presenting with heart failure symptoms [17]. The initial evaluation starts with a thorough history and physical examination, focusing on detection of hypertension, diabetes, dyslipidemia, valvular heart disease, vascular disease, rheumatic fever, mediastinal radiation, sleep-disordered breathing, exposure to cardiotoxic agents (including alcohol, illicit drugs, alternative therapies, or chemotherapy), exposure to sexually transmitted diseases, thyroid disorders, pheochromocytoma, or obesity. A family history of vascular disease, sudden cardiac death, skeletal myopathy or cardiomyopathy, conduction system disease, and arrhythmias is also useful. Laboratory evaluation should also be performed, including complete blood count, serum electrolytes, glycohemoglobin, lipid profile, tests of renal and hepatic function, and thyroid function tests. A chest radiograph is useful to detect cardiomegaly, fluid overload, and pulmonary disease. A 12-lead electrocardiogram is useful to detect abnormalities of cardiac rhythm and conduction, left ventricular hypertrophy, widened QRS duration, and evidence of myocardial ischemia or infarction. After this routine examination, the most useful test is a two-dimensional echocardiogram with Doppler flow studies to detect abnormalities of the myocardium, heart valves, or pericardium. Further studies aimed at identifying the cause of the cardiomyopathy, including coronary arteriography, endomyocardial biopsy, and specialized laboratory testing, may be performed depending on

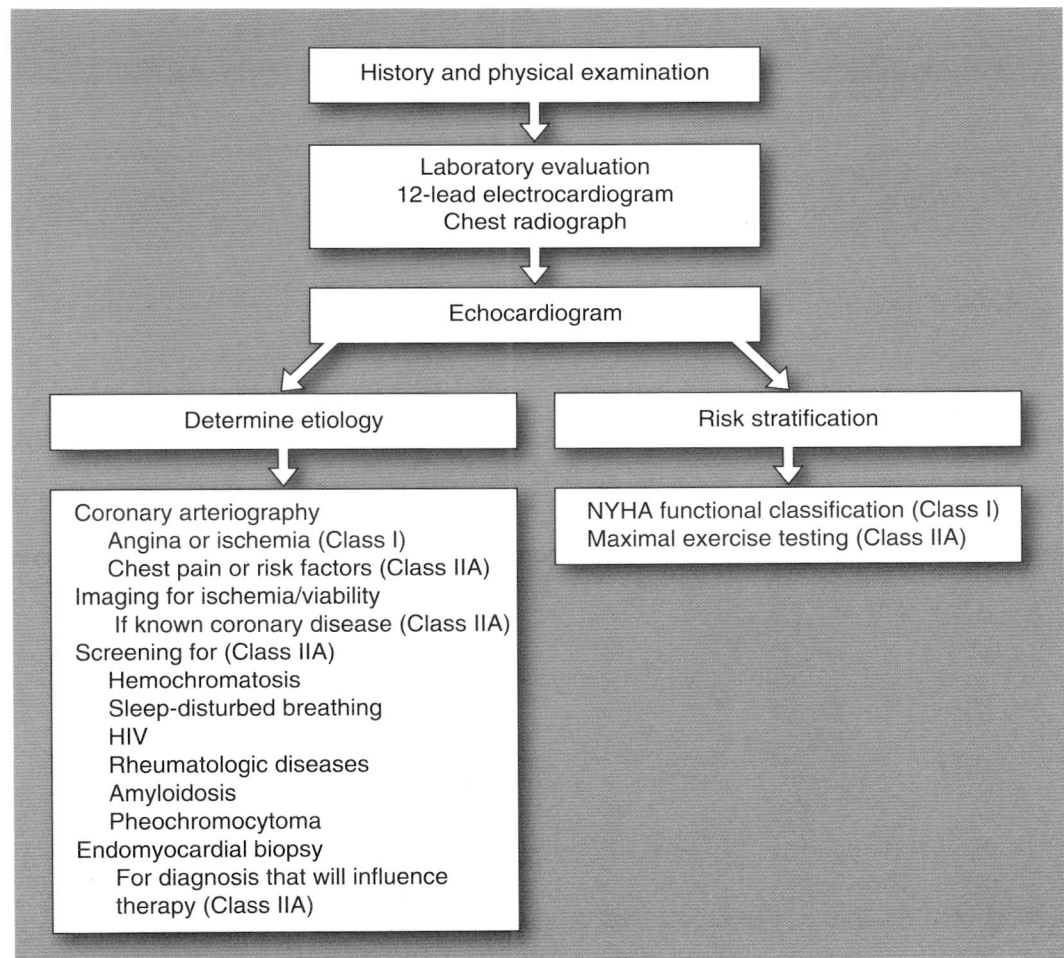

History and physical examination
↓
Laboratory evaluation
12-lead electrocardiogram
Chest radiograph
↓
Echocardiogram
↓ ↓
Determine etiology | Risk stratification
↓ | ↓
Coronary arteriography
  Angina or ischemia (Class I)
  Chest pain or risk factors (Class IIA)
Imaging for ischemia/viability
  If known coronary disease (Class IIA)
Screening for (Class IIA)
  Hemochromatosis
  Sleep-disturbed breathing
  HIV
  Rheumatologic diseases
  Amyloidosis
  Pheochromocytoma
Endomyocardial biopsy
  For diagnosis that will influence
  therapy (Class IIA)
                    | NYHA functional classification (Class I)
Maximal exercise testing (Class IIA)

information from the history and physical examination. Finally, it is essential to risk-stratify patients using the New York Heart Association (NYHA) classification, degree of decompensation, and, in selected patients, using maximal exercise testing with measurement of oxygen consumption.

Left Ventricular Failure Versus Right Ventricular Failure

	Left ventricular failure	Right ventricular failure
Etiology	Cardiomyopathy	Left ventricular failure
	Left-sided valvular disease	Right-sided valvular disease
		Pulmonary hypertension
		Constrictive pericarditis
Symptoms		
Dyspnea	++	+
Fatigue	++	++
Increasing abdominal girth	0	+
Anorexia	0	+
Signs		
Rales	+	0
Elevated JVP	+	++
Ascites	0	+
Dependent edema	+	++
Laboratory findings		
Chest radiography	Pulmonary vascular congestion, alveolar edema	Pleural effusions
Hepatic enzymes	Normal	Increased

Figure 5-21. Left ventricular failure versus right ventricular failure. Patients with systolic heart failure commonly have a combination of left and right ventricular failure, since the most common cause of right ventricular failure is left ventricular failure. Right ventricular failure is also seen in pulmonary hypertension and constrictive pericarditis. Patients with heart failure and preserved systolic function, on the other hand, present primarily with signs and symptoms of left ventricular failure. In left ventricular failure, cardiac output decreases and pulmonary venous pressure increases, causing extravasation of fluid into the interstitial space and alveoli, reducing pulmonary compliance and increasing the work of breathing even before marked pulmonary edema decreases arterial oxygenation. In right ventricular failure, systemic venous pressure increases, causing fluid extravasation and consequent edema, primarily in dependent tissues and abdominal viscera. Chronic venous congestion in the viscera can cause anorexia and malabsorption. The liver is affected most, but stomach and intestine also become congested and ascites can occur. Right ventricular failure commonly causes moderate hepatic dysfunction, with modest increases in bilirubin, prothrombin time, and hepatic enzymes. JVP—jugular venous pressure.

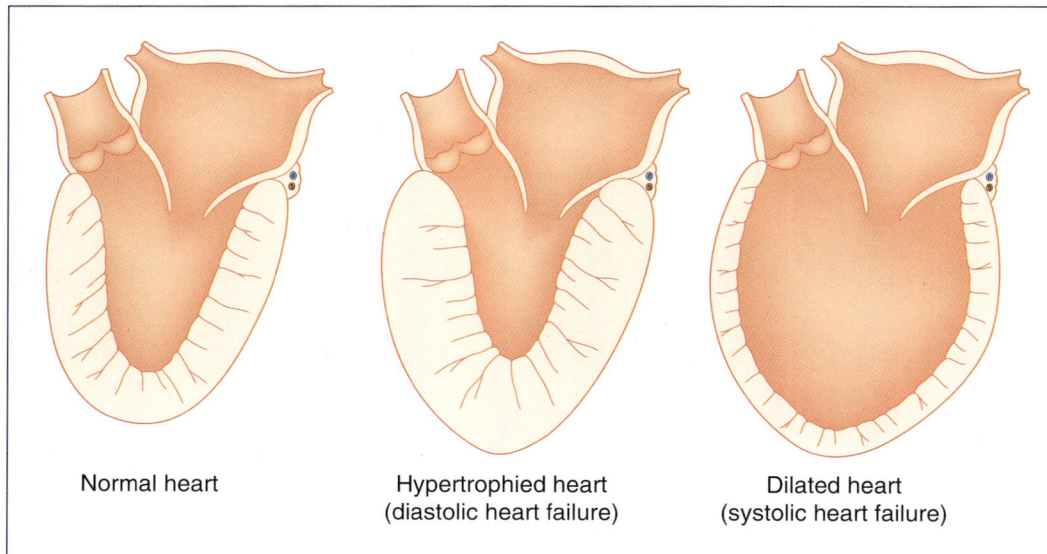

Normal heart

Hypertrophied heart (diastolic heart failure)

Dilated heart (systolic heart failure)

Figure 5-22. Pathophysiology of heart failure with preserved and reduced systolic function. In heart failure with preserved systolic function, ventricular remodeling results in a normal-sized left ventricular cavity with thickened walls and preserved systolic function. This classically results from conditions resulting in left ventricular hypertrophy, such as long-standing systemic hypertension, aortic stenosis, hypertrophic cardiomyopathy, or infiltrative cardiomyopathies like amyloidosis. In systolic heart failure, remodeling results in a globular heart with thinning of the left ventricular walls, a decrease in systolic function, and a distortion of the mitral valve apparatus, leading to mitral regurgitation. (*Adapted from* Jessup and Brozena [18].)

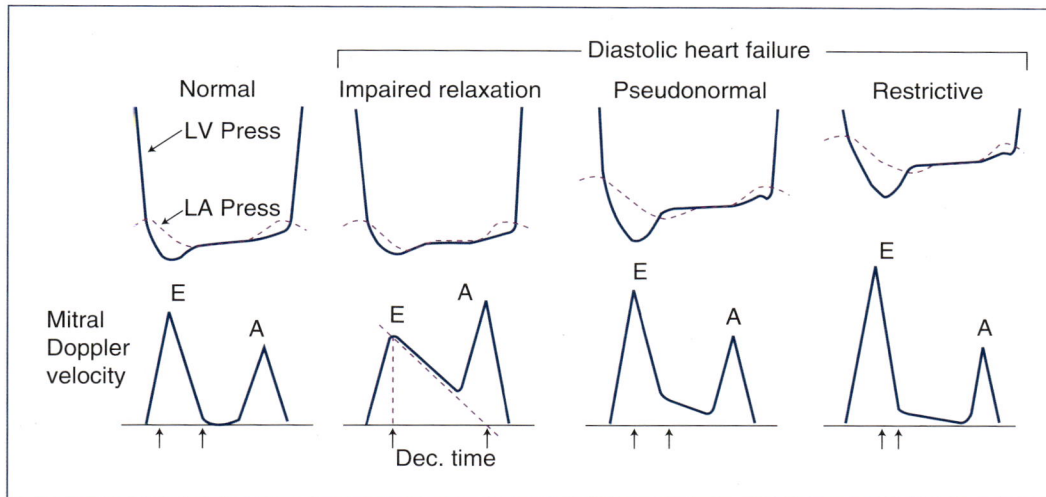

Figure 5-23. Echocardiographic flow signals across the mitral valve used to obtain a clinical impression of the extent to which abnormalities in diastolic function occur in diastolic and systolic heart failure. As shown, progressive changes occur in the pattern of the mitral inflow signals in diastole from normal (*left*) to restrictive (*right*). When there is a change in left ventricular (LV) chamber compliance and a greater dependence on left atrial (LA) contraction for filling, the pattern of E/A reversal is recorded. As pulmonary congestion occurs and pulmonary capillary wedge pressure increases, a pseudo-normal pattern is identified with a shortened deceleration (dec) time from the peak of the E wave. In severe heart failure, the restrictive pattern carries with it a poor outcome if it cannot be reversed with appropriate therapy. (*Adapted from* Zile and Brutsaert [19].)

Characteristics of Patients With Heart Failure With Preserved and Reduced Systolic Function

Characteristic	HF with PSF	Systolic HF
Age	Frequently elderly	All ages, typically 50–70 y
Sex	Frequently female	More often male
Left ventricular ejection fraction	40% or higher	Less than 40%
Left ventricular cavity size	Usually normal	Usually dilated
Left ventricular hypertrophy on echocardiography	Usually present	Sometimes present
Chest radiography	Congestion with or without cardiomegaly	Congestion and cardiomegaly
Gallop rhythm present	Fourth heart sound	Third heart sound
Coexisting conditions		
Hypertension	+++	++
Diabetes mellitus	+++	++
Previous MI	+	+++
Obesity	+++	+
Chronic lung disease	++	0
Sleep apnea	++	++
Long-term dialysis	++	+
Atrial fibrillation	+ (usually proxysmal)	+ (usually persistent)

Figure 5-24. Characteristics of patients with heart failure (HF) with preserved and reduced systolic function. In HF with preserved systolic function (PSF), although the left ventricle contracts normally, relaxation is impaired and cardiac output, especially during exercise, is limited by the abnormal filling characteristics of the ventricle. For a given ventricular volume, ventricular pressures are elevated, leading to pulmonary congestion, dyspnea, and edema identical to the manifestations in patients with systolic heart failure. However, while the symptoms may be similar, the demographic and clinical profiles of patients with HF with preserved and reduced systolic function do differ. Patients with systolic HF are more often male, and can be older since the most common cause of systolic heart failure is ischemic cardiomyopathy. However, patients with HF and PSF are typically elderly, female, and often obese with hypertension and diabetes. Patients with systolic HF often have a third heart sound on examination due to left ventricular dilation, while those with HF and PSF often have a fourth heart sound due to decreased compliance of the left ventricle. Sleep apnea and atrial fibrillation occur commonly in both conditions. MI—myocardial infarction. (*Adapted from* Jessup and Brozena [18].)

Ambulatory Management

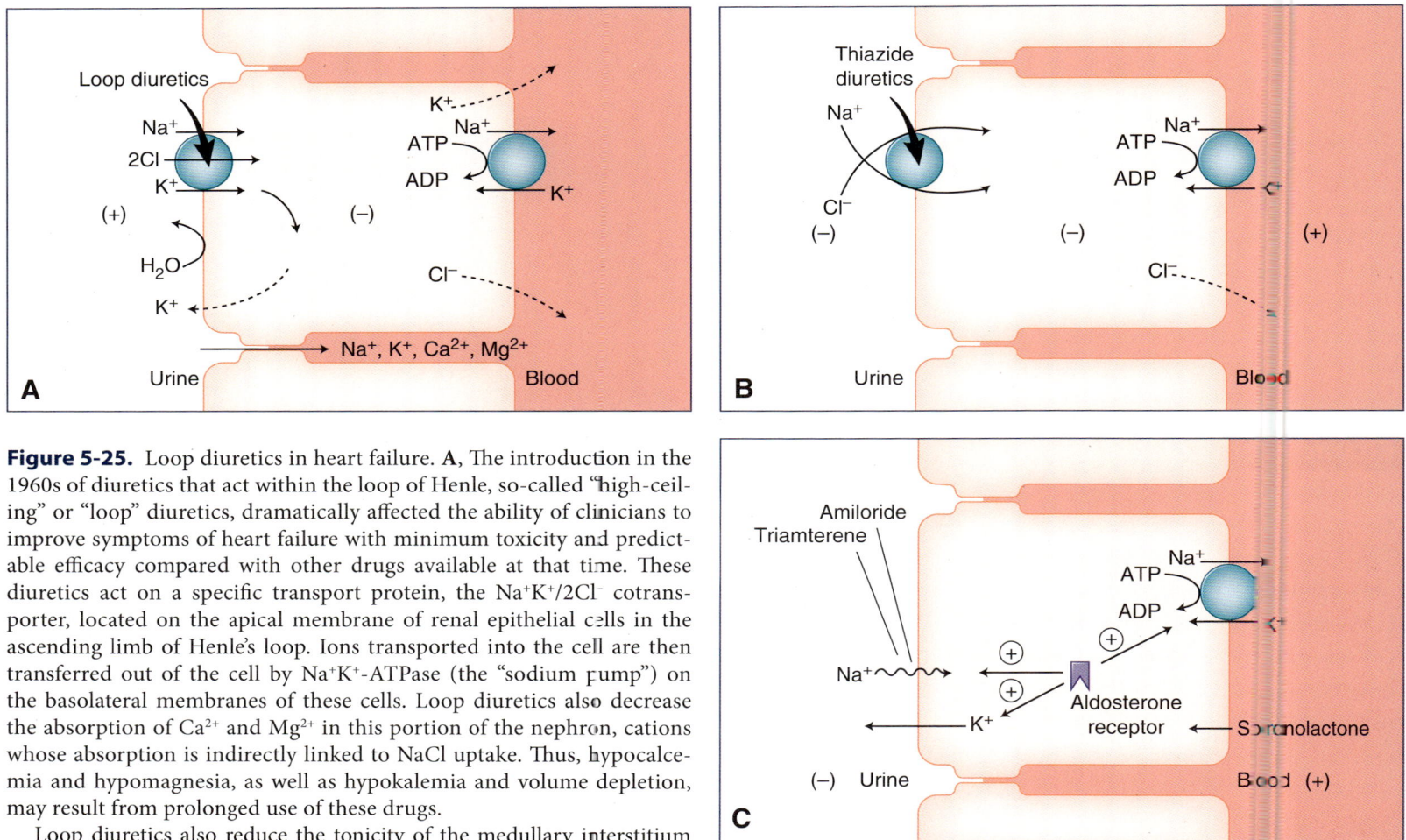

Figure 5-25. Loop diuretics in heart failure. **A,** The introduction in the 1960s of diuretics that act within the loop of Henle, so-called "high-ceiling" or "loop" diuretics, dramatically affected the ability of clinicians to improve symptoms of heart failure with minimum toxicity and predictable efficacy compared with other drugs available at that time. These diuretics act on a specific transport protein, the $Na^+K^+/2Cl^-$ cotransporter, located on the apical membrane of renal epithelial cells in the ascending limb of Henle's loop. Ions transported into the cell are then transferred out of the cell by Na^+K^+-ATPase (the "sodium pump") on the basolateral membranes of these cells. Loop diuretics also decrease the absorption of Ca^{2+} and Mg^{2+} in this portion of the nephron, cations whose absorption is indirectly linked to NaCl uptake. Thus, hypocalcemia and hypomagnesia, as well as hypokalemia and volume depletion, may result from prolonged use of these drugs.

Loop diuretics also reduce the tonicity of the medullary interstitium by preventing the normal uptake of solute in the absence of water in the thick ascending limb of Henle's loop. This limits the kidney's ability to concentrate the urine and may contribute to the development of hyponatremia. The loop diuretics are clearly the most useful diuretics as single agents for patients with decompensated heart failure, in large part because of the magnitude of the natriuresis that can be achieved over a short period, which can reach as high as 20% of the filtered load of sodium. Typically, the fraction of NaCl filtered at the glomerulus and reabsorbed in the ascending limb of the loop of Henle declines from about 20% to 13% with a loop diuretic, resulting in a 1% to 2% increase in the fractional excretion of sodium over 24 hours [19].

B, Thiazide diuretics. In general, the thiazide diuretics are not useful as single drugs for the therapy of volume retention in heart failure patients, largely because their site of action in the distal convoluted tubule permits rapid adjustment of water and solute absorption in other more proximal nephron segments. Interestingly, the target renal tubular protein of the thiazide class of diuretics, the electroneutral Na^+Cl^- cotransporter, has recently been cloned and sequenced. This is the last of the known diuretic-responsive renal epithelial cell transport proteins to be identified. Many other tissues also express this transport protein, which may have important implications for understanding the effectiveness of these drugs in the treatment of hypertension as well as their less desirable metabolic effects on lipid and glucose metabolism. Unlike loop diuretics, thiazides enhance calcium reabsorption but not that of magnesium, although magnesium wasting is much less pronounced than with loop diuretics [19].

C, Potassium-sparing diuretics. The potassium-sparing diuretics fall into two categories: agents such as amiloride and triamterene, which reduce Na^+ conductance through an apical membrane sodium channel; and aldosterone antagonists such as spironolactone, which, by inhibiting the actions of aldosterone at its intracellular receptor in renal epithelial cells of the distal collecting duct, reduce Na^+ uptake from the tubular lumen and decrease K^+ secretion by several mechanisms. Aldosterone antagonists also limit the kidney's ability to acidify the urine by inhibiting the action of aldosterone on a renal tubular proton pump. Although none of these diuretics is effective as a single agent in the treatment of heart failure, they play a useful role in diminishing renal K^+ wasting. When combined with loop or thiazide diuretics, the aldosterone antagonists also prevent Mg^{2+} depletion. Because ACE inhibitors increase the serum K^+ concentration, an effect that may be magnified by β-blockers and nonsteroidal anti-inflammatory drugs, potassium-sparing diuretics should be prescribed cautiously for patients who are already receiving vasodilators of this class [19]. ADP—adenosine diphosphate; ATP—adenosine triphosphate.

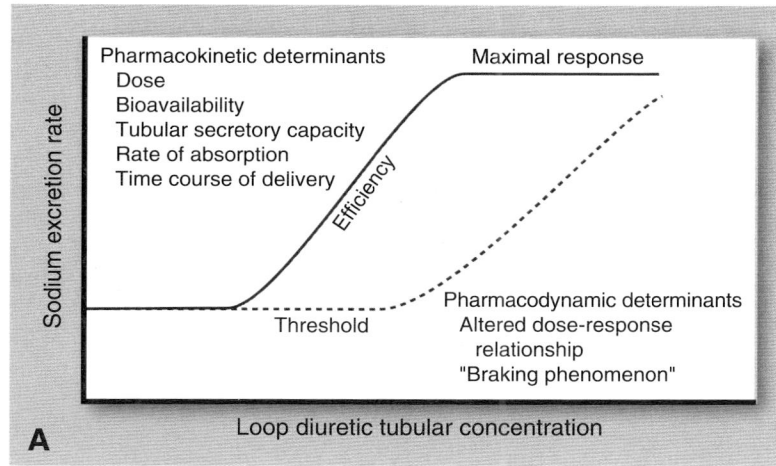

Figure 5-26. A, Pharmacokinetic and pharmacodynamic determinants of loop diuretic response. Loop diuretics are delivered to the site of action, the lumen of the tubule, by organic anion transporters located in the proximal tubule. The solid line demonstrates several important points. There is a clear threshold concentration of the loop diuretic, below which there is no effective excretion of sodium or water above baseline. There is also a clear plateau concentration above which no further excretion of sodium and water occurs. The dashed line represents an altered dose-response relationship, as is frequently encountered in diuretic resistant states such as heart failure and renal disease. The "braking phenomenon" refers to a commonly seen physiologic response to diuretic therapy beyond the first dose. As the extracellular fluid volume decreases, a complex series of neurohormonal hemodynamic and intrarenal changes occur that cause an avid state of post-diuretic sodium retention, which offsets the effectiveness of the initial diuresis. (*Adapted from* Sica and Deedwania [20].)

B, Pharmacokinetics of diuretic drugs, including oral bioavailability and elimination half-life. Of note, torsemide and bumetanide have an oral bioavailability that is consistently higher than that of furosemide, and with less variability. ND—not determined. (*Adapted from* Brater [21].)

Pharmacokinetics of Diuretic Drugs

Loop diurectics	Oral bioavailability, %	Elimination half-life, h	
		Normal subjects, %	Patients with heart failure, %
Furosemide	10–100	1.5–2	2.7
Bumetanide	80–100	1	1.3
Torsemide	80–100	3–4	6
Thiazide			
Chlorothiazide	30–50	1.5	ND
Hydrochlorothiazide	65–75	2.5	ND
Distal			
Spironolactone	Conflicting data	1.5	ND
Active metabolites of spironolactone		> 15	ND

B

Effect of Angiotensin-Converting Enzyme Inhibitors on Mortality in Heart Failure

Placebo-controlled studies							
Trial (patients, *n*)	NYHA	Agent	Mean follow-up, *mo*	Placebo, %	ACEI, %	Risk reduction, %	P value
Largely asymptomatic							
SOLVD-P (4228)	I–II	Enalapril	37	15.8	14.8	8	0.3
Munich Trial (170)	I–II	Captopril	30	25.3	26.5	−4.7	NS
Captopril-Digoxin (300)	I–III	Captopril	6	6	7.7	−28	NS
Moderate symptoms							
SOLVD-T (2569)	I–III	Enalapril	41	39.7	35.2	16	0.004
CMRG (92)	II–III	Captopril	3	9.5	0	100	NS
Severe symptoms							
CONSENSUS (253)	IV	Enalapril	6	54	39	27	0.003

Hydralazine/nitrate-controlled studies							
Trial (patients, *n*)	NYHA	Agent	Mean follow-up, *mo*	Hyd/N, %	ACEI, %	Risk reduction, %	P value
V-HeFT II (804)	II–III	Enalapril	24	25	18	28	0.016
Hy-C (117)	III–IV	Captopril	8	49	19	61	0.05

Figure 5-27. Effect of angiotensin-converting enzyme inhibitors (ACEIs) on mortality in heart failure. Placebo-controlled studies of the use of ACEIs in heart failure patients have assessed mortality endpoints in mild, moderate, and severe heart failure. Trials performed in patients largely asymptomatic, such as Studies of Left Ventricular Dysfunction–Prevention (SOLVD-P), the Munich trial, and the Captopril-Digoxin Trial, have not demonstrated an improvement in survival in these patients. The Studies of Left Ventricular Dysfunction–Treatment (SOLVD-T) trial, performed largely in patients with New York Heart Association (NYHA) class II and III symptoms, showed a 16% reduction in all-cause mortality using enalapril. A 27% reduction in all-cause mortality was observed in the CONSENSUS trial.

Continued on the next page

Figure 5-27. *(Continued)* This study was performed in patients with severe heart failure. ACEIs have also been shown to improve survival when compared with the combination of hydralazine and isosorbide dinitrate (Hyd/N). The V-HeFT II study showed a 28% reduction in all-cause mortality using enalapril versus Hyd/N in patients with NYHA class II and III symptoms. A 61% reduction in mortality was observed in the captopril or hydralazine plus isosorbide dinitrate (Hy-C) trial, a study of 104 patients with moderate to severe heart failure symptoms [22,23]. CMRG—Captopril MultiCenter Research Group; NS—not significant.

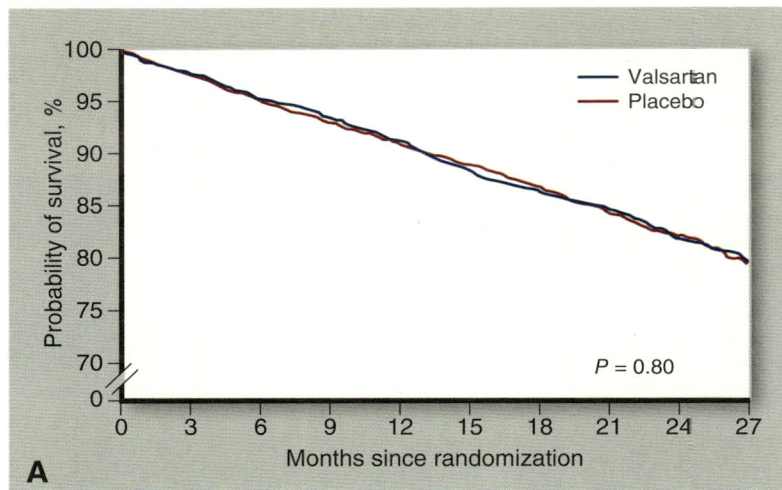

A

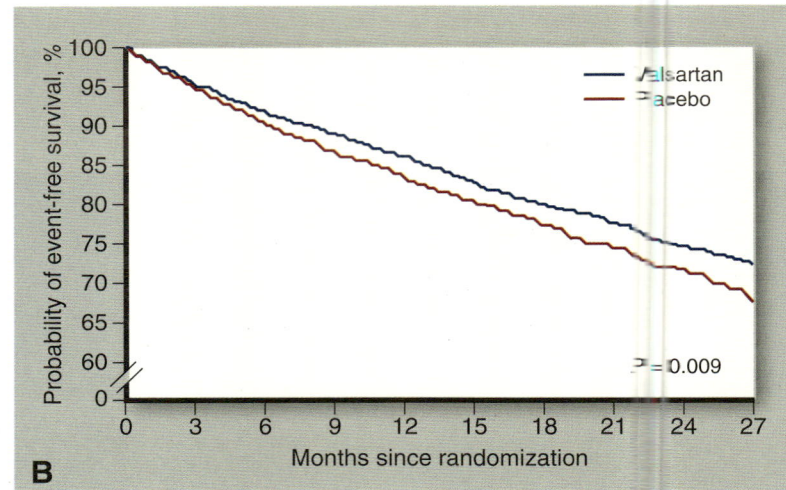

B

Effect of Angiotensin Receptor Blockade on Morbidity and Mortality in Addition to Standard Heart Falure Medications (Primary and Secondary Endpoints)

Variable	Placebo	Valsartan	RR (CI)	P value
Patients, *n*	2499	2511		
All-cause morality, *n* (%)	484 (19.4%)	495 (19.7%)	1.02 (0.90–1.15)	0.8
Mortality + hospitalization + sudden death + inotrope need, *n* (%)	801 (32.1%)	723 (28.8%)	0.87 (0.79–0.96)	0.009
Heart failure hospitalization, *n* (%)	455 (18.2%)	246 (13.8%)	0.73 (0.63–0.83)	0.001

C

Figure 5-28. The effects of angiotensin receptor blockade on morbidity and mortality in the Valsartan in Heart Failure Trial (Val-HeFT). This randomized, double-blind, placebo-controlled trial studied the clinical effect of the addition of valsartan to standard heart failure care that included angiotensin-converting enzyme (ACE) inhibitor therapy. This study enrolled 5010 patients and included two primary endpoints: all-cause mortality (**A**), and the composite endpoint of mortality, hospitalization, and the need for intravenous inotropes for greater than 4 hours (**B**). **C**, The patient population studied was largely New York Heart Association class II and III. The majority received an ACE inhibitor (93%), some received a β-blocker (35%), and only 5% received spironolactone. The addition of valsartan to standard heart failure care resulted in no improvement in all-cause mortality. However, the risk of reaching the composite endpoint was reduced by 13% with valsartan. The vast majority of the benefit found in this composite endpoint was through reduction in heart failure hospitalizations. Hospitalizations were reduced by 27.5% with the addition of valsartan, with a highly significant P value of 0.001. (*Adapted from* Cohn and Tognoni [24].)

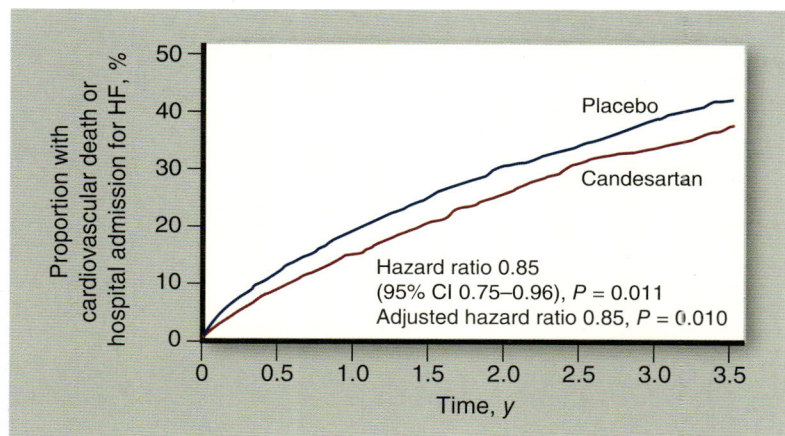

Figure 5-29. The effects of angiotensin receptor blockade on morbidity and mortality in the Candesartan in Heart failure Assessment of Reduction on Mortality and morbidity (CHARM-Added) trial. This randomized, double-blind, placebo-controlled trial studied the clinical effect of the addition of candesartan to standard heart failure care that included angiotensin-converting enzyme (ACE) inhibitor therapy. This study enrolled 2548 patients, the primary endpoint being cardiovascular death or hospitalization for heart failure. The patient population studied was largely New York Heart Association class II and III. The majority received an ACE inhibitor (99.9%), some received a β-blocker (55.5%), and 17.2% received spironolactone. The addition of candesartan to standard heart failure care resulted in a significant reduction in the primary outcome by 15%. All secondary outcomes were significantly reduced, as well. HF—heart failure. (*Adapted from* McMurray et al. [25].)

Results of Trials Using an Angiotensin Receptor Blocker in ACE Inhibitor—Naïve and Intolerant Patients: Effect on Mortality

Trial (patients, n)	Severity	Agents	Mean FU	Control, %	ARB, %	Risk reduction, %	P value
ELITE II (3152)	NYHA II-IV	Losartan vs captopril	18 mo	15.9	17.7	−13	0.16
RESOLVD (768)	NYHA II-IV	Candesartan vs enalapril	43 wk	6.4	13.1	−105	0.09
SPICE (270)	NYHA II-III	Candesartan vs placebo	12 wk	3.3	3.4	−4	NS
CHARM–Alternative (2028)	NYHA II-IV	Candesartan vs placebo	34 mo	29.2	26.2	10	0.033

Figure 5-30. The effect of angiotensin receptor blockade on mortality: results of trials using angiotensin-converting enzyme (ACE) inhibitor naive and intolerant patients. The Evaluation of Losartan in The Elderly (ELITE) study randomly assigned 722 patients 65 years of age or older with symptomatic left ventricular failure to receive 50 mg of losartan or captopril titrated to 50 mg three times per day. The primary endpoint of this initial study was an increase in serum creatinine. There were no differences seen in the incidence of increased creatinine. However, an unexpected 46% decrease in all-cause mortality was observed with losartan. Because of the limited power of this study to demonstrate this difference, a follow-up study was performed (ELITE-II). The ELITE-II trial was performed in 3152 patients with New York Heart Association (NYHA) class II to IV symptoms. This study failed to show a significant difference in all-cause mortality between losartan and captopril. There was a nonsignificant trend (P = 0.16) favoring captopril in this analysis. The Randomized Evaluation of Strategies for Left Ventricular Dysfunction (RESOLVD) trial enrolled 768 patients in one of three arms, which included candesartan, enalapril, and the combination of candesartan and enalapril. This study also showed a nonsignificant trend toward worsened survival in the candesartan arms. The Study of Patients Intolerant of Converting Enzyme Inhibition (SPICE) enrolled 270 patients who were previously found to be ACE inhibitor intolerant. This study followed patients over 12 weeks who had received either candesartan or placebo. There was no significant difference in mortality in this relatively low-risk population [26]. The Candesartan in Heart failure Assessment of Reduction on Mortality and morbidity (CHARM-Alternative) trial randomized 2028 patients with chronic heart failure and ejection fraction (EF) of 40% or less who were intolerant to ACE inhibition to candesartan versus placebo [27]. These patients were largely NYHA class II–III. There was a reduction in the combined endpoint of cardiovascular death or hospital admission for heart failure (P < 0.0001). Adjusted for covariates, there was also a reduction in all-cause mortality (P = 0.033). ARB—angiotensin receptor blocker.

Figure 5-31. Effect of spironolactone on survival in patients with heart failure. Patients with severe heart failure have been shown to have elevated levels of aldosterone compared with that of normal subjects. Treatment with angiotensin-converting enzyme (ACE) inhibitors reduces aldosterone release by limiting the production of angiotensin II. Because of non–ACE-dependent production of angiotensin II (serine protease pathways), aldosterone levels have been shown to rise over time in patients treated with recommended doses of ACE inhibitor. Aldosterone has direct effects on the kidney, leading to sodium retention and reduction in serum potassium concentration. Additionally, animal models of heart failure have shown that aldosterone may be responsible for myocardial fibrosis and myocyte hypertrophy seen with chronic heart failure. The Randomized Aldactone Evaluation Study (RALES) was performed in 1663 patients with ejection fraction of 35% or lower and New York Heart Association (NYHA) IV symptoms, or patients with NYHA IV symptoms who had experienced NYHA III symptoms within the past 6 months. Patients were randomly assigned to receive 25 to 50 mg of spironolactone daily versus placebo, delivered in a double-blind fashion. The survival plot demonstrates the effect of spironolactone on all-cause mortality, with a reduction of 30% compared with placebo. This reduction in the risk of death among patients in the spironolactone group was attributed to a lower risk of death from progressive heart failure and sudden cardiac death. The frequency of hospitalization for worsening heart failure was 35% lower in the spironolactone group than in the placebo group. Patients receiving spironolactone treatment should have close monitoring of the serum potassium level, particularly in the first month of therapy [28].

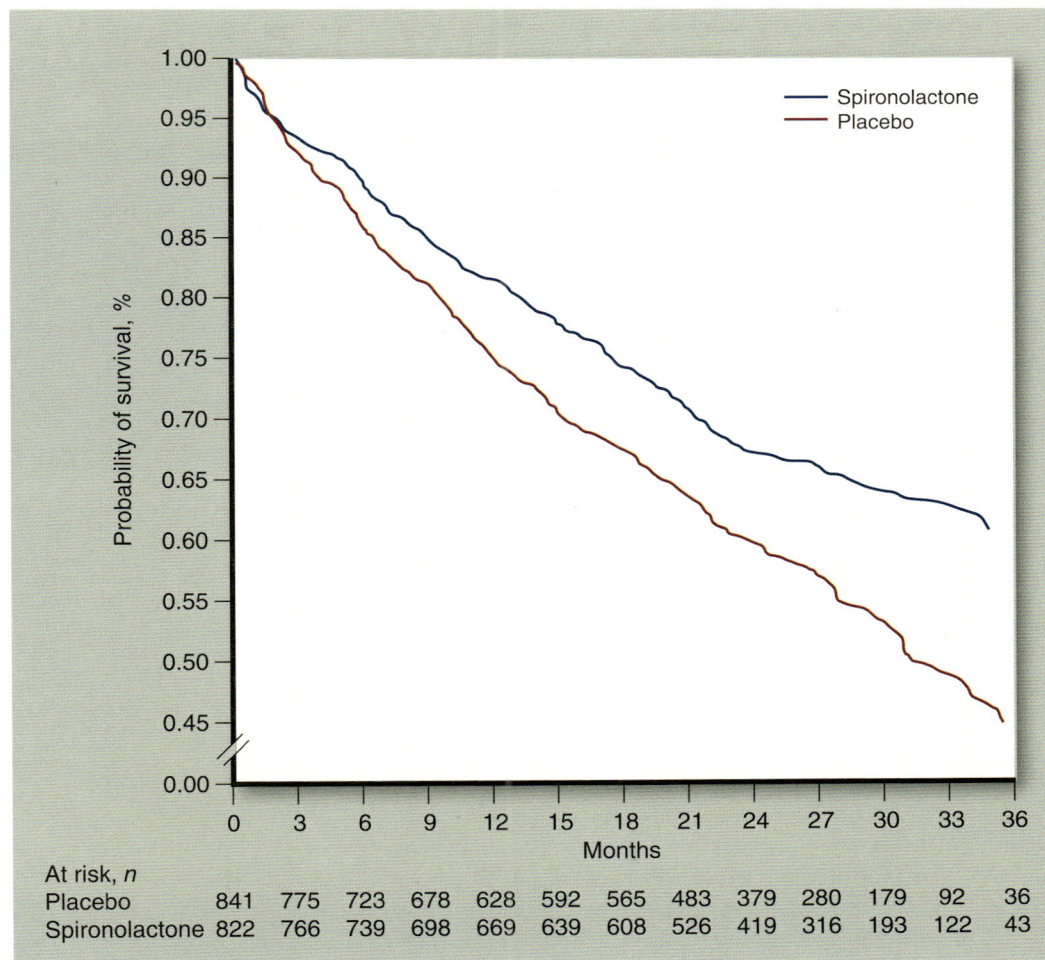

At risk, n

	0	3	6	9	12	15	18	21	24	27	30	33	36
Placebo	841	775	723	678	628	592	565	483	379	280	179	92	36
Spironolactone	822	766	739	698	669	639	608	526	419	316	193	122	43

Figure 5-32. Risk of serious hyperkalemia with aldosterone receptor blockade in heart failure. The Randomized Aldactone Evaluation Study (RALES) demonstrated that spironolactone reduced mortality by 30% in patients with severe heart failure [28]. Although the risk of serious hyperkalemia was not significantly different in the spironolactone-treated patients (2% versus 1% in placebo; $P = 0.42$), subjects were carefully selected for study entry and closely monitored. Juurlink *et al.* [29] hypothesized that life-threatening hyperkalemia might occur more frequently when these drugs were used together with angiotensin-converting enzyme (ACE) inhibitors in clinical practice. In this population-based time-series analysis linking prescription claims data and hospital admission records for more than 1.3 million older adults, the rate of in-hospital death from hyperkalemia rose significantly following the online publication of RALES from 0.3 per 1000 patients in 1994 to 2.0 per 1000 patients in 2001 ($P < 0.001$). Close laboratory monitoring and more judicious use of spironolactone is indicated to reduce serious adverse events. (*Adapted from* Juurlink *et al.* [29])

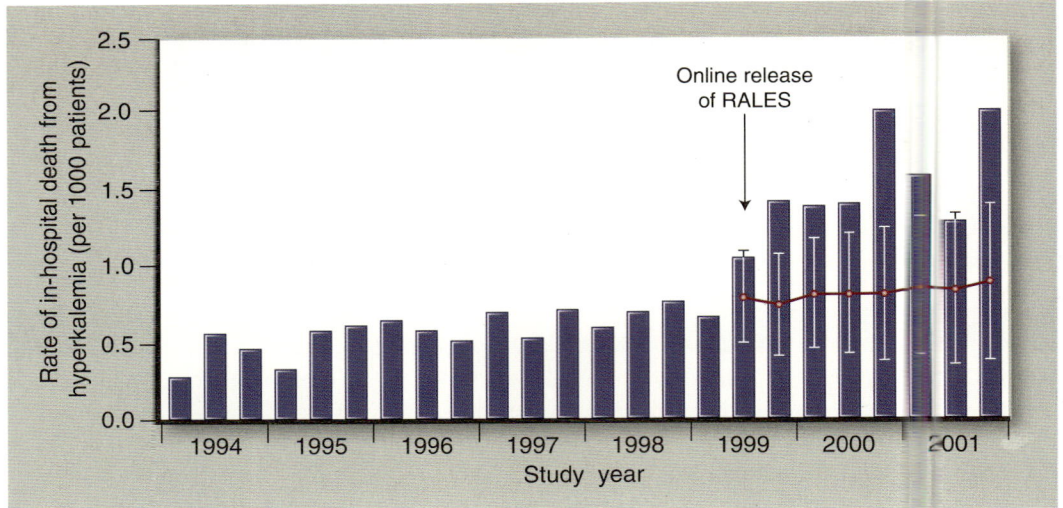

Figure 5-33. Major placebo-controlled trials of β-blockers in heart failure. The available randomized data overwhelmingly show that carvedilol, metoprolol CR/XL, and bisoprolol reduce morbidity (eg, all-cause hospitalization) and all-cause mortality in patients with mild to severe heart failure. SENIORS (Study of the Effects of Nebivolol Intervention on Outcomes and Rehospitalization in Seniors with Heart Failure) showed similar benefits with nebivolol in elderly patients with heart failure. BEST—Beta-blocker Evaluation of Survival Trial; COPERNICUS—Carvedilol Prospective Randomized Cumulative Survival study; MERIT-HF—Metoprolol CR/XL Randomized Intervention Trial in Heart Failure; NS—not significant. (*Adapted from* Gheorghiade *et al.* [30].)

Results From Major Placebo-Controlled Trials of β-Blockers in Heart Failure

Study	Drug	Heart failure severity	Mortality, %	Hospitalization, %
US Carvedilol	Carvedilol	Mild-moderate	↓ 65	↓ 27
CIBIS-II	Bisoprolol	Moderate-severe	↓ 34	↓ 20
MERIT-HF	Metoprolol CR/XL	Mild-moderate	↓ 34	↓ 18
BEST	Bucindolol	Moderate-severe	↓ 10 ($P = 0.13$)	↓ 8 ($P = 0.08$)
COPERNICUS	Carvedilol	Severe	↓ 35	↓ 20
SENIORS	Nebivolol	Mild-moderate	↓ 12 ($P = 0.21$)	↓ 10

Figure 5-34. β-Adrenergic antagonists in severe heart failure. The US Carvedilol Program and the Metoprolol CR/XL Randomized Intervention Trial in Heart Failure (MERIT-HF) study confirmed that β-blockers reduce morbidity and mortality in patients with mild-to-moderate heart failure. To test the efficacy of β-blockers in patients with severe heart failure, the Carvedilol Prospective Randomized Cumulative Survival (COPERNICUS) study randomly assigned 2289 patients with symptoms of heart failure at rest or on minimal exertion and a left ventricular ejection fraction (LVEF) less than 25% to carvedilol or placebo for a mean of 10.4 months. Patients were receiving standard therapy, including diuretics optimized to achieve euvolemia; they were excluded if they required intensive care or intravenous vasodilators or positive inotropes. The study was stopped early by the Data and Safety Monitoring Board because of the finding of a 35% decrease in the risk of death with carvedilol (95% CI, 19%–48%; $P = 0.00013$ unadjusted) (**A**).

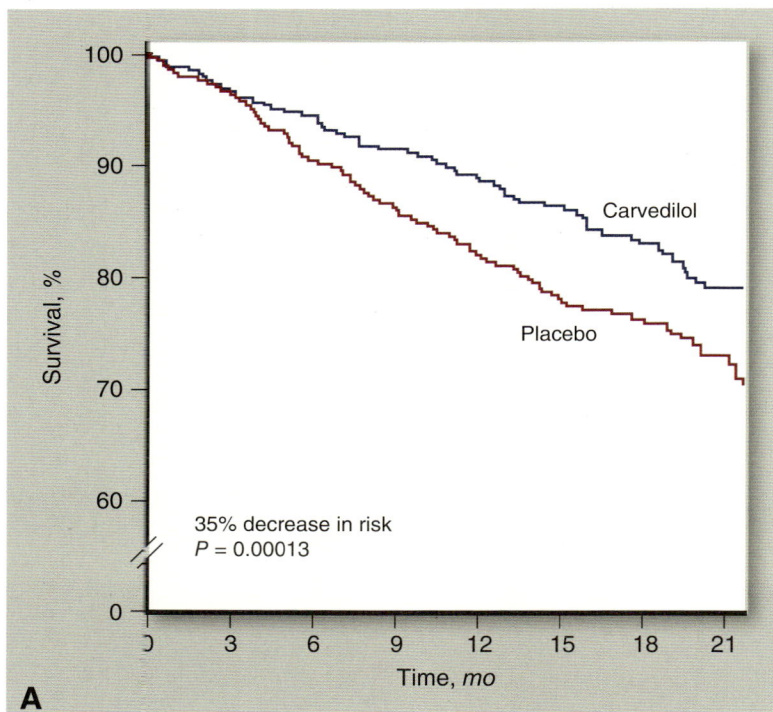

Continued on the next page

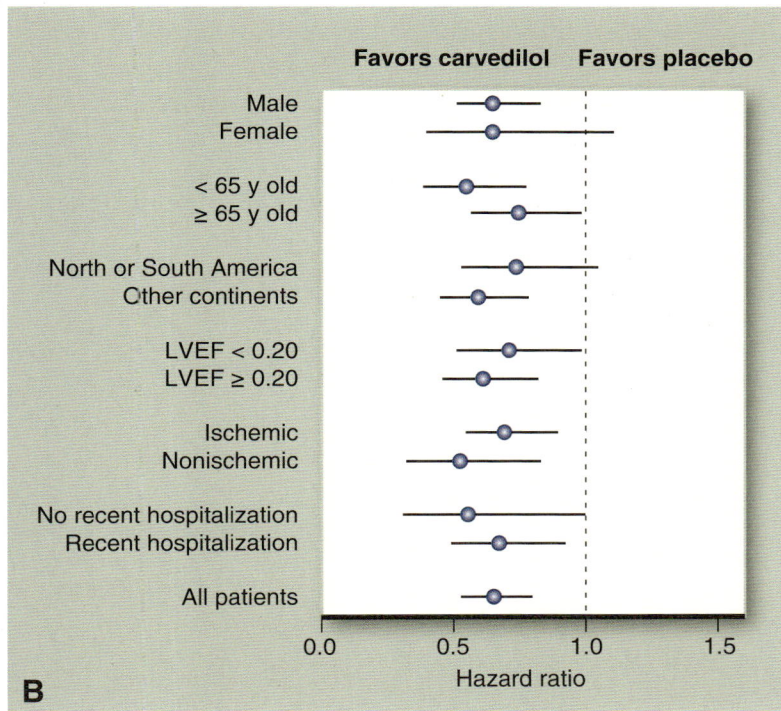

Figure 5-34. (Continued) The reduction in mortality was consistent across a range of subgroups defined according to sex, age, location of study center, LVEF, cause of heart failure, and history of recent heart failure hospitalization (B). Carvedilol was well tolerated in patients with severe heart failure as demonstrated by the fact that fewer patients in the carvedilol group were permanently withdrawn from study medication because of adverse effects (1-year withdrawal rate 18.5% in the placebo group vs 14.8% in the carvedilol group [P = 0.02]). (Adapted from Packer et al. [31].)

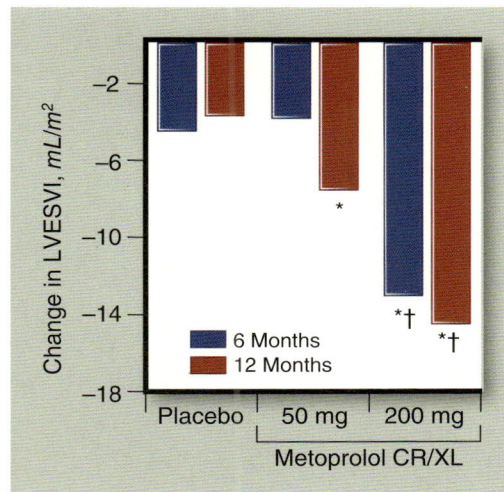

Figure 5-35. Reverse remodeling in asymptomatic left ventricular (LV) dysfunction. Previous studies showed that treatment with β-blockers reverses LV remodeling in patients with symptomatic heart failure due to reduced systolic function. The Reversal of Ventricular Remodeling with Toprol-XL (REVERT) trial was a multicenter, double-blind, placebo-controlled study designed to test the hypothesis that β-blockers slow or reverse remodeling in patients with asymptomatic LV dysfunction. A total of 149 β-blocker-naïve patients with New York Heart Association (NYHA) class I heart failure and an ejection fraction of less than 40% were randomly assigned to metoprolol CR/XL 25 mg titrated over 2 months to a target dose of 50 mg or 200 mg, or to placebo. At entry, 92% of patients were receiving renin-angiotensin system inhibitors and 65% were on diuretics. The primary endpoint of the study, mean change in LV end-systolic volume index (LVESVI) at 12 months, was significantly reduced in the 200 mg dose group compared with placebo (Asterisk indicates $P < 0.05$ vs baseline; dagger indicates $P < 0.05$ vs placebo). Metoprolol CR/XL also appeared to reduce LV end-diastolic volume index and increase ejection fraction in a dose- and time-dependent manner. The effects of β-blockers on morbidity and mortality in asymptomatic LV dysfunction have not been tested. (Adapted from Colucci et al. [32].)

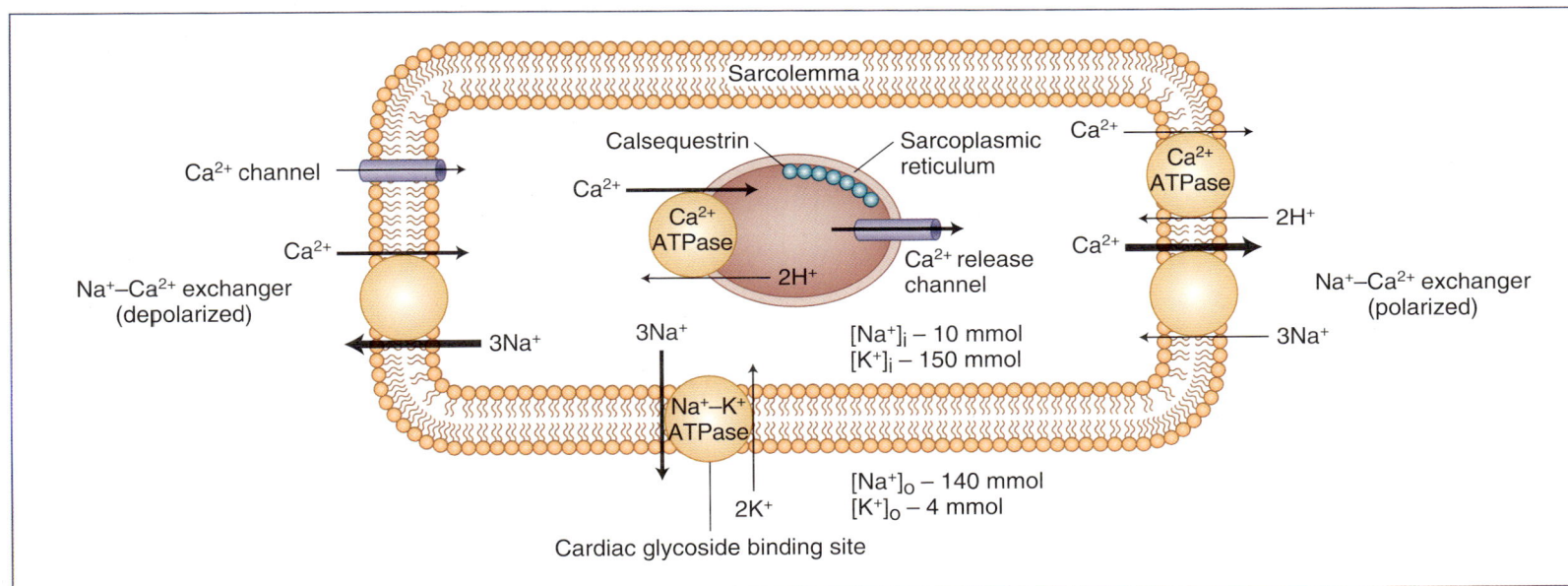

Figure 5-36. Sodium pump inhibition by cardiac glycosides. The present understanding of the mechanism by which the cardiac glycosides induce a positive inotropic effect in cardiac muscle is based on the specificity of these drugs for Na^+K^+-ATPase (or the "sodium pump"), a cell membrane protein responsible for the active (ie, ATP-consuming) transport of the monovalent cations Na^+ and K^+ [33]. Both Na^+ and Ca^{2+} ions enter cardiac muscle cells during each cycle of depolarization, contraction, and repolarization. Ca^{2+} is also released from internal stores in an intracellular compartment called the sarcoplasmic reticulum (SR), where it is bound to the protein calsequestrin. During cellular repolarization, Na^+ is actively extruded by Na^+K^+-ATPase, whereas Ca^{2+} is either pumped back into the SR by a Ca^{2+}-ATPase or is removed from the cell by a cell membrane transport protein that exchanges Na^+ for Ca^{2+}. This Na^+ for Ca^{2+} exchanger transports three Na^+ ions in for every Ca^{2+} ion out when the cell is polarized, using the favorable chemical and electrical potential of Na^+ to drive the exchange reaction.

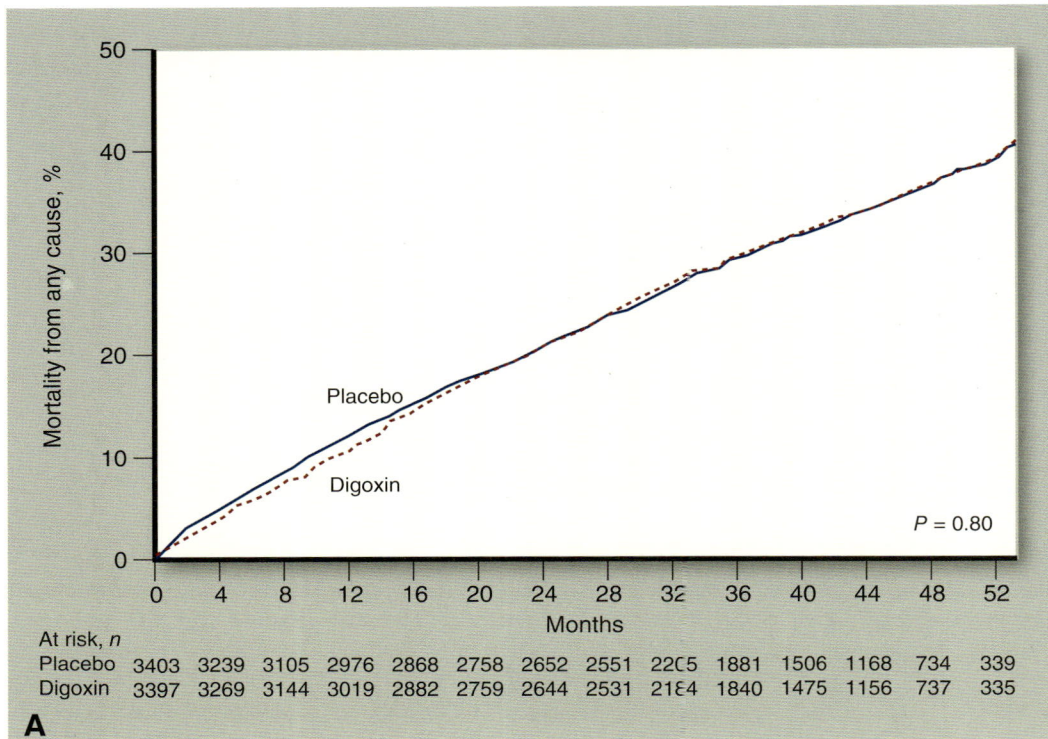

A

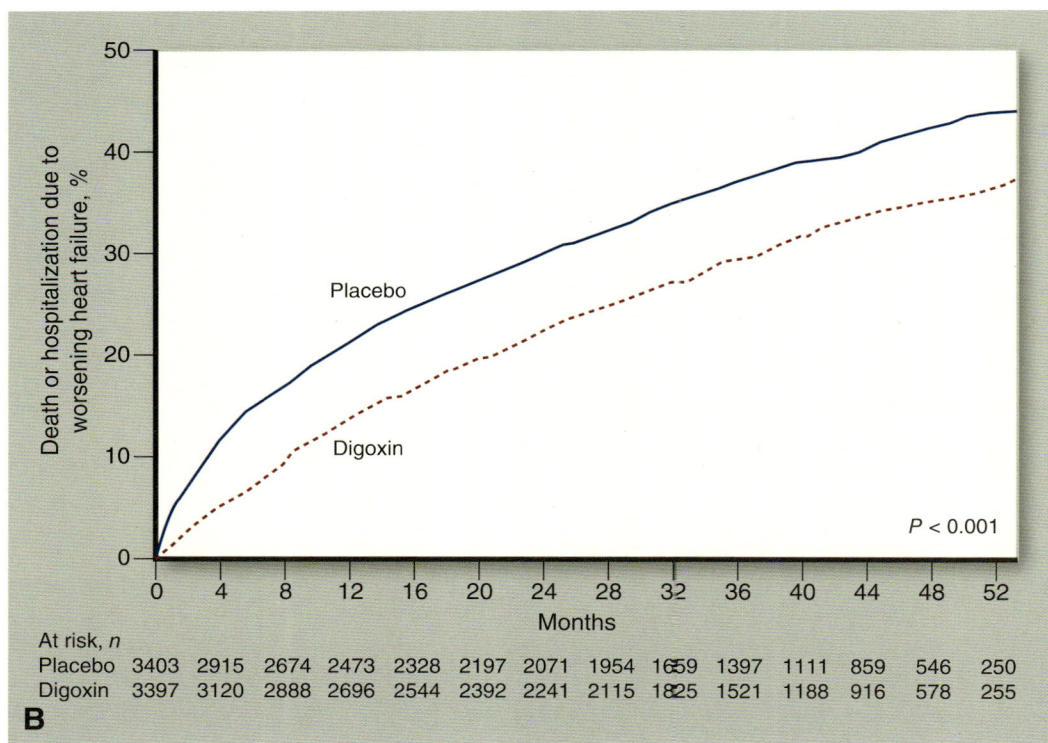

B

Figure 5-37. The Digitalis Investigation Group (DIG) trial evaluated the effects of digoxin on survival in 6800 patients [34]. The average follow-up was 37 months. Digoxin did not increase or decrease overall mortality (A). However, digoxin-treated patients had a reduction in the overall rate of hospitalization and also the rate of hospitalization for worsening heart failure (B). There was no increased risk of ventricular arrhythmias in the digoxin-treated group.

The question as to whether or not serum digoxin concentration (SDC) is important for outcomes in patients with heart failure has recently been addressed. In a post-hoc analysis of the DIG trial cohort, superior survival was observed in patients with SDCs in the range of 0.5 to 0.8 ng/mL compared with placebo [35]. Concentrations of greater than 1.2 ng/mL were associated with decreased survival compared with placebo. These findings persisted after multivariable adjustment for clinical variables associated with severity of illness. (*Adapted from* the Digitalis Investigation Group [34].)

Figure 5-38. Adjuvant treatment with hydralazine and nitrates in advanced heart failure. Retrospective analyses of prior heart failure studies strongly suggested that black patients have a clinically significant response to the combination of isosorbide dinitrate and hydralazine. The African American Heart Failure Trial (A-HeFT) randomly assigned 1050 self-identified blacks with moderate-severe heart failure and dilated ventricles to receive a fixed dose of isosorbide dinitrate plus hydralazine (target total daily doses 120 mg and 225 mg, respectively) or placebo in addition to standard therapy. The primary endpoint was a composite score made up of weighted values for death from any cause, a first hospitalization for heart failure, and change in quality of life. At baseline, patients were well treated with renin angiotensin system inhibitors (86%), β-blockers (74%), and spironolactone (39%). The study was stopped early by the data and safety monitoring board after a mean follow-up of 10 months due to a significantly higher mortality rate in the placebo group (10.2% versus 6.4% in the isosorbide dinitrate plus hydralazine group). As shown in the Kaplan-Meier analysis, there was a 43% improvement in survival (hazard ratio, 0.57; $P = 0.01$). Combination therapy also significantly reduced the rate of HF hospitalization by 33% and improved quality of life. (*Adapted from* Taylor *et al.* [36].)

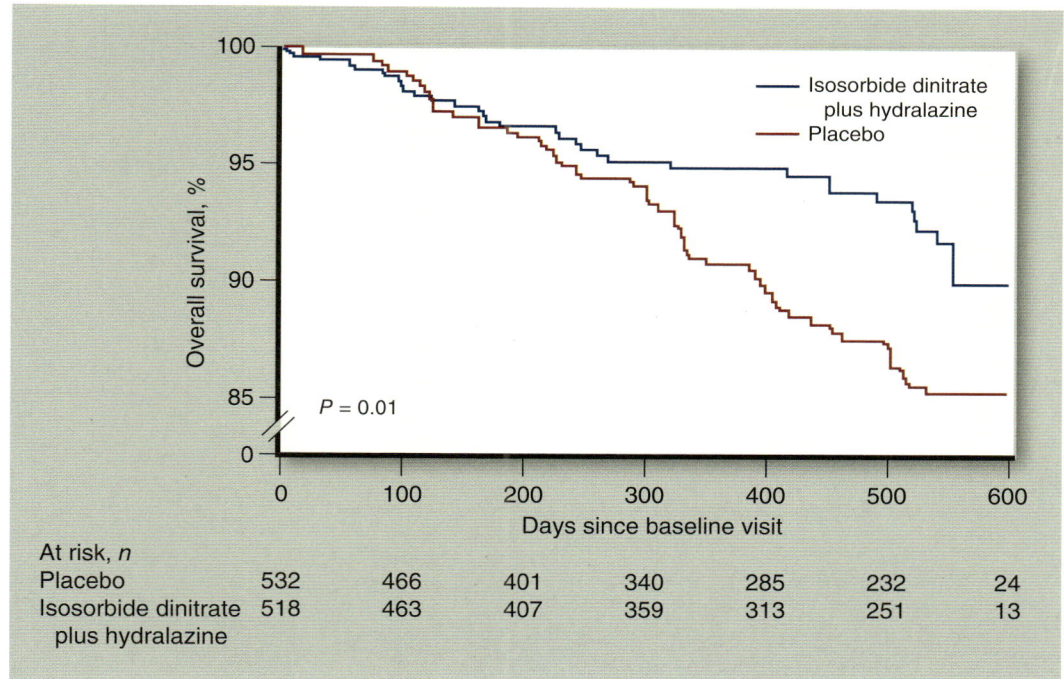

At risk, n						
Placebo	532	466	401	340	285	232	24
Isosorbide dinitrate plus hydralazine	518	463	407	359	313	251	13

Figure 5-39. American College of Cardiology/American Heart Association (ACC/AHA) guidelines for the treatment of patients with diastolic heart failure (DHF) [17]. Class I recommendations are those for which there is either consensus among an expert panel or scientific evidence to support the validity; class IIA and IIB recommendations are those for which there is conflicting evidence and/or divergence of opinion. Evidence A: there are data from multiple randomized controlled trials (RCTs) or meta-analyses. Evidence B: there are data from a single RCT or from nonrandomized studies. Evidence C: there are no data, only consensus of opinion among experts. The ACC/AHA guidelines suggest that treatment of patients with DHF (*top*) should focus on 1) control of arterial blood pressure, 2) control of heart rate, and 3) control of edema with diuretics.

Treatment of acutely decompensated DHF: acute pulmonary congestion or edema (*bottom*). Patients with DHF frequently have episodes of acute pulmonary edema, which may be life threatening. The treatment principles are outlined here. Pulmonary capillary wedge pressure (PCWP) can be reduced by vasodilators such as intravenous nitroglycerin, which may also relieve any ischemia that contributes to left ventricular (LV) stiffness. Rapidly acting diuretics, morphine, and other standard-care measures for treating pulmonary edema (*eg*, oxygen) are also helpful. If atrial fibrillation is present, an attempt should be made to restore normal sinus rhythm to preserve the atrial contribution to ventricular filling. Regardless of rhythm, any tachycardia should be controlled.

The stiff, noncompliant ventricle makes preload management difficult. A small increase in LV volume that would be tolerated without difficulty in a normally compliant left ventricle may result in a marked increase in PCWP in a stiff ventricle and thereby precipitate pulmonary edema. Conversely, the stiff left ventricle is abnormally sensitive to a lowering of filling pressure; because of its decreased distensibility and increased resistance to filling, the stiff left ventricle requires a higher-than-normal filling pressure to maintain an adequate diastolic volume and stroke volume. If initial preload reduction results in hypotension, a normal blood pressure can usually be restored by discontinuing the vasodilators and increasing LV volume by leg raising or infusion of a small amount of saline. ACE-Is—angiotensin-converting enzyme; AF—atrial fibrillation; ARB—angiotensin receptor blocker. (*Adapted from* Hunt *et al.* [17].)

ACC/AHA Treatment Guidelines for Diastolic Heart Failure

Class	Recommendation(s)	Evidence
I	Control systolic and diastolic blood pressure	A
	Control ventricular rate in AF	C
	Use diuretics to control edema	C
IIA	Coronary revascularization	C
IIB	Restore and maintain normal sinus rhythm	C
	β-blocker, ACE-Is, ARB, calcium antagonists, digitalis	C

Treatment of acutely decompensated diastolic heart failure: acute pulmonary congestion or edema

Reduce pulmonary capillary wedge pressure

Avoid hypotension from excessive preload reduction in stiff LV

Correct any hypertension

Restore normal sinus rhythm and/or control rapid heart rate

Relieve ischemia

Figure 5-40. Effect of candesartan on time to cardiovascular (CV) death or hospital admission for heart failure (HF) in patients with preserved ejection fraction (EF > 40%): the Candesartan in Heart Failure—Assessment of Reduction in Mortality and Morbidity (CHARM-PRESERVED) trial. A total of 3023 patients were randomly assigned to treatment with candesartan (32 mg once daily) or placebo in addition to standard HF medical therapy as prescribed by the patient's physicians. In addition to the assigned study treatment, most patients were also receiving one or more of the following drugs: ACE inhibitors, β-blockers, diuretics, spironolactone, digoxin, calcium antagonists, or other vasodilators. The primary endpoint of CHARM-PRESERVED was the composite of CV death or HF hospitalization. The addition of candesartan treatment resulted in a small reduction (11%) in the combined risk of CV death or hospital admission for HF. There was no significant effect of candesartan on CV death alone. The risk of admission for heart failure was reduced modestly, by 15% (*P* < 0.05), by candesartan over an average of 3.5 years of follow-up. HR—hazard ratio. (*Adapted from* Yusuf et al. [37].)

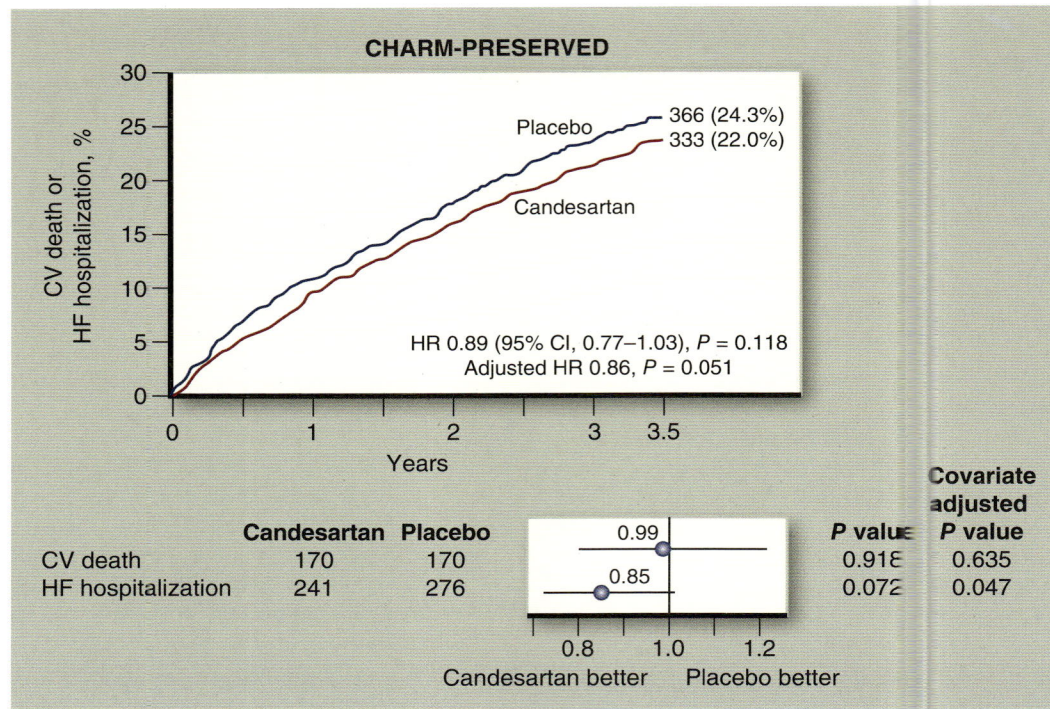

Hospital Management

Clinical Outcomes During Hospitalization for Patients With Heart Failure

Outcome	HF with preserved systolic function (n = 26,322)	Systolic HF (n = 25,856)
Mortality, %*	2.8	3.9
Length of hospitalization, d (median [IQR])*	4.9 (3.1–7.6)	5.0 (3.2–8.1)
Admitted to CU, %*	18.9	21.7
Length of ICU stay, d (median [IQR])*	2.7 (1.4–4.9)	3.0 (1.6–5.1)
Weight loss > 10 lbs, %*	26.9	33.4
Asymptomatic at discharge, %	55	55

*P < 0.0001

Figure 5-41. Clinical outcomes during hospitalization for patients with heart failure (HF) due to preserved or reduced systolic function. Data from over 50,000 hospitalizations from the Acute Decompensated Heart Failure National Registry (ADHERE) were analyzed to describe the clinical characteristics of patients hospitalized for acute decompensated HF. While in-hospital mortality was significantly lower for patients with HF and preserved systolic function compared with patients with systolic dysfunction, the mortality rates were similar in magnitude. Length of stay in the two groups was similar, but the need for intensive care unit management was lower in patients with HF with preserved systolic function. A similar proportion of patients in both groups lost over 10 lbs during hospitalization, and a similar and large number of patients in both groups were discharged with persistent HF symptoms. ICU—intensive care unit; IQR—interquartile range. (*Adapted from* Yancy et al. [38].)

Figure 5-42. Goals of in-patient therapy. The early goal of treatment is to improve symptoms while maintaining or improving the hemodynamic status. Progress may be tracked by following body weights and fluid intake and output while monitoring vital signs, electrolytes, and renal function. Consideration also should be given to identifying precipitating factors and etiology, and patients who may benefit from coronary revascularization. The strategy of using hemodynamic targets to tailor treatment has been shown to be effective at improving symptoms and allowing hospital discharge without surgery in patients evaluated for transplantation [39], but more recent data suggest no role for routine use of a pulmonary artery catheter (*see* Fig. 5-48). Franciosa *et al.* [40]

Goals of Treatment in Decompensated Heart Failure

Clinical goals	Hemodynamic goals
Resolution of dyspnea and orthopnea	Systolic blood pressure ≥ 80 mm Hg
Resolution of ascites and peripheral edema	Right atrial pressure ≤ 8 mm Hg
Jugular venous pressure ≤ 8 cm H_2O	Pulmonary capillary wedge pressure ≤ 16 mm Hg
Control of hypertension	Systemic vascular resistance ≤ 1200 dynes/s/cm-5
Minimize adverse effects of treatment, reduce duration and cost of stay	
Initiate treatments that improve long-term outcome	

showed that it is possible to reduce filling pressures to near normal levels (*eg*, pulmonary capillary wedge pressure 16 mm Hg or less) while maintaining or improving stroke volume in patients with heart failure.

Figure 5-43. Diuretics and therapeutic considerations. Diuretics are effective in managing symptoms of congestion in patients with heart failure. Loop diuretics are usually required in all but the mildest cases of volume overload. Diuretic regimens requiring greater than once-daily administration are frequently required for patients with diuretic resistance; an alternative is the concurrent administration of a thiazide diuretic, allowing a synergistic effect from dual loop of Henle and distal convoluted tubule blockade. Continuous intravenous (IV) infusions of a loop diuretic in the tubule lumen may be tried if bolus administration is ineffective [41,42].

Diuretic Strategies

Drug	Dosing	Comments
Loop diuretics		
Furosemide	Oral 20–240 mg per dose, one to three times per day	IV furosemide provides a more consistent response than oral
	IV bolus 20–200 mg per dose, once to three times per day	Continuous infusion may further augment diuresis
	IV infusion 10–40 mg/h	Higher risk of ototoxicity
Bumetanide	Oral 0.5–10 mg per dose, once to three time per day	Greater oral bioavailability than furosemide
Torsemide	Oral 10–100 mg per dose, once to three times per day	Greater oral bioavailability than furosemide
Thiazide diuretics		
Metolazone		
	Oral 2.5–5 mg per dose once to twice daily	Weak diuretic with monotherapy; potent synergistic diuresis when combined with a loop diuretic
Chlorothiazide	IV Bolus 250–500 mg per dose, once to twice daily	Moderate synergistic diuresis when combined with a loop diuretic

Figure 5-44. A practical working diagram of the cardiovascular support drugs commonly used in the initial short-term management of acute decompensated heart failure. It is assumed that patients who require these support drugs have adequate to high left ventricular end-diastolic filling pressure (18 mm Hg or greater) or clinical evidence of volume overload. Systemic hypoperfusion and hypotension in a patient without evidence of volume overload or with filling pressures of less than 18 mm Hg should be approached with a cautious fluid challenge or trial of dopamine.

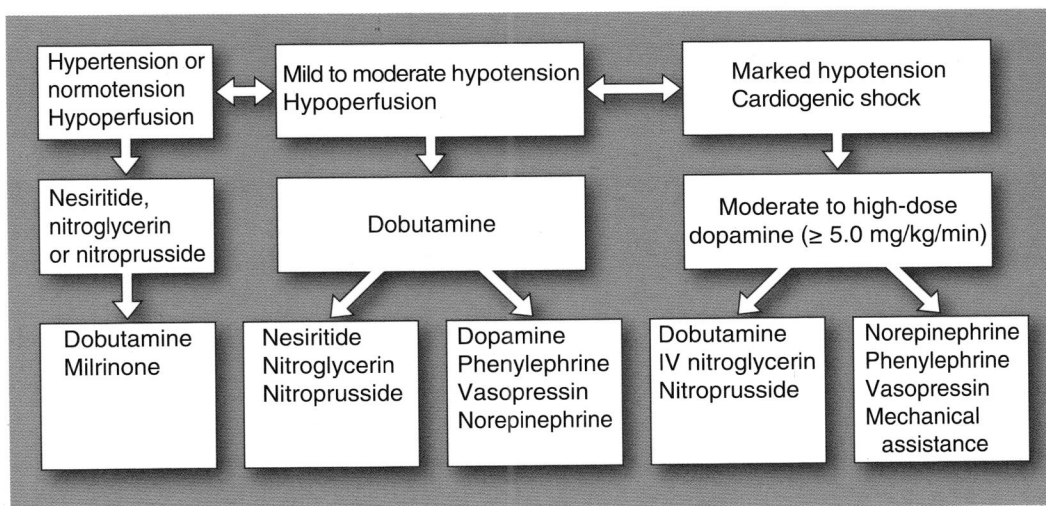

On the basis of the clinical presentation and the state of the systemic perfusion and blood pressure, the initial drug of choice is selected and its dosage increased until clinical or hemodynamic endpoints are achieved or adverse effects occur. At this point, inadequate improvement of clinical status and systemic perfusion usually require either the addition of a second agent as combination therapy or mechanical circulatory support. IV—intravenous.

Principal Preload- and Afterload-Reducing Drugs for Acute or Severe Heart Failure

Drug	Dosing	Potential advantages	Potential disadvantages
Nitroglycerin	Sublingual: 1 tablet (or 1–2 sprays) three or four times at 5-minute intervals; IV: 0.4 μg/kg/min initially (increase as needed)	Favorable effect on coronary vasculature and in myocardial ischemia/infarction; preload reduction > afterload	Tolerance during prolonged infusion; inadequate afterload reduction in catastrophic cardiovascular disorders (eg, acute valvular insufficiency, ventricular rupture)
Nitroprusside	IV: 0.1 μg/kg/min initially; increase as needed	Relatively powerful preload and afterload reduction	Less favorable effects on coronary vasculature and myocardial ischemia; administration must be closely monitored to avoid marked hypotension; thiocyanate or cyanide toxicity during high-dose or prolonged infusions, particularly in patients with renal or hepatic dysfunction
Nesiritide	0.005–0.01 μg/kg/min initially, ± bolus; increase as needed	Preload and afterload reduction; possible facilitative effect on diuresis	Hypotension; meta-analyses of clinical trials suggest adverse effects on mortality and renal function

Figure 5-45. Principal preload- and afterload-reducing drugs for acute decompensated heart failure. Nitroglycerin, nitroprusside, and nesiritide are the primary vasodilators used to reduce excessive preload and afterload in acute decompensated heart failure [43,44]. Nitroglycerin is used most often, particularly in heart failure due to acute coronary syndromes. Nitroprusside is the drug of choice when more aggressive afterload and preload reduction are needed; examples include catastrophic cardiovascular events (eg, acute, severe mitral, or aortic regurgitation), hypertensive emergencies (eg, aortic dissection, pulmonary edema), and inadequate response to nesiritide or nitroglycerin. Nitroprusside has also been used safely to stabilize patients with severe aortic stenosis [45].

Pharmacologic Properties and Therapeutic Considerations in Using Inotropic Agents

Pharmacologic feature	Dobutamine	Milrinone	Dopamine		Norepinephrine
			Low-dose	High-dose	
General description	Positive inotrope with mild balanced peripheral vascular effects	Positive inotrope with balanced peripheral vascular effects	Dopaminergic vasodilator, "renal" vasodilator	Vasopressor with some positive inotropic effects	Vasopressor
Dose, μg/kg/min					
Initial	2.5	0.25, ± bolus	2	5	0.01
Usual range	2.5–15	0.25–0.75	2–5	5–20	0.01–0.20
Most common adverse effects	Tachycardia; dysrhythmias; angina	Tachycardia; dysrhythmias; angina; hypotension	Tachycardia; dysrhythmias	Tachycardia; dysrhythmias; angina; increased cardiac filling pressures	Intense vasoconstriction; dysrhythmias; angina; increased cardiac filling pressures

A

Pharmacologic Properties and Therapeutic Considerations in Using Inotropic Agents

Pharmacologic feature	Dobutamine	Milrinone	Dopamine		Norepinephrine
			Low-dose	High-dose	
Receptor agonism					
α	+	0	+	+++	++++
β1	++++	0	+	++	+
β1	++	0	0	0	0
Dopaminergic	0	0	+++	++	0
Systemic vascular resistance	↓↓	↓↓↓	↓	↑↑	↑↑↑
Stroke volume and cardiac output	↑↑↑↑	↑↑↑↑	↑	↑↑	↑
Ability to increase systemic blood pressure	→ to ↑	→ to ↑	→	↑↑↑	↑↑↑
Ventricular filling pressure	↓↓	↓↓↓	↓ to →	↓ to ↑↑	→ to ↑↑
Heart rate	→ to ↑↑	→ to ↑↑	→ to ↑	→ to ↑↑↑	— to ↑
Myocardial oxygen demand/supply	→ to ↑	→ to ↓	→ to ↑	↑↑	↑↑

B

Figure 5-46. A and B, Principal pharmacologic properties and therapeutic considerations in the use of the major inotropic and vasopressor agents in acute decompensated heart failure [46,47].

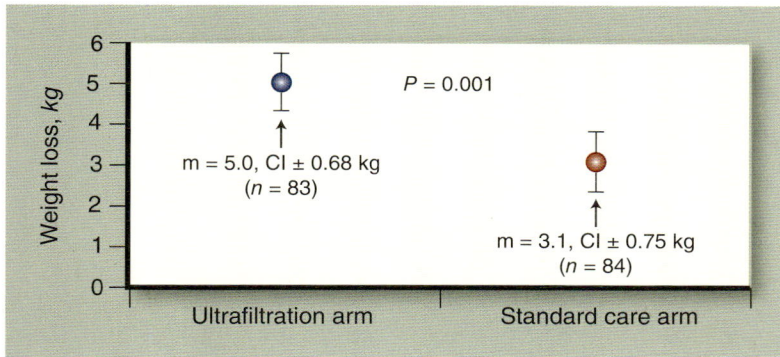

Figure 5-47. Ultrafiltration as a strategy for treatment of volume overload in heart failure. Diuretic use is associated with electrolyte and metabolic abnormalities, worsening renal function, and an increasing prevalence of diuretic resistance with prolonged use [41]. Venovenous ultrafiltration has emerged as a treatment strategy for management of volume overload. Using peripheral or central venous access, an ultrafiltration circuit and an extracorporeal blood pump mounted in a small console, fluid removal can be achieved at rates of up to 500 mL per hour. The use of such a device, the Aquadex System 100 (CHF Solutions, Brooklyn Park, MN), was studied in the UNLOAD trial [48]. Two hundred patients admitted with acute decompensated heart failure and significant volume overload were randomized to receive standard care including diuretics or to a peripheral ultrafiltration strategy. Patients receiving ultrafiltration had significantly greater weight loss at 48 hours compared with patients with standard care, without a significant difference in renal function. Interestingly, the risk of worsening heart failure at 90 days also was significantly reduced in patients receiving ultrafiltration.

Although the efficacy of ultrafiltration has been established in this and other studies, its optimal clinical role remains to be defined, whether it is used as an early alternative to diuresis or reserved for diuretic-resistant patients. Equally, the cost effectiveness of an ultrafiltration-based strategy for fluid removal has not yet been established. CI—confidence interval; M—mean. (*Adapted from* Costanzo *et al.* [48].)

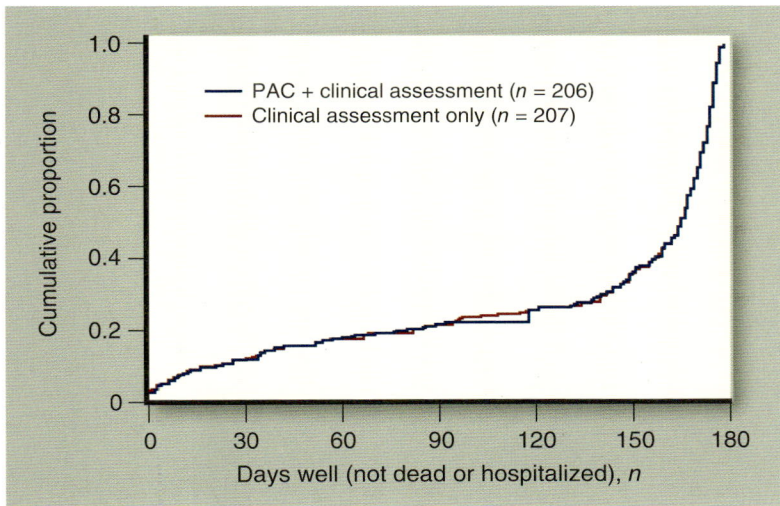

Figure 5-48. Evaluation Study of Congestive Heart Failure and Pulmonary Artery Catheter Effectiveness (ESCAPE). Four hundred thirty-three patients hospitalized for treatment of decompensated heart failure (HF) were randomized to pulmonary artery catheter (PAC)-directed therapy or to clinical management without a PAC [49]. Patients with a PAC were diuresed to a greater degree than the usual care group but had less deterioration in renal function and had lower discharge diuretic doses.

A greater incidence of adverse events was reported in the PAC group during their hospitalization. The primary endpoint of days alive and out of hospital over the next 6 months was identical in the two groups. On the basis of these results, PAC should not be used routinely in patients with decompensated HF. The reasons for the neutral results of this study remain unclear [50].

Cardiac Resynchronization Therapy

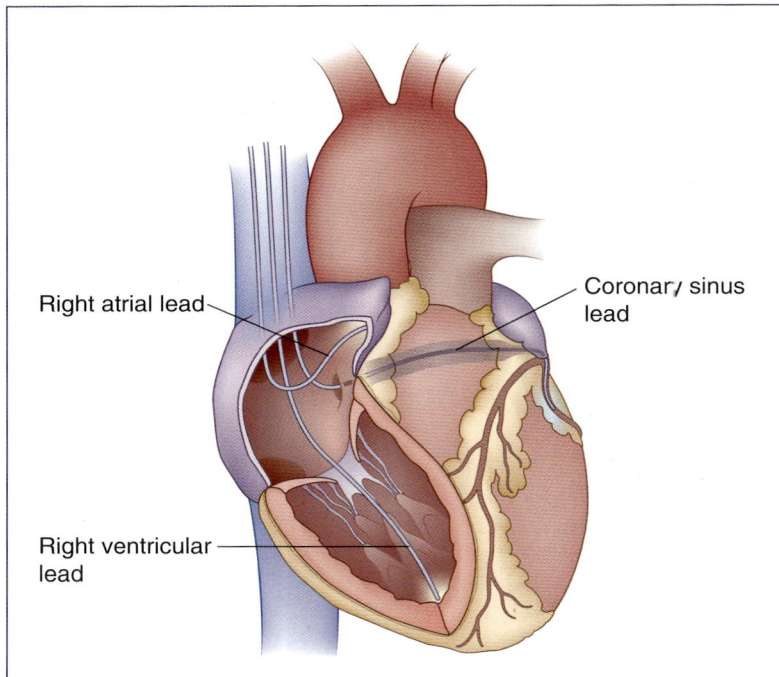

Figure 5-49. Biventricular pacing for cardiac resynchronization therapy. The use of cardiac pacing to synchronize contraction of the right and left ventricles is called cardiac resynchronization therapy (CRT). The implantation procedure involves insertion of the right atrial and right ventricular leads in the standard fashion in the right atrial appendage and right ventricular apex, respectively. The left ventricular (LV) lead is inserted into the coronary sinus and advanced into a cardiac vein ideally on the lateral wall of the left ventricle. Due to variable coronary venous anatomy, the location of a suitable vein differs from patient to patient. For patients in whom LV lead placement cannot be achieved percutaneously due to unsuitable anatomy or a procedural complication such as coronary sinus dissection, epicardial LV lead placement may be performed via thoracotomy or thoracoscopy, but carries a higher procedural risk [51]. (*Adapted from* Jarcho [52].)

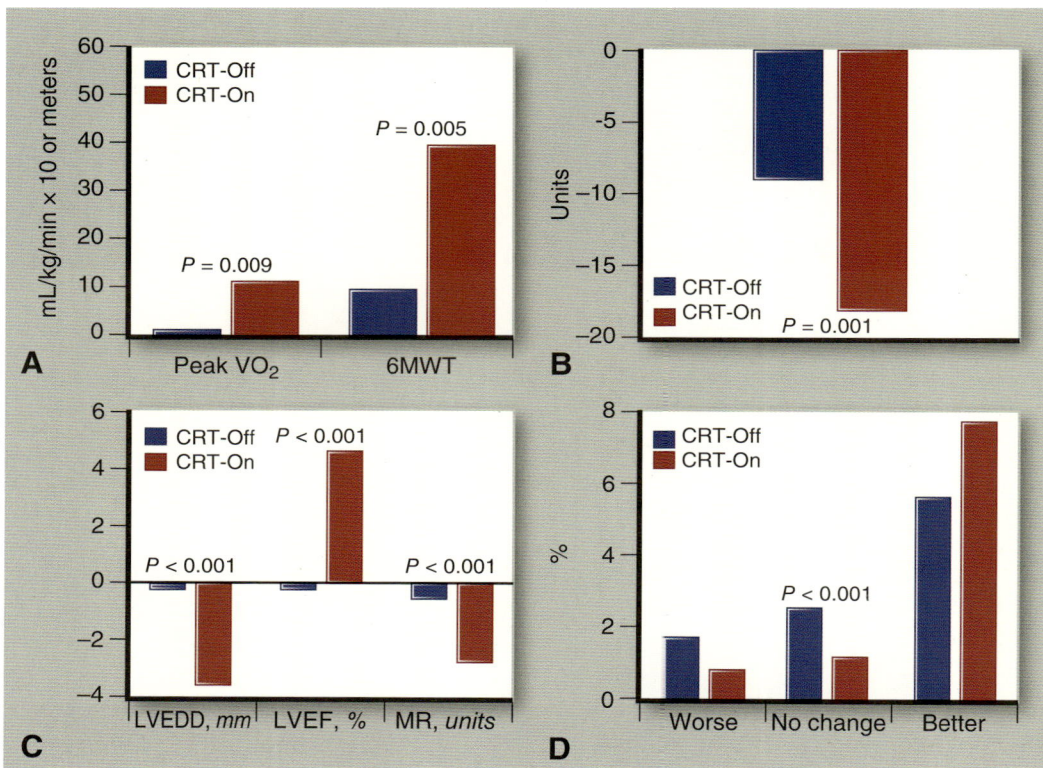

Figure 5-50. Multicenter InSync Randomized Clinical Evaluation (MIRACLE). The primary endpoints of the MIRACLE study were New York Heart Association class, quality-of-life score on the Minnesota scale, and the distance walked in 6 minutes (6MWT), all of which improved significantly ($P = 0.005$ or better) [53]. This study established cardiac resynchronization therapy (CRT) as an effective treatment for symptoms. Hospitalizations for heart failure were also reduced ($P < 0.05$). **A**, Exercise capacity. **B**, Quality of life based on the Minnesota Living With Heart Failure Questionnaire. Negative values mean greater benefit. **C**, Echocardiography. **D**, Global patient response. LVEDD—left ventricular end-diastolic dimension; LVEF—left ventricular ejection fraction; MR—mitral regurgitation.

Effect of CRT on Mortality

Study	Patients, n	Follow-up, mo	Hazard ratio (95% CI)	P value
MIRACLE [53]	453	6	0.73 (0.34–1.54)	0.4
COMPANION [54]	1520	12	0.76 (0.58–1.01)	0.06
CARE-HF [55]	813	29	0.64 (0.48–0.85)	< 0.002
Extension phase [56]		38	0.60 (0.47–0.77)	< 0.0001

Figure 5-51. Effect of cardiac resynchronization therapy (CRT) on all-cause mortality in patients with advanced heart failure, reduced ejection fraction and electrical dyssynchrony. The Multicenter InSync Randomization Clinical Evaluation (MIRACLE) and Comparison of Medical Therapy, Pacing, and Defibrillation in Chronic Heart Failure (COMPANION) studies [53, 54] demonstrated non-significant reductions in mortality of 27% and 24%, respectively. The Cardiac Resynchronization in Heart Failure (CARE-HF) trial [55] compared the effects of CRT ($n = 409$) with pharmacologic management alone ($n = 404$) using an unblinded, parallel-arm design. The study was completed according to plan (median follow-up, 29.4 months) and included an extension phase [56] to allow for analysis and presentation of results (median follow-up, 37.6 months). Both analyses revealed a highly significant reduction in mortality with the addition of CRT to optimal medical therapy.

Heart Transplant and Mechanical Assist

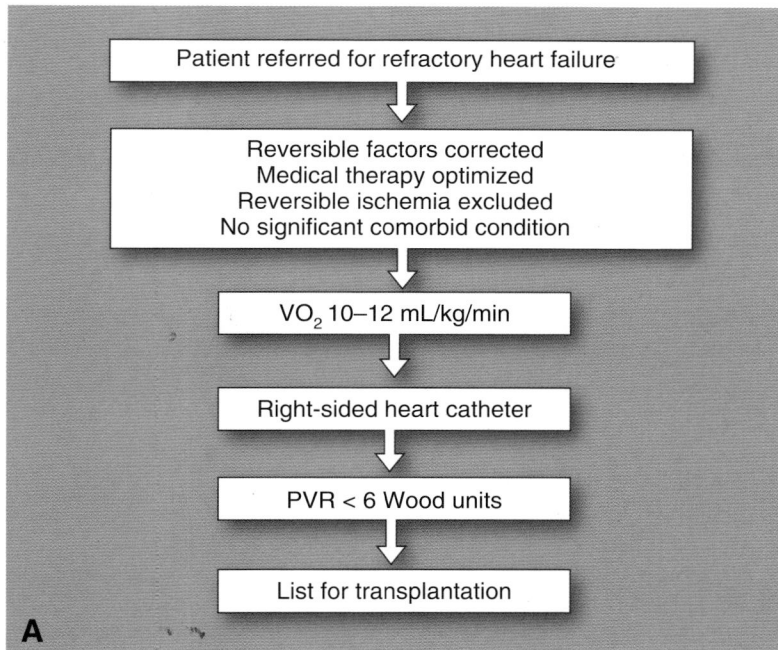

Relative or Absolute Contraindications to Cardiac Transplantation

Age > 65 years

Fixed PVR > 6 Wood units

Peptic ulcer disease or pulmonary infarct within 3 months

Brittle diabetes mellitus or diabetes with end-organ damage

Major debilitating comorbid disease

Symptomatic severe peripheral arterial or carotid disease

Symptomatic hypertension requiring multidrug therapy

Active infection

Renal insufficiency (creatinine level > 2.5 mg/dL or creatine clearance < 50 mL/min)

Severe liver dysfunction (bilirubin level > 2.5 mg/dL or transaminase level > two times normal)

Significant obstructive pulmonary disease (FEV_1 < 1 liter)

Significant intrinsic coagulation abnormalities

Active or recent malignancy (within 2 years)

HIV seroconversion

Amyloidosis

Excessive obesity (BMI > 35)

Evidence of active tobacco, alcohol, or drug abuse

History of severe mental illness or psychosocial instability

Figure 5-52. Proposed algorithm for cardiac transplantation recipient selection (**A**) and clinical contraindications to transplantation (**B**) [57]. All referred candidates should be New York Heart Association class III or IV after optimization of medical therapy. BMI—body mass index; FEV_1—1-second forced expiratory volume; PVR—pulmonary vascular resistance.

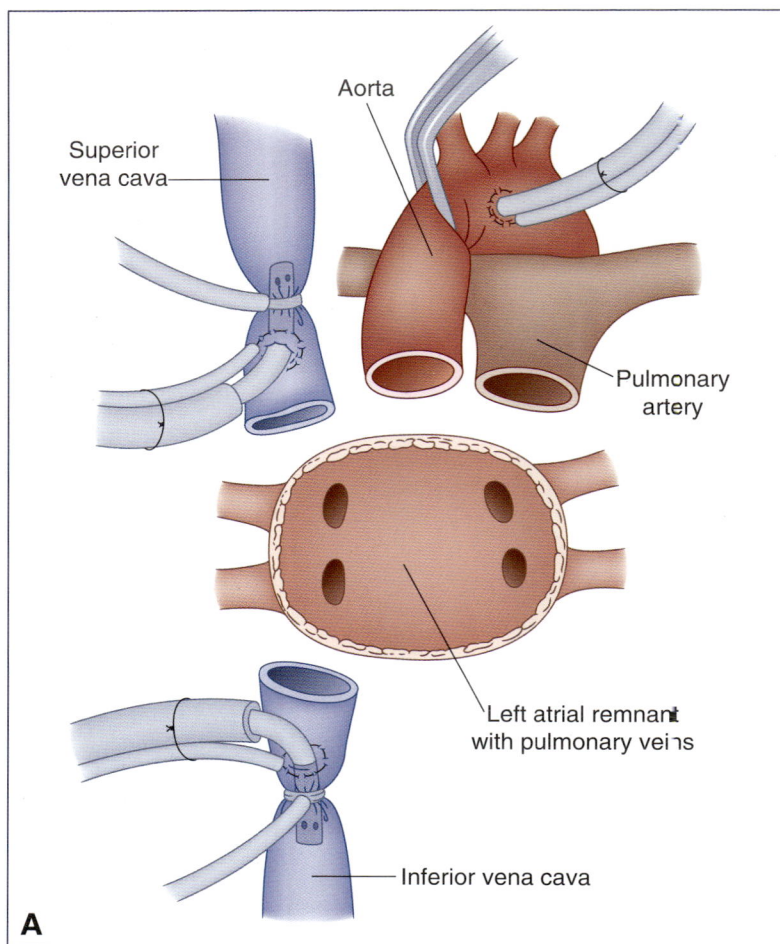

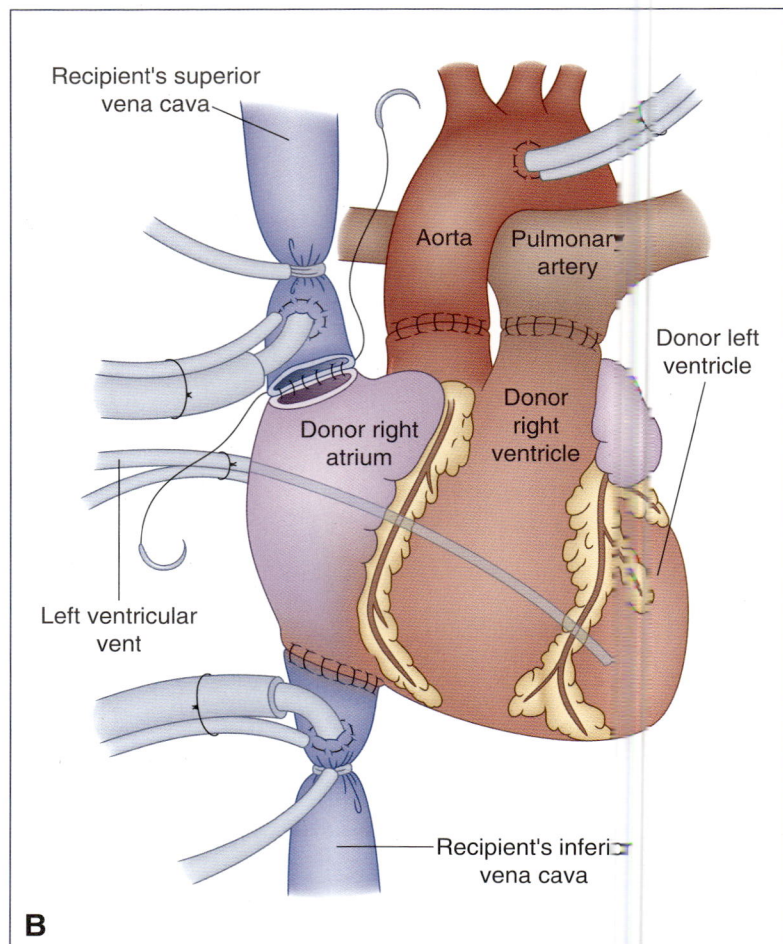

Figure 5-53. Surgical technique for orthotopic cardiac transplantation. **A**, Recipient heart explantation in preparation for bicaval anastamoses. The atrial septum and right atrium are resected with the ventricles of the diseased heart, leaving only a small cuff at the origin of the venae cavae. The left atrium is further resected, leaving a cuff of tissue around the ostia of the pulmonary veins.

B, The left atrial anastomosis is completed and a left ventricular vent is inserted through the suture line. After the recipient and donor pulmonary artery anastomosis is completed except for the anterior part the aortic anastomosis is completed. The heart is de-aired and modified reperfusion is instituted. During reperfusion the inferior vena caval anastomosis is performed. The heart is then de-aired and the cross-clamp is released. The superior vena caval anastomosis is then completed while the heart is beating. (*Adapted from Kapoor and Laks [58].*)

Figure 5-54. Typical regimen of medications four months after cardiac transplantation. In addition to immunosuppressive medications, approximately 75% of patients require drug therapy for hypertension, often with diltiazem, which decreases the metabolism and cost of cyclosporine and may decrease cardiac allograft vasculopathy, and/or an ACE inhibitor. A loop diuretic is required to control fluid retention in most patients during the first 6 months and is less commonly required thereafter. Omeprazole is commonly given to decrease gastrointestinal side effects of prednisone. Clotrimazole troches are used to decrease mucosal candidiasis during the first 3 months. Trimethoprim-sulfamethoxazole may be given every other day to decrease the incidence of Pneumocystis carinii pneumonia during the first 6 months. Both prophylactic antibiotics may be resumed briefly after subsequent therapy for rejection. There is general agreement in the importance of lipid-lowering therapy in transplant recipients, who respond well to HMG-CoA reductase inhibitors but require lower doses and careful monitoring to avoid rhabdomyolysis. Aspirin is often used to decrease platelet aggregation as a potential factor in the vasculopathy. Calcium and vitamin D are recommended in postmenopausal women and other patients with decreased bone density, which can result from cyclosporine and corticosteroid use. ACE—angiotensin-converting enzyme; HMG-CoA—hepatic hydromethylglutaryl coenzyme A.

Sample Regimen of Medications After Transplantation	
Cyclosporine or tacrolimus	Clotrimazole troches
Mycophenolate mofetil	Trimethoprim-sulfamethoxazole
Prednisone	HMG-CoA reductase inhibitor
Diltiazem or ACE inhibitor	Aspirin
Furosemide	Calcium carbonate
Omeprazole	Vitamin D

ISHLT Endomyocardial Grading System

Grade		Cellular rejection old system	Histologic description
0R	No acute rejection	0	Normal
1R	Mild low-grade rejection	1A, 1B, 2	Focal or diffuse perivascular or interstitial infiltrate with up to one focus of myocyte necrosis
2R	Moderate, intermediate rejection	3A	Two or more foci of myocyte necrosis with interstitial infiltrates
3R	Severe, high grade	3B, 4	Diffuse aggressive polymorphous infiltrate with necrosis ± edema, hemorrhage, vasculitis
Acute antibody-mediated rejection (AMR)			
AMR0	Negative	Negative	No histologic or immuno-pathologic features
AMR1	Positive	Positive	Histologic features: endothelial cell swelling, intravascular macrophage accumulation; interstitial edema, hemorrhage; positive immuno-fluorescence or immunoperoxidase staining for CD68 or C4d

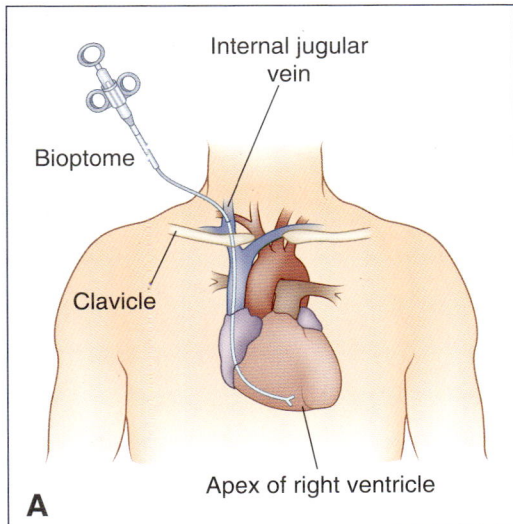

Figure 5-55. Histologic grading of allograft rejection remains the primary method for the diagnosis of rejection. **A,** Periodic endomyocardial biopsies are performed using a disposable bioptome. The bioptome is inserted through the internal jugular vein to the right ventricular portion of the interventricular septum under fluoroscopy. Three to four specimens containing at least 50% myocytes are required for 90% to 95% confidence in the interpretation. **B,** There has been a recent revision of the histologic biopsy grading system of the International Society for Heart and Lung Transplantation (ISHLT), which now includes criteria for both cellular and humoral rejection [59].

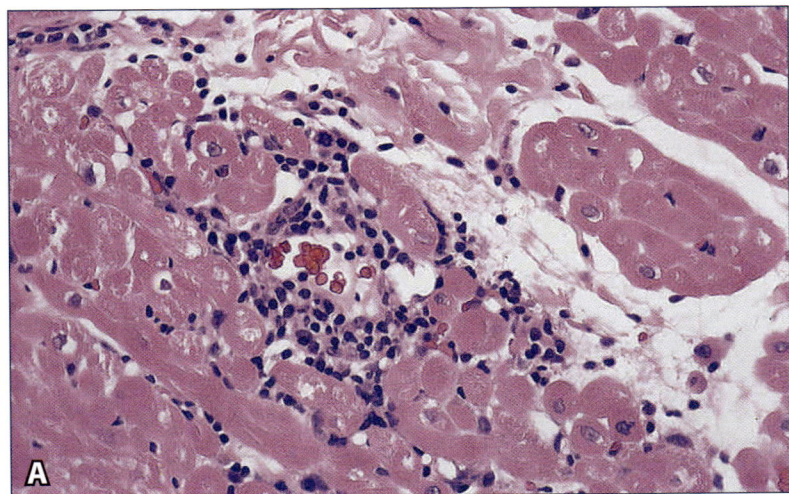

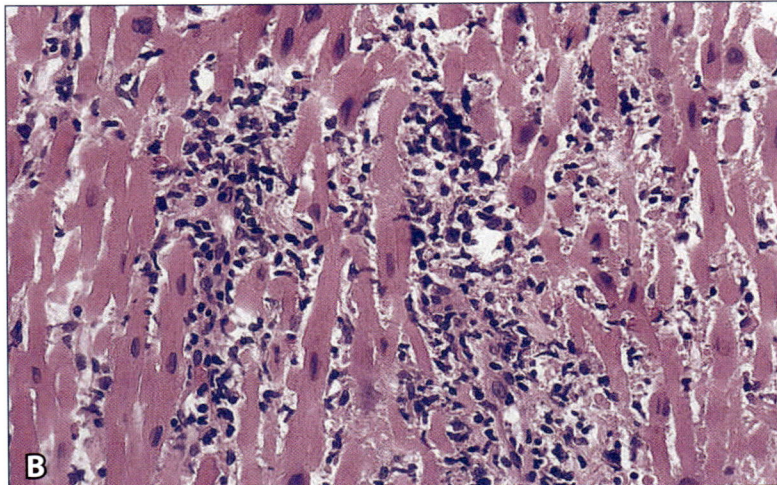

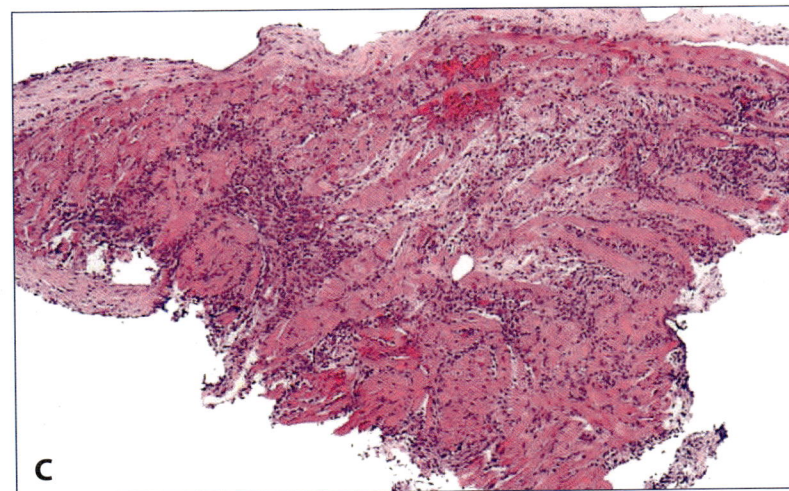

Figure 5-56. Hematoxylin and eosin staining of representative endomyocardial biopsies at a magnification of 100 × showing grade 1R (previous grade 1B) rejection with focal lymphocytic infiltrate without evidence of myocardial necrosis (**A**), grade 2R (previous grade 3A) rejection demonstrating more intensive lymphocytic infiltration and myocyte necrosis (**B**), and grade 3R (previous grade 4) allograft rejection with extensive lymphocyte infiltration, myocyte necrosis, and hemorrhage (**C**).

Recent developments in the area of genomics have been applied to noninvasive diagnosis of allograft rejection using gene expression profiling of peripheral blood mononuclear cells. Leukocyte microarrays from 252 candidate genes were screened and 11 identified as markers of allograft rejection [60]. Allomap testing is currently being investigated as a means to identify patients at high risk for rejection.

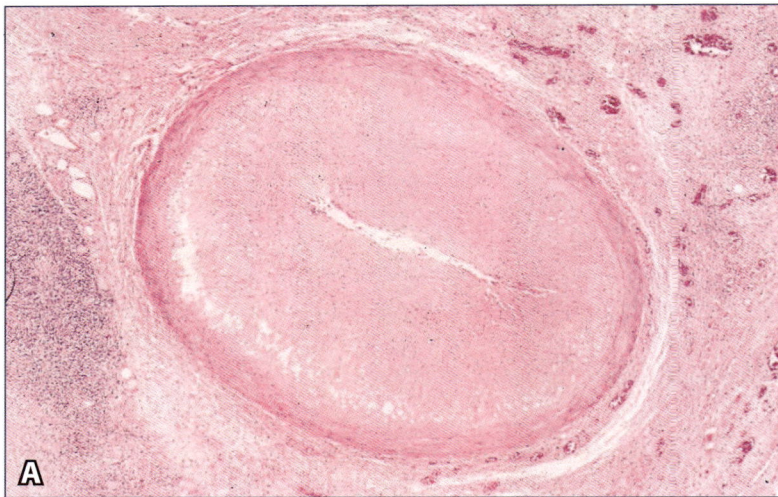

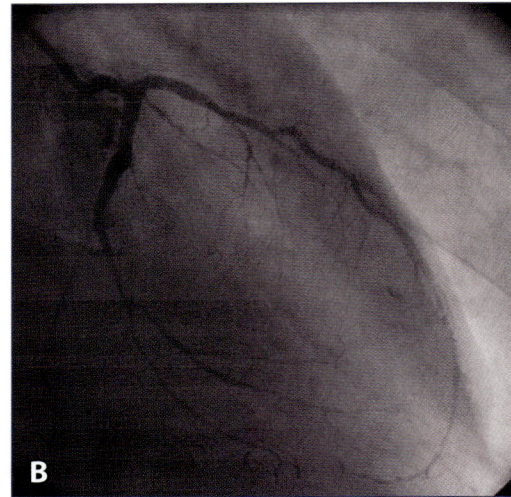

Figure 5-57. Cardiac allograft vasculopathy (CAV). The major cause of late death after cardiac transplantation is the development of CAV, a unique accelerated form of coronary artery disease. By 1 year post-transplantation, about 30% of patients demonstrate some CAV, and the incidence and severity continue to increase with time [61]. The pathogenesis of CAV is thought to begin with immunologic and non-immunologic injury to the arterial endothelium, with resultant loss of endothelial integrity. Microthrombi, cellular proliferation, and plasma lipids accumulate at the site of the injured intima.

A, This leads to further cellular proliferation and finally profound myointimal hyperplasia leading to diffuse coronary artery lumen narrowing [62]. (*Courtesy of* Richard Mitchell, MD, PhD, Boston, MA.)

B, Selective left coronary angiography from a patient with severe CAV, which shows diffuse tapering of the left anterior descending and circumflex arteries as well as pruning of all the secondary vessels. Intravascular ultrasound may be used to measure intimal thickening, which may be present even when the artery appears normal. Given the diffuse, concentric nature of this disease, percutaneous coronary intervention and coronary bypass grafting are not useful strategies for management [63]. Unfortunately, patients with CAV have a fivefold greater risk of cardiac events such as myocardial infarction, severe refractory heart failure, and sudden death.

C, Until recently, retransplantation was the only treatment for severe CAV despite reduced survival; however, a recent study described the effi-

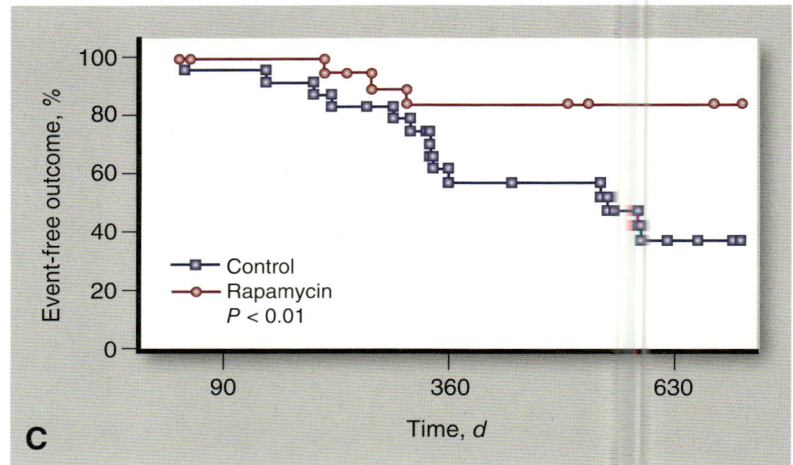

cacy of rapamycin to slow the progression of graft vasculopathy [64]. In this randomized prospective study of 46 patients with severe CAV, clinically significant adverse events such as death, myocardial infarction, need for revascularization, or worsening of a quantitative catheterization score were significantly reduced in the cohort receiving rapamycin. Similarly, cardiac hospitalizations were also reduced in the rapamycin-treated arm. Preventative strategies for CAV continue to be stressed. Hyperlipidemia management with HMG CoA (3-hydroxy-3-methylglutaryl coenzyme A) reductase inhibitors and routine aspirin use are two such approaches.

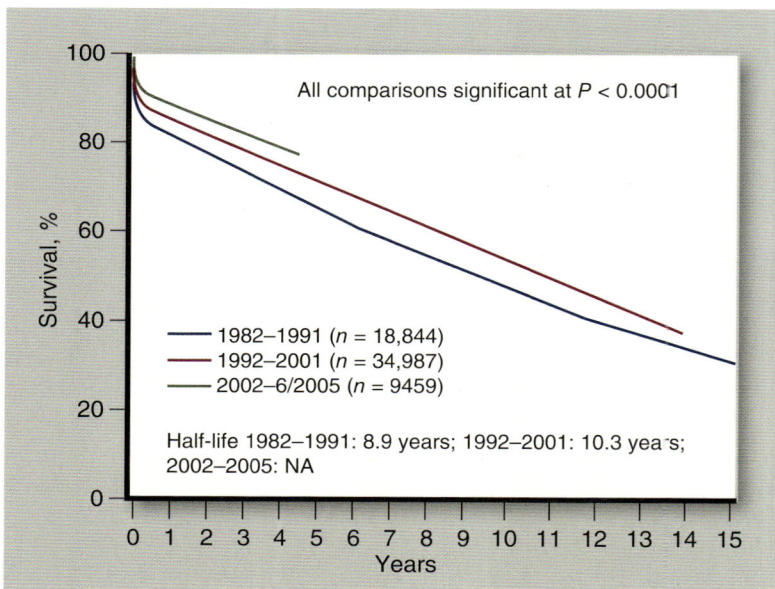

Figure 5-58. Long-term survival following orthotopic cardiac transplantation. Kaplan-Meier survival data for 63,290 heart transplants performed between January 1982 and June 2005 by era as observed in the Registry of the International Society for Heart and Lung Transplantation. The transplant half-life (the time at which 50% of those transplanted remain alive, or median survival) has increased steadily, with a projected half-life for the most recent era of approximately 11 years. Small, but significant improvement in survival over time has been attributed to progress in immunosuppression and better management of co-morbidities such as hypertension, dyslipidemia, and renal insufficiency. However, late survival continues to be limited by transplant vasculopathy, which has not decreased noticeably in the cyclosporine era. (*Adapted from* Taylor et al. [65].)

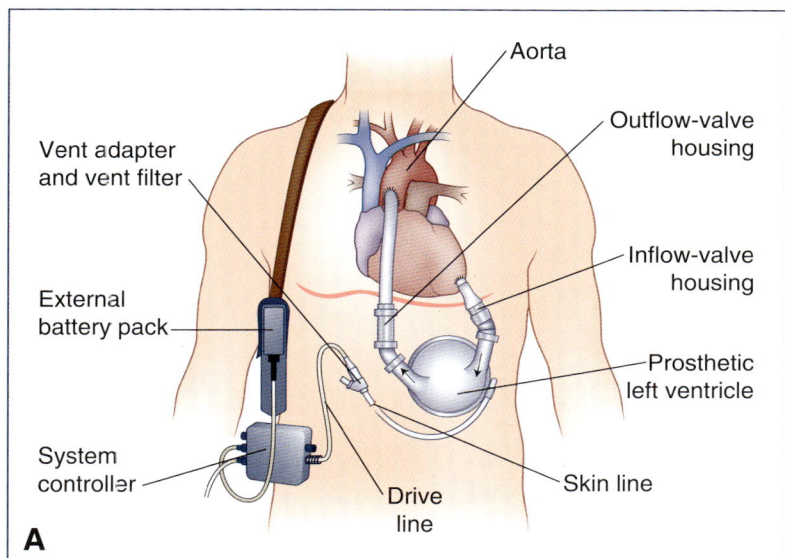

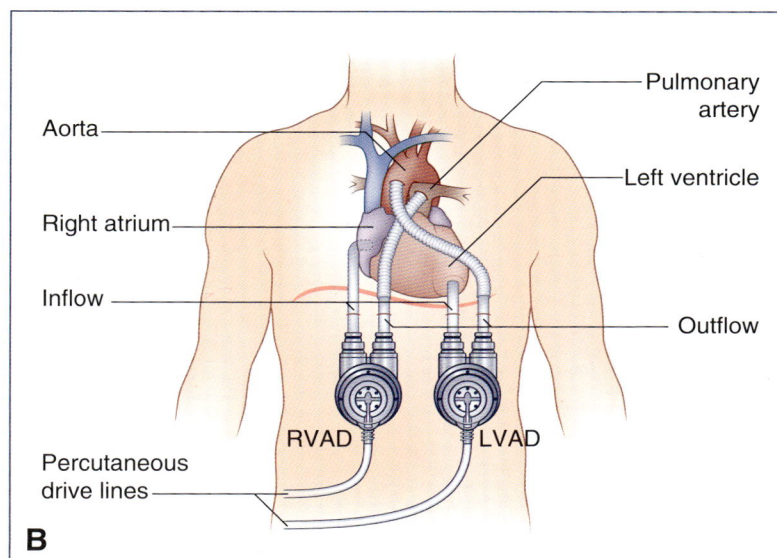

Figure 5-59. A, Thoratec HeartMate Vented Electric (Thoratec, Pleasanton, CA). This pulsatile implantable left ventricular assist device (LVAD), which is approved for bridge-to-transplantation and destination therapy [66,67] is designed to be portable and easy to operate. The inflow cannula is placed in the apex of the left ventricle with blood flow directed from the left ventricle through a porcine valve into the pump. Blood is then ejected by the electric motor positioned below the diaphragm through another porcine valve directing blood to the ascending aorta through a Dacron outflow graft. The pump is coated with a textured titanium surface that is thromboresistant and requires only a full strength aspirin for anticoagulation. An external vent equalizes the air pressure and permits emergency pneumatic actuation. The external system controller and batteries are small and lightweight, allowing the patient nearly unlimited mobility. The maximum blood flow using this device is approximately 10 L/min.

B, Anatomic configuration of the Thoratec paracorporeal ventricular assist device (VAD) (Thoratec, Pleasanton, CA). The Thoratec VAD is a pneu-

matically driven pulsatile device that is used to support patients with post-cardiotomy shock, acute cardiogenic shock from a myocardial infarction or myocarditis, or as a bridge to transplantation in patients with chronic heart failure [68]. Like all extracorporeal devices available, the system requires long-term anticoagulation to prevent clotting of the device. Depending on the configuration and the patient's needs, the device can provide right ventricular, left ventricular, or biventricular support. In patients who require long-term support as a bridge to transplantation, the left ventricular inflow cannula is usually placed in the apex of the left ventricle as opposed to the left atrium. An external drive console sends pressurized air to the pump, which compresses the polyurethane blood sac, resulting in ejection of blood from the device. Bjork-Shiley tilting disc valves within the inflow and outflow conduits ensure unidirectional blood flow through the device. The pump has a maximum flow of 6.5 L/min and can be operated in fixed-rate, volume, or synchronous modes. LVAD—left ventricular assist device; RVAD—right ventricular assist device. (*Adapted from* Farrar *et al.* [69].)

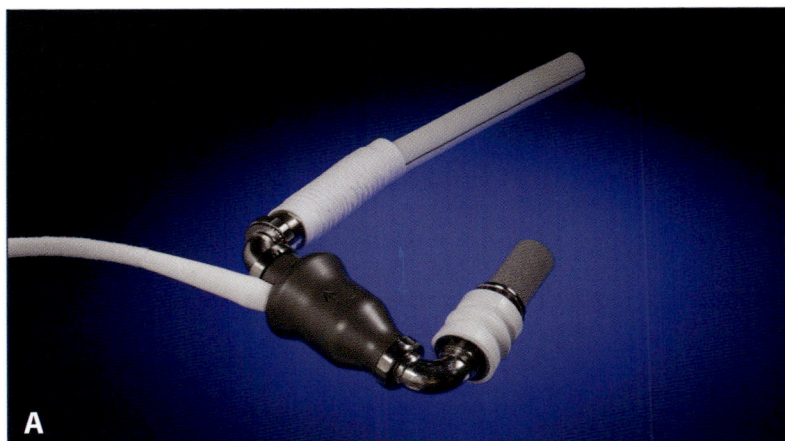

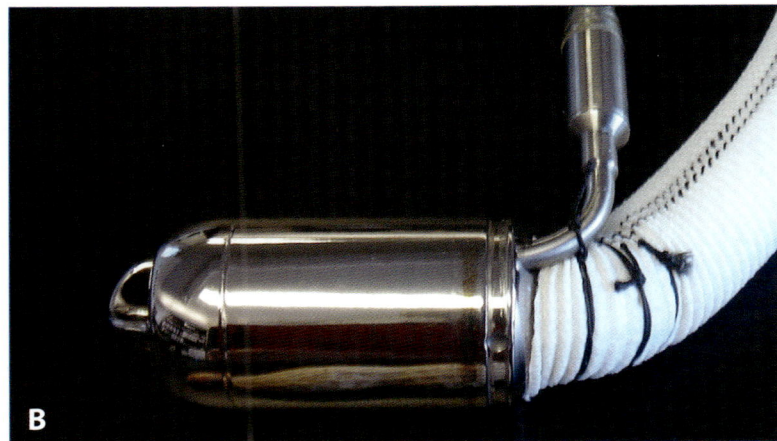

Figure 5-60. Axial flow pumps: HeartMate II (Thoratec, Pleasanton, CA) and Jarvik 2000 (Jarvik Heart, New York, NY) left ventricular assist devices (LVADs). The success of future long-term LVAD use will depend on smaller implantable, user-friendly blood pumps with less risk of infection and thromboembolism [70]. The HeartMate II (**A**) is a high-speed, axial flow, rotary blood pump [71]. Weighing only 12 ounces and measuring approximately 1.5 inches in diameter and 2.5 inches in length, the internal pump surfaces are smooth, polished titanium. Within the pump is a rotor that is rotated using electromotive force generated by the motor. The rotor propels the blood from the inflow cannula out to the natural circulation. The

pump speed can vary from 6000 rpm to 15,000 rpm, providing blood flow of up to 10 L/min. The Jarvik 2000 (**B**) is an axial flow ventricular assist device designed for bridge or destination therapy [72]. The device produces axial flow by means of a single rotating impeller, and is placed inside the left ventricle, providing flow from the left ventricle to the ascending or descending aorta. The device is power-driven by batteries connected to it by means of a percutaneous cable. The pump operating range is 8000 to 12,000 rpm, generating flows of up to 6 L/min. The HeartMate II device was recently approved for use as a bridge to transplantation. (*Courtesy of* Thoratec, Pleasanton, CA; and Jarvik Heart, New York, NY.)

References

1. American Heart Association. Heart Disease and Stroke Statistics, 2007 Update. American Heart Association, 2007.

2. Levy D, Larson MG, Vasan RS, *et al.*: The progression from hypertension to congestive heart failure. *JAMA* 1996, 275:1557–1562.

3. Rosamond W, Flegal K, Furie K, *et al.*: Heart disease and stroke statistics--2008 update: a report from the American Heart Association Statistics Committee and Stroke Statistics Subcommittee. *Circulation* 2008, 117:e25–e146.

4. Wang TJ, Evans JC, Benjamin EJ, *et al.*: Natural history of asymptomatic left ventricular systolic dysfunction in the community. *Circulation* 2003, 108:977–982.

5. Starling MR, Kirsh MM, Montgomery DG, *et al.*: Impaired left ventricular contractile function in patients with long-term mitral regurgitation and normal ejection fraction. *J Am Coll Cardiol* 1993, 22:239–250.

6. Grossman W, Carabello BA: Ventricular wall stress and the development of cardiac hypertrophy and failure. In *Perspectives in Cardiovascular Research: Myocardial Hypertrophy and Failure*, vol 7. Edited by Alpert NR. New York: Raven Press, 1993:1–15.

7. Olivetti G, Abbi R, Quaini F, *et al.*: Apoptosis in the failing human heart. *N Engl J Med* 1997, 336:1131–1141.

8. Floras JS: Clinical aspects of sympathetic activation and parasympathetic withdrawal in heart failure. *J Am Coll Cardiol* 1993, 22:72A–84A.

9. Anand IS, Fisher LD, Chiang YT, *et al.*: Changes in brain natriuretic peptide and norepinephrine over time and mortality and morbidity in the Valsartan Heart Failure Trial (Val-HeFT). *Circulation* 2003, 107:1278–1283.

10. Paganelli WC, Creager MA, Dzau VJ: Cardiac regulation of renal function. In *The International Textbook of Cardiology*. Edited by Cheng TO. New York: Pergamon Press, 1986:1010–1020.

11. Sun Y, Weber KT: Angiotensin converting enzyme and myofibroblasts during tissue repair in the rat heart. *J Mol Cell Cardiol* 1996, 28:851–858.

12. Sun Y, Weber KT: Angiotensin II receptor binding following myocardial infarction in the rat. Cardiovasc Res 1994, 28:1623–1628.

13. Wilkins MR, Redondo J, Brown LA: The natriuretic-peptide family. *Lancet* 1997, 349:1307–1310.

14. Tsutamoto T, Wada A, Maeda K, *et al.*: Attenuation of compensation of endogenous cardiac natriuretic peptide system in chronic heart failure: prognostic role of plasma brain natriuretic peptide concentration in patients with chronic symptomatic left ventricular dysfunction. *Circulation* 1997, 96:509–516.

15. Ho KK, Anderson KM, Kannel WB, *et al.*: Survival after the onset of congestive heart failure in Framingham Heart Study subjects. *Circulation* 1993, 88:107–115.

16. Farrell MH, Foody JM, Krumholz HM: β-Blockers in heart failure: clinical applications. *JAMA* 2002, 287:890–897.

17. Hunt SA, Abraham WT, Chin MH, *et al.*: ACC/AHA 2005 guideline update for the diagnosis and management of chronic heart failure in the adult: a report of the American College of Cardiology/American Heart Association Task Force on Practice Guidelines (Writing Committee to Update the 2001 Guidelines for the Evaluation and Management of Heart Failure): developed in collaboration with the American College of Chest Physicians and the International Society for Heart and Lung Transplantation: endorsed by the Heart Rhythm Society. *Circulation* 2005, 112:e154–e235.

18. Jessup M, Brozena S: Heart failure. *N Engl J Med* 2003, 348:2007–2018.

19. Zile MR, Brutsaert DL: New concepts in diastolic dysfunction and diastolic heart failure. Part I: diagnosis, prognosis, and measurements of diastolic function. *Circulation* 2002, 105:1387–1393.

20. Sica DA, Deedwania P: Pharmacotherapy in congestive heart failure: principles of combination diuretic therapy in congestive heart failure. *Congest Heart Fail* 1997, 3:29–38.

21. Brater DC: Diuretic therapy. *N Engl J Med* 1998, 339:387–395.

22. Fonarow GC, Chelimsky-Fallick C, Stevenson LW, *et al.*: Effect of direct vasodilation with hydralazine versus angiotensin-converting enzyme inhibition with captopril on mortality in advanced heart failure: the Hy-C trial. *J Am Coll Cardiol* 1992, 19:842–850.

23. Givertz MM, Cohn JN: Pharmacologic management of heart failure in the ambulatory setting. In *Cardiovascular Therapeutics: A Companion to Braunwald's Heart Disease*, edn 3. Edited by Antman EM. Philadelphia: Saunders Elsevier, 2007:331–362.

24. Cohn JN, Tognoni G: A randomized trial of the angiotensin-receptor blocker valsartan in chronic heart failure. *N Engl J Med* 2001, 345:1667–1675.

25. McMurray JJ, Ostergren J, Swedberg K, *et al.*: Effects of candesartan in patients with chronic heart failure and reduced left-ventricular systolic function taking angiotensin-converting-enzyme inhibitors: the CHARM-Added trial. *Lancet* 2003, 362:767–771.

26. Givertz MM: Manipulation of the renin-angiotensin system. *Circulation* 2001, 104:e14–e18.

27. Granger CB, McMurray JJ, Yusuf S, *et al.*: Effects of candesartan in patients with chronic heart failure and reduced left-ventricular systolic function intolerant to angiotensin-converting-enzyme inhibitors: the CHARM-Alternative trial. *Lancet* 2003, 362:772–776.

28. Pitt B, Zannad F, Remme WJ, *et al.*: The effect of spironolactone on morbidity and mortality in patients with severe heart failure. Randomized Aldactone Evaluation Study Investigators. *N Engl J Med* 1999, 341:709–717.

29. Juurlink DN, Mamdani MM, Lee DS, *et al.*: Rates of hyperkalemia after publication of the Randomized Aldactone Evaluation Study. *N Engl J Med* 2004, 351:543–551.

30. Gheorghiade M, Colucci WS, Swedberg K: Beta-blockers in chronic heart failure. *Circulation* 2003, 107:1570–1575.

31. Packer M, Coats AJ, Fowler MB, *et al.*: Effect of carvedilol on survival in severe chronic heart failure. *N Engl J Med* 2001, 344:1651–1658.

32. Colucci WS, Kolias TJ, Adams KF, *et al.*: Metoprolol reverses left ventricular remodeling in patients with asymptomatic systolic dysfunction: the REversal of VEntricular Remodeling with Toprol-XL (REVERT) trial. *Circulation* 2007, 116:49–56.

33. Gheorghiade M, Adams KF Jr, Colucci WS: Digoxin in the management of cardiovascular disorders. *Circulation* 2004, 109:2959–2964.

34. The Digitalis Investigation Group: The effect of digoxin on mortality and morbidity in patients with heart failure. *N Engl J Med* 1997, 336:525–533.

35. Rathore SS, Curtis JP, Wang Y, *et al.*: Association of serum digoxin concentration and outcomes in patients with heart failure. *JAMA* 2003, 289:871–878.

36. Taylor AL, Ziesche S, Yancy C, *et al.*: Combination of isosorbide dinitrate and hydralazine in blacks with heart failure. *N Engl J Med* 2004, 351:2049–2057.

37. Yusuf S, Pfeffer MA, Swedberg K, *et al.*: Effects of candesartan in patients with chronic heart failure and preserved left-ventricular ejection fraction: the CHARM-Preserved Trial. *Lancet* 2003, 362:777–781.

38. Yancy CW, Lopatin M, Stevenson LW, *et al.*: Clinical presentation, management, and in-hospital outcomes of patients admitted with acute decompensated heart failure with preserved systolic function: a report from the Acute Decompensated Heart Failure National Registry (ADHERE) database. *J Am Coll Cardiol* 2006, 47:76–84.

39. Stevenson LW, Dracup KA, Tillisch JH: Efficacy of medical therapy tailored for severe congestive heart failure in patients transferred for urgent cardiac transplantation. *Am J Cardiol* 1989, 63:461–464.

40. Franciosa JA, Dunkman WB, Wilen M, *et al.*: "Optimal" left ventricular filling pressure during nitroprusside infusion for congestive heart failure. *Am J Med* 1983, 74:457–464.

41. Ellison DH: Diuretic therapy and resistance in congestive heart failure. *Cardiology* 2001, 96:132–143.

42. Salvador DR, Rey NR, Ramos GC, *et al.*: Continuous infusion versus bolus injection of loop diuretics in congestive heart failure. *Cochrane Database Syst Rev* 2005:CD003178.

43. Publication Committee for the VMAC Investigators. Intravenous nesiritide vs nitroglycerin for treatment of decompensated congestive heart failure: a randomized controlled trial. *JAMA* 2002, 287:1531–1540.

44. Mullens W, Abrahams Z, Francis GS, *et al.*: Sodium nitroprusside for advanced low-output heart failure. *J Am Coll Cardiol* 2008, 52:200–207.

45. Khot UN, Novaro GM, Popovic ZB, *et al.*: Nitroprusside in critically ill patients with left ventricular dysfunction and aortic stenosis. *N Engl J Med* 2003, 348:1756–1763.

46. Leier CV, Binkley PF: Parenteral inotropic support for advanced congestive heart failure. *Prog Cardiovasc Dis* 1998, 41:207–224.

47. Givertz MM, Stevenson LW, Colucci WS: Strategies for management of decompensated heart failure. In *Cardiovascular Therapeutics: A Companion to Braunwald's Heart Disease*, edn 3. Edited by Antman EM. Philadelphia: Saunders Elsevier, 2007:385–409.

48. Costanzo MR, Guglin ME, Saltzberg MT, *et al.*: Ultrafiltration versus intravenous diuretics for patients hospitalized for acute decompensated heart failure. *J Am Coll Cardiol* 2007, 49:675–683.

49. Binanay C, Califf RM, Hasselblad V, *et al.*: Evaluation study of congestive heart failure and pulmonary artery catheterization effectiveness: the ESCAPE trial. *JAMA* 2005, 294:1625–1633.

50. Le Jemtel TH, Alt EU: Are hemodynamic goals viable in tailoring heart failure therapy? Hemodynamic goals are outdated. *Circulation* 2006, 113:1027–1032.

51. Shah RV, Lewis EF, Givertz MM: Epicardial left ventricular lead placement for cardiac resynchronization therapy following failed coronary sinus approach. *Congest Heart Fail* 2006, 12:312–316.

52. Jarcho JA: Resynchronizing ventricular contraction in heart failure. *N Engl J Med* 2005, 352:1594–1597.

53. Abraham WT, Fisher WG, Smith AL, *et al.*: Cardiac resynchronization in chronic heart failure. *N Engl J Med* 2002, 346:1845–1853.

54. Bristow MR, Saxon LA, Boehmer J, *et al.*: Cardiac-resynchronization therapy with or without an implantable defibrillator in advanced chronic heart failure. *N Engl J Med* 2004, 350:2140–2150.

55. Cleland JG, Daubert JC, Erdmann E, *et al.*: The effect of cardiac resynchronization on morbidity and mortality in heart failure. *N Engl J Med* 2005, 352:1539–1549.

56. Cleland JG, Daubert JC, Erdmann E, *et al.*: Longer-term effects of cardiac resynchronization therapy on mortality in heart failure [the CArdiac REsynchronization-Heart Failure (CARE-HF) trial extension phase]. *Eur Heart J* 2006, 27:1928–1932.

57. Kirklin JK, McGiffin DC, Pinderski LJ, *et al.*: Selection of patients and techniques of heart transplantation. *Surg Clin North Am* 2004, 84:257–287.

58. Kapoor AS, Laks H: *Atlas of Heart-Lung Transplantation*. New York: McGraw-Hill; 1994.

59. Stewart S, Winters GL, Fishbein MC, *et al.*: Revision of the 1990 working formulation for the standardization of nomenclature in the diagnosis of heart rejection. *J Heart Lung Transplant* 2005, 24:1710–1720.

60. Deng MC, Eisen HJ, Mehra MR, *et al.*: Noninvasive discrimination of rejection in cardiac allograft recipients using gene expression profiling. *Am J Transplant* 2006, 6:150–160.

61. Ventura HO, Mehra MR, Smart FW, *et al.*: Cardiac allograft vasculopathy: current concepts. *Am Heart J* 1995, 129:791–799.

62. Libby P, Pober JS: Chronic rejection. *Immunity* 2001, 14:387–397.

63. Mitchell RN, Libby P: Vascular remodeling in transplant vasculopathy. *Circ Res* 2007, 100:967–978.

64. Mancini D, Pinney S, Burkhoff D, *et al.*: Use of rapamycin slows progression of cardiac transplant vasculopathy. *Circulation* 2003, 108:48–53.

65. Taylor DO, Edwards LB, Boucek MM, *et al.*: Registry of the International Society for Heart and Lung Transplantation: twenty-fourth official adult heart transplant report—2007. *J Heart Lung Transplant* 2007, 26:769–781.

66. Oz MC, Argenziano M, Catanese KA, *et al.*: Bridge experience with long-term implantable left ventricular assist devices. Are they an alternative to transplantation? *Circulation* 1997, 95:1844–1852.

67. Rose EA, Gelijns AC, Moskowitz AJ, *et al.*: Long-term mechanical left ventricular assistance for end-stage heart failure. *N Engl J Med* 2001, 345:1435–1443.

68. Hunt SA, Frazier OH: Mechanical circulatory support and cardiac transplantation. *Circulation* 1998, 97:2079–2090.

69. Farrar DJ, Hill JD, Pennington DG, *et al.*: Preoperative and postoperative comparison of patients with univentricular and biventricular support with the thoratec ventricular assist device as a bridge to cardiac transplantation. *J Thorac Cardiovasc Surg* 1997,113:202-209.

70. Song X, Throckmorton AL, Untaroiu A, *et al.*: Axial flow blood pumps. *ASAIO J* 2003, 49:355–364.

71. Miller LW, Pagani FD, Russell SD, *et al.*: Use of a continuous-flow device in patients awaiting heart transplantation. *N Engl J Med* 2007, 357:885–896.

72. Siegenthaler MP, van de Loo A, *et al.*: Implantation of the permanent Jarvik-2000 left ventricular assist device: a single-center experience. *J Am Coll Cardiol* 2002, 39:1764–1772.

Cardiomyopathy, Myocarditis, and Pericardial Disease

6

Kenneth L. Baughman

Hypertrophic Cardiomyopathy

Hypertrophic cardiomyopathy (HCM) is characterized by left ventricular hypertrophy without apparent cause. Asymmetric hypertrophy and myocardial disarray are important pathologic features.

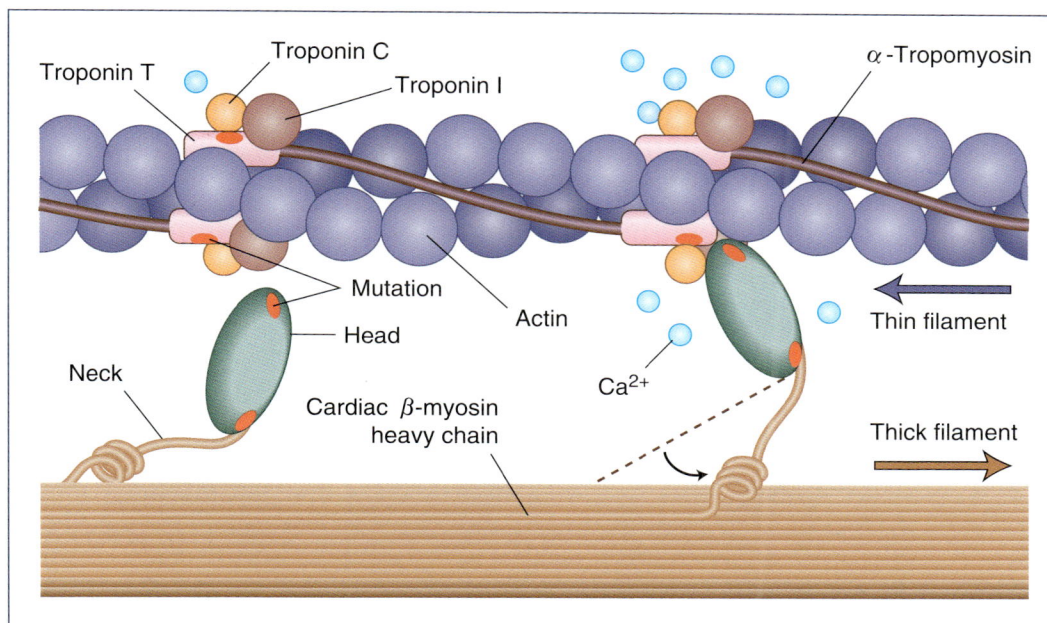

Figure 6-1. Components of the myofiber. Cardiac muscle is composed of myosin (thick filament) and actin (thin filament) layers as depicted in this illustration. Cardiac contraction occurs when calcium binds the troponin complex (subunits I, C, and T) and α-tropomyosin and releases the inhibition of the myosin-actin interactions maintained by troponin I. ATPase activity and binding of actin by the globular myosin head causes a conformational change that bends the neck (lever arm) of the thick filament, resulting in sliding of the thick filament in relation to the thin filament. This movement results in cardiac contraction. Genetic alterations in the sarcomeric proteins (including cardiac [beta] myosin heavy chain, troponin T, troponin I, α-tropomyosin, and cardiac myosin-binding protein C) may cause an enhancement of contractile function resulting in hypertrophic cardiomyopathy. Alternatively, mutations in the myosin or actin components may cause reduced production of contractile force by the sarcomere resulting in a genetic form of dilated cardiomyopathy [1].

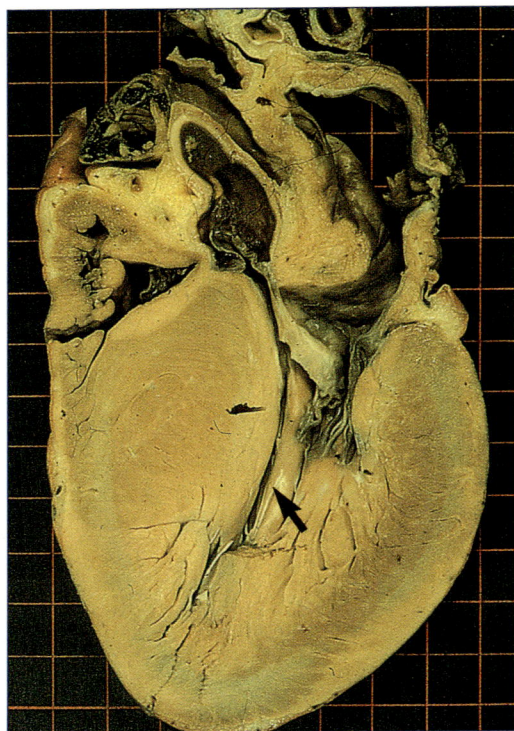

Figure 6-2. Asymmetric septal hypertrophy. Longitudinal section of the heart of a 32-year-old woman with subaortic obstructive hypertrophic cardiomyopathy who died suddenly while on propranolol therapy. Hemodynamic investigation confirmed subaortic obstruction as well as mitral regurgitation. The regurgitation was partially due to an abnormal mitral valve (insertion of an anomalous papillary muscle [*arrow*] onto the ventricular surface of the anterior mitral leaflet). Note the asymmetric hypertrophy with a grossly thickened ventricular septum. A narrowed outflow tract between the upper septum and the anterior mitral leaflet, which is thickened and fibrosed from repeated contact with the septum, can also be seen. There was microscopic evidence of extensive myocardial fiber disarray involving the septum and free wall of the left ventricle [2]. (*Courtesy of* L. Horlick.)

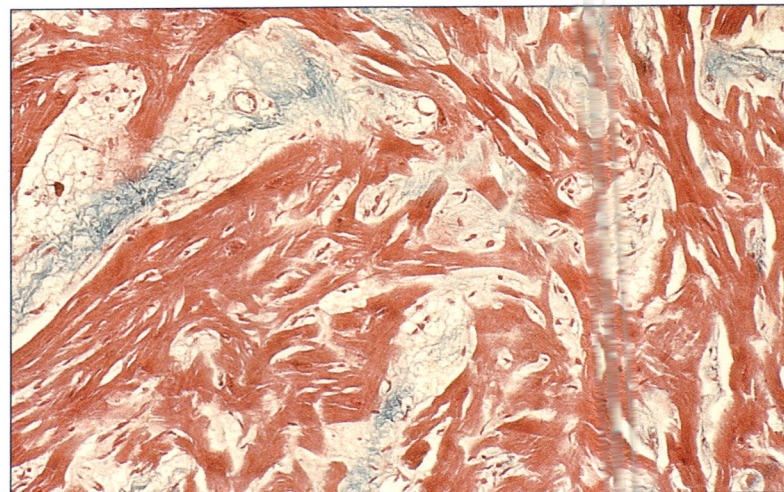

Figure 6-3. Myocardial fiber disarray. Microscopic section of the ventricular septum of a 28-year-old patient with hypertrophic cardiomyopathy who died while jogging. This section shows a typical area of myocardial fiber disarray. The muscle cells are short and plump, and the nuclei are large and hyperchromatic. Note the extensive amount of loose intercellular connective tissue that may become transformed into diffuse myocardial fibrosis late in the disease (magnification, × 100). (*From* Wigle *et al.* [2]; with permission.)

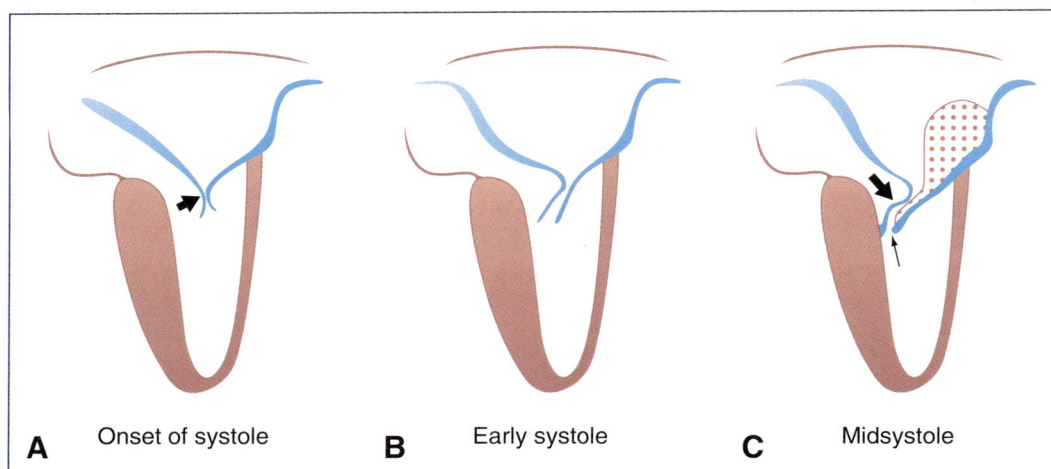

| A | Onset of systole | B | Early systole | C | Midsystole |

Figure 6-4. Functional anatomy of mitral leaflet systolic anterior motion and mitral regurgitation in subaortic obstructive hypertrophic cardiomyopathy. Drawing of a transesophageal echocardiogram (frontal long-axis plane) demonstrating the anterior and superior motion of the anterior mitral leaflet to produce mitral leaflet–septal contact and failure of leaflet coaptation in midsystole. **A,** At the onset of systole, the coaptation point (*arrow*) is in the body of the anterior and posterior leaflets rather than at the tip of the leaflets, as in normal subjects [3,4]. The portion of the leaflets beyond the coaptation point is referred to as the residual length of the leaflet [3,4]. During early systole (**B**) and midsystole (**C**) there is anterior and superior movement of the residual length of the anterior mitral leaflet (*thick arrow in C*), with septal contact and failure of leaflet coaptation (*thin arrow in C*) with consequent mitral regurgitation directed posteriorly into the left atrium (*dotted area*). (*Adapted from* Grigg *et al.* [4].)

Figure 6-5. Physical examination in subaortic obstructive hypertrophic cardiomyopathy (HCM). There are seven physical signs in subaortic obstructive HCM that are not found in nonobstructive HCM. On palpation, a spike-and-dome arterial pulse can often be felt in the carotid artery or in a peripheral pulse. On palpation of the left ventricular (LV) apex, there may be a triple apex beat caused by a palpable left atrial gallop and a double systolic impulse—one impulse comes before the onset of obstruction and the other after. On auscultation, at or just medial to the LV apex, there is a late onset, diamond-shaped systolic murmur of grade 3 to 4/6 in intensity. This murmur is caused by both the subaortic obstruction and the concomitant mitral regurgitation, causing the murmur to radiate to both the left sternal border and to the axilla. Because of the mitral regurgitation, there is often a short diastolic inflow murmur after the third heart sound. Rarely, a mitral leaflet–septal contact (ML–SC) sound may be heard preceding the systolic murmur at the apex. Finally, if there is severe subaortic obstruction, reversed splitting of the second heart sound may occur. In nonobstructive HCM, there is often a third or fourth heart sound at the apex, depending on the type of diastolic dysfunction. If the fourth heart sound is palpable, there will be a double apex beat, which is quite different in timing and significance from the double systolic apex beat that occurs in subaortic obstructive HCM. In nonobstructive HCM, there is either no apical systolic murmur or at most a grade 1 to 2/6 murmur of mitral regurgitation. In any type of HCM, a grade 1 to 3/6 systolic ejection murmur at or below the pulmonary area may be heard. This murmur may reflect obstruction to right ventricular (RV) outflow. Examining the jugular venous pulse frequently reveals a prominent a-wave that rises on inspiration, depending on the degree of RV diastolic dysfunction. Rarely, this is accompanied by an RV fourth heart sound.

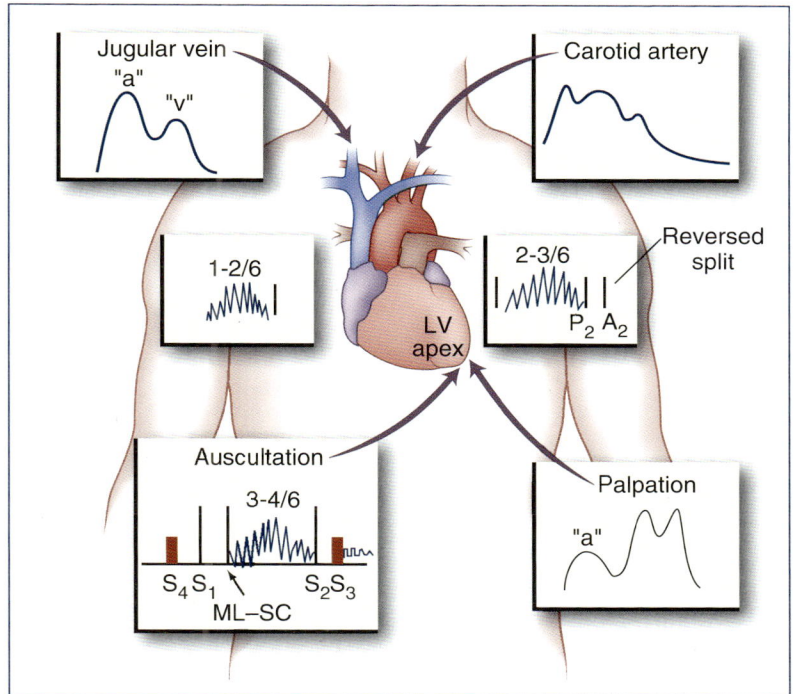

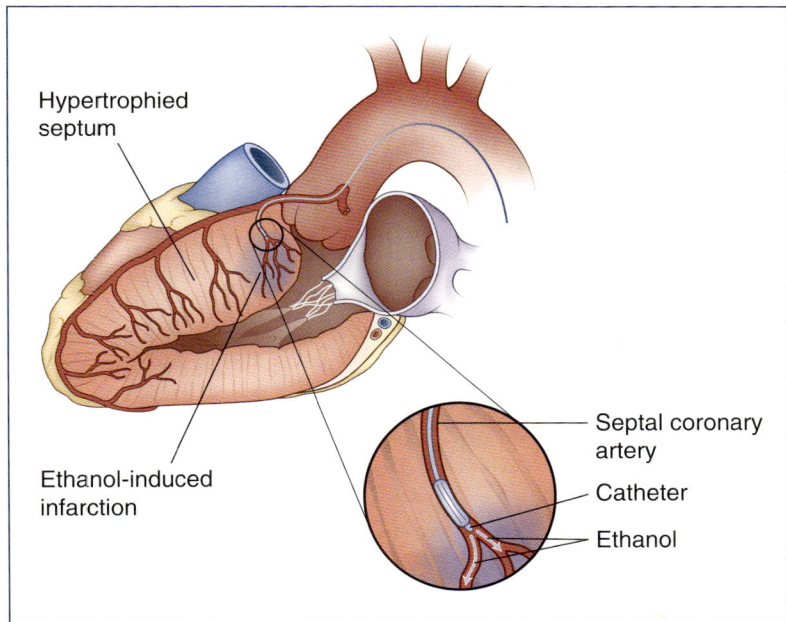

Figure 6-6. Alcohol septal ablation. A catheter is inserted into the left anterior descending artery and directed into the septal branch that supplies blood to the hypertrophied portion of the septum. The septal artery catheter balloon is inflated preventing backwash of alcohol into the remainder of the coronary tree. Through a distal port on the balloon-tipped catheter, ethanol is injected into the septal artery, resulting in a controlled myocardial infarction [5].

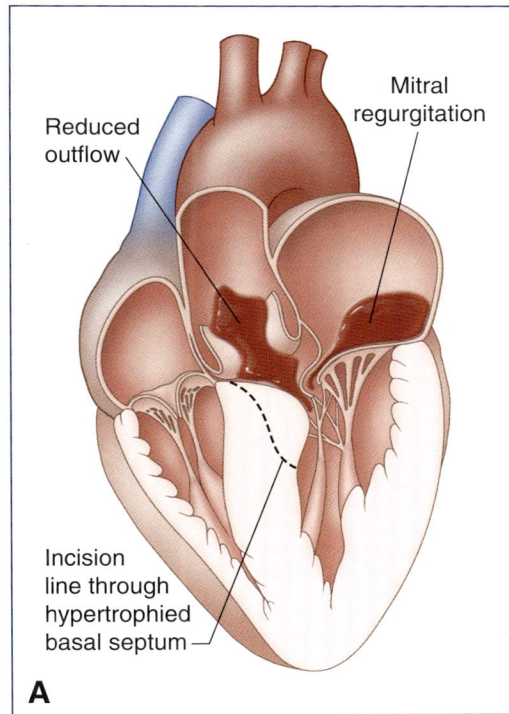

Figure 6-7. Illustration of surgical septal myectomy. **A,** Before surgical intervention the severe septal hypertrophy and systolic anterior motion of the mitral valve result in mitral regurgitation and outflow obstruction.

Continued on the next page

B

Septal
myectomy

C

Increased
outflow

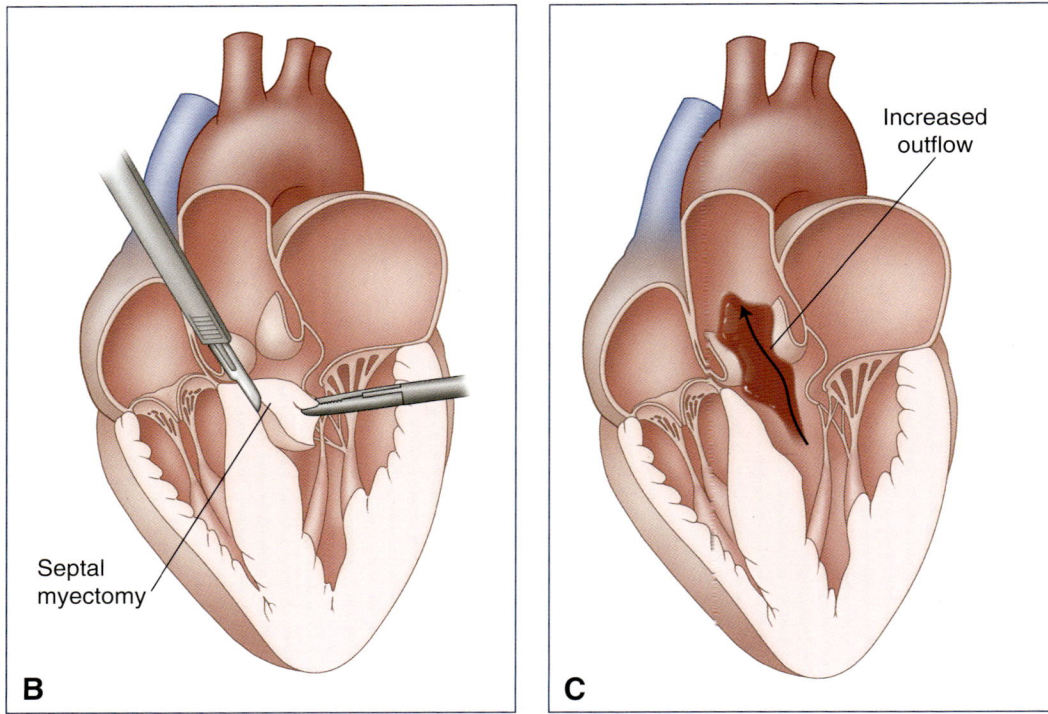

Figure 6-7. *(Continued)* **B,** In surgical myectomy the septal hypertrophy is surgically reduced. **C,** This surgical ablation reduces the outflow obstruction and often eliminates mitral regurgitation [6].

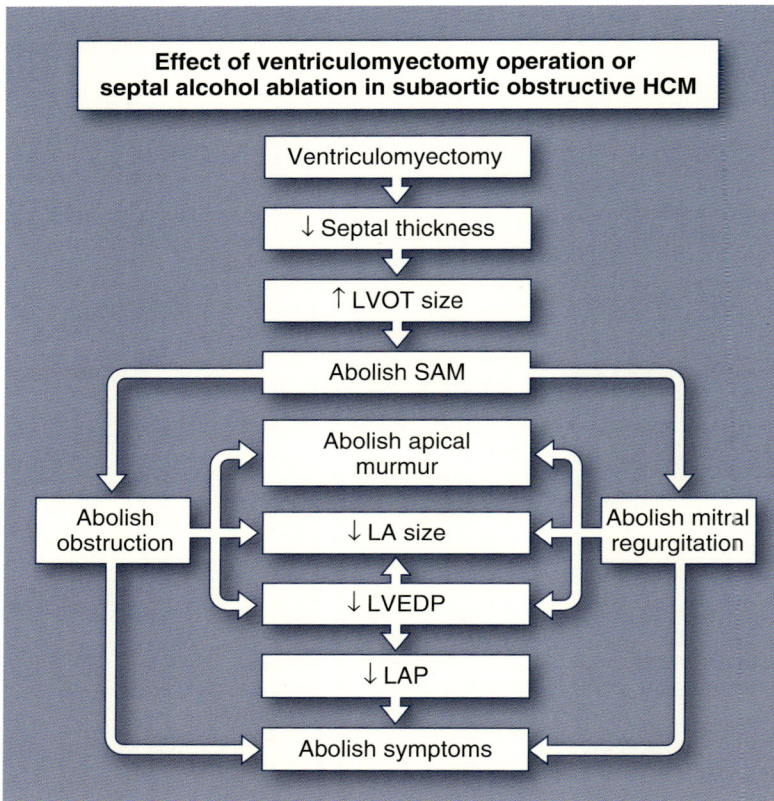

Effect of ventriculomyectomy operation or septal alcohol ablation in subaortic obstructive HCM

Ventriculomyectomy

↓ Septal thickness

↑ LVOT size

Abolish SAM

Abolish apical murmur

Abolish obstruction

↓ LA size

Abolish mitral regurgitation

↓ LVEDP

↓ LAP

Abolish symptoms

Figure 6-8. Management of obstructive hypertrophic cardiomyopathy (HCM) that does not respond to medical therapy. When patients with obstructive HCM are unresponsive to medical therapy, or are dissatisfied by the disease-imposed limitations or the side effects of medication, atrioventricular sequential pacemaker therapy, alcohol septal ablation, or surgery may be considered. Ventricular pacing from the right ventricular apex may cause a rightward septal shift and alleviation of the subaortic obstruction with resultant symptomatic improvement in some patients. This form of therapy is not, however, effective in all patients. The obstruction in some patients is not completely relieved, and up to 25% of patients require atrioventricular nodal ablation to achieve ventricular capture [7,8]. Ventriculomy-ectomy surgery, however, has been performed for more than 30 years, and a number of centers have had extensive experience (and good to excellent results) [9–12]. The mechanisms of benefit of this procedure are illustrated. Myectomy thins the ventricular septum and widens the left ventricular outflow tract (LVOT), which abolishes mitral leaflet systolic anterior motion (SAM). This in turn abolishes the obstruction and mitral regurgitation. These effects eliminate the apical murmur and decrease the left ventricular end-diastolic pressure (LVEDP) as well as left atrial pressure (LAP) and size. Symptoms are dramatically relieved by these mechanisms. Myectomy is also indicated in recurrent atrial fibrillation to decrease left atrial size and restore normal sinus rhythm. The procedure should be performed in patients with obstructive HCM with unexplained syncope or cardiac arrest.

Alcohol ablation attempts to reduce the subaortic gradient by creation of myocardial dysfunction. Alcohol is injected into the septal branch or branches of the left anterior descending artery that supply the hypertrophied septum. If successful, the myocardial infarction decreases septal contraction and reduces the outflow gradient.

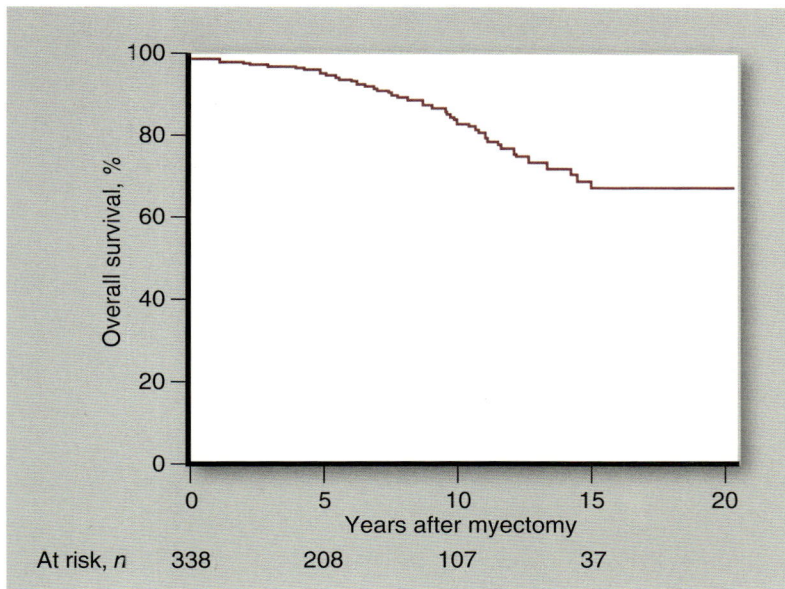

Figure 6-9. Kaplan-Meier survival curve for 338 adult patients who underwent myectomy at a single institution. Survival at 1 year is 98%, 95% at 5 years, and 83% at 10 years after this procedure. In long-term follow up, 83% of patients had improvement to functional class I or II. Predictors of late cardiovascular events include female gender, history of atrial fibrillation before surgery, and a left atrial diameter greater than 46 mm. Surgical myectomy by an experienced surgeon is associated with excellent long-term results [13].

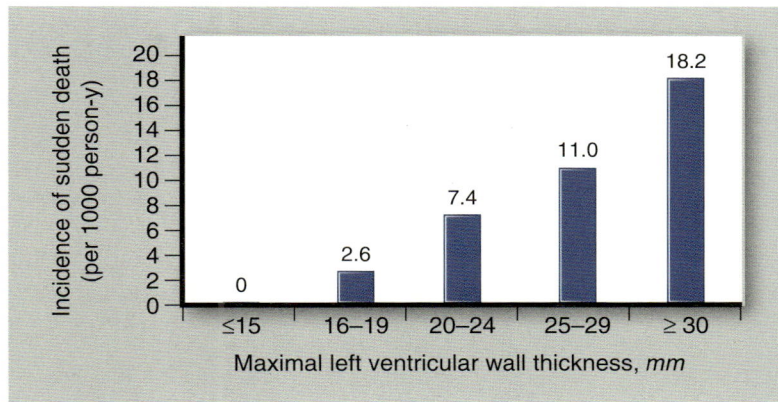

Figure 6-10. Patients with asymmetric septal hypertrophy die of progressive heart failure or sudden cardiac death. The risk of sudden death appears to correlate with the maximal left ventricular wall thickness. Severe hypertrophy may be present in young patients with mild or no symptoms [14]. (*Adapted from* Spirito *et al.* [14].)

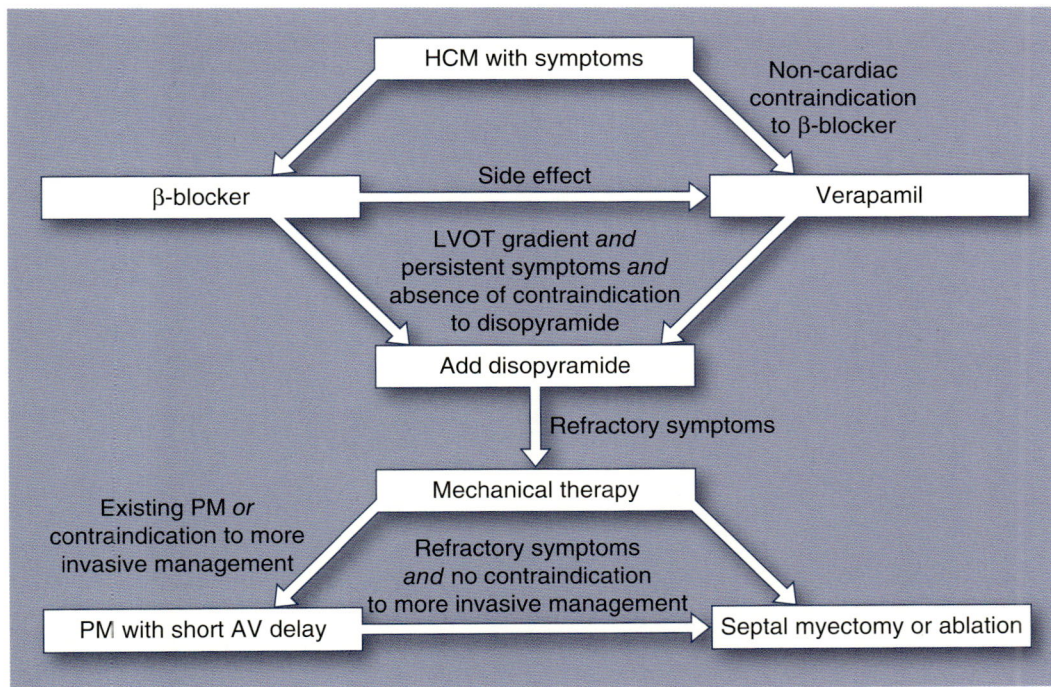

Figure 6-11. Proposed algorithm for the medical, mechanical, and surgical/interventional ablative treatment of patients with hypertrophic cardiomyopathy. Only 20% to 30% of patients with hypertrophic cardiomyopathy have outflow obstruction and would be candidates for the addition of disopyramide pacemaker therapy, or septal ablation [15]. AV—atrial ventricular; HCM—hypertrophic cardiomyopathy; LVOT—left ventricular outflow tract; PM—pacemaker.

Idiopathic Dilated Cardiomyopathy

According to the World Health Organization, idiopathic dilated cardiomyopathy is characterized by dilatation of the left, right, or both ventricles with impaired systolic function and is of unknown cause.

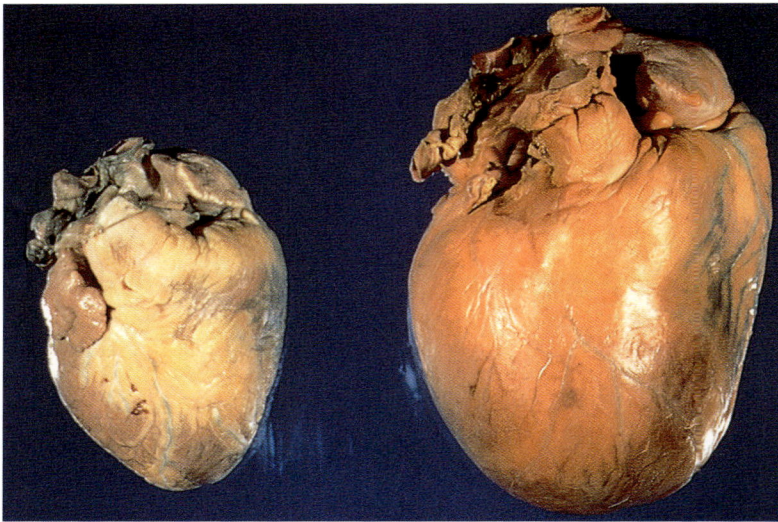

Figure 6-12. Gross pathology. In contrast to the normal heart (*left*), the heart in idiopathic dilated cardiomyopathy (*right*) is characterized by biventricular hypertrophy and four-chamber enlargement. The weight is often 25% to 50% above normal. Enlargement of the heart can be seen easily on chest radiography or cardiac echocardiography.

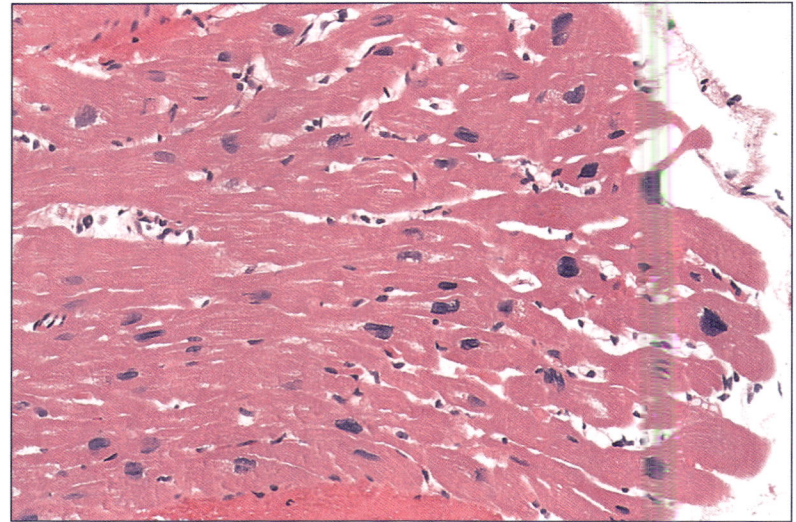

Figure 6-13. Endomyocardial biopsy from a patient with idiopathic cardiomyopathy. Large, irregularly shaped hyperchromatic nuclei are present, consistent with myocyte hypertrophy. The interstitium is cellular, but this should not be confused with myocarditis. These features, although nonspecific, support the diagnosis of idiopathic dilated cardiomyopathy. A completely normal endomyocardial biopsy does not support a diagnosis of idiopathic dilated cardiomyopathy and should suggest a focal cause, such as sarcoidosis, which requires further investigation [16].

Specific Heart Muscle Diseases

Heredofamilial	Sensitivities and toxic reactions
Familiar cardiomyopathy	Ethanol
Muscular dystrophies	Anthracycline
Infectious	Cocaine
Bacterial	Cobalt
Viral	Catecholamines
Human immunodeficiency virus	Corticosteroids
Other	Lithium
Metabolic	Radiation
Endocrine	Heavy metal
Nutritional	Scorpion sting
Storage diseases	Other
Myocarditis	Uremia
Neoplastic	Anemia
Peripartum	Leukemia
Systemic	Obesity
Infiltrative	
Connective tissue disease	

Figure 6-14. Specific causes of dilated cardiomyopathy. These are also called secondary cardiomyopathies or specific heart muscle diseases. Almost any disease process can involve cardiac muscle, as can be seen from this list. Multiple factors may actually play a causative role in any single patient. (*Adapted from* Abelmann [17].)

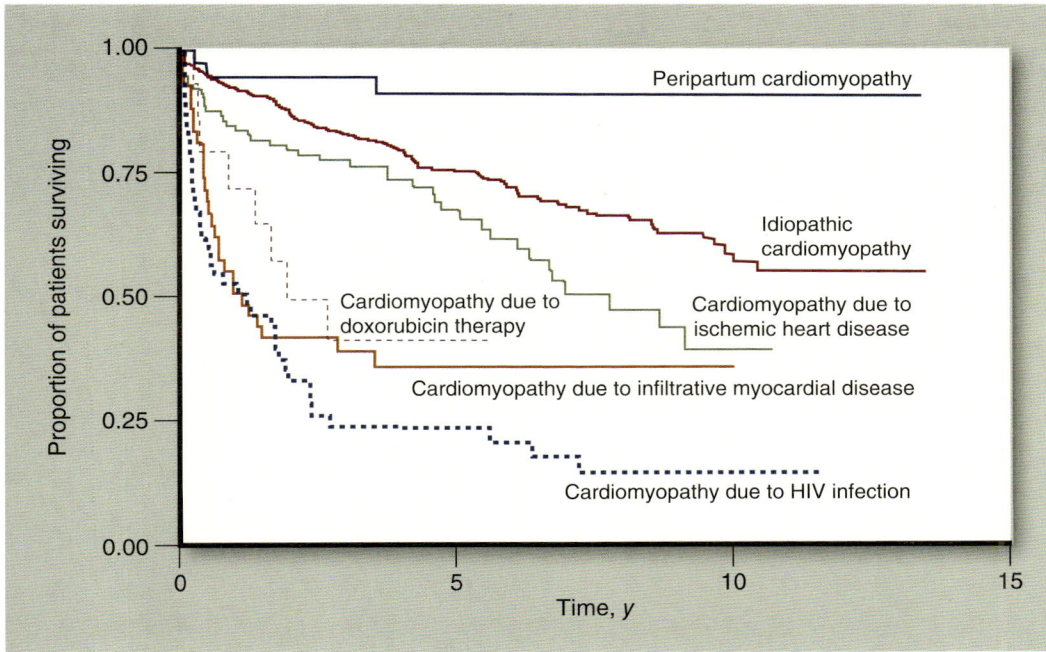

Figure 6-15. Although the prognosis in patients with heart failure is poor, it is dramatically influenced by the etiology of the left ventricular compromise [18]. (*Adapted from* Felker *et al.* [18].)

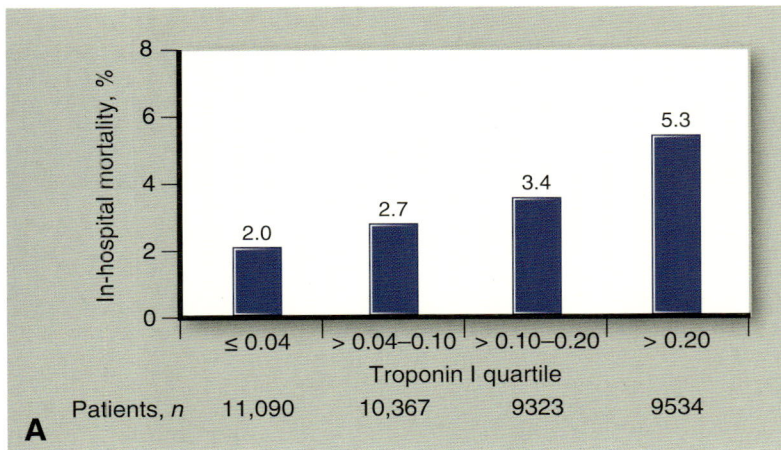

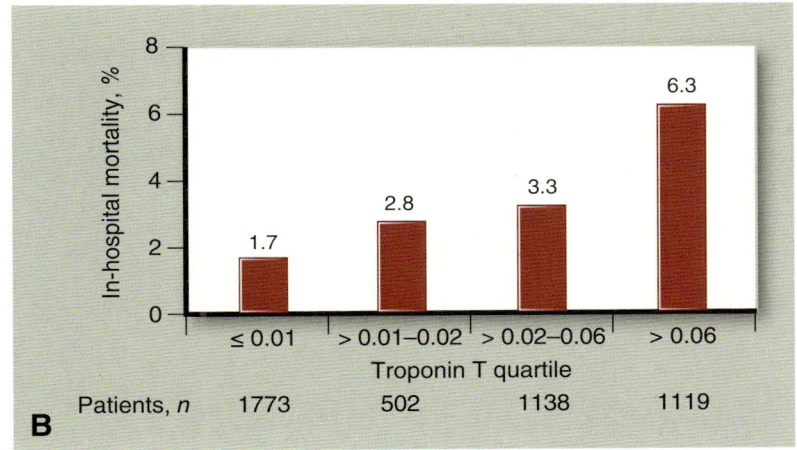

Figure 6-16. Hospital mortality related to troponin I (**A**) and troponin T (**B**) quartile in hospitalized heart failure patients. Cardiac troponin I was measured in 61,379 patients and cardiac troponin T in 7880 patients, with creatinine levels less than 2.0 mg/dL. Patients were admitted for acute decompensated heart failure. Of these patients, 4240 (6.2%) were positive for troponin. Troponin-positive patients had hospital mortality of 8% versus 2.7% in those without this biomarker elevation and the risk of in-hospital mortality increases with increasing troponin levels. Therefore, myocardial muscle loss, presumably due to increased myocardial oxygen demand from wall stress and decreased myocardial perfusion due to low diastolic blood pressure and elevated left ventricular diastolic pressure is associated with poor prognosis for patients admitted with decompensated heart failure [19].

Biomarkers in Heart Failure

Inflammation[*,†,‡]	Neurohormones[*,¯,§]	Myocyte stress[*,†,§,¶]
C-reactive protein	Norepinephrine	Brain natriuretic peptide
Tumor necrosis factor α	Renin	N-terminal pro–brain natriuretic peptide
Fas (APO-1)	Angiotensin II	Midregional fragment of proadrenomedullin
Interleukins 1, 6, and 18	Aldosterone	ST2
Oxidative stress[*,†,§]	Arginine vasopressin	**New biomarkers[†]**
Oxidized low-density lipoproteins	Endothelin	Chromogranin
Myeloperoxidase	**Myocyte injury[*,†,ä]**	Galectin 3
Urinary biopyrins	Cardiac-specific troponins I and T	Osteoprotegerin
Urinary and plasma isoprostanes	Myosin light-chain kinase I	Adiponectin
Plasma malondialdehyde	Heart-type fatty-acid protein	Growth differentiation factor 15
Extracellular-matrix remodeling[*,†,§]	Creatine kinase MB fraction	
Matrix metalloproteinases		
Tissue inhibitors of metalloproteinases		
Collagen propeptides		
Propeptide procollagen type I		
Plasma procollagen type III		

*Biomarkers in this category aid in elucidating the pathogenesis of heart failure.
†Biomarkers in this category provide prognostic information and enhance risk stratification.
‡Biomarkers in this category can be used to identify subjects at risk for heart failure.
§Biomarkers in this category are potential targets of therapy.
¶Biomarkers in this category are useful in the diagnosis of heart failure and in monitoring therapy.

A

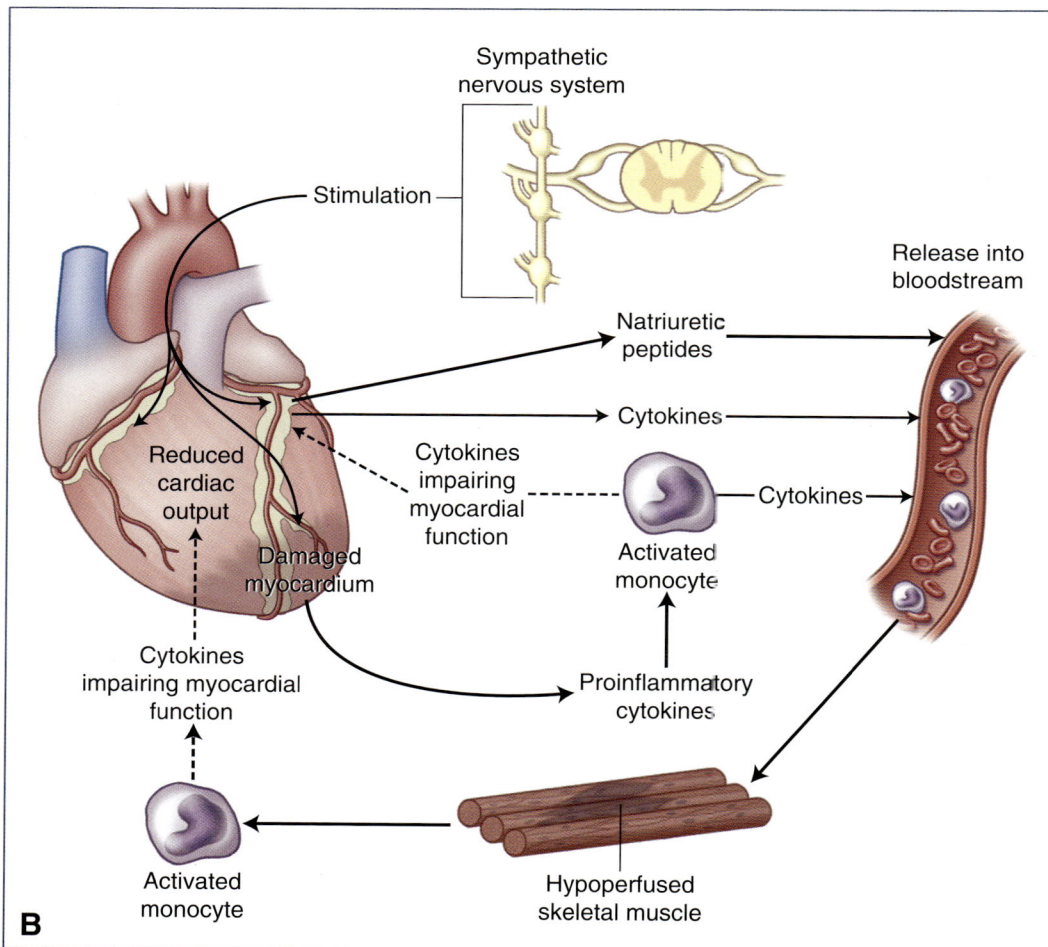

B

Figure 6-17. A, Biomarkers currently being used that are under investigation, measure inflammation, oxidative stress, extracellular matrix/remodeling, myocyte injury, myocyte stress, or elevation of novel noncardiac biomarkers. Clinically applicable biomarkers should be available to the clinician at an affordable cost, and should provide supplemental data, not routinely acquired, that impact medical therapy.

B, The figure shows an example of the effect of a cytokine (an inflammatory marker) on the heart and vasculature in a patient with heart failure. Proinflammatory cytokines produced by the damaged myocardium depress myocardial function and alter vascular tone. These effects are enhanced by sympathetic nervous system stimulation. The cytokines are produced by both skeletal and cardiac tissue in response to underperfusion [20].

Specific Heart Muscle Disease

Lyme Disease

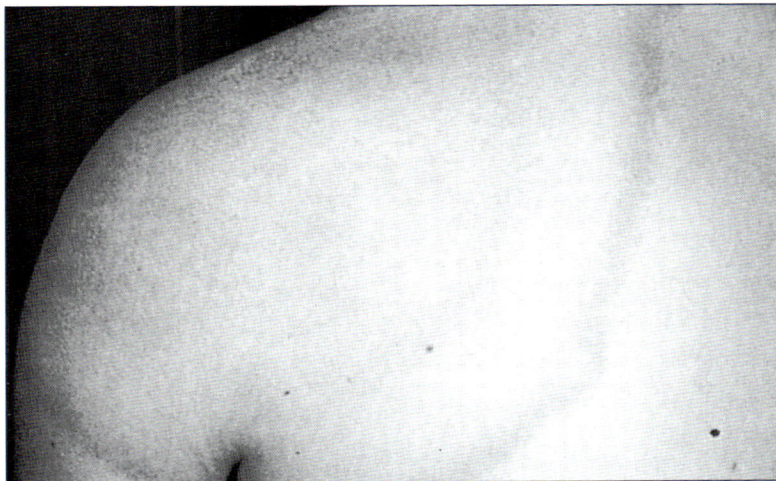

Figure 6-18. Erythema chronicum migrans (ECM). Lyme disease is usually contracted during the summer and is heralded by the appearance of a pathognomonic skin lesion, ECM. The appearance of ECM is generally annular, with a sharply demarcated outer border, and it is erythematous or bluish, warm to the touch, flat, and minimally tender or nontender. This unique cutaneous lesion is the best clinical marker of Lyme disease. ECM is followed in weeks to months by joint, neurologic, or cardiac involvement. However, in perhaps one third of cases, the skin lesion is absent or missed and patients present with symptoms of disseminated disease. (*From* Fitzpatrick *et al.* [21]; with permission.)

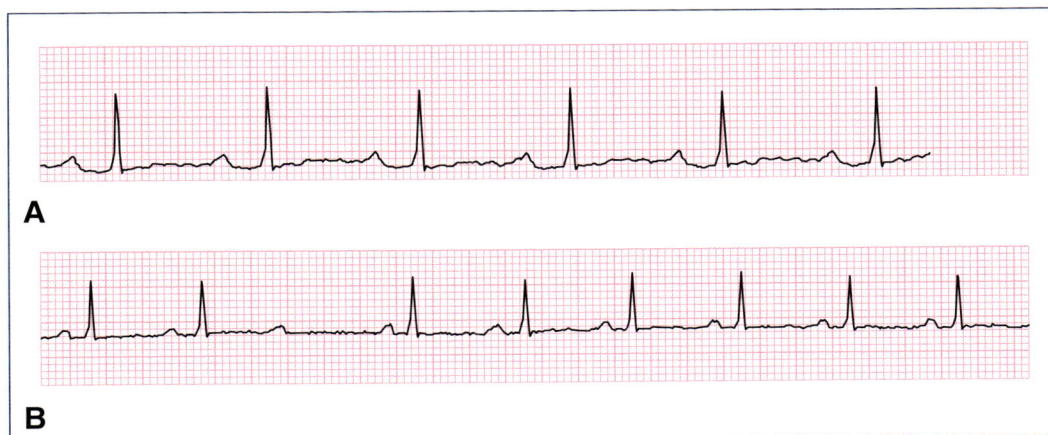

Figure 6-19. Development of first- and second-degree heart block in Lyme disease. About 10% of patients with Lyme disease develop evidence of transient cardiac involvement. The most common cardiac manifestation is variable degrees of atrioventricular (AV) block [22,23]. First-degree heart block (**A**) may progress to second-degree (**B**) or complete heart block over hours. According to some authorities, the risk for progression to complete heart block is much higher when the P-R interval exceeds 0.3 seconds. Syncope from complete heart block is common with cardiac involvement, as there is often associated depression of ventricular escape rhythm. McAlister *et al.* [22], in reviewing 52 reported cases of Lyme carditis, noted that 45 (87%) of these patients had documented AV block and 28 experienced either complete or high-grade AV block and were almost always symptomatic. When AV block of unknown origin develops suddenly, Lyme carditis should be considered, especially in younger patients who live in an area in which the vector is endemic [22,23].

Cardiac Sarcoidosis

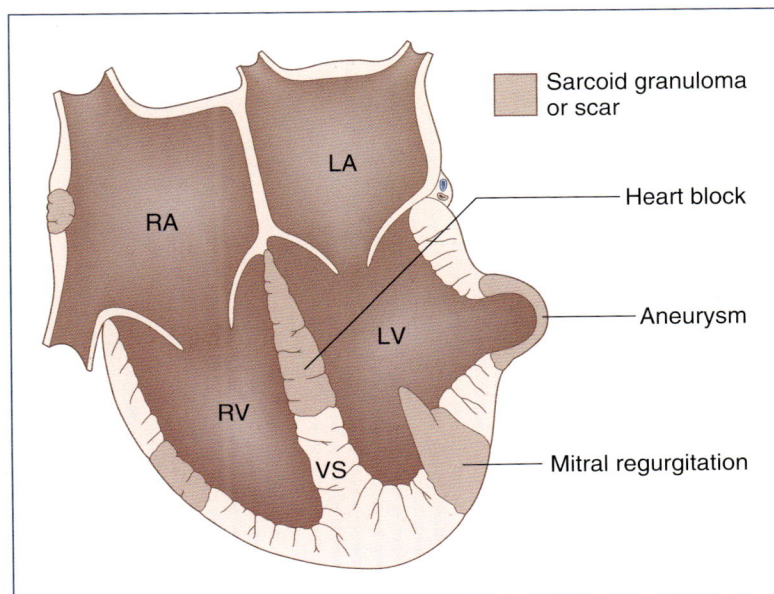

Figure 6-20. Distribution and consequences of sarcoid granulomas in sarcoid heart disease. In an autopsy series of 26 patients reported by Roberts *et al.* [24], cardiac granulomas were observed grossly in 25 hearts. Sarcoid granulomas were present in the left ventricular (LV) free wall of all 25 patients, in the right ventricular (RV) septum in 19, in the RV wall in 12, in the right atrial (RA) wall in three patients, and in the left atrial (LA) wall in two. Involvement of the cephalad portion of the muscular ventricular septum was associated with complete heart block. Important consequences of the involvement of the LV wall were aneurysm formation and mitral regurgitation. VS—ventricular septum. (*Adapted from* Roberts *et al.* [24].)

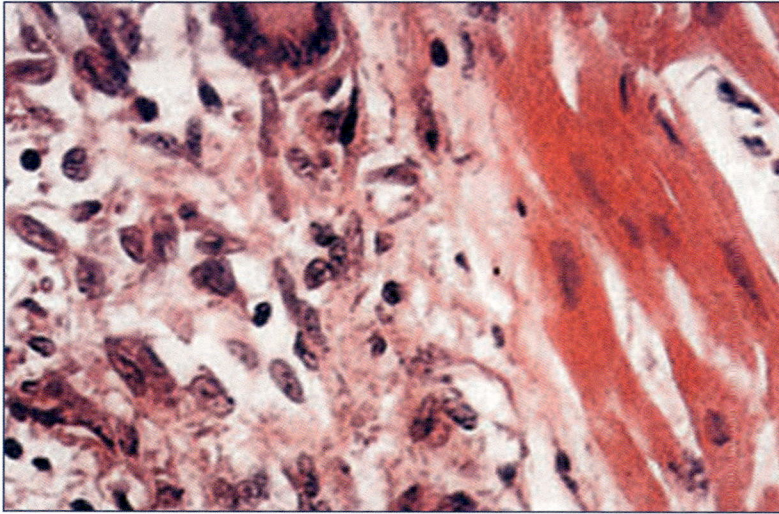

Figure 6-21. Endomyocardial biopsy sample demonstrating a sarcoid granuloma. Endomyocardial biopsy is the only technique that allows definitive diagnosis of myocardial sarcoidosis during life [25,26]. The depicted histologic specimen, obtained from the left ventricle, shows a typical noncaseating granuloma, that is characteristic of sarcoidosis (magnification × 250). In some series, demonstration of sarcoid granulomas on endomyocardial biopsy is possible in only a small percentage of patients with probable myocardial sarcoidosis. This seeming discrepancy may relate to the patchy, diffuse nature of granulomatous involvement. Support for this concept is provided by the observations of Sekiguchi *et al.* [27], who simulated endomyocardial biopsy at different sites in both the left and right ventricles of the autopsied hearts of seven patients with fatal myocardial sarcoidosis. All seven hearts exhibited gross sarcoid involvement. Despite this, the sensitivity of biopsy was only 50% in the right ventricle and 47% in the left ventricle. Therefore, nonspecific biopsy findings do not exclude the diagnosis of myocardial sarcoidosis in clinically suspected cases. (*From* Uretsky [26]; with permission.)

Cardiac Amyloidosis

Clinical Presentations of Cardiac Amyloidosis	
Restrictive cardiomyopathy	Congestive heart failure due to systolic dysfunction
Jugular venous distention	Orthostatic hypotension
Narrow pulse pressure	Abnormalities of cardiac impulse formation and conduction (resulting in arrhythmias and conduction disturbances)
Protodiastolic gallop	
Hepatomegaly	
Peripheral edema	

Figure 6-22. In amyloidosis associated with an immunocyte dyscrasia (primary amyloidosis), pathologic evidence of cardiac involvement is virtually the rule. However, clinically apparent heart disease is present in only one third to one half of patients [28,29]. The most common clinical presentation of cardiac amyloidosis is that of a restrictive cardiomyopathy, in which right-sided findings dominate the clinical picture [29]. A second common presentation is congestive heart failure due to systolic dysfunction. Much less commonly, patients may present with orthostatic hypotension or with symptoms caused by abnormalities of cardiac impulse formation and conduction.

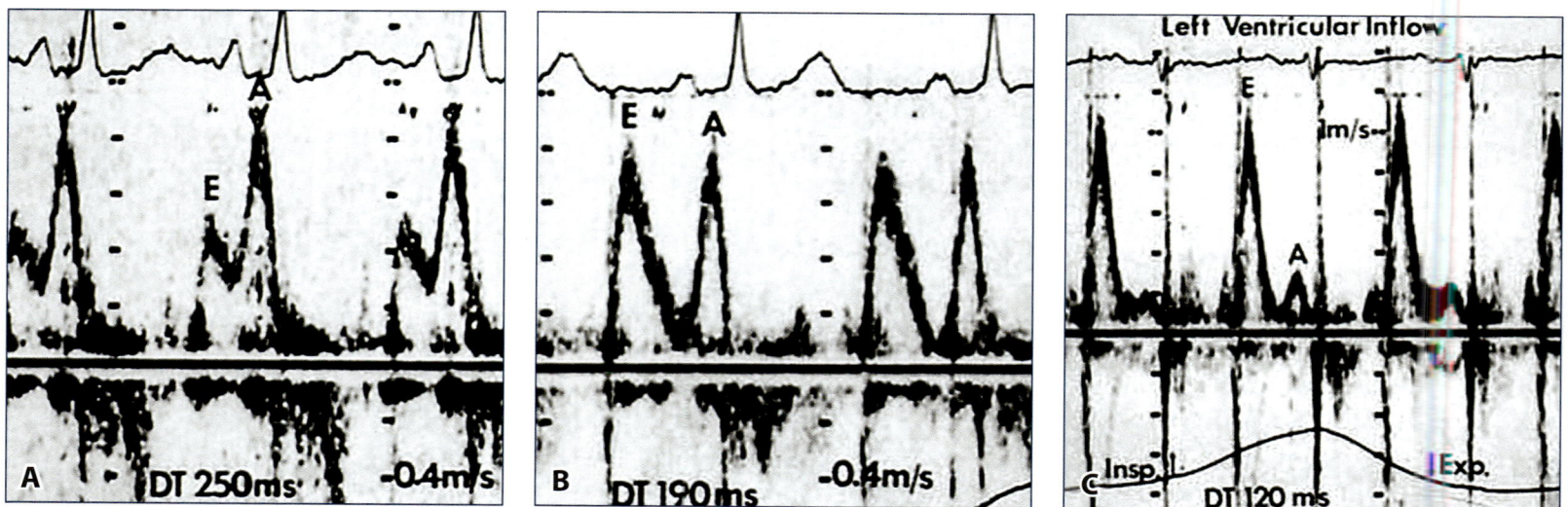

Figure 6-23. The spectrum of abnormal Doppler echocardiographic patterns in cardiac amyloidosis. Echocardiography is of considerable value in the diagnosis of infiltrative amyloid heart disease [30]. Typical features on two-dimensional echocardiography include a granular appearance of the myocardium and increased thickness of the myocardial walls. A number of studies have clearly shown that diastolic dysfunction in cardiac amyloidosis exhibits a spectrum of abnormalities that can be followed up serially by Doppler echocardiography. **A,** In earlier stages of amyloid heart disease, abnormal relaxation is the Doppler pattern seen. The E wave is of lower magnitude than the a-wave and the deceleration time is prolonged. As the disease progresses, a pseudonormalization Doppler pattern may emerge. **B,** The same patient as in *panel A,* taken 6 months later. **C,** Eventually, a restrictive pattern emerges. As shown in this example (pulsed-wave Doppler recording of a left ventricular inflow profile), there is increased E/A ratio (3.7) and short deceleration time (DT; 120 ms). (*Adapted from* Klein *et al.* [30].) Exp—expiration; Insp—inspiration.

Summary of the Main Forms of Amyloidosis That Affect the Heart

Nomenclature	Precursor of amyloid fibril	Organ involvement	Treatment	Comment
AL	Immunoglobulin light chain	Heart, kidney, liver, peripheral/autonomic nerves, soft tissue, gastrointestinal system	Chemotherapy	Plasma cell dyscrasia related to (but usually not associated with) multiple myeloma; heart disease occurs in 1/3 to 1/2 of AL patients; heart failure tends to progress rapidly and has a very poor prognosis
ATTR (familial)	Mutant transthyretin	Peripheral/autonomic nerve, heart	Liver transplantation? New pharmacologic strategies to stabilize the TTR	Autosomal dominant; amyloid derived from a mixture of mutant and wild-type TTR; if present before, cardiac amyloid may progress despite liver transplantation
AApoA1	Mutant apolipoprotein	Kidney, heart	Liver transplantation?	Kidney disease is the most common presentation; heart involvement is rare
Senile systemic amyloid	Wild-type transthyretin	Heart	Supportive? New pharmacologic strategies to stabilize the TTR	Almost exclusively found in elderly men; slowly progressive symptoms
AA	Serum amyloid A	Kidney, heart (rarely)	Treat underlying inflammatory process	Heart disease rare and, if present, rarely clinically significant
AANP	Atrial natriuretic peptide	Localized to the atrium	None required	Very common; may increase risk of atrial fibrillation and/or be deposited in greater amounts in the fibrillating atrium

A

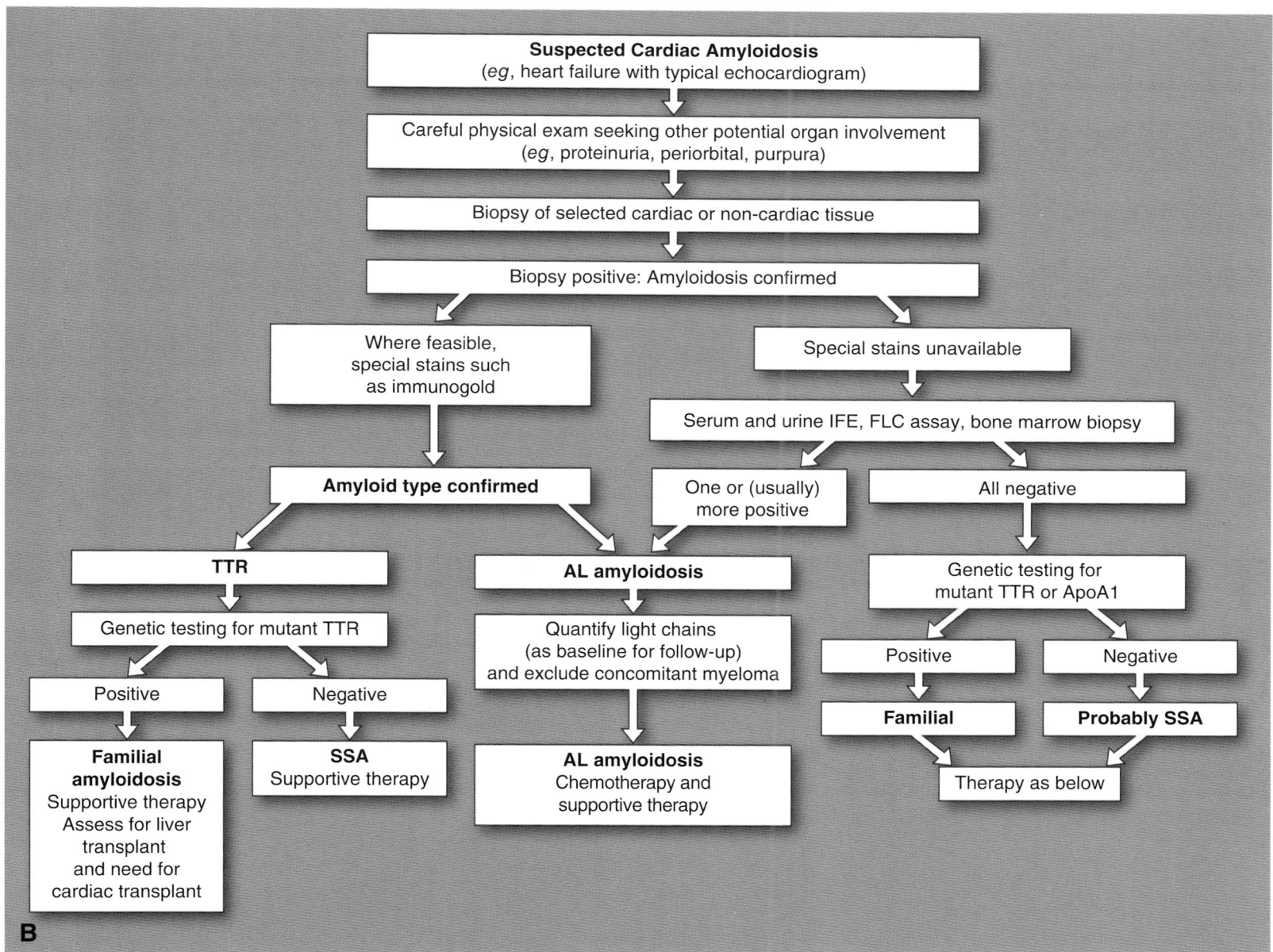

B

Figure 6-24. A, The table indicates the main forms of amyloidosis that affect the heart. The precursor, or amyloid fibril, organ involvement and potential treatment are listed for each form of amyloidosis. **B,** The figure demonstrates a proposed algorithm for the evaluation of patients with suspected cardiac amyloidosis. A tissue diagnosis is mandatory. If the heart is involved, the biopsy will demonstrate not only the amyloidosis, but allow determination of the responsible amyloid fibril. This requires a special staining, including analysis for free-light chains (FLC) in some cases [31]. IFE—immunofixation; SSA—senile systemic amyloidosis; TTR— transthyretin.

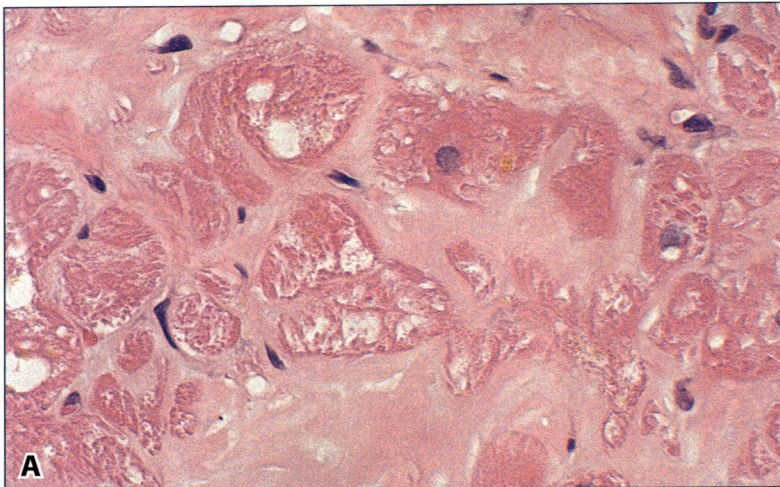

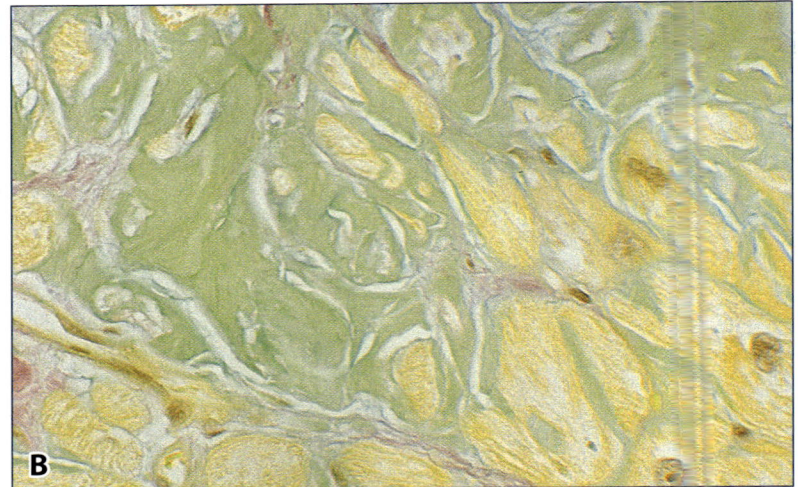

Figure 6-25. Appearance of myocardial tissue obtained at endomyocardial biopsy in cardiac amyloidosis. Endomyocardial biopsy may provide a definitive diagnosis in cardiac amyloidosis [26]. The depicted images are those of myocardium obtained at endomyocardial biopsy in a 53-year-old woman with rapidly progressive heart failure, in whom neither cardiac amyloidosis nor a blood dyscrasia was suspected prior to biopsy.

A, Hematoxylin and eosin staining shows pink eosinophilic deposits of amyloid. **B,** Sulfated Alcian blue staining demonstrates apple green staining of the deposits. (*Courtesy of* Vijaya Reddy, Maywood, IL.)

Restrictive Cardiomyopathy and Hypereosinophilic Heart Disease

In restrictive cardiomyopathy, the stiff ventricle has difficulty filling and manifestations of diastolic heart failure are evident. The most important conditions causing restrictive cardiomyopathy are sarcoidosis (*see* Figs. 6-20 and 6-21), hemochromatosis, amyloidosis (*see* Figs. 6-22 and 6-23), radiation heart disease, glycogen storage disease, and familial neuromuscular disorders (*see* Figs. 6-29 to 6-31). Restrictive cardiomyopathy may also be idiopathic.

Classification of Types of Restrictive Cardiomyopathy According to Cause

Myocardial	
Noninfiltrative	
Idiopathic cardiomyopathy*	Scleroderma
Familial cardiomyopathy	Pseudoxanthoma elasticum
Hypertrophic cardiomyopathy	Diabetic cardiomyopathy
Infiltrative	
Amyloidosis*	Hurler's disease
Sarcoidosis*	Fatty infiltration
Gaucher's disease	
Storage diseases	
Hemochromatosis	Glycogen storage disease
Fabry's disease	
Endomyocardial	
Endomyocardial fibrosis*	Radiation
Hypereosinophilic syndrome	Toxic effects of anthracycline*
Carcinoid heart disease	Drugs causing fibrous endocarditis (serotonin, methysergide, ergotamine, mercurial agents, bisulfan)
Metastatic cancers	
This condition is more likely than the others to be encountered in clinical practice.	

Figure 6-26. The etiology of heart failure can virtually always be identified in patients with restrictive cardiomyopathy. The causes include sarcoidosis and amyloidosis, which have already been described [32]. (*Adapted from* Kushwaha *et al.* [32].)

Idiopathic Restrictive Cardiomyopathy

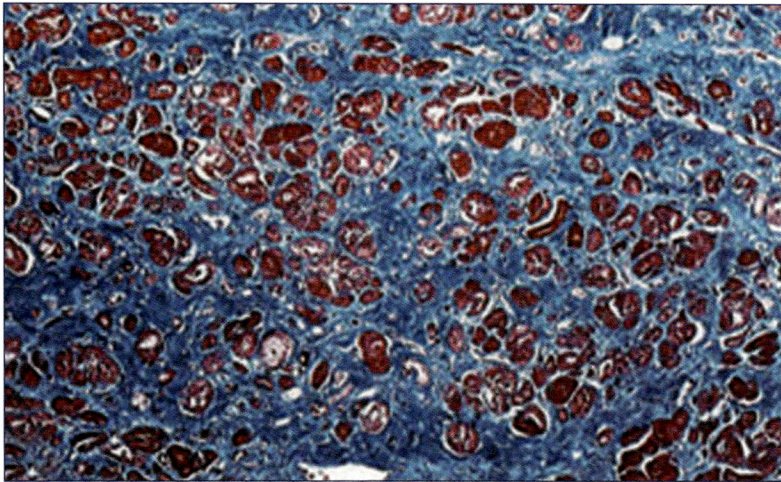

Figure 6-27. Idiopathic restrictive cardiomyopathy. Cross-sectional view of myocytes surrounded by fibrous tissue (Mallory-azan stain). Whereas severe interstitial fibrosis is seen here, fibrous tissue surrounds each myocyte (predominantly endomysial fibrosis).

Hypereosinophilic Heart Disease (Löffler's Syndrome)

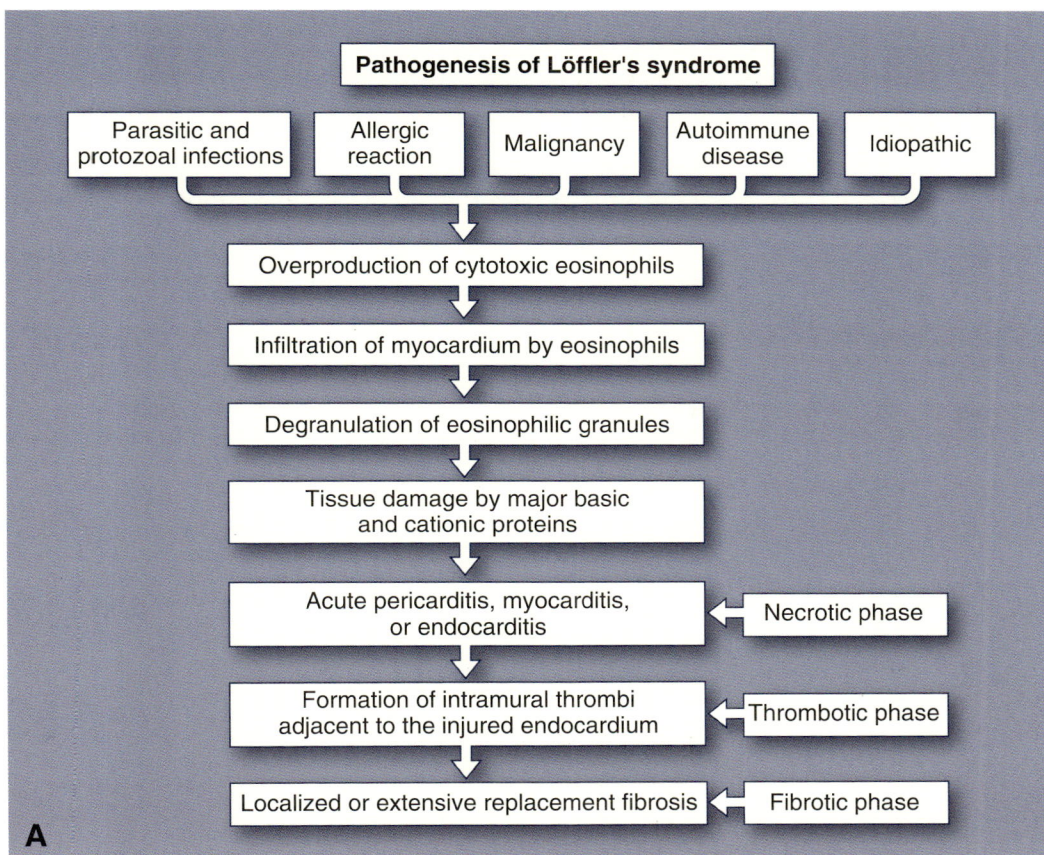

Pathogenesis of Löffler's syndrome

Parasitic and protozoal infections | Allergic reaction | Malignancy | Autoimmune disease | Idiopathic

↓

Overproduction of cytotoxic eosinophils

↓

Infiltration of myocardium by eosinophils

↓

Degranulation of eosinophilic granules

↓

Tissue damage by major basic and cationic proteins

↓

Acute pericarditis, myocarditis, or endocarditis ← Necrotic phase

↓

Formation of intramural thrombi adjacent to the injured endocardium ← Thrombotic phase

↓

Localized or extensive replacement fibrosis ← Fibrotic phase

A

Clinical Manifestations

Necrotic phase
  Manifestations of acute endo-, myo-, or pericarditis with hypereosinophilia
Thrombotic phase
  Cavity obliteration with intramural thrombi with or without hypereosinophilia (common in the tropics and rare in the temperate zone)
Fibrotic phase
  Atrioventricular block
  Valvular regurgitation
  Heart failure with restrictive physiology (ranging from diastolic dysfunction to endomyocardial fibrosis) or systolic dysfunction
Absence of hypereosinophilia

B

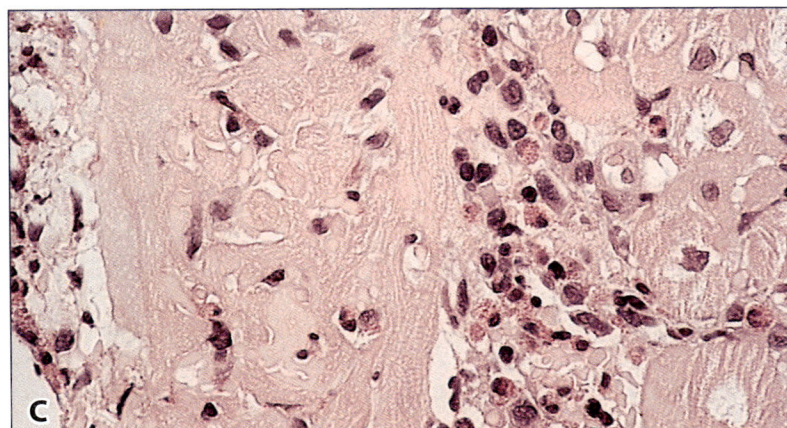

C

Figure 6-28. A, The pathogenesis of Löffler's syndrome. Tissue damage is caused by major basic and cationic proteins derived from cytotoxic eosinophils [33–37]. These cytotoxic proteins may stay in the myocardium for a prolonged period and produce continuous tissue damage. At the fibrotic phase, various types of heart diseases, such as endomyocardial fibrosis, dilated cardiomyopathy, atrioventricular block, or valvular regurgitation can be seen according to the difference of the most dominantly involved site.

B, The clinical manifestations of Löffler's syndrome and endomyocardial fibrosis [33,36]. The necrotic phase is acute, lasting for months. The thrombotic phase is subacute, lasting for months to 2 years. The fibrotic phase is chronic, and lasts for years.

C, Histologic view of a biopsy specimen shows massive infiltration of eosinophils in the myocardium as well as in the endocardium (hematoxylin and eosin).

Clinical Manifestations With Cardiac Involvement

Muscular Dystrophy

A

Figure 6-29. A, The posterolateral (infra-atrial) involvement of the left ventricle in Duchenne dystrophy. **B,** Posterobasal portion of the left ventricular wall. In contrast to the posterobasal wall, which shows extensive connective tissue proliferation with scattered islands of myocardial fibers, no fibrous scars are present in the ventricular septum (hematoxylin and eosin, × 25). A reduction in or loss of electromotive force caused by the location of myocardial dystrophy in the posterobasal and contiguous lateral left ventricular walls is believed to be responsible for the characteristic scalar electrocardiogram, and is represented by tall right precordial R waves and deep but narrow Q waves in leads 1, augmented voltage left (aVL), and the left precordium. Duchenne dystrophy emerges as a unique form of heart disease characterized by a genetically determined predilection for specific regions of myocardium.

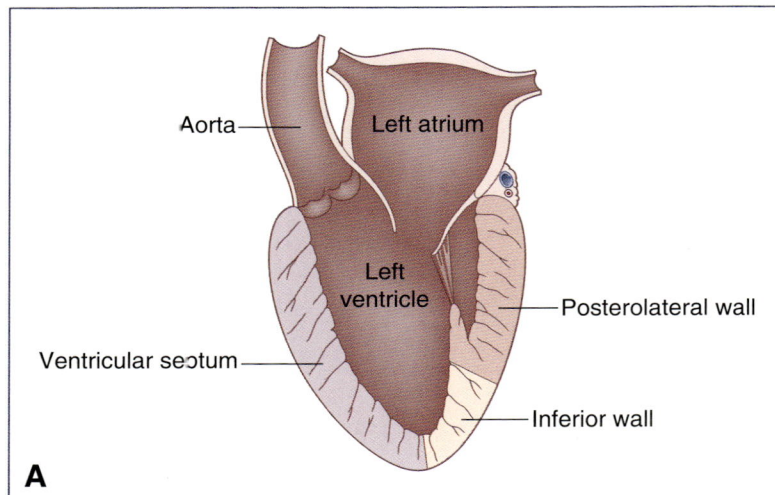

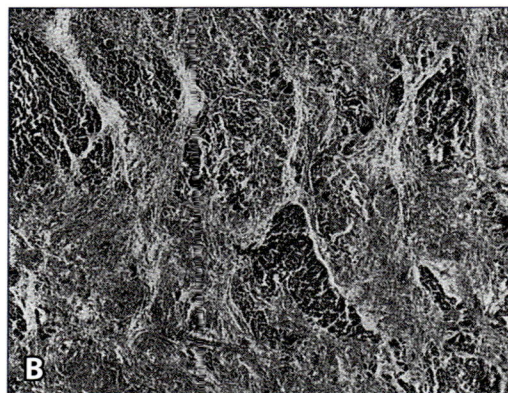

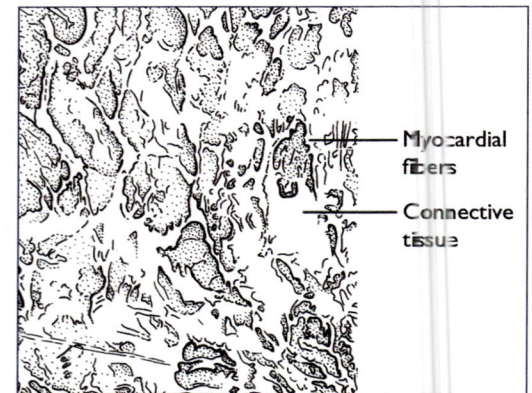

B

Figure 6-30. Typical electrocardiogram of Duchenne muscular dystrophy in a 10-year-old boy. The P-R interval is short (0.10 seconds in lead 2). The QRS complex shows an anterior shift in the right precordial leads (tall R waves) and deep but narrow Q waves in leads 1, augmented voltage left (aVL), and V4-6. A reduction in or loss of electromotive force caused by myocardial dystrophy in the postero-basal and contiguous lateral left ventricular walls is believed to be responsible for the QRS pattern. The standard scalar electrocardiogram is the simplest and most reliable tool for detecting cardiac involvement in Duchenne dystrophy. Abnormal electrocardiograms are present even in early childhood. Tall right precordial R waves and increased R:S amplitude ratios, together with deep Q waves in leads 1, aVL, and V5-6, are characteristic of classic, rapidly progressive X-linked Duchenne dystrophy.

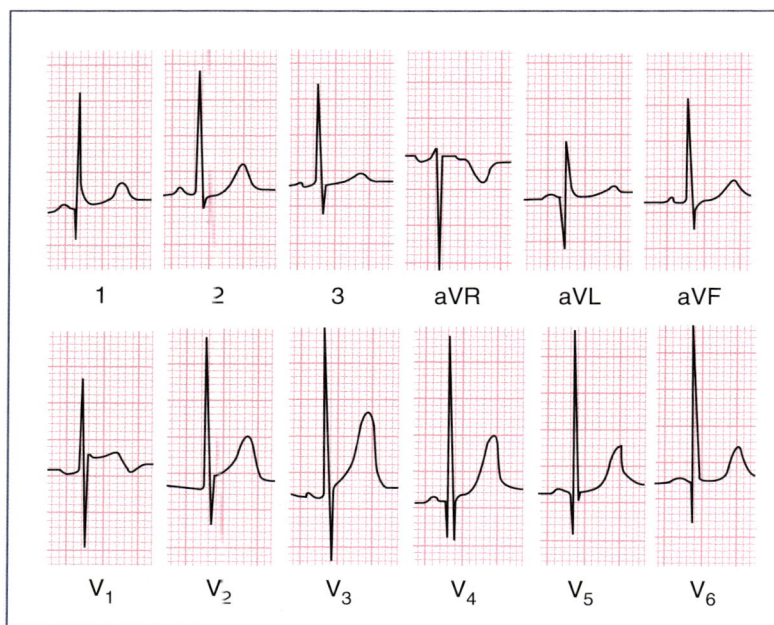

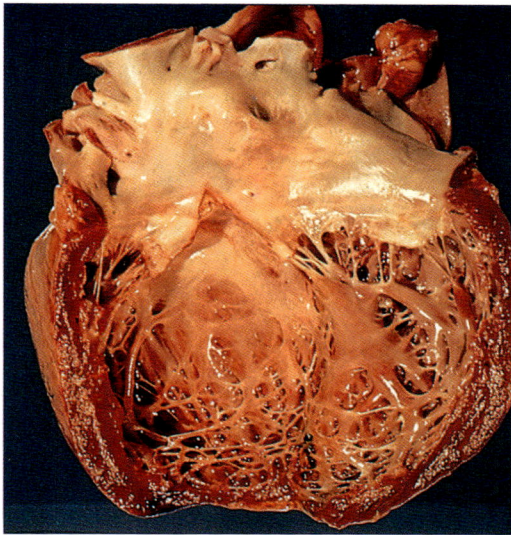

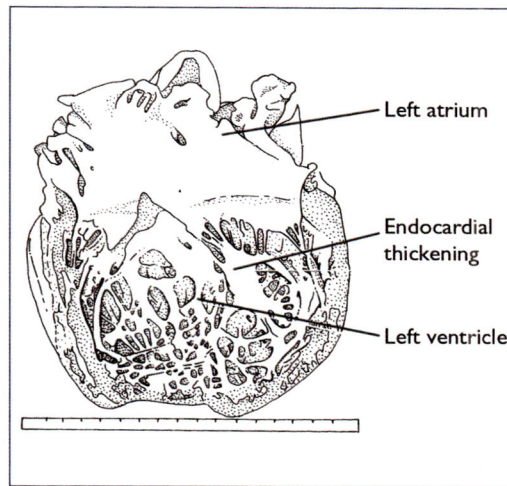

Figure 6-31. Gross and microscopic cardiac pathologic specimen from a 45-year-old man with late-onset, slowly progressive Becker muscular dystrophy. The left atrium was also dilated. No significant coronary artery disease was identified. In Becker dystrophy, the protein product of the gene is present but is abnormal in molecular weight, whereas in Duchenne dystrophy the protein product is absent or scanty but of normal molecular weight. In contrast to Duchenne dystrophy, cardiac involvement in Becker dystrophy involves all four chambers, with dilatation and failure of the ventricles in addition to abnormalities of the His bundle and infranodal conduction that express themselves as fascicular block and complete heart block.

Genetic and Inherited Disorders

Gene Mutations Causing Dilated Cardiomyopathy

Chromosome	Protein	Disease	Inheritance
1p1–q21	Lamins A and C	Dilated cardiomyopathy	Autosomal dominant
1q11–21	Unknown	Dilated cardiomyopathy*†	Autosomal dominant
1q11–23	Lamins A and C	Autosomal dominant Emery-Dreifuss muscular dystrophy	Autosomal dominant
1q32	Unknown	Dilated cardiomyopathy	Autosomal dominant
2q11–22	Unknown	Dilated cardiomyopathy	Autosomal dominant
2q31	Unknown	Dilated cardiomyopathy	Autosomal dominant
3p22–25	Unknown	Dilated cardiomyopathy	Autosomal dominant
6q23	Unknown	Dilated cardiomyopathy*	Autosomal dominant
9q13–22	Unknown	Dilated cardiomyopathy	Autosomal dominant
10q21–23	Unknown	Dilated cardiomyopathy	Autosomal dominant
10q22	Metavinculin	Dilated cardiomyopathy	Unknown
15q14	Actin	Dilated cardiomyopathy	Autosomal dominant
17q12–21.33	alpha-Sarcoglycan (adhalin)	Dilated cardiomyopathy*	Autosomal recessive
Xp28	Emerin	Emery-Dreifuss muscular dystrophy	X-linked
Xp21	Dystrophin	X-linked dilated cardiomyopathy	X-linked
Xp21	Dystrophin	Becker type muscular dystrophy	X-linked
Xp21	Dystrophin	Duchenne type muscular dystrophy	X-linked

*This form is associated with limb-girdle muscular dystrophy.
†Although the loci on chromosome 1q are similar to those for Emery-Dreifuss muscular dystrophy, the disease form is distinct.

Figure 6-32. Specific genetic mutations are increasingly being associated with both hypertrophic and dilated cardiomyopathy. Familial (genetic) dilated cardiomyopathy may account for 20% of all patients presenting with cardiomyopathy [38].

Myocarditis

Etiology and Epidemiology

Etiologies of Human Myocarditis: Infectious

Viral	**Protozoal and metazoal**
Coxsackievirus (A and B)	Trypanosomiasis
Parvovirus	Toxoplasmosis
Echovirus	Malaria
Influenza	Schistosomiasis
Cytomegalovirus	Trichinosis
Hepatitis	**Bacterial**
Mumps	Diphtheria
Herpes simplex	Tuberculosis
Rabies	Legionella
EBV	Brucella
HIV	Clostridium
Rickettsial	Salmonella/shigella
Q fever	Meningococcus
Rocky Mountain spotted fever	Yersinia
Scrub typhus	**Spirochetal**
Fungal	Borrelia (Lyme)
Cryptococcus	
Candidiasis	
Histoplasmosis	
Aspergillus	

Figure 6-33. Infectious causes of myocarditis. Strictly speaking, the Dallas criteria are confined to cases of idiopathic myocarditis rather than cases secondary to specific infectious or noninfectious causes. The presence of cardiotropic viruses is rarely confirmed, however, and the clinical significance of such viruses is still debated. Thus, most cases of myocarditis are clinically idiopathic and likely represent the largest subgroup of cases of human myocarditis [39]. EBV—Epstein-Barr virus.

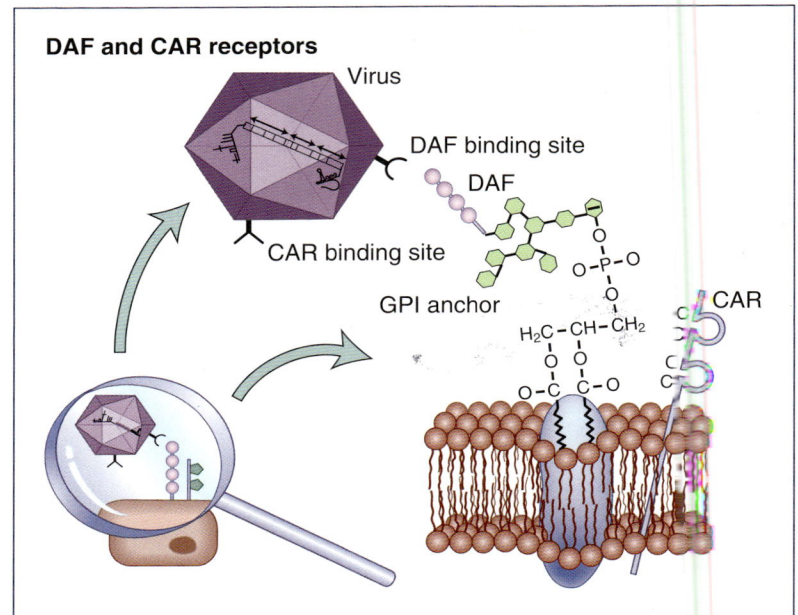

Figure 6-34. Viral receptors on myocardial cells. Viruses enter the heart cells through receptors on the myocyte membrane. This is best characterized with the coxsackie adenoviral receptor (CAR), immunoglobulins that colocalize in target cell membranes. The CAR binds to the virus, and in the presence of co-receptors, such as decay accelerating factor (DAF), facilitates virus entry into the cell [40]. GPI—glycosylphosphatidylinositol.

Histopathology and Immunohistology

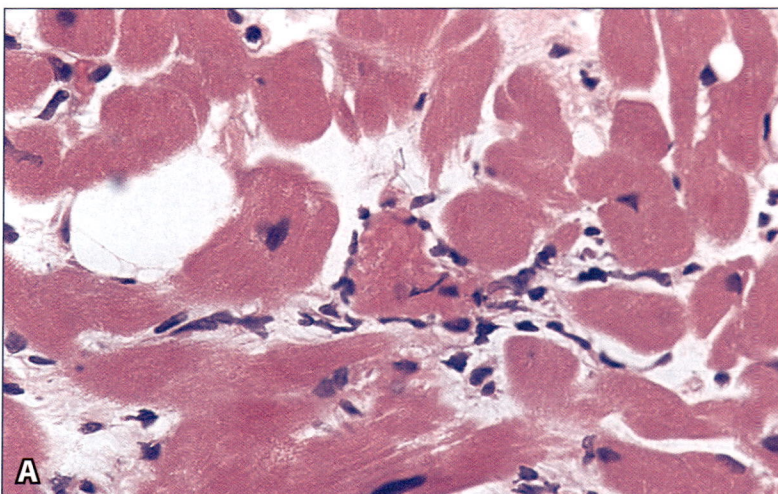

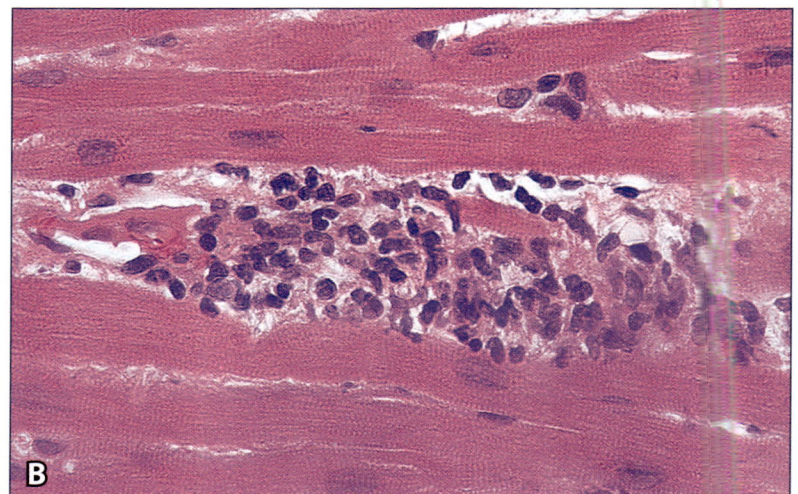

Figure 6-35. Histopathologic features of endomyocardial biopsy samples from patients with myocarditis. **A,** High-power photomicrograph of an endomyocardial biopsy sample stained with hematoxylin and eosin, highlighting one isolated necrotic myocyte surrounded by a mixed inflammatory infiltrate.

B, A small cluster of longitudinally oriented myocytes engulfed in a dense inflammatory infiltrate composed primarily of mononuclear cells. Typically, outside the focus of active myocarditis, the adjacent myocardium appears relatively preserved. Interstitial inflammatory cells surround the myocytes, which no longer have crisp cellular outlines.

Continued on the next page

Figure 6-35. *(Continued)* The interstitial space between affected myocytes contains granular basophilic material that contains fibrin and fibrinogen, a likely consequence of microvascular injury. The inflammatory cells extend from the central core of necrotic myocytes into the adjacent myocardium. In 1986 and 1987, Aretz *et al.* [40,41], in an attempt to establish a uniform histologic classification for the diagnosis of myocarditis on endomyocardial biopsy, published a classification proposed by eight cardiac pathologists (the Dallas panel). Two separate classifications were described, one for the first biopsy and one for subsequent biopsies. On the first biopsy, active myocarditis was defined as a process characterized by an inflammatory infiltrate of the myocardium with necrosis or degeneration of adjacent myocytes not typical of the ischemic damage associated with coronary artery disease. The diagnosis of active myocarditis therefore requires the presence of myocardial inflammation as well as adjacent myocyte damage.

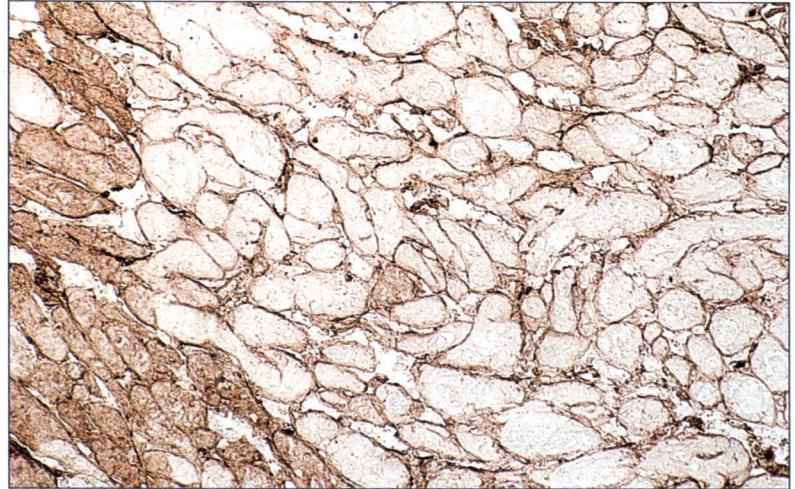

Figure 6-36. Myocardial immunoglobulin G deposition 14 days after coxsackie-virus B3 infection. The diffuse reactivity on myocyte sarcolemmal membranes suggests that in the setting of induced expression of major histocompatibility complex (MHC) antigens (either by primary viral infection or by secondary release of cytokines by cardiac-infiltrating cells), antibodies bind to self-peptides on the myocyte cell surface. Investigative studies have shown that in addition to myosin, other intracellular proteins (such as the two mitochondrial proteins known to be autoantigens in human myocarditis: the adenine nucleotide translocator [ANT] and the branched-chain ketoacid dehydrogenase [BCKD] complex) are transported to the myocyte cell surface during the course of chronic myocarditis. These proteins are thus presented to the immune system in the context of MHC [42]. Studies by Huber and Moraska [43] have raised the possibility that nonviral insults that produce myocarditis may similarly induce cardiac-specific autoimmunity. Adriamycin-treated mice developed myocarditis and cytolytic T lymphocytes, as well as antibodies specifically reactive to only drug-treated myocytes. Thus, the antigenicity of a myocyte may change sufficiently to induce immune reactivity to new antigenic epitopes regardless of the type of toxic insult. Whether these autoantibodies are directly involved in the pathogenesis of cardiac injury or whether they represent an epiphenomenon of ongoing myocardial injury is still the subject of debate. In addition, whether autoantibodies recognize intracellular proteins (such as myosin, ANT, and BCKD) transported to the surface of myocytes and expressed as peptides that have been part of the MHC or normal membrane constituents, which cross-react with antigenic epitopes of these intracellular proteins, is not known.

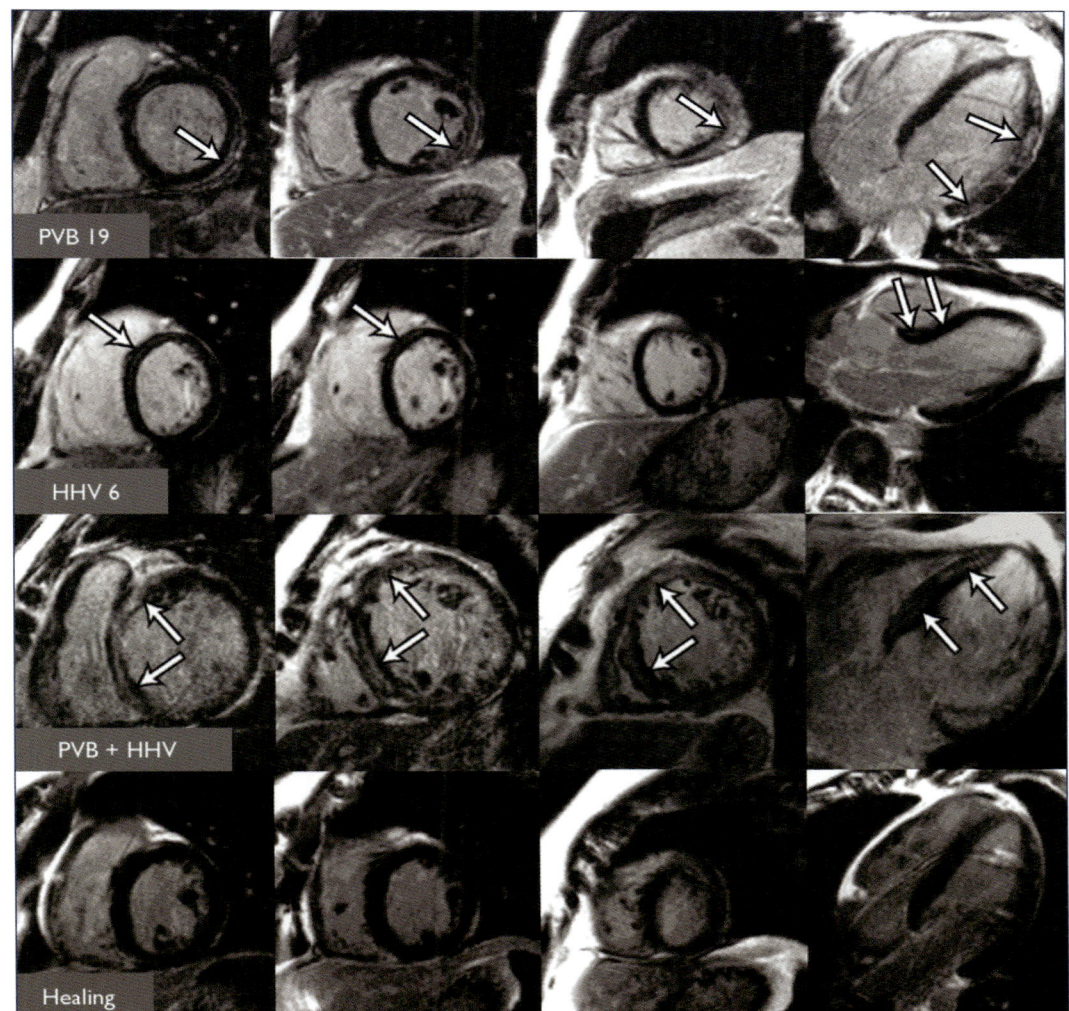

Figure 6-37. Contrast cardiovascular magnetic resonance images in patients with myocarditis. These authors identified 87 patients with myocarditis of 128 patients who met their clinical criteria of myocarditis. Parvovirus B19 was found in 19, and human herpes virus 6 in 16 with combined infection in 15. The authors believe that those with parvovirus B19 (PVB19) demonstrate subepicardial lateral wall gadolinium enhancement whereas human herpesvirus 6 (HHV6) patients display septal enhancement. (*Arrows* indicate areas of contrast enhancement in the myocardium, which appears to correlate with myocardial infarction.) These data suggest that cardiovascular magnetic resonance imaging may be of benefit to diagnose patients with myocarditis, particularly when the involvement is in areas that cannot be reached by routine right ventricular endomyocardial biopsy. The issue of geographic localization as an identifying feature for a specific virus must be validated [44]. (*See* Ch. 16.)

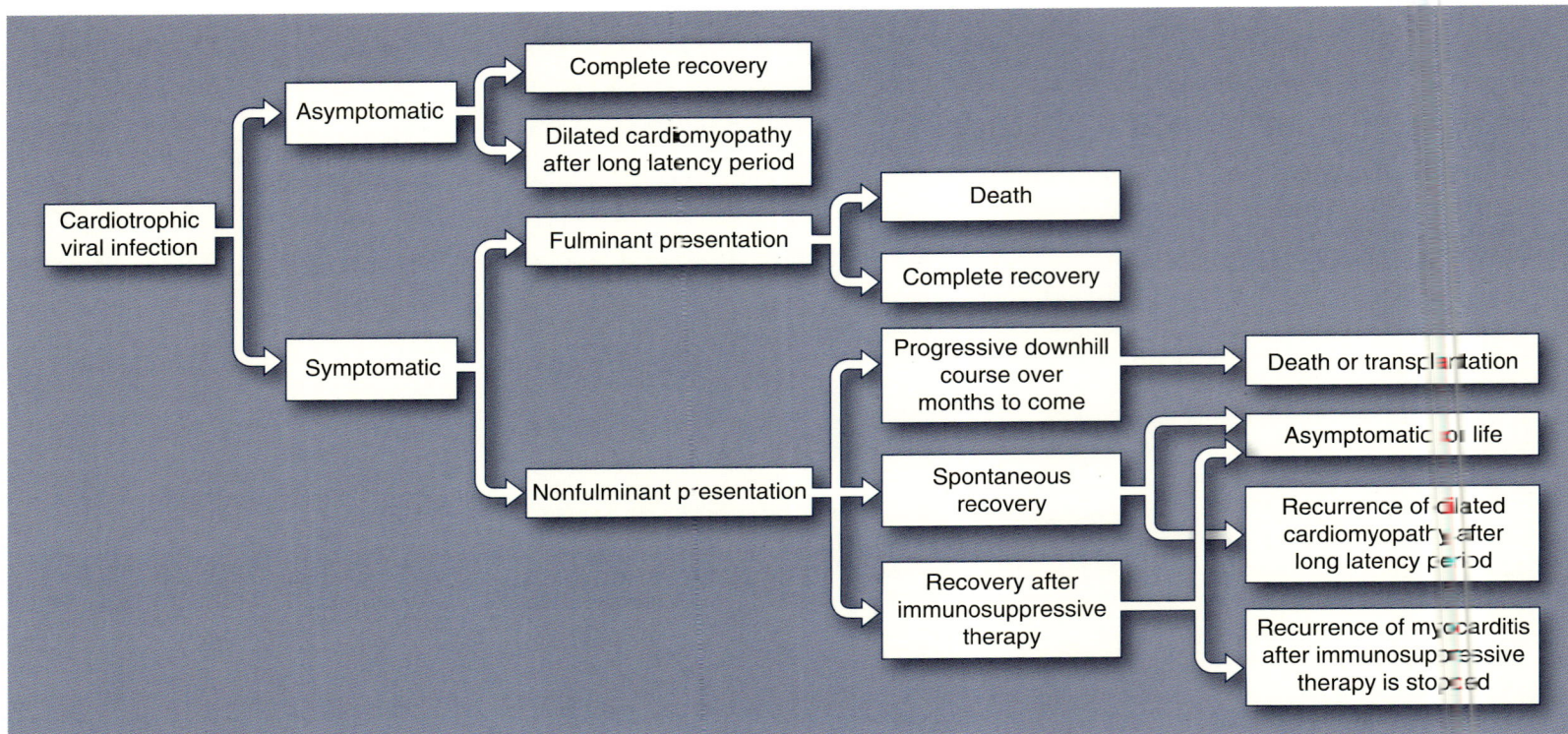

Figure 6-38. The natural history of human myocarditis. Most patients with mild symptoms of acute myocarditis are not seen by cardiologists and most of these patients appear to recover fully. Of the patients with symptomatic heart disease typically seen by cardiologists, a small number have fulminant presentations and either die in the acute stage or appear to recover fully. Of the remaining patients with myocarditis, a few are characterized by a progressive downhill course over a period of months to years that ends in death from heart failure or intractable arrhythmias [45,46]. Some spontaneously recover and remain asymptomatic for life and others have an asymptomatic period followed by development of dilated cardiomyopathy. The heterogeneity of clinical presentations and natural history in human myocarditis probably reflect the genetic predisposition of the individual, the virulence of the cardiotropic virus, and environmental factors. With the advent of molecular viral probes, it will be critical to relate the presence of persistent enterovirus RNA with the patterns of the natural history of myocarditis.

The Role of Endomyocardial Biopsy in 14 Clinical Scenarios

Scenario number	Clinical scenario	Class of recommendation	Level of evidence
1	New onset heart failure of < 2 weeks' duration associated with a normal-sized or dilated left ventricle and hemodynamic compromise	I	B
2	New onset heart failure of 2 weeks' to 3 months' duration associated with a dilated left ventricle and new ventricular arrhythmias, second- or third-degree heart block, or failure to respond to usual care within 1–2 wk	I	B
3	Heart failure of > 3 months' duration associated with a dilated left ventricle and new ventricular arrhythmias, second- or third-degree heart block, or failure to respond to usual care within 1 to 2 weeks	IIa	C
4	Heart failure associated with a DCM of any duration associated with suspected allergic reaction and/or eosinophilia	IIa	C
5	Heart failure associated with suspected anthracycline cardiomyopathy	IIa	C
6	Heart failure associated with unexplained restrictive cardiomyopathy	IIa	C
7	Suspected cardiac tumors	IIa	C
8	Unexplained cardiac tumors	IIb	C
9	New onset heart failure of 2 weeks' to 3 months' duration associated with a dilated left ventricle, without new ventricular arrhythmias or second- or third-degree heart block, that responds to usual care within 1–2 wks	IIb	C
10	Heart failure of > 3 months' duration associated with a dilated left ventricle and new ventricular arrhythmias, second- or third-degree heart block, that responds to usual care within 1–2 wk	IIb	C
11	Heart failure associated with unexplained HCM	IIb	C
12	Suspected ARVD/C	IIb	C
13	Unexplained ventricular arrhythmias	IIb	C
14	Unexplained atrial fibrillation	III	C

Figure 6-39. *Continued on the next page*

Figure 6-39. *(Continued)* The role of endomyocardial biopsy in the management of cardiovascular disease clinical scenarios are presented followed by the class of recommendation and level of evidence supporting the recommendation. Class I level of recommendations are conditions for which there is conflicting evidence or there is general agreement that a given procedure is beneficial, useful, and effective. Class II are conditions for which there is conflicting evidence and/or a divergence of opinion about usefulness/efficacy of a procedure or treatment. Class IIa are conditions for which the weight of evidence/opinion is in favor of the usefulness/efficacy and Class IIb are conditions for which the usefulness/efficacy is less well established by evidence/opinion. Level of evidence includes level A (multiple randomized clinical trails), level B (limited number of randomized trails, nonrandomized studies, and registries), and level C (primarily expert consensus). The scenarios described in I and II are compatible with the clinical presentation of fulminant myocarditis, giant cell myocarditis, and necrotizing eosinophilic myocarditis (scenario I) and giant cell myocarditis (scenario II). Patients presenting with these clinical manifestations should undergo endomyocardial biopsy [47]. ARVD/C—arrhythmogenic right ventricular dysplasia/cardiomyopathy; DCM—dilated cardiomyopathy; HCM—hypertrophic cardiomyopathy.

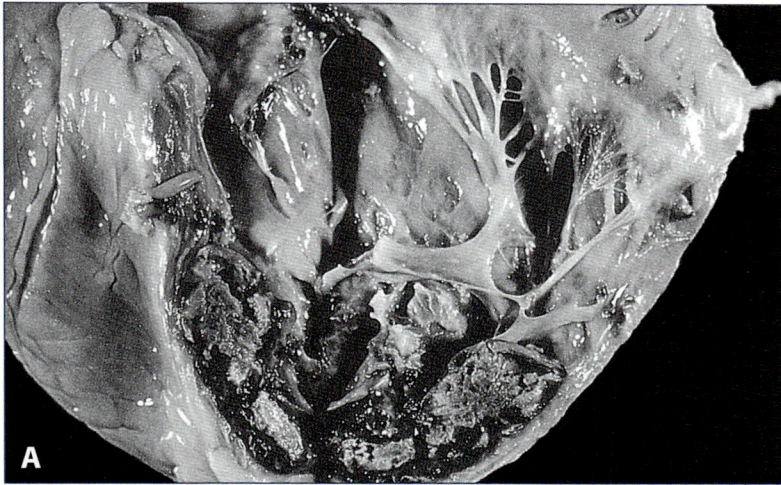

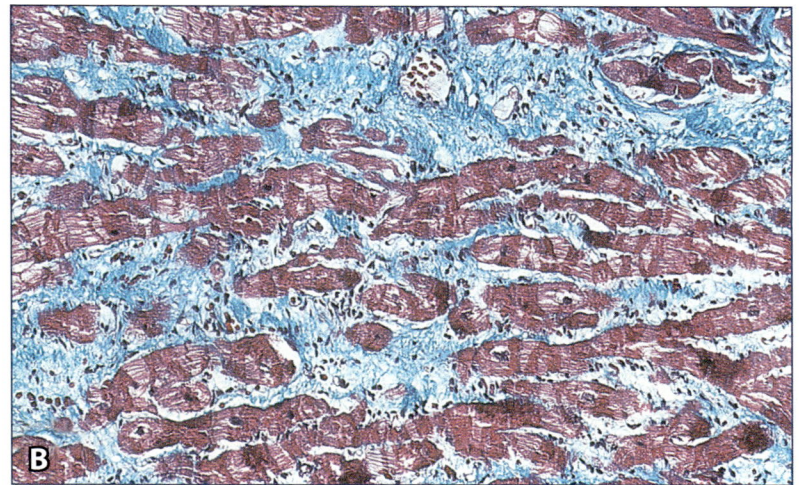

Figure 6-40. A, Gross autopsy specimen of a heart with fulminant myocarditis. The right ventricle is cut along the long axis to demonstrate an apical mural thrombus. Fulminant myocarditis is characterized by a nonspecific, severe influenza-like illness and the distinct onset of cardiac involvement. The patient's condition deteriorates rapidly, and the disorder frequently results in profound hemodynamic compromise and multisystem failure. Endomyocardial biopsies from fulminant myocarditis patients demonstrate unequivocal active myocarditis and are particularly notable for very extensive inflammatory infiltrates and numerous foci of myocyte necrosis. Within 1 month, the patients usually recover left ventricular function completely or die [48]. In contrast, acute myocarditis describes the clinical spectrum of the largest group of patients with active or borderline myocarditis. These patients have minimally dilated, hypokinetic left ventricles on presentation. The onset of cardiac symptoms is frequently indistinct, and some patients provide a vague history consistent with (but not diagnostic of) an antecedent viral illness. Active or borderline myocarditis is present on initial (but not subsequent) endomyocardial biopsies. Some patients in this group appear to respond to immunosuppressive therapy [49], whereas others experience either partial recovery of ventricular function or continue to deteriorate to end-stage dilated cardiomyopathy.

B, Masson's trichrome (which stains collagen blue) of an endomyocardial biopsy of a patient with chronic active myocarditis. Note the extensive collagen deposition characteristically seen in end-stage dilated cardiomyopathy. Patients with chronic active myocarditis usually have a vague clinical presentation. Such patients have a slowly progressive course that inevitably deteriorates but may be punctuated by brief, often dramatic but unsustained responses to immunosuppressive therapy. Serial endomyocardial biopsies demonstrate ongoing myocarditis with the development of extensive interstitial fibrosis. Inflammatory infiltrates in this subgroup of myocarditis patients may contain multinucleated giant cells.

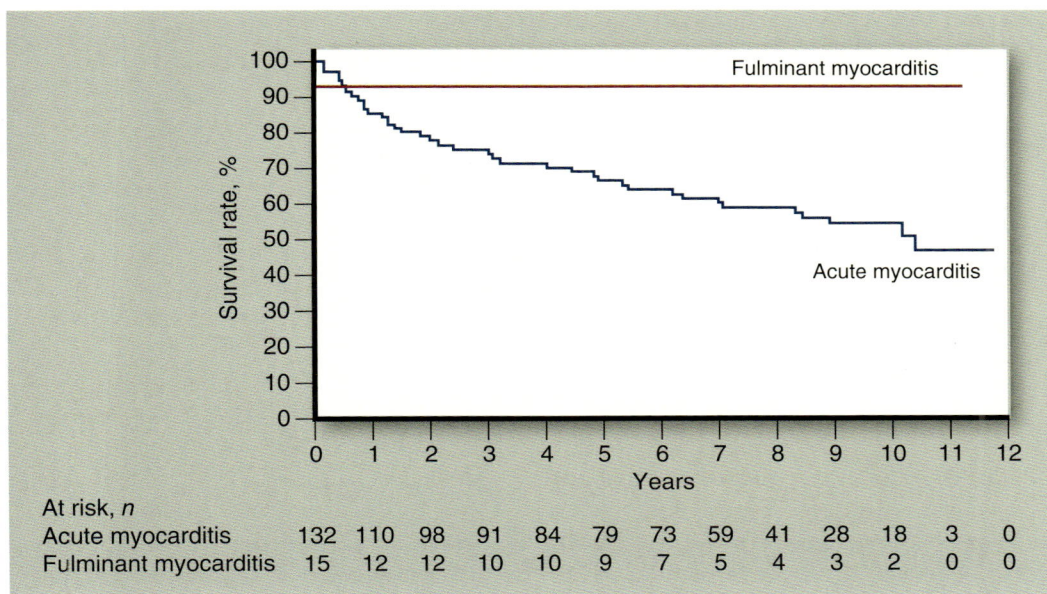

Figure 6-41. The outcome of patients with fulminant versus acute myocarditis is dramatically different. Those with fulminant myocarditis die acutely or survive without additional evidence of left ventricular compromise or symptoms of congestive heart failure. Patients with acute myocarditis display a progressive mortality rate that is similar to that of patients with idiopathic dilated cardiomyopathy [50].

At risk, n												
Acute myocarditis	132	110	98	91	84	79	73	59	41	28	18	3	0
Fulminant myocarditis	15	12	12	10	10	9	7	5	4	3	2	0	0

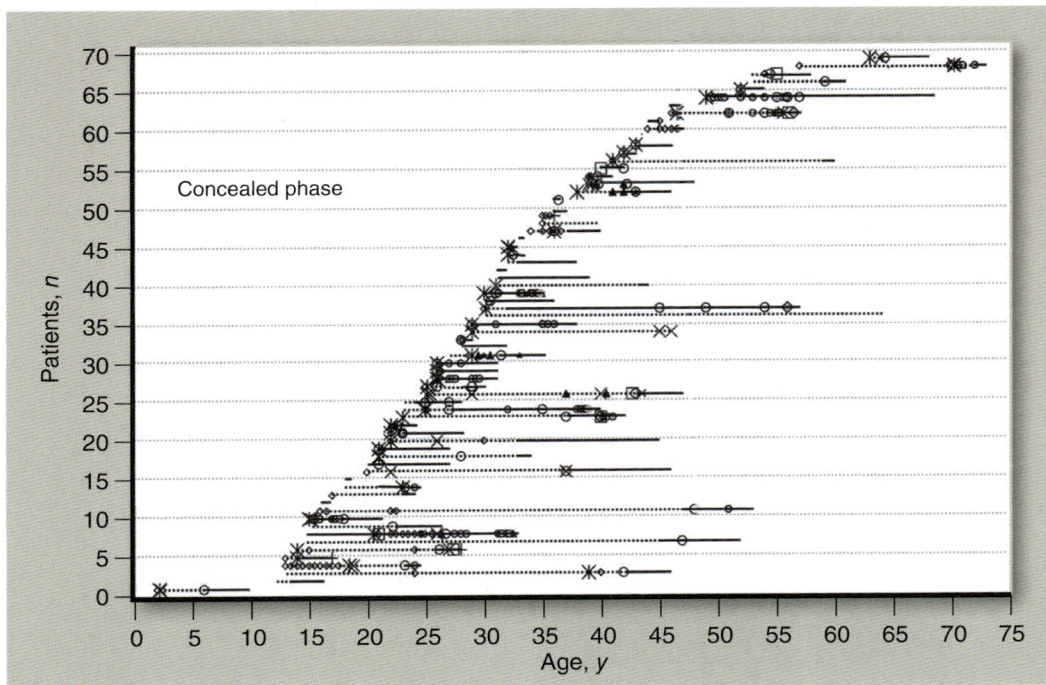

Figure 6-42. The clinical course of 69 patients with arrhythmogenic right ventricular dysplasia (ARVD) is outlined. Each patient's course is characterized by a straight line with plotted events and the age at which they occurred. The line initiates at symptomatic presentation and ends at death or a censoring event. Events include syncope (*diamond*), first documented ventricular tachyarrhythmia (VT; *asterisk*), termination of VT by cardioversion externally (*X*), catheter ablation of VT (*small black triangle*), implantable cardioverter defibrillators (ICD; *light-shaded circle*), appropriate ICD therapy (*black dot*), onset of heart failure (*white square*), heart transplant (*shaded diamond*), and death (*plus sign*). These data indicate that patients usually present in their second to fifth decade, the diagnosis is often delayed, and the course varies widely. Also noted is the long preclinical phase preceding clinical recognition [51].

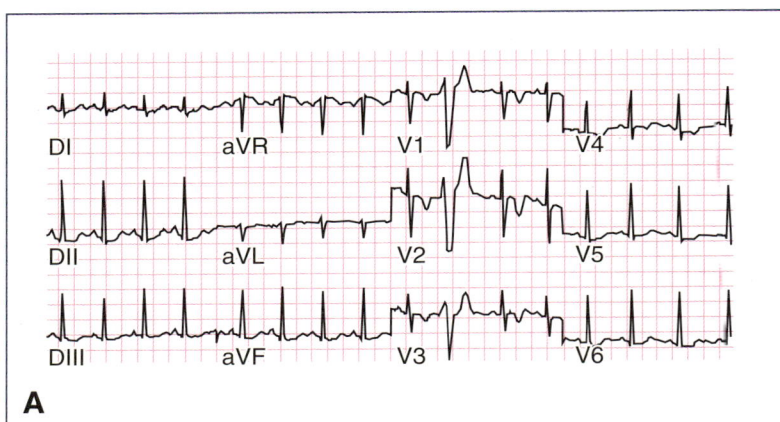

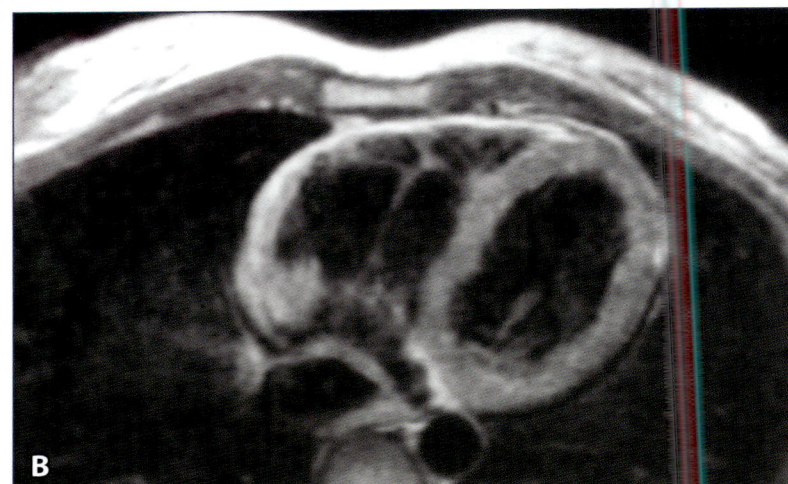

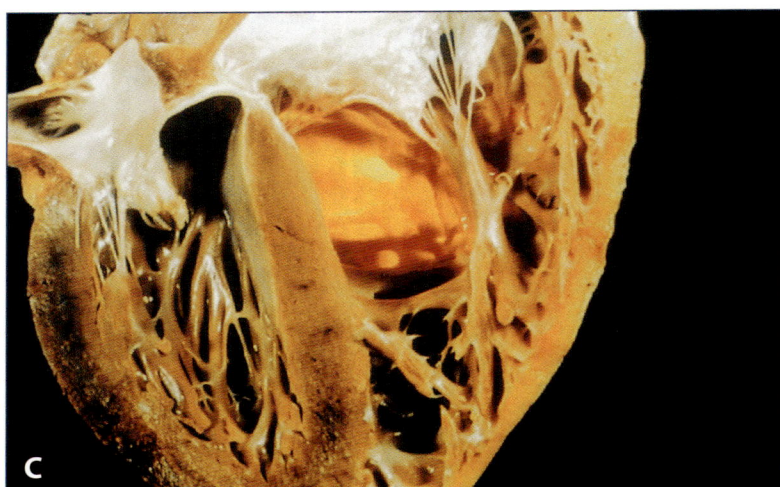

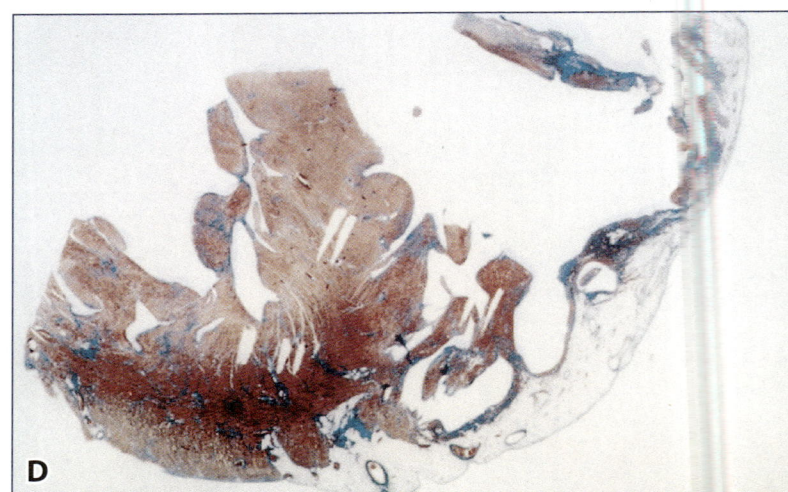

Figure 6-43. Means of diagnosing arrhythmogenic dysplasia. **A,** Electrocardiogram. Note the typical abnormalities consisting of inverted T waves in V1 to V4 and isolated premature ventricular contractions with a left bundle branch block morphology. **B,** Magnetic resonance imaging. The right ventricle is dilated with bright signals from the thinned and fatty infiltrated right ventricular free wall. **C,** Histologic confirmation. Transmural fibrofatty replacement of the right ventricular free wall. Morphologic features in a 25-year-old man who died sud- denly from arrhythmogenic right ventricular cardiomyopathy. This is a four-chamber view cut of the heart specimen showing the transmural fatty replacement of the right ventricular free wall and the translucent infundibulum. **D,** Panoramic histologic section of the heart noted in C, displaying myocardial atrophy in the right ventricle primarily affecting the free wall. Increased fat or fibrous material, beyond normal limits, helps to establish the diagnosis in those submitted to right ventricular endomyocardial biopsy [52]. (*See* Ch. 16.)

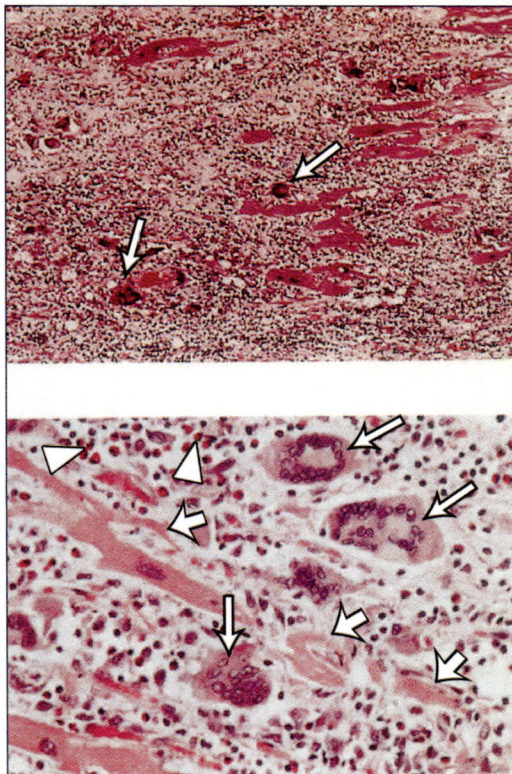

Figure 6-44. Giant cell myocarditis. Multinucleated giant cells (*long arrows*) are seen adjacent to degenerating myocytes (*short arrows*). The cellular infiltrate contains lymphocytes, histiocytes, and collections of eosinophils (*arrowheads*) (hematoxylin and eosin, × 400) [53,54].

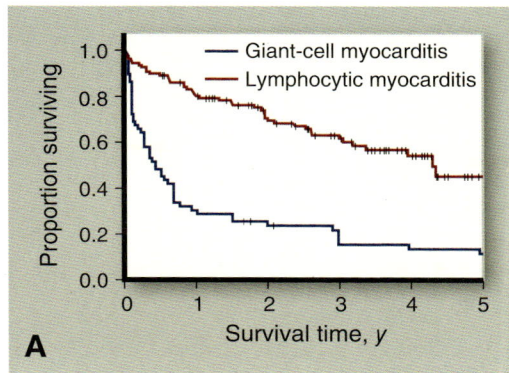

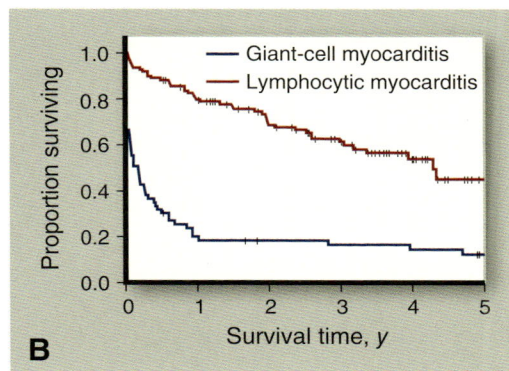

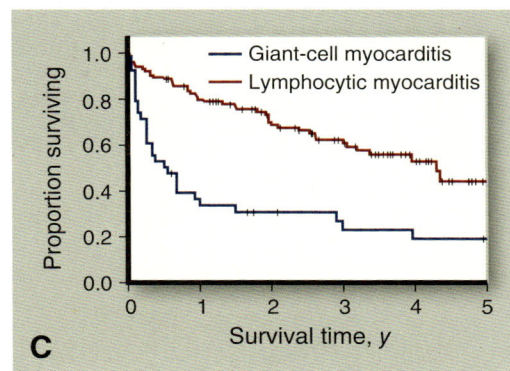

Figure 6-45. Kaplan-Meier survival curves for patients with giant cell myocarditis. Panel A shows the duration of survival from the onset of symptoms; panel B shows the duration of survival from the time of presentation at the referring institution; and panel C shows the duration of survival among 38 patients in whom giant cell myocarditis was diagnosed by endomyocardial biopsy or by examination of a section of the ventricular apex. In each case, survival was significantly longer among patients with lymphocytic myocarditis.

Cardiac Tamponade

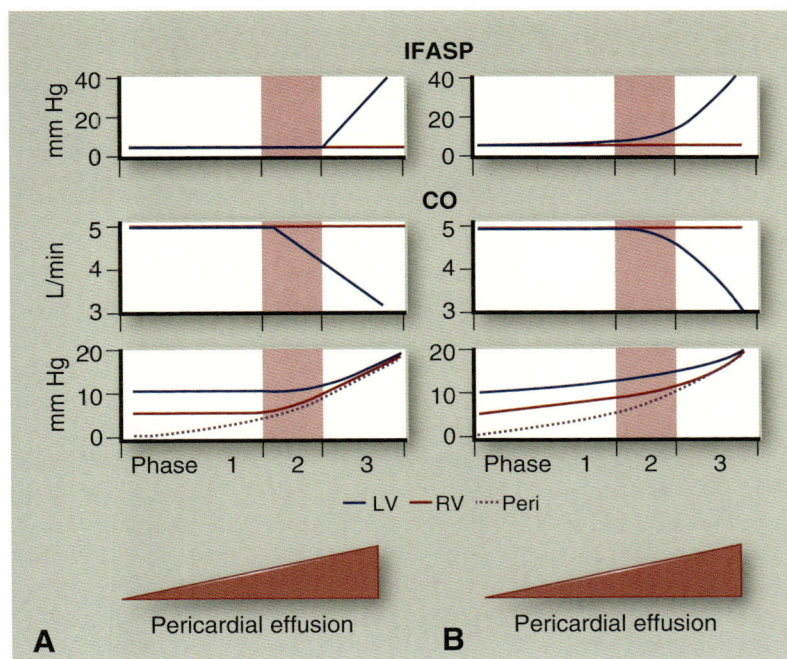

Figure 6-46. Hemodynamic changes in cardiac tamponade, including pericardial (Peri), right ventricular (RV), and left ventricular (LV) pressures and the inspiratory fall in arterial systolic pressure (IFASP) and cardiac output (CO), with increasing pericardial effusion in any given patient depicted by the increasing height of the triangle from left to right. Shaded vertical area indicates phase 2. **A,** The original concept. **B,** The revised concept, in which LV diastolic pressure does not equilibrate with RV diastolic pressure and pericardial pressure until phase 3. In phase 1, pericardial pressure rises but does not equilibrate with RV and LV diastolic pressures. There is no pulsus paradoxus. In phase 2, RV diastolic pressures equilibrate but not with LV diastolic pressure, which remains higher. Pulsus paradoxus is often present. In phase 3, left and right diastolic pressures equilibrate with pericardial pressure, and pulsus paradoxus is nearly always present. (*Adapted from* Reddy *et al.* [54].)

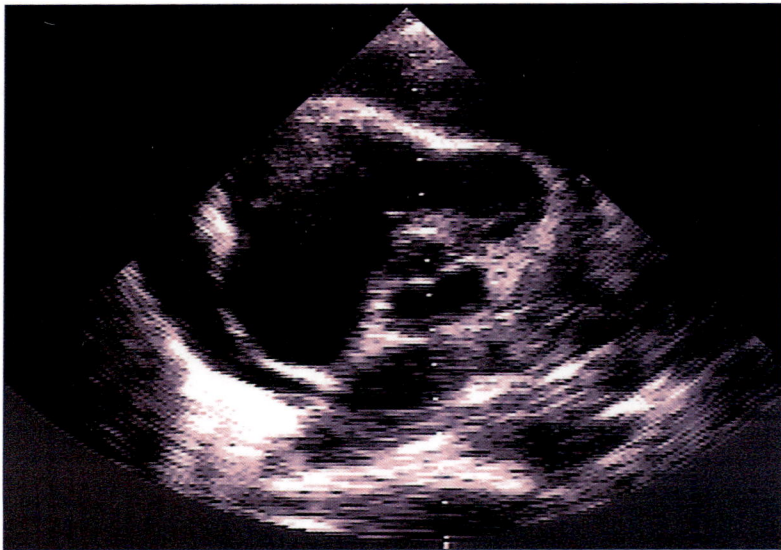

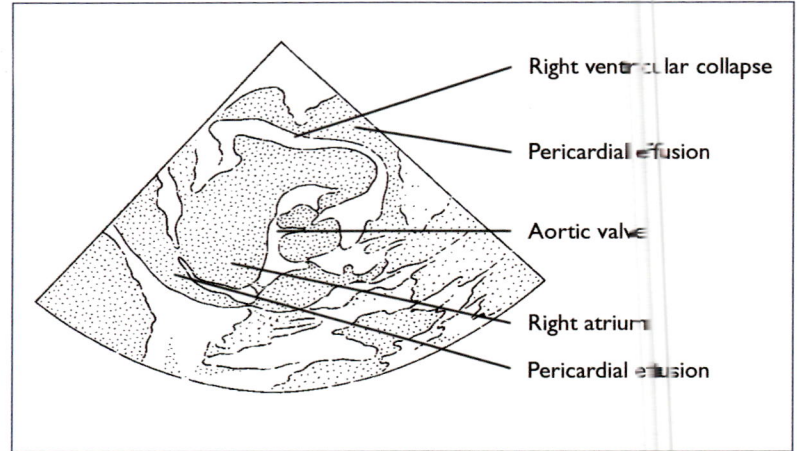

Figure 6-47. Two-dimensional echocardiogram, parasternal short-axis view, showing right ventricular diastolic collapse in a patient with a large pericardial effusion and cardiac tamponade. (*Courtesy of* Brian Hoit, MD.)

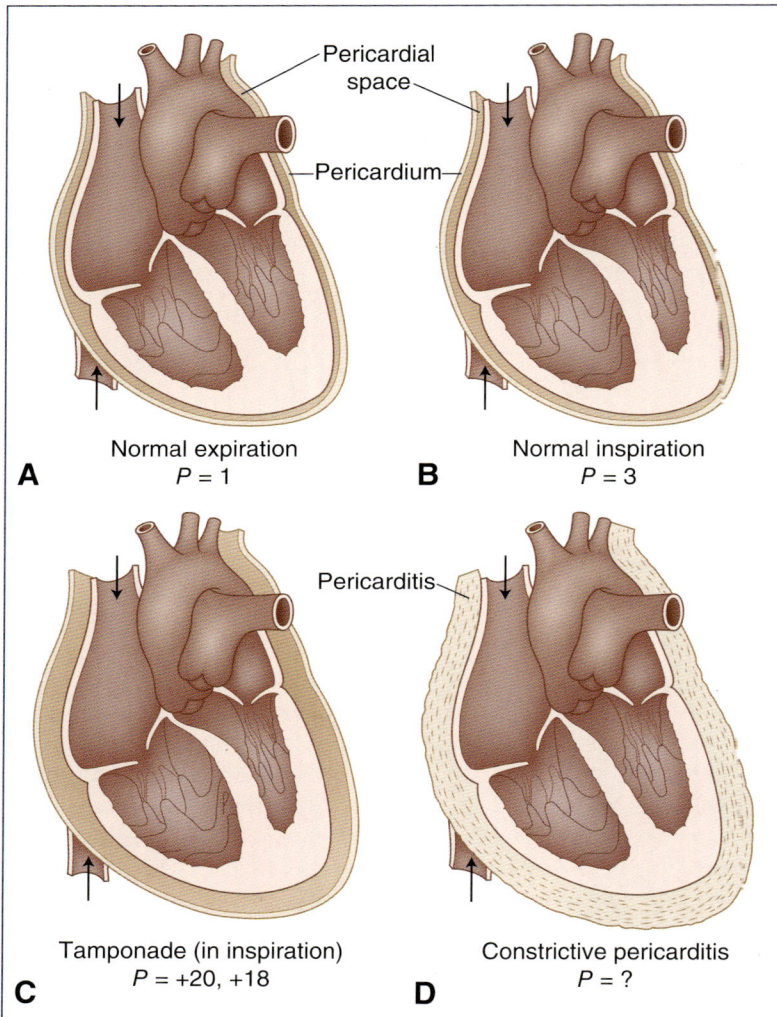

Figure 6-48. A comparison of the hemodynamic effects and the effects of respiration on cardiac tamponade compared with constrictive pericarditis. **A** and **B,** Normal physiology. In *A, arrows* in the venae cavae indicate systemic venous return. During inspiration, intrathoracic pressure declines, causing the pericardial pressure (P) to fall from 1 to -3 mm Hg. Venous return increases (*arrows* in *B*), causing an increase in the size of the right heart at the expense of the left ventricle, which becomes smaller. The latter effect is caused in part by bowing of the interventricular septum from right to left. The upper lead lines indicate the parietal pericardium; the lower ones indicate the pericardial space, which normally may contain up to 25 mL of pericardial fluid. **C** and **D,** Compressive cardiac disorders. During inspiration in cardiac tamponade (*C*), venous return increases (*arrows*) and pericardial pressure falls from 20 to 18 mm Hg. Right heart volume increases slightly because of septal bulging. In constrictive pericarditis (*D*), inspiration does not increase venous return (*arrows*). The pericardial space is obliterated and therefore intrathoracic pressure changes are not transmitted to the heart. During inspiration, the septum does not bow toward the left. (*Adapted from* Shabetai [55].)

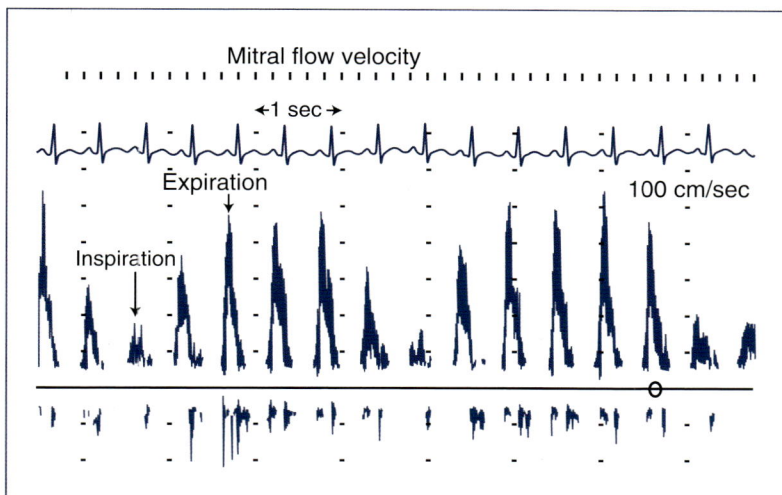

Figure 6-49. Doppler echocardiogram demonstrating abnormal inspiratory decrease in mitral flow velocity in cardiac tamponade. The normal decrease is less than 15%. Abnormal inspiratory decreases in mitral flow velocity also occur in constrictive pericarditis, right ventricular infarction, and chronic obstructive airway disease. (*Adapted from* Hoit [56].)

Acute Pericarditis

Causes of Acute Pericarditis

Malignant tumor

Idiopathic pericarditis

Uremia

Bacterial infection

Anticoagulant therapy

Dissecting aortic aneurysm

Diagnostic procedures

Connective tissue disease

Postpericardiotomy syndrome

Trauma

Tuberculosis

Others

  Radiation

  Drugs inducing lupuslike syndrome

  Myxedema

  Chylopericardium

  Postmyocardial infarction syndrome (Dressler's)

  Fungal infections

  AIDS-related pericarditis

A

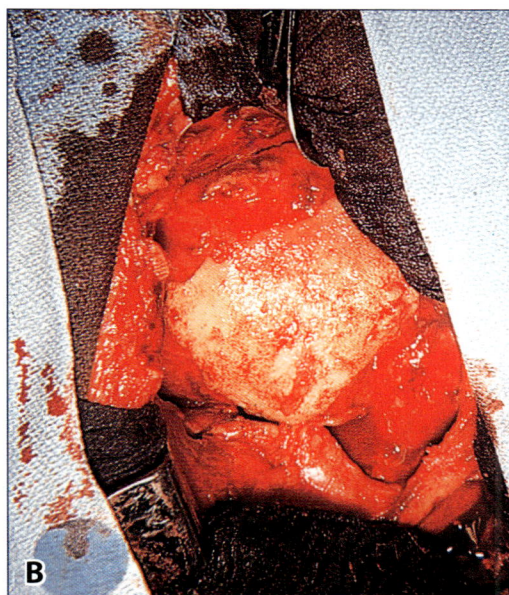

B

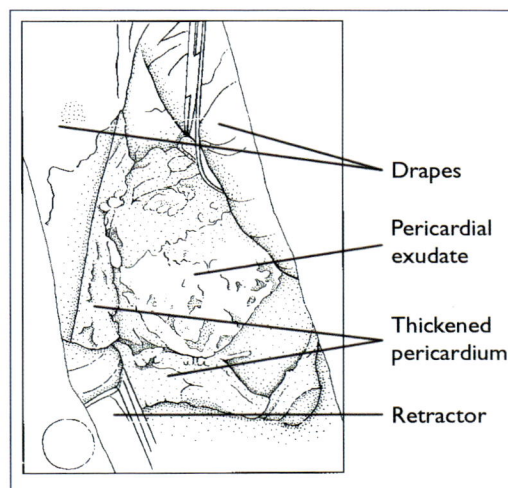

- Drapes
- Pericardial exudate
- Thickened pericardium
- Retractor

Figure 6-50. A, In most hospital series, malignant tumors are the most common cause of acute pericarditis, and idiopathic pericarditis is the second most common. These two causes, together with chronic renal failure, infection, and connective tissue disease, comprise about 50% of cases. In some inner-city hospitals, acquired immunodeficiency syndrome (AIDS)–related pericarditis has become one of the most common causes [57]. **B,** The exposed heart of a patient with pneumococcal pericarditis, showing purulent exudate and thickened pericardium.

Presenting Features of Acute Pericarditis

Chest pain of pleuropericardial quality	Cardiac tamponade with elevated venous pressure
Dull, oppressive chest pain	Incidental finding on electrocardiogram, echocardiogram, or chest radiogram
Pericardial rub	
Dyspnea or tachycardia	
Unexplained fever or toxicity	

Figure 6-51. Acute pericarditis is usually recognized by the presenting findings of chest pain or pericardial rub, but may be first recognized by echocardiographic evidence of pericardial effusion or changes on the chest radiogram or electrocardiogram. Some cases present with cardiac tamponade, dyspnea, tachycardia, and elevated venous pressure, simulating congestive heart failure.

Figure 6-52. Hazard ratios for complications of pericarditis in the Cox proportional hazard model. Indicators of poor prognosis in acute pericarditis. Hazard ratios are listed for complications in a Cox proportional hazard model for patients with acute pericarditis. These data represent the experience with 453 patients 17 to 90 years old with acute pericarditis, excluding postmyocardial infarction pericarditis. A specific cause was identified in only 16.8% of this population. After 31 months, complications occurred in 21% of the patient cohort, including tamponade in 3.1%, and constriction in 1.5%. The hazard ratios represent the increased risk after multivariable analysis, including age, female gender, fever greater than 38° centigrade, subacute course, immunodepression, trauma, oral anticoagulants, rise in cardiac troponin I, large pericardial fusion or cardiac tamponade, aspirin or nonsteroidal anti-inflammatory failure, and corticosteroid use [58]. ASA—acetylsalicylic acid; NSAID—nonsteroidal anti-inflammatory drug.

Hazard Ratios for Complications of Pericarditis			
Feature	HR	95% CI	P
Female gender	1.65	1.08–2.52	0.02
Large effusion/tamponade	2.51	1.37–4.61	0.003
ASA or NSAID failure	5.5	3.56–8.51	< 0.001

Figure 6-53. Two-dimensional echocardiogram (parasternal long-axis view) in a patient with pericardial and pleural effusions. A large pericardial effusion (PE) is present posterior to the left ventricle (LV) and left atrium (LA). A left pleural effusion (PL EFF) is seen as an echo-free space posterior to the pericardial effusion and partitioned from it by a linear echo (X) representing the pericardium. The most important landmark in distinguishing pleural from pericardial effusions is the descending thoracic aorta (*outlined, arrow*). Pericardial fluid accumulates anterior to the pericardial border, insinuating itself between the aorta and the heart; the left pleural effusion, conversely, resides exclusively posterior to the descending aorta. RV—right ventricle. (*From* Fowler [59]; with permission.)

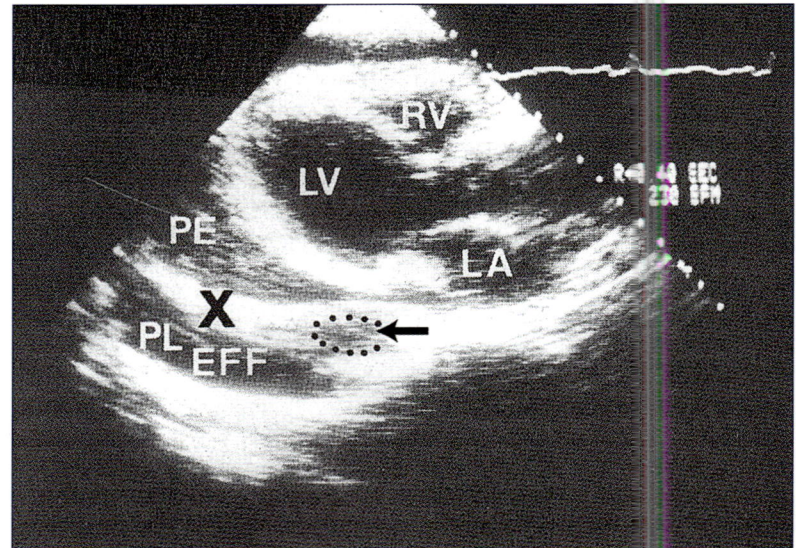

Figure 6-54. Chest radiographs of a patient with relapsing idiopathic pericarditis [60]. **A,** Enlarged cardiopericardial silhouette with a left pleural effusion. **B,** Essentially normal radiograph made during a remission following prednisone therapy. Pleural effusions occur commonly in idiopathic pericarditis and usually are either on the left or bilateral.

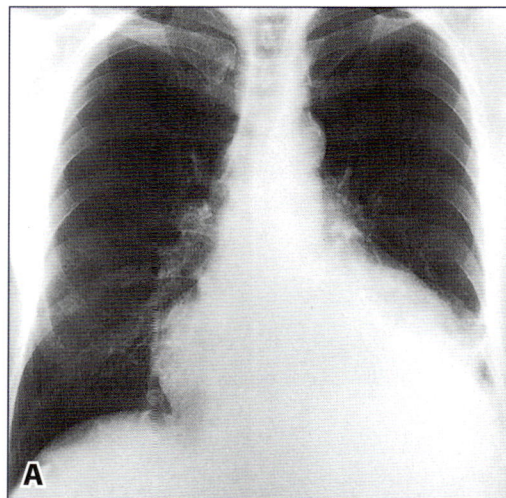

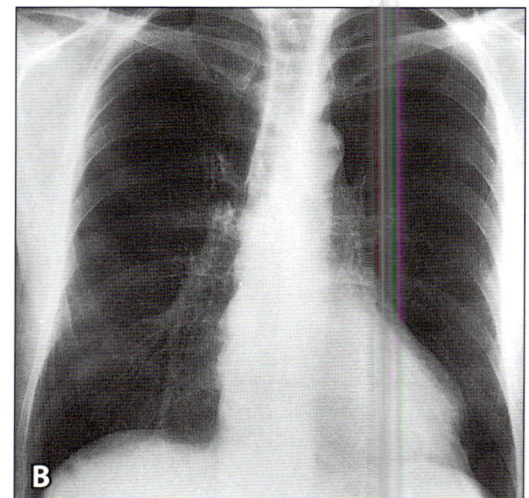

Constrictive Pericarditis

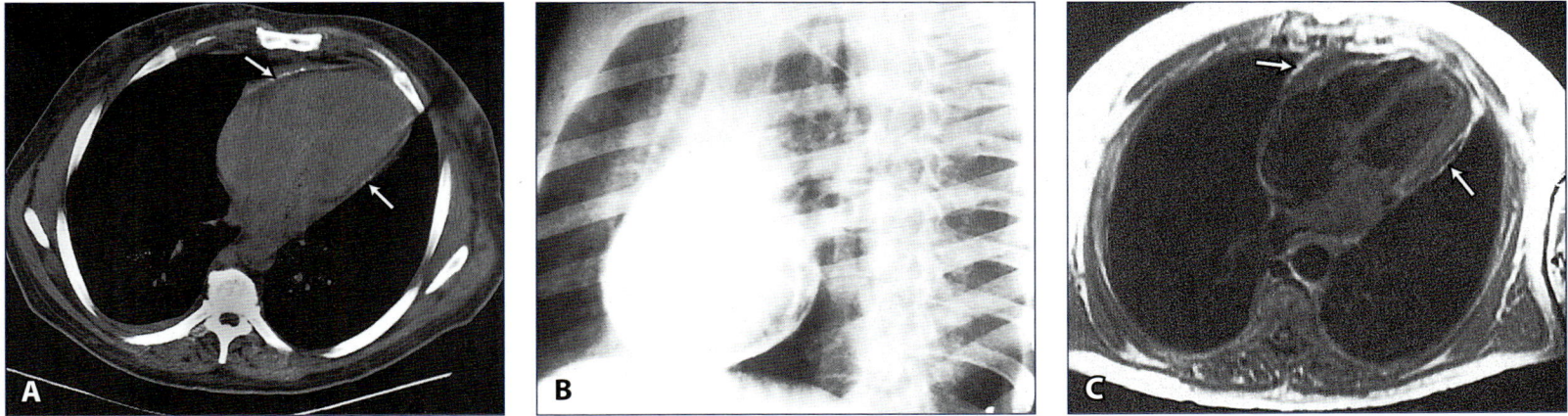

Figure 6-55. A, Computed tomography of the chest showing thickened pericardium and calcification (*arrows*) in a patient with constrictive pericarditis. **B,** Extensive pericardial calcification may occur with chronic pericarditis without constriction. The typical hemodynamic pattern must also be present to make the diagnosis of constrictive pericarditis. **C,** MRI from a patient with constrictive pericarditis. Note a dark area of thickened pericardium over the left ventricle (*arrow*) and a light area of pericardial fat over the right ventricle (*arrow*). (*Part A from* Fowler [57]; with permission.)

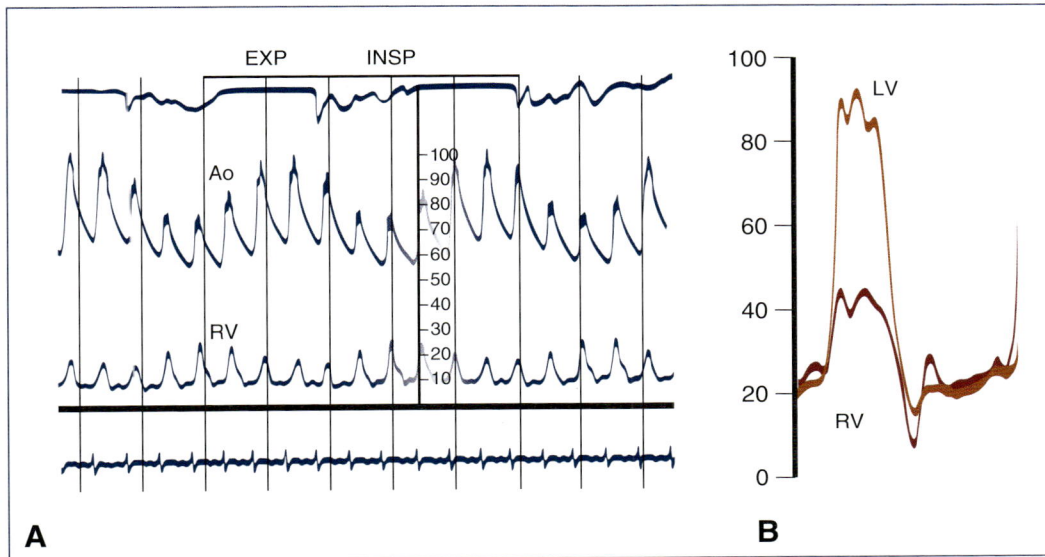

Figure 6-56. Contrasting pattern of a ventricular pressure pulse recording in cardiac tamponade (**A**) and in constrictive pericarditis (**B**) [61]. In constrictive pericarditis, there is a dip and plateau pattern (*square-root sign*) in both ventricular pressure pulse tracings with equalization of right ventricular (RV) and left ventricular (LV) end-diastolic pressures. In cardiac tamponade, there is no pronounced diastolic dip in the RV pressure pulse. The patient with cardiac tamponade demonstrates a pronounced inspiratory decline of aortic pressure (Ao). Pressure scale is in mm Hg. EXP—expiration; INSP—inspiration. (*Adapted from* Shabetai *et al.* [62].)

References

1. Kamisago M, Sharma SD, DePalma SR, *et al.*: Mutations in sarcomere protein genes as a cause of dilated cardiomyopathy. *N Engl J Med* 2000, 343:1688–1696.

2. Wigle ED, Sasson Z, Henderson MA, *et al.*: Hypertrophic cardiomyopathy. The importance of the site and the extent of hypertrophy: a review. *Prog Cardiovasc Dis* 1985, 28:1–85.

3. Shah PM, Taylor RD, Wong M: Abnormal mitral valve coaptation in hypertrophic obstructive cardiomyopathy: proposed role in systolic anterior motion of mitral valve. *Am J Cardiol* 1981, 48:258–262.

4. Grigg LE, Wigle ED, Williams WG, *et al.*: Transesophageal Doppler echocardiography in obstructive hypertrophic cardiomyopathy: clarification of pathophysiology and importance in intraoperative decision making. *J Am Coll Cardiol* 1992, 20:42–52.

5. Braunwald E: Hypertrophic cardiomyopathy: the benefits of a multidisciplinary approach. *N Engl J Med* 2002, 347:1306–1307.

6. Nishimura RA, Holmes DR: Hypertrophic obstructive cardiomyopathy. *N Engl J Med* 2004, 350:1320–1327.

7. McDonald K, McWilliams E, O'Keeffe B, *et al.*: Functional assessment of patients treated with permanent dual chamber pacing as a primary treatment for hypertrophic cardiomyopathy. *Eur Heart J* 1988, 9:893–898.

8. Fananapazir L, Cannon RO, Tripodi D, *et al.*: Impact of dual-chamber permanent pacing in patients with obstructive hypertrophic and cardiomyopathy with symptoms refractory to verapamil and beta-adrenergic blocker therapy. *Circulation* 1992, 85:2149–2161.

9. Wigle ED, Chrysohou A, Bigelow W: Results of ventriculomyotomy in muscular subaortic stenosis. *Am J Cardiol* 1963, 11:572–586.

10. Maron BJ, Epstein SE, Morrow AG: Symptomatic status and prognosis of patients after operation for hypertrophic obstructive cardiomyopathy: efficacy of ventricular septal myotomy and myectomy. *Eur Heart J* 1983, 4:175–185.

11. Beahrs MM, Tajik AJ, Seward JB, *et al.*: Hypertrophic obstructive cardiomyopathy: 10–21 year follow-up after partial septal myectomy. *Am J Cardiol* 1983, 51:1160–1166.

12. Williams WG, Wigle ED, Rakowski H, *et al.*: Results of surgery for idiopathic hypertrophic obstructive cardiomyopathy (IHSS). *Circulation* 1987, 76:V104–V108.

13. Woo A, Williams WG, Choi R, *et al.*: Clinical and echocardiographic determinants of long-term survival after surgical myectomy in obstructive hypertrophic cardiomyopathy. *Circulation* 2005, 111:2033–2041.

14. Spirito P, Bellone P, Harris KM, *et al.*: Magnitude of left ventricular hypertrophy and risk of sudden death in hypertrophic cardiomyopathy. *N Engl J Med* 2000, 342:1778–1785.

15. Fifer MA, Vlahakes GJ: Management of symptoms in hypertrophic cardiomyopathy. *Circulation* 2008, 117:429–439.

16. Manolio TA, Baughman KL, Rodeheffer R, *et al.*: Prevalence and etiology of idiopathic dilated cardiomyopathy. *Am J Cardiol* 1992, 69:1458–1466.

17. Abelmann WH: Classification and natural history of primary myocardial disease. *Prog Cardiovasc Dis* 1985, 127:73–94.

18. Felker GM, Thompson RE, Hare JM, *et al.*: Underlying causes and long-term survival in patients with initially unexplained cardiomyopathy. *N Engl J Med* 2000, 342:1077–1084.

19. Peacock FW IV, De Marco T, Fonarow GC, *et al.*: Cardiac Troponin and outcome in acute heart failure. *N Engl J Med* 2008, 358:2117–2126.

20. Braunwald E: Biomarkers in heart failure. *N Engl J Med* 2008, 358:2148–2159.

21. Fitzpatrick TB, Eisen AZ, Wolff K, *et al.*: *Dermatology in General Medicine*, vol 2, ed 4. New York: McGraw-Hill; 1993:2412.

22. McAlister HF, Klementowicz PT, Andrews C, *et al.*: Lyme carditis: an important cause of reversible heart block. *Ann Intern Med* 1989, 110:339–345.

23. van der Linde MR, Crijns HJCM, de Konig J, *et al.*: Range of atrioventricular disturbances in Lyme borreliosis: a report of four cases and review of other published reports. *Br Heart J* 1990, 63:162–168.

24. Roberts WC, McAlister HA, Ferrano VJ: Sarcoidosis of the heart. *Am J Med* 1977, 63:86–108.

25. Shammas RL, Movahed A: Sarcoidosis of the heart. *Clin Cardiol* 1993, 16:462–472.

26. Uretsky BF: Diagnostic considerations in the adult patient with cardiomyopathy or congestive heart failure. In *Cardiovascular Clinics.* Edited by Shaver JA. Philadelphia: FA Davis; 1988:35–56.

27. Sekiguchi M, Numao Y, Nunoda S, *et al.*: Clinical histopathological profile of sarcoidosis of the heart and acute idiopathic myocarditis: concepts through a study employing endomyocardial biopsy. *Jpn Circ J* 1980, 44:249–263.

28. Gertz MA, Kyle RA: Primary systemic amyloidosis: a diagnostic primer. *Mayo Clin Proc* 1989, 64:1505–1519.

29. Falk RH: Cardiac amyloidosis. In *Progress in Cardiology.* Edited by Zipes DP, Rowlands DJ. Philadelphia: Lea & Febiger; 1989:143–153.

30. Klein AL, Hatle LK, Burstow DJ, *et al.*: Doppler characterization of left ventricular diastolic function in cardiac amyloidosis. *J Am Coll Cardiol* 1989, 13:1017–1026.

31. Falk R: Diagnosis and management of the cardiac amyloidosis. *Circulation* 2005, 112:2047–2060.

32. Kushwaha SS, Fallon JT, Fuster V: Restrictive cardiomyopathy [review]. *N Engl J Med* 1997, 336:267–276.

33. Spry CJF, Tai PC: Clinical studies on endomyocardial fibrosis in patients with hypereosinophilia: a historical review. In *Cardiomyopathy Update 3. Restrictive Cardiomyopathy and Arrhythmias.* Edited by Olsen EGJ, Sekiguchi M. Tokyo: University of Tokyo Press; 1990:81–98.

34. Vijayaraghavan G, Sadanandan S, Cherian G: Endomyocardial fibrosis in India: an overview. In *Cardiomyopathy Update 3. Restrictive Cardiomyopathy and Arrhythmias.* Edited by Olsen EGJ, Sekiguchi M. Tokyo: University of Tokyo Press; 1990:9–20.

35. Nakayama Y, Kohriyama T, Yamamoto S, *et al.*: Electron microscopic and immunohistochemical studies on endomyocardial biopsies from a patient with eosinophilic endomyocardial disease. *Heart Vessel* 1985, 1:250–255.

36. Olsen EGJ: Morphological overview and pathogenetic mechanism in endomyocardial fibrosis associated with eosinophilia. In *Cardiomyopathy Update 3. Restrictive Cardiomyopathy and Arrhythmias.* Edited by Olsen EGJ, Sekiguchi M. Tokyo: University of Tokyo Press; 1990:1–8.

37. Andy JJ: The relationship of microfilaria and other helminthic worms to tropical endomyocardial fibrosis: a review. In *Cardiomyopathy Update 3. Restrictive Cardiomyopathy and Arrhythmias.* Edited by Olsen EGJ, Sekiguchi M. Tokyo: University of Tokyo Press; 1990:21–34.

38. Graham RM, Owens WA: Pathogenesis of inherited forms of dilated cardiomyopathy. *N Engl J Med* 1999, 341:1759–1762.

39. Liu PP, Mason JW: Advances in the understanding of myocarditis. *Circulation* 2001, 104:1076–1082.

40. Aretz HT: Myocarditis: the Dallas criteria. *Hum Pathol* 1987, 18:619–624.

41. Aretz HT, Billingham ME, Edwards WD, *et al.*: A histopathologic definition and classification. *Am J Cardiovasc Pathol* 1986, 1:3–14.

42. Neumann DA, Rose NR, Ansari AA, *et al.*: Induction of heart auto-ant bodies in mice with coxsackievirus B3- and cardiac myosin-induced autoimmune myocarditis. *J Immunol* 1994, 152:343–350.

43. Huber SA, Moraska A: Cytolytic T lymphocytes and antibodies to myocytes in adriamycin-treated BALB/c mice. *Am J Pathol* 1992, 140:233–242.

44. Mahrholdt H, Wagner A, Deluigi CC, *et al.*: Presentation, patterns of myocardial damage, and clinical course of viral myocarditis. *Circulation* 2006, 114:1581–1590.

45. Strain JE, Grose RM, Factor SM, *et al.*: Results of endomyocardial biopsy in patients with spontaneous ventricular tachycardia but without apparent structural heart disease. *Circulation* 1983, 68:1171–1181.

46. Smith WG: Coxsackie B myopericarditis in adults. *Am Heart J* 1980, 80:34–36.

47. Cooper LT, Baughman KL, Feldman AM, *et al.*: The role of endomyocardial biopsy in the management of cardiovascular disease. *Circulation* 2007, 116:2216–2233.

48. Rockman HA, Adamson RM, Dembitsky WP, *et al.*: Acute fulminant myocarditis: long-term follow-up after circulatory support with left ventricular assist device. *Am Heart J* 1991, 121:922–926.

49. Jones SR, Herskowitz A, Hutchins GM, *et al.*: Effects of immunosuppressive therapy in biopsy-proved myocarditis and borderline myocarditis on left ventricular function. *Am J Cardiol* 1991, 68:370–376.

50. McCarthy RE, Boehmer JP, Hruban RH, *et al.*: Long-term outcome of fulminant myocarditis as compared with acute (nonfulminant) myocarditis. *N Engl J Med* 2000, 342:690–695.

51. Dalal D, Nasir K, Bomma C, *et al.*: Arrhythmogenic right ventricular dysplasia: a United States experience. *Circulation* 2005, 112:3823–3832.

52. Cooper LT Jr, Berry GJ, Shabetai R: Idiopathic giant-cell myocarditis—natural history and treatment. Multicenter Giant Cell Myocarditis Study Group Investigators. *N Engl J Med* 1997, 336:1860–1866.

53. Menghini VV, Savcenko V, Olson LJ, *et al.*: Combined immunosuppression for the treatment of idiopathic giant cell myocarditis. *Mayo Clin Proc* 1999, 74:1221–1226.

54. Reddy PS, Curtiss EI, Uritsky BF: Spectrum of hemodynamic changes in cardiac tamponade. *Am J Cardiol* 1990, 66:1487–1491.

55. Shabetai R: *The Pericardium.* New York: Grune and Stratton; 1981.

56. Hoit BD: Imaging the pericardium. In *Diseases of the Pericardium. Cardiology Clinics,* vol 8. Philadelphia: WB Saunders; 1990:587–600.

57. Fowler NO: Pericardial disease. *Heart Dis Stroke* 1992, 1:85–94.

58. Imazio M, Cecchi E, Demichelis B, *et al.*: Indicators of poor prognosis of acute pericarditis. *Circulation* 2007, 115:2739–2744.

59. Fowler NO: *The Pericardium in Health and Disease.* Mount Kisco, NY: Futura Publishing Co; 1985.

60. Fowler NO: Recurrent pericarditis. In *Diseases of the Pericardium. Cardiology Clinics,* vol 8. Edited by Shabetai R. Philadelphia: WB Saunders; 1990:621–626.

61. Goldschlager N, Epstein A, Grubb BP, *et al.*: Etiologic considerations in the patient with syncope and an apparently normal heart. *Arch Intern Med* 2003, 163:151–162.

62. Shabetai R, Fowler NO, Guntheroth WG: The hemodynamics of cardiac tamponade and constrictive pericarditis. *Am J Cardiol* 1970, 26:480–489.

7

Arrhythmias

Laurence M. Epstein, William G. Stevenson, Daniel Steven,
Jens Seiler, Kurt C. Roberts-Thomson, and Vincent Y. See

Conduction and Excitation: Normal Pathway of Electrical Conduction

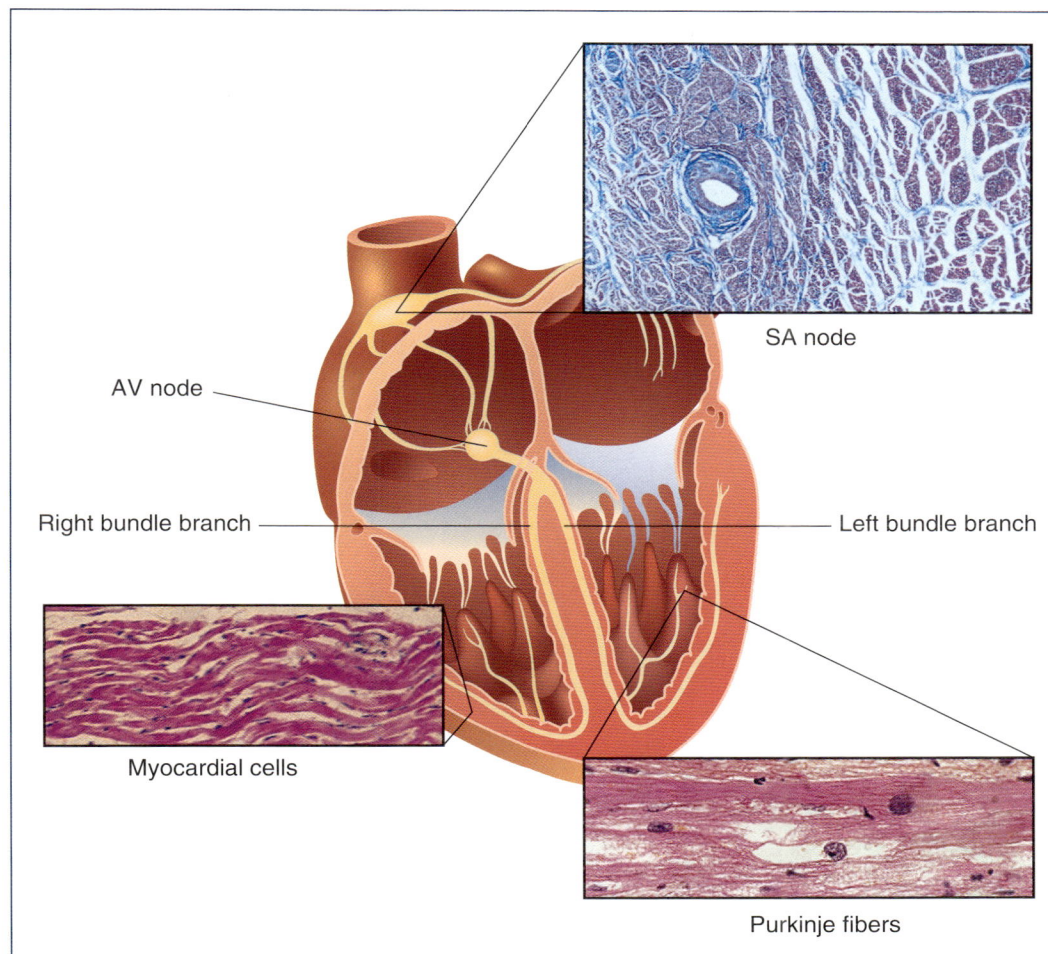

Figure 7-1. Normal pathway of electrical conduction in the heart. Note the differences between the conductive and the contractile tissue of the heart (*insets*). The sinus nodal cells are smaller and interwoven to form a network of cells grouped together by the surrounding fibrous matrix. They contain relatively few myofilaments compared with "working" myocardial cells. The Purkinje fibers are composed of short, cylindrical cells that are irregularly shaped. The ultrastructure of an irregularly shaped cell, which increases cell-to-cell contact, and the large gap junctions at both the ends and sides of the cells provide the membrane properties of rapid impulse conduction. AV—atrioventricular; SA—sinoatrial.

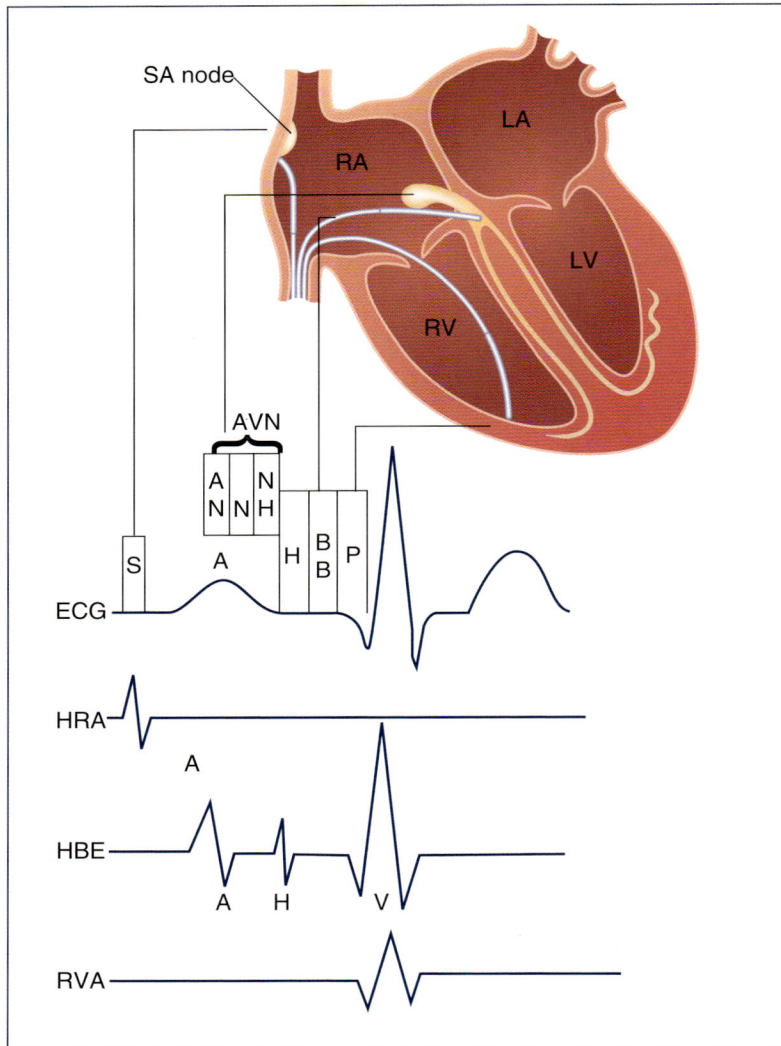

Figure 7-2. Sequence of activation through the conduction system relative to surface electrocardiogram (ECG) events and intracardiac electrograms. The intracardiac catheters are positioned in the high right atrium (RA; to record atrial intracardiac ECGs), the low atrioseptal RA (to record the His bundle ECG), and the right ventricular (RV) apex (to record the ventricular intracardiac ECG). Note the activation of the sinoatrial (SA) node before the onset of the P-wave. Conduction through the atrioventricular (AV) node begins well before atrial depolarization is completed, while conduction through the His-Purkinje system precedes contraction of the ventricles (reflected as the QRS complex). Intracardiac ECGs confirm the activation sequence and timing of the conduction system. Note that the atrial activity in the atrial intracardiac ECG precedes the atrial activity in the His bundle recording, as atrial conduction begins high in the SA node. A—atrial conduction; AN—nodal conduction; AVN—AV nodal conduction; BB—bundle branch conduction; H—His bundle conduction; HBE—His-bundle ECG; HRA—high RA intracardiac ECG; LA—left atrium; LV—left ventricle; N—nodal conduction; NH—nodal–His conduction; P—Purkinje fiber conduction; RVA—RV apex ECG; S—SA node conduction; V—ventricular conduction. (*Adapted from* Marriot and Conover [1].)

Cellular Electrophysiology

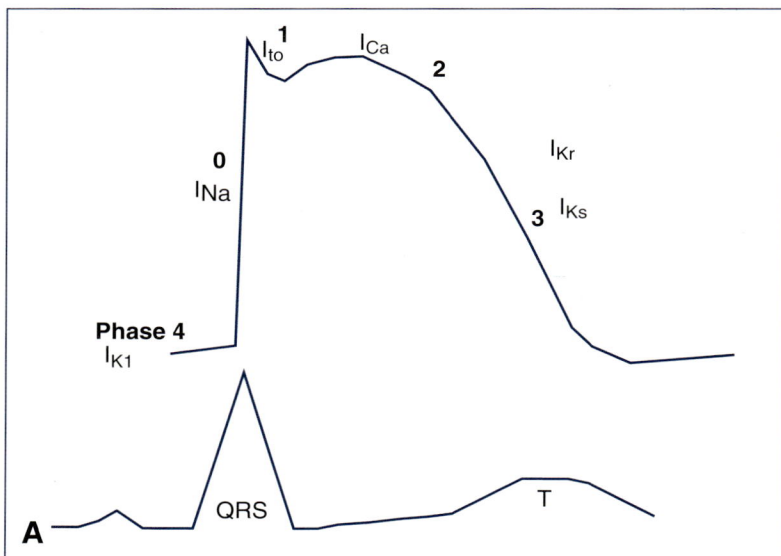

Figure 7-3. A, Phases of the ventricular action potential and ionic currents. Phase 0 is the upstroke that is due to rapid inward sodium (I_{Na}) current. Activation of a transient potassium current Ito causes the phase 1 notch in the action potential. The plateau phase 2 is maintained by the I_{Na} and calcium (I_{Ca}) currents. Repolarization is due to activation of the delayed rectifier potassium currents comprised of rapid (I_{Kr}) and slowly activating (I_{Ks}) currents. The resting membrane potential during phase 4 is maintained by the inward rectifier potassium current (I_{K1}).

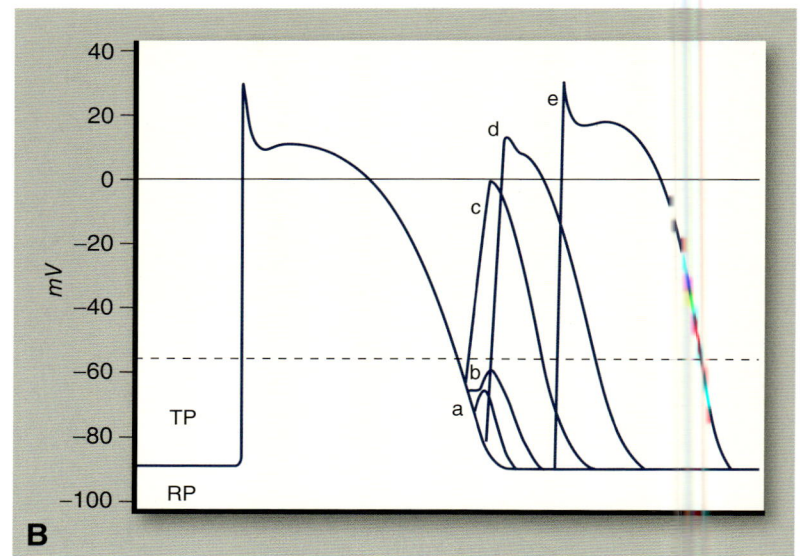

B, A normal action potential and its relative refractory period (RP). This diagram represents a normal action potential and the responses elicited by stimuli applied at different stages of repolarization. The amplitude and upstroke velocity of the elicited responses are directly related to the membrane potential stimuli applied early during repolarization. As *a* and *b* are from low amplitude stimuli during the relative refractory period, they do not generate a propagated response.

Continued on the next page

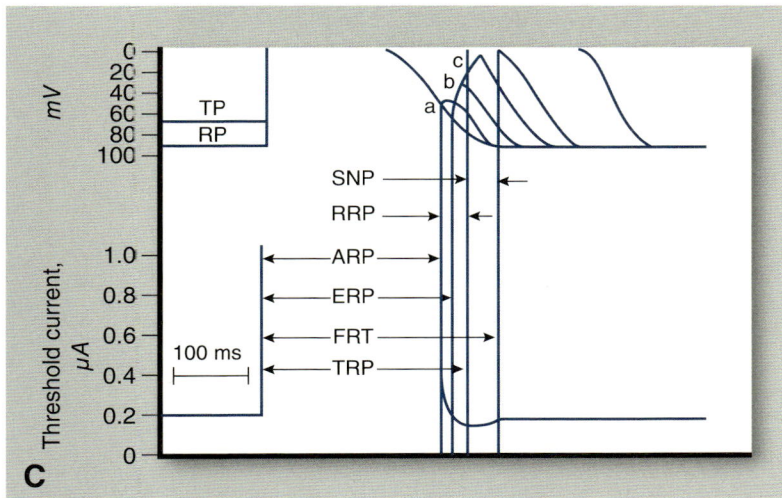

C

Figure 7-3. *(Continued)* The earliest propagated action potential is response *c*, which defines the end of the effective refractory period (ERP). However, response *c* propagates slowly due to its low amplitude and low upstroke velocity. Response *d* is elicited during the supernormal period (SNP) of excitability and its rates of rise and amplitude are greater than those of *c* because it arises from a higher membrane potential. However, it still propagates more slowly than the normal response *e*, which occurs after complete repolarization and therefore has a normal rate of depolarization and amplitude. Response *e* propagates rapidly [2].

C, The refractory periods in respect to the action potential. The fiber becomes inexcitable beginning with the inscription of phase 0 of the action potential. Recovery of excitability progresses slowly during phase 3 of repolarization. A period of supernormal excitability, in which a submaximal stimulus can elicit a propagated action potential, occurs at the terminal portion of phase 3. The diagram also illustrates the absolute refractory period (ARP), ERP, relative RP (RRP), total refractory period (TRP), full recovery time (FRT), and the SNP of excitability. The threshold currents are indicated in microamperes (μA). *Vertical lines* demonstrate the relationship of the refractory period to the elicited responses during repolarization. This diagram demonstrates the time course relationships among repolarization, refractoriness, and excitability. RP—rest potential; TP—test potential.

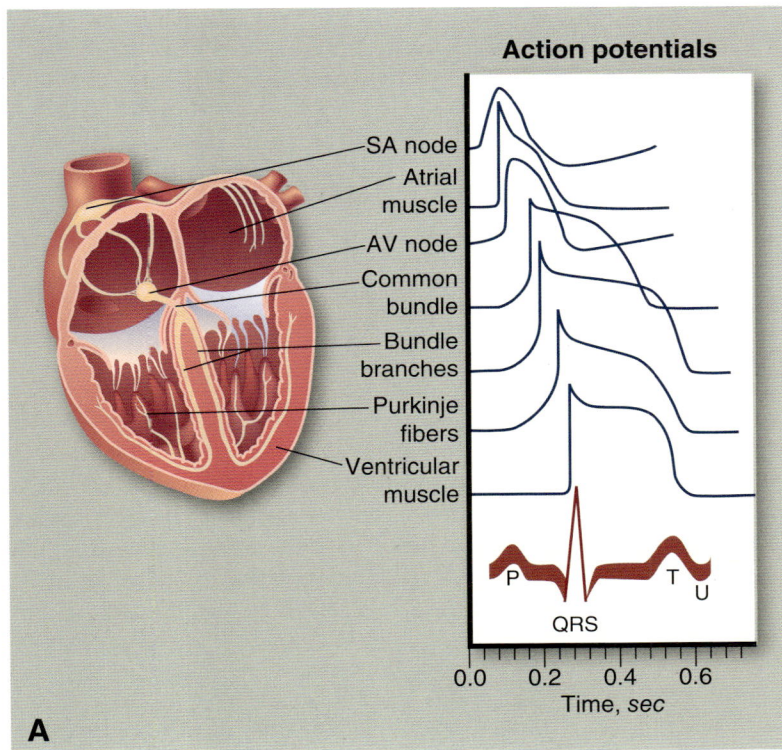

A

Figure 7-4. A, Localized variations in the action potential of the heart's electrical system. Cardiac action potentials from different locations in the heart have different shapes, leading to different electrophysiologic properties. Compared with other cardiac tissue, the sinoatrial (SA) and atrioventricular (AV) nodes have a less-negative resting membrane potential and depolarize due to the slow inward current of calcium (Ca^{2+}) and sodium (Na^+), resulting in slower propagation. All other cardiac cells depolarize in response to the rapid inward current of sodium ions. Note the progressive increase in the action potential duration beginning at the AV node and reaching its maximum in the Purkinje fiber. The specialized cells of the sinus and AV nodes and Purkinje tissue exhibit spontaneous depolarization during phase 4, resulting in spontaneous automaticity, whereas atrial and ventricular muscle does not.

Continued on the next page

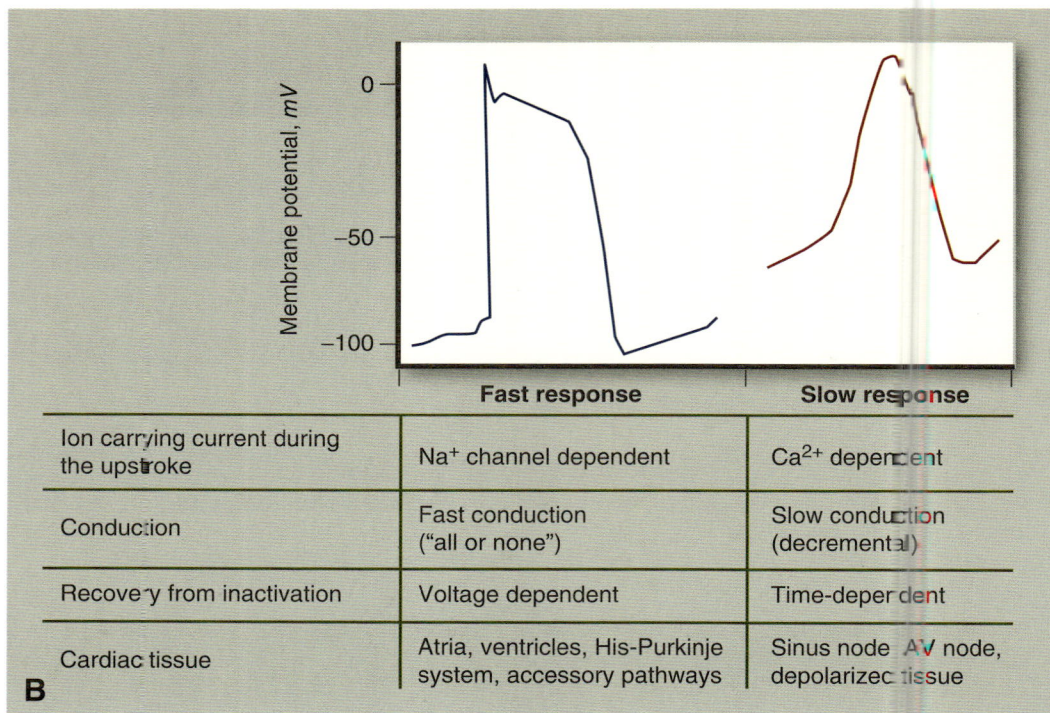

	Fast response	Slow response
Ion carrying current during the upstroke	Na+ channel dependent	Ca^{2+} dependent
Conduction	Fast conduction ("all or none")	Slow conduction (decremental)
Recovery from inactivation	Voltage dependent	Time-dependent
Cardiac tissue	Atria, ventricles, His-Purkinje system, accessory pathways	Sinus node, AV node, depolarized tissue

B

Figure 7-4. *(Continued)* **B**, Summary of the differences between the fast and slow response action potential in the heart. (**A**, *adapted from* CIBA Pharmaceutical Company Division of CIBA-GEIGY Corporation [3].)

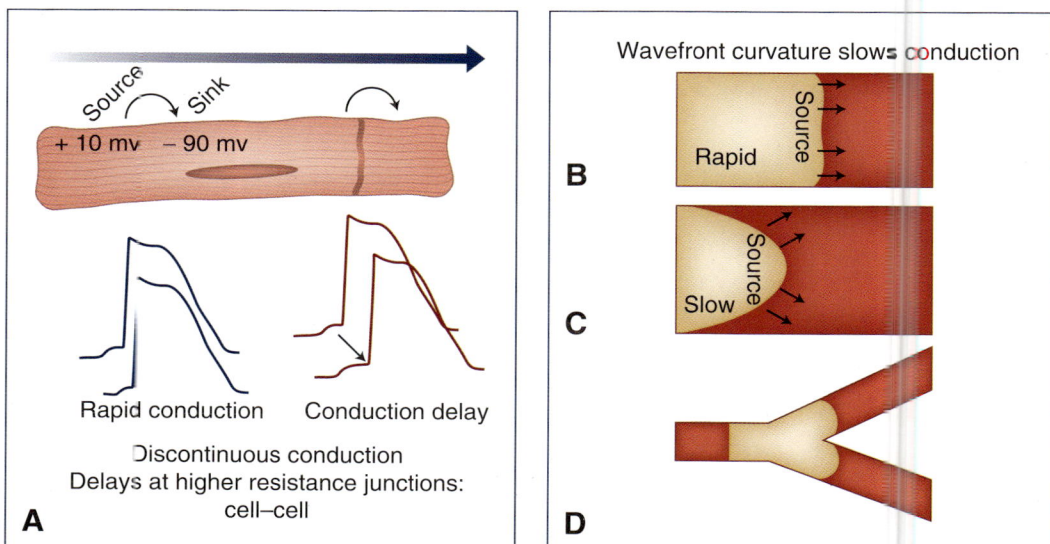

Figure 7-5. Current sources and sinks in the myocardial syncytium have an important impact on conduction velocity. **A**, Propagation along a myocyte. As the action potential moves from left to right, the membrane that is depolarized must supply sufficient current to bring the membrane to its right threshold to produce an action potential. This propagation is rapid as schematically indicated by the short interval between two action potentials below the myocyte. The increased resistance between cells at their borders results in an increase in the time required for the depolarizing membrane to bring the adjacent cell to threshold, hence producing a delay in propagation and slowing conduction (*arrow*). This effect may be magnified when cell-to-cell coupling is reduced in diseased myocardium, such as in hypertrophy and infarct regions. **B**, **C**, and **D** show the important effect of the propagation wavefront geometry and tissue geometry on conduction in multicellular myocardial strands. In each panel, propagation is from left to right. The depolarization wavefront is the *yellow* end of the wave, the *darker* portion is repolarizing. Propagation is most rapid for planar or near planar wavefronts that have little curvature (**B**). Conduction velocity slows for curved wavefronts (**C**). The depolarized cells must supply current to a larger area of cells as the propagation wavefront expands. **D**, Branching tissue architecture importantly influences conduction velocity. Velocity slows where a single strand branches. The interplay of these factors is responsible for slow conduction in the infarct border zone and areas of scar in myopathic ventricles and is an important factor promoting reentry [4].

Mechanism of Arrhythmias

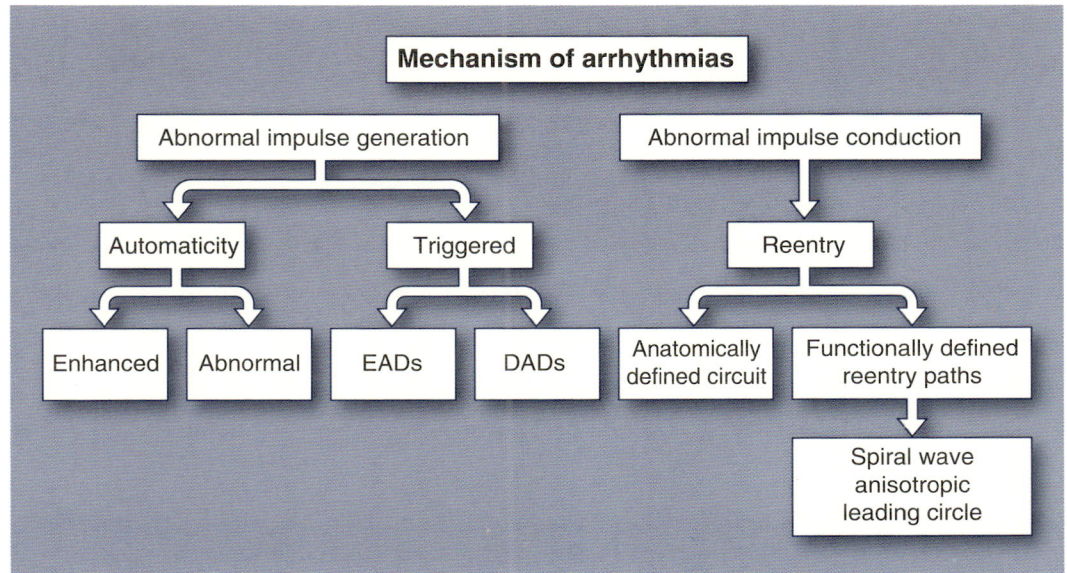

Figure 7-6. Mechanism of arrhythmias. Tachyarrhythmias can be separated into those due to abnormal impulse generation (automaticity) and those due to abnormal impulse conduction (reentry). Reentry can occur over an anatomically defined reentry path, such as in the Wolff-Parkinson-White Syndrome, or in many scar-related reentry circuits. Reentry can also occur around areas of block that are functional in nature, or can follow a spiraling path (spiral wave reentry or rotors). DAD—delayed after-depolarization; EAD—early after-depolarization.

Triggered Arrhythmias

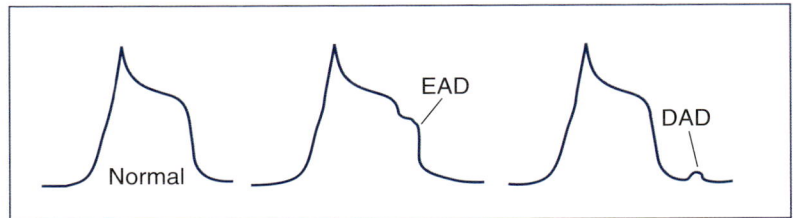

Figure 7-7. Triggered activity (also know as triggered automaticity) is due to after-depolarizations, which are membrane depolarizations that occur during the action potential (early after-depolarization [EAD]) or after the action potential (delayed after-depolarization [DAD]). DADs are due to intracellular calcium overload, such as can be caused by digitalis intoxication. The membrane depolarization can elicit a subsequent action potential or repetitive action potentials causing tachycardia. Atrial and ventricular tachycardias due to digitalis intoxication and multifocal atrial tachycardia are likely due to this mechanism. EADs are due to action potential prolongation that allows reactivation of depolarizing currents. EADs can occur during phase 2 or phase 3 of repolarization. They can further prolong action potential duration or elicit premature beats or repetitive beats that degenerate to polymorphic ventricular tachycardia (VT). EADs are involved in initiation of polymorphic VTs in the acquired and congenital long QT syndromes. In the congenital and acquired long QT syndromes, a membrane defect prolongs repolarization, most commonly by diminishing repolarizing potassium currents. EADs lead to triggered arrhythmias.

Reentry

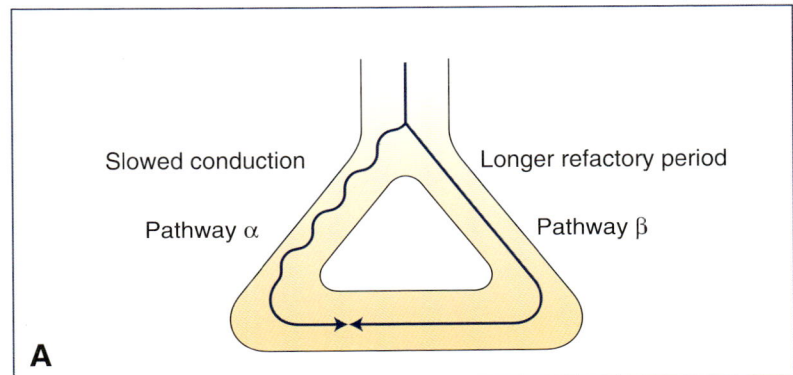

Figure 7-8. Prerequisites for anatomically defined reentry arrhythmias include 1) an anatomic circuit with two pathways (α and β) joined at the proximal and distal ends; 2) the two pathways have different electrophysiologic properties such that a wavefront can block in the β-pathway alone because it has a longer refractory period than the α-pathway; and 3) the reentry path has sufficient length and a sufficiently slow conduction to allow recovery of each point after depolarization at each point in the circuit. **A,** During sinus rhythm, the sinus excitation impulse enters both pathways and collides, preventing reentry.

Continued on the next page

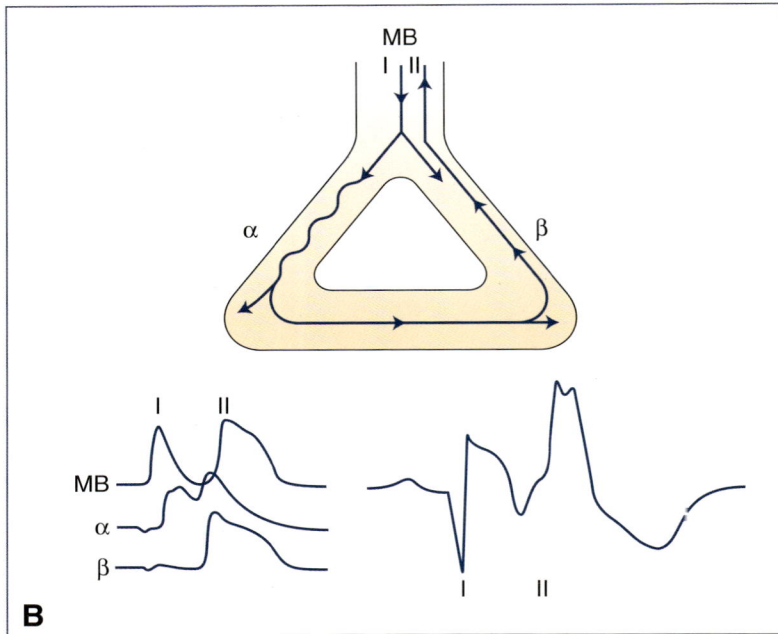

Figure 7-8. *(Continued)* **B,** This panel shows the initiation of reentry when a premature beat or change in cycle length results in conduction block in the β-pathway only. Conduction through the α-pathway occurs entering the β-pathway in the retrograde (known as *antidromic*) direction. Slow conduction in the α-pathway, indicated by the sinuous portion of the arrow, allows time for the initial region of conduction block in the β-pathway to recover, and the wavefront propagates in the antidromic direction through the area of initial block, producing the reentry beat. If the wavefront continues circulating through the circuit, a tachycardia occurs [5]. MB—myocardial bridge.

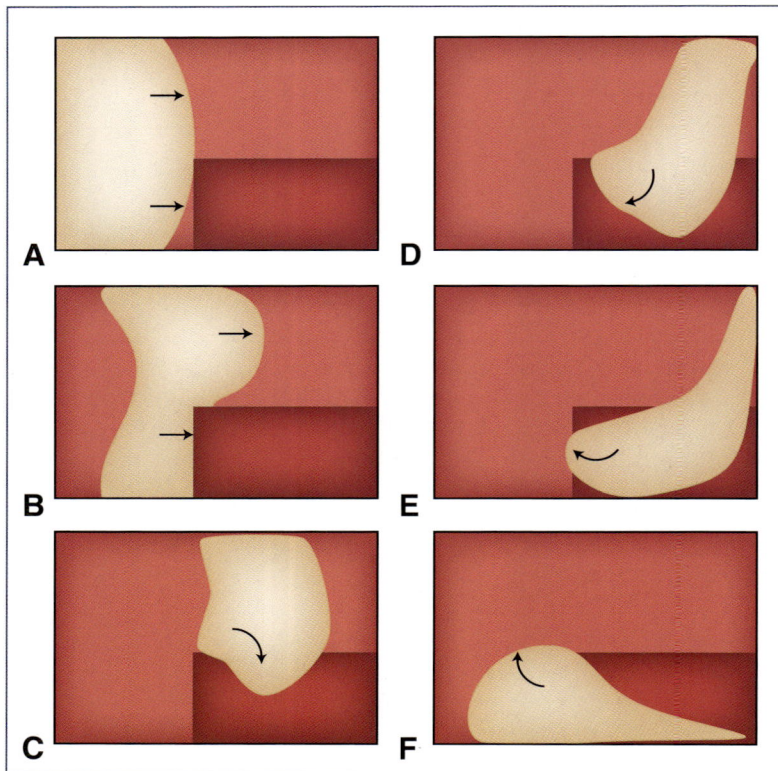

Figure 7-9. Initiation of spiral wave reentry. The schematic represents a region of myocardium with a segment (*darker red*) in the lower right portion that has a longer recovery time than the adjacent tissue. **A,** An excitation wave propagating from left to right initially blocks (**B**) at the region of longer refractoriness. **C,** The wavefront propagates along the border of the refractory tissue until it reaches a region that has recovered and propagates inferiorly into the region. **D, E,** and **F,** The wavefront continues through the longer refractory period region from left to right, reentering the normal region and continuing its propagation along the same path. Thus, a curved wavefront is established that continuously propagates around a point of singularity at its core. Spiral wave reentry can be elicited in normal or abnormal myocardium and can wander through the tissue causing polymorphic ventricular tachycardia or break into multiple wavelets causing ventricular fibrillation [4].

Antiarrhythmic Drugs

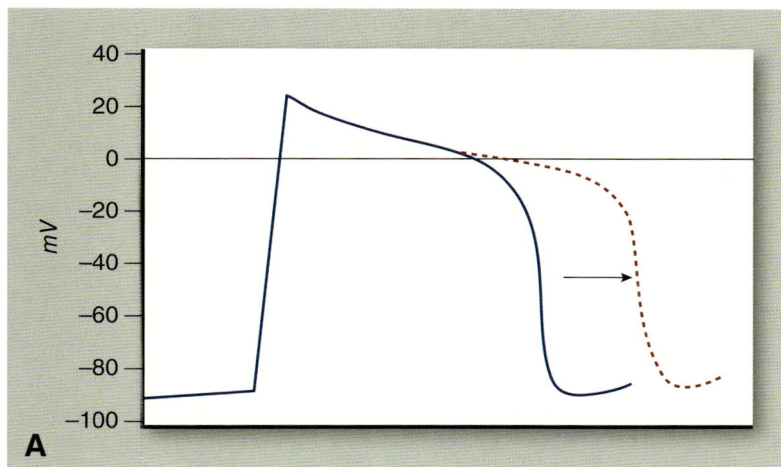

A

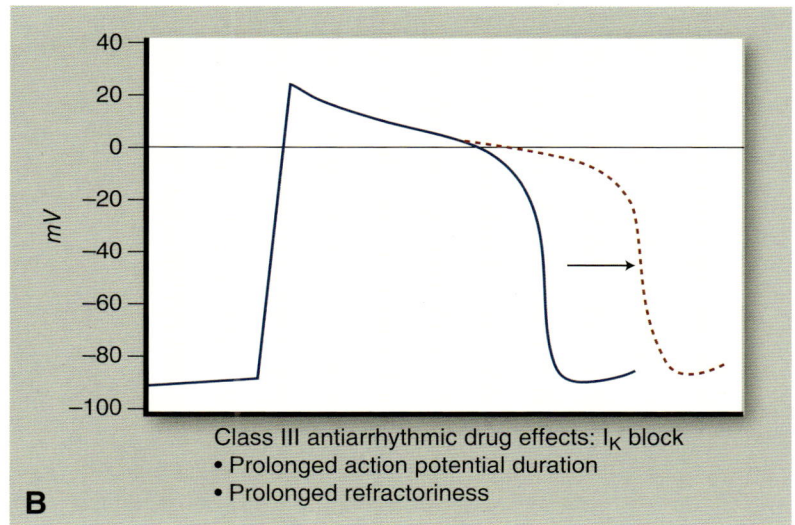

Class III antiarrhythmic drug effects: I$_K$ block
• Prolonged action potential duration
• Prolonged refractoriness

B

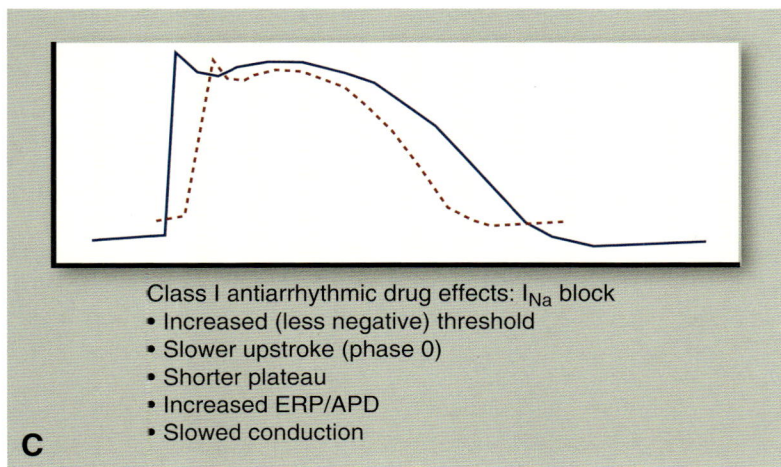

Class I antiarrhythmic drug effects: I$_{Na}$ block
• Increased (less negative) threshold
• Slower upstroke (phase 0)
• Shorter plateau
• Increased ERP/APD
• Slowed conduction

C

Figure 7-10. Effects of Class III and Class I antiarrhythmic drugs on Purkinje fibers. **A** and **B**, Class III drug effects are due to block of the delayed rectifier outward potassium (I$_K$) currents, most specifically block I$_{Kr}$, the rapidly activating component of the delayed rectifier current, prolonging action potential duration and refractoriness. The diagrams represent a normal action potential of a Purkinje cell (*solid line*) and the effects of D-sotalol (*dotted line*) on the action potential duration. **C**, Class I antiarrhythmic drug effect due to block of the rapid inward sodium (I$_{Na}$) current. Slowing of phase 0, the upstroke of the action potential, slows conduction velocity and failure of conduction may occur.

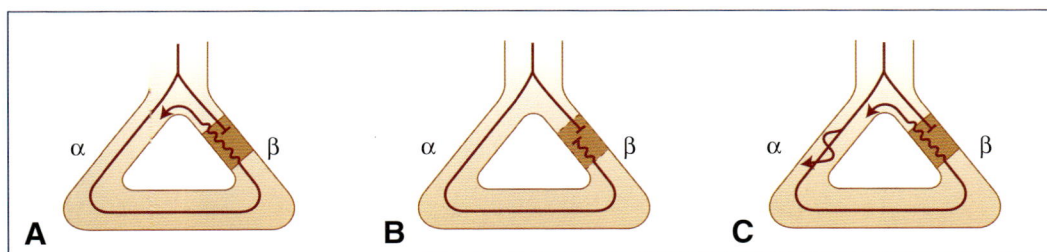

A **B** **C**

Figure 7-11. Potential effects of antiarrhythmic drugs on reentrant arrhythmias. **A**, Initiation of reentry following unidirectional block and slow conduction in the β-pathway. The *shaded area* represents tissue with prolonged refractoriness in which conduction block occurs. Antiarrhythmic drugs can eliminate reentry tachyarrhythmias by further prolonging refractoriness or suppressing conduction so that the wavefront blocks in the circuit (**B**). If the drug slows conduction without causing block it may facilitate reentry causing a slower or different tachycardia, which may be more frequent or difficult to control (**C**). This effect is known as "proarrhythmia." Antiarrhythmic drugs can also reduce the frequency of arrhythmias by suppressing automaticity and premature beats that initiate reentry.

Sinus Node Disorders

Figure 7-12. Sinus node dysfunction. Sinus node dysfunction can be manifest as sinus bradycardia (defined as sinus rhythm < 60 beats per minute [BPM]) or sinus pauses. Simultaneous leads V5 (*top*) and V1 (*bottom*) of a Holter recording from an 85-year-old woman with a history of syncope. Sinus bradycardia (38 BPM) is followed by sinus arrest (4.2-sec pause) with a junctional escape rhythm. Sinus bradycardia and pauses can be normal during sleep or in people with high vagal tone, such as trained athletes. Sinus bradycardia is clinically significant only if it results in failure to meet the patient's metabolic demands, in which case it may cause signs and symptoms due to hypotension or congestive heart failure. Symptoms include fatigue, dyspnea, exercise intolerance, angina, lightheadedness, or syncope. Aging and all cardiac disease can be associated with sinus node dysfunction. It is also important to exclude hypothyroidism and hyperkalemia. β-Adrenergic blockers, calcium channel blockers, and many antiarrhythmic drugs aggravate sinus node dysfunction, but cannot always be withdrawn. Implantation of a dual chamber (atrial and ventricular) or, when atrioventricular conduction is well preserved, a single chamber atrial pacemaker is effective treatment for symptomatic sinus node dysfunction that is not due to a correctable cause. (*Adapted from* Evans [6].)

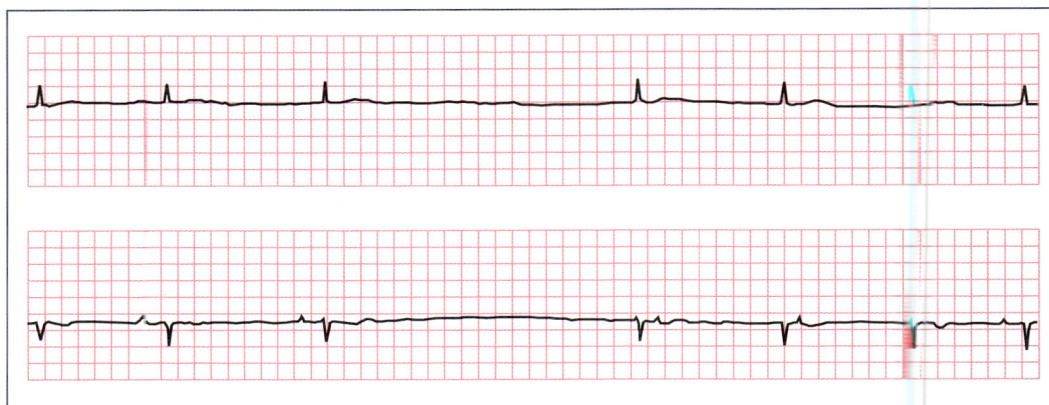

Supraventricular Tachycardias

Figure 7-13. Electrocardiographic (ECG) patterns of regular supraventricular tachycardias that have a one-to-one relation between QRS and P-wave. The most important clue to the likely mechanism of a narrow complex tachycardia is the relationship of the P-wave to the QRS complex. No visible P-wave often means that the P-wave is buried in the QRS complex. This is usually due to typical atrioventricular (AV) nodal reentry, which often has a portion of the P-waves visible at the beginning or end of the QRS complex, giving a QRS pattern in leads II, III, or aVF, or rSR' pattern in V_1. With a simultaneous P-wave and QRS AV reentry, using an accessory pathway is excluded, but atrial tachycardia with a long PR interval is still possible. When the P-wave follows the QRS and is located closer to the previous QRS complex than the following QRS, it is identified as a short-RP tachycardia (RP < PR). This is often seen with AV reentry due to an accessory pathway with the P-wave due to retrograde atrial activation from conduction over the accessory pathway. Atypical AV nodal reentry and atrial tachycardia are also possible. Finally, the P-wave may also be far from the previous QRS complex, and is identified as a long-RP tachycardia. Atrial tachycardia is the most likely cause, but atypical AV nodal reentry and AV reentry using an accessory pathway with a long conduction time from ventricle to atrium are also possible. Analysis of P-wave morphology and other features may allow distinction among these possibilities [7]. AT—atrial tachycardia, AVNRT—atrioventricular nodal reentry tachycardia.

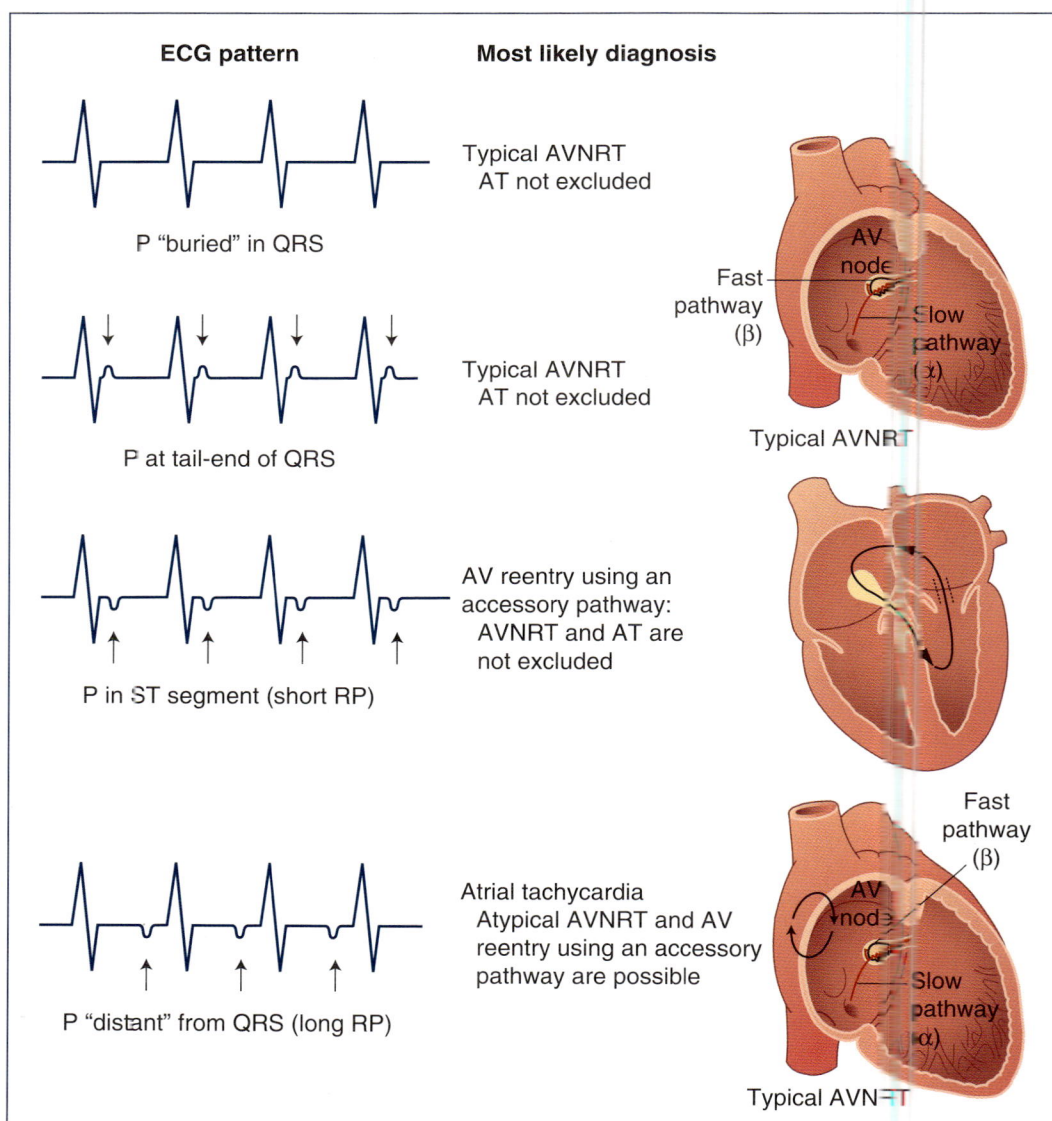

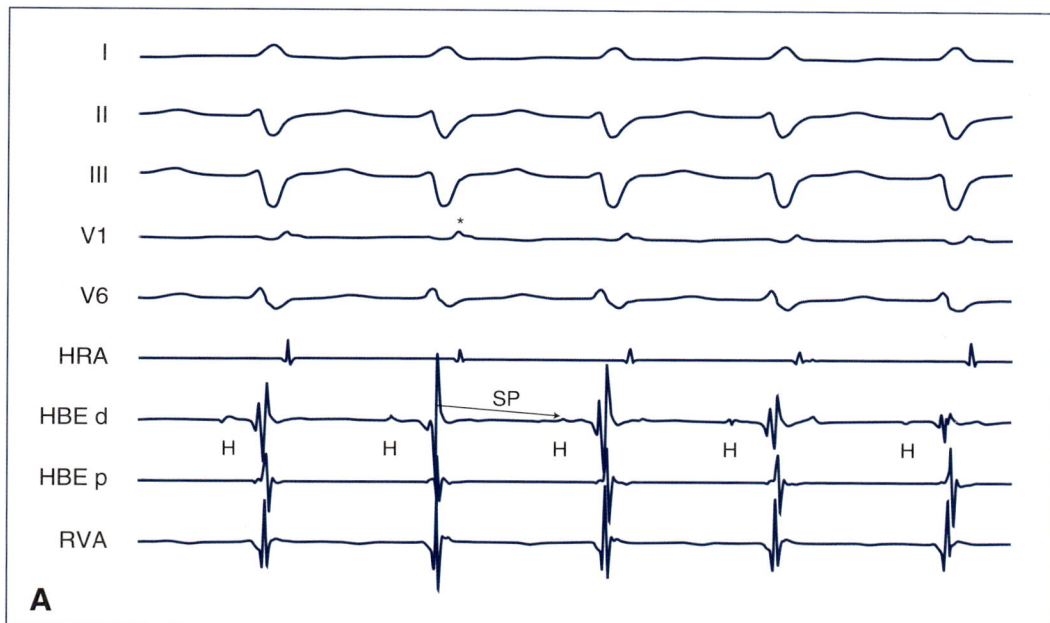

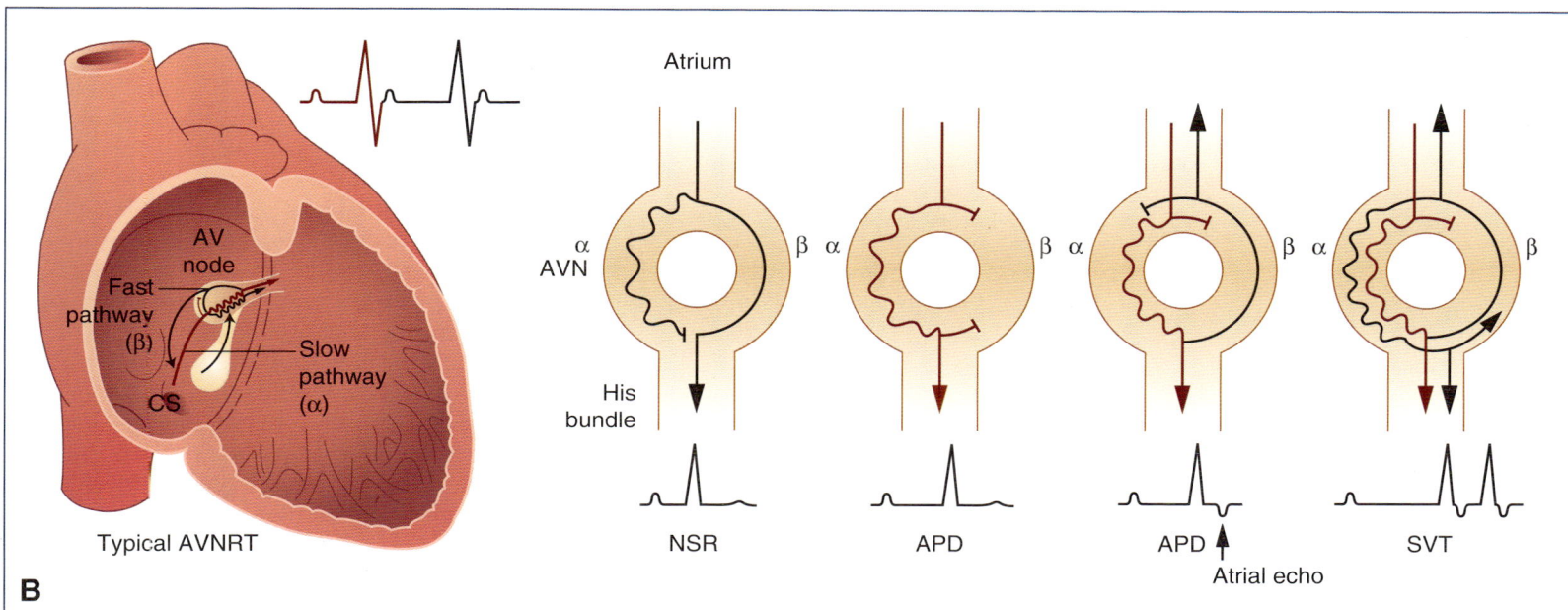

Figure 7-14. Atrioventricular nodal reentry tachycardia (AVNRT) is the most common paroxysmal supraventricular tachycardias (SVT) in adults. **A,** Surface leads and intracardiac recordings from SVT due to atrioventricular nodal reentry. Intracardiac electrograms are recorded from catheters placed in the high right atrium (HRA), the His bundle (HBE d = distal electrode pair, HBE p = proximal electrode pair), and right ventricular apex (RVA). Note the narrow complex QRS morphology with 1:1 ventricular-to-atrial relationship. Note that in the surface electrocardiogram, the P-wave is buried at the end of the QRS complex. In the His bundle recordings, the atrial electrogram is not visible because it is inscribed during the larger ventricular electrogram. The timing of atrial activation can be seen in the HRA recording, where the electrogram occurs at the end of the QRS. *Arrow* indicates the conduction time over the slow AV nodal pathway (SP).

B, The mechanism of the common form of AVNRT. A lobe of the AV node extends inferiorly along the tricuspid annulus, anterior to the coronary sinus os, which functions as a slowly conducting pathway. During AVNRT-conduction occurs from inferior to superior through the slow pathway, then through the compact portion of the AV node to the His bundle

and retrograde through this superior portion of the AV node to the atrium. The path from the compact AV node back down to the slow pathway may involve musculature around the coronary sinus, within the atrium, or may be largely confined to the AV node. Initiation of AV nodal reentry is shown in schematics on the *right* in which α is the slow AV nodal pathway and β is the fast pathway. During normal sinus rhythm (NSR), an impulse from the atrium enters the AV node and travels down both the slow and fast pathways with the impulse from the fast pathway reaching the His bundle first and activating the ventricles with a short PR interval. Collision of fast pathway and slow pathway impulses in the distal portion of the AV node prevents reentry. An atrial premature depolarization (APD) that blocks in the fast pathway (β) allows conduction of the impulse down the slow pathway to the ventricles, thus a longer PR interval. If this impulse blocks in the distal fast pathway, no reentry occurs. However, an APD can produce an atrial echo beat if the fast pathway has recovered allowing the impulse to continue retrogradely in the fast pathway back to the atrium. If the slow pathway has recovered to allow conduction, the impulse may continue circulating as supraventricular tachycardia (SVT).

Continued on the next page

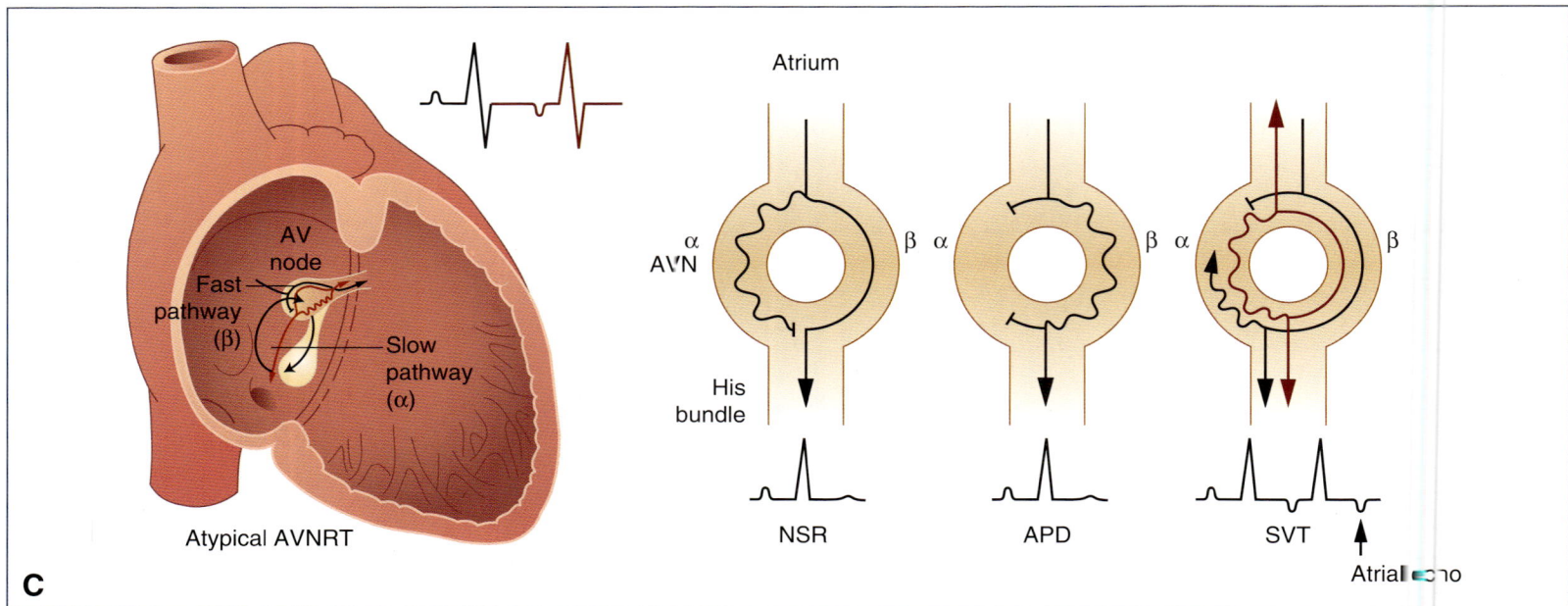

C Atypical AVNRT

Atrium

α AVN β   α β   α β

His bundle

NSR   APD   SVT

Atrial echo

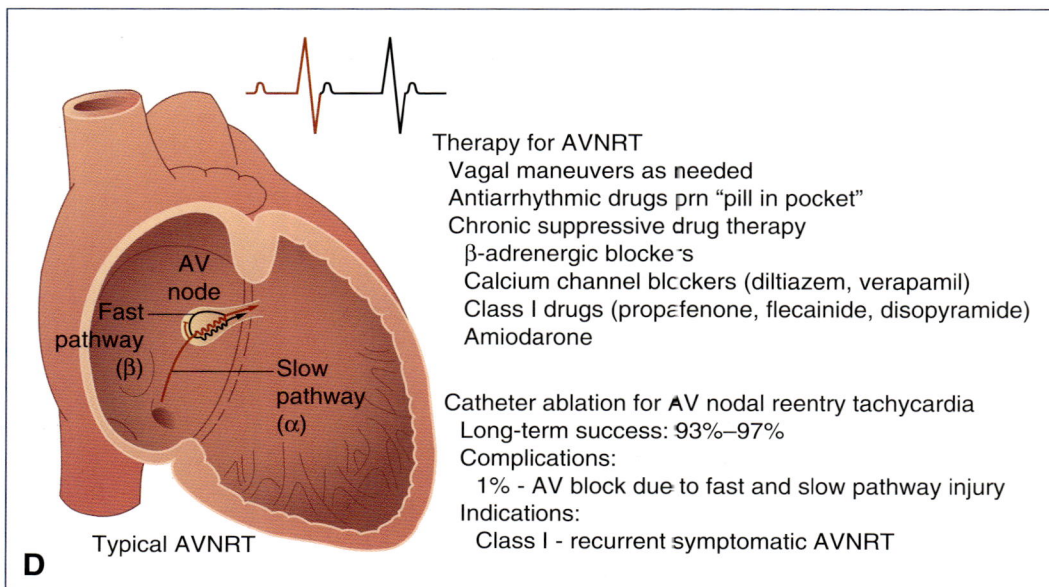

D Typical AVNRT

Therapy for AVNRT
  Vagal maneuvers as needed
  Antiarrhythmic drugs prn "pill in pocket"
  Chronic suppressive drug therapy
    β-adrenergic blockers
    Calcium channel blockers (diltiazem, verapamil)
    Class I drugs (propafenone, flecainide, disopyramide)
    Amiodarone

Catheter ablation for AV nodal reentry tachycardia
  Long-term success: 93%–97%
  Complications:
    1% - AV block due to fast and slow pathway injury
  Indications:
    Class I - recurrent symptomatic AVNRT

Figure 7-14. *(Continued)* **C** demonstrates that when the circuit is reversed, as during typical AV node reentry, antegrade conduction occurs over the fast pathway and retrograde conduction over the slow pathway. In typical AV node reentry, an APD is conducted over the fast pathway. The PR interval remains short. If there is retrograde activation over the slow pathway to the atrium, then SVT may be initiated. The QRS complex remains narrow because activation of the ventricle is still via the normal HPS. Retrograde atrial activation over the slow pathway takes longer compared with conduction over the fast pathway, resulting in a long-RP interval. **D**, Therapeutic options for AVNRT [7]. In more than 96% of patients, the slow pathway can be ablated in this location between the coronary sinus and the tricuspid valve annulus without injury to the fast AV nodal pathway.

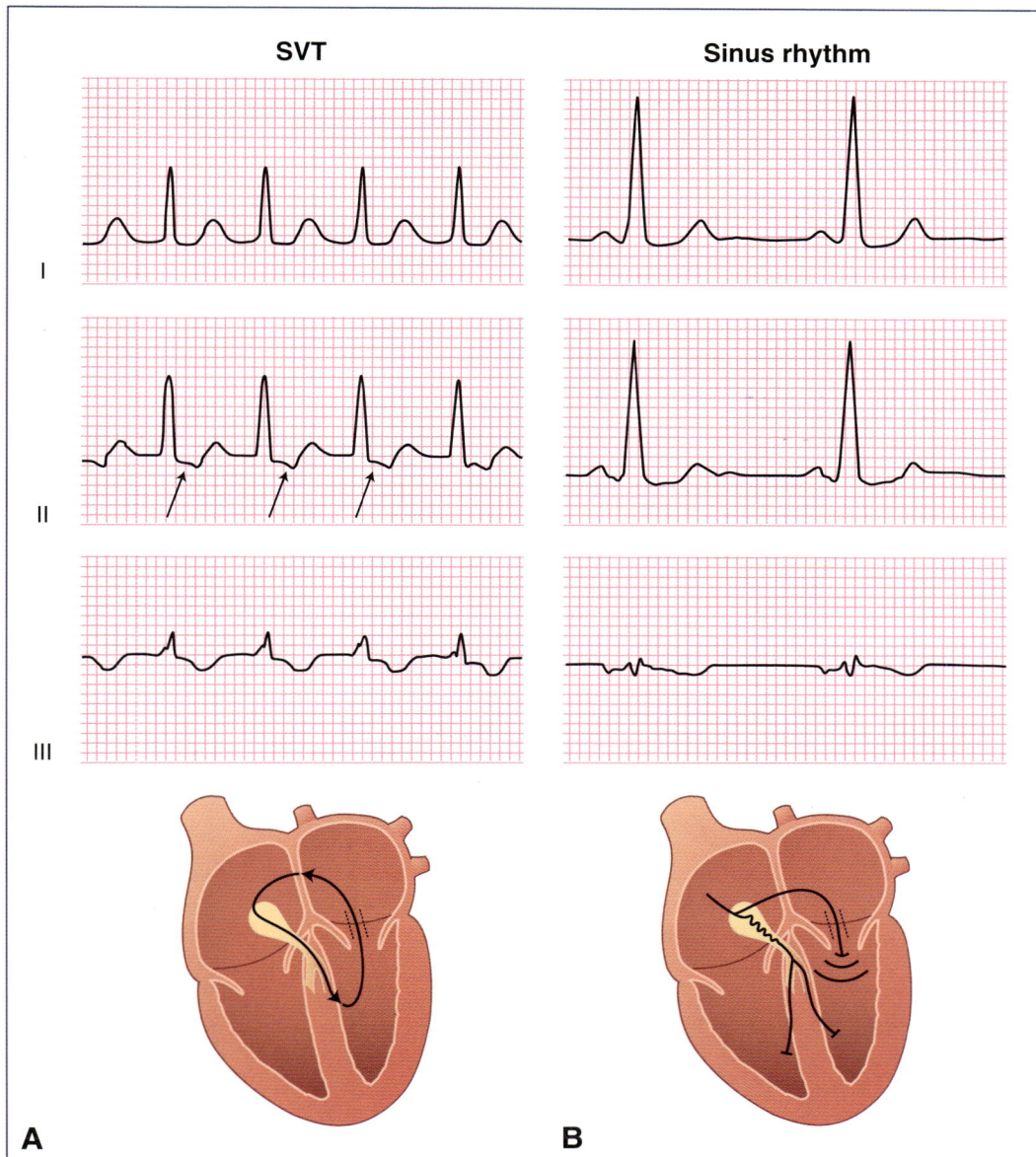

Figure 7-15. Atrioventricular (AV) reentry due to an accessory pathway. Three lead electrocardiograms (ECGs) during supraventricular tachycardia (SVT) (**A**) and following restoration of sinus rhythm (**B**) by administration of intravenous adenosine. **A,** During tachycardia, a narrow QRS indicates activation of the ventricles from the His-Purkinje system. The timing of P-waves, seen as notches deforming the ST-segment (*arrows*) indicate a short R-P tachycardia. The mechanism of tachycardia is shown at the *bottom* of the figure. The reentry circuit involves conduction over the AV node and retrograde to the atrium over an accessory pathway. **B,** Sinus rhythm is now present. The sinus impulse conduction over the AV node to the ventricles and also from atrium to ventricle over the accessory pathway. Thus, ventricular beats are fused between these two wavefronts. Conduction over the accessory pathway occurs without delay and activates a portion of the ventricles before conduction over the His-Purkinje system, causing the short PR interval and slurred upstroke (delta wave) and widening of the QRS complex.

Continued on the next page

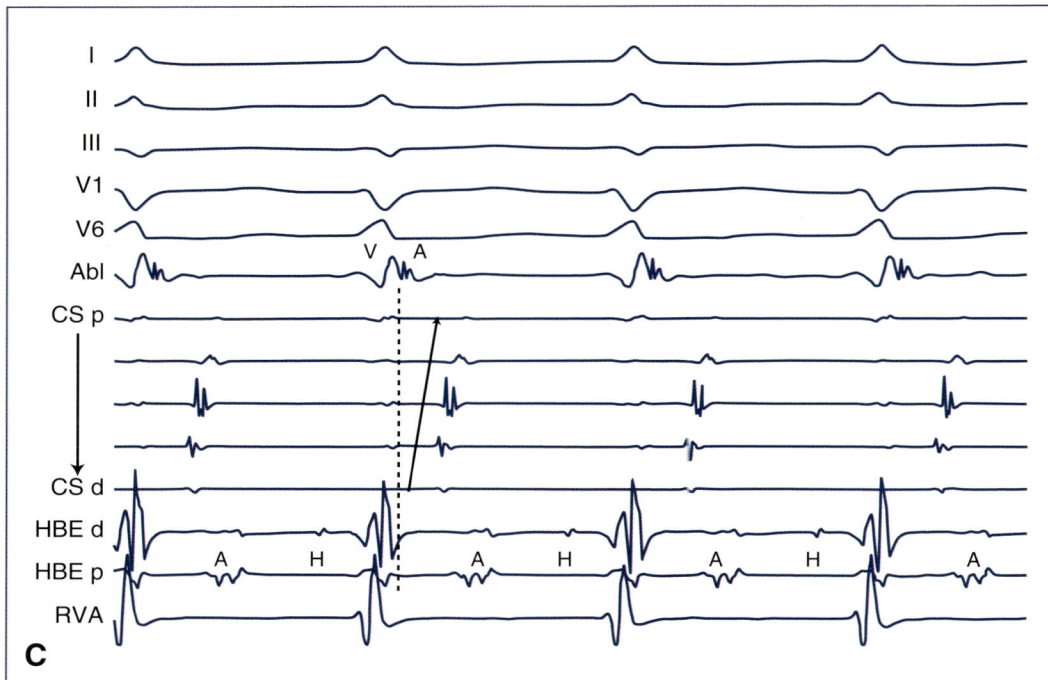

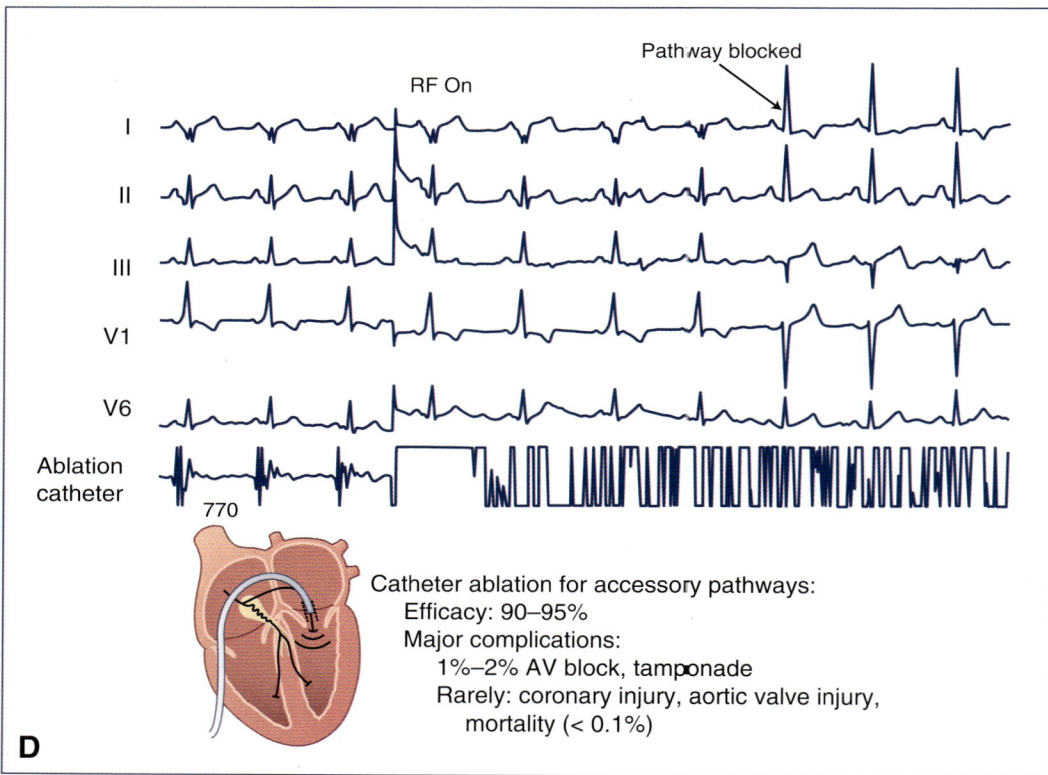

Figure 7-15. *(Continued)* **C,** Intracardiac tracings recorded during AV reentry tachycardia that uses a left lateral accessory pathway. Intracardiac electrograms are recorded from catheters placed at the lateral mitral annulus (Abl), in the coronary sinus, at the His bundle (HBE), and right ventricular apex (RVA). Note the narrow complex QRS morphology with 1:1 ventricular to atrial relationship. Activation proceeds from the atrium (A) down the AV node, through the His bundle (H), to the ventricle (V). Earliest retrograde activation of the atrium occurs at the ablation catheter (Abl) with the distal coronary sinus (CS d) activated before the proximal coronary sinus (CS p). The latest atrial activation occurs at the His bundle. This is consistent with orthodromic AV reentrant tachycardia due to a left lateral accessory pathway.

Ablation at this site terminated tachycardia and resulted in abolition of the accessory pathway. **D,** The effect of catheter ablation of an accessory pathway on the ECG in a patient with the Wolff-Parkinson-White syndrome. Sinus rhythm with a cycle length of 770 ms is present. Preexcitation is evident from the wide-slurred QRS complexes and short PR interval. The ablation catheter is positioned at the accessory pathway on the mitral annulus. Radiofrequency (RF) energy is applied starting after the third beat. After four beats, an abrupt change in the QRS occurs, with narrowing of the QRS complex and prolongation of the PR interval, indicating block in conduction over the accessory pathway. Catheter ablation for accessory pathways is summarized at the *bottom* of the figure [7].

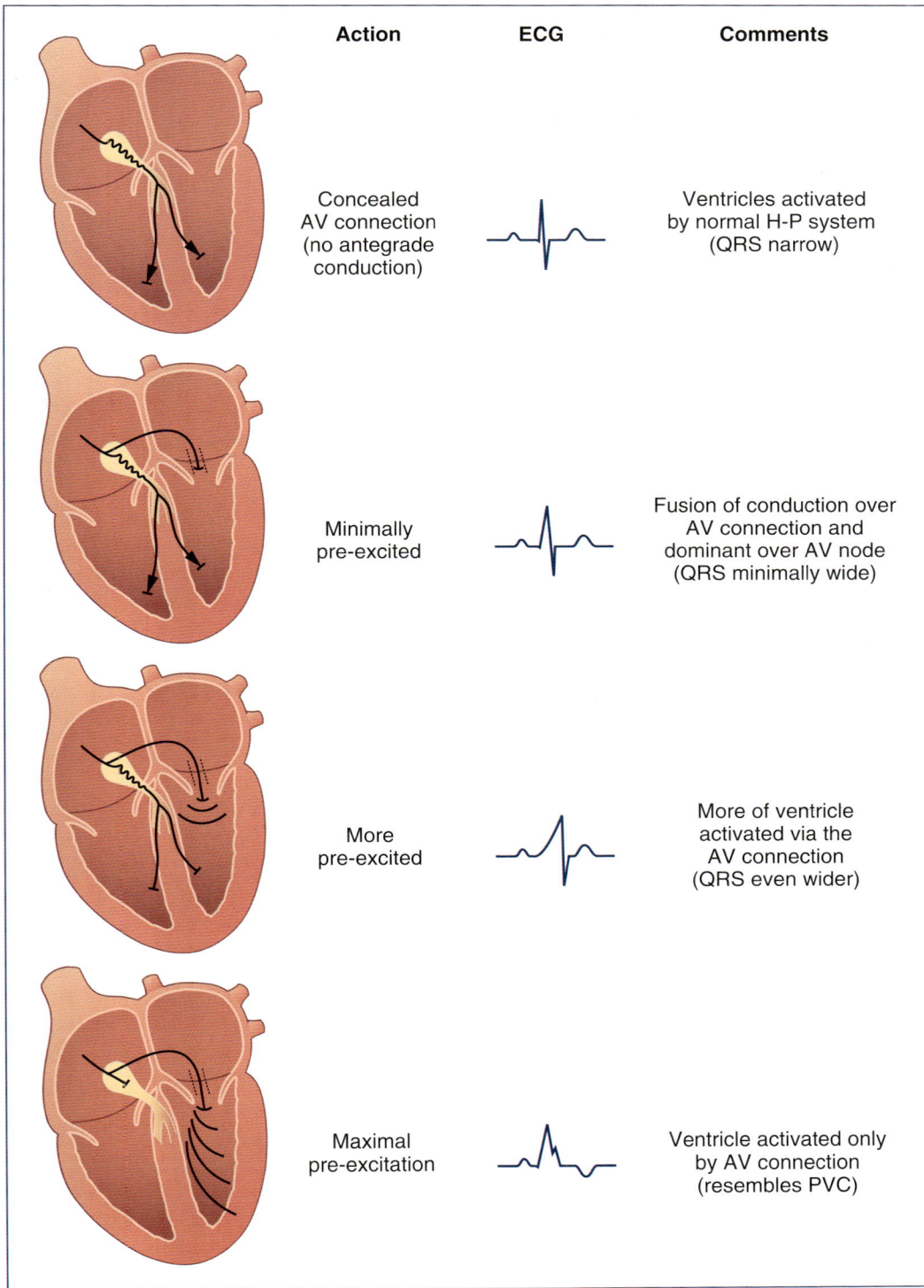

Action	ECG	Comments
Concealed AV connection (no antegrade conduction)		Ventricles activated by normal H-P system (QRS narrow)
Minimally pre-excited		Fusion of conduction over AV connection and dominant over AV node (QRS minimally wide)
More pre-excited		More of ventricle activated via the AV connection (QRS even wider)
Maximal pre-excitation		Ventricle activated only by AV connection (resembles PVC)

Figure 7-16. Conduction over an accessory pathway during sinus rhythm causing QRS fusion compared with absence of an accessory (*top*). The morphology of a QRS complex in patients with an accessory pathway (AP) is an excellent example of fusion between the wavefront conducting over the atrioventricular (AV) node and the wavefront that conducts over the pathway. Conduction over an AP is influenced by drugs, sympathetic states, and its location along the AV annulus. If there is no anterograde conduction over the AP (which is common), the AP may still conduct in the retrograde direction and cause supraventricular tachycardia, but is considered concealed, because it is not apparent on the electrocardiogram (ECG). When conduction over the AP is minimal and AV node conduction predominates, the QRS is created by fusion of conduction over the AV node—His-Purkinje (H-P) system and the AP. When conduction to the ventricle over the AP predominates, a larger portion of the ventricle is activated by the AP, such that the QRS is even wider. If ventricular activation is only over the AP, as with maximally preexcited tachycardias, it is difficult to distinguish the complex from ventricular tachycardia. PVC—premature ventricular complex.

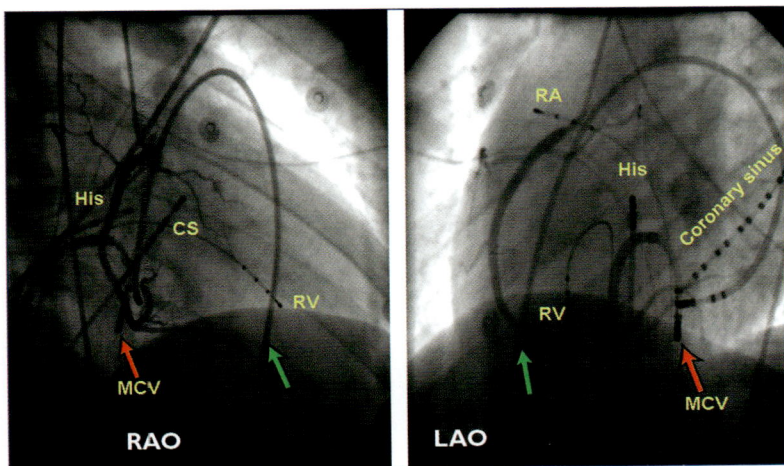

Figure 7-17. Right anterior oblique (RAO) (*left*) and left anterior oblique (LAO) (*right*) images during right coronary angiography showing catheter positions during mapping of an unusual accessory pathway that was located in the fat in the posteroseptal region of the heart. Four electrode catheters that enter the heart from the inferior vena cava are positioned at the His-bundle region (His), high right atrium (RA), and right ventricle (RV), and in the middle cardiac vein near the os of the coronary sinus (MCV) (*red arrow*). A catheter has been inserted into the pericardial space (*green arrow*) via a subxiphoid percutaneous approach for epicardial mapping. The right coronary artery is located 3 to 4 mm above the catheter in the middle cardiac vein where the accessory pathway was located. Posteroseptal accessory pathways can be difficult to locate and ablate. Epicardial mapping is rarely required. These pathways can be located in close proximity to the continuation of the right coronary artery in the atrioventricular groove, necessitating precautions to avoid coronary arterial injury.

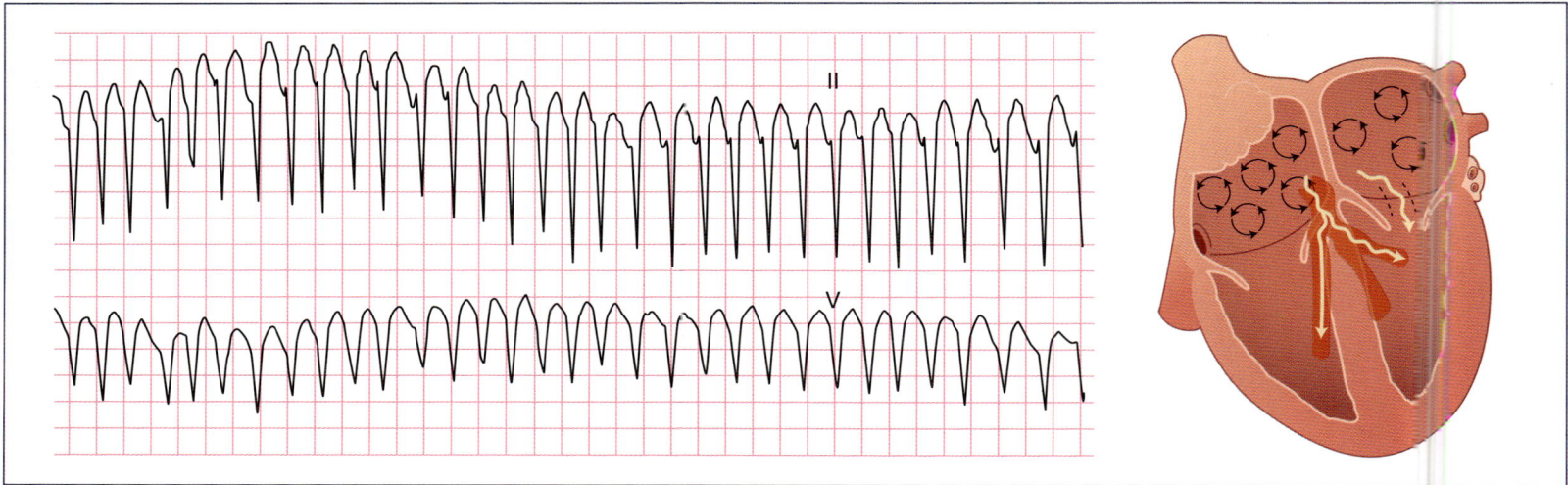

Figure 7-18. Atrial fibrillation in the Wolff-Parkinson-White syndrome (WPW). Two leads of an electrocardiogram are shown. A rapid irregular wide complex rhythm is present. The mechanism is shown at *right*. Atrial fibrillation is present with conduction of impulses predominantly over an accessory pathway. Approximately 25% of accessory pathways are capable of dangerously rapid conduction that can lead to hemodynamic collapse and ventricular fibrillation, which is the mechanism of rare sudden deaths that occur in patients with WPW. Urgent cardioversion is often needed. Intravenous administration of procainamide or ibutilide will slow the ventricular rate. Administration of calcium channel blockers, digoxin, or β-adrenergic blockers or adenosine alone will not slow conduction over the accessory pathway and may precipitate cardiac arrest. Catheter ablation is indicated [7].

Figure 7-19. Mechanisms of atrial tachycardia. Atrial tachycardias may originate from a small focus of either reentry or automaticity [8], or may be due to a large macroreentrant circuit [7,9]. As atrial tachycardia is not dependent on the atrio-ventricular (AV) node or ventricular myocardium for maintenance, the presence of AV block strongly suggests atrial tachycardia, although AV nodal reentry is not absolutely excluded. Focal atrial tachycardia originates from a point source with centrifugal activation away from this source. Macroreentrant atrial tachycardias, sometimes referred to as atrial flutter, have a defined reentry circuit around a fixed obstacle

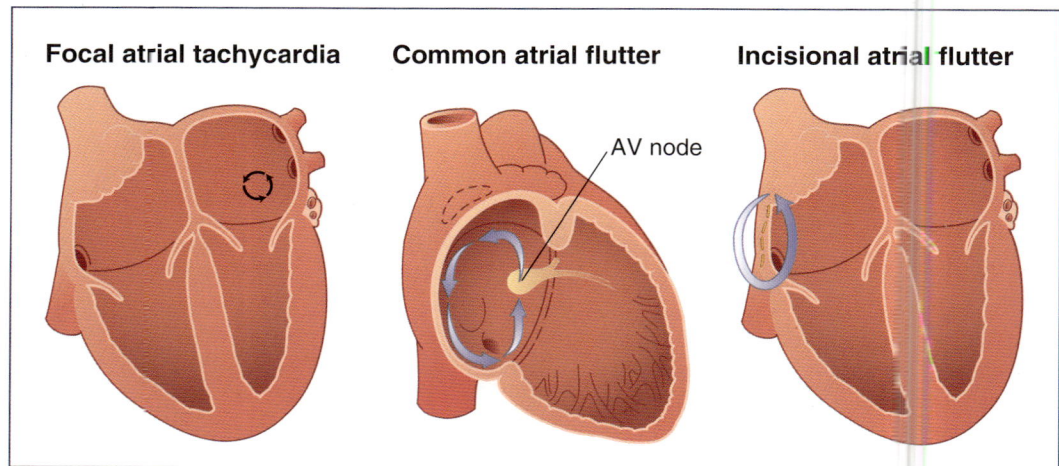

Focal atrial tachycardia   **Common atrial flutter**   **Incisional atrial flutter**

AV node

or area of conduction block, such as a valve annulus or an area of scar. Areas of scar can be idiopathic, but are most commonly incisions from prior cardiac surgery or catheter ablation lesions, often from ablation of atrial fibrillation. Repair of congenital heart disease and mitral valve surgery are common causes. The most common macroreentrant atrial tachycardia is typical atrial flutter, in which a wavefront rotates around the tricuspid annulus in either a counterclockwise (as viewed from the left anterior oblique perspective) or counterclockwise direction. Common atrial flutter is dependent on conduction through an isthmus between the tricuspid annulus and the inferior vena cava, and are also referred to as "isthmus-dependent." Catheter ablation of this isthmus interrupts the circuit and is curative in more than 90% of patients [7]. The mechanism of atrial tachycardia usually can be determined from the 12-lead electrocardiogram. Continuous undulation without an isoelectric interval suggests macroreentry, whereas a discrete P-wave with an intervening isoelectric interval suggests focal atrial tachycardia.

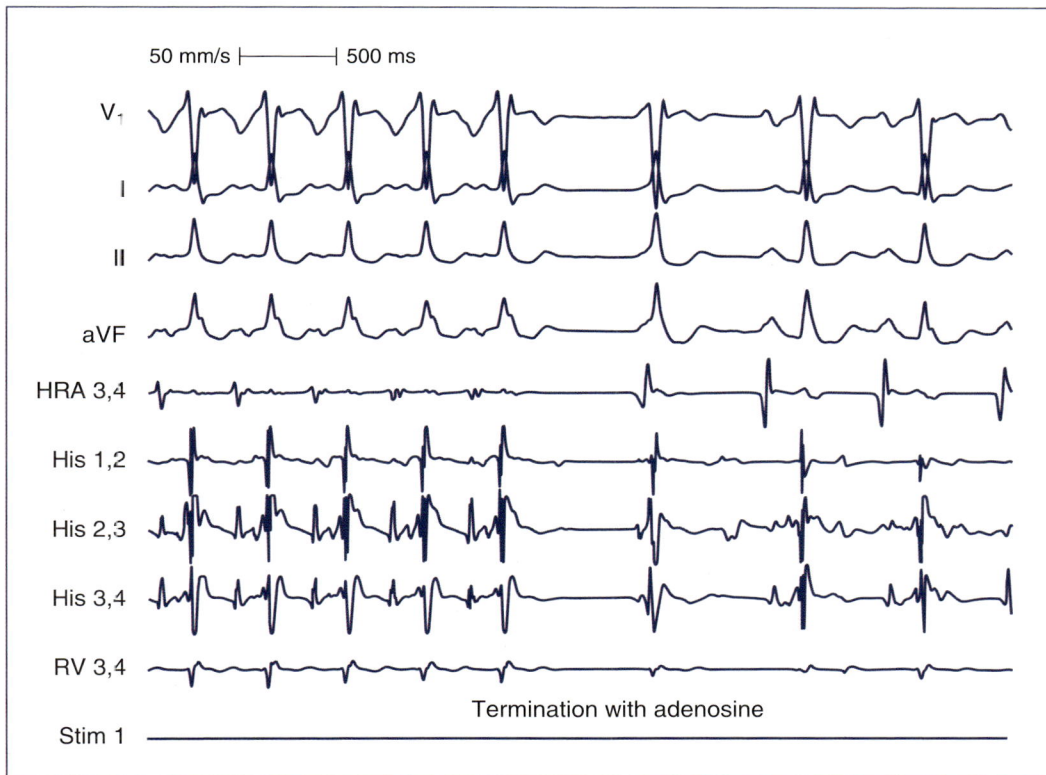

Figure 7-20. Atrial tachycardia. The surface electrocardiogram leads show regular tachycardia at 130 beats per minute with P-waves preceding the QRS (long R-P tachycardia). Examination of the intracardiac tracings confirms a one-to-one ventricular relationship, with atrial activity seen well in the right atrium (HRA 3,4). A large His bundle deflection is present in the His bundle recordings (His 1,2–His 3,4). The tracing was obtained during administration of intravenous adenosine. After five beats, tachycardia terminates, followed by a junctional beat, and then sinus rhythm. Although adenosine effects the atrioventricular (AV) node and is widely appreciated to terminate AV nodal dependent arrhythmias, it also terminates arrhythmias that are dependent on cyclic adenosine monophosphate–mediated triggered activity. Adenosine often terminates focal atrial tachycardias, suggesting that this mechanism is operative. Adenosine does not terminate macroreentrant atrial tachycardias, but does increase the degree of AV block, facilitating observation of the P-wave [10].

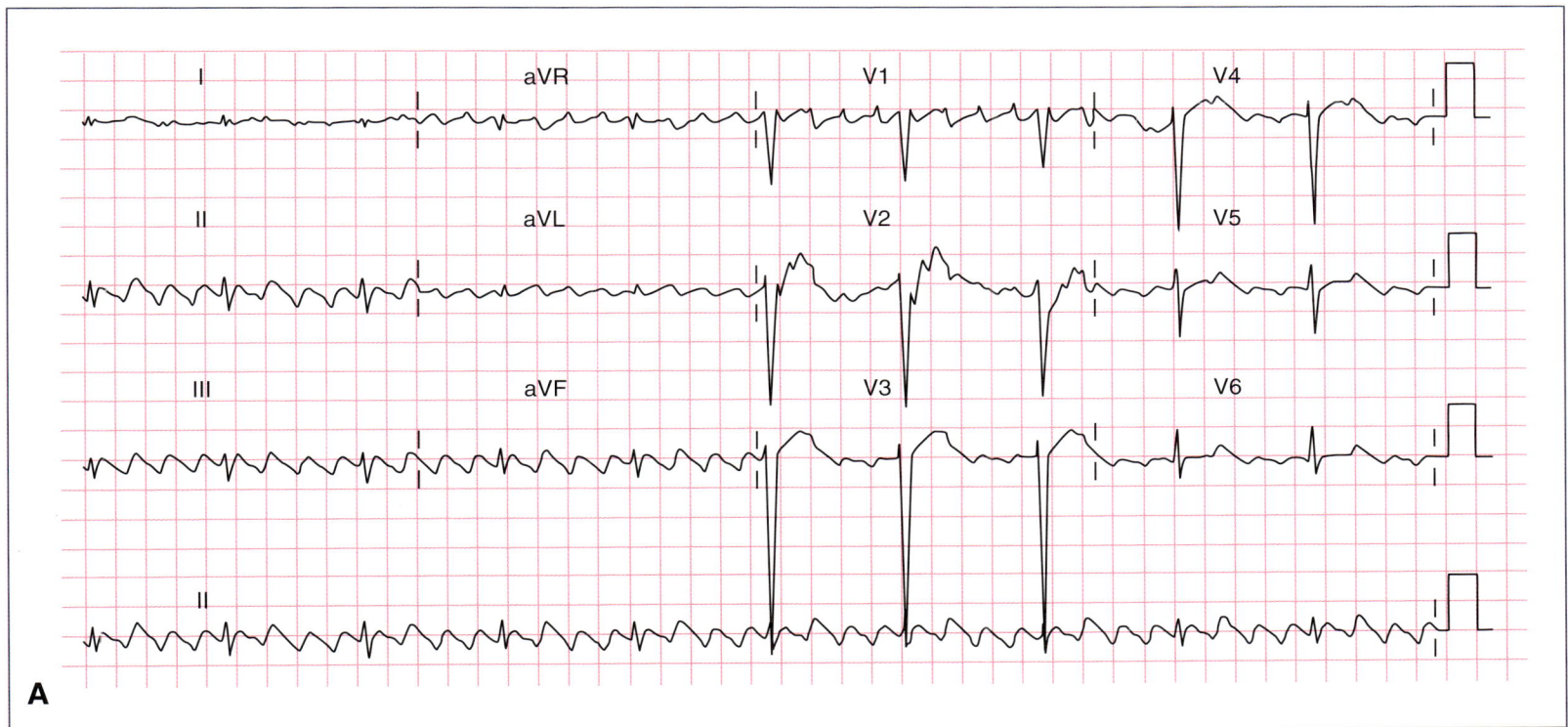

Figure 7-21. Macroreentrant atrial tachycardias. **A,** 12-Lead electrocardiogram (ECG) of common counterclockwise atrial flutter. Note the typical sawtooth P-waves in leads II, III, and aVF. **B,** 12-Lead ECG of atrial tachycardia late after repair of an atrial septal defect. The atrial rate is relatively rapid and P-waves have some variability that suggests coarse atrial fibrillation. Despite these findings, the tachycardia was found to be due to a macroreentrant circuit in the lateral right atrial free wall and was successfully ablated. **C** and **D,** Findings from macroreentrant atrial tachycardia late after mitral valve repair and atrial maze surgery. **C** shows the 12-lead ECG. The P-waves are low amplitude in the limb leads, but a prominent biphasic P-wave is evident in lead V1 (*arrows*) where an atrial rate of 200/min is evident with 2:1 conduction to the ventricles. A single premature ventricular contraction is present after the ninth QRS. Although the P-wave morphology is unusual, this arrhythmia was found to be dependent on conduction through the right atrial subeustachian isthmus, consistent with common counterclockwise atrial flutter.

Continued on the next page

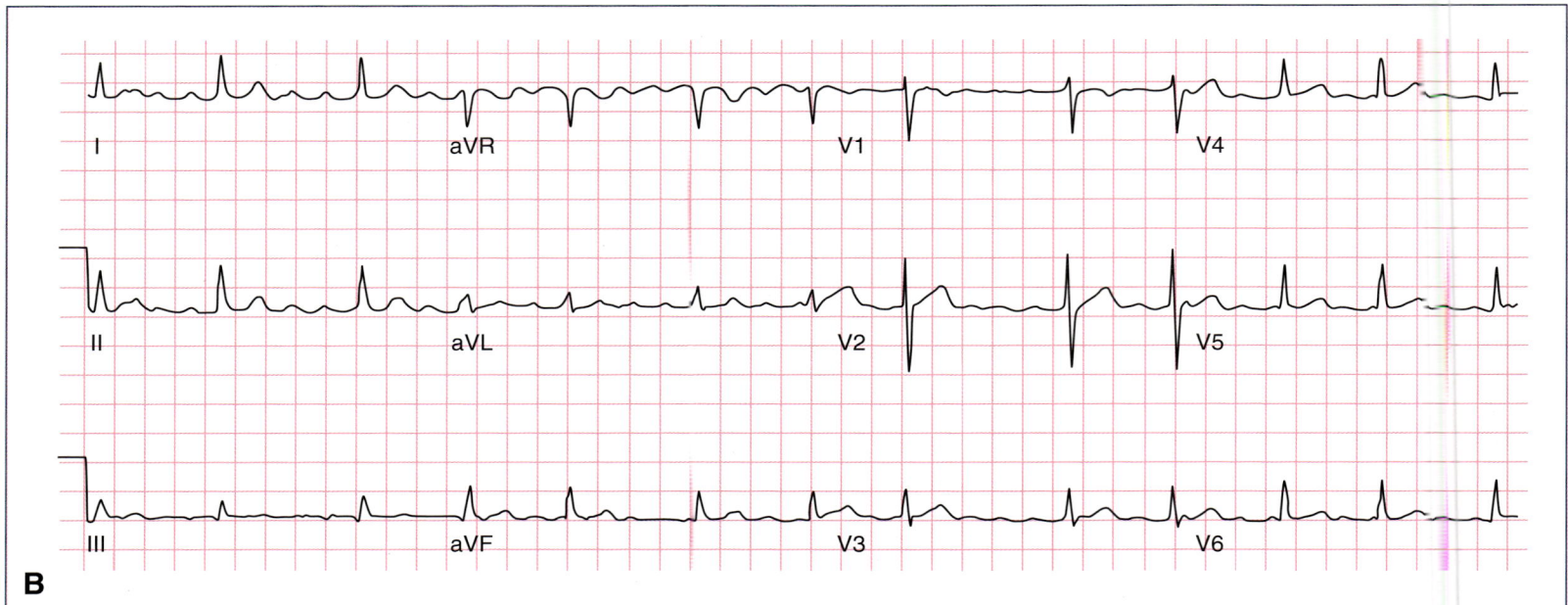

B

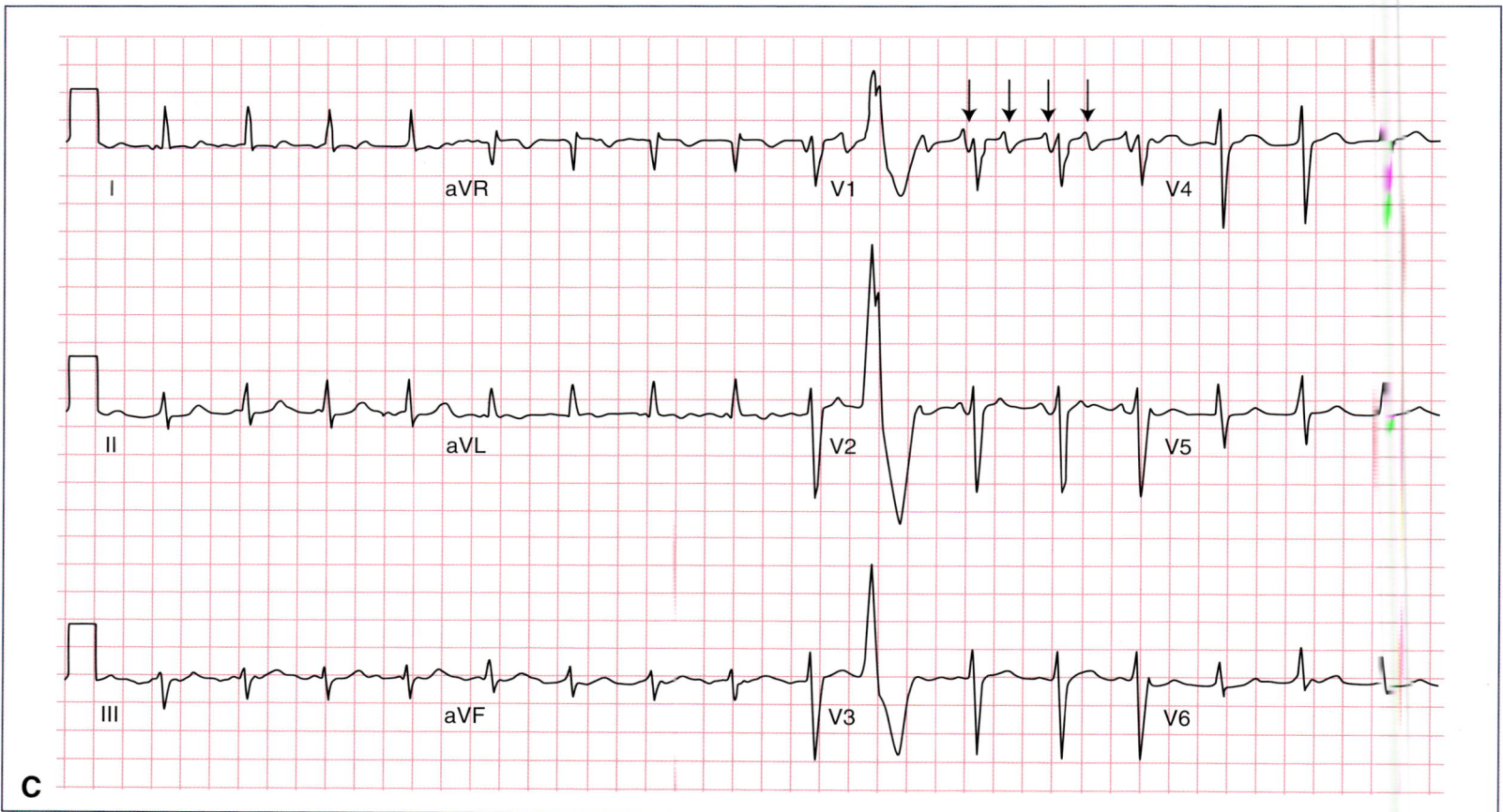

C

Figure 7-21. (*Continued*) Intracardiac tracings from this tachycardia are shown (**D**) during radiofrequency (RF) ablation. From the top are surface ECG leads I, II, III, V1, and V5, followed by intracardiac electrograms from a 20-electrode catheter positioned with its tip (electrodes 1–2) in the coronary sinus, and proximal electrodes along the lateral right atrium as indicated in a left anterior oblique radiograph. Tachycardia is present and activation precedes down the lateral atrial wall, through the isthmus between the tricuspid annulus and inferior vena cava. RF ablation terminates the arrhythmia (*arrows*). RF ablation is applied near electrode 9–10, between the tricuspid valve and inferior vena cava and terminates atrial flutter with block prior to electrodes 9–10. Following extensive atrial surgery or ablation for atrial fibrillation, the P-wave morphology of common flutter can be misleading due to the reduced contribution of left atrial signal to the P-wave and regions of conduction block in the atria [11].

Continued on the next page

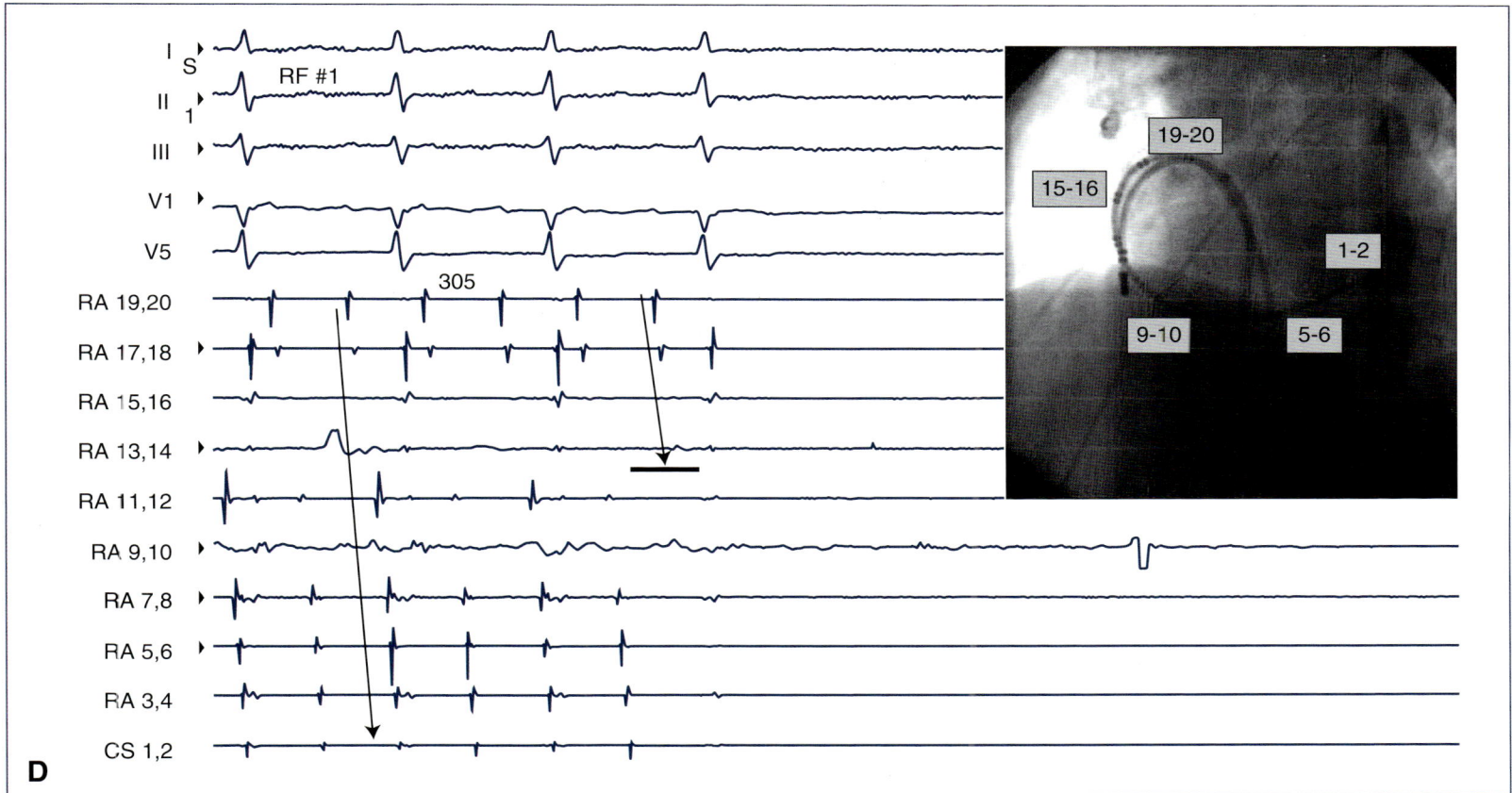

Figure 7-21. (Continued)

Atrial Fibrillation

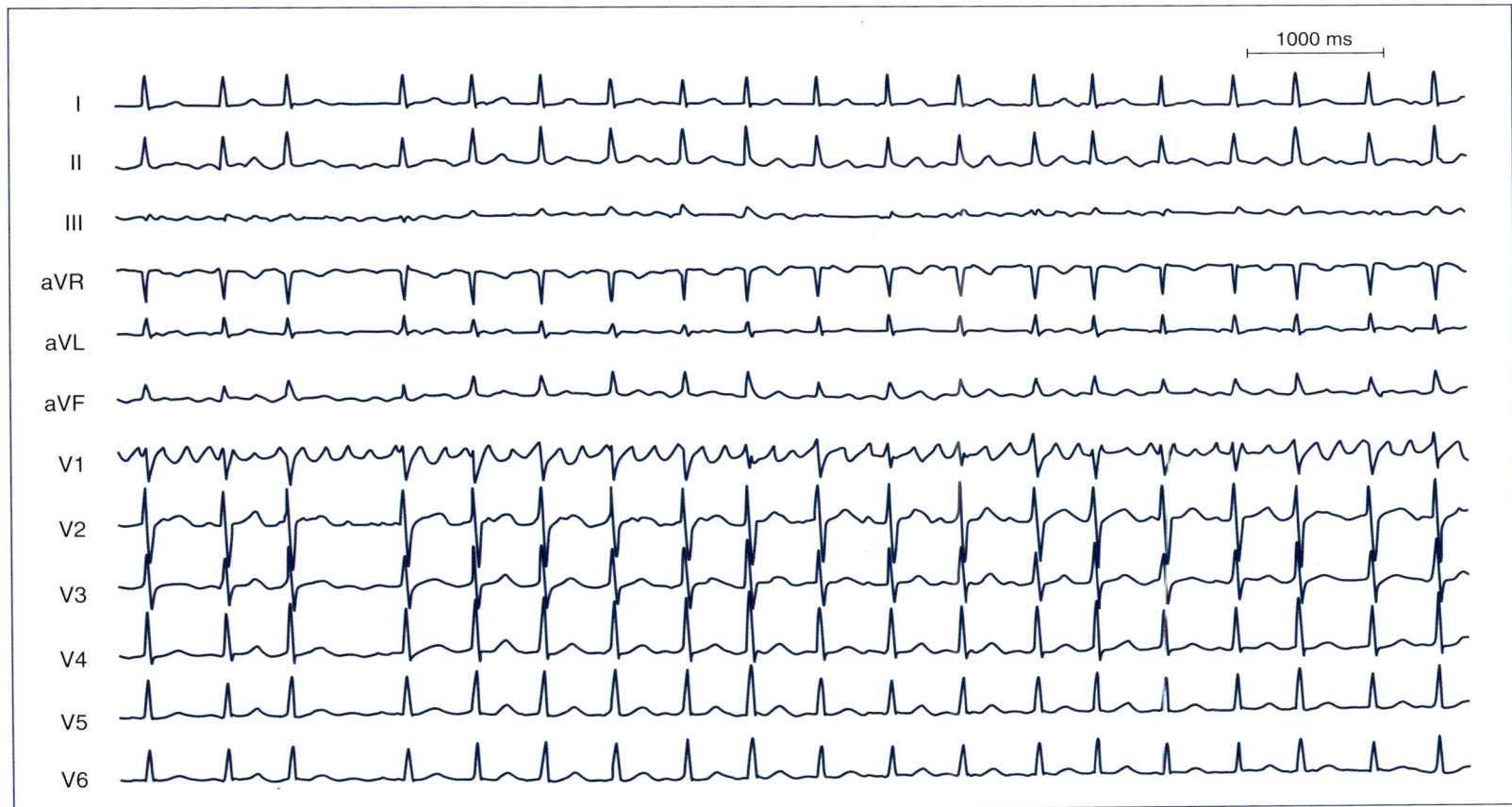

Figure 7-22. Atrial fibrillation (AF) 12-lead surface electrocardiogram. AF is the most common sustained arrhythmia and is particularly prevalent in the elderly. Characteristic of AF is an irregular ventricular response and rapid irregular oscillations or fibrillatory waves that vary in shape, amplitude, and timing [12].

Figure 7-23. Mechanisms of atrial fibrillation (AF). **A,** Initiation and maintenance of AF is dependent on triggers (typically rapidly firing foci) and the presence of the substrate for reentry in the atrium. It is likely that there are multiple mechanisms for AF. **B, C,** and **D** show a magnetic resonance image of the left atrium viewed from the posterior aspect, such that the left superior pulmonary vein is at the upper left and the right superior pulmonary vein is at the upper right. *Starbursts* indicate foci that can fire rapidly to initiate AF and *arrows* indicate propagating wavefronts. **B,** A focus (*lower-left starburst*) firing rapidly in the left inferior pulmonary vein produces wavefronts that propagate across the atrium. Other potential triggering foci are usually present in the other veins, as well (*other three starbursts*).

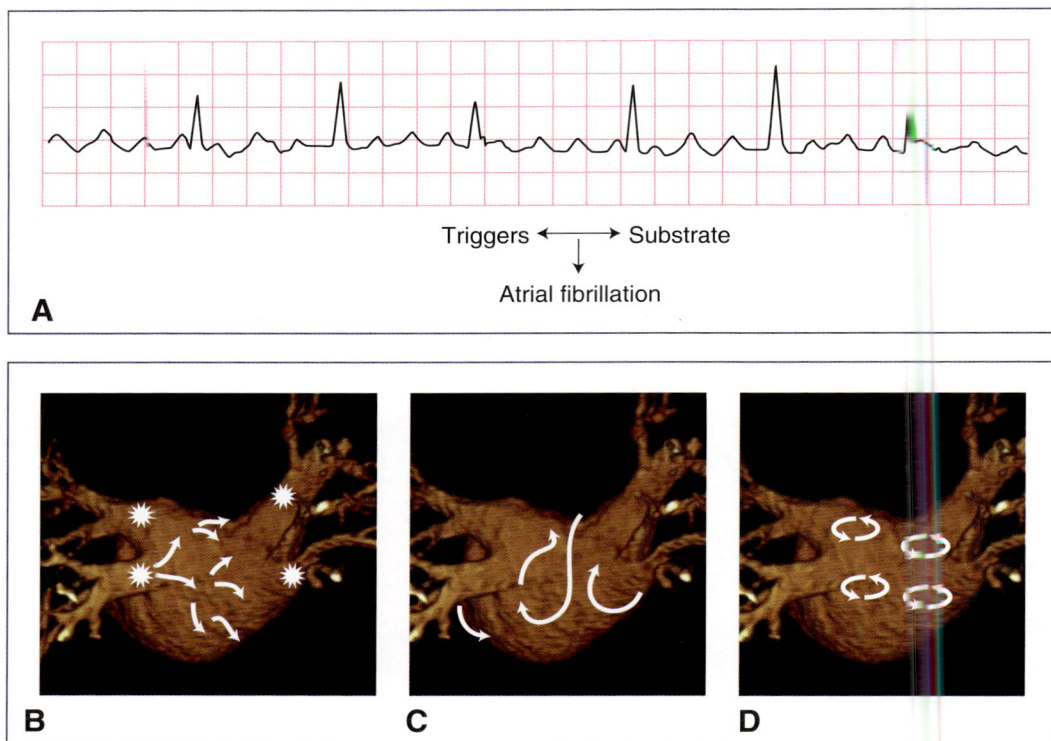

With very rapid firing, the wavefronts break up or "fractionate," producing an electrocardiographic pattern of AF. Alternatively, the wave breaks initiate reentry, which continues in the atrium after the trigger has stopped firing (**C** and **D**). Reentry may take different forms. **C,** A few wavefronts wander through the atrium. **D,** Multiple rapid reentry circuits are present and may wander through the atrium or remain relatively anchored [12–14].

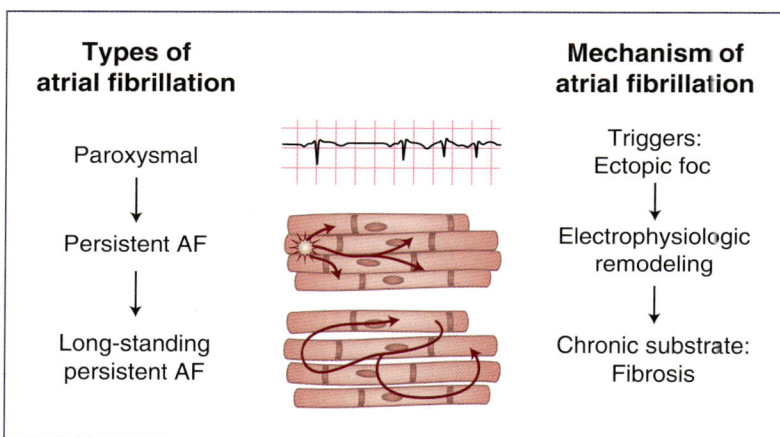

Figure 7-24. Classification and progression of atrial fibrillation (AF). Recurrent self-terminating episodes of AF are designated paroxysmal AF; in persistent AF, episodes are sustained longer than 7 days [13]. Long-standing persistent AF lasts for more than 12 months. After the initial diagnosis of paroxysmal AF, many patients experience a slow progression to chronic AF [12]. Electrophysiologic remodeling (alterations in ion currents, cellular calcium handling, and connexin function) and structural remodeling (atrial fibrosis) accompany this process and create a functional and structural basis for reentry and the perpetuation of the arrhythmia. In general, paroxysmal AF in structurally healthy hearts is typically initiated by rapid firing of foci involving the pulmonary vein regions, whereas chronic AF in structural heart disease is largely related to substrate changes with fibrosis involving the atria [14].

Chronic Treatment for Atrial Fibrillation

Prevention of thromboembolism

Aspirin or no therapy for CHADS$_2$ score of 0 or 1, dose-adjusted warfarin to INR 2–3 for CHADS$_2$ > 1

Aspirin or warfarin may be used for CHADS$_2$ > 1

Pharmacologic rate control with AV nodal blocking agents

β-Blockers, calcium channel blockers, digoxin, rarely amiodarone

Pharmacologic rhythm control to maintain sinus rhythm with membrane-active antiarrhythmic drugs

Class IA: procainamide, disopyramide, quinidine

Class IC: flecainide, propafenone

Class III: amiodarone, sotalol, dofetilide

Nonpharmacologic rate control

AV node ablation and pacemaker implantation

Nonpharmacologic rhythm control

Electrical cardioversion

Catheter ablation

Surgical Maze procedures

A

Figure 7-25. A, Treatment options for atrial fibrillation (AF). Treatment of AF includes antithrombotic therapy, rate control, and rhythm control. Depending on the presence of clinical risk factors assessed from the CHADS$_2$ (Congestive heart failure; history of Hypertension; Age ≥ 75 years; Diabetes; prior Stroke or transient ischemic attack [TIA]) score [12], antithrombotic therapy with aspirin or dose-adjusted warfarin is warranted. Rate control or rhythm control can be achieved by pharmacologic and nonpharmacologic therapy. The therapeutic goal of rate control is a resting heart rate of 60 to 80 beats per minute (BPM) and a heart rate of 90 to 115 BPM during moderate exercise. The aim of rhythm control is the restoration and maintenance of sinus rhythm.

Continued on the next page

The CHADS₂ INDEX

Risk Factor	Points
Congestive heart failure	1
Hypertension	1
Age ≥ 75 years	1
Diabetes mellitus	1
Prior stroke or TIA	2

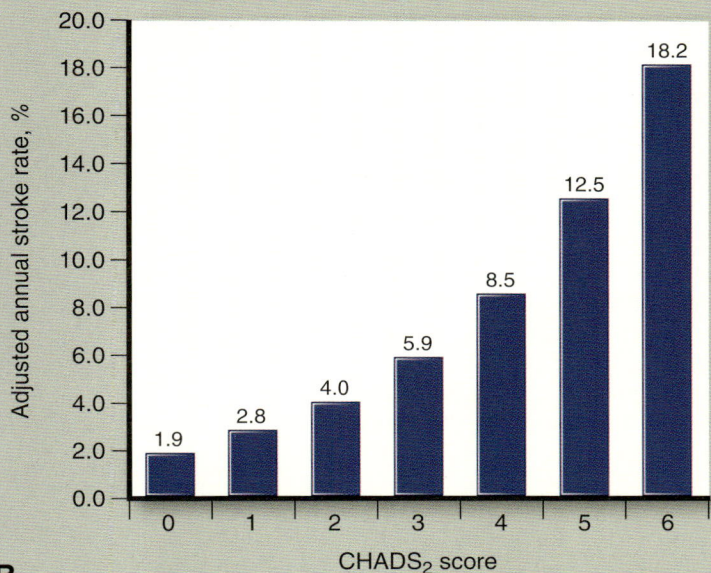

B

Figure 7-25. (*Continued*) Patients treated with rhythm control spend more days in hospital and do not have better survival than those treated with rate control. Therapy is therefore guided by symptoms. Acute cardioversion can be attempted by electrical or pharmacologic means. Atrioventricular (AV) node ablation and placement of a permanent pacemaker can be performed when rhythm and pharmacologic rate control fail, but this measure renders patients pacemaker-dependent. Catheter ablation of atrial fibrillation is usually considered for symptomatic patients who failed at least one antiarrhythmic drug. Surgical Maze procedures or a modified Maze procedure using alternative energy sources (radiofrequency energy, cryothermal energy, ultrasound, laser) are often combined with other required cardiac surgery, such as mitral valve repair, but is an alternative for symptomatic patients [12]. **B**, The CHADS₂ index estimates the annual risk of stroke in patients with nonrheumatic AF not taking warfarin based on clinical risk factors. The CHADS₂ score is calculated by adding one point for each risk factor and two points for prior stroke or TIA. The graph shows the annual risk of stroke increases from 1.9% with a CHADS₂ score of 0 points to 18.2% with a CHADS₂ score of 6 points [12]. INR—international normalized ratio.

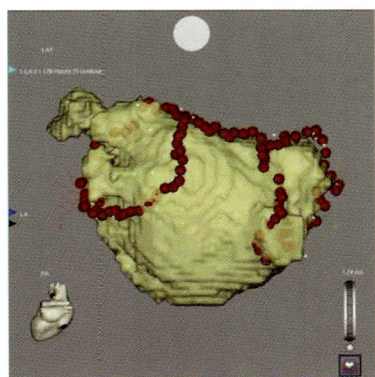

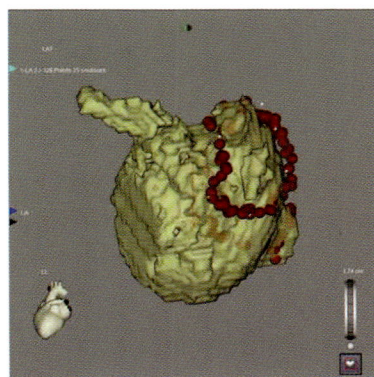

A **B**

Figure 7-26. Radiofrequency (RF) catheter ablation of atrial fibrillation (AF). There are a variety of ablation techniques for AF. Most are based on the recognition that the pulmonary veins and the antral regions around the veins are involved in promoting AF either because they contain ectopic foci that trigger AF or contain regions of substrate that promote reentry for persistent AF. **A**, Left atrial ablation with antral circumferential linear ablation lesions around the ostia of the left- and right-sided pulmonary veins. Electrical isolation, with conduction block is the most common end point for the ablation procedure. The yellow shell represents the three-dimensional reconstruction of the left atrium obtained from magnetic resonance imaging before the procedure. This anatomic image was imported into the mapping system and used along with intra-cardiac ultrasound (Cartosound and Cartomerge; Biosense Webster, Diamond Bar, CA) to guide ablation. The four pulmonary veins are truncated approximately 0.5 to 1 cm after the origin in the left atrium. The prominent anterolateral structure represents the left atrial appendage. Ablation lesions are represented as brown dots. *Left panel* shows a posterior-anterior view; *right panel* shows a left lateral view. RF lines of lesions encircle the pulmonary venous antra. Additional ablation lesions are often placed for patients with persistent or longstanding persistent AF. **A**, An additional ablation line was placed at the left atrial roof, connecting the circumferential lines. **B**, Mapping of a pulmonary vein and assessment of complete conduction block into the vein often uses a circumferential mapping catheter placed into the ostium of the vein.

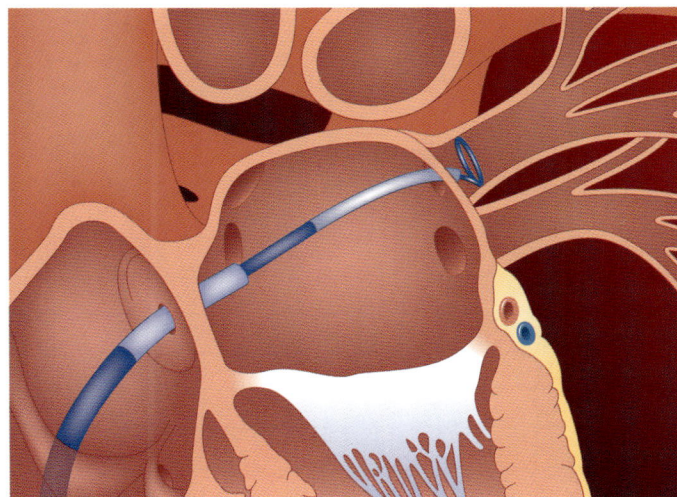

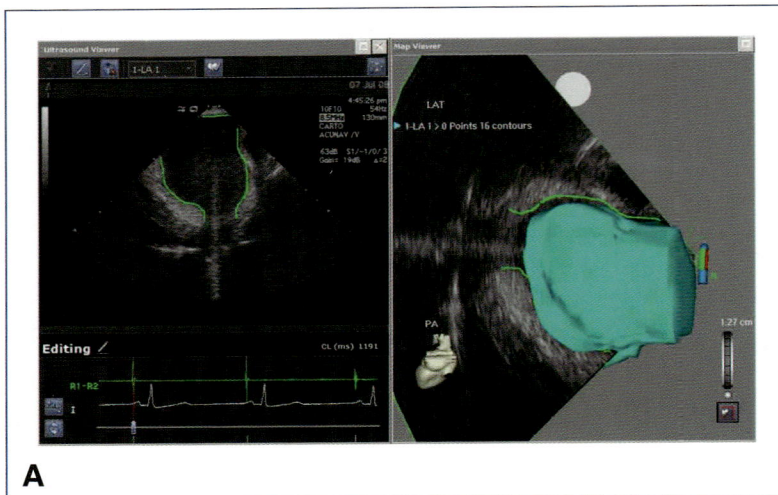

A

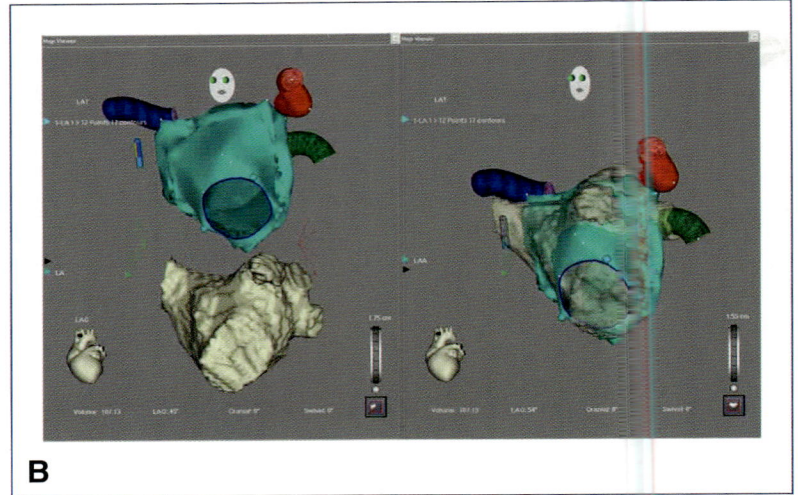

B

Figure 7-27. Three-dimensional mapping and image integration using intracardiac ultrasound for atrial fibrillation (AF) ablation. The ablation process can be facilitated by the three-dimensional reconstruction of the left atrium using three-dimensional mapping systems and image integration. **A,** Creation of a three-dimensional map of the left atrium using intracardiac echocardiography. The ultrasound probe is located in the right atrium. In the ultrasound image (*left*), the endocardial border of the left atrium (*green line*) is marked. Multiple ultrasound slices create a shell of the left atrium (*right*). **B,** Integration of a magnet resonance image of the left atrium (*yellow shell*) into a three-dimensional map of the left atrium, left anterior oblique view. The multicolored icon represents the ultrasound probe. The *blue*, *red*, and *green* tubes represent the right superior, left superior, and left inferior pulmonary veins, respectively. The Cartomerge and Cartosound system (Biosense Webster, Diamond Bar, CA) was used for image integration.

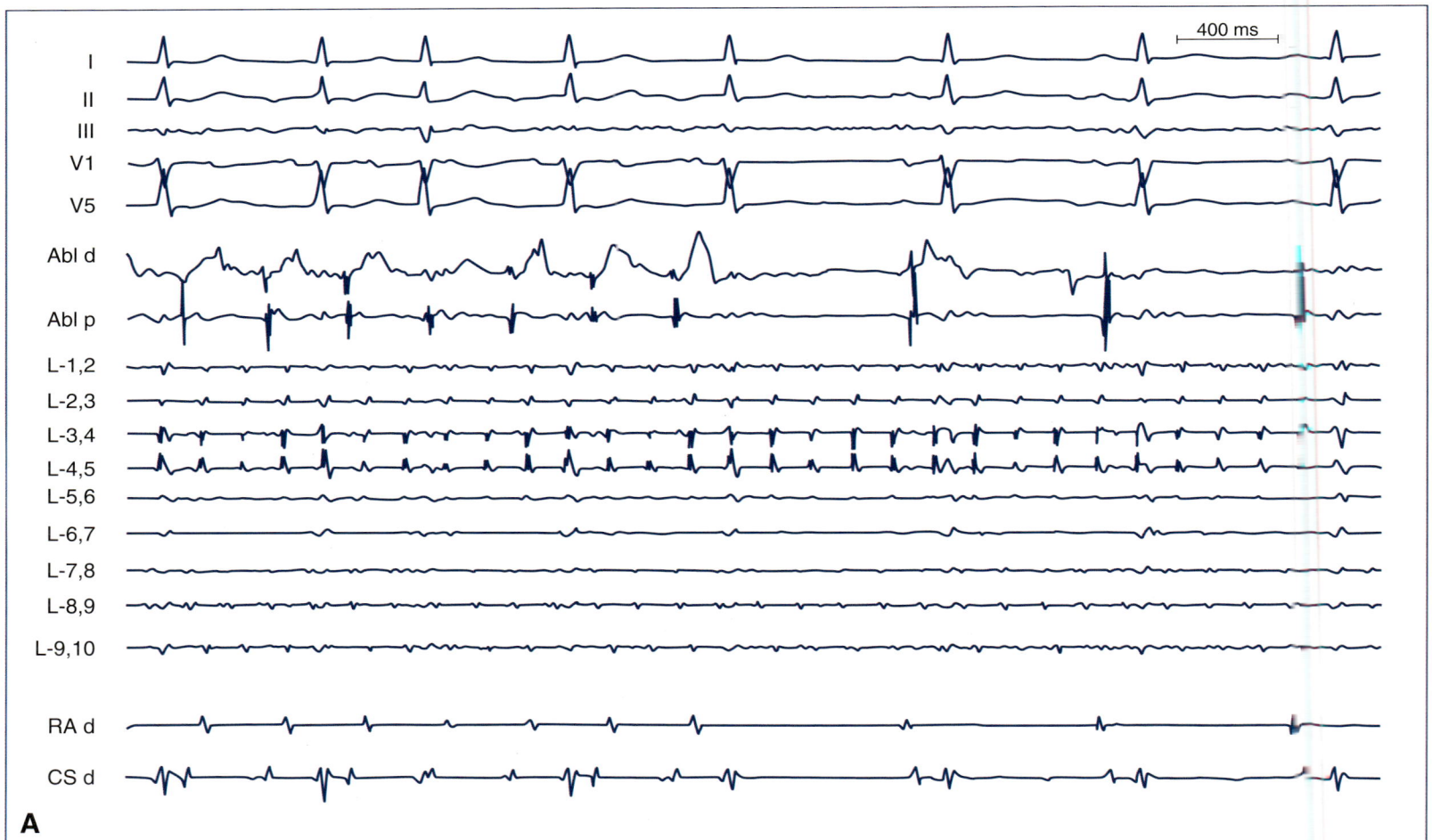

A

Figure 7-28. Catheter ablation of atrial fibrillation (AF). **A,** The tracing was obtained during radiofrequency catheter ablation. Surface electrocardiogram (ECG) and intracardiac tracings are shown. A circumferential mapping catheter (L) is in the common ostium of the left pulmonary veins revealing rapid pulmonary vein tachycardia with a mean cycle length of 160 ms. The ablation catheter (Abl) is positioned in the antrum of the left pulmonary veins. On the left side of the image, there is 2:1 conduction block from the left pulmonary veins to the antrum of left atrium producing an ECG appearance of coarse AF. With ongoing radiofrequency energy application, complete isolation of the left pulmonary veins is achieved. The patient converts to sinus rhythm (note the P-waves in the surface ECG), although the pulmonary vein tachycardia persists.

Continued on the next page

Catheter Ablation for Atrial Fibrillation

Primary indication: symptomatic AF refractory or intolerant to at least one Class 1 or 3 AAD

Left atrial thrombus is a contraindication

Efficacy

Paroxysmal AF

Single procedure: ≥ 60%

Multiple procedures: 80%

Persistent AF:

Single procedure: 22%–45%

Multiple procedures: 37%–88%

Risks

Any major complication: 2%–6%

Tamponade: 1%–3%

Stroke or TIA: 0.5%–2%

Phrenic nerve injury: 0.5%

Fatal atrio-esophageal fistula: rare

Ablation proarrhythmia

Transient AF or tachycardia in the first 2 months after ablation is common

Left atrial tachycardia or flutter requiring repeat ablation: 7%–20%

Caveats

Reported series are biased toward younger patients with less structural heart disease than the overall population of AF patients

Long-term follow-up data beyond 1–2 years is limited

The procedure is technically challenging with a significant learning curve

B

Figure 7-28. (*Continued*) **B**, Catheter ablation for treatment of AF [13–15]. AAD—antiarrhythmic drugs; Abl d—ablation distal dipole; Abl p—ablation proximal dipole; CS d—distal coronary sinus; RA d—low lateral right atrium; TIA—transient ischemic attack.

Pharmacologic Approach to Rhythm Control

Drug	Class	Route	Use in AF	Potential Major Adverse Effects	Remarks
Disopyramide	IA	PO, IV	Cardioversion; facilitation of DC cardioversion; maintenance of SR	QT prolongation, TdP, myocardial depression, glaucoma, urinary retention, hypoglycemia	Should not be initiated out of hospital; use for maintenance of SR in hypertrophic cardiomyopathy
Procainamide	IA	PO, IV	Cardioversion; facilitation of DC cardioversion; maintenance of SR	QT prolongation, TdP, hypotension, lupus-like syndrome	Should not be initiated out of hospital; use for cardioversion in Wolff-Parkinson-White syndrome
Quinidine	IA	PO	Conversion of AF; maintenance of SR	QT prolongation, TdP, fast ventricular response in AF or atrial flutter, hypotension, Chinoism	Should not be initiated out of hospital
Propafenone	IC	PO	Conversion of AF; facilitation of DC conversion; maintenance of SR	Hypotension, heart failure, atrial flutter with fast ventricular response, ventricular tachycardia	Usually used in combination with AV nodal blocking agent; non-selective beta-blocker activity
Flecainide	IC	PO, IV	Conversion of AF; facilitation of DC conversion; maintenance of SR	QT prolongation; hypotension; heart failure; atrial flutter with fast ventricular response; ventricular tachycardia	Usually used in combination with AV nodal blocking agent
Amiodarone	III	PO, IV	Conversion of AF; facilitation of DC conversion; maintenance of SR	Hypotension (IV); bradycardia; QT prolongation; TdP (rare), photosensitivity; pulmonary toxicity; liver toxicity; thyroid dysfunction; eye complications; polyneuropathy	Recommended for maintenance of SR in HF, CAD or in hypertension with severe LVH; can be used to rate control
Sotalol	III	PO, IV	Facilitation of DC cardioversion; maintenance of SR	QT prolongation, TdP, heart failure, bradycardia, exacerbation of chronic obstructive or bronchospastic lung disease	Dose adjustment for renal function; recommended for patients with CAD
Ibutilide	III	IV	Conversion of AF; facilitation of DC conversion	QT prolongation; TdP	Use of cardioversion in Wolff-Parkinson-White syndrome
Dofetilide	III	PO	Conversion of AF, facilitation of DC conversion, maintenance of SR	QT prolongation; TdP	In-hospital initiation of therapy mandatory; dose adjustment for renal function, body size, and age; recommended for maintenance of SR if HF and CAD
Dronedarone	III	PO	Investigational drug; potentially: maintenance of SR	QT prolongation, elevation of serum creatinine	Low potential for TdP; significantly slows ventricular rate in AF
Tedisamil	III	IV	Investigational drug; potentially: cardioversion	QT prolongation; ventricular tachycardia	–
Vernakalant	–	PO, IV	Investigational drug; potentially: cardioversion, maintenance of SR	QT prolongation, hypotension, cardiogenic shock, heart block	–

Figure 7-29. Drugs for pharmacologic approach to rhythm control. As general class effects, class IA and class III antiarrhythmic drugs prolong the QT interval and can exhibit proarrhythmic effects including torsades de pointes (TdP). Risk factors for TdP with these drugs include hypokalemia, female gender, the presence of heart failure, and renal failure. Class IA antiarrhythmic drugs are usually considered as second- or third-line choices. Class IC antiarrhythmic drugs should be avoided in patients with structural heart disease [12,16,17]. AV—atrioventricular; CAD—coronary artery disease; HF—heart failure; IV—intravenous; LVH—left ventricular hypertrophy; PO—oral; SR—sinus rhythm.

Ventricular Tachycardia

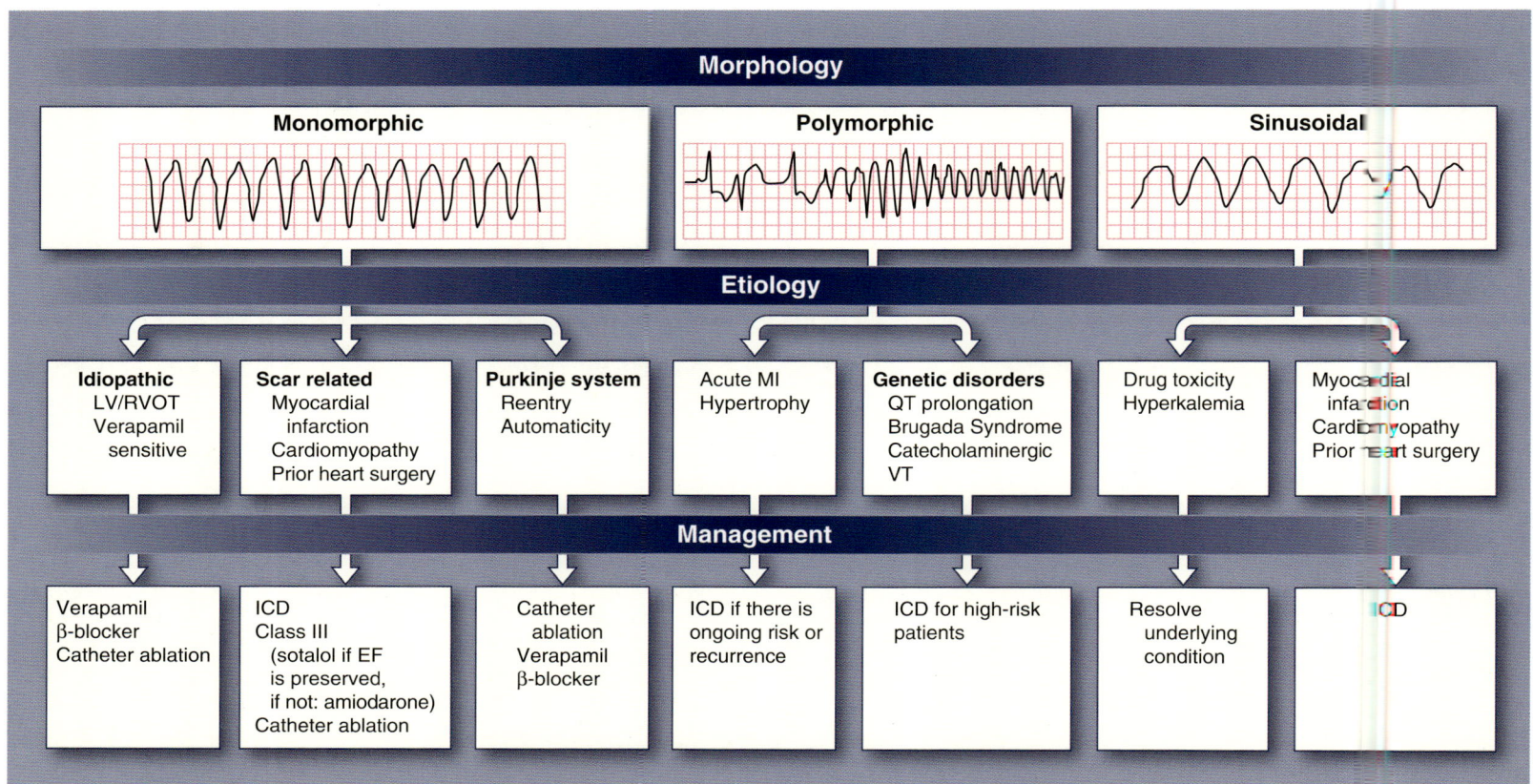

Figure 7-30. Ventricular tachycardia (VT) types, etiologies, and management. Sustained VTs require an intervention, such as cardioversion or administration of an antiarrhythmic drug for termination or if they are sufficiently long and rapid to produce severe symptoms, such as syncope, before terminating spontaneously. Monomorphic VTs have the same ventricular activation sequence from beat to beat, indicating repetitive initial depolarization from a fixed location or reentry through a fixed arrhythmia substrate, most commonly an area of ventricular scar, but can also originate from an arrhythmogenic focus in the absence of structural heart disease (idiopathic VT). Polymorphic VTs have a continuously changing QRS configuration due to changing ventricular activation sequence from beat to beat. These tachycardias do not require the presence of an anatomic, fixed arrhythmia substrate. Acute myocardial infarction is the most common cause, but cardiac ion channel abnormalities that can be genetic or acquired are also causes. Treatment options depend on the risk of sudden death, which is largely determined by underlying heart disease, and susceptibility to pharmacologic and ablation therapies. An implantable cardioverter defibrillator (ICD) is considered for those VTs associated with a sudden death risk [18]. Class III—Class III antiarrhythmic agent; LV—left ventricular; RVOT—right ventricular outflow tract.

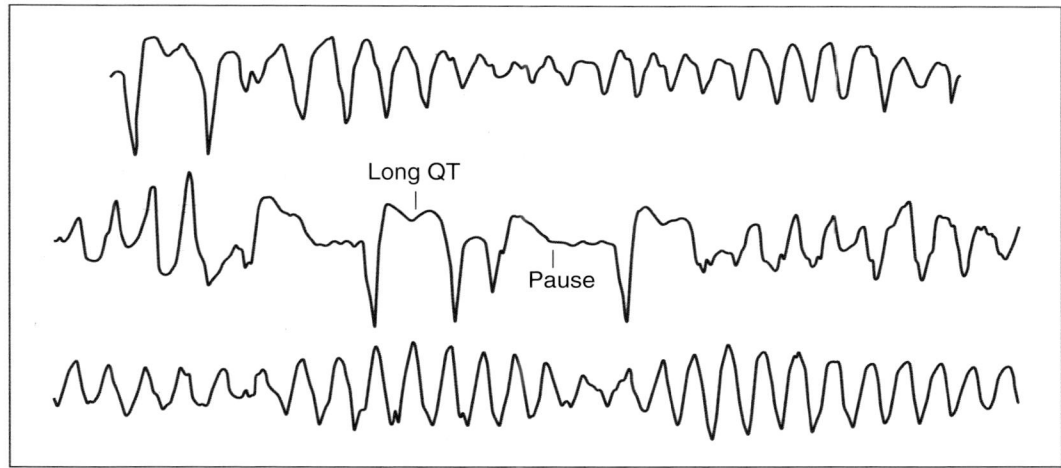

Figure 7-31. The polymorphic ventricular tachycardia torsades de pointes. The waxing and waning QRS amplitude gives rise to the "twisting about the points" designation. When viewed in a single lead, torsades de pointes may appear monomorphic, thus multiple simultaneous leads should be obtained if possible. This tachycardia is associated with prolonged QT interval and may be due to a genetic ion channel abnormality or acquired due to a drug (*eg,* dofetilide, ibutilide, sotalol, methadone, and many others), toxin, or electrolyte disturbance (hypokalemia, hypomagnesemia, hypocalcemia). In the *top strip,* a polymorphic ventricular tachycardia seems to undulate around a fixed baseline and is continued in the *middle strip.* Note that the arrhythmia self-terminates, a frequent characteristic of torsades de pointes. However, it is reinitiated after a characteristic pause followed by a shortly coupled premature ventricular complex.

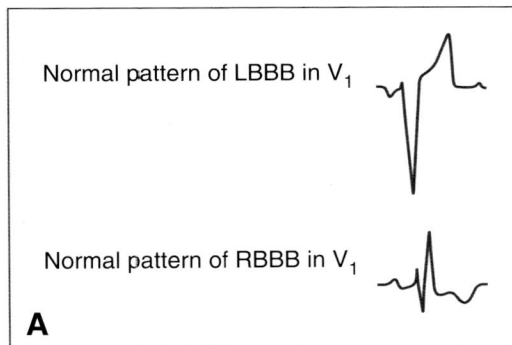

A

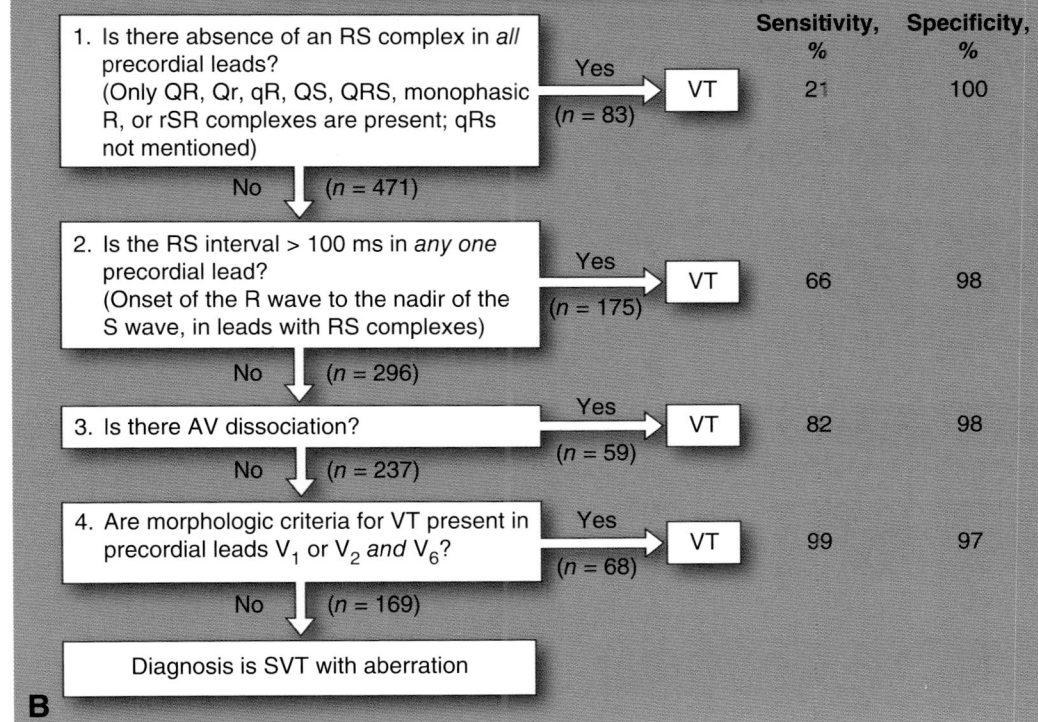

B

Figure 7-32. The 12-lead electrocardiogram in the differential diagnosis of sustained monomorphic ventricular tachycardia (VT) versus supraventricular tachycardia (SVT) with aberrancy. Brugada *el al.* [19] analyzed 384 cases of sustained monomorphic VT and 170 cases of SVT with aberrancy, representing 554 patients with tachycardia (those taking antiarrhythmic medications were excluded). They then devised a systematic approach for diagnosing regular, wide QRS complex tachycardia. **A,** The first step is to access the possibility of sinus tachycardia or atrial tachycardia with right bundle branch block (RBBB) or left bundle branch block (LBBB), which is usually a long RP tachycardia (the RP interval is longer than the PR interval) such that the P-wave is seen shortly preceding the QRS complex. A typical sinus P-wave in that location supports the diagnosis of sinus tachycardia. If sinus tachycardia is not evident further assessment of QRS morphology and P-waves can often determine if tachycardia is supraventricular with bundle branch aberration or ventricular. **B,** Steps in diagnosis of VT versus SVT with aberration. A "yes" answer at any point indicates a likely diagnosis of VT and no further steps in the algorithm need to be taken. When the answer is no, proceed to the next step. The cumulative sensitivity using this method is 97% and specificity is 99%.

Continued on the next page

C

ECG lead
V_1 only

Monophasic R wave

qR or Rs

ECG lead
V_6

QS or qR

R/S < 1
(seen with LAD)

D

V_1 or V_2

1. R wave width > 30 ms

2. Notched S wave

Any of the three criteria

3. > 60 ms to nadir of S wave

V_6

qR   QS

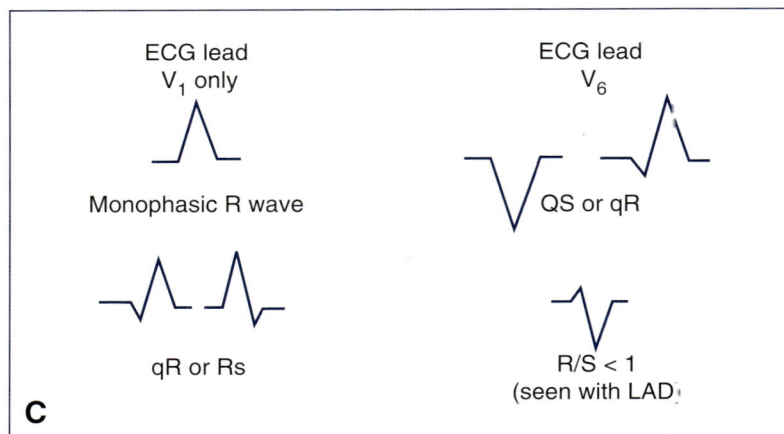

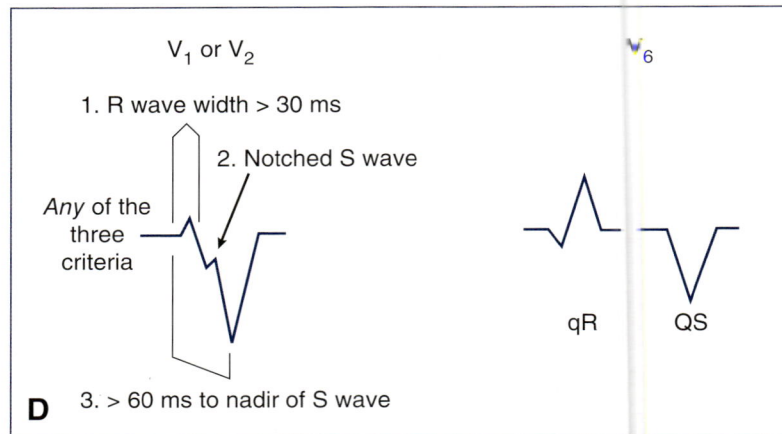

Figure 7-32. *(Continued)* **C,** Morphologic criteria favoring diagnosis of VT in the presence of RBBB–type QRS complexes (dominant positive in V_1). Both leads must meet these criteria in order to diagnose VT. **D,** Morphologic criteria used to diagnose VT in the presence of LBBB-type QRS complexes (dominant negative in V_1). Both leads must meet these criteria to diagnose VT. These QRS morphology criteria are probably less reliable in the presence of severe cardiac disease or antiarrhythmic drugs. ECG—electrocardiogram; LAD—left anterior descending. *(Adapted from Brugada et al* [19]*.)*

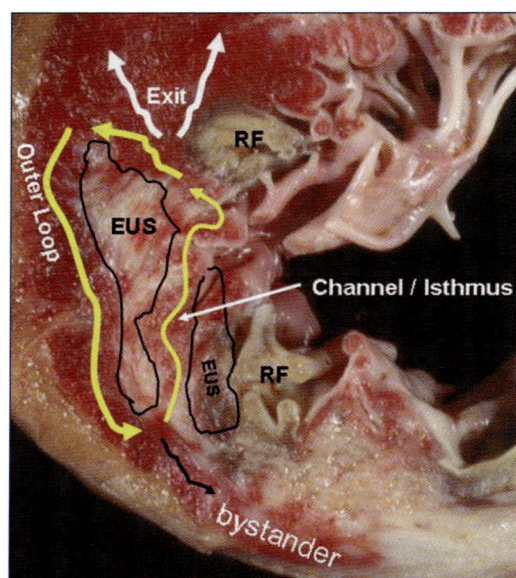

Figure 7-33. An autopsy specimen from a patient who died of uncontrollable ventricular tachycardia (VT) late after myocardial infarction showing the anatomic basis of a potential reentry circuit causing scar-related monomorphic VT. The cross-section of the left ventricle shows areas of fibrosis (*white regions*) due to prior inferior wall infarction. Dense fibrosis is electrical unexcitable scar (EUS) that creates the borders of channels (also called "isthmuses") of surviving myocardium. Conduction through these regions is slowed by uncoupling of myocyte bundles by intervening microscopic fibrosis that forces the wavefront to take a zigzag course through the region [20]. *Yellow arrows* indicate potential reentry paths. The wavefront from the channel reaches the exit from the channel in the border of the infarct, from which activation spreads across the ventricles producing the QRS complex. The location of this exit from the channel determines the myocardial activation sequence and hence, the resulting QRS morphology [21]. The wavefront continues along the border of the scar (*outer loop*) to reach the entrance to the channel. The QRS morphology of VT is often an indication of the location of the scar containing the reentry circuit and the exit of the reentry channel. These channels and exits can be targeted for catheter and surgical ablation procedures. Identification can be challenging due to varied locations, multiple potential circuits, and bystander regions of abnormal conduction that can mimic electrophysiologic features of channels. Sites of radiofrequency (RF) current application are depicted as RF in the figure, but were not successful in controlling the VT. In this case, failure of ablation was likely related to portions of the reentry circuits located within the myocardium beyond the reach of current ablation technology.

Bundle branch morphology (dominant deflection in V1)
Exit location

Right	left ventricle
Left	right ventricle/septum

Frontal plane axis
  Superior   inferior wall or inferior septum
  Inferior   anterior wall or anterior septum

Dominant deflection in V3–V4
  R-wave: basal (near the mitral or tricuspid annulus)
  S-wave: apical LV or RV

Slurred QRS upstroke: epicardial origin

A

B

C

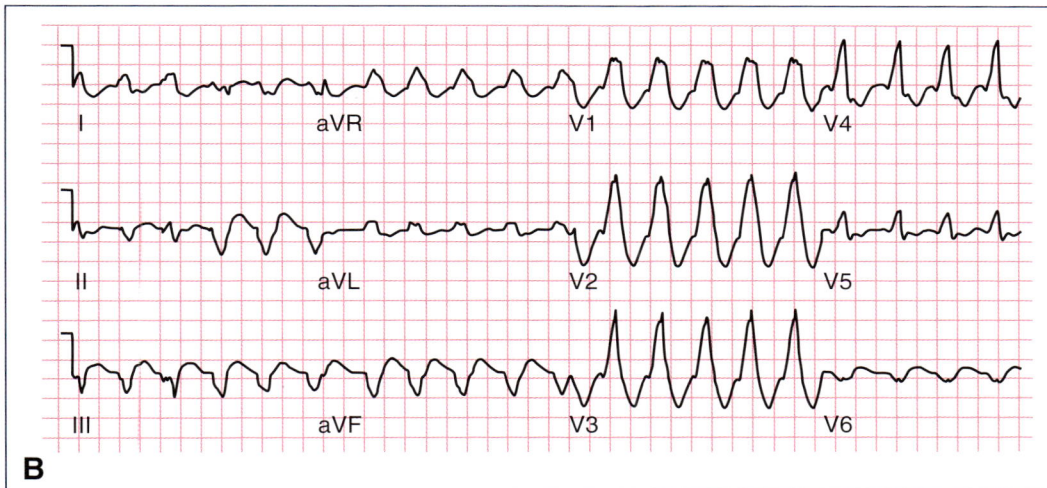

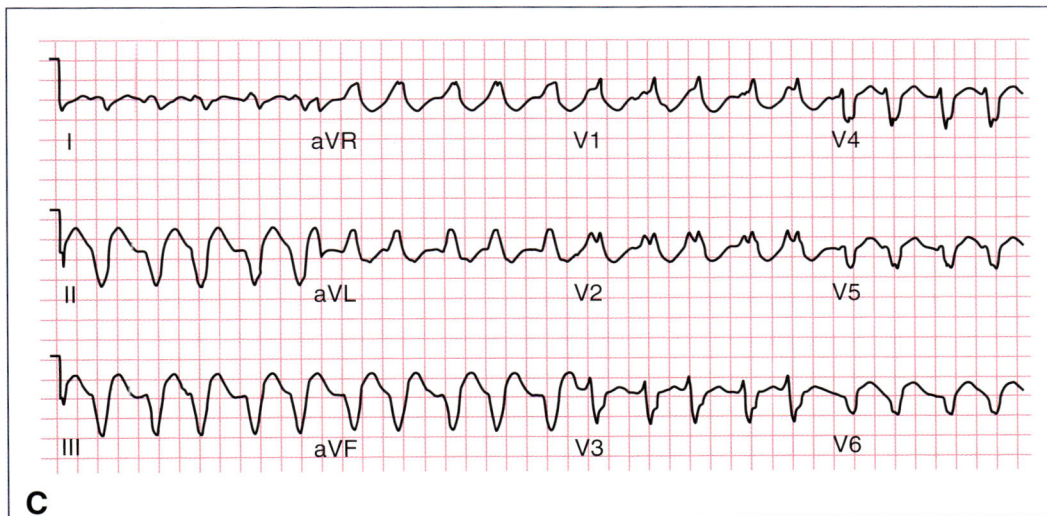

Figure 7-34. A, The location of a ventricular tachycardia (VT) focus or exit from a scar is suggested by the QRS morphology of the VT [20]. A dominant S-wave in V_1 suggests a right ventricular (RV) or septal exit. A dominant R wave in V_1 usually indicates a left ventricular (LV) origin. The frontal plane axis can be used to determine whether the VT exit is more likely to be inferior or anterior. It should be noted that the 12-lead electrocardiogram morphology can be misleading when extensive scarring is present in diseased ventricles. **B** and **C,** Monomorphic VTs in a patient with an old inferior wall myocardial infarction. Most patients with monomorphic VT due to a prior infarction have multiple morphologies of VT that are inducible with programmed stimulation in the electrophysiology laboratory, indicating different potential reentry circuits within the infarct region. **B,** VT has a right bundle branch block configuration and superiorly directed frontal plan axis, suggesting an exit on the inferior wall of the LV. Dominant R-waves are present in V_3–V_4, suggesting that the exit is located close to the mitral annulus. **C,** A second VT in the same patient has an RS configuration in V_1 and a superiorly directed frontal plane axis suggesting an inferior wall exit close to the septum. Dominant S-waves are present in V_3–V_4, suggesting an exit closer to the apex.

Secondary prevention ICD
Shocks for VT: 40%–60%
> 3 shocks in 24 h: 20%
Need for AADs: 20%

Primary prevention ICD
Shocks for VT: 2%–5% y
Inappropriate shocks: 2.5%/y
Need for AADs: 14%

Symptomatic VT after ICD

Antiarrhythmic Drugs
Risk of recurrent VT
β-blocker: 40%
Sotalol: 24%
Amiodarone + β-blocker: 10%

Catheter ablation
Freedom from recurrent VT: 75%–50%
Reduction in VT frequency in > 67%
Control of incessant VT or VT storm in 80% of patients
Procedure mortality 3% (usually due to uncontrollable VT when procedure fails)

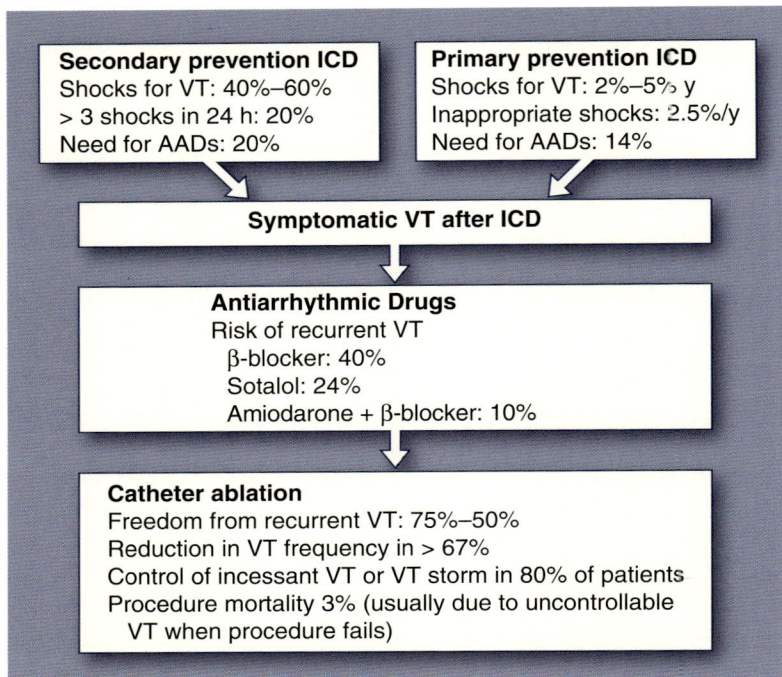

Figure 7-35. Therapies to prevent recurrent arrhythmias in patients with implantable cardioverter defibrillators (ICDs). ICDs terminate ventricular tachycardia (VT) or ventricular fibrillation (VF) when it occurs but do not prevent the arrhythmia. Spontaneous episodes of arrhythmias decrease quality of life by causing symptoms or eliciting painful shocks from the ICD and are a marker for increased mortality, likely indicating progression of underlying heart disease [22]. Recurrent VT or VF usually mandates additional therapy despite effective termination of the arrhythmia by the ICD. VT is more likely to occur in patients who have had spontaneous VT, rather than in those who receive an ICD for primary prevention of sudden death. A significant number of patients experience "VT storm," defined as three or more separate episodes of VT in a 24-hour period. Antiarrhythmic drugs (AADs) are generally used to reduce VT episodes [23]. When pharmacologic therapy is ineffective, tolerated, or not desirable, catheter ablation should be considered [18,21].

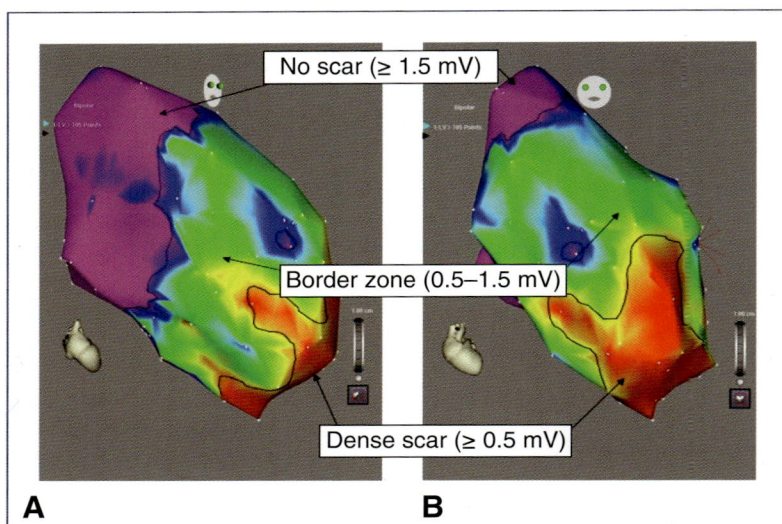

A **B** **C**

Figure 7-36. Electroanatomic bipolar voltage maps to identify scar during ventricular tachycardia (VT) catheter ablation procedures. Areas of infarction scar are the most common source of sustained monomorphic VT. Catheter mapping techniques have been developed to locate these scars based on electrogram characteristics. **A** and **B**, Maps from a patient with a large anterior wall infarction. During catheter mapping of the endocardium, a mapping catheter was introduced via the femoral artery into the left ventricle (LV). These maps were constructed by moving a catheter point by point around the ventricle and sampling the electrogram amplitude at each point [24].

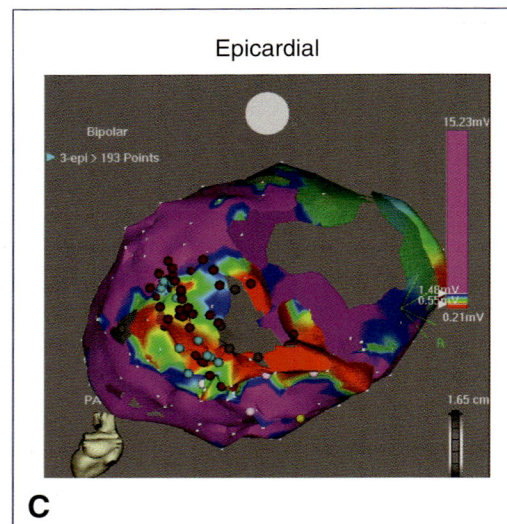

Continued on the next page

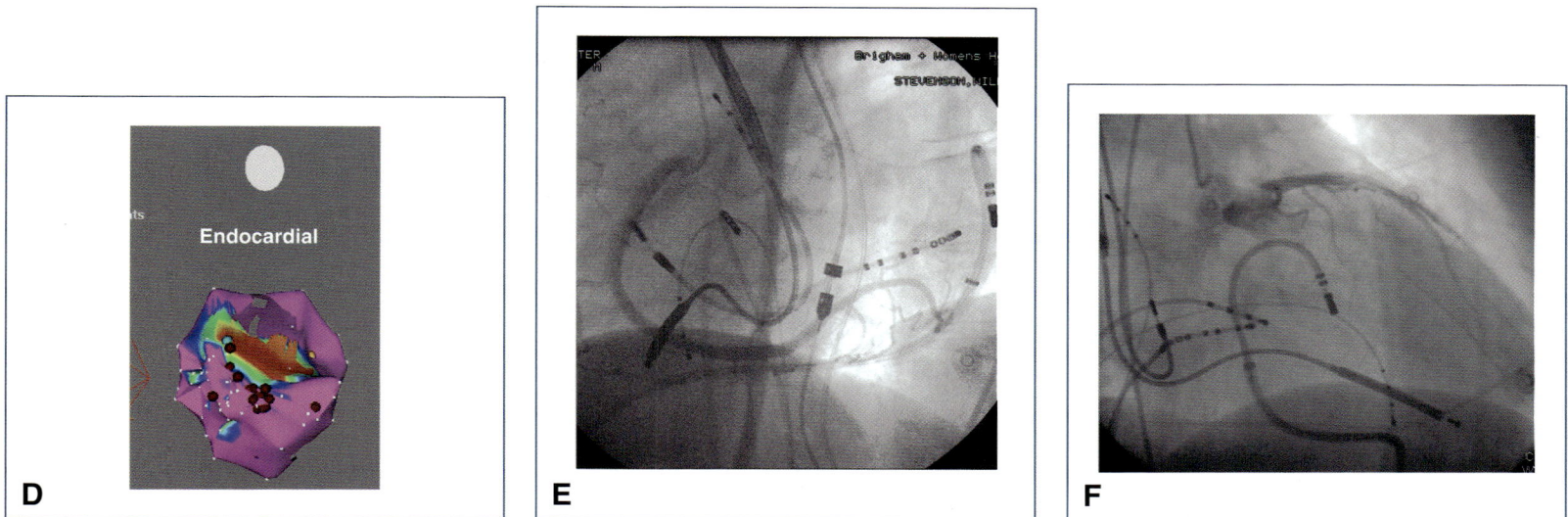

Figure 7-36. *(Continued)* **A** shows a right anterior oblique (RAO) view, **B** shows an anterior–posterior (AP) view of the LV. Areas of ventricular scar are detected as regions with reduced electrogram amplitude. *Purple* indicates areas of normal electrogram voltage (> 1.5 mV). Voltage is progressively smaller, moving from *blue* to green to *yellow* to *red*. This large anteroseptal infarct contained multiple reentry circuits, giving rise to multiple morphologies of inducible monomorphic VT that were targeted for catheter ablation. **C, D, E,** and **F** show findings from a patient with nonischemic cardiomyopathy and VT. In contrast to most infarct-related VTs that are subendocardial in location, VT in nonischemic cardiomyopathy often originates from scars that involve the epicardium [25]. Percutaneous pericardial puncture is used to insert a mapping catheter into the epicardial space for mapping and ablation [26]. **C,** A voltage map from the epicardium viewed from the left posterior oblique projection. A region of low voltage scar is present, extending from the basal LV near the mitral annulus toward the apex. *Brown circles* represent sites where ablation lesions were placed to transect reentry pathways giving rise to multiple morphologies of VT. **D** shows the corresponding endocardial map. The size of the endocardial low voltage area was substantially smaller than that observed on the epicardium. **E** and **F** show radiograph images from the procedure with the epicardial mapping catheter with its tip positioned over the epicardial scar. Coronary angiography was performed (right coronary injection in left anterior oblique view [**E**]; left coronary injection in RAO [**F**]) to avoid ablation injury to an epicardial coronary artery.

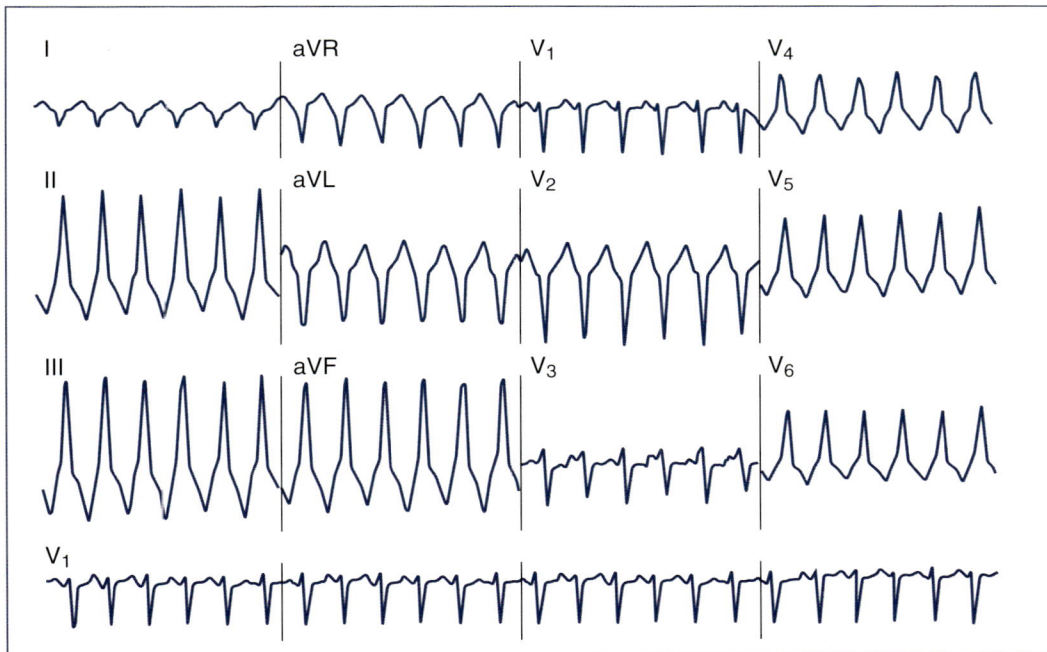

Figure 7-37. Idiopathic sustained monomorphic ventricular tachycardia (VT) originating from the right ventricular outflow tract (RVOT). This 12-lead electrocardiogram from a healthy 22-year-old woman who experienced frequent palpitations with exercise shows a left bundle branch block–type pattern in V_1, with an inferior axis consistent with origin in the RVOT. This is the most common type of idiopathic VT [21]. Focal idiopathic VTs occur in patients with structurally normal hearts and are often due to cAMP-mediated triggered activity. They may be exercise-induced or occur at rest. They are frequently adenosine-sensitive. These VTs are important to recognize because they do not require implantation of a cardioverter defibrillator. Many respond to β-adrenergic blockers or nondihydropyridine calcium channel blockers. More than 80% can be cured by radiofrequency ablation, with failures due to the inability to initiate VT in the electrophysiology laboratory or difficult anatomic locations, such as the epicardium. It is important to exclude underlying heart disease and causes of VT associated with right ventricular scar-related VTs, such as arrhythmogenic right ventricular dysplasia, which can cause VT and ventricular fibrillation leading to sudden death. Idiopathic VTs may also arise from the left ventricular outflow tract, aortic annulus, mitral annulus, and left ventricular septum, which have different QRS configurations reflecting their respective origins [27].

Sudden Cardiac Death

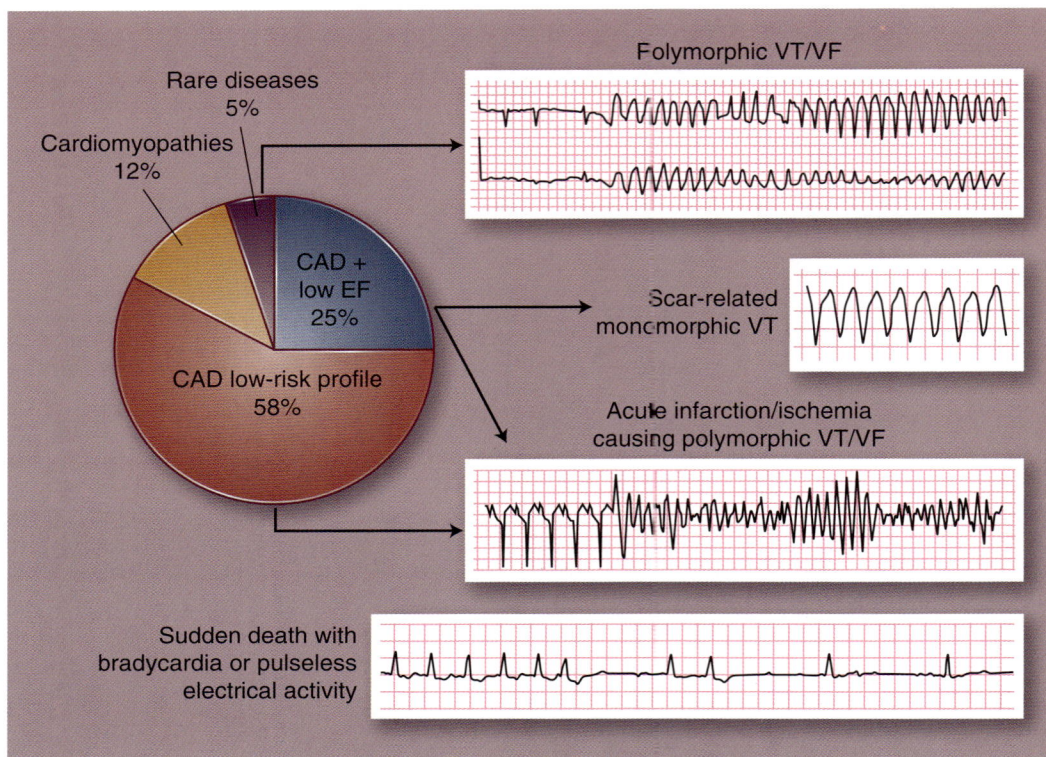

Figure 7-38. Sudden cardiac death. There are 150,000 to 300,000 sudden, out-of-hospital, cardiac deaths annually in the United States. The majority occur in patients with coronary artery disease, and most have preserved ventricular function, suggesting that acute myocardial ischemia causing polymorphic ventricular tachycardia (VT)/ventricular fibrillation (VF) is a likely cause. In approximately half of patients with coronary artery disease (CAD), sudden death is the first recognized manifestation of the disease. A small fraction of sudden deaths occur in patients with ventricular scars due to an old infarction or a cardiomyopathic process that can cause monomorphic VT that may degenerate to VF. Genetic diseases of cardiac ion channels, such as the long QT syndrome and Brugada syndrome, or hypertrophic cardiomyopathy, typically present with polymorphic VT. The initial rhythm at the time of sudden death is often asystole or pulseless electrical activity. This may be due to deterioration after VT/VF or caused by another catastrophic event, such as stroke, ruptured aneurysm, or pulmonary embolism [18]. EF—ejection fraction.

Genetic Syndromes Causing Sudden Death

Inherited Arrhythmia Disorders Associated With Sudden Cardiac Death

QT Interval	Gene	Protein/Subunit	Function	Chromosome	Arrhythmia Triggers/ Syndrome/Phenotype	Heritance	Incidence	Therapy—Sudden Cardiac Death Prevention
Long QT								
LQT1	KCNQ1	Kv7.1α	$\downarrow I_{KS}$/KvLQT1	11p15.5	TdP induced by exercise, swimming, strong emotion, rarely auditory stimuli	Dominant/ recessive	30%–35%	β-Blockers: ~90% effective; ICD if high risk
LQT2	KCH2	Kv11.1α	$\downarrow I_{KR}$/HERG	7q35	TdP from auditory stimuli, abrupt arousal from sleep	Autosomal dominant	25%–30%	β-Blockers: ~80% effective; ICD if high risk
LQT3	SCN5A	NAv1.5α	$\uparrow$ INA	3p21	TdP during sleep, not commonly exercise related	Autosomal dominant	5%–10%	β-Blockers: < 70% effective; ICD if high risk
LQT4	ANK2	Ankyrin-B	$\downarrow 1_{NA,K}, I_{NCX}$: trafficking	4q25	TdP: exertion, emotional stress	Autosomal dominant	1%–2%	Lifestyle, β-blockers, ICD if high risk
LQT5	KCNE1	minK β	$\downarrow I_{KS}$	21q22.1	TdP: auditory stimuli, abrupt arousal from sleep	Dominant/ recessive	1%–2%	Lifestyle, β-blockers, ICD if high risk
LQT6	KCNE2	MiRP1 β	$\downarrow I_{KS}$	21q22.1	TdP: Anderson-Tawil Syndrome: periodic paralysis, micrognathia, dental abnormalities, clinodactyly, widely spread eyes	Autosomal dominant	Rare	Lifestyle, β-blockers, ICD if high risk
LQT7	KCNJ2	Kir2.1 α	$\downarrow I_{K1}$	17q23	Timothy Syndrome: VT, AF, bradycardia	Autosomal dominant	Unknown	Lifestyle, β-blockers, ICD if high risk
LQT8	CAC-NA1C	Cav1.2α1C	$I_{ca,L}$	2p13.3	Autism, syndactaly hands and feet, musculoskeletal	Autosomal dominant	Unknown	Lifestyle, β-blockers, ICD if high risk
LQT9	CAV3	Caveolin-3	$\uparrow I_{NA}$	3p25	Nonexertional syncope, SCD in sleep	Unknown	Rare	Lifestyle, β-blockers, ICD if high risk
LQT10	SCN4B	NAv1.5 β4	$\uparrow I_{NA}$	11q23	TdP, Jervell-Lange-Nielson: homozygous mutations with LQT1 or LQT5 with sensorineural hearing loss; Romano-Ward Syndrome: heterozygous mutations in LQT1-10	Unknown	Rare	Lifestyle, β-blockers, ICD if high risk
Short QT								
SQT1	KCNH2	Kv11.1α	$\downarrow I_{KR}$/HERG	7q35	QT < 320–360 ms, syncope, paroxysmal AF, VF, PMVT	Autosomal dominant	Unknown	Quinidine, class III agents?
SQT2	KCNQ1	Kv7.1α	$\downarrow I_{KS}$/KvLQT1	11p15.5	QT < 320–360 ms, syncope, paroxysmal AF, VF, PMVT	Autosomal dominant	Unknown	Unknown, ICD if high risk
SQT3	KCNJ2	Kir2.1 α	$\uparrow I_{K1}$	17q23	QT < 320–360 ms, syncope, paroxysmal AF, VF, PMVT	Autosomal dominant	Unknown	Unknown, ICD if high risk
Brugada								
BrS1	SCN5A	Nav1.5 α	$\downarrow I_{Na}$	3p21	Syncope, PMVT, VF—often nocturnal	Autosomal dominant	~15%	ICD if high risk
BrS2	GPD1L	Glycerol 3-phosphate; dehydrogenase 1-like	$\downarrow I_{Na}$	3p24	Syncope, VT, conduction disease; low sensitivity to procainamide, relatively better prognosis	Autosomal dominant	< 1%	ICD if high risk
BrS3	CAC-NA1C	Cav1.2α1C	$I_{ca,L}$	12p13.3	Repolarization abnormalities with short QTc	Autosomal dominant	Rare	ICD if high risk
BrS4	CAC-NB2B	Cavβ2B	$I_{ca,L}$	10p12.33	Repolarization abnormalities with short QTc	Autosomal dominant	Rare	ICD if high risk

Figure 7-39. Inherited arrhythmia disorders associated with sudden cardiac death (SCD). Mutations in ion channel function, trafficking, or cytoskeletal organization result in "channelopathies," such as long QT syndrome (LQTS), short QT syndrome (SQTS), and Brugada syndrome with repolarization abnormalities that predispose to SCD with variable penetrance and severity. The incidence of LQT1, LQT2, and LQT3 mutations is approximately 75% of genotyped LQTS patients. LQT1 and LQT5 associated with hearing loss with homozygous mutations are known as the Jervel-Lange-Nielson Syndrome. LQT1-10 without hearing loss and heterozygous genotypes are referred to collectively as Romano-Ward syndrome. Disorders of Ca²⁺ handling in the sarcoplasmic reticulum have been identified as causes of catecholaminergic polymorphic ventricular tachycardia (CPVT). Mutations in genes required for development of the cardiac conduction system may result in conduction block and SCD.
Continued on the next page

QT Interval	Gene	Protein/Subunit	Function	Chromosome	Arrhythmia Triggers/ Syndrome/Phenotype	Heritance	Incidence	Therapy—Sudden Cardiac Death Prevention
Catecholaminergic polymorphic VT (CPVT)								
CPVT1	*RYR2*	RyR2 α	↑ SR Ca²⁺ leak	1q42	Stress-induced VT, bidirectional VT, polymorphic VT	Autosomal dominant	~50%–60%	β-Blockers ICD if high risk
CPVT2	*CSQ2*	Calsequestrin	↑ SR Ca²⁺ leak/ ↓ Ca²⁺ buffer	1p13.3	–	Autosomal recessive	< 5%	
	KCNJ2	Kir2.1 α	↑ IK1	17q23		Autosomal dominant	Rare/unknown	
	ANK2	Ankyrin-β	SR Ca²⁺ leak	4q25		Autosomal dominant	Rare/unknown	
Conduction disease								
	LMNA	Lamin A/C	Nuclear structure, gene expression	1q21	Dilated cardiomyopathy, AV block, progeria syndromes	Dominant/ recessive	Rare/unknown	Pacemaker ± defibrillator
	NKX2.5	NKX2.5 Transcription factor	Cardiac morphogenesis	5q34	Septation, AV block, sudden death	Autosomal dominant	Rare/unknown	Pacemaker
	TBX5	TBX5 Transcription factor	Cardiac development/maturation	12q24	Holt-Oram Syndrome: SAN & AVN block, AV canal defects	Autosomal dominant	Rare/unknown	Pacemaker
	SCN5A	Nav1.5α	↓ I_Na	3p21	Lenegre-Lev Syndrome–His Purkinje degeneration	Autosomal dominant	Rare	Pacemaker
Structural heart disease; hypertrophic cardiomyopathy		β-Myosin, heavy chain (β-MHC, α-MHC), cardiac myosin binding protein C (cMYBPC), Cardiac troponin C (cTnC), a-Tropomyosin (TPM1), Myosin essential light chain (MYL3), Myosin regulatory light chain (MYL2), a-Actin (ACTC), Titin (TTN), muscle LIM protein (MLP)		Sarcomeropathy	Most common cause of SCD in young athletes in USA. Heterogenous penetrance, phenotype	Autosomal dominant	1/500 in US population	Lifestyle modification, septal reduction, β-blockers or calcium channel blockers, ICD
Arrhythmogenic right ventricular dysplasia/ cardiomyopathy		Plakophilin-2 (PKP2), desmoglein-2 (DSG-2), desmocollin-2 (DSC2), transforming grown factor β-3 (TGF β3), plakoglobin (JUP), Ryanodine receptor (RYR2), transmembrane protein 43 (TMEM43)		Desmosome abnormalities	LBBB configuration VT often exercise-induced or VF/Naxos syndrome (Plakoglobin)	Autosomal dominant	1/5000 population	Lifestyle modification, β-blockers, ICD, antiarrhythmic drugs, catheter ablation
Glycogen storage	*PRKAG2*	AMP kinase γ-submit 2	Cellular energy sensor	7q35	Multiple accessory pathways, hypertrophy phenocopy, AV block	Autosomal dominant	Rare	Unknown catheter ablation for WPW
Danon-type storage disease	*LAMP2*	Lysosome-associated membrane protein 2	Autophagy	Xq24	Preexcitation, HCM phenocopy, AV block	X-linked recessive	Rare	Pacing catheter ablation of WPW
Fabry disease	*GLA*	α-galactosidase A	Glycosphingolipid storage	Xq22	Preexcitation, AV block, VT, AF, HCM phenocopy	X-linked recessive	Rare	Transplant, pacing, enzyme stabilization/ replacement
Pompe disease	*GLA*	α-glucosidase	Lysosome glycogenolysis	17q25	Preexcitation, conduction disease, HCM phenocopy	Autosomal recessive	Rare	Pacing enzyme replacement

Figure 7-39. *(Continued)* Inherited structural cardiomyopathies including hypertrophic cardiomyopathy (HCM) and arrhythmogenic right ventricular cardiomyopathy/dysplasia (ARVC/D) frequently manifest ventricular tachycardia (VT) and are the most common cause of SCD in competitive athletes in the United States and Italy, respectively. More than 400 mutations of various components of the sarcomere are associated with HCM. ARVC/D is a disease of the desmosome, resulting in fibrofatty replacement of the right ventricular myocardium. Rare glycogen storage, metabolic/infiltrative, and lysosomal disorders include cardiac manifestations of ventricular preexcitation, atrioventricular (AV) conduction defects, and ventricular arrhythmias [18,28]. AF—atrial fibrillation; ICD—implantable cardioverter defibrillator; LBBB—left bundle branch block; PMVT—polymorphic VT; TdP—torsade de pointes; VF—ventricular fibrillation; WPW—Wolff-Parkinson-White.

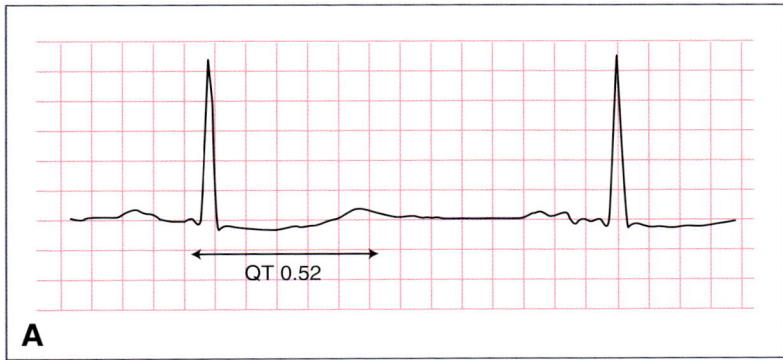

A

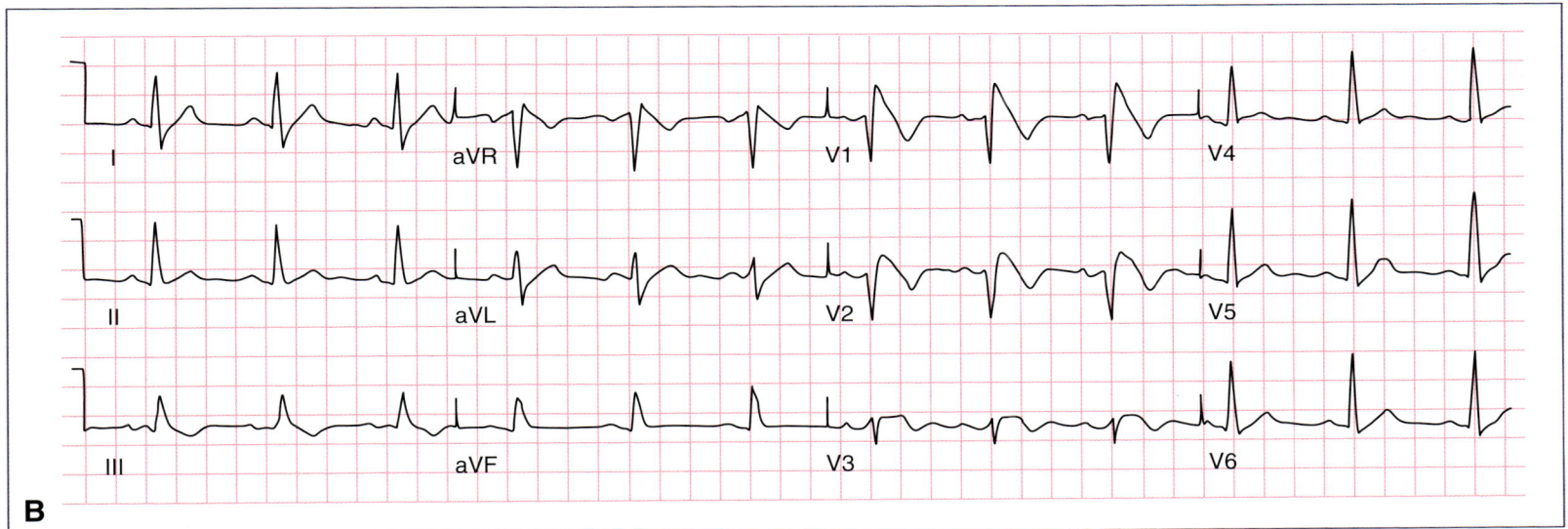

B

Figure 7-40. Familial sudden death syndromes. Electrocardiogram (ECG) findings in two different patients, both of whom have had first-degree relatives suddenly, unexpectedly die. **A,** The QT interval is prolonged to 0.52 seconds in the absence of any medications that prolong the QT. These findings are consistent with the long QT syndrome. **B,** The ECG is typical of a Brugada-type ECG, with J-point elevation exceeding 2 mm in V1 to V3 and flat ST segments.

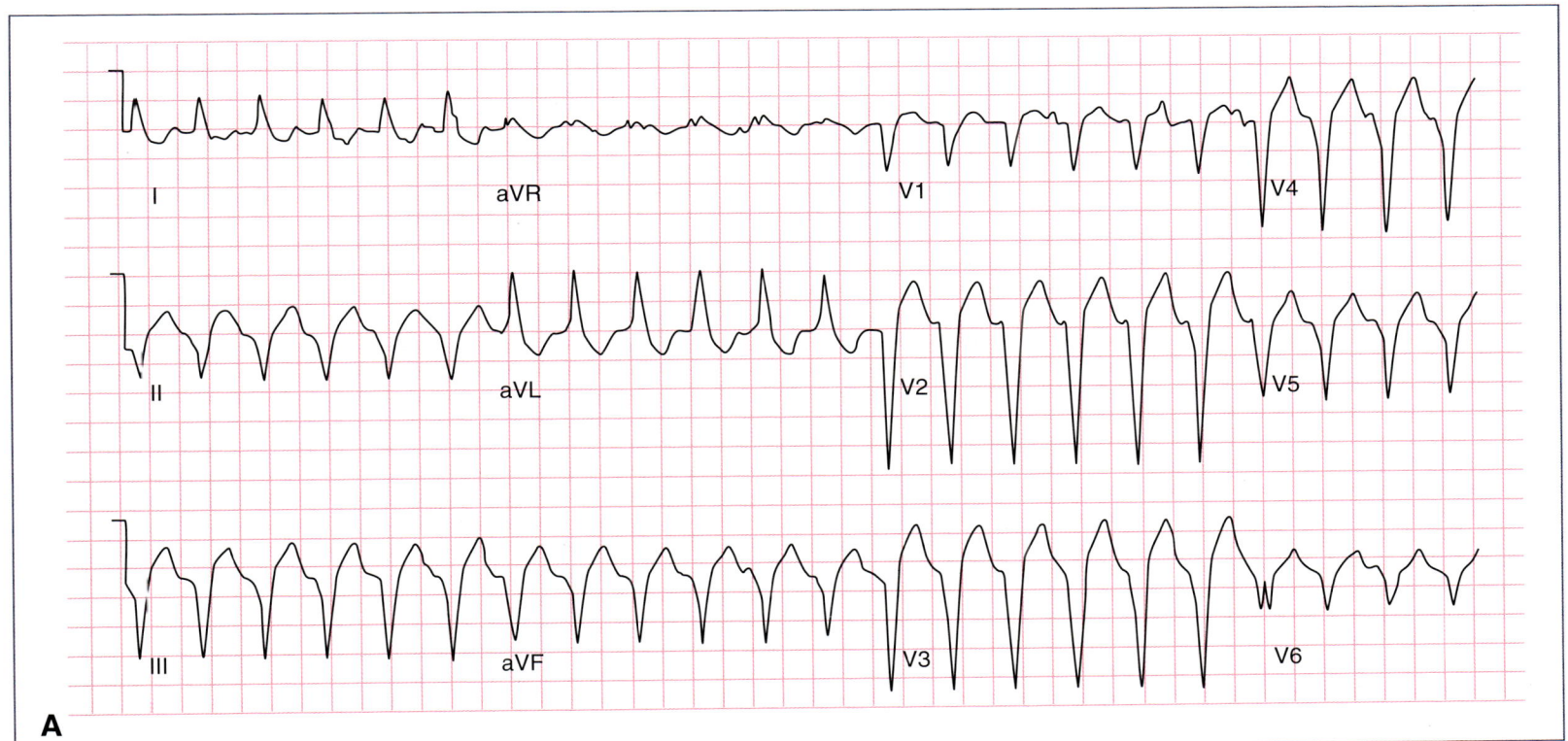

A

Figure 7-41. *Continued on the next page*

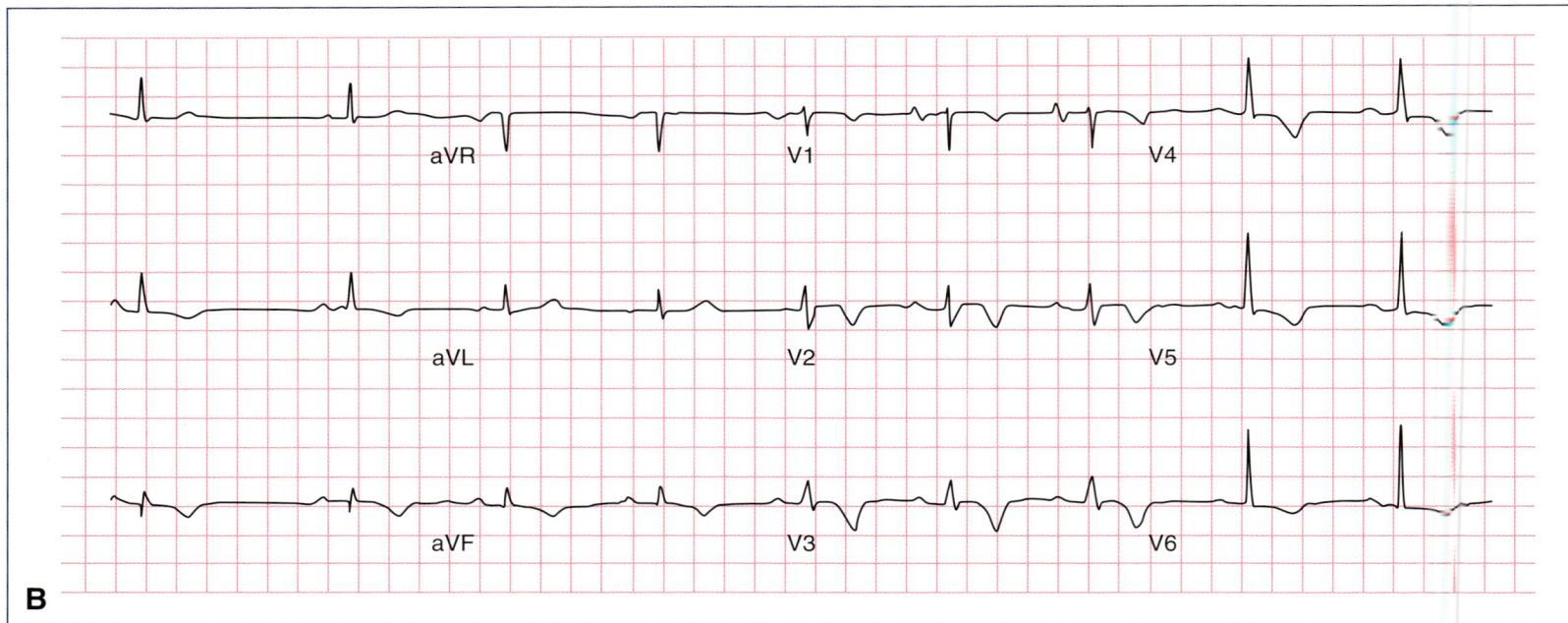

B

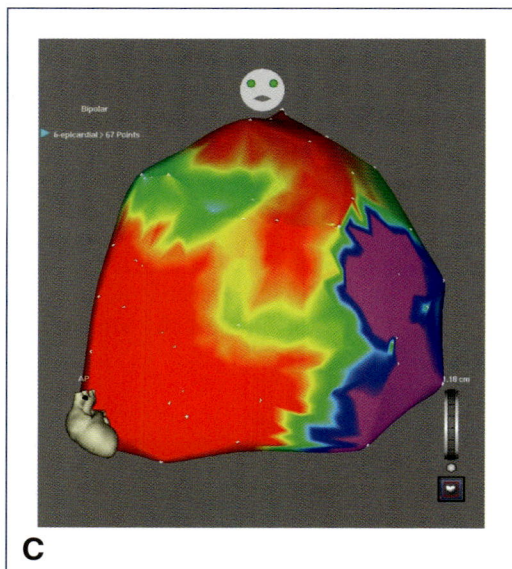

C

Figure 7-41. *(Continued)* Arrhythmogenic right ventricular dysplasia/cardiomyopathy. **A,** The patient presented with sustained monomorphic ventricular tachycardia, which had a left bundle branch block configuration, consistent with an origin from the right ventricle (RV). Atrioventricular dissociation is present. The frontal plane axis is directed superiorly, indicating an exit on the inferior wall, in contrast to the most common idiopathic RV tachycardias that originate in the RV outflow tract. **B,** Following conversion, the sinus rhythm electrocardiogram is usually abnormal, most frequently showing T-wave inversions in leads V1 to V3, and often a slurred upstroke to the S-wave in V2 as is present here. **C,** At electrophysiologic study, RV mapping demonstrated that the septum had normal voltage, more than 1.5 mv *(purple)*, but the free wall of the RV had extensive low-voltage regions consistent with scar. Magnetic resonance imaging often shows scar in these patients, as well. Multiple ventricular tachycardias are common and, in contrast to idiopathic RV tachycardias, there is risk of sudden death, such that an implantable cardioverter defibrillator should be considered [18,29].

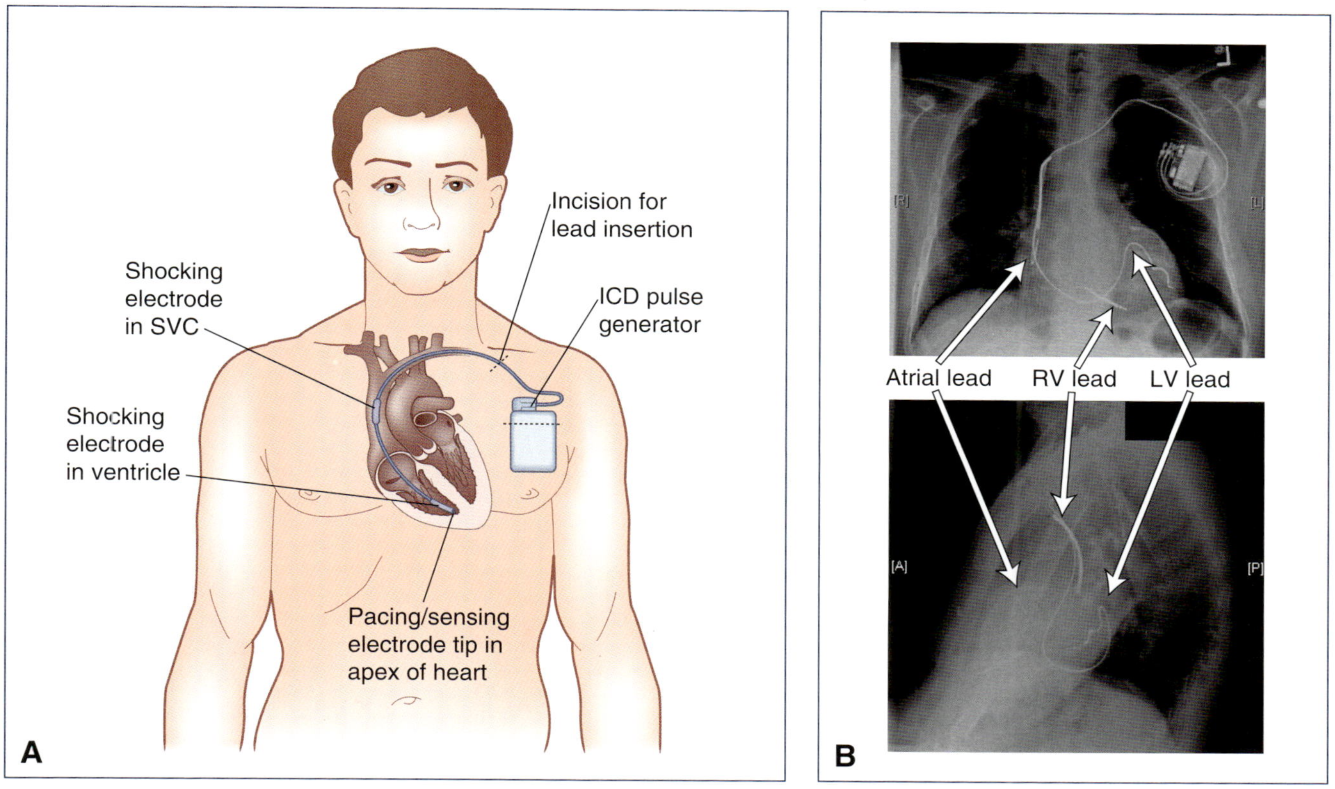

Implantable Defibrillators for Preventing Sudden Death

Figure 7-42. Implantable cardioverter defibrillator (ICD). **A**, The simple ICD system consists of a right ventricular (RV) lead and pulse generator. Pacing is provided from the RV and high voltage shocks for defibrillation or cardioversion are applied between the coil electrode in the RV and the titanium casing of the pulse generator, and sometimes to an additional coil in the superior vena cava (SVC), or an electrode array placed subcutaneously in the chest wall (not shown). Vascular access for the ICD leads is usually obtained via the left axillary, subclavian, or cephalic vein. **B**, Posteroanterior (*top*) and lateral (*bottom*) chest radiograph of an ICD system that incorporates atrial and biventricular (RV and left ventricle [LV]) pacing.

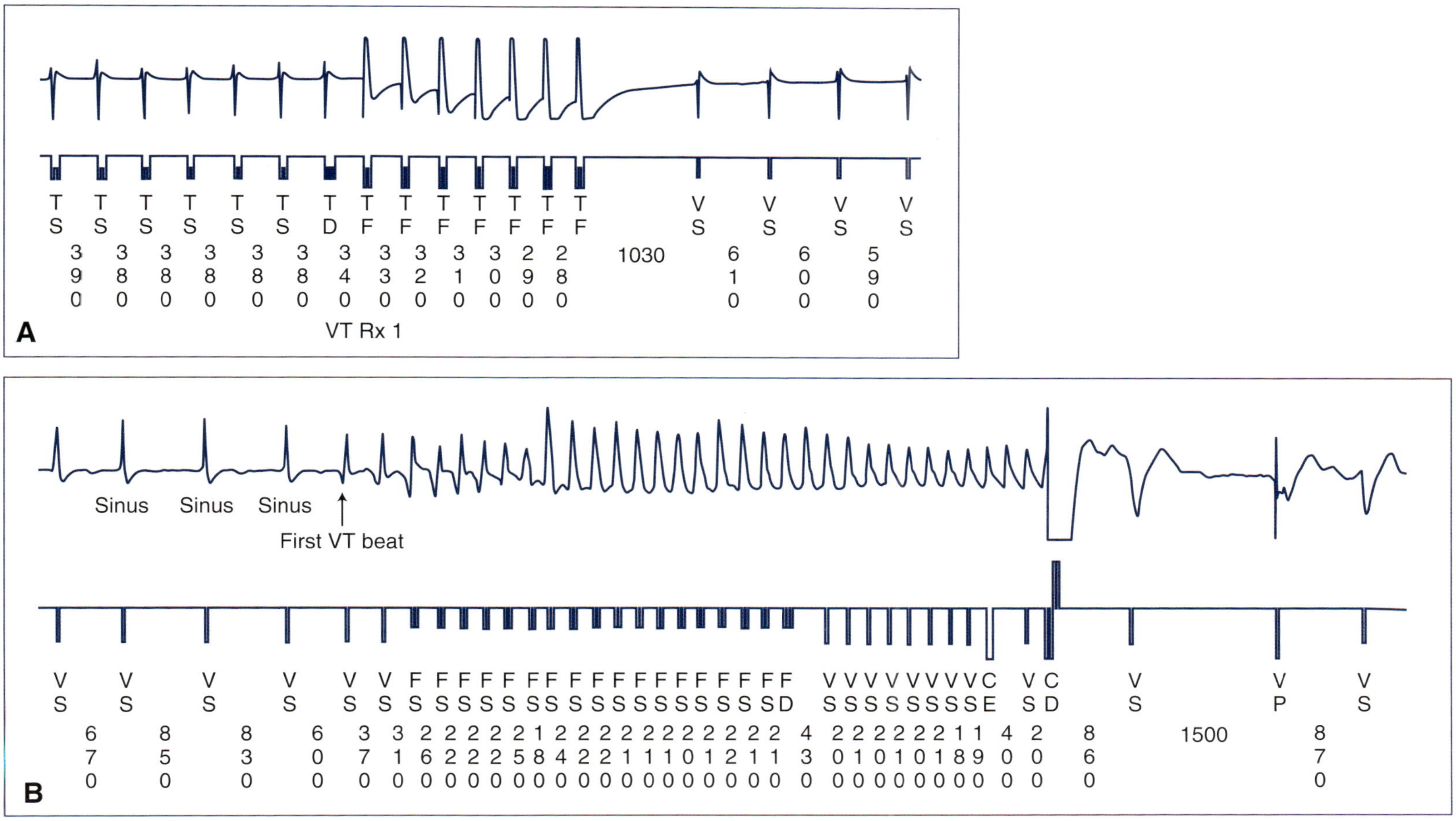

Figure 7-43. *Continued on the next page*

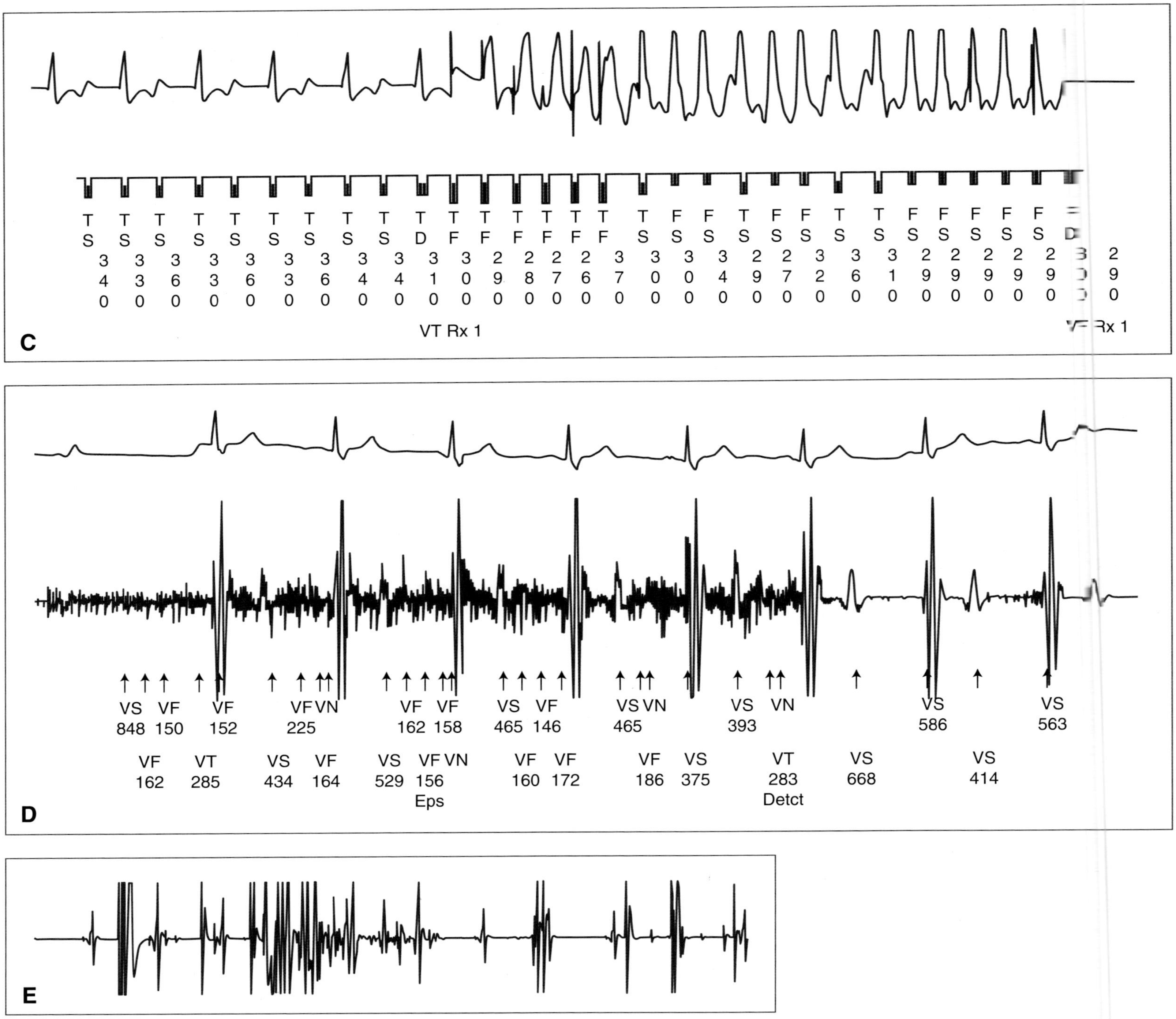

C

VT Rx 1

VF Rx 1

D

| VS | VF | | VF | VF VN | | VF | VF | | VS | VF | | VS VN | | VS | VN | | VS | | VS |
| 848 | 150 | 152 | | 225 | | 162 | 158 | | 465 | 146 | | 465 | | 393 | | | 586 | | 563 |

VF	VT		VS	VF		VS	VF VN		VF	VF		VF	VS		VT		VS		VS
162	285		434	164		529	156		160	172		186	375		283		668		414
							Eps								Detct				

E

Figure 7-43. Implantable cardioverter defibrillator (ICD) stored electrograms showing ICD function and malfunction. ICDs record electrograms of arrhythmia events. **A,** Information obtained from an ICD interrogation of an episode of sustained monomorphic ventricular tachycardia (VT) (cycle length 380–390 ms) successfully terminated by "ramp" antitachycardia pacing (ATP) (progressively shortening the cycle length from 340–280 ms). At the top of the tracing is the electrogram recorded from the right ventricular (RV) electrodes, followed by a marker channel provided by the device that indicates the device function. Termination of VT by pacing is referred to as ATP. **B,** Detection and termination of ventricular fibrillation. In this tracing from an ICD interrogation, sinus rhythm is followed by a premature ventricular contraction (PVC) that initiates a rapid irregular ventricular rate consistent with VF that has a cycle length varying between 180 and 220 ms. After 32 beats, a high-voltage shock (CD) is applied that terminates VF. The patient recovers with a slow rhythm treated with ventricular pacing (VP).

C, D, and **E,** Examples of T-wave oversensing, ICD lead malfunction, and ICD oversensing, respectively. During sinus rhythm, double counting of R and T waves led to VT detection, triggering therapy with ATP (C) ATP initiates VF, which was detected and treated with a single shock (not shown). Oversensing of diaphragmatic myopotentials (D). The patient received multiple shocks while having a bowel movement. Interrogation showed sensing of diaphragmatic myopotentials (rapid potentials) with Valsalva maneuvers, sensed by the ICD as VF. Lead fracture (E). Electrical noise (large, sharp spikes) was detected as VF. In this case, the shock was aborted when decreased noise at a later strip allowed for detection of sinus rhythm. Lead malfunctions are the most common cause of ICD system malfunction. Lead fractures or insulation fractures require replacement of the ICD lead. TS—sensed event that meets tachycardia cycle length; TP—tachycardia pacing to terminate the arrhythmia; VS—ventricular sensed event after VT is terminated. (*Adapted from* Maisel and Kramer [30].)

Randomized Trials of ICD Versus Drug Therapy

Trial	Treatment groups	Patients	Results
AVID	Amiodarone or EP-guided sotalol therapy vs ICD	SCD survivors, VT + syncope + EF ≤ 40%	Lower mortality with ICD
CASH	Amiodarone vs β-blocker vs propafenone vs ICD	SCD survivors with inducible VT/VF	Lower mortality with ICD
CIDS	Amiodarone vs ICD	SCD survivors, VT + syncope; symptomatic VT + EF ≤ 35%	No mortality benefit for ICD
CABG-Patch	CABG alone vs CABG + ICD	Elective CABG, positive SAECG, EF ≤ 35%	No mortality benefit for ICD
MADIT	Medical therapy vs ICD	NSVT, QWMI, EF ≤ 35%, inducible VT/VF at EP study	Lower mortality with ICD
MUSTT	No therapy vs ICD vs drugs	CAD, asymptomatic NSVT, EF ≤ 40%	Lower mortality with ICD
MADIT II	Medical therapy vs ICD	CAD, LVEF ≤ 0.30	Lower mortality with ICD
DEFINITE	Medical therapy vs ICD	Nonischemic CM, LVEF, < 0.36, NSVT	Nonsignificant lower mortality with ICD
SCD-HeFT	Amiodarone vs placebo vs ICD	Heart failure, LVED ≤ 35%, NYHA II/III	Lower mortality with ICD
DINAMIT	Medical therapy vs ICD	< 42 days after acute MI, LVEF	No ICD benefit

Figure 7-44. Randomized trials of implantable cardioverter defibrillator (ICD) versus medical therapy. Several large-scale prospective trials (AVID, CAD, CASH, CIDS) have compared ICD therapy with medical therapy for secondary prevention of sudden death after survival of cardiac arrest or sustained ventricular tachycardia (VT); or for primary prevention of sudden death in high-risk subjects who have not yet experienced a life-threatening arrhythmia. AVID—Antiarrhythmic Versus Implantable Defibrillator; CABG—coronary artery bypass graft; CAD—coronary artery disease; CASH—Cardiac Arrest Hamburg Study; CIDS—Canadian Implantable Defibrillator Study; CM—cardiomyopathy; DEFINITE—Defibrillators in Nonischemic Cardiomyopathy Treatment Evaluation; DINAMIT—Defibrillator in Acute Myocardial Infarction Trial; EF—ejection fraction; EP—electrophysiology; LVEF—left ventricular ejection fraction; MADIT and MADIT II—Multicenter Automatic Defibrillator Implantation Trials; MI—myocardial infarction; MUSTT—Multicenter Unsustained Tachycardia Trial; NYHA—New York Heart Association; NSVT—nonsustained VT; QWMI—Q-wave myocardial infarction; SAECG—signal averaged electrocardiogram; SCD—sudden cardiac death; SCD-HeFT—Sudden Cardiac Death in Heart Failure Trial; VT—ventricular tachycardia [18,31–37].

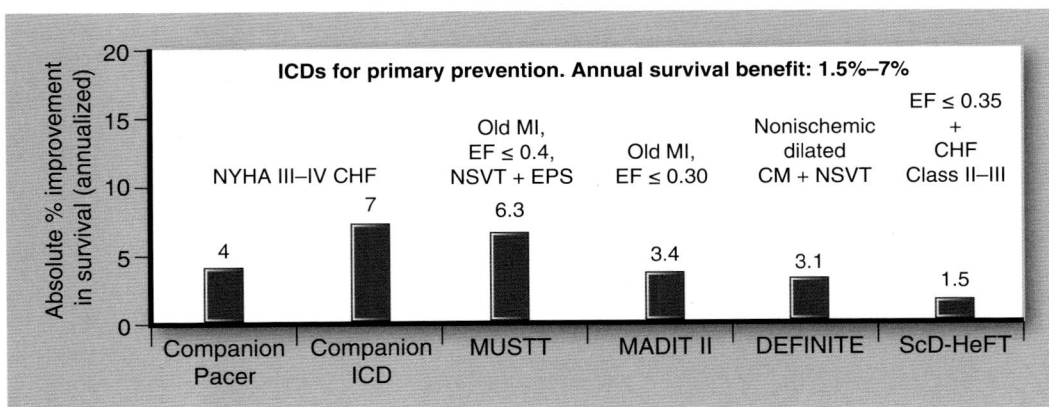

Figure 7-45. Mortality benefit of implantable cardioverter defibrillators (ICDs) for primary prevention of sudden death. The annual reduction in mortality is summarized for trials of biventricular pacing, biventricular ICD, and ICDs in the risk groups shown. In these studies, one can estimate that devices save 1.5 to seven lives per year for every 100 ICDs implanted. Benefit increases with longer follow-up, provided that competing causes of mortality, such as heart failure, do not intervene [31,33–35,37,38]. CHF—congestive heart failure; CM—cardiomyopathy; DEFINITE—Defibrillators in Nonischemic Cardiomyopathy Treatment Evaluation; EF—ejection fraction; EPS—electrophysiologic study; MADIT II—Multicenter Automatic Defibrillator Implantation Trial II; MI—myocardial infarction; NVST—nonsustained ventricular tachycardia; NYHA—New York Heart Association; ScD-HeFT—Sudden Cardiac Death in Heart Failure.

Guidelines for Selecting Patients for ICDs

Class I: ICD implantation is indicated:

VF or hemodynamically unstable VT not due to a transient or reversible cause

Spontaneous sustained VT with structural heart disease

Syncope of undetermined origin with clinical relevant, hemodynamically significant sustained VT or VF induced at electrophysiological study

Status post-MI (> 40 days) with LVEF < 35% at NYHA class II or III

Nonischemic dilative cardiomyopathy with LVEF ≤ 35% at NYHA class II or III

Status post-MI (> 40 days) with LVEF < 30% who are NYHA class I

Nonsustained VT, prior MI with LVEF < 40% and sustained VT or VF induced at EP study

Class IIa: ICD implantation is reasonable:

Unexplained syncope, significant LV dysfunction in nonischemic dilated cardiomyopathy

Sustained VT with normal or near-normal LVEF

Hypertrophic cardiomyopathy with a major risk factor for SCD

ARVD with a major risk factor for SCD

Long-QT syndrome with syncope or VT while receiving β-blocker

Patients on heart transplant waiting list who are out of hospital

Brugada syndrome with syncope or VT

Catecholaminergic polymorphic VT with syncope or sustained VT while receiving β-blocker

Cardiac sarcoidosis, Chagas disease, or giant cell myocarditis

Class IIb: ICD may be considered:

Nonischemic cardiomyopathy with LVEF ≤ 35% in functional class I

Long-QT syndrome and risk factors for SCD

Syncope of unclear cause after investigation in the setting of advanced structural heart disease

Familial cardiomyopathy associated with SCD

LV noncompaction

Class II: ICD is not indicated

Life expectancy < 1 y even if ICD criteria specified above is met

Incessant VT of VF

Psychiatric illness potentially aggravated by the ICD/precluding follow-up

Drug refractory NYHA class IV heart failure who are not candidates for transplantation or CRT implantation

Syncope of undetermined cause without structural heart disease with no VT inducible at EP study

VT or VF is amenable to surgical or catheter ablation cure (AF with WPW syndrome, idiopathic or fascicular VT without structural heart disease)

Figure 7-46. Recommendations for using implantable cardiac devices (ICDs) to prevent sudden death. Class I: evidence and general agreement is present that treatment is useful. Class II: usefulness is less well established or evidence is conflicting (IIa, consensus favors; IIb, less well established). Class III: evidence or general agreement is that the therapy is not useful or is harmful. All indications require that the patients have an acceptable prognosis and quality of life for 1 year [18,31]. AF—atrial fibrillation; ARVD—arrhythmogenic right ventricular dysplasia; EP—electrophysiology ICD—implantable cardioverter defibrillator; LVEF—left ventricular rejection fraction; MI—myocardial infarction; MUSTT—Multicenter Unsustained Tachycardia Trial; NYHA—New York Heart Association; SCD—sudden cardiac death; VF—ventricular fibrillation; VT—ventricular tachycardia; WPW—Wolf-Parkinson-White.

Cardiac Pacing

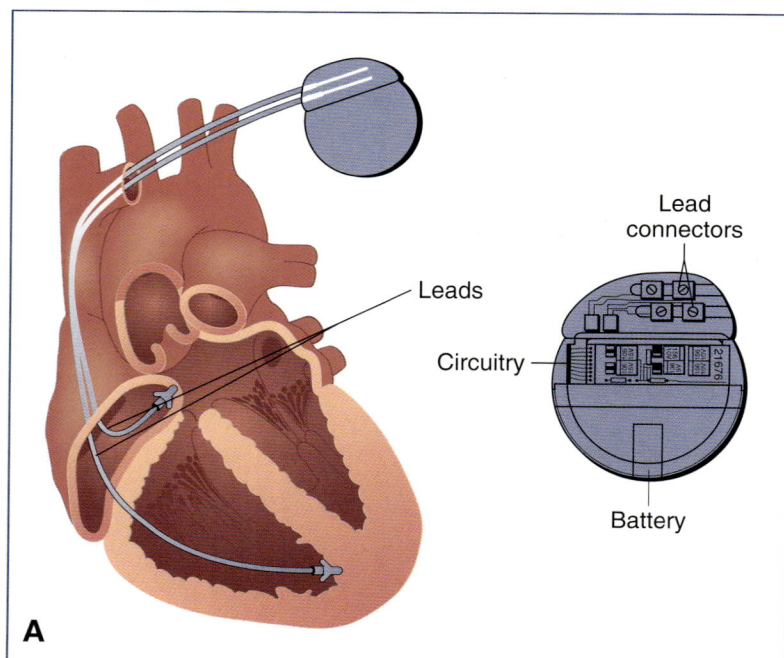

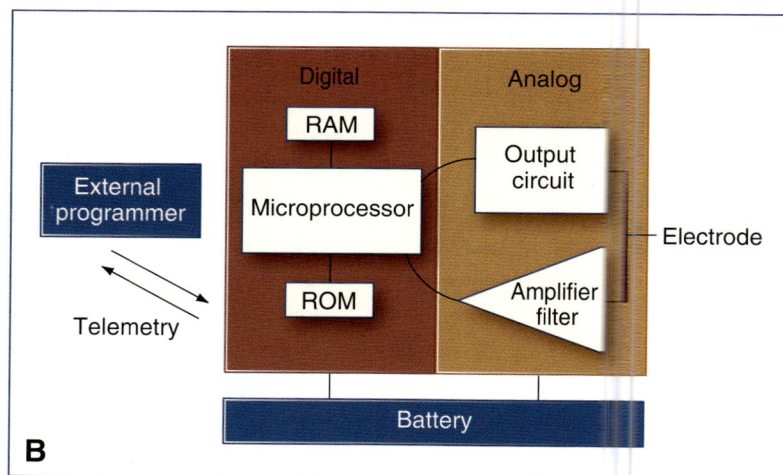

Figure 7-47. **A,** A dual chamber cardiac pacemaker. The pulse generator contains circuits and microprocessors that perform the logic chores of the pacemaker, including storage of programmable settings and interpretation and response to various sensed and paced cardiac electrical events, as well as the control of radiofrequency telemetry communications with external programmers.

Continued on the next page

Figure 7-47. *(Continued)* The microprocessor is dependent on a highly precise timer circuit based on a crystal oscillator. Many devices (**B**) employ both "read-only memory" (ROM), which contains the pacing algorithm, and "read and write memory" (RAM) for data, including programmed settings, device identification, and storage of a wide array of measured data values. While the pacing algorithm and memory functions of the pacemaker represent the digital side of the device, certain analog elements, including filters and amplifiers for detecting intrinsic cardiac activity and controlling pacing output levels at appropriate intervals as instructed by the microprocessor, are necessary components as well. All of these components are mounted on a circuit board and placed along with the battery within a hermetically sealed container, usually a titanium canister.

NASPE/BPEG Generic (NBG) Pacemaker Code*

Position	I	II	III	IV	V
Category	Chamber(s) paced	Chamber(s) sensed	Response to sensing	Programmability rate modulation	Antitachyarrhythmia functions
	O = none	O = none	O = none	O = none	O = none
	A = atrium	A = atrium	T = triggered	P = simple programmable	P = pacing (antitachyarrhythmia)
	V = ventricle	V = ventricle	I = inhibited	M = multiprogrammable	S = shock
	D = dual (A + V)	D = dual (A + V)	D = dual (T + I)	C = communicating	D = dual (P + S)
	S = single (A or V)†	S = Single (A or V)†		R = rate modulation	

*Positions I through III are used exclusive for antibradyarrhythmia functions.
†Manufacturer's designation only.

Figure 7-48. Modes of cardiac pacing. The mode of cardiac pacing refers to the way in which the pacemaker interacts with the underlying cardiac rhythm. The various modes may be described by the shorthand code suggested by the North American Society of Pacing and Electrophysiology (NASPE) and the British Pacing and Electrophysiology Group (BPEG) Pacemaker Code, 1987. A—atrial channel events; P—pace event; S—sensing event; V—ventricular channel events. (*Adapted from* Bernstein *et al.* [39].)

Pacing for Cardiac Resynchronization Therapy

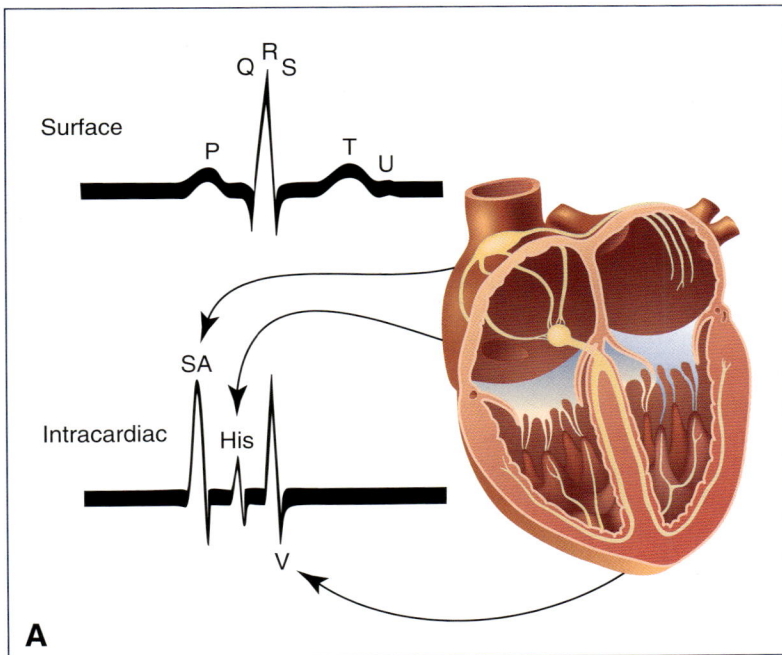

Figure 7-49. The importance of the sequence of ventricular activation. **A**, The intact specialized interventricular conduction system results in the rapid, ordered, and precisely timed activation of both left and right cardiac chambers and regional (septal) segments, as well as the natural repolarization sequence, resulting in optimal stroke volume. Documentation of various pacing methods has highlighted the importance of the ventricular activation sequence and the potential limitations inherent with long-term pacing from the right ventricular apex. Pacing modes that allow for ventricular activation using the native specialized conduction system (AAI and DDD) result in greater cardiac output at rest and exercise (**B**), perhaps largely due to intact septal activation and right-left heart synchrony [31]. AAI—atrial pacing, sensing, inhibition; DDD—dual chamber pacing; His—His bundle; SA—sinoatrial node; VVI—ventricular pacing, sensing, inhibition.

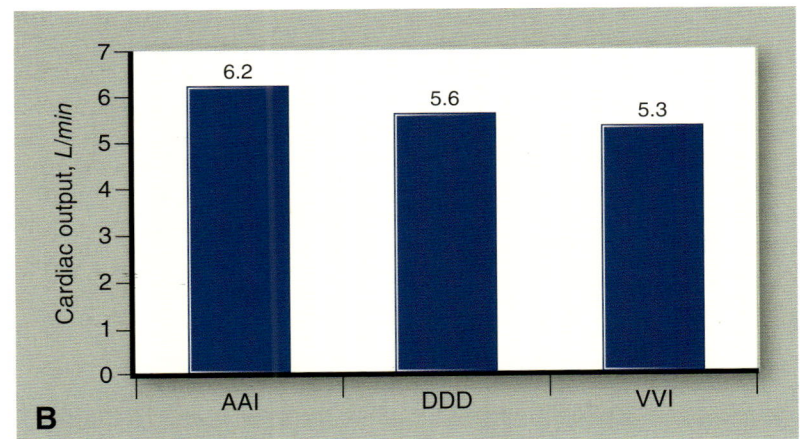

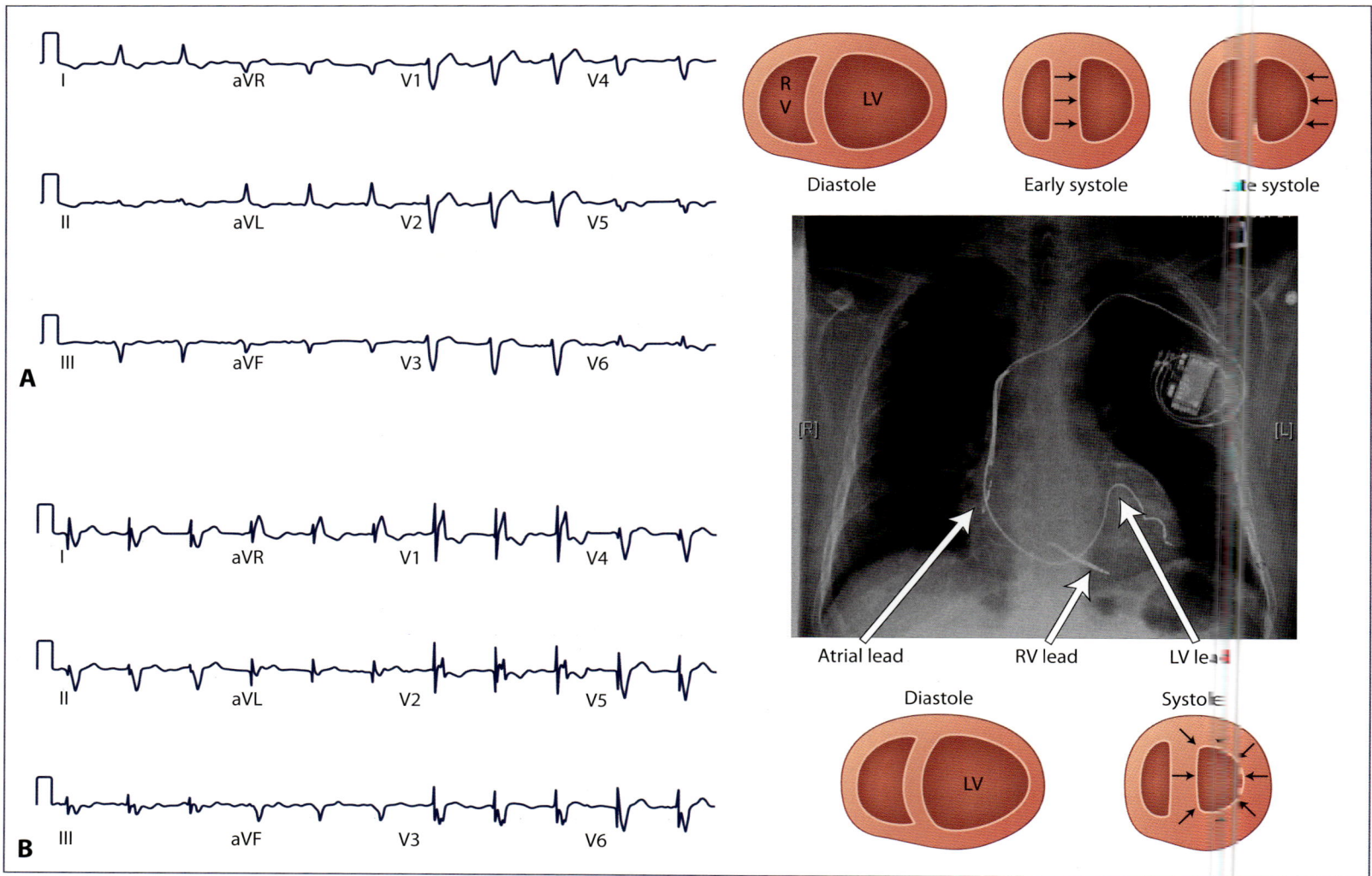

Figure 7-50. Biventricular pacing to improve cardiac function. **A,** Left bundle branch block produces interventricular conduction delay and dyschronous cardiac contraction as shown in the schematics of the heart as viewed from the left anterior oblique perspective (*right*). In early systole, the septum contracts before the lateral left ventricle (LV) wall. The lateral wall is passive and may move away from the septum, inefficiently absorbing the septal force of contraction. Later in systole, the lateral wall contracts after the septum has completed contraction. Dyschrony reduces mechanical efficiency of the heart. Dyschrony is also produced by pacing from the right ventricular (RV) apex. In patients with ventricular dysfunction, RV apical pacing was associated with increased mortality and heart failure hospitalizations [40]. Therefore, pacemakers and implantable cardioverter defibrillators should generally be programmed to minimize the amount of RV apical pacing applied when atrioventricular conduction is intact, particularly if the conducted QRS complex is narrow. **B,** Resynchronization by pacing simultaneously from the RV and lateral LV attempts to restore simultaneous contraction of the septum and lateral LV wall, improving efficiency. Cardiac resynchronization therapy is implemented by implanting pacing devices with a lead in the right atrium, RV, and a lateral branch of the coronary sinus or directly into the epicardium at cardiac surgery to allow pacing of the LV. The lead positions are shown in the chest radiogram. Cardiac resynchronization therapy improves acute hemodynamics and may reduce mitral regurgitation and result in ventricular remodeling. Of patients with QRS duration longer than 130 ms who have heart failure, approximately two thirds have an improvement in cardiac function and symptoms with this therapy. Following resynchronization, electrocardiogram often shows a shift in the QRS axis rightward and anteriorly and may narrow. Approximately 30% of patients with chronic heart failure have LV conduction delays [31]

813 Patients

Dilated heart failure   (38% ischemic)
LV EF ≤ 35%   (Median EF 25%)
NYHA class   III (93%) or IV (7%)
QRS > 120 ms or dyssynchrony by echo (median QRS 160 ms)
Sinus rhythm

Randomized

CRT pacemaker   Medical therapy

HR = 0.63 CI (0.51–0.77) CRT reduced the primary endpoint:
death + unanticipated hospitalization for major cardiac events

	2-year mortality	Sudden death
CRT	18%	7%
Medical	25%	9%

A

1520 Patients

55% Ischemic cardiomyopathy
NYHA III or IV   (86% Class III)
EF ≤ 35%   (22%)
QRS ≥ 120 ms   (160 ms)
Sinus rhythm

Control group "optimal medical management" n = 308	Cardiac resynchronization pacemaker "CRT" n = 617	Cardiac resynchronization defibrillator "CRT-D" n = 595

| Primary endpoint: | 68%* | 58%* HR = 0.81 CI (0.69–0.96) | 56% HR = 0.80 CI (0.68–0.01) |
| Death + hospitalizations | | | |

* For 1 year of follow-up

B

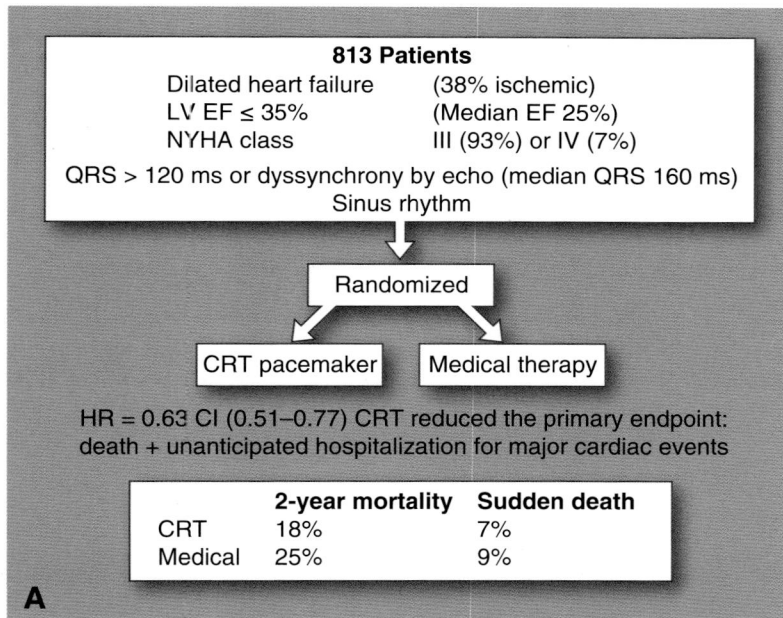

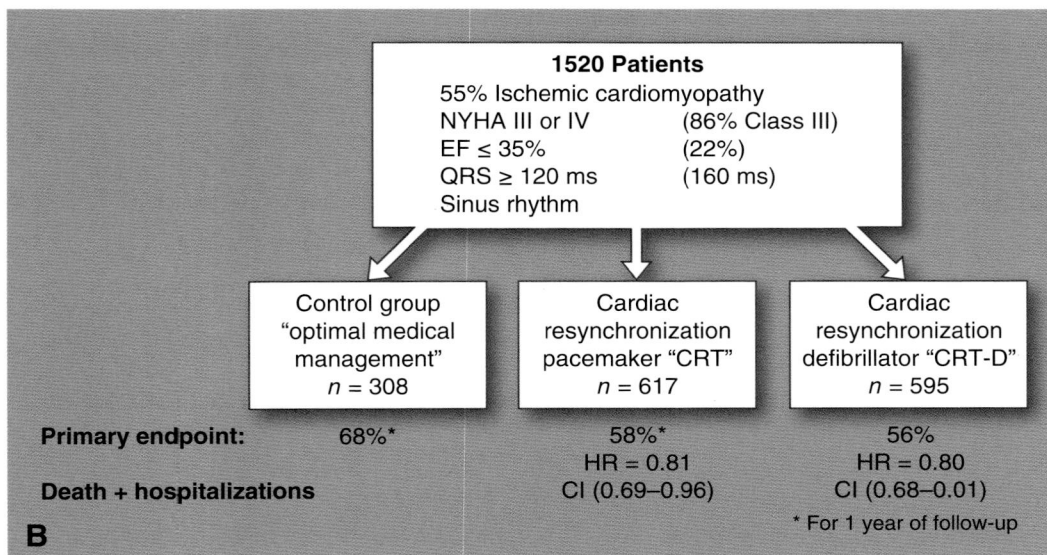

Figure 7-51. Major trials of cardiac resynchronization therapy (CRT). **A,** CARE-HF (Cardiac Resynchronization-Heart Failure) trial. In this trial, 813 patients with heart failure (New York Heart Association [NYHA] class III/IV; left ventricular ejection factor [LVEF] < 35%) and left ventricular dyschrony were randomly assigned to medical therapy alone or medical therapy with CRT with a biventricular pacemaker that did not incorporate tachycardia therapy (no implantable cardioverter defibrillator capability). Biventricular pacing significantly reduced the primary endpoint of death and hospitalization for major cardiac events. Cardiac resynchronization also improved LVEF and quality of life [41]. **B,** The COMPANION (Comparison of Medical Therapy, Pacing, and Defibrillation in Chronic Heart Failure) trial randomly assigned 1520 patients who had an LVEF of less than 35%, NYHA class III or IV heart failure from either ischemic or nonischemic cause, and QRS duration greater than 120 ms to 1) medical treatment alone or medical treatment combined with 2) biventricular pacing device or 3) biventricular implantable defibrillator. The combined endpoint of death or hospitalization was reduced by 20% in the device groups compared with the medical treatment group. In this study, the addition of a defibrillator did not result in further benefit in the primary endpoint compared with resynchronization therapy with pacing without an implantable coronary device, but the addition of ICD therapy decreased the risk of death by 36% compared with the medical treatment group [37].

References

1. Marriot HJC, Conover MH: *Advanced Concepts in Arrhythmias.* St Louis: CV Mosby; 1983.

2. Singer DH, Ten Eick RE: Pharmacology of cardiac arrhythmias. *Prog Cardiovasc Dis* 1969, 11:488–514.

3. Corporation CPCDoC-G: *The CIBA Collection of Medical Illustrations by Frank H. Netter, MD*: CIBA-Geigy; 1969.

4. Kleber AG, Rudy Y: Basic mechanisms of cardiac impulse propagation and associated arrhythmias. *Physiol Rev* 2004, 84:431–488.

5. Wit AL, Bigger JT: Possible electrophysiologic mechanism for lethal arrhythmias accompanying myocardial ischemia and infarction. *Circulation* 1975, 3(Suppl 51,52):96.

6. Evans TS: *Electrocardiographic Test Set: Basic Electrocardiography and Cardiac Arrhythmias,* edn 2. Thomas Evans; 1993.

7. Blomstrom-Lundqvist C, Scheinman MM, Aliot EM, et al.: ACC/AHA/ESC guidelines for the management of patients with supraventricular arrhythmias—executive summary: a report of the American College of Cardiology/American Heart Association Task Force on Practice Guidelines and the European Society of Cardiology Committee for Practice Guidelines (Writing Committee to Develop Guidelines for the Management of Patients With Supraventricular Arrhythmias). Circulation 2003, 108:1871–1909.

8. Kistler PM, Roberts-Thomson KC, Haqqani HM, et al.: P-wave morphology in focal atrial tachycardia: development of an algorithm to predict the anatomic site of origin. J Am Coll Cardiol 2006, 48:1010–1017.

9. Saoudi N, Cosio F, Waldo A, et al.: Classification of atrial flutter and regular atrial tachycardia according to electrophysiologic mechanism and anatomic bases: a statement from a joint expert group from the Working Group of Arrhythmias of the European Society of Cardiology and the North American Society of Pacing and Electrophysiology. J Cardiovasc Electrophysiol 2001, 12:852–866.

10. Iwai S, Markowitz SM, Stein KM, et al.: Response to adenosine differentiates focal from macroreentrant atrial tachycardia: validation using three-dimensional electroanatomic mapping. Circulation 2002, 106:2793–2799.

11. Chugh A, Latchamsetty R, Oral H, et al.: Characteristics of cavotricuspid isthmus-dependent atrial flutter after left atrial ablation of atrial fibrillation. Circulation 2006, 113:609–615.

12. Fuster V, Ryden LE, Cannom DS, et al.: ACC/AHA/ESC 2006 Guidelines for the Management of Patients with Atrial Fibrillation: a report of the American College of Cardiology/American Heart Association Task Force on Practice Guidelines and the European Society of Cardiology Committee for Practice Guidelines (Writing Committee to Revise the 2001 Guidelines for the Management of Patients With Atrial Fibrillation): developed in collaboration with the European Heart Rhythm Association and the Heart Rhythm Society. Circulation 2006, 114:e257–e354.

13. Calkins H, Brugada J, Packer DL, et al.: HRS/EHRA/ECAS Expert Consensus Statement on catheter and surgical ablation of atrial fibrillation: recommendations for personnel, policy, procedures, and follow-up. A report of the Heart Rhythm Society (HRS) Task Force on catheter and surgical ablation of atrial fibrillation. Heart Rhythm 2007, 4:816–861.

14. Peters NS, Schilling RJ, Kanagaratnam P, Markides V: Atrial fibrillation: strategies to control, combat, and cure. Lancet 2002, 359:593–603.

15. Oral H, Chugh A, Ozaydin M, et al.: Risk of thromboembolic events after percutaneous left atrial radiofrequency ablation of atrial fibrillation. Circulation 2006, 114:759–765.

16. Savelieva I, Camm J: Anti-arrhythmic drug therapy for atrial fibrillation: current anti-arrhythmic drugs, investigational agents, and innovative approaches. Europace 2008, 10:647–665.

17. Singh BN, Connolly SJ, Crijns HJ, et al.: Dronedarone for maintenance of sinus rhythm in atrial fibrillation or flutter. N Engl J Med 2007, 357:987–999.

18. Zipes DP, Camm AJ, Borggrefe M, et al.: ACC/AHA/ESC 2006 guidelines for management of patients with ventricular arrhythmias and the prevention of sudden cardiac death: a report of the American College of Cardiology/American Heart Association Task Force and the European Society of Cardiology Committee for Practice Guidelines (Writing Committee to Develop Guidelines for Management of Patients With Ventricular Arrhythmias and the Prevention of Sudden Cardiac Death). J Am Coll Cardiol 2006, 48:e247–e346.

19. Brugada P, Brugada J, Mont L, et al.: A new approach to the differential diagnosis of a regular tachycardia with a wide QRS complex. Circulation 1991, 83:1649–1659.

20. de Bakker JM, van Capelle FJ, Janse MJ, et al.: Slow conduction in the infarcted human heart. "Zigzag" course of activation. Circulation 1993, 88:915–926.

21. Stevenson WG, Soejima K: Catheter ablation for ventricular tachycardia. Circulation 2007, 115:2750–2760.

22. Moss AJ, Greenberg H, Case RB, et al.: Long-term clinical course of patients after termination of ventricular tachyarrhythmia by an implanted defibrillator. Circulation 2004, 110:3760–3765.

23. Connolly SJ, Dorian P, Roberts RS, et al.: Comparison of beta-blockers, amiodarone plus beta-blockers, or sotalol for prevention of shocks from implantable cardioverter defibrillators: the OPTIC Study: a randomized trial. JAMA 2006, 295:165–171.

24. Marchlinski FE, Callans DJ, Gottlieb CD, Zado E: Linear ablation lesions for control of unmappable ventricular tachycardia in patients with ischemic and nonischemic cardiomyopathy. Circulation 2000, 101:1288–1296.

25. Soejima K, Stevenson WG, Sapp JL, et al.: Endocardial and epicardial radiofrequency ablation of ventricular tachycardia associated with dilated cardiomyopathy: the importance of low-voltage scars. J Am Coll Cardiol 2004, 43:1834–1842.

26. Zei PC, Stevenson WG: Epicardial catheter mapping and ablation of ventricular tachycardia. Heart Rhythm 2006, 3:360–363.

27. Tada H, Ito S, Naito S, et al.: Idiopathic ventricular arrhythmia arising from the mitral annulus: a distinct subgroup of idiopathic ventricular arrhythmias. J Am Coll Cardiol 2005, 45:877–886.

28. Roden DM: Clinical practice. Long-QT syndrome. N Engl J Med 2008, 358:169–176.

29. Dalal D, Nasir K, Bomma C, et al.: Arrhythmogenic right ventricular dysplasia: a United States experience. Circulation 2005, 112:3823–3832.

30. Maisel WH, Kramer DB: Implantable cardioverter-defibrillator lead performance. Circulation 2008, 117:2721–2723.

31. Epstein AE, DiMarco JP, Ellenbogen KA, et al.: ACC/AHA/HRS 2008 Guidelines for Device-Based Therapy of Cardiac Rhythm Abnormalities: a report of the American College of Cardiology/American Heart Association Task Force on Practice Guidelines (Writing Committee to Revise the ACC/AHA/NASPE 2002 Guideline Update for Implantation of Cardiac Pacemakers and Antiarrhythmia Devices) developed in collaboration with the American Association for Thoracic Surgery and Society of Thoracic Surgeons. J Am Coll Cardiol 2008, 51:e1–e62.

32. Moss AJ, Hall WJ, Cannom DS, et al.: Improved survival with an implanted defibrillator in patients with coronary disease at high risk for ventricular arrhythmia. Multicenter Automatic Defibrillator Implantation Trial Investigators [see comments]. N Engl J Med 1996, 335:1933–1940.

33. Moss AJ, Zareba W, Hall WJ, et al.: Prophylactic implantation of a defibrillator in patients with myocardial infarction and reduced ejection fraction. N Engl J Med 2002, 346:877–883.

34. Kadish A, Dyer A, Daubert JP, et al.: Prophylactic defibrillator implantation in patients with nonischemic dilated cardiomyopathy. N Engl J Med 2004, 350:2151–2158.

35. Bardy GH, Lee KL, Mark DB, et al.: Amiodarone or an implantable cardioverter-defibrillator for congestive heart failure. N Engl J Med 2005, 352:225–237.

36. Hohnloser SH, Kuck KH, Dorian P, et al.: Prophylactic use of an implantable cardioverter-defibrillator after acute myocardial infarction. N Engl J Med 2004, 351:2481–2488.

37. Buxton AE, Lee KL, DiCarlo L, et al.: Electrophysiologic testing to identify patients with coronary artery disease who are at risk for sudden death. Multicenter Unsustained Tachycardia Trial Investigators. N Engl J Med 2000, 342:1937–1945.

38. Bristow MR, Saxon LA, Boehmer J, et al.: Cardiac-resynchronization therapy with or without an implantable defibrillator in advanced chronic heart failure. N Engl J Med 2004, 350:2140–2150.

39. Bernstein AD, Camm AJ, Fletcher RD, et al.: The NASPE/BPEG generic pacemaker code for antibradyarrhythmia and adaptive-rate pacing and antitachyarrhythmia devices. Pacing Clin Electrophysiol 1987, 10:794–799.

40. Wilkoff BL: The Dual Chamber and VVI Implantable Defibrillator (DAVID) Trial: rationale, design, results, clinical implications, and lessons for future trials. Card Electrophysiol Rev 2003, 7:468–472.

41. Cleland JG, Daubert JC, Erdmann E, et al.: The effect of cardiac resynchronization on morbidity and mortality in heart failure. N Engl J Med 2005, 352:1539–1549.

Hypertension

8

Norman K. Hollenberg and Peter Libby

Epidemiology of Hypertension

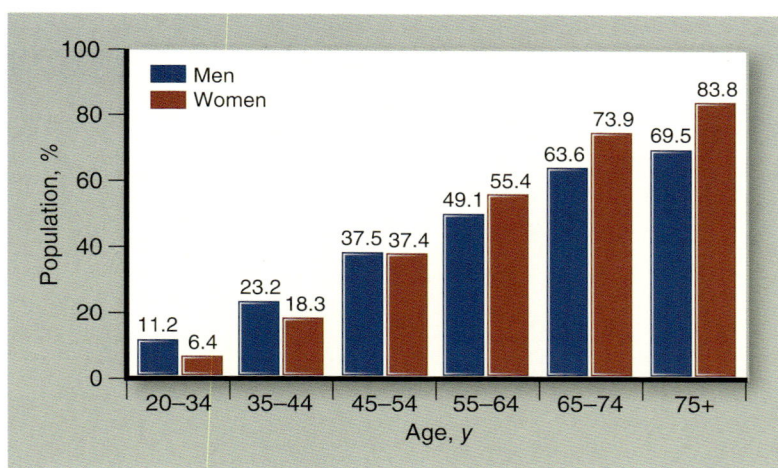

Figure 8-1. This chart shows the prevalence of hypertension in Americans age 20 years and older by age and sex [1].

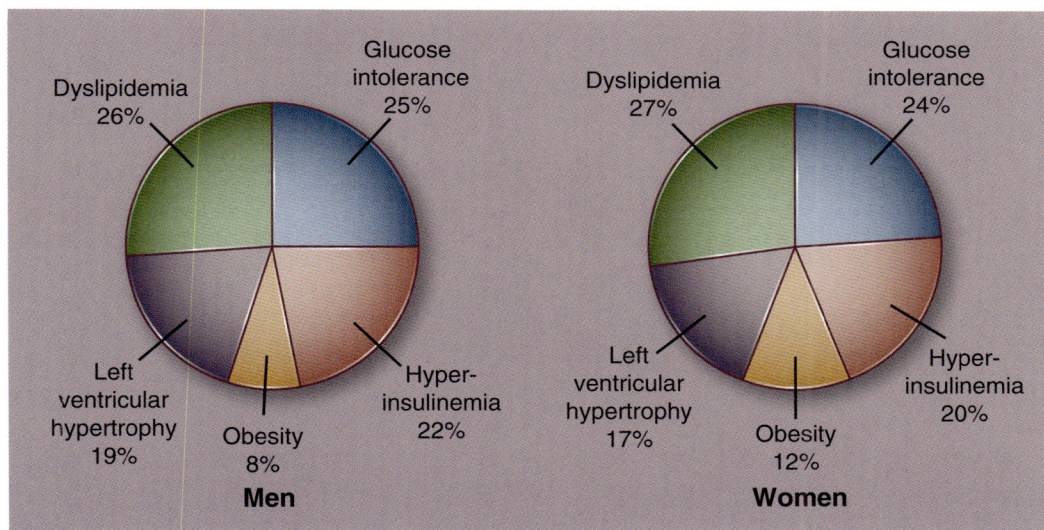

Figure 8-2. According to data from the Framingham Study, elevated blood pressure has a tendency to present with other major risk factors for coronary artery disease, including obesity, dyslipidemia, glucose intolerance, and left ventricular hypertrophy. More than half of patients with hypertension will experience a cluster of two or more risk factors, a frequency twice that expected by chance. Clusters of three or more occur at four times the expected rate. The absence of one or more of the following—dyslipidemia, glucose intolerance, hyperinsulinemia, obesity, and left ventricular hypertrophy—accounts for less than 20% of hypertension [2].

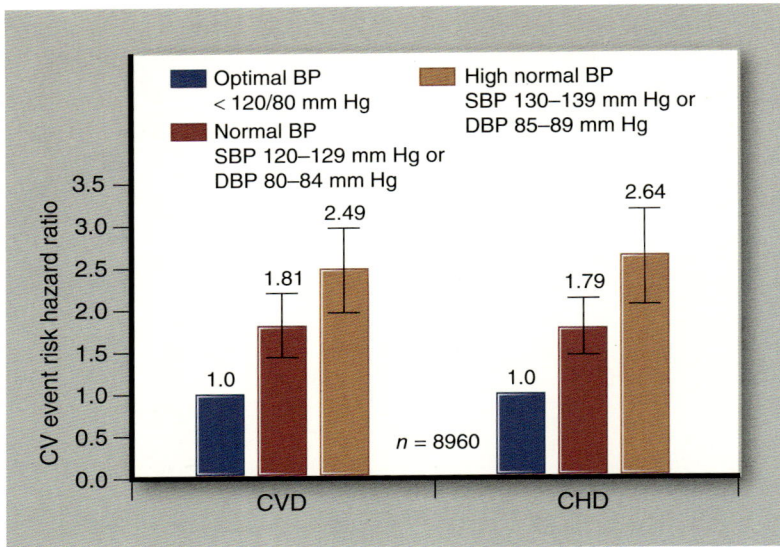

Figure 8-3. Blood pressure (BP) usually considered normal is associated with elevated risk for cardiovascular disease (CVD). The Atherosclerosis Risk in Communities study, a prospective epidemiologic study of the etiology and natural history of atherosclerotic diseases in patients 45 to 64 years of age, used a prospective cohort analysis among 8960 middle-aged adults to reveal a more direct association between CVD and prehypertension. The study controlled for study site, age, sex, and race. BP levels served as exposure variables: high-normal BP (systolic BP [SBP] 130–139 mm Hg or diastolic BP [DBP] 85–89 mm Hg) and normal BP (SBP 120–129 mm Hg or DBP 80–84 mm Hg). The outcome was incident CVD defined as fatal/nonfatal coronary heart disease (CHD), cardiac procedure, silent myocardial infarction, or ischemic stroke. Analyzed subgroups included blacks, individuals with diabetes, individuals 55 to 64 years of age, individuals with renal insufficiency, and those with a range of low-density lipoprotein cholesterol levels and body mass index scores.

The baselines for optimal, normal, and high-normal BP were 106/67 mm Hg, 123/75 mm Hg, and 132/79 mm Hg, respectively. At a mean follow-up of 11.6 years, normal BP and high-normal BP was associated with a 69% and 133% greater risk of incident CVD, respectively, compared with optimal BP [3].

Pathogenesis of Hypertension

Genetic and Environmental Factors

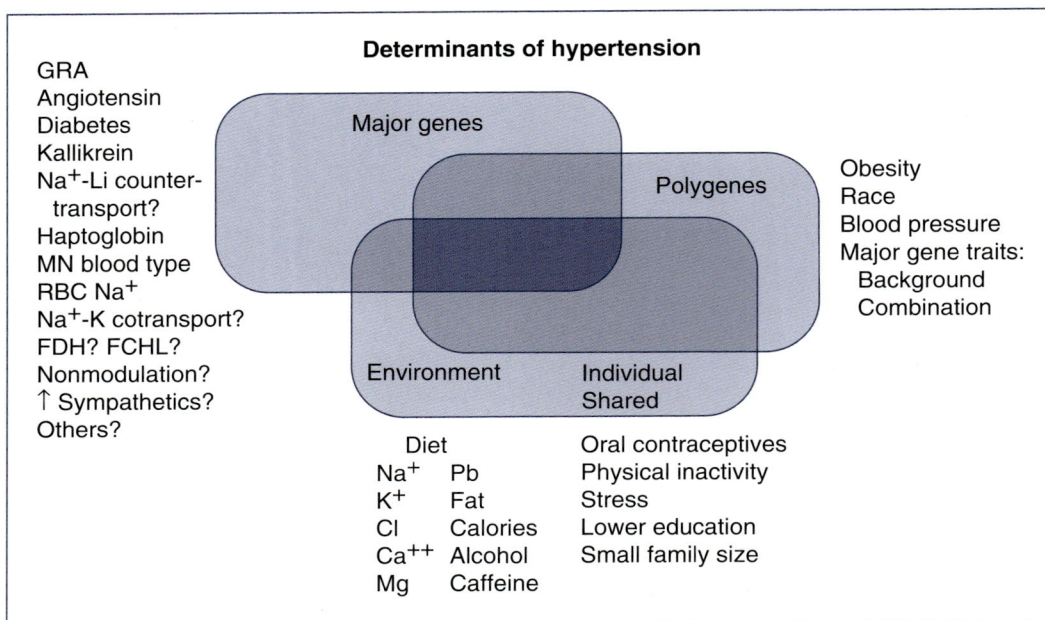

Figure 8-4. A model indicating the mechanisms by which essential hypertension could result from the combined effects of individual major genes that have a large impact on blood pressure, blended polygenes with small individual contributions, and environmental effects operating on individuals or within families. FCHL—familial combined hyperlipidemia; FDH—familial dyslipidemic hypertension; GRA—glucocorticoid-remediable aldosteronism; RBC—red blood cell. (*Courtesy of* Roger R. Williams, MD.)

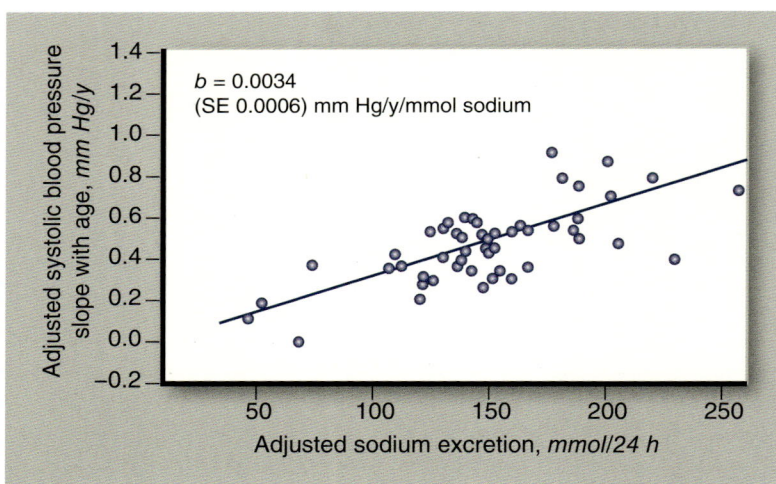

Figure 8-5. Averages for urinary sodium excretion and blood pressure rise with age in the INTERSALT Study. The INTERSALT Study [4] was undertaken to determine the relationship between urinary sodium excretion, which reflects dietary sodium intake, and blood pressure. Two hundred individuals were studied at each of 52 international centers. Averages for urinary sodium excretion (adjusted for age, sex, body mass index, and alcohol consumption) and blood pressure rise with age are shown. Each point represents one center. From the slope of the regression line (0.0034 ± mm Hg/y/mmol Na$^+$) the magnitude of the effect of urinary sodium excretion can be estimated; reduction of sodium intake by 100 mmol/d could reduce the rise in systolic blood pressure by 3.4 mm Hg for 10 years [4].

Figure 8-6. Hypothetical sequence of events demonstrating the role of sodium retention in cases of hypertension. An underlying genetic lesion may be expressed as a deficiency of sodium excretion, which becomes more apparent as sodium intake increases. The reduction in sodium excretion may initially cause a transient increase in total blood volume and a rise in intrathoracic blood volume. This change stimulates the hypothalamus to secrete a circulating sodium transport inhibitor, which adjusts renal sodium excretion, returning the sodium balance to normal. This balance is sustained only by a continuously high circulating sodium transport inhibitor, which raises the tone and reactivity of vascular smooth muscle. As a result, arterial pressure rises and venous compliance diminishes. Increased venous tone shifts blood from the periphery to the central vascular bed and thus raises intra-thoracic pressure and perpetuates the stimulus for greater secretion of the sodium transport inhibitor. Total blood volume may be normal or low. (*Adapted from* de Wardener and MacGregor [5].)

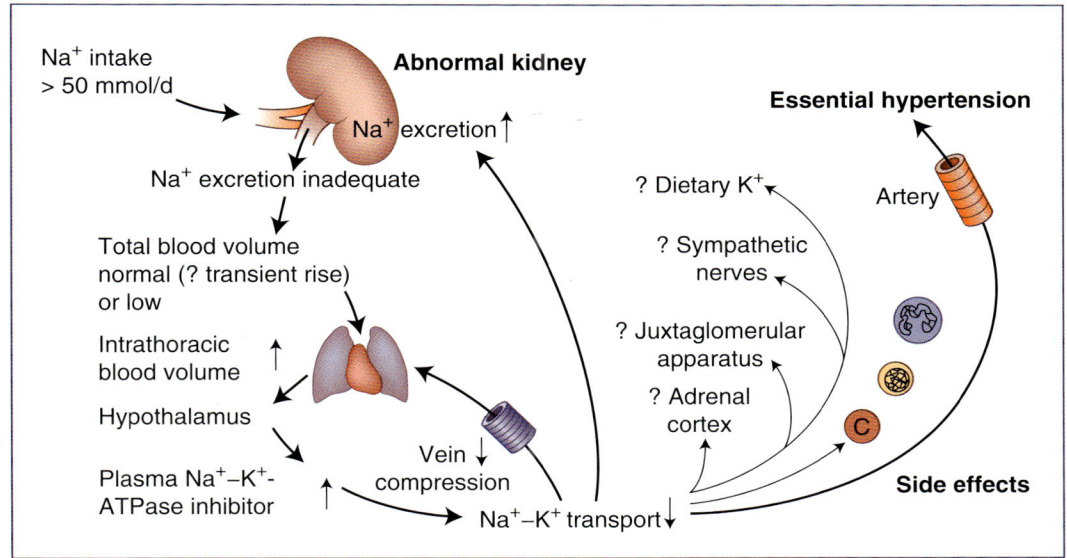

Figure 8-7. A, Dietary potassium intake is inversely related to systolic blood pressure. Displayed are values for systolic blood pressure and daily intake of potassium, as determined from dietary recall by participants in the National Health and Nutrition Examination Survey I cohort (a national population–based sample) [6]. **B,** Several dietary factors may interact to promote hypertension. The effect of dietary sodium and potassium on blood pressure may be conditioned by the contemporaneous intake of calcium. In this survey, continuous and graded relationships between blood pressure, dietary calcium, and the ratio of dietary sodium to potassium intake (numbers inside each bar) were found. Low calcium intake and an increased ratio of sodium to potassium intake were both associated with higher systolic blood pressure; the combination of both dietary habits was associated with the highest systolic blood pressure. (**B,** *adapted from* Gruchow *et al.* [7].)

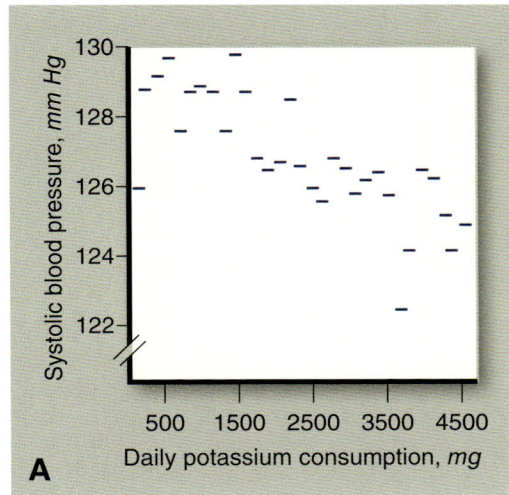

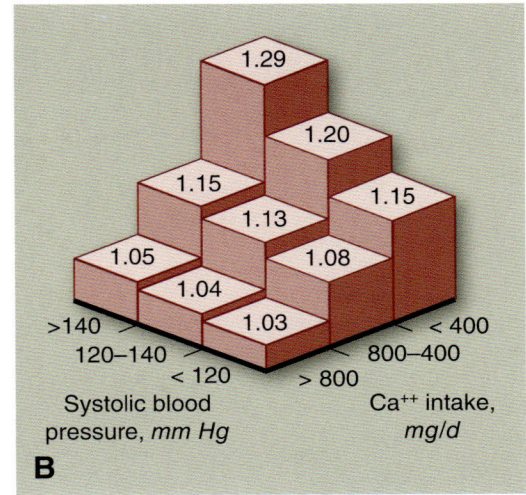

Figure 8-8. A final common pathway for the pathogenesis of hypertension. All inherited and acquired forms of hypertension share increased net salt balance as an inciting factor. Increased intravascular volume and volume delivery to the heart augment cardiac output and therefore blood pressure. The resulting tissue perfusion exceeds metabolic demand, leading to autoregulation of blood flow via increased vasoconstriction, resulting in a steady-state hemodynamic pattern of elevated blood pressure with increased systemic vascular resistance and normal cardiac output [8].

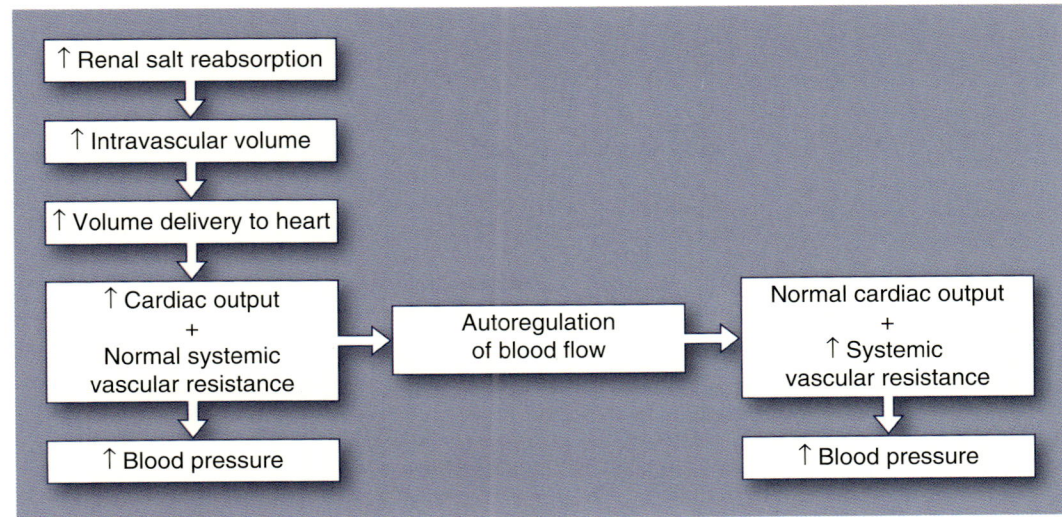

Adrenergic Nervous System

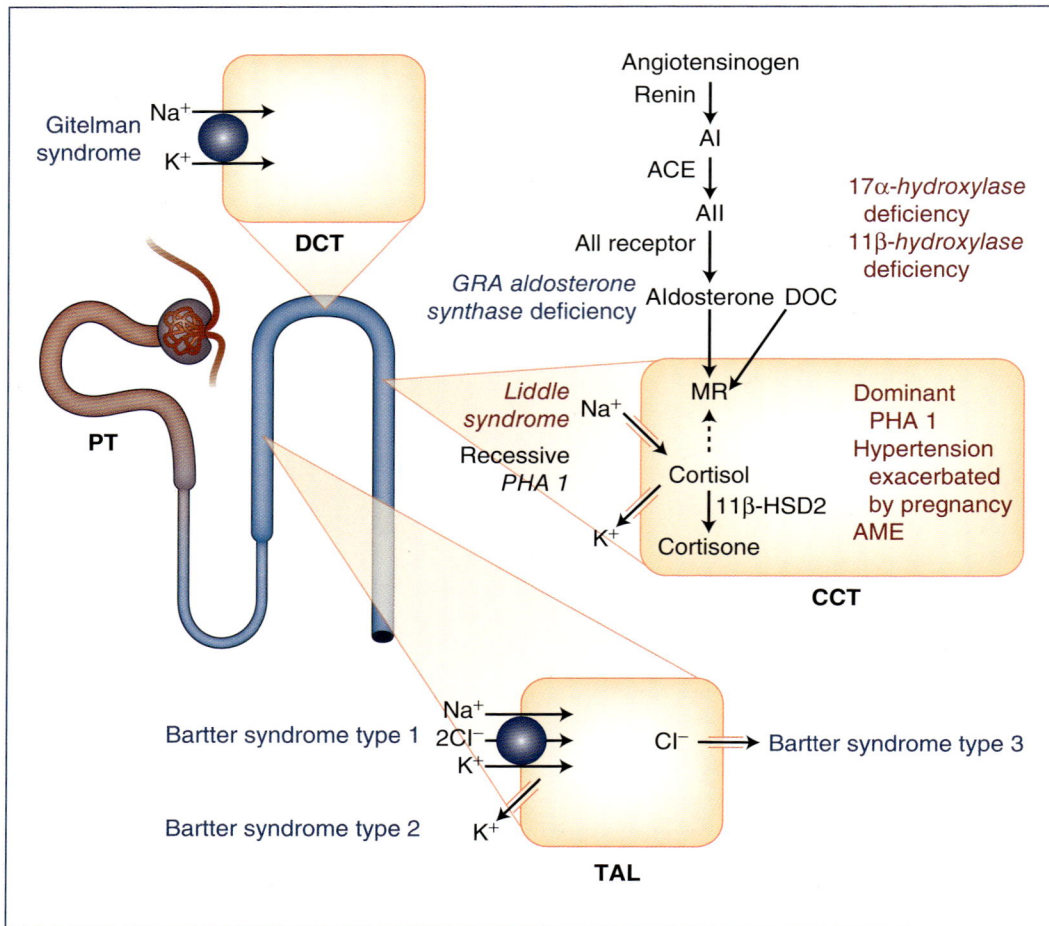

Figure 8-9. Mutations altering blood pressure in humans point to the critical role of renal salt and water metabolism in hypertension. A diagram of a nephron, the filtering unit of the kidney, is shown. The elucidation of the molecular bases of rare monogenic forms of hypertension focuses attention on the importance of salt handling by the kidney and provides strong genetic support for the pathogenic model for common forms of hypertension depicted in Figure 8-8. The molecular pathways mediating NaCl reabsorption in individual renal cells in the thick ascending limb of the loop of Henle (TAL), distal convoluted tubule (DCT), and the cortical collecting tubule (CCT) are indicated, along with the pathway of the renin-angiotensin system, the major regulator of renal salt reabsorption. Inherited diseases affecting these pathways are indicated with hypertensive disorders in *red* and hypotensive disorders in *blue*. 11β-HSD2—11β-hydroxysteroid dehydrogenase-2; AI—angiotensin I; AII—angiotensin II; ACE—angiotensin-converting enzyme; AME—apparent mineralocorticoid excess; DOC—deoxycorticosterone; GRA—glucocorticoid-remediable aldosteronism; MR—mineralocorticoid receptor; PHA 1—pseudohypoaldosteronism type 1; PT—proximal tubule [8].

The Renin-Angiotensin-Aldosterone System

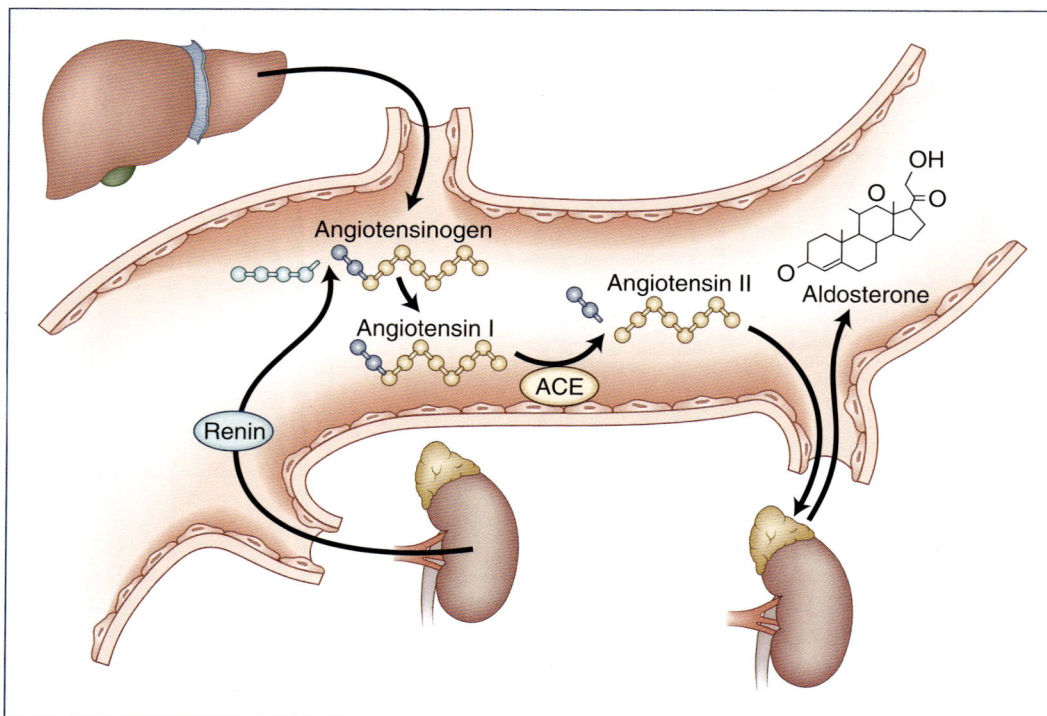

Figure 8-10. To regulate the homeostasis of salt and water in mammals, sensors and controls operate in a negative feedback loop. Renin, released by the juxtaglomerular cells, and the adrenal gland–produced aldosterone work together to control the renin-angiotensin-aldosterone system (RAAS). Renin cleaves four amino acids from circulating angiotensinogen to form angiotensin, the angiotensin-peptide precursor made by the liver, to form the biologically inert decapeptide angiotensin I (AI). Bound to the plasma membrane of endothelial cells, an angiotensin-converting enzyme (ACE) then cleaves two amino acids from AI to form angiotensin II (AII). Promoting constriction of the arterioles and reabsorption of sodium in the nephron, AII maintains circulatory homeostasis and stimulates the secretion of aldosterone, which absorbs potassium and promotes the reabsorption of sodium into the nephron, the colon, and the salivary and sweat glands.

The amount of renin secretion varies as a result of the changing intake of sodium and water, as absorption of salt and water inhibits renin secretion. In response to salt and water deprivation, which can occur with prolonged sweating, the RAAS works to sustain circulatory homeostasis [9].

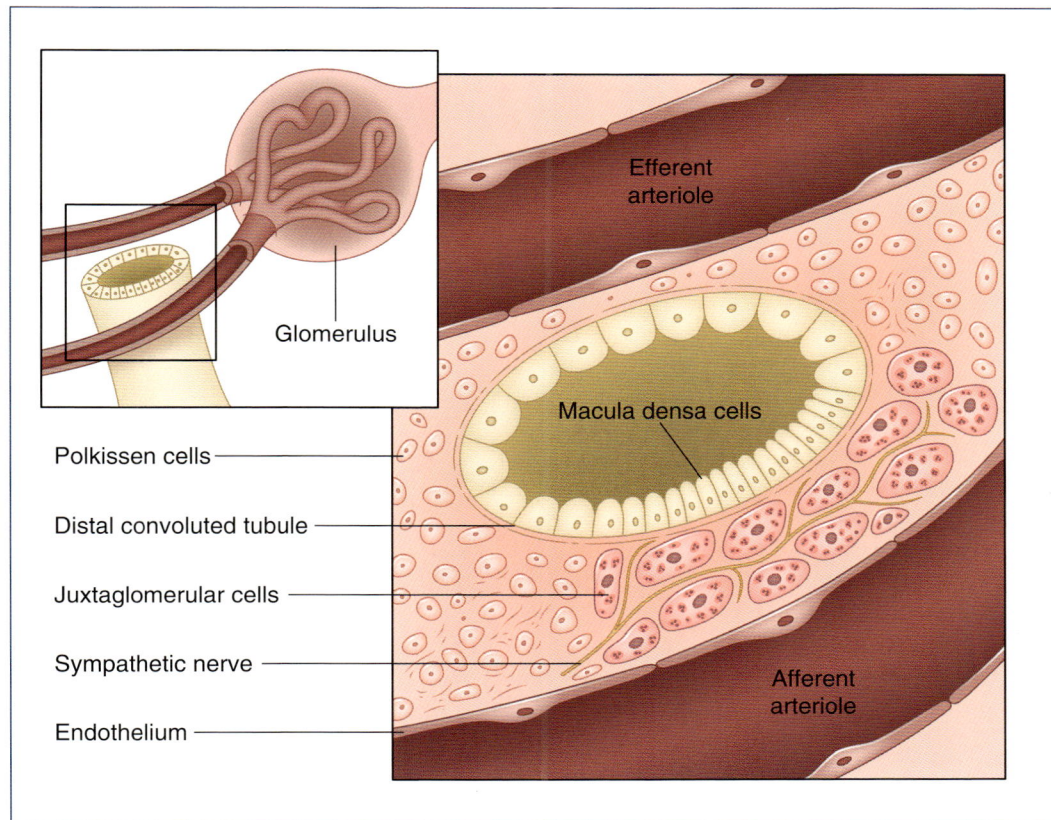

Figure 8-11. The juxtaglomerular apparatus, illustrating tubular and vascular components. The tubular component consists of 1) a specialized region of the distal convoluted tubule, which bends between the afferent and efferent arterioles, and 2) the macula densa, which contains cells that are sensitive to sodium chloride flux and control renin secretion. The macula densa cells can be identified by the proximity of their nuclei to each other. The vascular component consists of the afferent and efferent arterioles as well as the extraglomerular mesangium. The extraglomerular mesangium is a collection of small cells with pale nuclei, called Polkissen cells, the function of which is unknown. The juxtaglomerular cells, in which renin is synthesized, stored, and secreted, are vascular smooth muscle cells modified by the presence of secretory and lysosomal granules; juxtaglomerular cells are absent from the efferent arteriole. The macula densa cells have no basement membrane, allowing intimate contact of the juxtaglomerular cells with tubular cells. Renin is stored in and secreted from the granules of the juxtaglomerular cells. The vascular and tubular components are innervated by sympathetic nerves. Renal nerve stimulation increases renin secretion by norepinephrine-induced stimulation of β-adrenergic receptors. Juxtaglomerular cells also have angiotensin II receptors, the stimulation of which leads to inhibition of renin secretion.

Figure 8-12. Major mechanisms of renin release. Three major mechanisms are thought to govern renin release: 1) signals at the individual nephron, 2) signals involving the entire kidney, and 3) local effectors. Individual nephron signals include decreased sodium chloride load at the macula densa, which is the specialized group of distal tubular cells in approximation to the juxtaglomerular apparatus, and decreased afferent arteriolar pressure, which is probably mediated by a cellular stretch mechanism. Whole kidney signals include negative-feedback inhibition by angiotensin II at the juxtaglomerular cell, β_1-adrenergic receptor stimulation at the juxtaglomerular cell, and other hormonal factors. Local effectors include the prostaglandins E_2 and I_2, nitric oxide, adenosine, dopamine, and arginine vasopressin. The angiotensin II inhibitory feedback loop is thought to be the predominant and overriding mechanism that controls renin release in humans.

Major Mechanisms of Renin Release

Individual nephron signals
  Low macula densa sodium chloride (stimulates)
  Decreased afferent arteriolar pressure (stimulates)
Whole kidney modulating signals
  Angiotensin II negative feedback (inhibits)
  β-1 receptor stimulation (stimulates)
  Other humoral factors
    Vasopressin (inhibits)
    Atrial natriuretic peptide (inhibits)
    Dopamine DA-1 receptor (stimulates)
Local effectors
  Prostaglandins (stimulate)
  Nitric oxide (inhibits)
  Adenosine (inhibits)
  Kinins (stimulate)

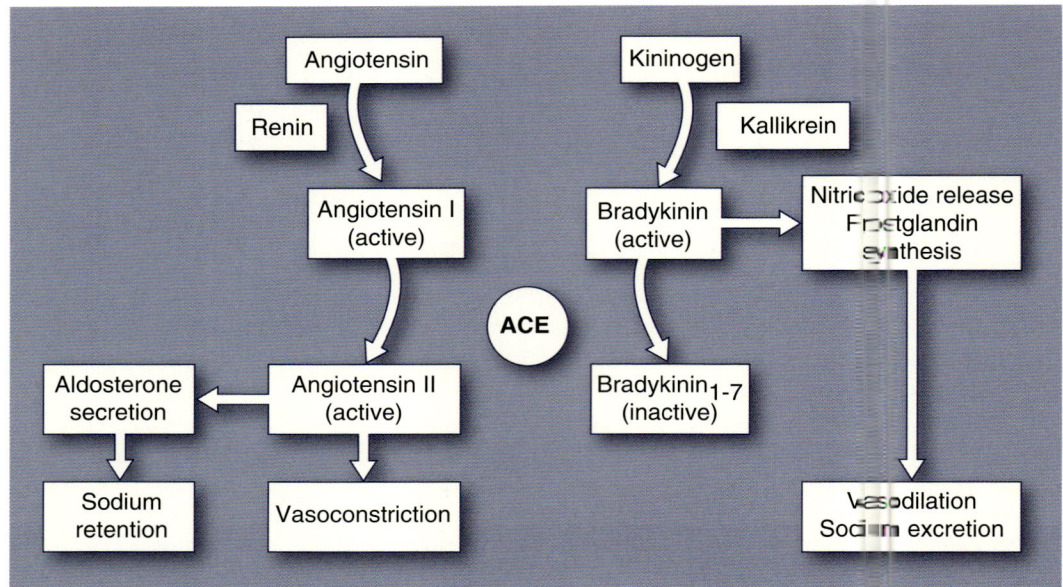

Figure 8-13. The actions of angiotensin-converting enzyme (ACE). The *left side* of the figure demonstrates how the enzyme converts inactive angiotensin I to active angiotensin II. The *right side* depicts how ACE metabolizes bradykinin, an active vasodilator and natriuretic substance, to bradykinin$_{1-7}$, an inactive metabolite. ACE therefore increases production of a potent vasoconstrictor, angiotensin II, while promoting the degradation of a vasodilator, bradykinin. Both actions of ACE increase vasoconstriction, and inhibition of ACE leads to vasodilation and natriuresis. Bradykinin is formed by the action of the enzyme kallikrein on the substrate kininogen. Bradykinin acts as a vasodilator and natriuretic substance by releasing nitric oxide (an endothelium-derived relaxing factor) and stimulating formation of prostaglandins E$_2$ and I$_2$.

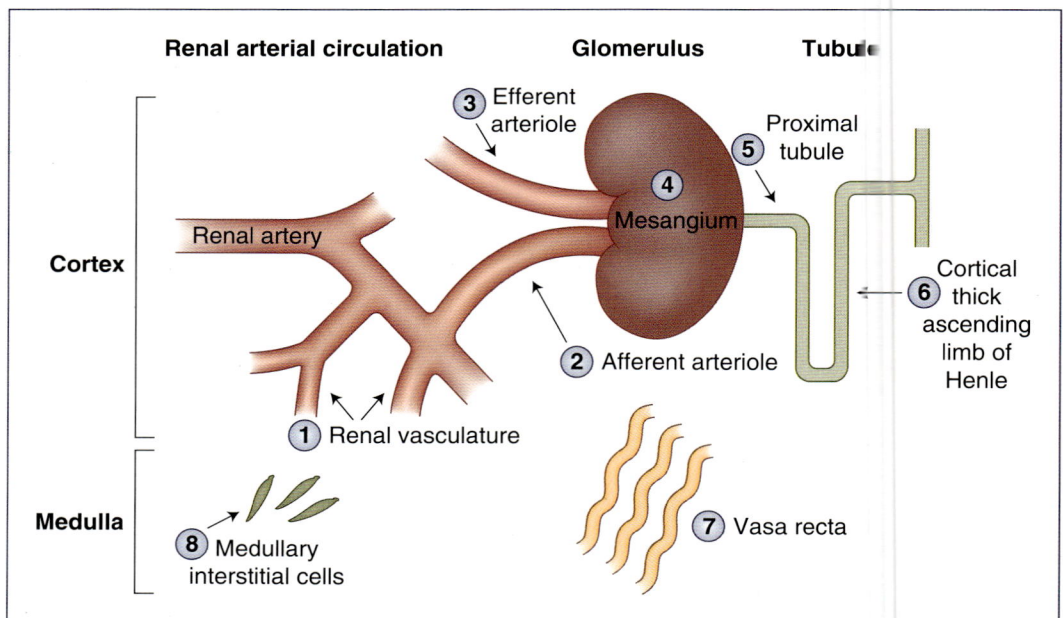

Figure 8-14. The renal tissue localization of angiotensin II receptors and the physiologic action stimulated by these receptors. Vasoconstriction occurs when angiotensin II acts at receptors in the arcuate and interlobular arteries, the afferent and efferent arterioles, and the medullary vasa recta. Angiotensin II preferentially constricts the efferent arteriole, thereby increasing glomerular filtration pressure; however, angiotensin II also acts on mesangial cell receptors to produce cellular contraction and reduce glomerular filtration. Angiotensin II receptors also are localized to the proximal tubule and the cortical thick ascending loop of Henle cells, which cause sodium resorption. Angiotensin II receptors have been found on renomedullary interstitial cell membranes, but the physiologic significance of these receptors is still unknown. 1—vasoconstriction; 2—limited vasoconstriction, and inhibition of renin synthesis and release; 3—preferential vasoconstriction; 4—contraction; 5 and 6—sodium reabsorption; 7—vasoconstriction; 8—unknown action.

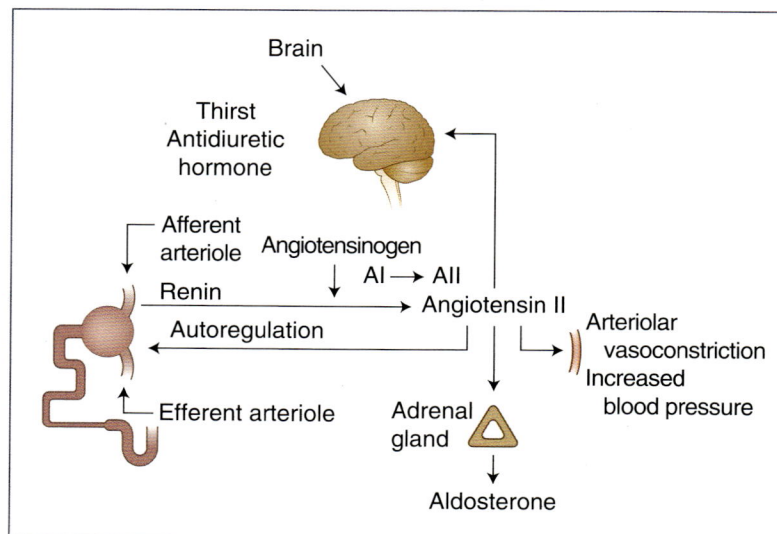

Figure 8-15. Effects of angiotensin II. Angiotensin II has three major effects: 1) arteriolar vasoconstriction; 2) renal sodium retention; and 3) increased aldosterone biosynthesis, all of which result in sodium retention. These effects work together to maintain arterial blood pressure as well as blood volume. Angiotensin II also stimulates the sympathetic nervous system, particularly the thirst center in the hypothalamus.

Vascular Mechanisms

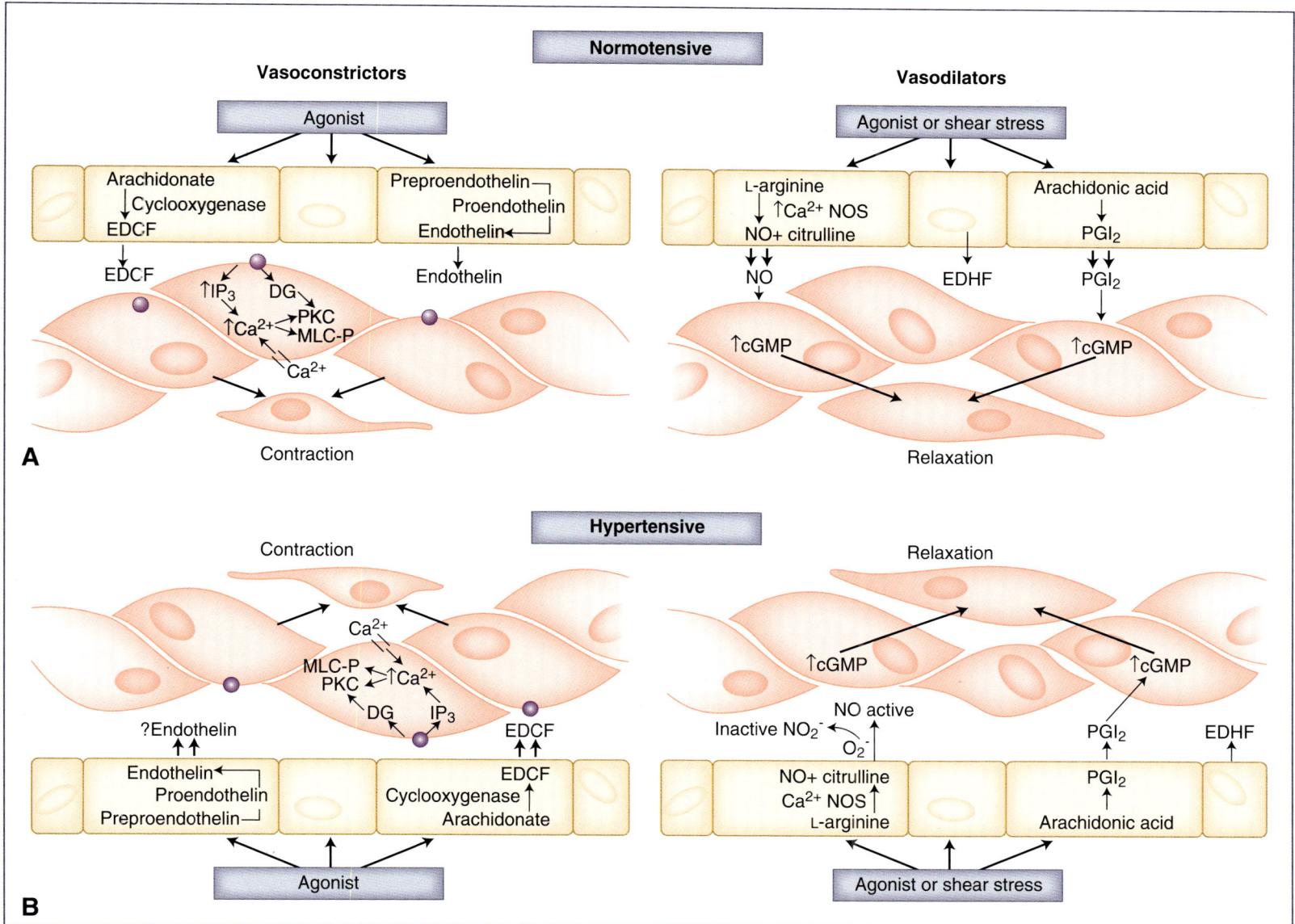

Figure 8-16. Endothelium-dependent vasodilator and vasoconstrictor mechanisms: modification in hypertension. Normal endothelial cells secrete both vasodilators, the most prominent of which are nitric oxide (NO), prostacyclin (PGI$_2$), and endothelium-derived hyperpolarizing factor (EDHF), and vasoconstrictors, including endothelin and endothelium-derived contracting factor (EDCF) [10]. Vessel tone is dependent on the balance between these factors and on the ability of the smooth muscle cell to respond to them.

A, In normotensive vessels there is a predominance of vasodilator secretion. These substances may also contribute to the inhibition of smooth muscle cell growth or hypertrophy. The relative concentrations of the vasoconstricting/vasodilating agents are indicated by the relative size of the arrows.

B, In hypertension, release of vasoconstrictor substances may predominate [11]. In addition, vasodilator release may be decreased or, alternatively, the vasodilator itself may be inactivated by superoxide anion. Under certain circumstances, endothelin can also be growth-promoting, thereby contributing to smooth muscle cell hypertrophy or hyperplasia and intimal thickening. The biochemical pathways activated by endothelial agonists and by contracting and relaxing factors acting on smooth muscle can also be affected in hypertension. NO, produced by the conversion of L-arginine to citrulline, traverses the endothelial cell membrane, and activates the smooth muscle cell guanylate cyclase to generate intracellular cyclic guanosine monophosphate. PGI$_2$ and EDCF are produced via cyclooxygenase action on arachidonic acid. PGI$_2$ relaxes vessels by increasing smooth muscle cell cyclic adenosine monophosphate; the mechanism of action of EDCF is unknown. Endothelin is made and modified by endothelium. It then stimulates the phospholipase C pathway in smooth muscle to produce the second messengers inositol trisphosphate (IP$_3$) and diacylglycerol (DG), which in turn activate the Ca^{2+} and protein kinase C (PKC) signaling pathways. This leads to phosphorylation of the myosin light chain (MLC-P), causing contraction. Alterations of any of these signals could easily augment contraction or decrease the ability of the vessel to dilate.

Secondary Hypertension

Renovascular Hypertension

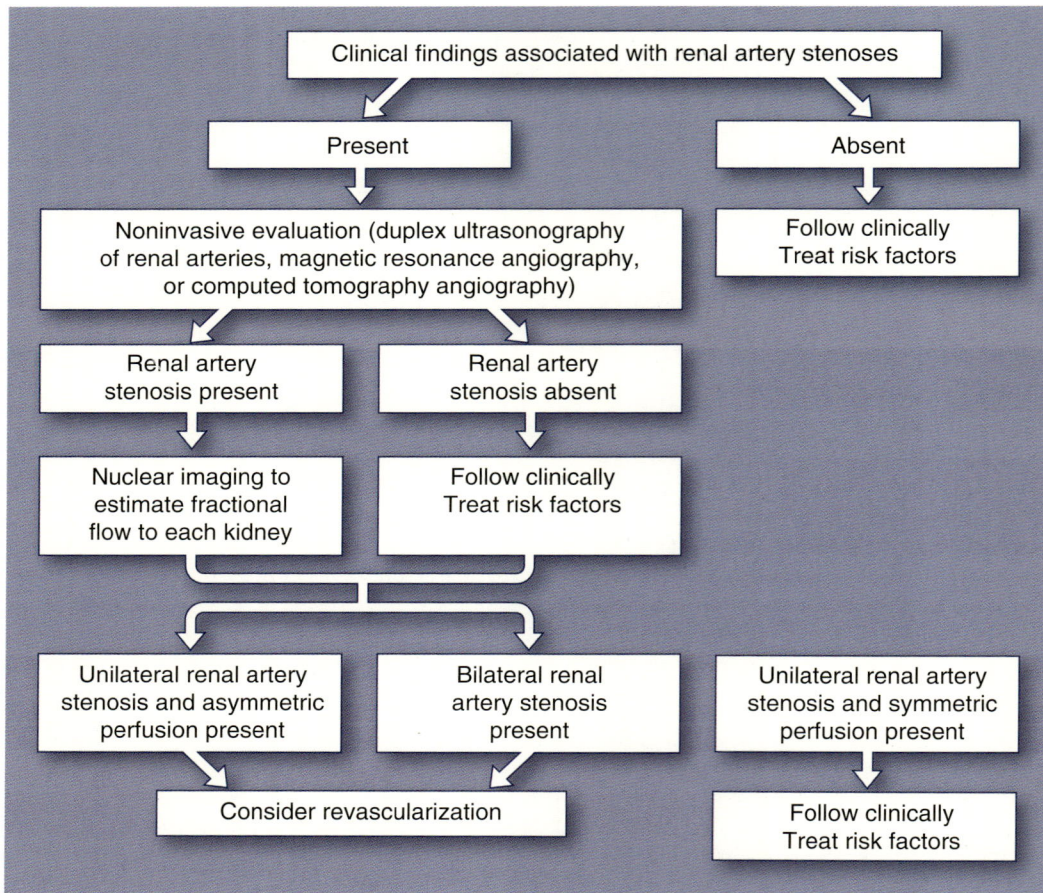

Clinical findings associated with renal artery stenoses

Present → Noninvasive evaluation (duplex ultrasonography of renal arteries, magnetic resonance angiography, or computed tomography angiography)

Absent → Follow clinically / Treat risk factors

Renal artery stenosis present → Nuclear imaging to estimate fractional flow to each kidney

Renal artery stenosis absent → Follow clinically / Treat risk factors

Unilateral renal artery stenosis and asymmetric perfusion present

Bilateral renal artery stenosis present

Unilateral renal artery stenosis and symmetric perfusion present

Consider revascularization

Follow clinically / Treat risk factors

Figure 8-17. Algorithm for evaluating patients with suspected renal artery stenosis. Clinical follow-up includes periodic reassessment with duplex ultrasonography, magnetic resonance angiography, and nuclear imaging to estimate fractional blood flow to each kidney. The treatment of risk factors includes smoking cessation and the use of aspirin, lipid-lowering agents, and antihypertensive therapy [12].

Performance Characteristics and Advantages/ Disadvantages of Four Common Screening Tests for Renovascular Hypertension

Screening test	Captopril scintigraphy	Doppler ultrasound	Magnetic resonance angiogram	Computed tomography
Publications, *n*	56	39	23	11
Patients/arteries, *n*	4295	3470	1788	1485
Sensitivity	0.79	0.82	0.88	0.86
Specificity	0.82	0.9	0.88	0.94
Advantages	Noninvasive; not expensive; may predict BP results after revascularization	Noninvasive; inexpensive; predicts BP results after revascularization	No contrast needed; excellent image quality	Excellent image quality
Disadvantages	Less accurate in renal impairment, bilateral disease, obstructive uropathy	Operator-dependent; less useful in obesity, bowel gas, branch lesions, FMD	Expensive; poor images with stents or distal stenoses (*eg*, FMD); overcalls moderate stenoses	Expensive; time-consuming to process and interpret; not widely available; large amount of contrast sometimes needed

Figure 8-18. Performance characteristics (weighted averages of the world's literature, 1990–2004) and advantages and disadvantages of four commonly used screening tests for renovascular hypertension [13]. BP—blood pressure; FMD—fibromuscular dysplasia.

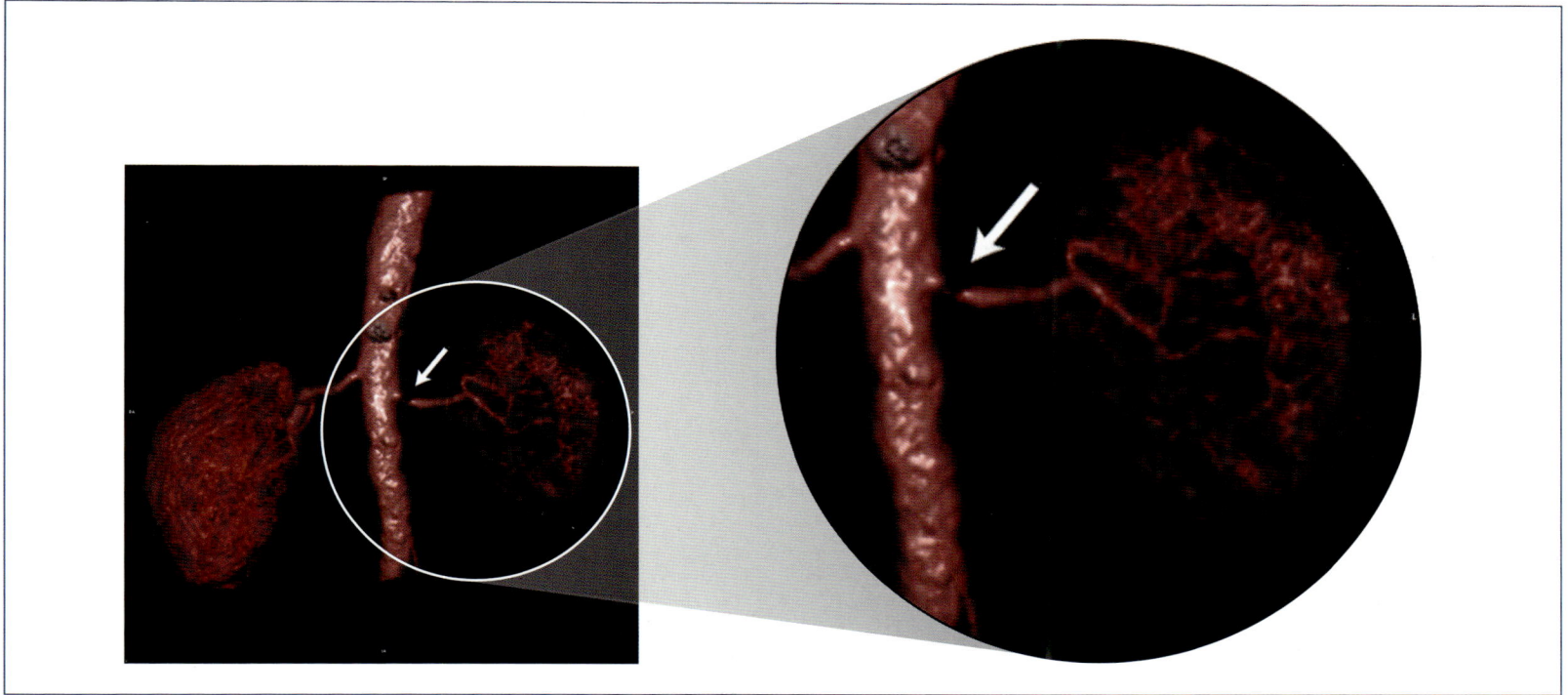

Figure 8-19. Computed tomographic image demonstrating a right renal artery stenosis in a three-dimensional reconstruction. (*Courtesy of* Drs. Frank Rybicki and Raymond Kwong, Brigham and Women's Hospital.)

Hypertensive Syndromes Secondary to Cortisol Excess

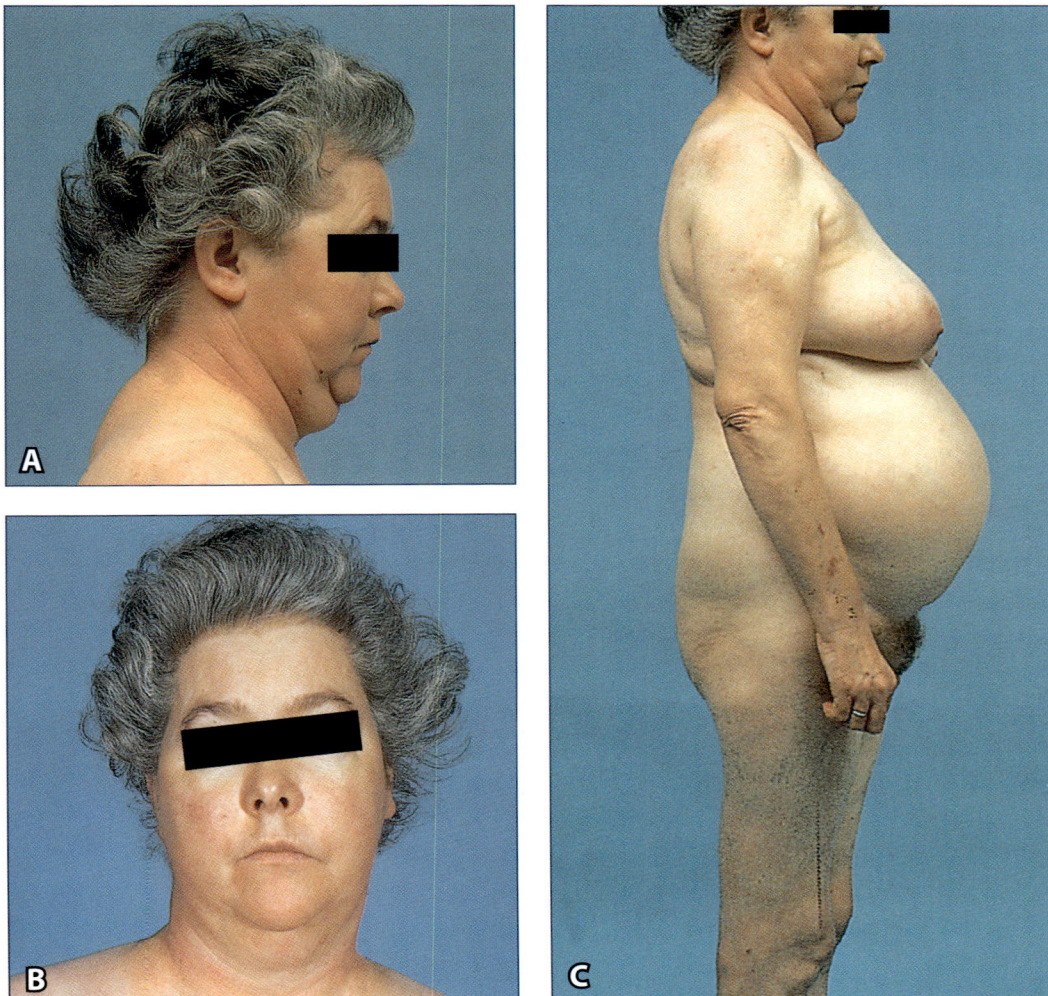

Figure 8-20. Physical features of Cushing's syndrome. The recognizable causes of Cushing's syndrome include Cushing's disease (72%), ectopic adrenocorticotropic hormone (ACTH) excess (12%), adrenal adenoma (8%), carcinoma (6%), and hyperplasia (4%). The typical clinical presentation of Cushing's syndrome includes truncal obesity, moon facies, hypertension, plethora, muscle weakness and fatigue, hirsutism, emotional disturbances, and typical purple skin striae. Carbohydrate intolerance or diabetes, amenorrhea, loss of libido, easy bruising, and spontaneous fracture of ribs and vertebrae may also be encountered. Patients with ectopic ACTH excess may not have the typical manifestations of cortisol excess but may present with hyperpigmentation of the skin, severe hypertension, and marked hypokalemic alkalosis.

These images show the physical features of Cushing's syndrome. **A,** Side view of the patient revealing a buffalo hump. **B,** Facial features show the characteristic moon facies with a malar flush. Also obvious are the full supraclavicular fat pads. **C,** There is centripetal distribution of fat associated with significant atrophy of the thigh muscles.

Figure 8-21. Differential diagnosis of Cushing's syndrome. Although cumbersome to perform, the determination of 24-hour urinary free cortisol is the best available test for documenting endogenous hypercortisolism. A level above 100 µg/24 h suggests excessive cortisol production. There are virtually no false-negative results. False-positive results may, however, be obtained in non-Cushing's hypercortisolemic states (*eg*, stress, chronic strenuous exercise, psychiatric states, glucocorticoid resistance, and malnutrition). If differentiation between pituitary and ectopic sources cannot be made based on plasma levels alone, pharmacologic manipulation of adrenocorticotropic hormone (ACTH) secretion should be performed (*ie*, high-dose dexamethasone suppression test or inferior petrosal sinus sampling for ACTH after corticotropin-releasing hormone administration).

The overnight dexamethasone suppression test requires only a blood collection for serum cortisol the morning after the patient has taken a 1.0-mg dose of dexamethasone at 11 PM the previous evening. In normal subjects, cortisol levels at 8 AM will be suppressed to 5.0

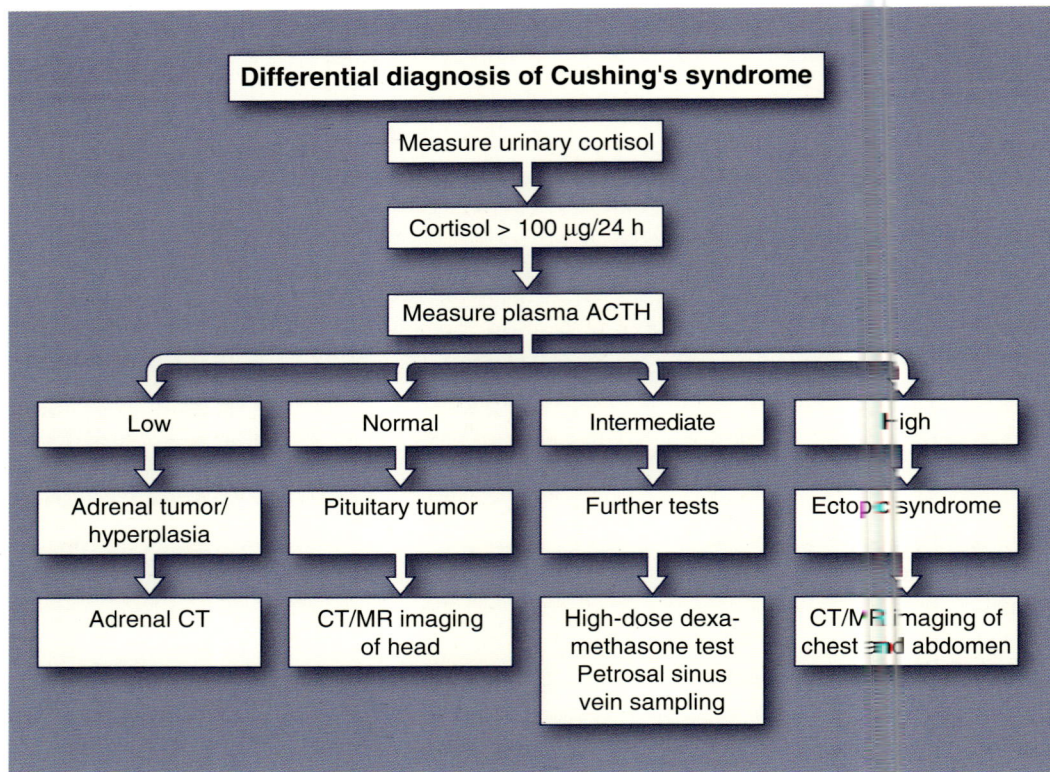

Differential diagnosis of Cushing's syndrome

Measure urinary cortisol → Cortisol > 100 µg/24 h → Measure plasma ACTH →

- Low → Adrenal tumor/hyperplasia → Adrenal CT
- Normal → Pituitary tumor → CT/MR imaging of head
- Intermediate → Further tests → High-dose dexamethasone test / Petrosal sinus vein sampling
- High → Ectopic syndrome → CT/MR imaging of chest and abdomen

µg/dL or less. When the presence of the syndrome has been verified by appropriate biochemical testing, the cause must be identified. Radio-immunoassay of plasma ACTH is the procedure of choice for pinpointing the basis of hypercortisolism. In patients with ACTH-independent Cushing's syndrome, ACTH levels have usually been suppressed to less than 5 pg/mL. In contrast, patients with the ACTH-dependent form tend to have either normal or elevated levels, usually greater than 10 pg/mL. In patients with Cushing's disease, ACTH release can be inhibited only at much higher doses of dexamethasone (2 mg every 6 hours for 2 days). The established criterion for the test is that suppression of the 24-hour urine and plasma steroids to less than 50% of baseline indicates pituitary Cushing's syndrome. Failure to suppress to less than 50% of baseline is considered consistent with an ectopic source of ACTH or ACTH-independent Cushing's syndrome.

Surgical resection of a pituitary or ectopic source of ACTH or of a cortisol-producing adrenocortical tumor is the treatment of choice for Cushing's syndrome. For pituitary Cushing's syndrome, transsphenoidal pituitary adenomectomy is the treatment of choice but total hypophysec-

tomy may be required in patients with diffuse hyperplasia or large pituitary tumors. Bilateral adrenalectomy for Cushing's disease is universally successful in alleviating the hypercortisolemic state; however, 10%–38% of individuals may later develop pituitary tumors and hyperpigmentation (Nelson's syndrome). Radiotherapy (*ie*, external pituitary irradiation, seeding the pituitary bed with yttrium or gold) has also been used with occasionally good results. The long-acting analogue SMS 201-995 (octreotide or sandostatin) has been used with varied success to treat ectopic ACTH syndromes; some benefit has been reported in Cushing's disease and Nelson's syndrome. Cyproheptadine has had limited success in the treatment of Cushing's disease. Ketoconazole, an inhibitor of several steroid biosynthetic pathways, has been used for rapid correction of hypercortisolism awaiting definitive intervention. Mitotane (o,p'-DDD), an insecticide derivative, induces destruction of the zonae reticularis and fasciculata with relative sparing of the zona glomerulosa. Mitotane has been used to treat Cushing's syndrome associated with adrenal carcinoma or to suppress cortisol secretion in Cushing's disease. CT—computed tomography; MR—magnetic resonance.

Hypertensive Syndromes Secondary to Hypersecretion of Aldosterone

Figure 8-22. Algorithmic approach to suspected mineralocorticoid-induced hypertension, which is usually associated with spontaneous hypokalemia. Although hypokalemia is often simply a side effect of diuretics, evaluation is recommended under the following circumstances: diuretic therapy results in serum potassium less than 3.0 mEq/L even if levels normalize when diuretics are withdrawn; oral potassium supplementation and potassium-sparing agents fail to maintain serum potassium values greater than 3.5 mEq/L in a patient on diuretics; or serum potassium levels fail to normalize after 4 weeks of diuretic abstinence.

The initial assessment and subsequent studies should be designed to answer three questions: Is potassium loss renal or extrarenal? If renal, is it steroid or nonsteroid-dependent? If steroid-dependent, what is its cause? A 24-hour urinary potassium excretion greater than 30 mEq/24 h when the serum potassium is equal to or less than 3.0 mEq/L usually reflects renal potassium wasting. Correction of hypokalemia, especially in the face of continued high dietary sodium, by short-term administration (3–5 days) of the specific aldosterone-receptor antagonist, spironolactone, indicates that the renal potassium wasting is steroid-dependent.

Specific diagnostic tests should then be performed to confirm the diagnosis. Serum potassium levels of 3.4 mEq/L or less associated with urinary potassium excretion greater than 30 mEq/24 h indicates renal wasting, while lower excretion rates suggest extrarenal loss caused by diarrhea, vomiting, or laxative abuse. Renal wasting should be investigated further after adequate repletion of total body potassium with oral chloride potassium supplementation. Salt-loading (oral sodium of 250 mEq/24 h for 5–7 days) that results in hypokalemia with renal potassium wasting suggests an exaggerated exchange mechanism of sodium for potassium at distal tubular sites mediated by inappropriate secretion of electrolyte-active steroids. An exception to this rule is Liddle's syndrome, a familial, non–steroid-dependent renal potassium wasting disorder associated with hypokalemia and hypertension. Response to spironolactone (50 mg four times daily for 3–5 days) can demonstrate conclusively whether renal potassium wasting is truly mineralocorticoid-dependent. If spironolactone produces an elevation in the serum potassium level with concomitant reduction in urinary excretion, potassium wasting is probably mediated by electrolyte-active steroids.

The determination of dexamethasone responsiveness is the final step in the evaluation, to be undertaken if the physician suspects familial primary aldosteronism. This glucocorticoid-responsive aldosteronism should be suspected in patients with a family history of aldosteronism when imag-

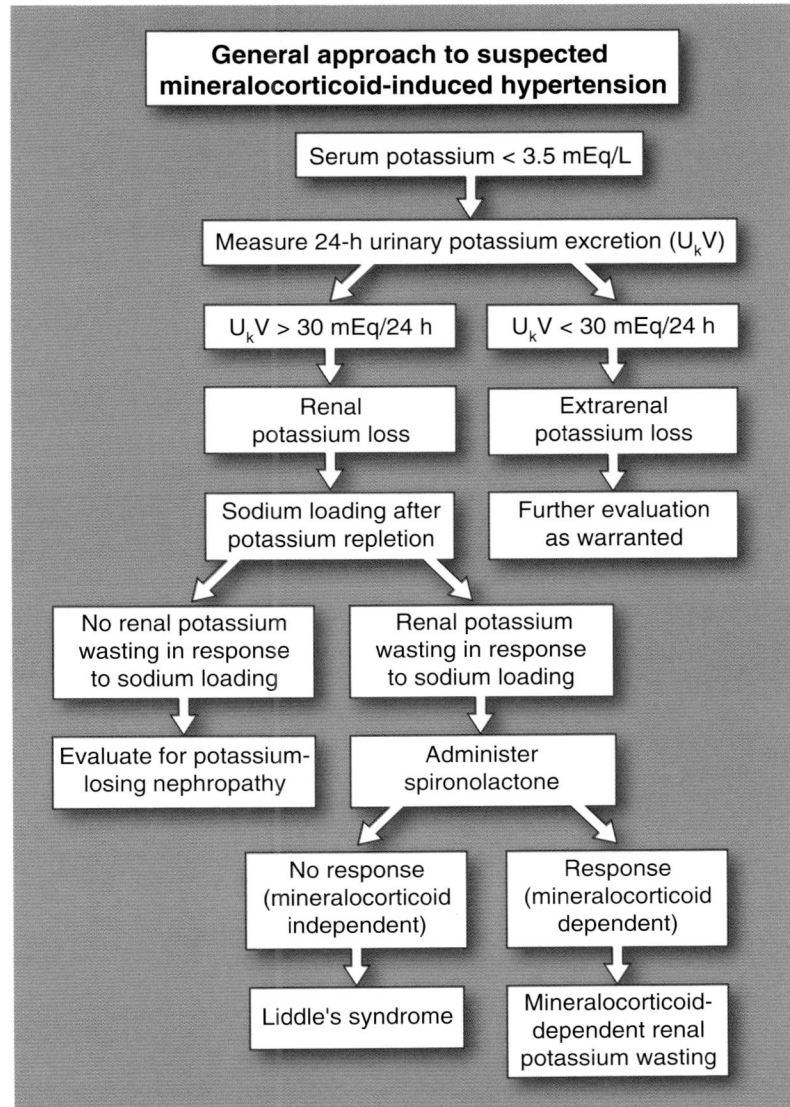

General approach to suspected mineralocorticoid-induced hypertension

ing techniques fail to reveal anatomic abnormalities in the adrenal glands. Administration of dexamethasone, in doses of 0.5 mg four times daily, usually results in remission of hypertension and hypokalemia in 10 to 14 days. (*Adapted from* Bravo [14].)

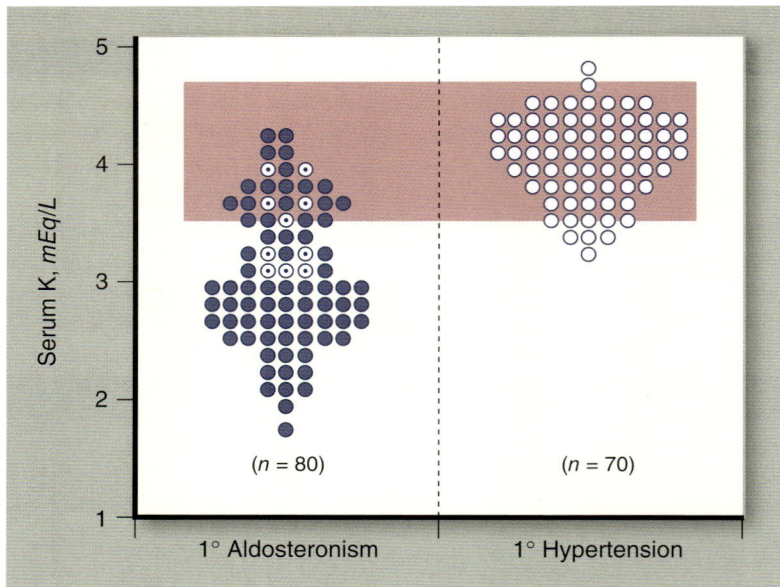

Figure 8-23. Serum potassium concentrations in cases of primary aldosteronism and essential hypertension. Patients were age- and sex-matched. No medication had been given for at least 2 weeks, and the patients were on an isocaloric diet containing 110 mEq of sodium and 80 mEq of potassium per day for 5 days. Blood was drawn between 8 AM and 9 AM after an overnight fast and at least 30 minutes of supine rest. Each point represents the mean of at least three determinations. For patients with primary aldosteronism, *solid circles* represent adenomas (*n* = 70) and *open circles with dotted centers* represent hyperplasia (*n* = 10). The *shaded area* represents 95% confidence intervals (3.5 to 4.6 mEq/L) of values obtained from 60 healthy subjects.

Twenty-two patients (27.5%) with primary aldosteronism (17 with tumors and five with hyperplasia) had fasting serum potassium values of 3.5 mEq/L or greater, while four (5.7%) subjects with essential hypertension (*open circles*) had values below 3.5 mEq/L. Serum potassium values below 3.0 mEq/L were usually associated with the presence of a tumor. Ten patients (six of 17 with tumors and four of five with hyperplasia) remained persistently normokalemic, despite intake of high dietary sodium for 3 days. (*Adapted from* Bravo [14].)

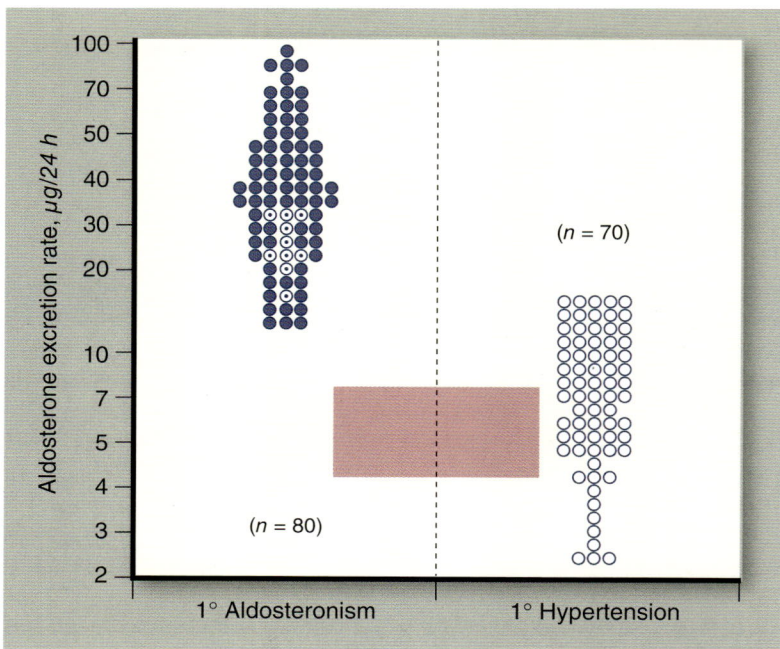

Figure 8-24. Aldosterone excretion rate after 3 days of high dietary sodium intake. Urine was collected on the third day of high sodium intake. The level of aldosterone in the urine was measured by a radioimmunoassay technique as the pH 1.0 conjugate 18-glucuronide metabolite. The *shaded area* represents the mean (4.0 μg/24 h) and +2 SD (8.0 μg/24 h) of values obtained from 47 healthy subjects. No patient with primary aldosteronism (*solid circles*) had a value within the 95% normal range. Ten patients (14%) with primary hypertension (*open circles*) had values that fell within the range obtained in patients with primary aldosteronism. Using a reference value of greater than 14 μg/24 h after a high sodium intake for 3 days, the sensitivity and specificity of the test were 96% and 93%, respectively. (*Adapted from* Bravo [14].)

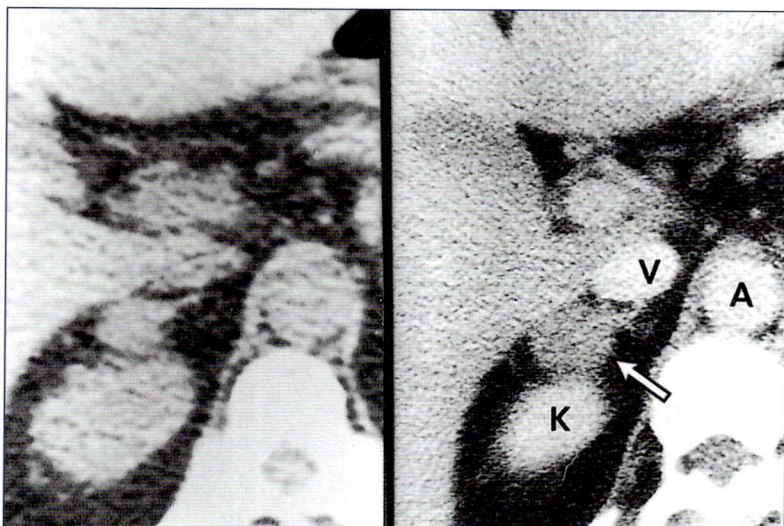

Figure 8-25. Computed tomography scan of a right adrenal tumor (*arrow*) before (*left*) and after (*right*) contrast injection. The tumor is located between the vena cava (V) and the upper pole of the kidney (K). A— aorta.

Pheochromocytoma

Important Facts About Pheochromocytoma

About 30% of pheochromocytomas reported in the literature are found either at autopsy or at surgery for an unrelated problem

Thirty-five percent to 76% of pheochromocytomas discovered at autopsy are clinically unsuspected during life

The average age of diagnosis in those whose disease was discovered before death was 48.5 y, while the average in those diagnosed at autopsy was 65.8 y

Death was usually attributed to cardiovascular complications

Figure 8-26. Facts about pheochromocytoma. Pheochromocytoma is a tumor of neuroectodermal origin that produces excessive quantities of catecholamines, thereby causing hypertension with a constellation of signs and symptoms that can mimic several other acute medical and surgical disorders. Early recognition, accurate localization, and appropriate management of benign pheochromocytomas nearly always result in complete cure. If unrecognized, these tumors cause lethal disease that can lead to significant cardiovascular morbidity and mortality and particularly to sudden death during surgical and obstetric procedures.

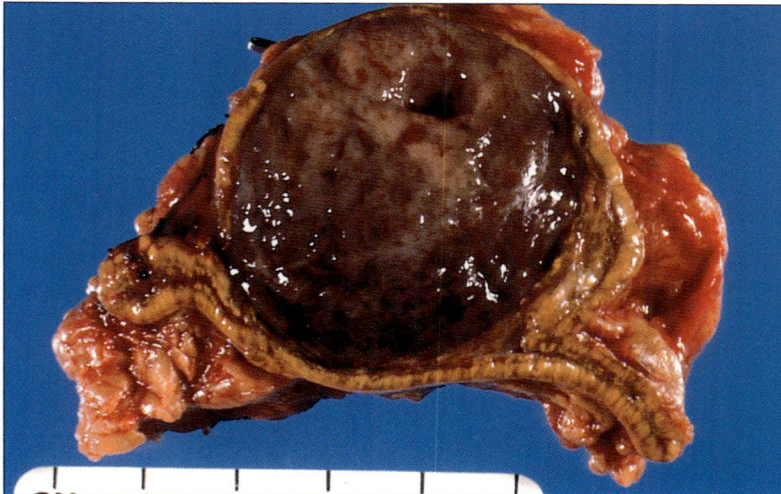

Figure 8-27. Typical gross pathologic features of an adrenal pheochromocytoma. The specimen is ovoid and encapsulated, surrounded by a rim of yellow tissue grossly resembling adrenal cortex. The lesion is rubbery to moderately firm and is pale gray to dusky brown. Pheochromocytomas have a strong affinity for chromium salts. Immersion in chromium salt fixative (Zenker's or potassium dichromate solution) changes the tumor from the usual pale-gray appearance to a dark-black color as cytoplasmic catecholamines are oxidized.

Priorities for Detection of Pheochromocytoma

Patients with the triad of episodic headaches, tachycardia, and diaphoresis (with or without associated hypertension)

Family history of pheochromocytoma

"Incidental" suprarenal masses

Patients with a multiple endocrine adenomatosis syndrome, neurofibromatosis, or von Hippel-Lindau disease

Adverse cardiovascular responses to anesthesia, to any surgical procedure, or to certain drugs (eg, guanethidine, tricyclics, thyrotropin-releasing hormone, naloxone, or anti-dopaminergic agents)

Figure 8-28. Priorities for detection of pheochromocytoma. The detection of pheochromocytoma requires a high degree of clinical alertness. Pheochromocytoma usually occurs as a sporadic event. These tumors, have, however, been associated with other clinical syndromes, such as von Recklinghausen's disease, von Hippel-Lindau disease, Werner's syndrome (MEN type I), Sipple's syndrome (MEN type IIA), mucocutaneous neuroma (MEN type IIB), acromegaly, and Cushing's syndrome. Most patients present with labile hypertension, diaphoresis, headaches, and tachycardia with or without palpitations; however, as many as 30% of all reported cases were unsuspected during life and the tumors were found either at autopsy or during surgery for an unrelated condition.

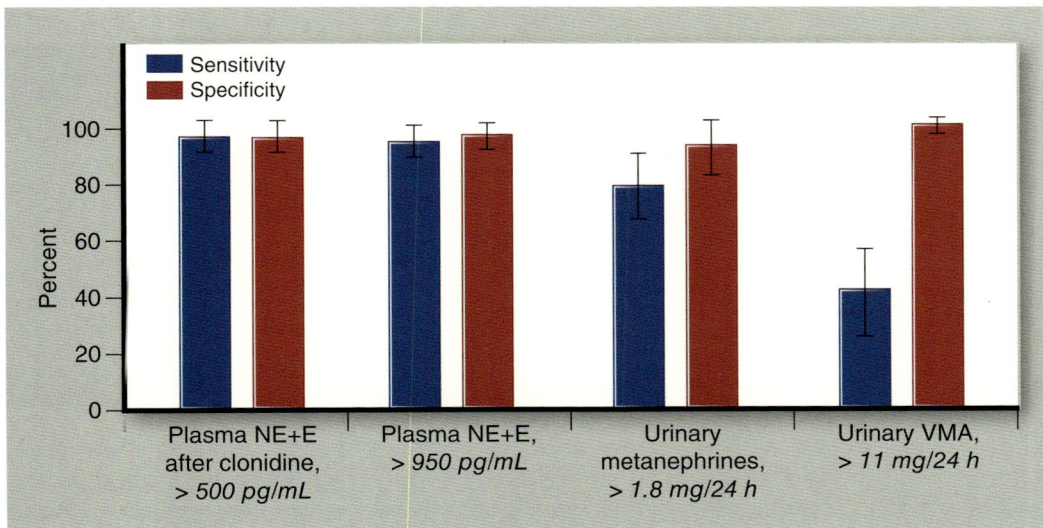

Figure 8-29. Sensitivity and specificity of various tests for pheochromocytoma. Measurement of plasma catecholamines appears to be the most sensitive test, and measurement of urinary vanillylmandelic acid (VMA) seems to be the least sensitive. When levels of catecholamines are elevated, all three tests provide excellent specificity. A combination test of plasma catecholamines and 24-hour urinary metanephrines provides nearly 100% accuracy (sensitivity and selectivity) in the diagnosis of pheochromocytoma. All values are mean ± 2 SE. NE+E—norepinephrine plus epinephrine.

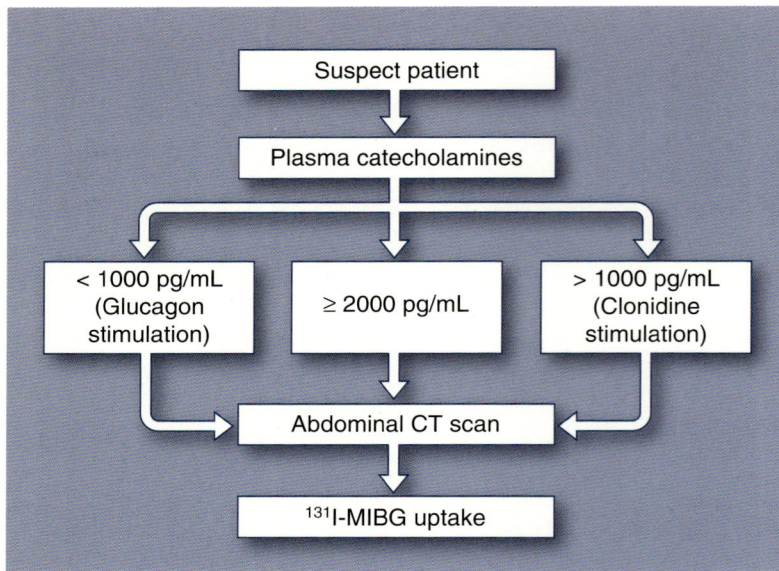

Figure 8-30. Diagnostic strategies in pheochromocytoma. Priority of evaluation is given to patients with the signs and symptoms detailed in Figure 8-28. Concentrations of plasma norepinephrine and epinephrine are measured after the patient has rested in a supine position for at least 30 minutes. Caffeine and nicotine are prohibited for at least 3 hours before testing. Values of 2000 pg/mL or greater are considered pathognomonic for pheochromocytoma. Values between 1000 and 2000 pg/mL require a clonidine suppression test. Abdominal computed tomography (CT) or magnetic resonance imaging is then performed in patients with clinical and biochemical features suggestive of pheochromocytoma. Approximately 5% of patients may have plasma catecholamines of 1000 pg/mL or less. If the clinical presentation strongly suggests pheochromocytoma in these patients, further evaluation should be performed. Such evaluation may include measurement of urinary catecholamine metabolites or a glucagon stimulation test. For patients with arterial pressure greater than 160/100 mm Hg or if coexistent medical problems make sudden increases in blood pressure risky, pretreatment with 10 mg of oral nifedipine, 30 minutes before testing, will attenuate any increases in blood pressure without interfering with catecholamine release. MIBG—meta-iodobenzylguanidine.

Nonpharmacologic Therapy

In most patients with hypertension, therapy should begin with or certainly include nonpharmacologic therapy.

Trial Results on Efficacy of Interventions for Primary Prevention of Hypertension

Documented efficacy	Limited or unproved efficacy
Weight loss	Stress management
Reduced sodium intake	Potassium (pill management)
Reduced alcohol consumption	Fish oil (pill supplementation)
Exercise	Calcium (pill supplementation)
	Macronutrient alteration
	Fiber supplementation

Figure 8-31. Trial results on the efficacy of interventions for the primary prevention of hypertension. It is ideal to prevent hypertension from becoming clinically evident in genetically susceptible people. We have not yet learned how to select our own genes, but it is possible to manipulate our environment. Not surprisingly, the methods for primary prevention of hypertension are quite similar to those for nonpharmacologic treatment of established hypertension [15].

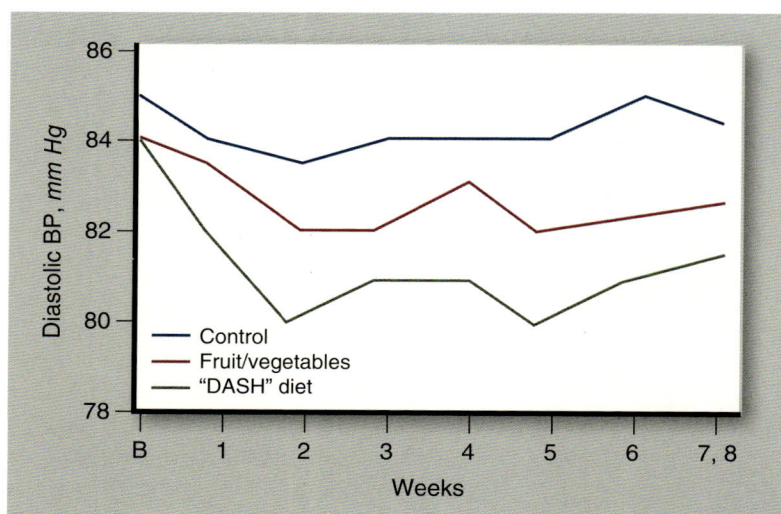

Figure 8-32. Blood pressure by week during the Dietary Approaches to Stop Hypertension (DASH) feeding study on three diets: controlled diet; fruits and vegetables diet; and the DASH Diet. The DASH Diet was relatively high in potassium and phosphorous and had a high protein content [16].

Nonpharmacologic (Nutritional-Hygienic) Therapy

Advantages
May reduce blood pressure substantially without drugs
Enhances efficacy of drug therapy
May prevent or mitigate adverse drug effects (*eg*, hypokalemia, hyperlipidemia)
May regress left ventricular hypertrophy

Disadvantages
Labor-intensive, expensive
Requires high patient and provider motivation
Requires continuous monitoring and reinforcement
May not protect against coronary artery disease and cardiovascular disease, including stroke, as effectively as the addition of drugs

Figure 8-33. Nutritional-hygienic therapy. Nonpharmacologic (nutritional-hygienic) therapy is of great potential value. However, there are disadvantages to its use, as well.

Clinical Trials of Drug Therapy

Hypertension Detection and Follow-up Program

Figure 8-34. Importance of lowering blood pressure. This figure shows a meta-regression analysis performed by Staessen *et al.* [17] that examined 30 clinical trials involving close to 150,000 randomized patients. It examined the long-term efficacy and safety of old and new classes of antihypertensive drugs. The trials included nine actively controlled trials (including MIDAS, CAPPP, NICS, STOP2, INSIGHT, NORDIL, VHAS, and UKPDS); the HOT trial, which investigated three levels of diastolic blood pressure; three placebo-controlled trials in isolated systolic hypertension (SHEP, Syst-China, Syst-Eur); six placebo-controlled trials in normotensive or hypertensive patients with high cardiovascular (CV) risk (including HOPE, PART2, and SCAT); and 11 trials testing the efficacy of antihypertensive drugs versus no treatment or placebo (including HEP, ATMH, EWPHE, MRC1, MRC2, and STONE).

The data shown indicate that when comparing the experimental treatment group with the reference treatment group, the greater the difference in systolic blood pressure reduction, the greater the reduction in CV mortality. *Red circles* indicate actively controlled trials. *Blue circles* indicate placebo-controlled studies or trials with an untreated control group. *Negative values* indicate tighter blood pressure control on reference treatment [17]. ATMH—Australian Trial in Mild Hypertension; CAPPP—Captopril Prevention Project; EWPHE—European Working Party in the Elderly; HEP—Hypertension Evaluation Project; HOPE—Hypertension Outreach Prevention Education; HOT L vs H—Hypertension Optimal Treatment 80 mm Hg vs 90 mm Hg as target diastolic pressure; HOT M vs H—Hypertension Optimal Treatment 85 mm Hg vs 90 mm Hg as target diastolic pressure; INSIGHT—Intervention as a Goal in Hypertension Treatment; MRC—Medical Research Council trial of treatment of mild hypertension; MIDAS—Myocardial Infarction Data Acquisition System; NICS—National Intervention Cooperative Study in Elderly Hypertensives Study Group; NORDIL—Nordic Diltiazem; PART2—Prevention of Atherosclerosis with Ramipril Treatment-2; RCT70-80—combined results of four randomized, controlled trials between 1970 and 1980; SBP—systolic blood pressure; SCAT—Simvastatin/Enalapril Coronary Atherosclerosis Trial; SHEP—Systolic Hypertension in the Elderly Program; STONE—Shanghai Trial of Hypertension in the Elderly; STOP2/ACEIs—Swedish Trial in Old Patients with Hypertension-2: Angiotensin-Converting Enzyme Inhibitors; STOP2/CCBs—Swedish Trial in Old Patients with Hypertension-2: Calcium Channel Blocks; Syst-China—Systolic Hypertension in China trial; Syst-Eur—Systolic Hypertension in Europe trial; UKPDS C vs A—United Kingdom Prospective Diabetes Study: Captopril vs Atenolol; UKPDS L vs H—United Kingdom Prospective Diabetes Study: Low vs High On-Treatment Blood Pressure; VHAS—Verapamil-Hypertension Atherosclerosis Study.

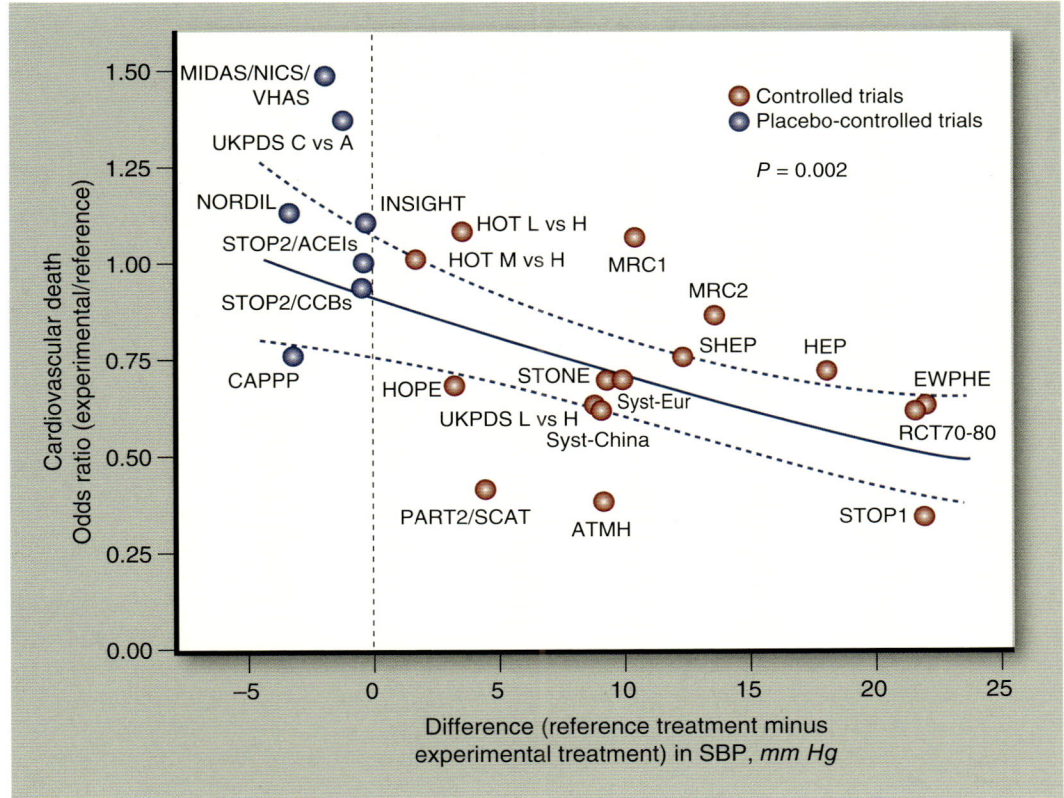

Figure 8-35. Effects of treatment in patients with mild-to-severe hypertension. Stroke reduction in the Hypertension Detection and Follow-up Program was greatest in the more severe hypertensives, especially for nonfatal stroke, but was demonstrable at all levels of hypertension. For those with a diastolic blood pressure of less than 100 mm Hg, the benefit was statistically significant. *Bracketed percentages* represent the percent reduction in the endpoints of nonfatal or fatal stroke. RC—referred care; SC—stepped care. (*Adapted from* the Hypertension Detection and Follow-up Program Cooperative Group [18].)

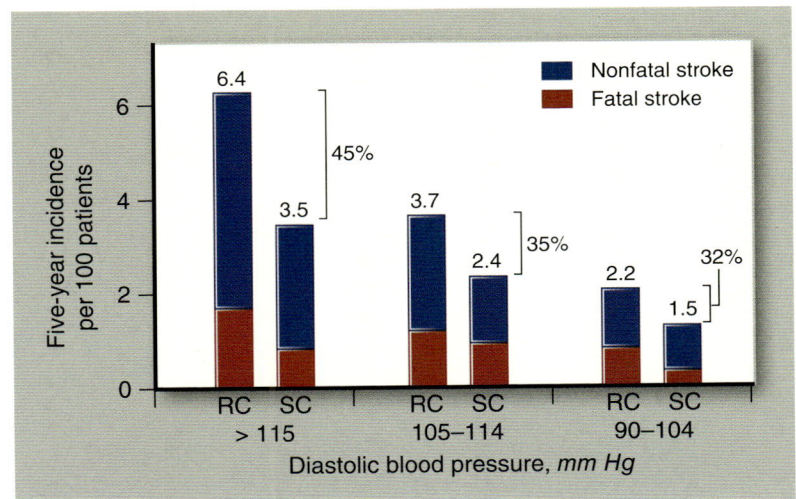

Summary of Trials

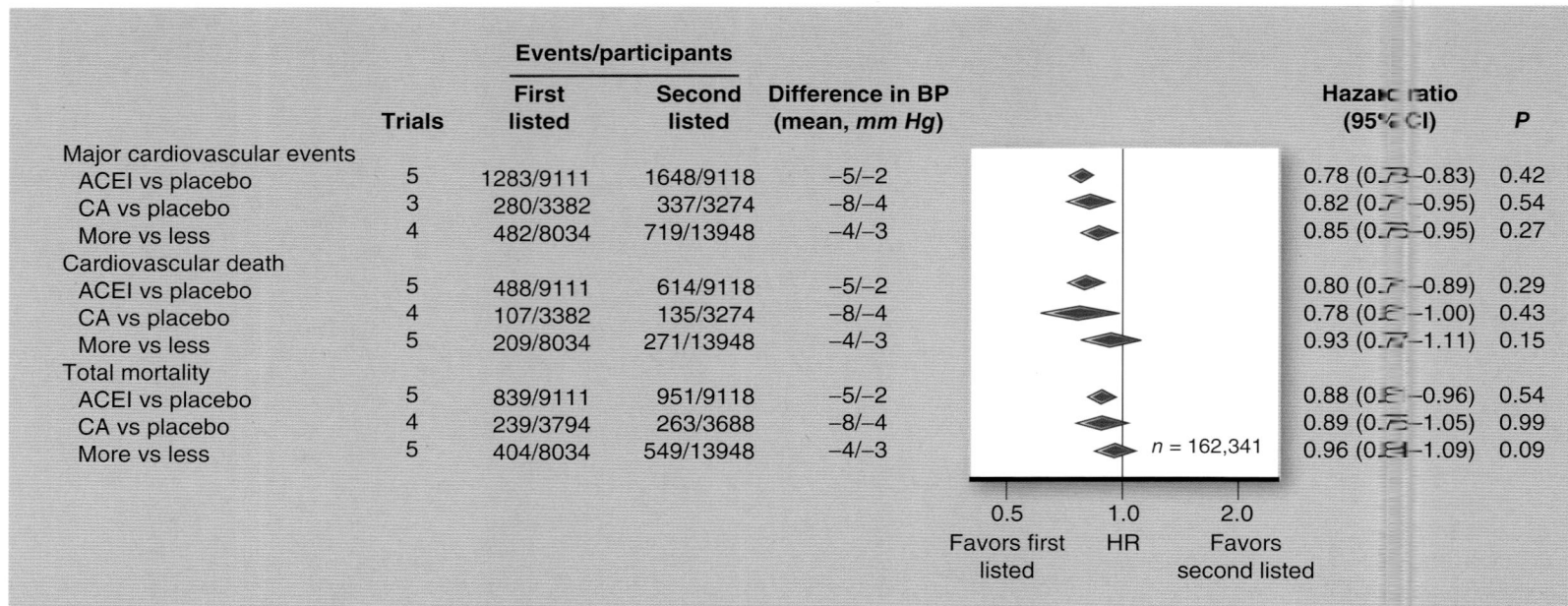

| | | Events/participants | | | | Hazard ratio | |
	Trials	First listed	Second listed	Difference in BP (mean, *mm Hg*)		(95% CI)	*P*
Major cardiovascular events							
ACEI vs placebo	5	1283/9111	1648/9118	−5/−2		0.78 (0.73–0.83)	0.42
CA vs placebo	3	280/3382	337/3274	−8/−4		0.82 (0.7–0.95)	0.54
More vs less	4	482/8034	719/13948	−4/−3		0.85 (0.75–0.95)	0.27
Cardiovascular death							
ACEI vs placebo	5	488/9111	614/9118	−5/−2		0.80 (0.7–0.89)	0.29
CA vs placebo	4	107/3382	135/3274	−8/−4		0.78 (0.6–1.00)	0.43
More vs less	5	209/8034	271/13948	−4/−3		0.93 (0.77–1.11)	0.15
Total mortality							
ACEI vs placebo	5	839/9111	951/9118	−5/−2		0.88 (0.8–0.96)	0.54
CA vs placebo	4	239/3794	263/3688	−8/−4		0.89 (0.75–1.05)	0.99
More vs less	5	404/8034	549/13948	−4/−3	*n* = 162,341	0.96 (0.84–1.09)	0.09

```
        0.5            1.0            2.0
   Favors first        HR          Favors
       listed                   second listed
```

Figure 8-36. This meta-analysis sought to estimate the effects of strategies based on different drug classes (angiotensin-converting enzyme inhibitors [ACEIs], calcium antagonists [CAs], angiotensin II receptor blockers [ARBs], and diuretics or β-blockers) or those targeting different blood pressure (BP) goals on the risks of major cardiovascular (CV) events and death. It included seven sets of prospectively designed overviews with data from 29 randomized trials (*n* = 162,341).

The study included the following criteria: 1) randomization of patients to either a BP-lowering drug or placebo; 2) randomization of patients to receive regimens based on different BP goals; 3) randomization of patients to regimens based on different classes of BP-lowering drugs.

This analysis compared ACEI-based regimens versus placebo, CA-based regimens versus placebo, and regimens targeting different BP goals. Comparisons of regimens based on ACEI and CAs with placebo both indicated reductions in the composite of all major CV events with active treatment, though not significant (*P* = 0.42 and *P* = 0.54, respectively). Compared with placebo, ACEI-based regimens reduced the risk of CV death, yet not significantly (*P* = 0.29). CA-based regimens trended toward fewer deaths but no clear evidence emerged of a reduction in risk with regimens targeting low BP goals. In trials comparing ACEI-based regimens with placebo, active treatment reduced the risk of death. Using a more intensive BP-lowering regimen commonly reduced the risk of total mortality (*P* = 0.09).

Figure 8-37. Clinical trial evidence shows that reaching the Seventh Report of the Joint National Committee on Prevention, Detection, Evaluation, and Treatment of High Blood Pressure (JNC 7)–recommended blood pressure (BP) levels (130/82 mm Hg) and National Kidney Foundation (NKF)–recommended BP levels (130/80 mm Hg) may require multiple antihypertensive drugs. In the trials listed, patients with diabetes or renal impairment were titrated to either JNC 7- or NKF-recommended treatment goals. To reach treatment goals, patients needed a mean of 3.2 antihypertensive medications daily. AASK—African-American Study of Kidney Disease and Hypertension; ABCD—Appropriate Blood Pressure in NIDDM; ALLHAT—Antihypertensive and Lipid-lowering Treatment to Prevent Heart Attack Trial; HOT—Hypertension Optimal Treatment; IDNT—Irbesartan in Diabetic Nephropathy Trial; MDRD—Modification of Diet in Renal Disease; RENAAL—Reduction of Endpoints in NIDDM With the Angiotensin II Antagonist Losartan Study; SBP—systolic blood pressure; UKPDS—United Kingdom Prospective Diabetes Study.

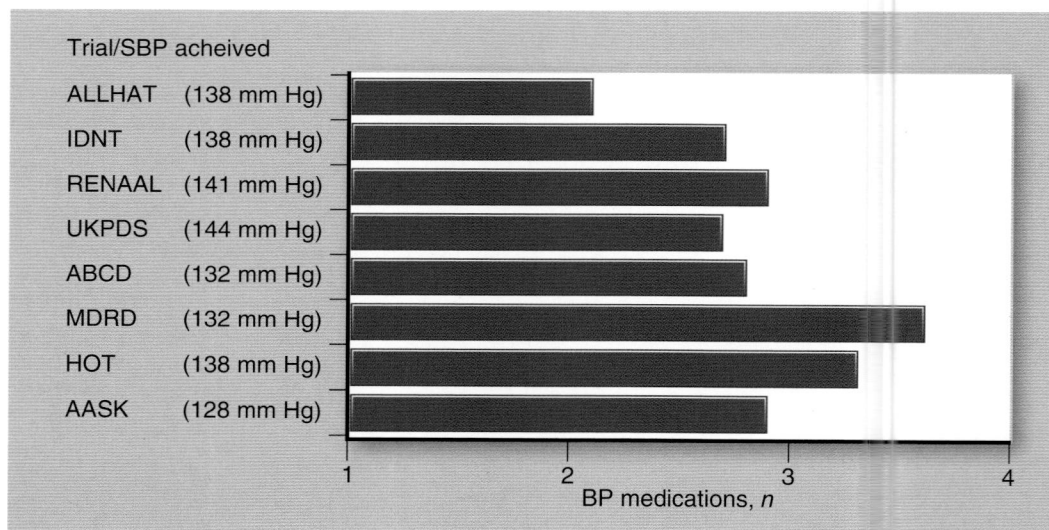

Trial/SBP acheived

ALLHAT	(138 mm Hg)
IDNT	(138 mm Hg)
RENAAL	(141 mm Hg)
UKPDS	(144 mm Hg)
ABCD	(132 mm Hg)
MDRD	(132 mm Hg)
HOT	(138 mm Hg)
AASK	(128 mm Hg)

BP medications, *n*

Effects of Therapy in Older Hypertensive Patients

	HDFP	EWPHE	SHEP	HYVET	Australian	Coope and Warrender	STOP	MRC
Patients, *n*	2374	840	4736	3845	582	884	1627	4396
Age, *y*	60–69	> 60	60 to ≥ 80	> 80	60–69	60–79	70–84	65–74
Mean entry blood pressure, *mm Hg*	170/101	182/101	170/77	173/91	165/101	197/100	195/102	185/91
Relative risk of event (treated vs control)								
Stroke	0.56*	0.64	0.67*	0.7	0.67	0.58*	0.53*	0.75*
CHD	0.85*	0.8	0.73*	0.72	0.82	1.03	0.87	0.81
CHF	–	0.78	0.45*	0.36	–	0.68	0.49*	–
All CVD	0.84*	0.71*	0.68*	0.77	0.69	0.76*	0.60*	0.83*

Figure 8-38. The results of eight clinical trials of antihypertensive therapy in the elderly. All showed a reduction in stroke, which was statistically significant in five of the trials. Although coronary heart disease (CHD) was reduced in seven trials, statistical significance was achieved only in the Hypertension Detection and Follow-up Program (HDFP) [18] and Systolic Hypertension in the Elderly Program (SHEP) [19] trials. Whether hypertension in the elderly differs from hypertension in younger patients in terms of the relative weight of cardiovascular risk factors is unknown. This consideration might bear on the importance of the metabolic side effects of diuretics and β-blockers, making them more significant for younger hypertensives. *Asterisks* indicate statistical significance. Australian—Australian National Therapeutic Trial in Mild Hypertension; CHF—congestive heart failure; CVD—cardiovascular disease; EWPHE—European Working Party on High Blood Pressure in the Elderly; HYVET—Hypertension in the Very Elderly Trial; MRC—Medical Research Council; STOP—Swedish Trial in Old Patients with hypertension.

Recommendations for the Treatment of Hypertension

Classification and Management of Blood Pressure

BP classification	SBP, *mm Hg*	DBP, *mm Hg*
Normal	< 120	and < 80
Prehypertension	120–139	or 80–89
Stage 1 hypertension	140–159	or 90–99
Stage 2 hypertension	≥ 160	≥ 100

DBP—diastolic blood pressure; SBP—systolic blood pressure.

Figure 8-39. The Seventh Report of the Joint National Committee on Prevention, Detection, Evaluation, and Treatment of High Blood Pressure (JNC 7) classifies blood pressure (BP) in adults on the basis of an average of two or more accurate BP readings at two or more office visits. Stage 1 hypertension remains 140–159/90–99 mm Hg and stage 2 hypertension ≥ 160/100 mm Hg. Patients in these categories should begin lifestyle modifications and pharmacologic therapy (if compelling indications accompany stage 1). Patients with stage 2 hypertension should begin a two-drug combination.

Prehypertension represents BP of 120–139/80–89 mm Hg, and patients in this category are more likely to progress to hypertension. Specifically, those in the 130–139/80–89 mm Hg BP range have twice the risk for developing hypertension as those with lower BP levels. DBP—diastolic blood pressure; SBP—systolic blood pressure.

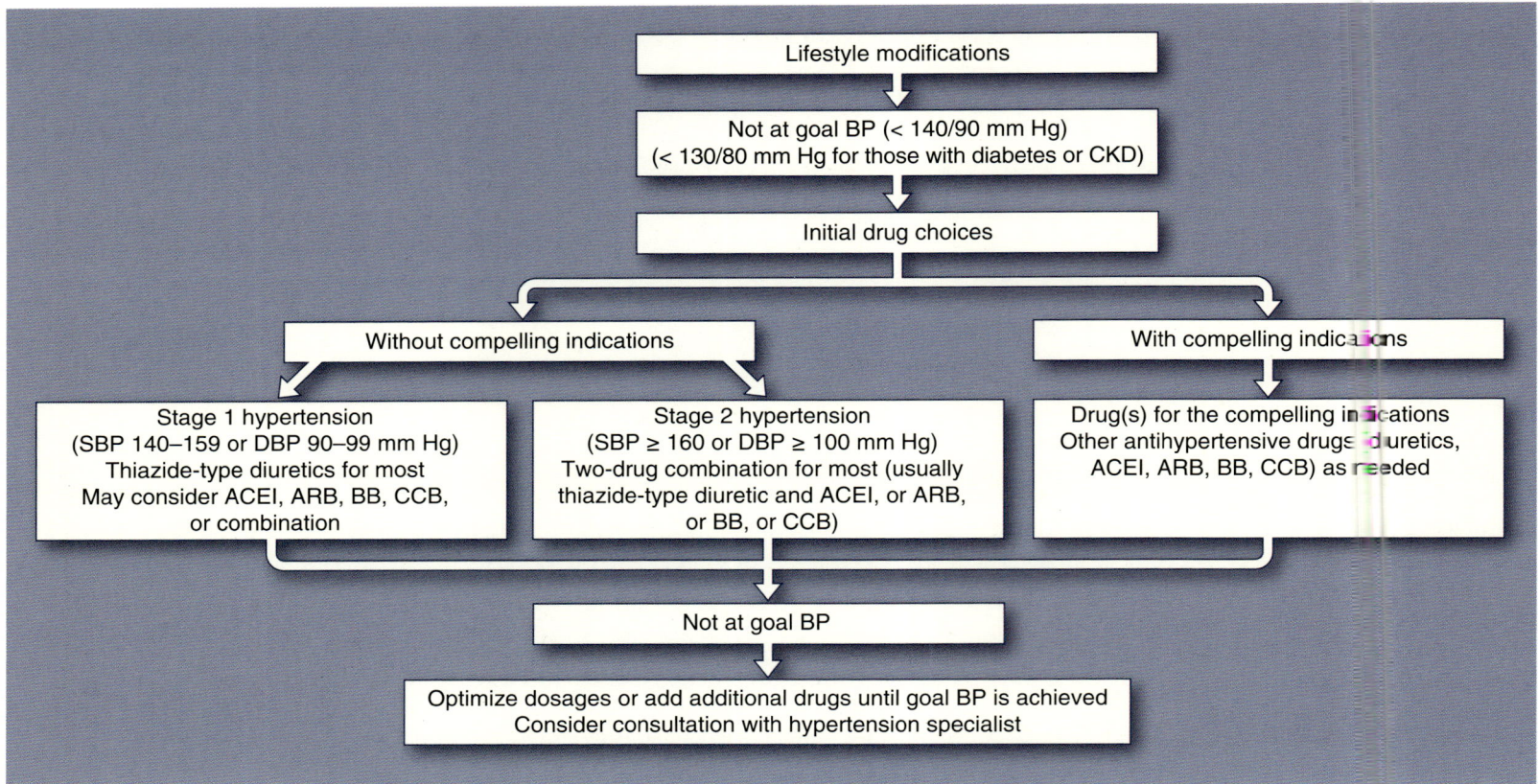

Figure 8-40. Lifestyle modifications constitute the first step in treating hypertension. If the patient has not reached the desired blood pressure (BP) of < 140/90 mm Hg (< 130/80 mm Hg for those diagnosed with diabetes or chronic kidney disease [CKD]), the next step is pharmacologic therapy. Initially, most patients with stage 1 hypertension should use a thiazide diuretic. Stage 2 hypertension usually requires a combination therapy utilizing two drugs. When the use of one drug fails to achieve the desired BP, a second drug from a different class should be initiated. A thiazide diuretic along with an angiotensin-converting enzyme inhibitor (ACEI), an angiotensin II receptor blockers (ARB), a β-blocker (BB), or a calcium channel blocker (CCB) often serves as an ideal two-drug combination.

Compelling indications (*eg*, post–myocardial infarction, heart failure, diabetes) require specific antihypertensives.

Even after following the treatment algorithm, the patient still may not reach the desired BP goal. In this case, optimize the patient's dosages, initiate additional drugs, or consult with a hypertension specialist [20]. DBP—diastolic blood pressure; SBP—systolic blood pressure.

Situations In Which Automated Noninvasive Ambulatory Blood Pressure Monitoring Devices May Be Useful

"Office" or "white-coat" hypertension: blood pressure repeatedly elevated in office setting but repeatedly normal out of office

Evaluation of drug resistance

Evaluation of nocturnal blood pressure changes

Episodic hypertension

Hypotensive symptoms associated with antihypertensive medications or autonomic dysfunction

Carotid sinus syncope and pacemaker syndromes

Figure 8-41. Situations in which automated noninvasive ambulatory blood pressure monitoring devices may be useful. For carotid sinus syncope and pacemaker syndromes, electrocardiographic monitoring should also be employed.

Special Situations in the Management of Hypertension

Hypertension in Pregnancy

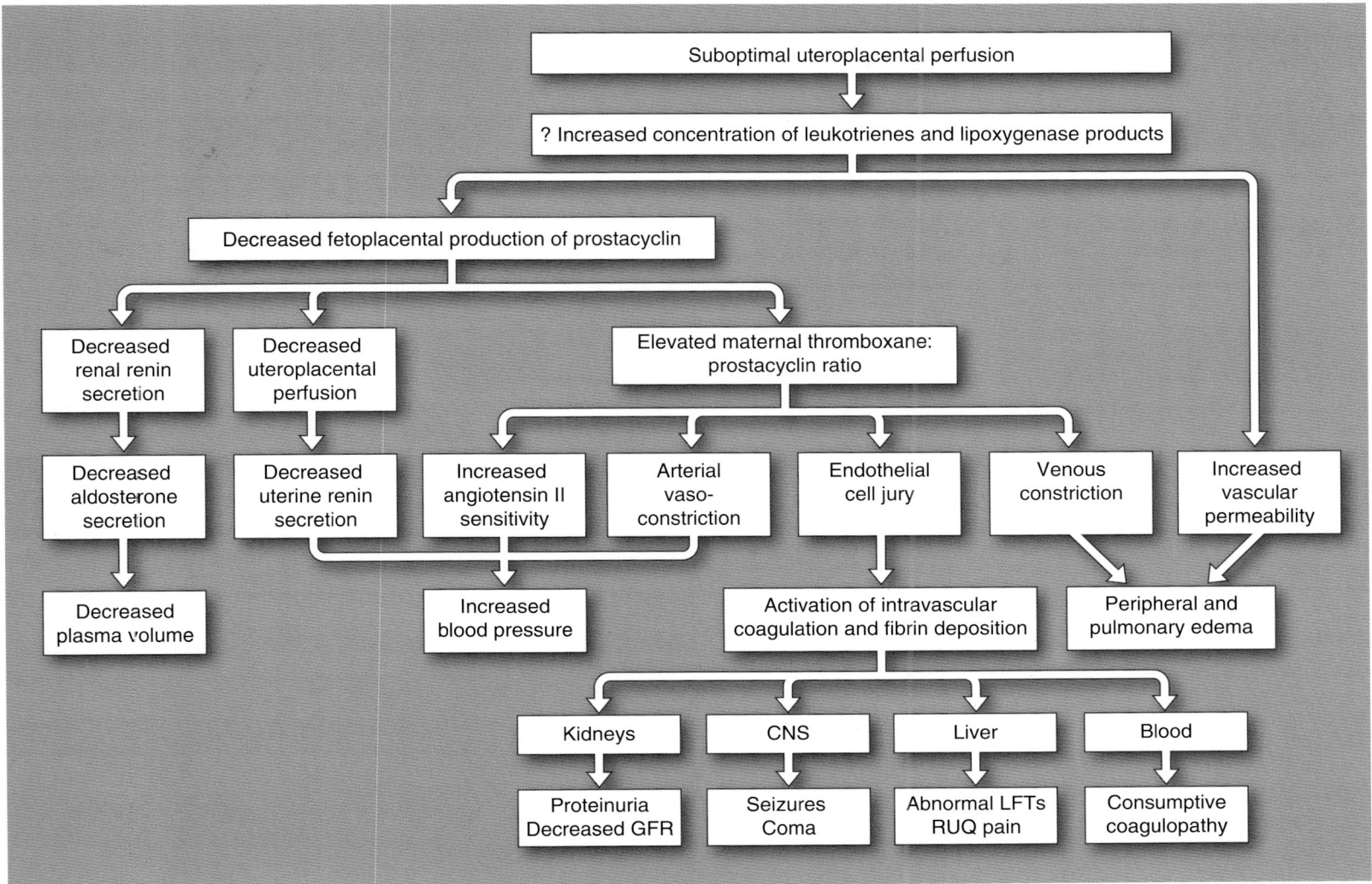

Figure 8-42. Scheme proposed to explain some of the pathophysiologic factors thought to be operative in preeclampsia and their consequences [21]. Note that hypertension is only one feature of this complex illness. CNS—central nervous system; GFR—glomerular filtration rate; LFTs—liver function tests; RUQ—right upper quadrant.

Hypertension in Blacks

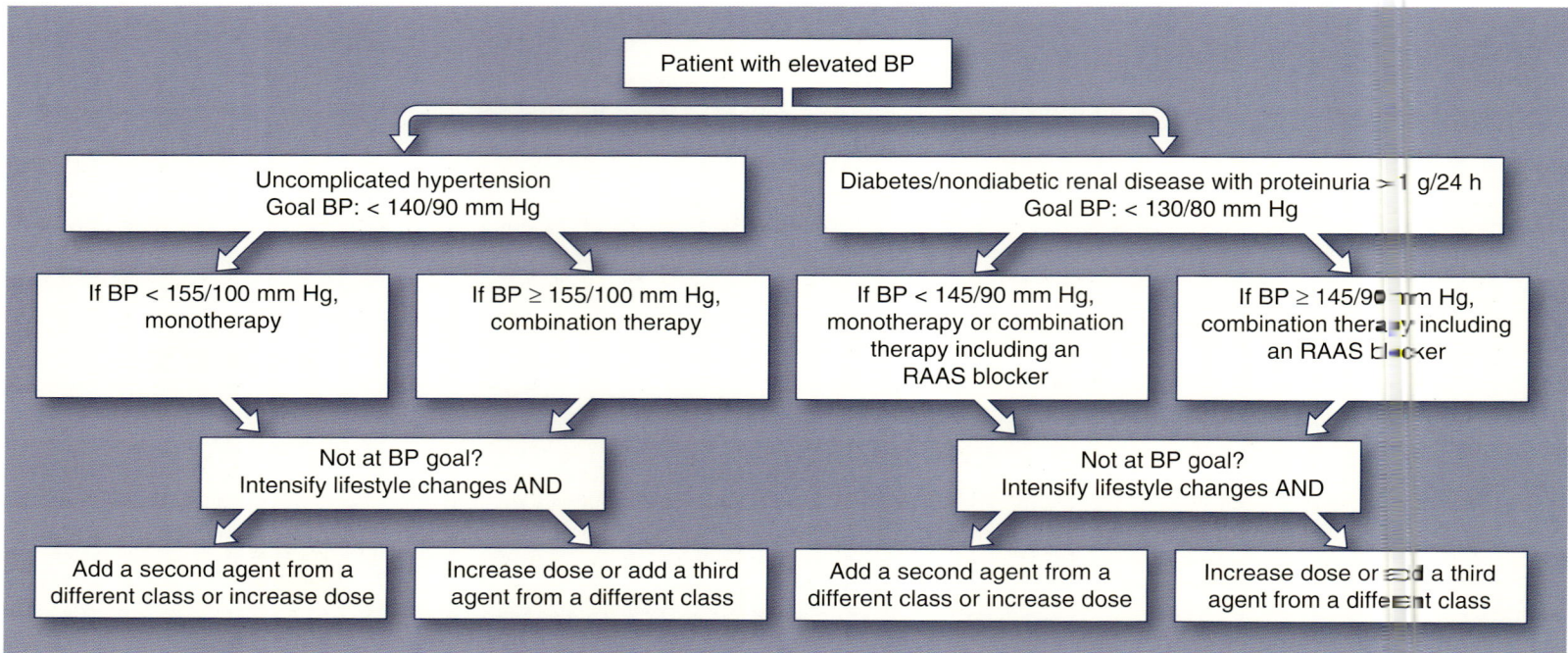

```
                        ┌──────────────────────────┐
                        │  Patient with elevated BP │
                        └──────────────────────────┘
```

| Uncomplicated hypertension Goal BP: < 140/90 mm Hg | Diabetes/nondiabetic renal disease with proteinuria > 1 g/24 h Goal BP: < 130/80 mm Hg |

| If BP < 155/100 mm Hg, monotherapy | If BP ≥ 155/100 mm Hg, combination therapy | If BP < 145/90 mm Hg, monotherapy or combination therapy including an RAAS blocker | If BP ≥ 145/90 mm Hg, combination therapy including an RAAS blocker |

| Not at BP goal? Intensify lifestyle changes AND | Not at BP goal? Intensify lifestyle changes AND |

| Add a second agent from a different class or increase dose | Increase dose or add a third agent from a different class | Add a second agent from a different class or increase dose | Increase dose or add a third agent from a different class |

Figure 8-43. This figure depicts the clinical algorithm for achieving blood pressure (BP) goals in hypertensive black patients. For patients with uncomplicated hypertension, the Hypertension in African Americans Working Group of the International Society on Hypertension in Blacks suggests monotherapy for blood pressure (BP) < 155/100 mm Hg and combination therapy for BP ≥ 155/100 mm Hg. In patients with diabe- tes or nondiabetic renal disease with BP < 145/90 mm Hg, the Working Group recommends initial monotherapy or combination therapy includ- ing a renin-angiotensin-aldosterone system (RAAS) blocker. Patients with diabetes or nondiabetic renal disease and BP ≥ 145/90 mm Hg, the Work- ing Group suggests combination therapy including an RAAS blocker. Most patients will require combination therapy to reach their goal [22].

Hypertensive Emergencies

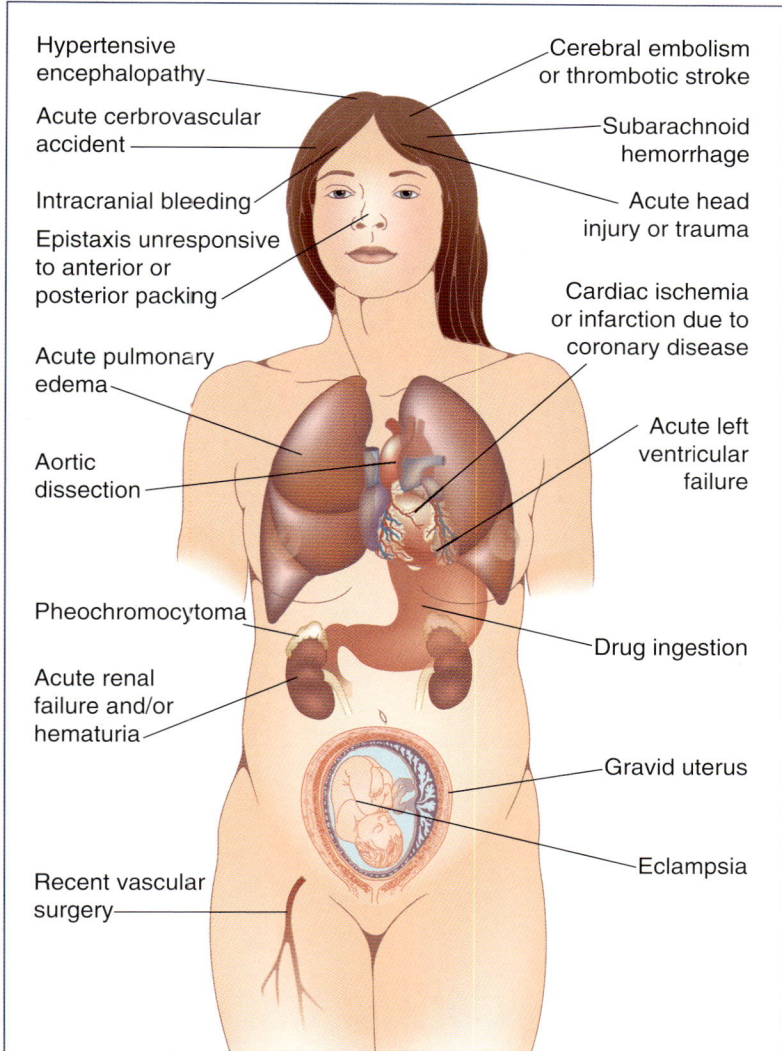

Figure 8-44. Common clinical conditions that are often considered hypertensive emergencies. Severe acute target organ damage is the major distinguishing factor between emergencies and urgencies.

Isolated Systolic Hypertension

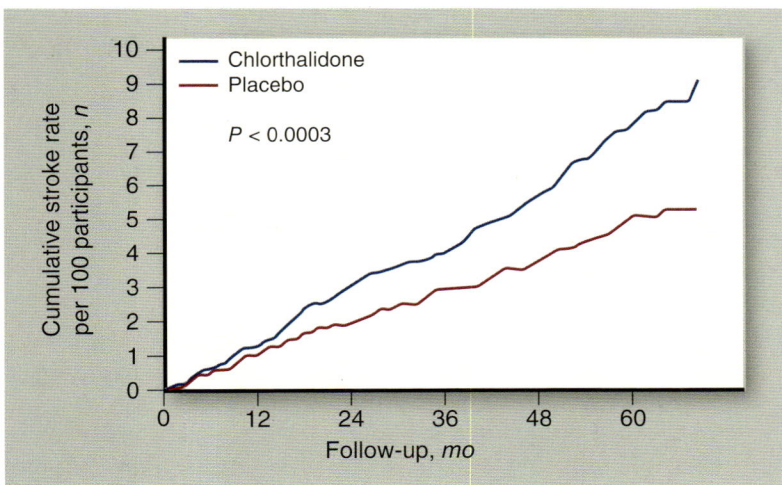

Figure 8-45. The occurrence of fatal and nonfatal strokes (the primary outcome measure) during the Systolic Hypertension in the Elderly Program [19]. In these elderly patients, compared with placebo, low-dose chlorthalidone therapy was statistically associated with decreased risk of stroke after an average of 4.5 years of therapy.

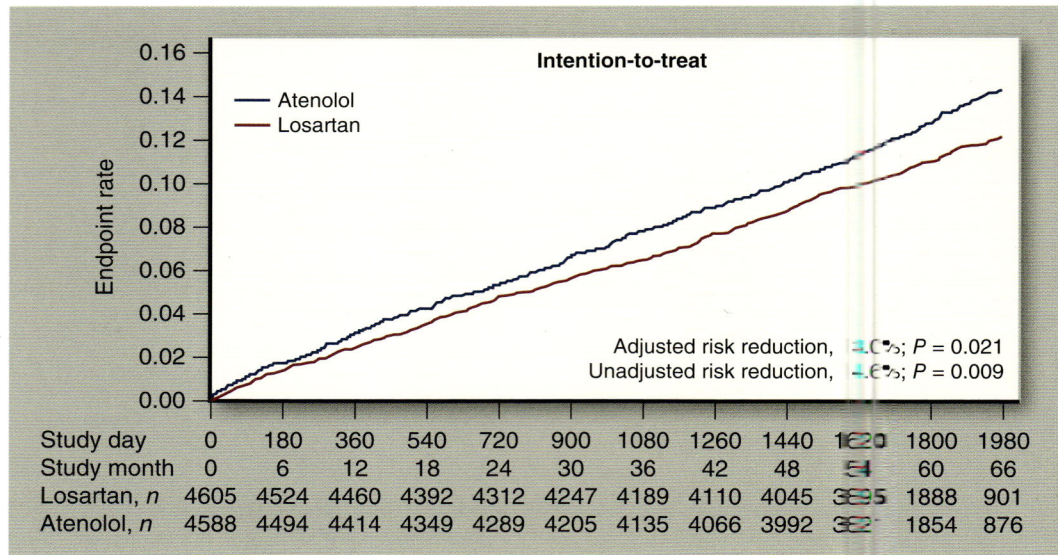

Figure 8-46. The Losartan Intervention for Endpoint reduction (LIFE) in hypertension study randomly assigned 9110 patients to receive either a β-blocker or angiotensin II receptor blocker as the baseline therapy (diuretics were allowed as add-on therapy). In this cohort of primarily older Scandinavian hypertensive subjects with left ventricular hypertrophy (LVH), there was an overall 16% reduction in combined cardiovascular disease events over the 4 years of follow-up. Interestingly, despite these subjects having higher risk of coronary events (all had LVH), the benefit was driven by reduction in stroke rather than heart disease [23].

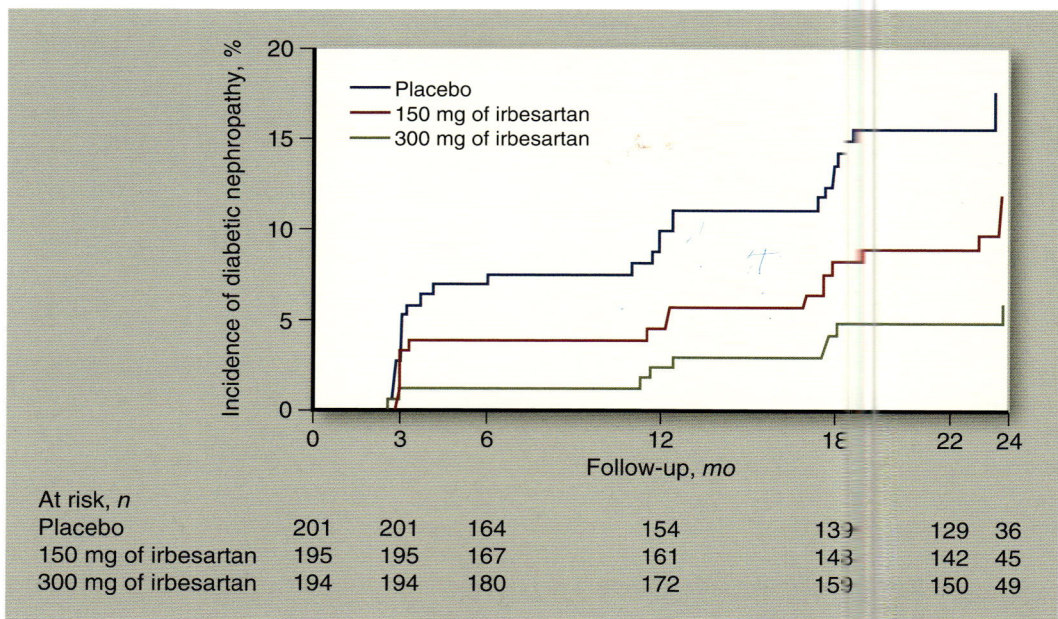

Figure 8-47. Advantages of antihypertensive regimens in preventing progression to clinical proteinuria. A total of 590 patients with hypertension (153/90 mm Hg), type 2 diabetes, microalbuminuria (56 μg/min), and normal renal function (serum creatinine 1.1 mg/dL) were randomly assigned to placebo plus conventional therapy, irbesartan 150 mg plus conventional therapy, or irbesartan 300 mg plus conventional therapy to see if there was an advantage of a specific antihypertensive regimen in preventing progression to clinical proteinuria (300 μg/min) over a 2-year period. The average follow-up blood pressure during the course of the study was approximately 143/83 mm Hg for the three groups. In this figure, one can appreciate the incidence of diabetic nephropathy based on the three therapies. Ten of 94 patients in the 300-mg irbesartan group (5.2%) and 19 of the 195 patients in the 150-mg irbesartan group (9.7%) reached clinical proteinuria, as compared with 30 of 201 patients in the placebo group: 14.9% (hazard ratios, 0.30; 95% CI, 0.14–0.61; $P < 0.001$) and 0.61% (95% CI, 0.34–1.09; $P = 0.08$), respectively. The angiotensin II receptor blocker irbesartan retards the progression to clinical proteinuria in hypertensive patients with type 2 diabetes and microalbuminuria independent of blood pressure [24].

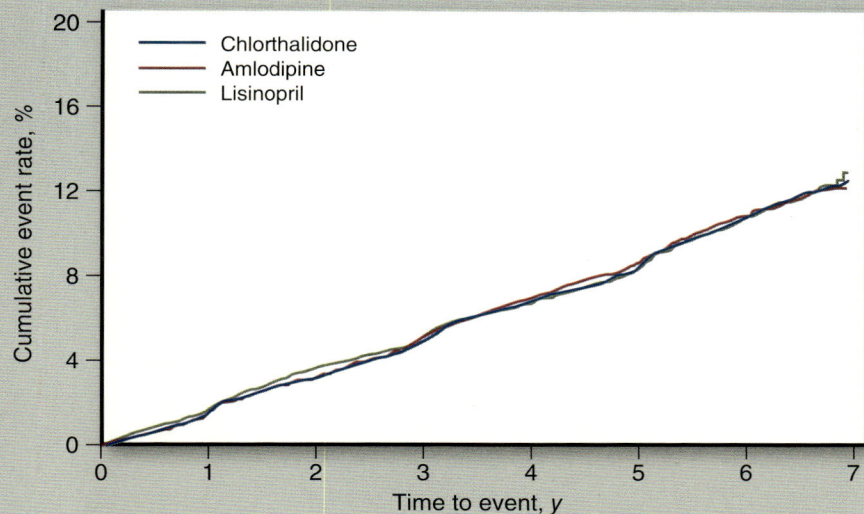

Figure 8-48. Cumulative event rate for the primary outcome in the Antihypertensive and Lipid-lowering Treatment to Prevent Heart Attack Trial (ALLHAT), which compared chlorthalidone, amlodipine, and lisinopril. The primary endpoint was fatal coronary heart disease or nonfatal myocardial infarction. There were no significant differences in the treatment groups [25].

At risk, n								
Chlorthalidone	15,255	14,477	13,820	13,102	11,362	6340	2956	209
Amlodipine	9848	8576	8218	7843	6824	3870	1878	215
Lisinopril	9854	8535	8123	7711	6662	3832	1770	195

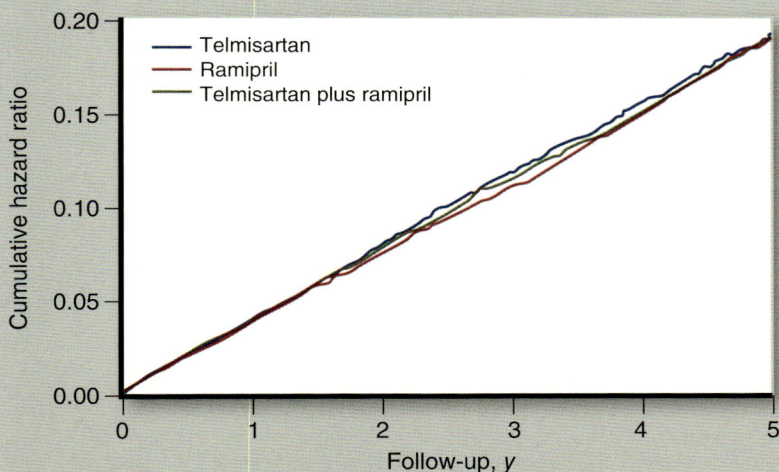

Figure 8-49. The recent ONTARGET study tested whether a combination of angiotensin-converting enzyme inhibitor and angiotensin-receptor blocker would provide incremental event reduction in hypertensive patients. The composite primary outcome was death from cardiovascular causes, myocardial infarction, stroke, or hospitalization for heart failure. There was no difference in more than 25,000 patients treated with telmisartan, ramipril, or the combination [26].

At risk, n					
Telmisartan	8542	8177	7778	7420	7051	1687
Ramipril	8576	8214	7832	7472	7093	1703
Telmisartan plus ramipril	8502	8133	7738	7375	7022	1718

Acknowledgments

Contributors to this chapter in previous editions were R. Wayne Alexander, John Amerena, Henry R. Black, Emmanuel L. Bravo, Hans R. Brunner, Robert M. Carey, William J. Elliott, Kathy K. Griendling, Randolph A. Hennigar, Stevo Julius, Barry J. Materson, Kenneth Jamerson, Helmy M. Siragy, Bernard Waeber, Alan B. Weder, Matthew R. Weir.

References

1. American Heart Association/American Stroke Association: *Heart Disease and Stroke Statistics*. Dallas: American Heart Association; 2008.

2. Kannel WB: Update on cardiovascular disease: recent findings and newest therapeutic choices. *Am J Hypertens* 2007, 3S–10S.

3. Kshirsagar AV, Carpenter M, Ban H, *et al.*: Blood pressure usually considered normal is associated with an elevated risk of cardiovascular disease. *Am J Med* 2006, 119:133–141.4.

4. INTERSALT Cooperative Research Group: INTERSALT: an international study of electrolyte excretion and blood pressure: results for 24 hour urinary sodium and potassium excretion. *BMJ* 1988, 297:319–328.

5. de Wardener HE, MacGregor GA: Natriuretic hormone and essential hypertension as an endocrine disease. In *Essential Hypertension as an Endocrine Disease*. Edited by Edwards CRW, Carey RM. London: Butterworths; 1985:132–157.

6. McCarron DA, Morris CD, Henry HJ, *et al.*: Blood pressure and nutrient intake in the United States. *Science* 1984, 224:1392–1398.

7. Gruchow HW, Sobocinski KA, Barboriak JJ: Calcium intake and the relationship of dietary sodium and potassium to blood pressure. *Am J Clin Nutr* 1988, 48:1463–1470.

8. Lifton RP, Gharavi AG, Geller DS: Molecular mechanisms of human hypertension. *Cell* 2001, 104:545–556.

9. Weber KT: Aldosterone in congestive heart failure. *N Engl J Med* 2001, 345:1689-1697.

10. Griendling KK, Alexander RW: Cellular biology of blood vessels. In *Hurst's The Heart*. Edited by Schlant RC, Alexander RW, O'Rourke R, *et al.*: New York: McGraw-Hill; 1994:31–45.

11. Lüscher TF, Vanhoutte PM: Endothelium-dependent contraction to acetylcholine in the aorta of the spontaneously hypertensive rat. *Hypertension* 1986, 8:344–348.

12. Victor RG, Kaplan NM: Systemic hypertension: mechanisms and diagnosis. In *Braunwald's Heart Disease*. Edited by Libby P, Bonow RO, Mann DL, Zipes DP. Philadelphia: Saunders Elsevier; 2007:1027–1048.

13. Elliott WJ: Renovascular Hypertension. In *Hypertension*. Edited by Black HR and Elliott WJ. Philadelphia: Saunders Elsevier; 2007:93–105.

14. Bravo EL: What to do when potassium is low or high. *Diagnosis* 1988, 10:1–6.

15. National High Blood Pressure Education Program Working Group: National High Blood Pressure Education Program working group report on primary prevention of hypertension. *Arch Intern Med* 1993, 153:186–208.

16. Appel LJ, Moore TJ, Obarzanek E, *et al.*: A clinical trial on the effects of dietary patterns on blood pressure: DASH Collaborative Research Group. *N Engl J Med* 1997, 336:1117–1124.

17. Staessen J, Li Y, Thijs L, *et al.*: Blood pressure reduction and cardiovascular prevention: an update including the 2003–2004 Secondary Prevention Trials. *Hypertens Res* 2005, 28:385–407.

18. Hypertension Detection and Follow-up Program Cooperative Group: Five-year findings of the Hypertension Detection and Follow-up Program: I. Reduction in stroke incidence among persons with high blood pressure. *JAMA* 1982, 247:633–638.

19. SHEP Cooperative Research Group: Prevention of stroke by antihypertensive treatment in older persons with isolated systolic hypertension: final results of the Systolic Hypertension in the Elderly Program (SHEP). *JAMA* 1991, 265:3255–3264.

20. Chobanian AV, Bakris GL, Black HR, *et al.*: The Seventh Report of the Joint National Committee on Prevention, Detection, Evaluation and Treatment of High Blood Pressure. *JAMA* 2003, 289:2560–2571.

21. Friedman SA: Preeclampsia: a review of the role of prostaglandins. *Obstet Gynecol* 1988, 71:122–137.

22. Douglas JG, Bakris GL, Epstein M, *et al.*: Management of high blood pressure in African Americans: Consensus Statement of the Hypertension in African Americans Working Group of the International Society of Hypertension in Blacks. *Arch Intern Med* 2003, 163:525–541.

23. Dahlöf B, Devereux BB, Kjeldsen SE, *et al.*, for the LIFE study group: Cardiovascular morbidity and mortality in the Losartan Intervention For Endpoint reduction study (LIFE): a randomised trial against atenolol. *Lancet* 2002, 359:995–1003.

24. Parving HH, Lenhert H, Brochner-Mortensen J, *et al.*: The effect of irbesartan on the development of diabetic nephropathy in patients with type 2 diabetes. *N Engl J Med* 2001, 345:870–878.

25. Major outcomes in high-risk hypertensive patients randomized to angiotensin-converting enzyme inhibitor or calcium channel blocker vs diuretic: the Antihypertensive and Lipid-lowering Treatment to Prevent Heart Attack Trial (ALLHAT). *JAMA* 2002, 288:2981–2997.

26. The ONTARGET investigators: telmisartan, ramipril, or both in patients at high risk for vascular events. *N Engl J Med* 2008, 358:1547–1559.

Valvular Heart Disease

9

Patrick T. O'Gara

Moderate-to-severe valvular heart disease (VHD) affects some 2.5% of U.S. adults and its prevalence increases significantly with age for men and women [1]. Bicuspid aortic valve disease is a common congenital defect, occurring in approximately 1% of the population with a 4:1 male predominance. Recent investigations have demonstrated that acquired, degenerative aortic valve disease shares many metabolic and cellular pathways in common with atherosclerosis [2]. Myxomatous degeneration of the mitral valve apparatus, with prolapse or flail leaflet, is the most common cause of isolated mitral valve disease for which surgery is required. Whereas the incidence of rheumatic fever has declined significantly in developed countries, infection with group A beta-hemolytic *Streptococcus* in a susceptible individual remains an important cause of VHD in less developed and impoverished regions. Infective endocarditis is an important source of morbidity and mortality. Its epidemiology and natural history have changed considerably with the emergence of virulent, antibiotic-resistant organisms on a substrate of increasing numbers of intracardiac devices [3].

The diagnosis of VHD begins with the appreciation of a cardiac murmur, the characteristics of which may delineate the etiology and severity of the lesion. The history and physical examination allow a more informed appreciation of natural history and help to direct clinical decision making. Transthoracic echocardiography has become the preferred, initial noninvasive means by which to assess valve morphology and function, as well as ventricular size, wall thickness, and systolic function, and to estimate pulmonary artery pressures. When indicated, transesophageal and/or three-dimensional echocardiographic imaging can supplement the initial findings on a transthoracic study. Cardiac magnetic resonance imaging provides more precise measures of ventricular volumes and function. Quantitative characterization of lesion severity is critical to the management of individual patients, especially those who are asymptomatic but approaching recommended thresholds for elective surgery.

The management of patients with VHD has evolved empirically over the past several decades; there are very few randomized controlled trial data on which to rely [4]. Medical therapy often aims to ameliorate the complications of VHD, such as atrial fibrillation or heart failure, or to prevent infective endocarditis when indicated by current guidelines. The most dramatic advances in the treatment of patients with VHD have related to the improvements in surgical repair techniques and long-term outcomes. Acceptance of the recommendation to intervene surgically at an earlier time point in the natural history of both aortic and mitral disease, primarily to prevent ventricular dysfunction and heart failure, has accelerated in recent years. Valve repair—both mitral and aortic—has been adopted more widely and percutaneous techniques are emerging. Balloon dilatation for mitral stenosis has become the procedure of first choice for anatomically appropriate candidates. Prosthetic heart valve replacement remains necessary in a large segment of the VHD population an intervention that engenders a consideration of the trade-offs between anticoagulation and the durability of the prosthesis.

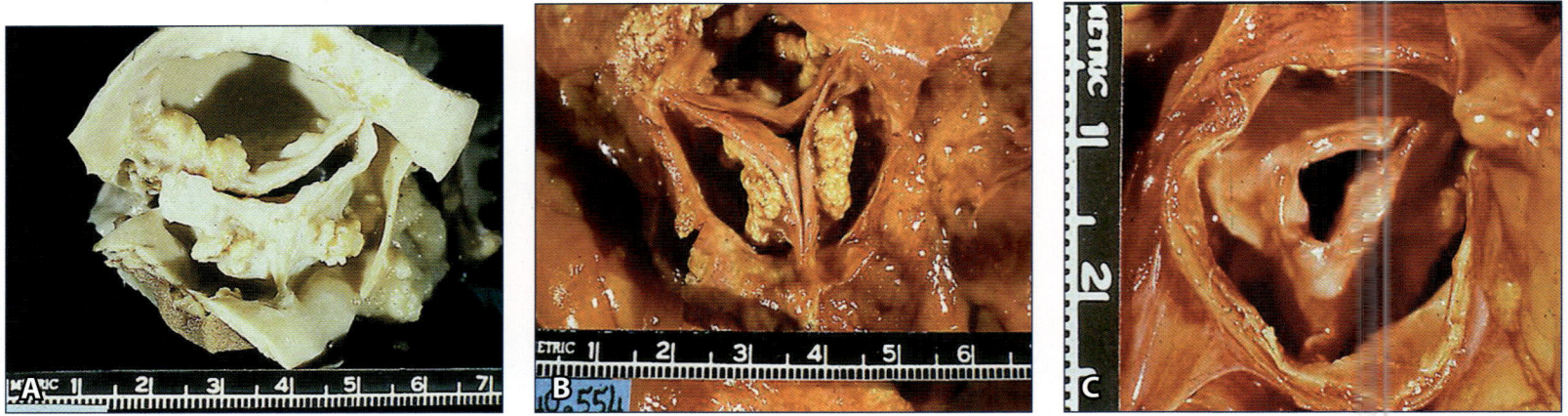

Figure 9-1. Dominant causes of aortic stenosis (AS). **A,** Congenitally bicuspid aortic valve disease, and its variants such as unicuspid valve disease, account for most cases of AS for which aortic valve replacement is performed. In this postmortem specimen, the bicuspid valve is thickened and heavily calcified with a horizontal commissure and rudimentary raphé at 6 o'clock. **B,** Trileaflet aortic valve with dense clumps of calcium adherent to the aortic surfaces, occupying the valve sinuses. Previously termed *senile, calcific AS*, this appearance is sometimes referred to as *atherosclerotic AS*. **C,** Rheumatic AS with thickening and contracture of the leaflets and commissures, resulting in a narrowed and incompetent orifice.

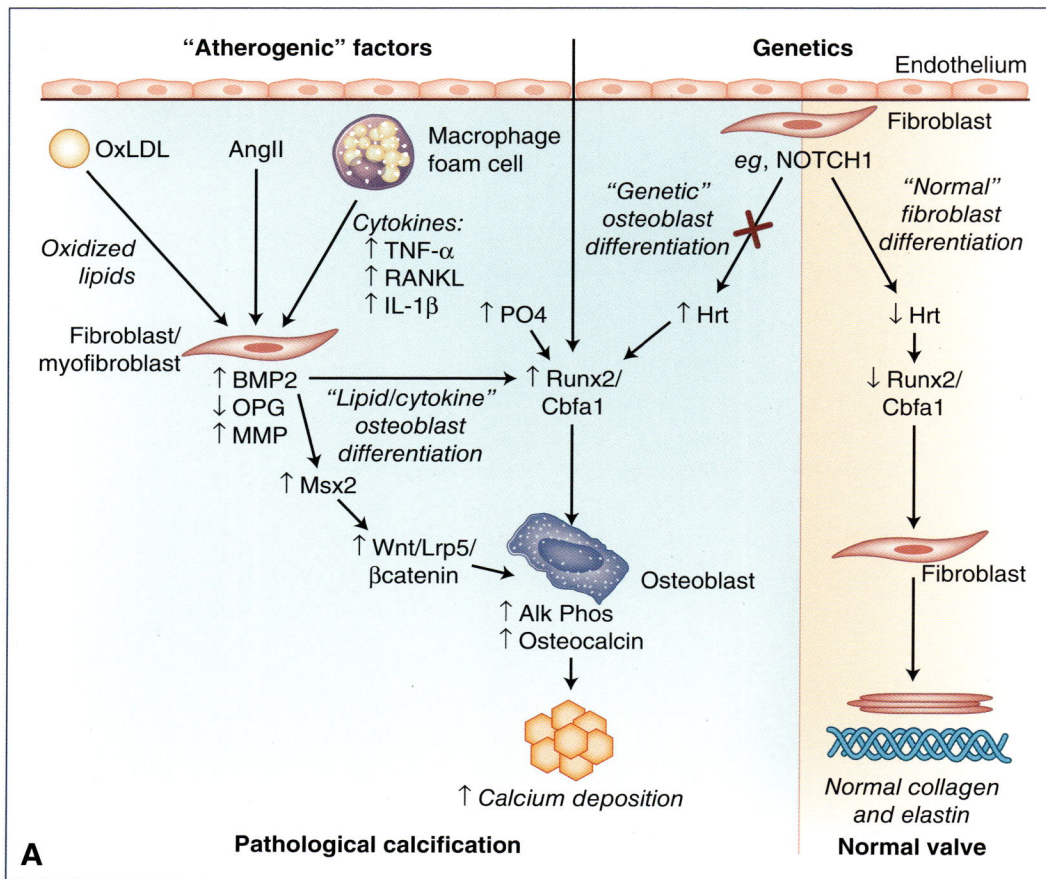

Figure 9-2. Pathogenesis of aortic stenosis. **A,** The cellular and metabolic processes that lead to pathological aortic valve calcification share many features in common with atherosclerosis. Endothelial injury or dysfunction facilitates the subintimal interplay among oxidized low-density lipoprotein (OxLDL), inflammatory cells, cytokines, and growth factors, leading eventually to differentiation of myofibroblasts along osteoblastic lines with bone protein production, deposition, and dystrophic calcification. On the *right* is an example of the possible contribution of genetic factors that may promote this process. NOTCH1 mutations have been described in only two families to date, but can lead to osteoblastic differentiation via lack of suppression of the Hrt and Runx2/Cbfa1 transcription pathways. AngII—angiotensin II; IL—interleukin; TNF—tumor necrosis factor. (*Adapted from* O'Brien [2].)

Continued on the next page

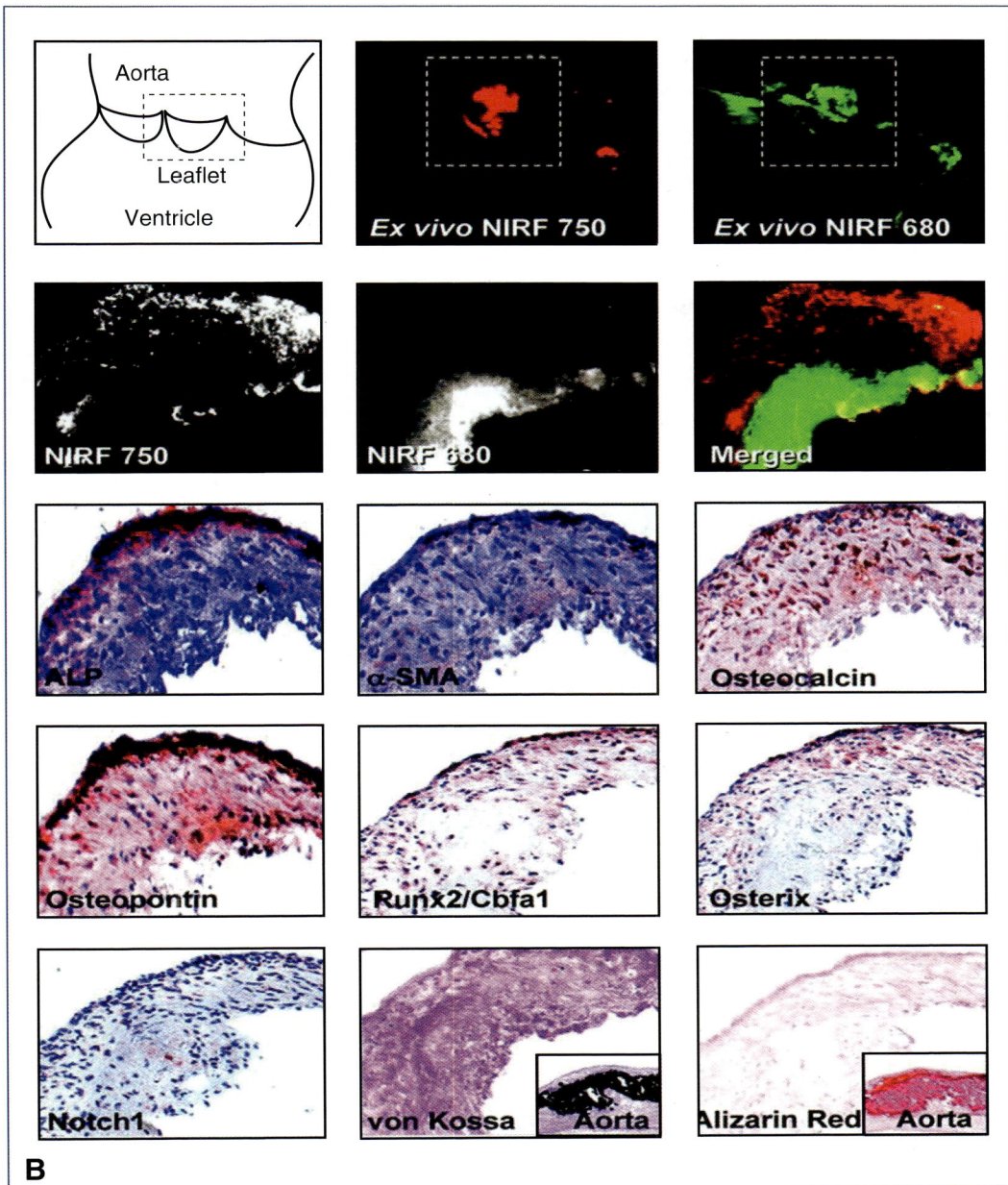

Figure 9-2. *(Continued)* **B,** Multimodality molecular imaging visualizes osteoblastic activity in the early stages of aortic valve stenosis. *Red* in the top row, middle panel, and second row, right panel, indicates osteogenesis; *green* in the top and second row, right panels, denotes inflammation. Lower three rows show colocalization of osteogenic activity with alkaline phosphatase, osteocalcin, osteopontin, and the osteogenic transcription factors Runx2/Cbfa1 and Osterix, and cleaved NOTCH 1. ALP—alkaline phosphatase; NIRF—near infrared fluorescent; α-SMA—α smooth muscle actin. (*Adapted from* Aikawa *et al.* [5].)

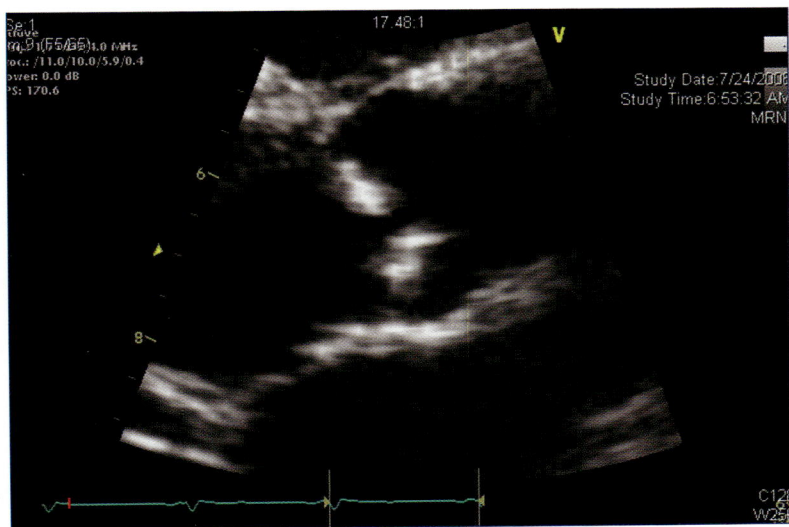

Figure 9-3. Heavily calcified, thickened aortic valve leaflets with reduced systolic opening as visualized in an echocardiographic parasternal long-axis view in a patient with bicuspid disease.

Valvular Heart Disease **215**

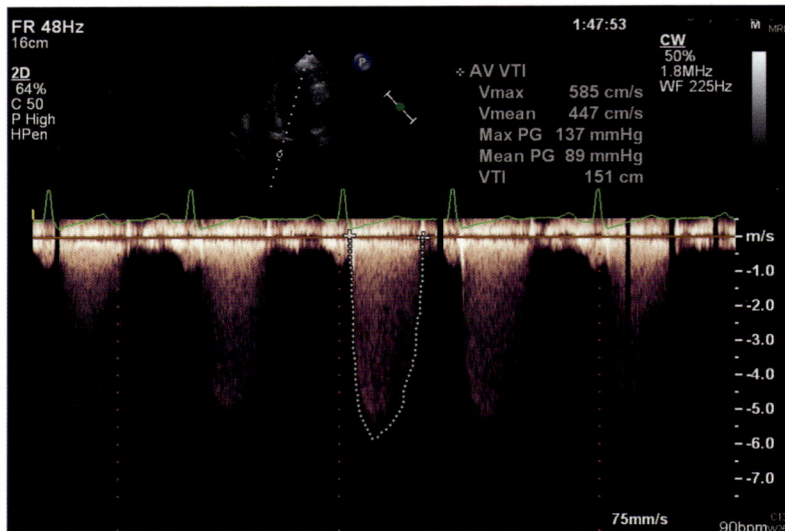

Figure 9-4. Continuous wave Doppler velocity profile obtained from the apical five-chamber view. In the velocity envelope outlined, the maximal velocity is 5.85 m/sec. By the modified Bernoulli equation, the estimated peak instantaneous gradient is 137 mm Hg; the mean pressure gradient is calculated at 89 mm Hg. These values are consistent with severe aortic stenosis, which by convention is also defined by a calculated valve area of less than 1.0 cm². There is a very strong correlation between Doppler and catheter-derived aortic valve gradients (*see* Chapter 13).

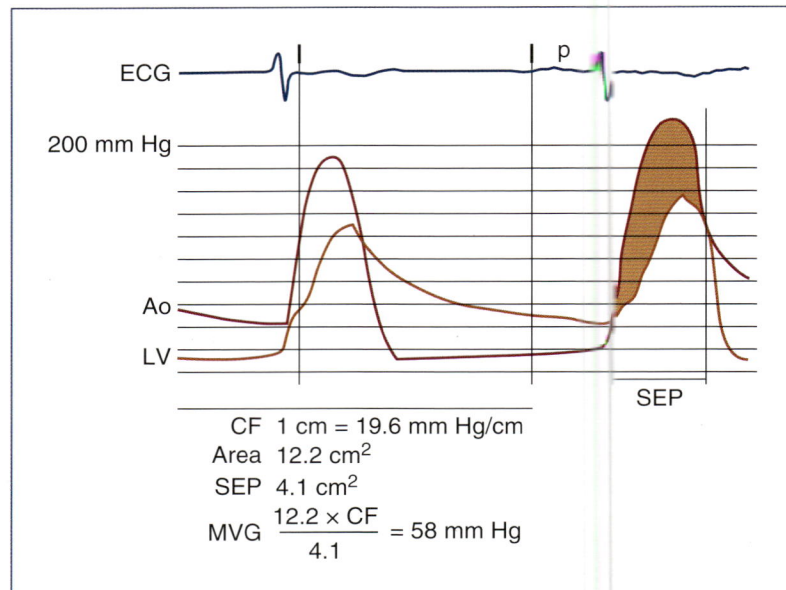

Figure 9-5. Hemodynamic study in a patient with aortic stenosis. *Orange* indicates the left ventricle (LV)–aortic (Ao) gradient. The planimetered area in this example is 58 mm Hg. The mean valve gradient (MVG) is used in the Gorlin formula to calculate valve area. CF—correction factor for planimetry calculation for the aortic orifice; ECG—electrocardiogram; SEP—systolic ejection period. (*Adapted from* Kern [6].)

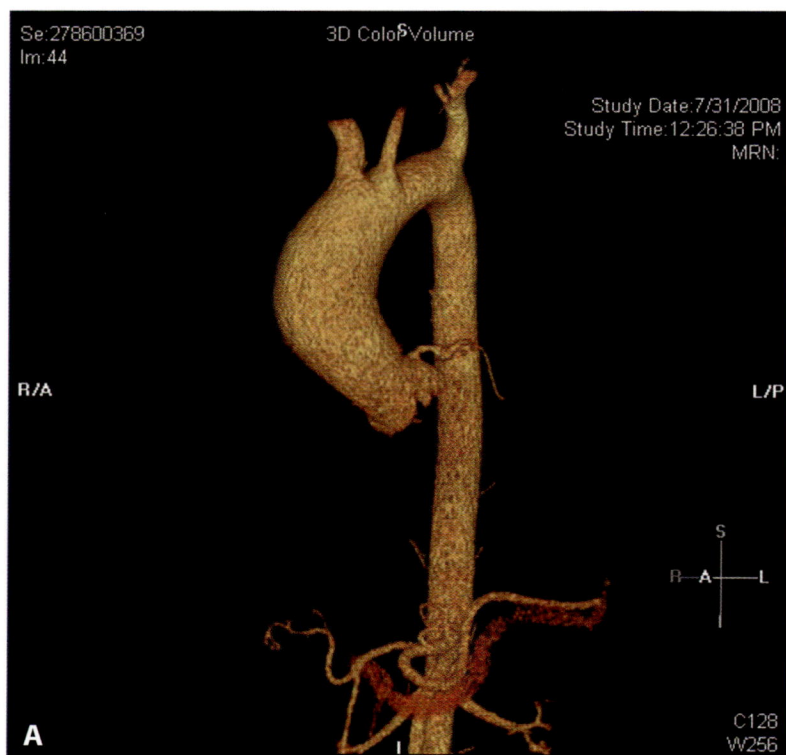

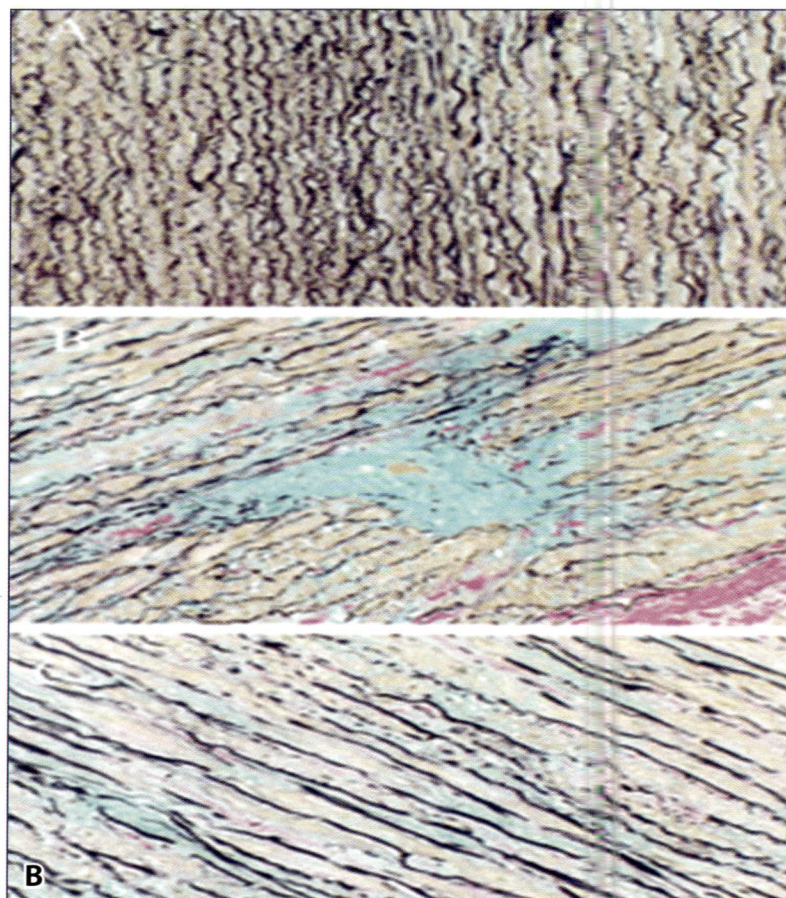

Figure 9-6. A, A 5.1-cm ascending aortic aneurysm in a 37-year-old man with bicuspid aortic valve disease and only moderate aortic stenosis (valve area, 1.2 cm²). Patients with bicuspid disease frequently develop aneurysms of the ascending aorta independent of the severity of hemodynamic valvular impairment, and are at risk for aortic dissection. Resection is indicated for maximal aneurysm size larger than 5.0 cm, an increase in aneurysm size of more than 0.5 cm/y, or at the time of aortic valve replacement if the aneurysm size exceeds 4.5 cm [4]. **B,** Histopathologic changes within the wall of aortic aneurysms in patients with Marfan syndrome (*middle*) and bicuspid aortic valve disease (*lower*), compared with normal aortic tissue from a control patient (*top*). In both pathological examples, there are areas of elastic lamellar degradation and cystic medial degeneration, more marked in the case of Marfan syndrome. (*Adapted from* Nataatmadja *et al.* [7].)

Indications for Aortic Valve Replacement for Aortic Stenosis

Severe aortic stenosis (peak jet velocity > 4 m/sec, mean gradient > 40 mm Hg, aortic valve area < 1.0 cm²)

1. Symptoms

2. Left ventricular ejection fraction < 0.5

3. Need for aortic, coronary, or other cardiac surgery

Moderate aortic stenosis (peak jet velocity, 3.0–4.0 m/sec, mean gradient 25–40 mm Hg, aortic valve area 1.0–1.5 cm²)

1. Need for aortic, coronary, or other cardiac surgery.

Figure 9-7. Indications for aortic valve replacement in patients with aortic stenosis [4].

Aortic Regurgitation

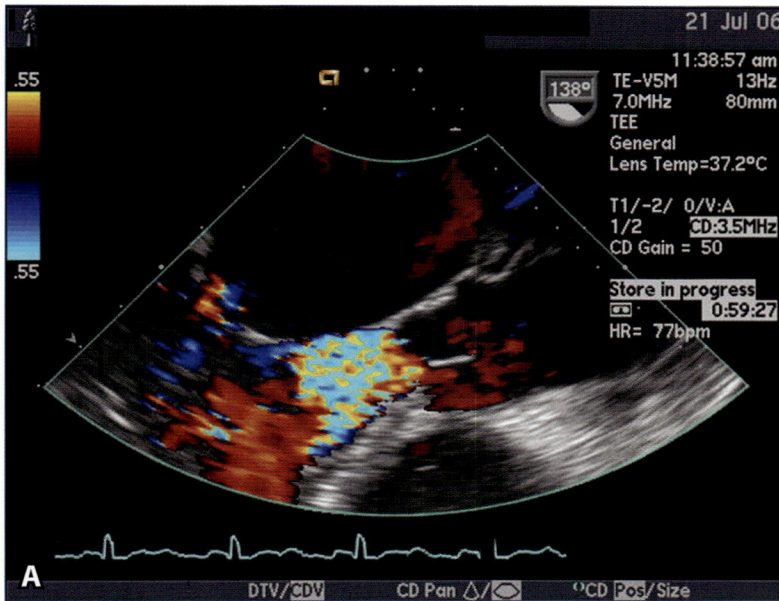

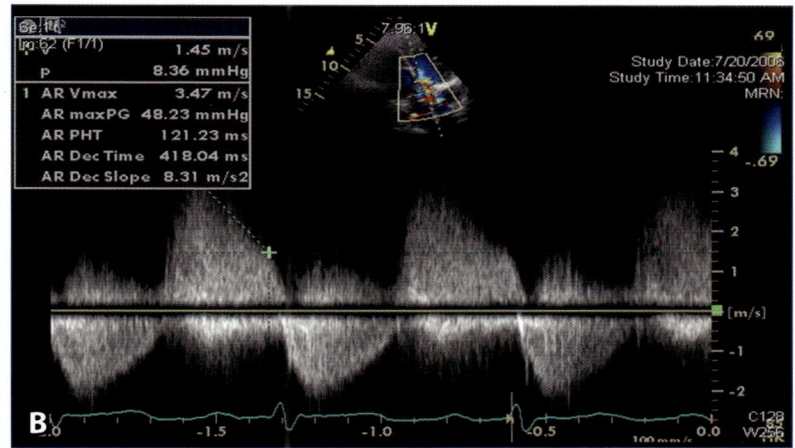

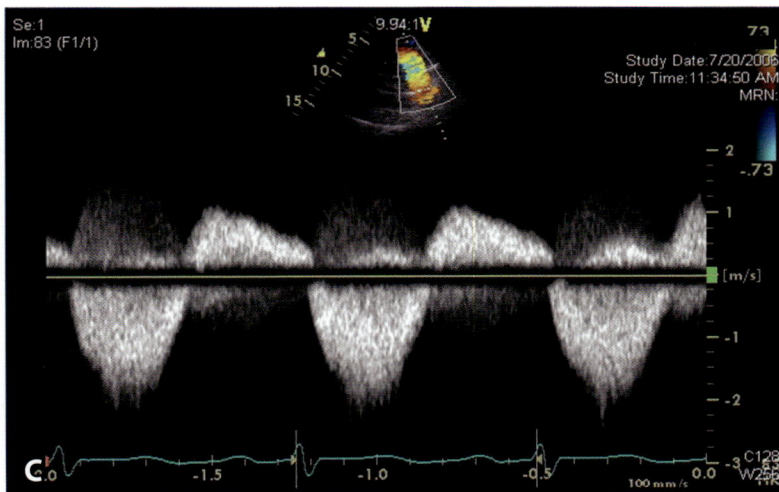

Figure 9-8. Acute severe aortic regurgitation (AR). The most common causes of acute severe aortic regurgitation are infective endocarditis, type A aortic dissection, and blunt chest wall trauma. The unprepared, noncompliant left ventricle operates on the steep portion of its pressure volume relationship and diastolic pressure rises precipitously, to the extent that the mitral valve closes prematurely. Forward stroke volume plummets and the heart rate increases to maintain cardiac output. Emergency aortic valve and/or root surgery is indicated. **A,** Color-flow Doppler image from a transesophageal echocardiogram (138° orientation) in a patient with *Staphylococcus aureus* infective endocarditis demonstrates a broad jet of severe AR that occupies the entire left ventricle outflow tract. **B,** Doppler recording from a transthoracic apical five-chamber view from the same patient shows a steep pressure half-time (AR PHT < 250 m/sec), reflecting the rapid rise in left ventricle diastolic pressure and its equilibration with aortic diastolic pressure (diastasis). **C,** Doppler recording from the descending thoracic aorta in the same patient shows dramatic diastolic reversal of flow, indicative of severe AR.

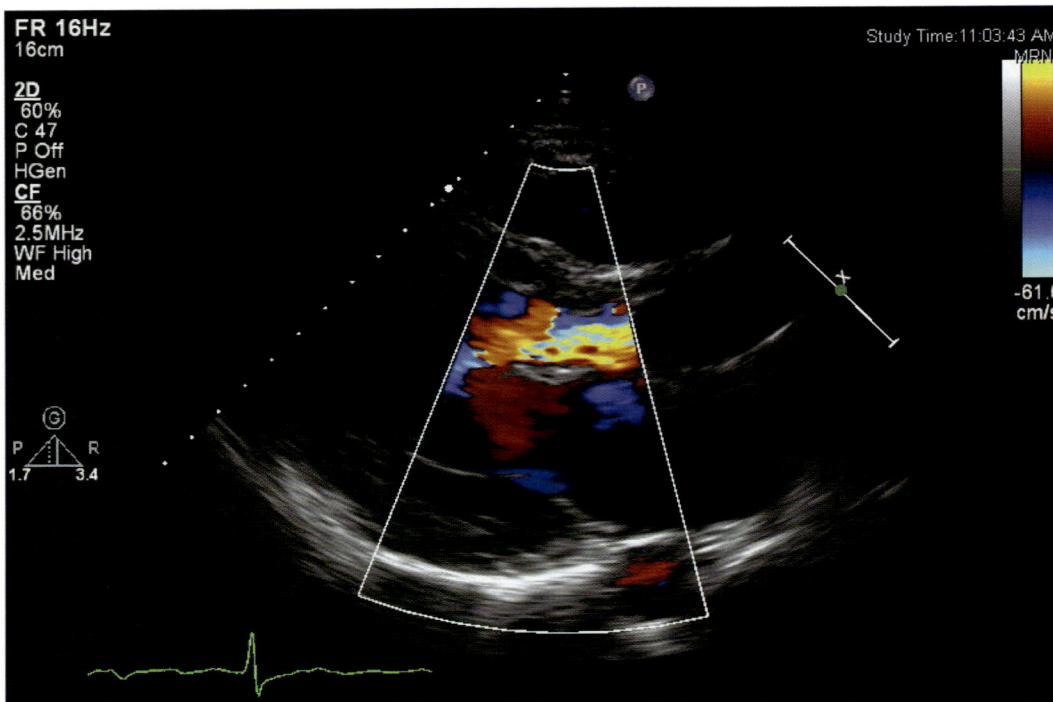

Figure 9-9. Chronic severe aortic regurgitation (AR). Color-flow Doppler image from the parasternal long-axis view in a 38-year-old man with bicuspid aortic valve disease followed conservatively for 20 years. Echocardiographic criteria for severe AR include a central jet occupying more than 65% of the left ventricular (LV) outflow tract, a regurgitant volume more than 60 mL/beat, a regurgitant fraction more than 50%, a regurgitant orifice area more than 0.30 cm², and LV cavity enlargement [8]. The LV end-diastolic dimension in this patient was measured at 6.5 cm.

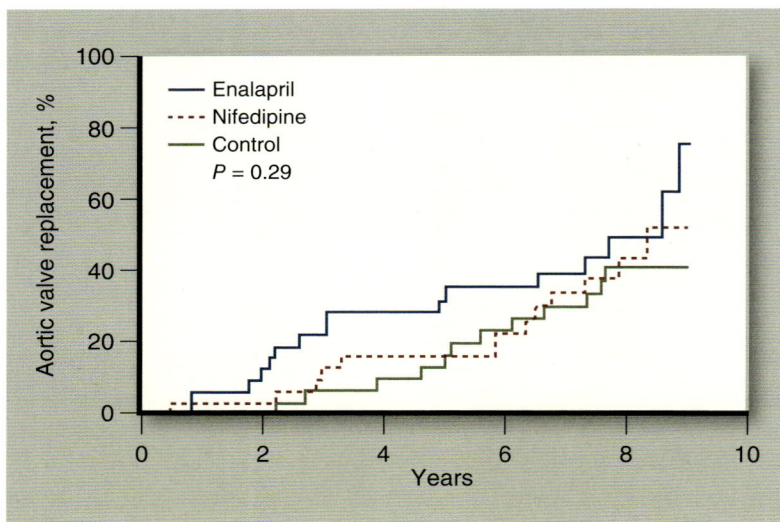

Figure 9-10. Lack of effect of vasodilators in chronic severe aortic regurgitation (AR). Ninety-five patients with asymptomatic, chronic severe AR, and normal left ventricular (LV) systolic function were randomly assigned to receive enalapril, nifedipine, or placebo. After a mean of 7 years, the rate of aortic valve replacement was similar among the three groups and there were no differences in echocardiographic indices of AR severity, LV size, or LV systolic function [9]. Vasodilators are recommended for treatment of hypertension, but not to extend the compensated phase of AR [4].

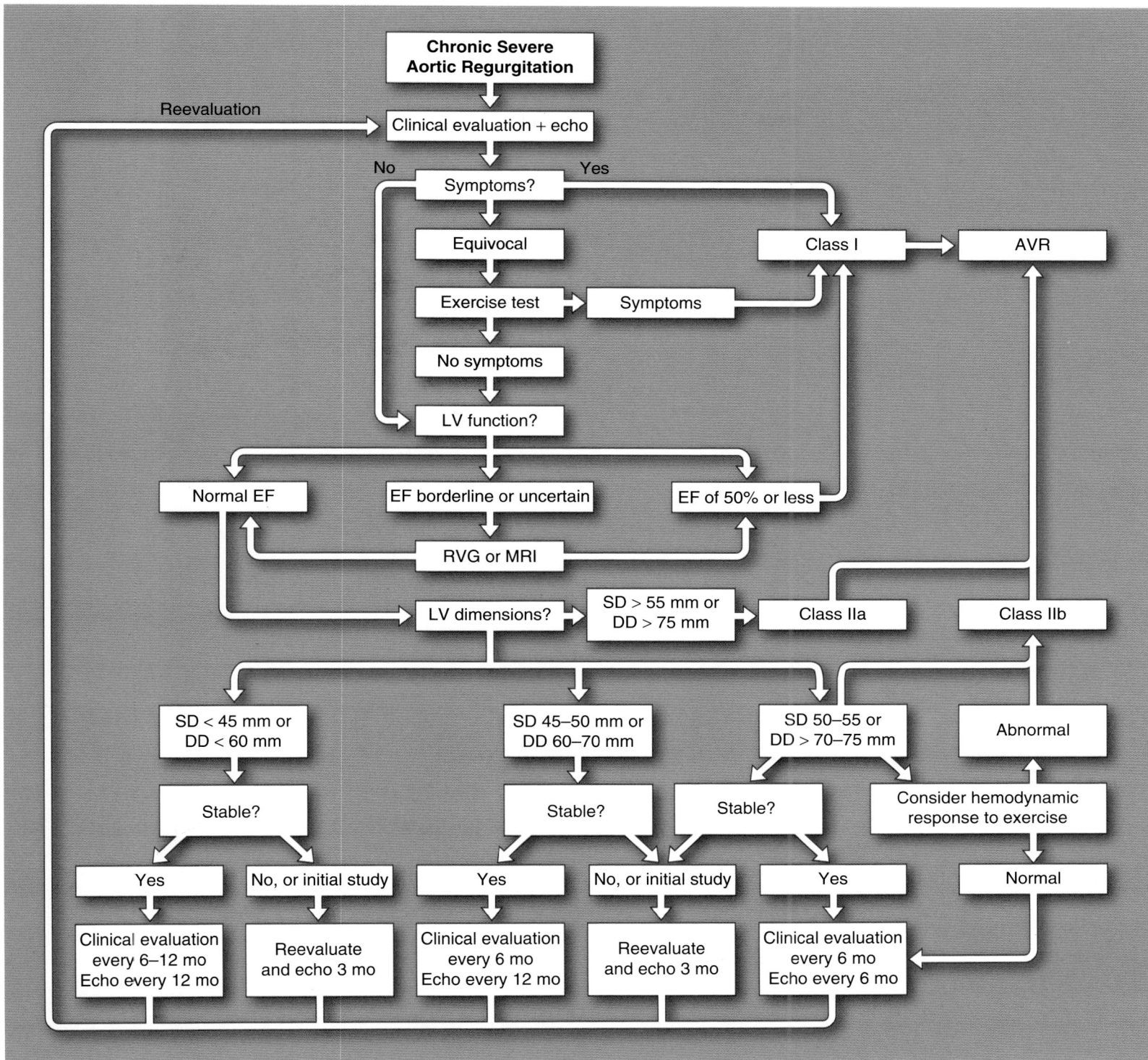

Figure 9-11. Management of chronic severe aortic regurgitation. Class recommendations (I, IIa, IIb) are according to American College of Cardiology/American Heart Association management guidelines. *Class I* indicates that there is general agreement that the intervention is useful and effective. *Class IIa* indicates that the recommendation is reasonable. *Class IIb* indicates that the recommendation can be condisered. AVR—aortic valve replacement; DD—end-diastolic dimension; echo—echocardiography; EF—ejection fraction; LV—left ventricle; MRI—cardiac magnetic resonance study; RVG—radionuclide ventriculogram; SD—end-systolic dimension. (*Adapted from* Bonow *et al.* [4].)

Mitral Stenosis

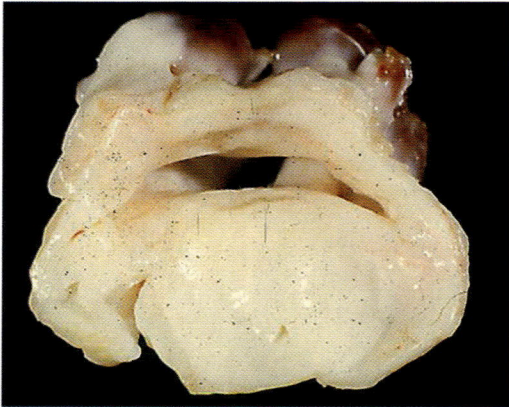

Figure 9-12. Operative specimen of a severely deformed, rheumatic mitral valve showing leaflet thickening, fusion of the commissures, thickening and foreshortening of the chordal apparatus, and extension of fibrosis and scarring onto the tips of the papillary muscles. Rheumatic fever, which remains prevalent in developing countries, is the dominant cause of mitral stenosis.

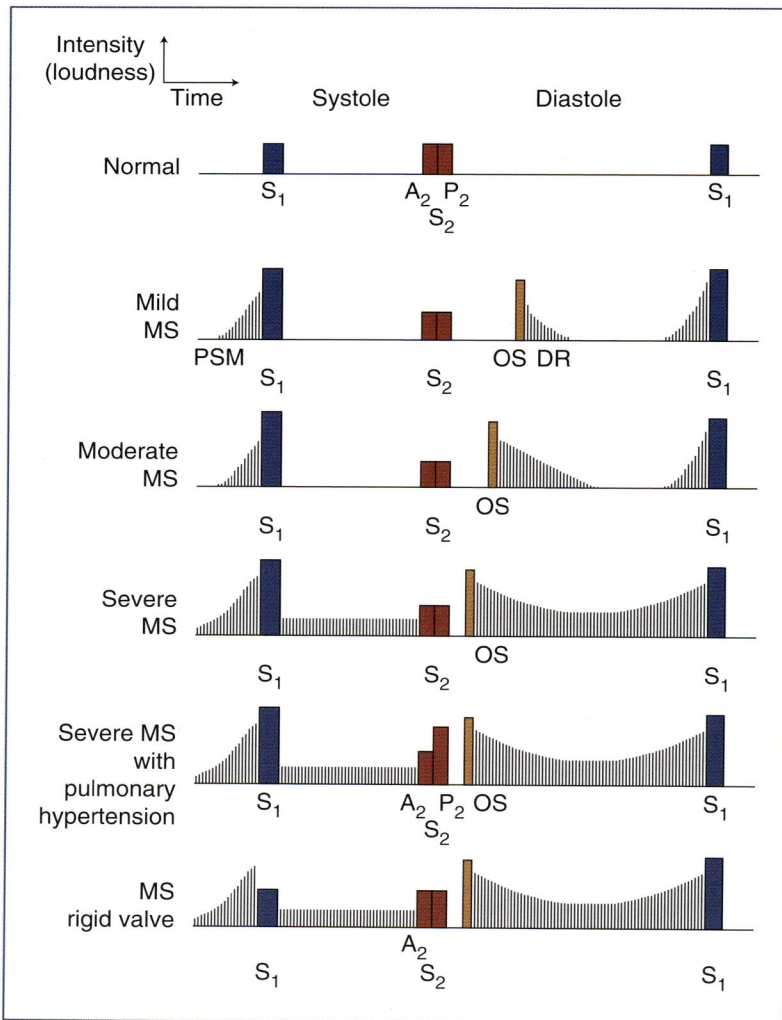

Figure 9-13. Auscultatory findings in mitral stenosis (MS) and sinus rhythm. Presystolic accentuation of the diastolic murmur is absent with atrial fibrillation. DR—diastolic closure rate; OS—opening snap; PSM—presystolic murmur

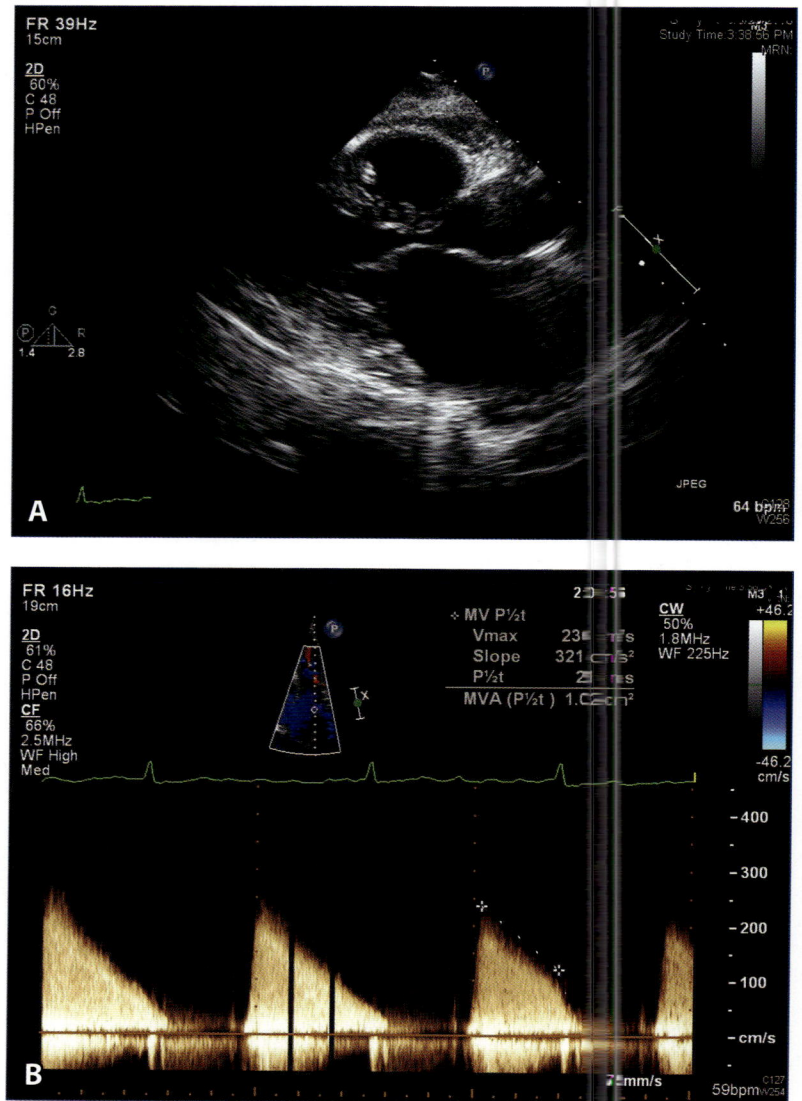

Figure 9-14. **A,** Parasternal long-axis image from a patient with rheumatic mitral stenosis showing classic "hockey-stick" deformity of the anterior mitral valve leaflet with tethering of the tip. The left atrium is dilated. **B,** Continuous-wave Doppler mitral inflow pattern from same patient demonstrating an elevated early peak velocity (2.36 m/sec), gradual velocity decay (pressure half-time [PHT] 215 m/sec), and calculated valve area (220/PHT) of 1.02 cm^2, consistent with severe mitral stenosis.

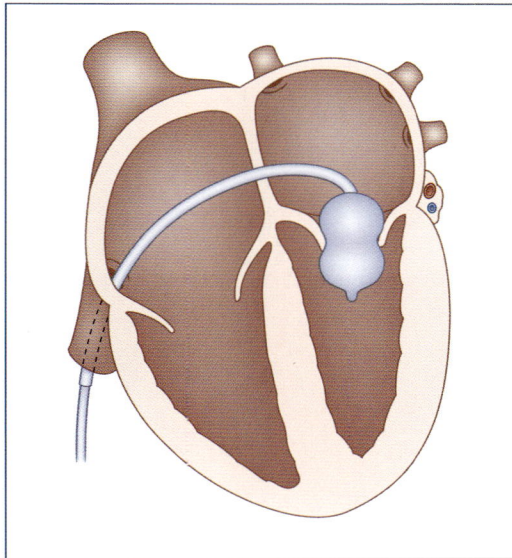

Figure 9-15. Inoue technique for percutaneous mitral balloon valvotomy (PMBV). The balloon catheter is sized to the annular diameter and delivered across the mitral valve via transseptal puncture, where it is inflated to split the commissures [10]. Indications for PMBV include the presence of moderate-to-severe mitral stenosis (valve area < 1.5 cm²) with appropriate anatomy and symptoms or pulmonary artery (PA) hypertension (PA systolic pressure > 50 mm Hg at rest or > 60 mm Hg with exercise). The systolic PA pressure can be estimated from the regurgitant tricuspid jet velocity on transthoracic echocardiogram. Contraindications to PMBV include the presence of left atrial thrombus or more than 2+ mitral regurgitation [4]. Short- and intermediate-term results are excellent and comparable to surgical commissurotomy for appropriately selected patients.

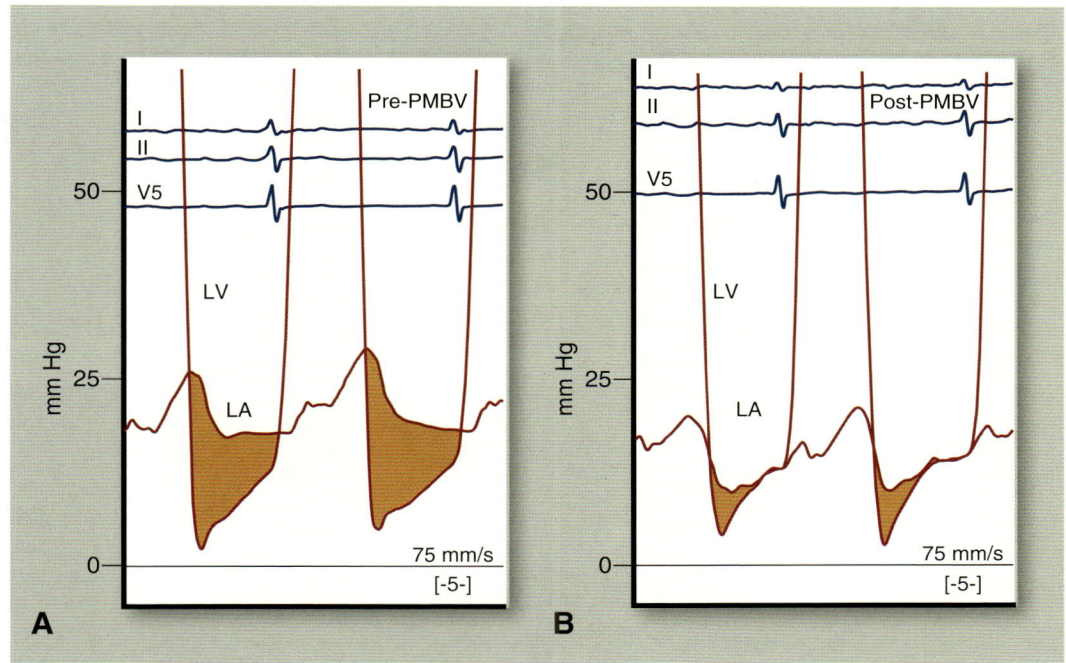

Figure 9-16. Left ventricular (LV) and left atrial (LA) pressure tracings before (**A**) and after (**B**) percutaneous mitral balloon valvotomy (PMBV). At baseline, the mean valve gradient was 11 mm Hg and valve area 1.1 cm². After balloon valvotomy, the mean gradient fell to 3 mm Hg and the valve area increased to 3.5 cm². A successful PMBV is characterized by a 50% reduction in mean gradient, a doubling of the valve area, and 0 to 1+ mitral regurgitation.

Mitral Regurgitation

Common Causes of Mitral Regurgitation
Acute
Infective endocarditis
Post–myocardial infarction papillary muscle rupture
Blunt chest trauma
Rupture of chordae
Chronic
Myxomatous degeneration of leaflets, chordae (mitral valve prolapse)
Ischemic (left ventricular modeling, apical displacement of papillary muscles, leaflet tethering)
Dilated cardiomyopathy
Mitral annular calcification
Hypertrophic obstructive cardiomyopathy
Rheumatic

Figure 9-17. Common causes of mitral regurgitation. Mitral regurgitation is a complex disease that can derive from abnormalities or dysfunction at any one or more of the multiple levels of the mitral apparatus (leaflets, annulus, chordae, papillary muscles, subjacent left ventricle).

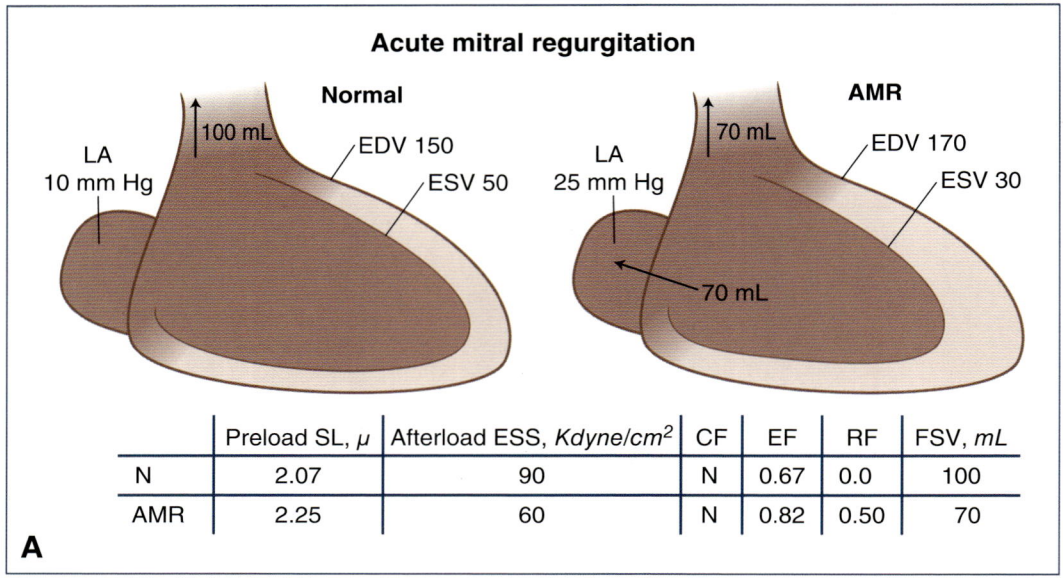

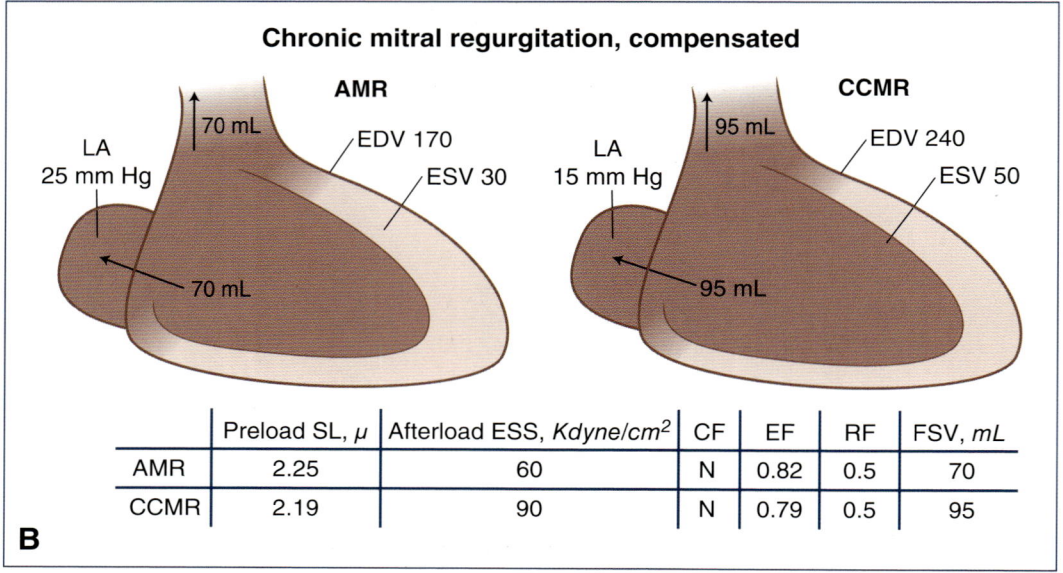

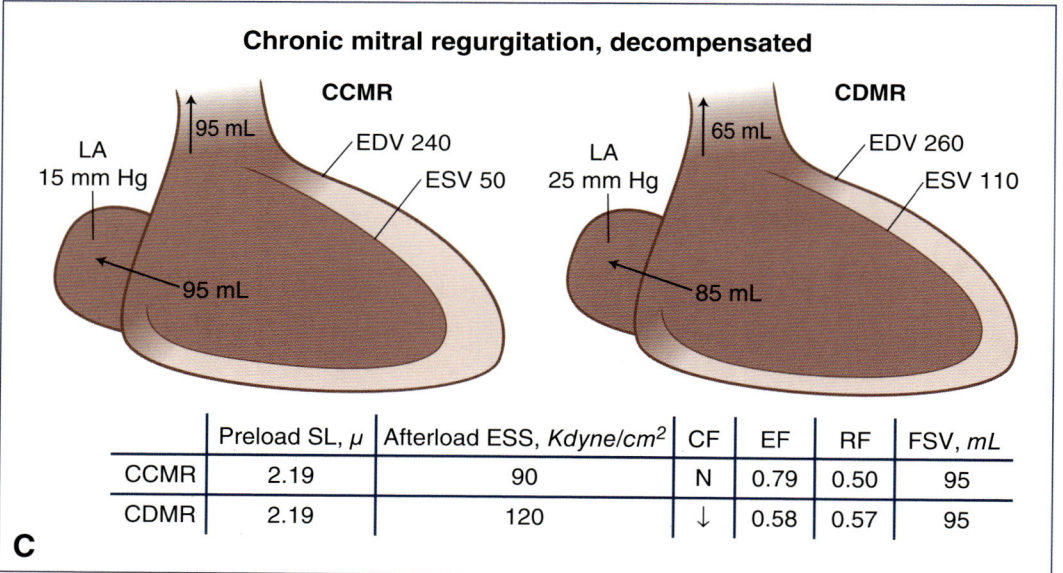

Figure 9-18. Pathophysiology of acute mitral regurgitation (AMR) and chronic mitral regurgitation (CMR). **A,** AMR. Left ventricular (LV) sarcomere length (SL) is increased, but afterload (as estimated by end-systolic stress [ESS]) is initially reduced, as the LV ejects into the low impedance left atrium (LA). Contractile function (CF) is unchanged, but ejection fraction (EF) increases. The regurgitant fraction (RF) in this example is 50%. Forward stroke volume (FSV) is reduced from 100 to 70 mL. Pressure in the unprepared and relatively noncompliant LA rises abruptly to 25 mm Hg. **B,** CMR, compensated phase (CCMR). The major compensatory changes are eccentric LV hypertrophy and chamber enlargement with an increase in LV end-diastolic volume (EDV). Afterload is higher because of the larger chamber radius. CF and EF are preserved. In addition, the LA has dilated and become more compliant, attenuating the rise in LA pressure. This phase may be clinically tolerated for years. **C,** CMR, decompensated phase (CDMR). Eventually, with uncorrected chronic severe mitral regurgitation, LV will deteriorate. EF falls and ESV increases with a reduction in FSV and rises in both LV diastolic and LA pressures [11]. It is important to intervene with surgical correction of chronic mitral regurgitation before the onset of contractile dysfunction.

The tables within the figure read:

A — Acute mitral regurgitation

	Preload SL, μ	Afterload ESS, Kdyne/cm²	CF	EF	RF	FSV, mL
N	2.07	90	N	0.67	0.0	100
AMR	2.25	60	N	0.82	0.50	70

B — Chronic mitral regurgitation, compensated

	Preload SL, μ	Afterload ESS, Kdyne/cm²	CF	EF	RF	FSV, mL
AMR	2.25	60	N	0.82	0.5	70
CCMR	2.19	90	N	0.79	0.5	95

C — Chronic mitral regurgitation, decompensated

	Preload SL, μ	Afterload ESS, Kdyne/cm²	CF	EF	RF	FSV, mL
CCMR	2.19	90	N	0.79	0.50	95
CDMR	2.19	120	↓	0.58	0.57	95

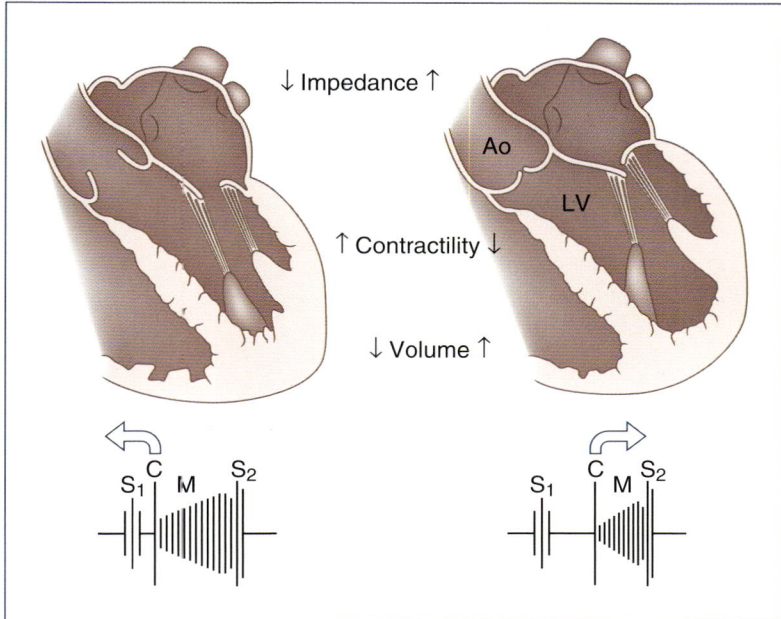

Figure 9-19. Classic auscultatory findings in a patient with mitral valve prolapse. The mid-systolic click occurs after the onset of the carotid upstroke. Maneuvers that decrease left ventricular (LV) volume, such as rapid standing from a squatting position or Valsalva, will cause the click/murmur complex to move closer to the first heart sound. Manuevers that increase LV volume or impedance, such as squatting from a standing position, will cause the click/murmur complex to move away from the first heart sound. Ao—aorta. (*Adapted from* O'Rourke and Crawford [12].)

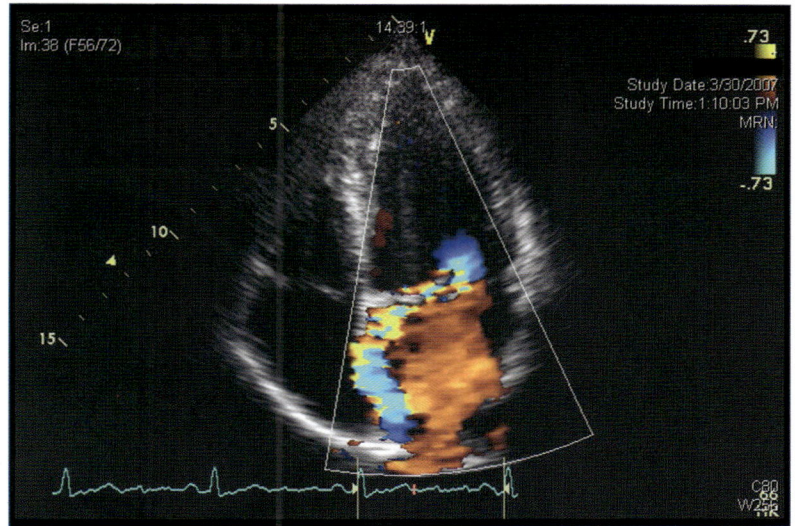

Figure 9-20. Color-flow Doppler image from apical four-chamber view of a 56-year-old woman with myxomatous degeneration and posterior mitral valve prolapse showing a wall-impinging jet of severe mitral regurgitation (MR) directed anteromedially against the inter-atrial septum. Eccentric jets of this type are common with prolapse and/or flail leaflet and are directed opposite from the involved leaflet. The associated systolic murmur tracks in parallel fashion. Quantitation of eccentric jets can be difficult. Severe nonischemic MR is defined echocardiographically by vena contracta width greater than 0.7 cm with a large central jet or a wall impinging jet of any size swirling in the left atrium (LA), regurgitant volume more than 60 mL/beat, regurgitant fraction more than 50%, effective regurgitant orifice (ERO) area more than 0.4 cm², and LA and left ventricular enlargement [8]. Ischemic MR is defined by an ERO of more than 0.3 cm².

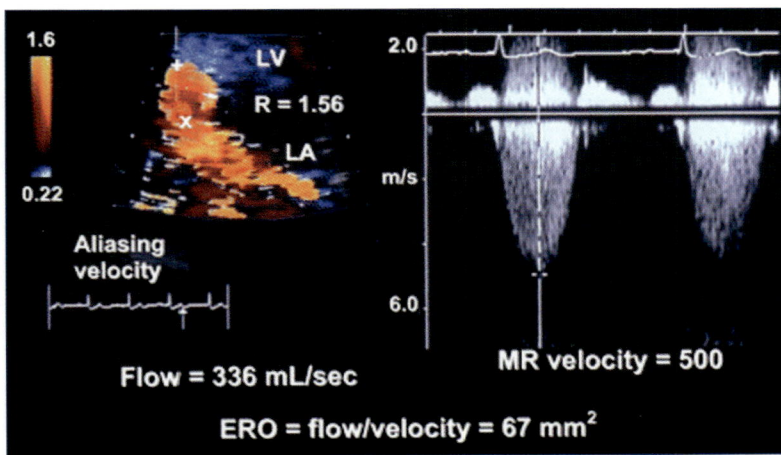

Figure 9-21. Calculation of mitral effective regurgitant orifice (ERO) area according to the proximal isovelocity surface area technique. The *left side* of the image is a zoomed view of the flow convergence zone with color-flow imaging and down-shifting of the baseline to an aliasing velocity of 22 cm/sec. The radius (R) of the flow convergence is measured using the two crosses shown and the flow is calculated at 336 mL/sec. The right side of the image shows continuous-wave Doppler measurement of the peak regurgitant velocity (MR velocity). The ERO area is calculated at 67 mm² or 0.67 cm², as the ratio of flow to velocity. LA—left atrium; LV—left ventricle. (*Adapted from* O'Gara *et al.* [13].).

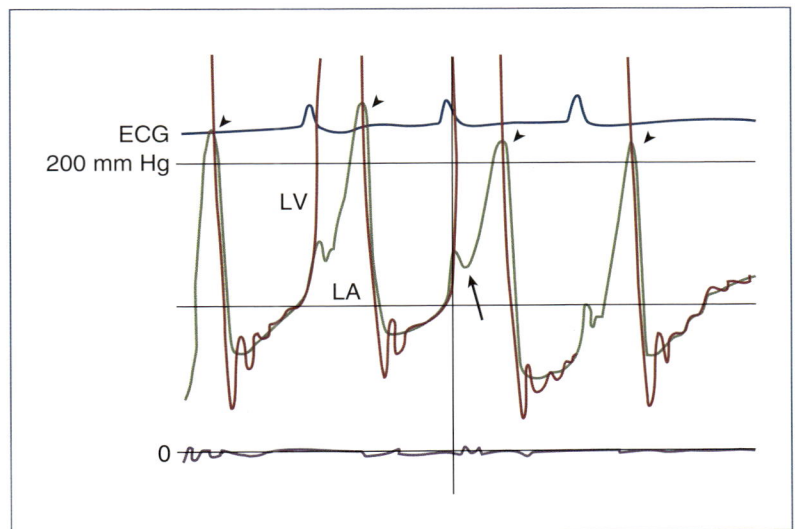

Figure 9-22. The "V" wave of mitral regurgitation. This tracing shows a large left atrial "V" wave (*arrowheads*) occurring at the end of systole in a patient with atrial fibrillation. Following the "V" wave, there is a rapid fall in left atrial (LA) pressure, along the course of the declining left ventricular (LV) pressure. In diastole, LA and LV pressures are equalized. The *arrow* indicates a "C" wave deflection [14]. Giant "V" waves are defined by a more than 10 mm Hg increase above the mean pressure. They are not pathognomonic of mitral regurgitation and are typically blunted in patients with a large and compliant left atria. ECG—electrocardiogram.

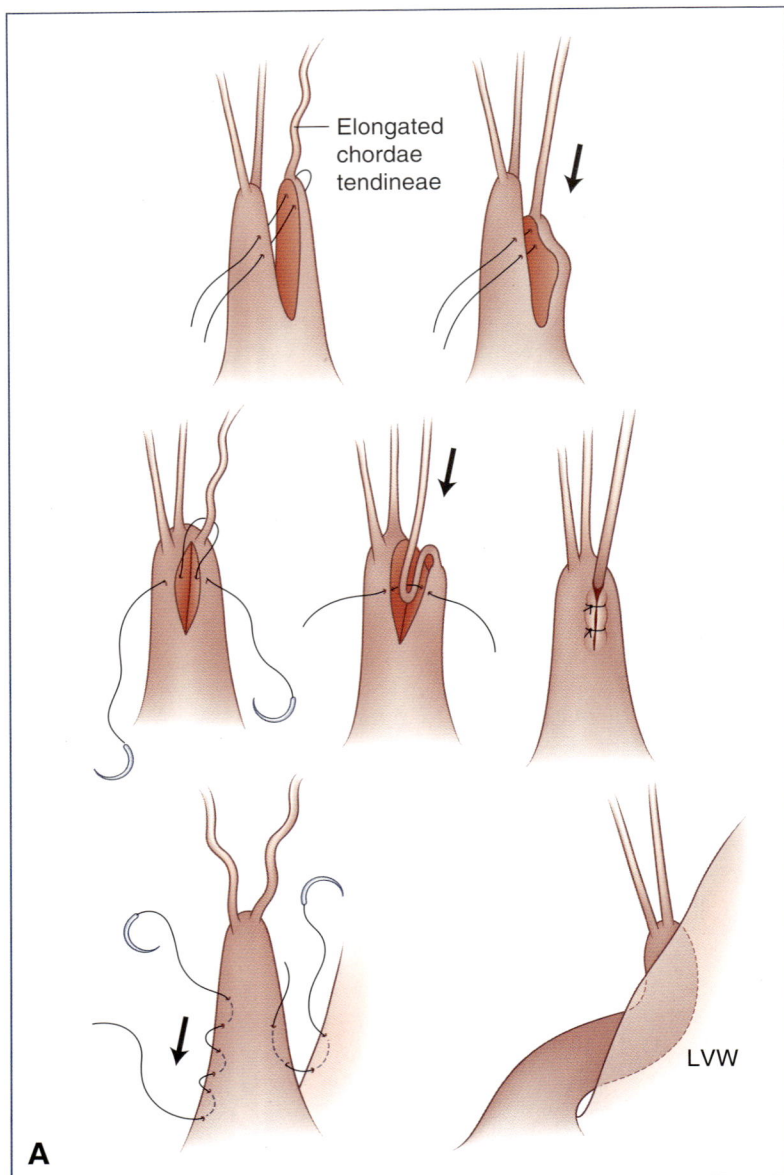

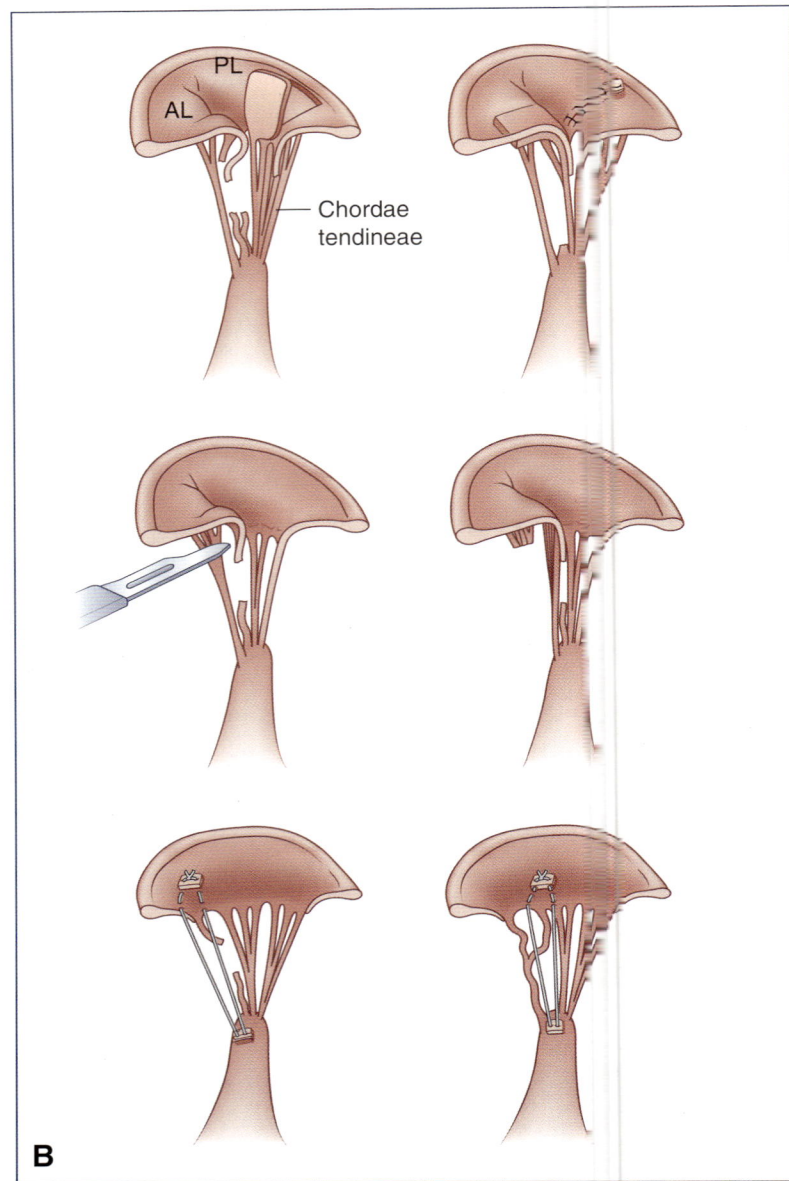

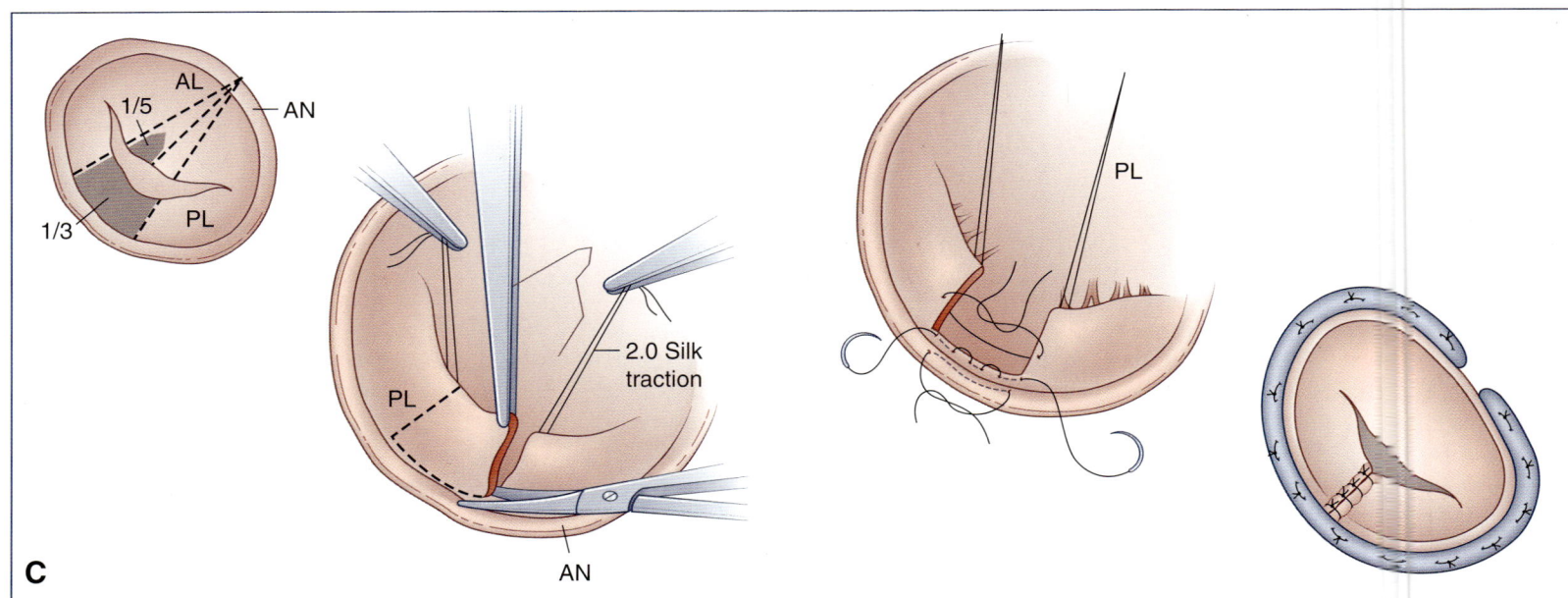

Figure 9-23. Mitral valve repair techniques. **A,** Shortening of elongat- ed chordae. Techniques include sliding the papillary muscle head (*top*), chordal plasty (*middle*), and shortening the papillary muscle (*bottom*). LVW—left ventricular wall. **B,** Management of ruptured chordae. Transpo- sition of posterior chordae (PL) to anterior mitral leaflet (AL; *top*), transfer of anterior chordae (*middle*), and construction of neo chordae (*bottom*) [15]. **C,** The most common approach to posterior mitral leaflet prolapse involves a quadrangular resection of the involved area (usually the middle scallop of the posterior leaflet), sliding annuloplasty (AL), suture closure of the defect, and implantation of an annuloplasty ring.

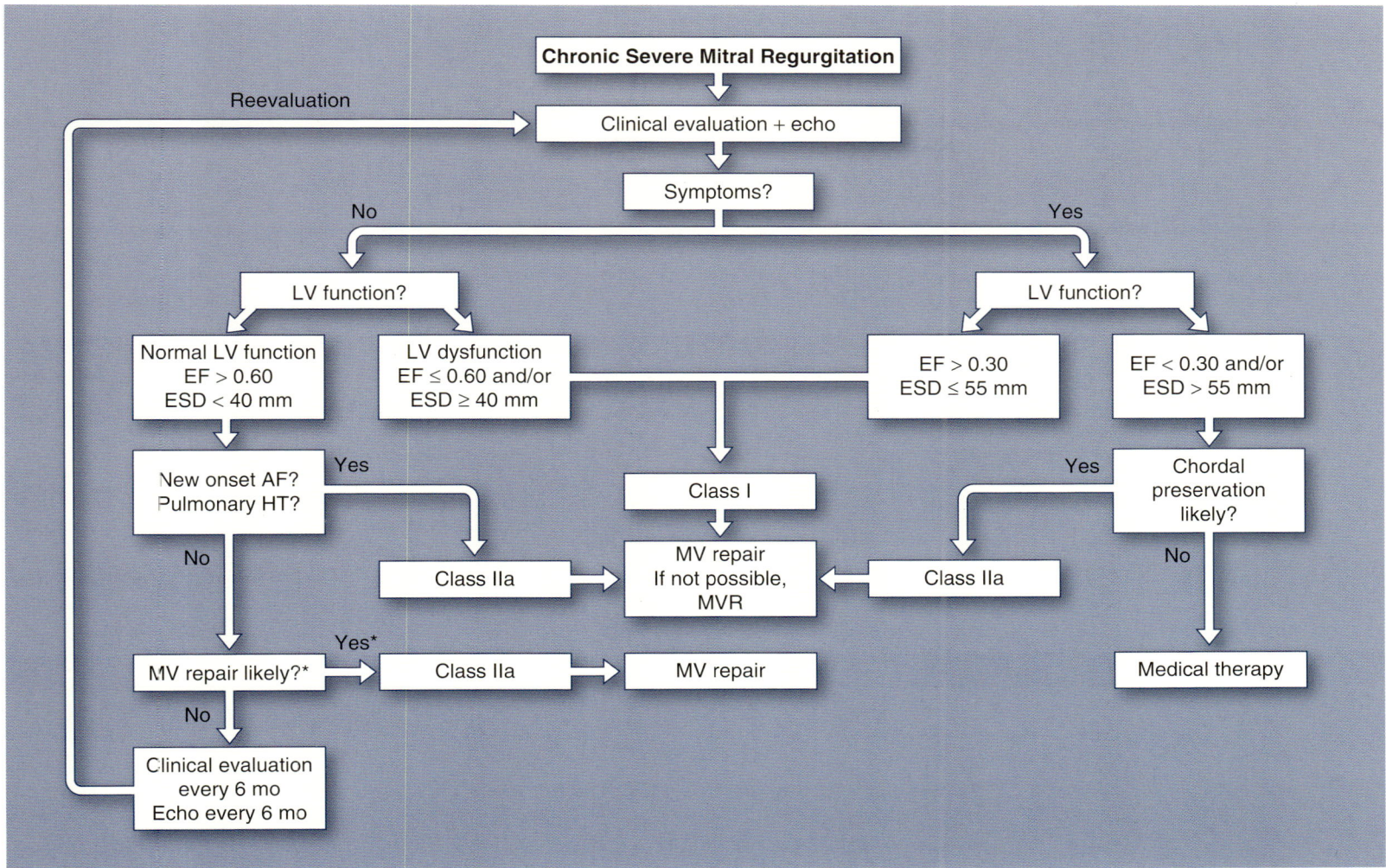

Figure 9-24. Management of chronic nonischemic mitral regurgitation (MR). There is no role for routine vasodilator therapy in patients with normal left ventricular (LV) systolic function (ejection fraction [EF] > 0.60) without systemic hypertension (HT) [4]. Critical thresholds in the asymptomatic patient include LVEF less than 0.60 or LV end-systolic dimension (ESD) more than 4.0 cm. Repair is strongly preferred over replacement whenever feasible for better preservation of LV function and avoidance of a prosthetic valve device. Left or biatrial maze procedures or pulmonary vein isolation for management of atrial fibrillation (AF) are commonly performed at the same time. Class recommendations are according to American College of Cardiology/American Heart Association management guidelines. Decisions regarding surgery for coronary artery disease and ischemic MR, as well as for MR with dilated cardiomyopathy, are more complex and must be individualized. echo—echocardiography; MV—mitral valve; MVR—mitral valve replacement.

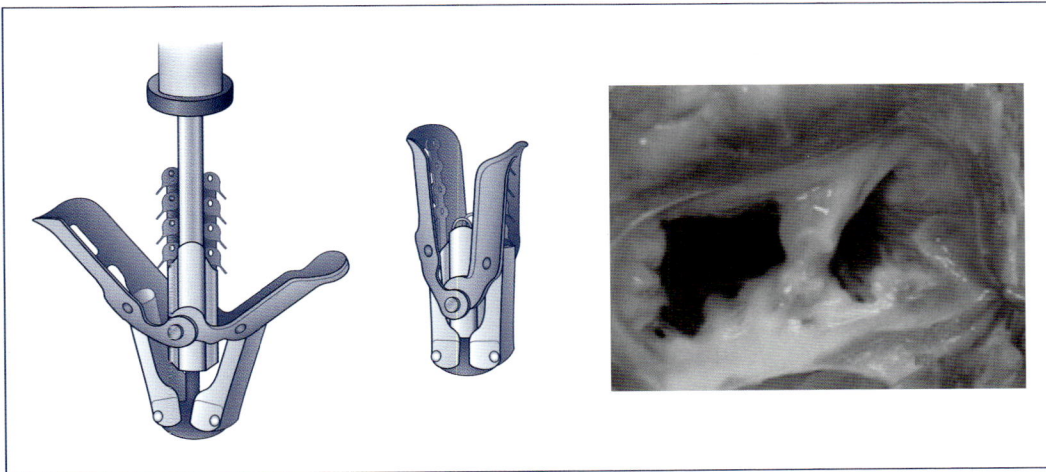

Figure 9-25. Percutaneous mitral valve repair for mitral regurgitation. One method involves the edge-to-edge technique that recapitulates the Alfieri stitch repair. Via a transseptal approach, a clip (*left*) can be positioned across the mitral valve under fluoroscopic and transesophageal guidance, then pulled back, catching the edges of the anterior and posterior leaflets, before it is closed. Once deployed, it results in a double orifice mitral valve with amelioration of the severity of mitral regurgitation. The *right image* shows the endothelialized appearance of a clip after long-term implantation in an animal model. (*Adapted from* Davidson and Baim [16].)

Tricuspid Valve Disease

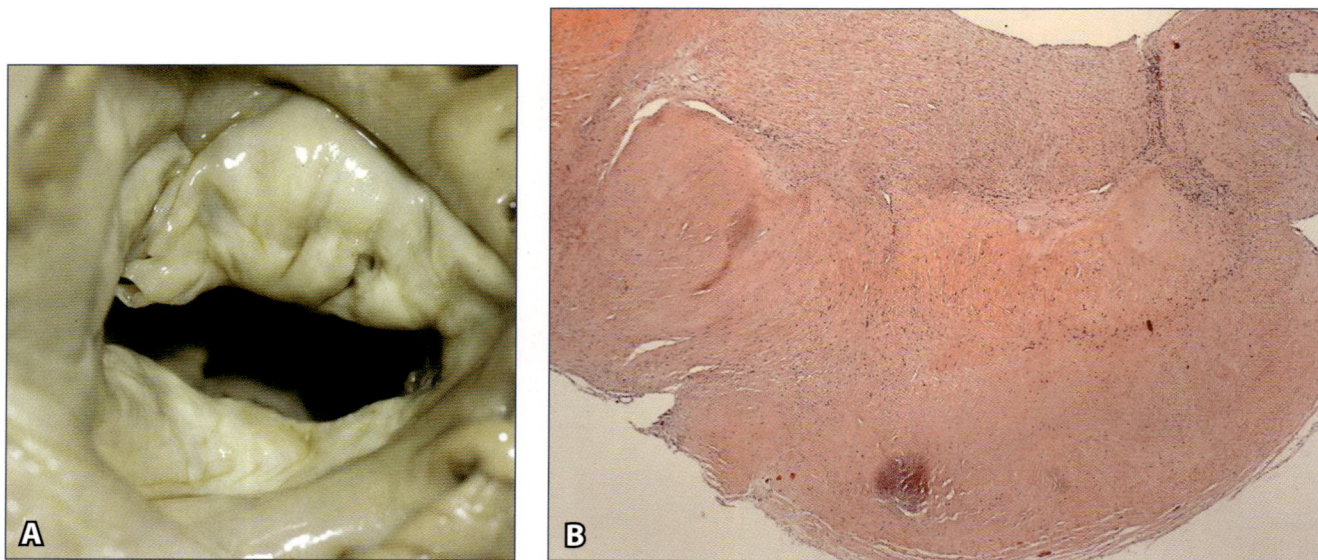

Figure 9-26. Gross (**A**) and microscopic (**B**) postmortem specimens of the tricuspid valve in a patient with metastatic carcinoid disease of small bowel origin. Carcinoid is one of the relatively few causes of primary tricuspid valve disease seen in adult patients. Other causes include tricuspid valve prolapse, infective endocarditis (especially with injection drug use), blunt chest wall trauma, Ebstein's anomaly, and chordal disruption during transvenous right ventricular endomyocardial biopsy in transplant recipients. In the gross example, the leaflets of the tricuspid valve appear thickened and retracted, creating an incompetent orifice. In the microscopic section, a thick, plaque-like mass (*bottom*) adheres densely to normal leaflet tissue (*top*).

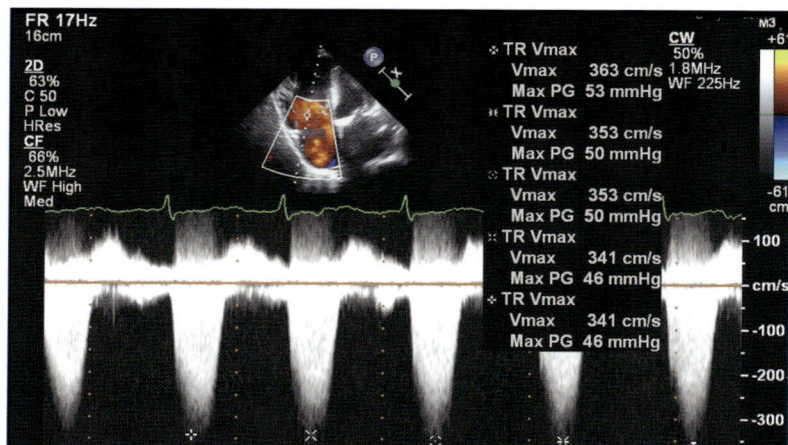

Figure 9-27. Secondary tricuspid regurgitation (TR). Continuous-wave tricuspid valve Doppler velocity profile from the apical four-chamber view in a patient with left-sided heart disease, pulmonary artery (PA) hypertension, right ventricular dilatation, and severe TR. The peak PA systolic pressure can be estimated from the maximal jet velocity by applying the modified Bernoulli equation and adding the estimated right atrium (RA) pressure. In this example, the maximum TR jet velocity varies from 3.4 to 3.6 m/sec. The peak instantaneous right ventricle–RA pressure gradient is then estimated as $4v^2$ or $4(3.5)^2$ = 49, plus estimated RA pressure = 59–64 mm Hg (assuming RA pressure 10–15 mm Hg, in this example).

Endocarditis

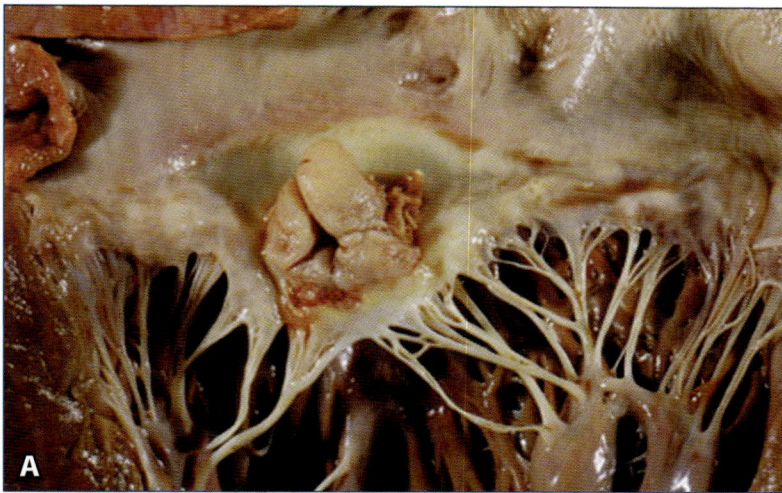

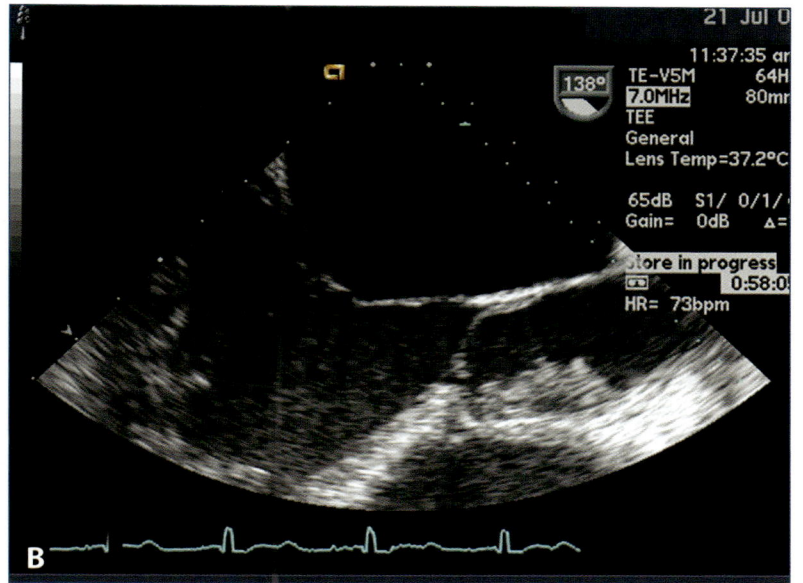

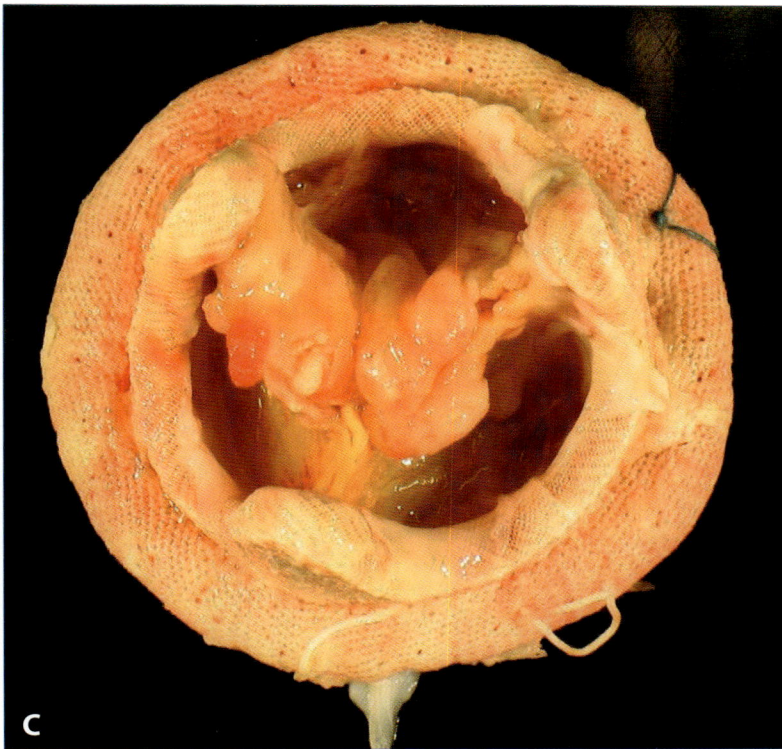

Figure 9-28. Infective endocarditis. **A,** Large, multilobulated vegetation on the anterior leaflet of the mitral valve from a patient with *Staphylococcus lugdunensis* endocarditis who died of a rupture mycotic cerebral aneurysm [3]. **B,** Transesophageal echocardiographic image (from same patient in Fig. 9–7) showing a cluster of vegetative material adherent to and above the anterior leaflet of the aortic valve. TEE is more sensitive than transthoracic echocardiogram (TTE) for the detection and characterization of vegetation and abscess in patients with suspected infective endocarditis. **C,** Gross operative specimen from a patient with prosthetic valve endocarditis affecting the valve leaflets, but sparing the sewing ring.

Revised Recommendations for the Use of Antibiotics to Prevent Infective Endocarditis

Prophylaxis against infective endocarditis is reasonable for the following patients at highest risk for adverse outcomes from infective endocarditis who undergo dental procedures that involve manipulation of either gingival tissue or the periapical region of teeth or perforation of the oral mucosa.

Patients with prosthetic cardiac valves or prosthetic material used for cardiac valve repair

Patients with previous infective endocarditis

Patients with congenital heart disease (CHD)

Unrepaired cyanotic CHD, including palliative shunts or conduits

Completely repaired congenital heart defect repaired with prosthetic material or device, whether placed by surgery or by catheter intervention, during the first six months after the procedure

Figure 9-29. Revised recommendations for the use of antibiotics to prevent infective endocarditis. The use of prophylactic antibiotics is considered reasonable for high-risk patients before dental procedures that involve manipulation of either gingival tissue or the periapical region of the teeth or perforation of oral mucosa. High-risk patients are those with underlying cardiac conditions associated with the highest risk of adverse outcomes from endocarditis and not simply highest risk for acquisition of endocarditis. Prophylaxis is no longer recommended for gastrointestinal or genitourinary procedures in the absence of an active infection.

In recognition that these revised guidelines may cause consternation and concern for patients and clinicians who have become accustomed to following the previous recommendations, the use of prophylaxis can be considered for patients with bicuspid aortic valve or coarctation of the aorta, severe mitral valve prolapse, or hypertrophic obstructive cardiomyopathy. In these settings, the clinician should determine that the risks associated with antibiotics are low before continuing a prophylaxis regimen [17].

Prosthetic Heart Valves

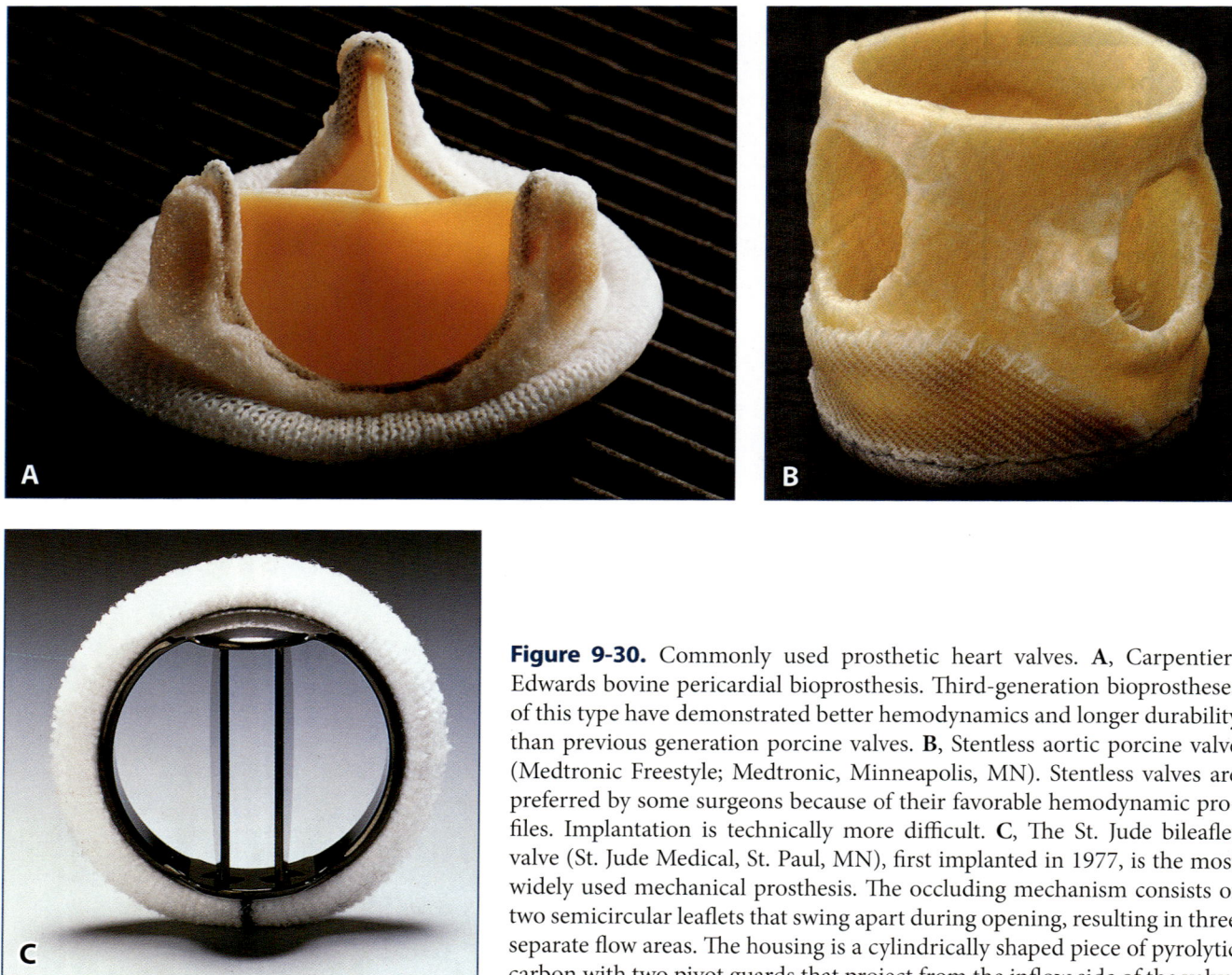

Figure 9-30. Commonly used prosthetic heart valves. **A,** Carpentier-Edwards bovine pericardial bioprosthesis. Third-generation bioprostheses of this type have demonstrated better hemodynamics and longer durability than previous generation porcine valves. **B,** Stentless aortic porcine valve (Medtronic Freestyle; Medtronic, Minneapolis, MN). Stentless valves are preferred by some surgeons because of their favorable hemodynamic profiles. Implantation is technically more difficult. **C,** The St. Jude bileaflet valve (St. Jude Medical, St. Paul, MN), first implanted in 1977, is the most widely used mechanical prosthesis. The occluding mechanism consists of two semicircular leaflets that swing apart during opening, resulting in three separate flow areas. The housing is a cylindrically shaped piece of pyrolytic carbon with two pivot guards that project from the inflow side of the valve.

Acknowledgment

The author wishes to acknowledge the contributions of Dr. Shahbudin Rahimtoola whose original efforts in previous editions of the text established the framework for the current chapter.

References

1. Nkomo VT, Gardin JM, Skelton TN, *et al.*: Burden of valvular heart diseases: a population-based study. *Lancet* 2006, 368:1005–1011.

2. O'Brien KD: Pathogenesis of calcific aortic valve disease: a disease process comes of age (and a good deal more). *Arterioscler Thromb Vasc Biol* 2006, 26:1721–1728.

3. Haldar SM, O'Gara PT: Infective endocarditis. In *Hurst's The Heart*, edn 12. Edited by Fuster V, O'Rourke RA, Walsh RA, Poole-Wilson PA. New York: McGraw-Hill; 2007:1975–2004.

4. Bonow RO, Carabello BA, Kanu C, *et al.*: ACC/AHA 2006 guidelines for the management of patients with valvular heart disease: a report of the American College of Cardiology/American Heart Association Task Force on Practice Guidelines (writing committee to revise the 1998 Guidelines for the Management of Patients With Valvular Heart Disease): developed in collaboration with the Society of Cardiovascular Anesthesiologists: endorsed by the Society for Cardiovascular Angiography and Interventions and the Society of Thoracic Surgeons. *Circulation* 2006, 114:e84–e231.

5. Aikawa E, Nahrendorf M, Sosnovik D, *et al.*: Multimodality molecular imaging identifies proteolytic and osteogenic activities in early aortic valve disease. *Circulation* 2007, 115:377–386.

6. Kern MJ: *The Cardiac Catheterization Handbook*, edn 2. St. Louis: Mosby-Year Book; 1994.

7. Nataatmadja M, West M, West J, *et al.*: Abnormal extracellular matrix protein transport associated with increased apoptosis of vascular smooth muscle cells in Marfan syndrome and bicuspid aortic valve thoracic aortic aneurysm. *Circulation* 2003, 108:II329–II334.

8. Zoghbi WA, Enriquez-Sarano M, Foster E, *et al.*: Recommendations for the evaluation of the severity of native valvular regurgitation with 2-dimensional and Doppler echocardiography. *J Am Soc Echocardiogr* 2003, 16:77–802.

9. Evangelista A, Tornos P, Sambola A, *et al.*: Long-term vasodilator therapy in patients with severe aortic regurgitation. *N Engl J Med* 2005, 353:1342–1349.

10. Inoe K, Owaki T, Nakamura T, *et al.*: Clinical application of transvenous mitral commissurotomy by a new balloon catheter. *J Thorac Cardiovasc Surg* 1984, 87:394–402.

11. Carabello BA: Mitral regurgitation: basic pathophysiologic principles. Part 1. *Mod Concepts Cardiovasc Dis* 1988, 57:53–58.

12. O'Rourke RA, Crawford MH: The systolic click-murmur syndrome: clinical recognition and management. *Curr Prob Cardiol* 1976, 1:9–60.

13. O'Gara PT, Sugene L, Lang R, *et al.*: The role of imaging in chronic degenerative mitral regurgitation. *J Am Coll Cardiol Img* 2008, 1:221–237.

14. Kern MJ: *Hemodynamic Rounds: Interpretation of Cardiac Pathophysiology From Pressure Wave Form Analysis*. New York: Wiley-Liss; 1993.

15. Cosgrove DM: Surgery for degenerative mitral valve disease. *Semin Thoracic Cardiovasc Surg* 1989, 1:183–193.

16. Davidson M Ji, Baim D Si: Percutaneous catheter-based mitral valve repair. In *Cardiac Surgery in the Adult*. Edited by Cohn LH. New York: McGraw-Hill; 2008:1101–1108.

17. Nishimura RA, Carabello BA, Faxon DP, *et al.*: ACC/AHA 2008 Guideline Update on Valvular Heart Disease: Focused Update on Infective Endocarditis. A Report of the American College of Cardiology/American Heart Association Task Force on Practice Guidelines. *Circulation* 2008, 52:676–685.

Addult Congenital Heart Disease

Adult Congenital Heart Disease

Adult Congenital Heart Disease

10

Anne Marie Valente, Michael J. Landzberg, and Andrew J. Powell

Congenital heart disease occurs in approximately 1% of all live births [1]. Advances in diagnosis and treatment have led to improved survival so that now 85% to 90% of infants born with congenital heart disease will reach adulthood [2]. There are more than 1 million adults with congenital heart disease in the United States [2,3] and this population increases by approximately 5% each year [4]. This chapter illustrates some of the more common congenital heart lesions, with a focus on anatomy, pathophysiology, and treatment options. The American College of Cardiology and American Heart Association have recently developed guidelines for managements of adults with congenital heart disease [5].

Acyanotic Lesions

Atrial Septal Defect

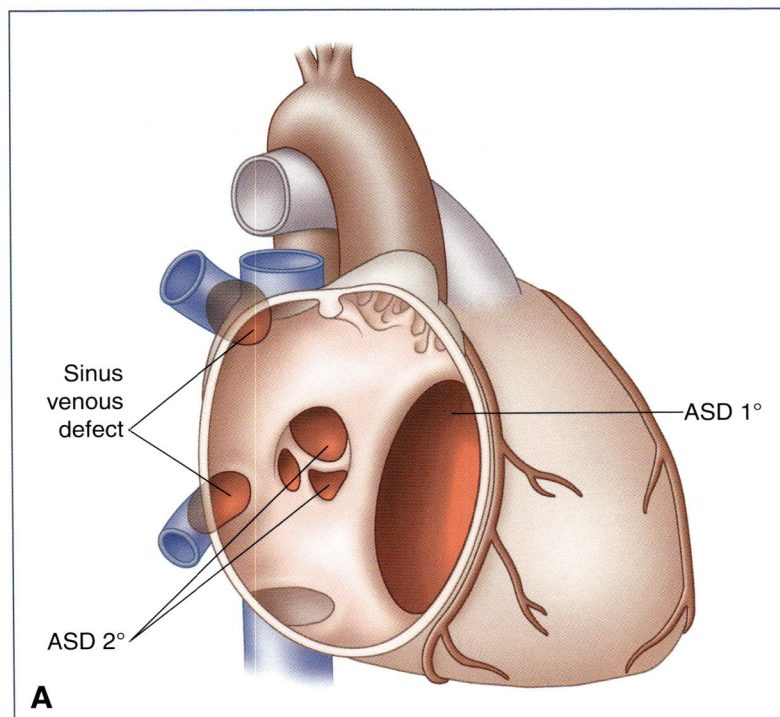

Figure 10-1. A, Diagrammatic representation of the locations of various atrial septal defects (ASD) [6]. ASDs are common congenital anomalies and are one of the few congenital heart lesions that are more prevalent in women. Defects that are large may present in childhood; however, many ASDs are not identified until adult life when patients develop exercise intolerance, atrial arrhythmias, or dyspnea. The long-term prognosis after closure for patients younger than 25 years is comparable to that of the general population [7]. Patients corrected at an older age, particularly those older than age 40, may have decreased long-term survival and experience higher rates of sequelae including atrial arrhythmias, pulmonary hypertension, and right heart failure [7]. Secundum ASDs (ASD 2°) can often be closed with occluder devices placed percutaneously. The other types of ASDs require surgical closure. (*Adapted from* Keane *et al.* [6]; with permission; *adapted from an illustration provided by* Emily Flynn McIntosh.)

Continued on the next page

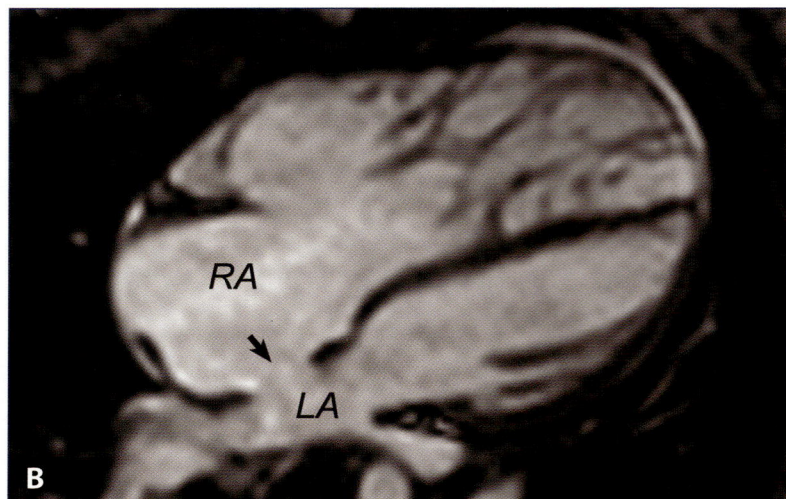

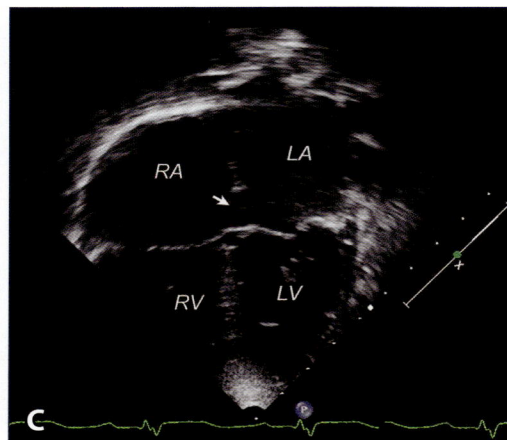

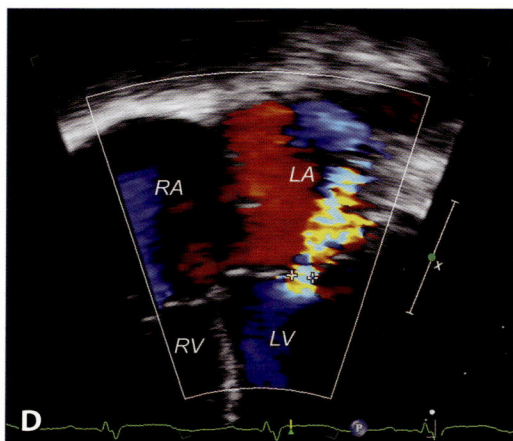

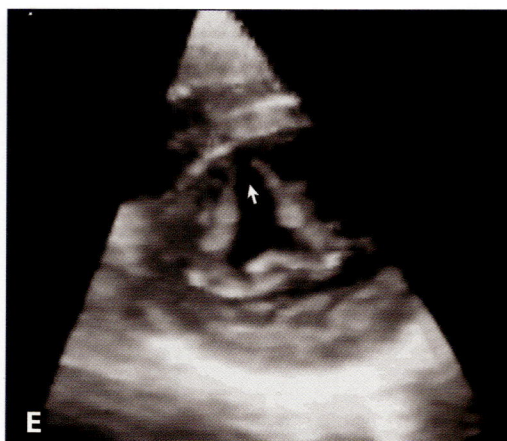

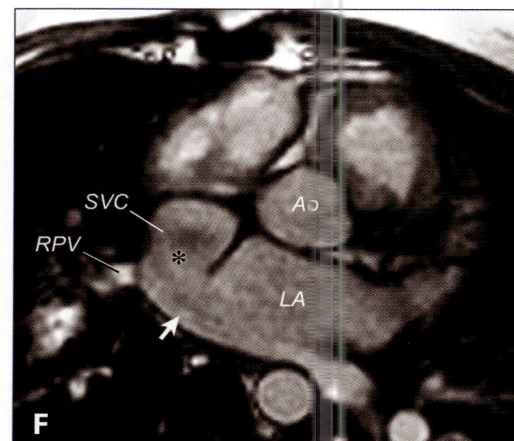

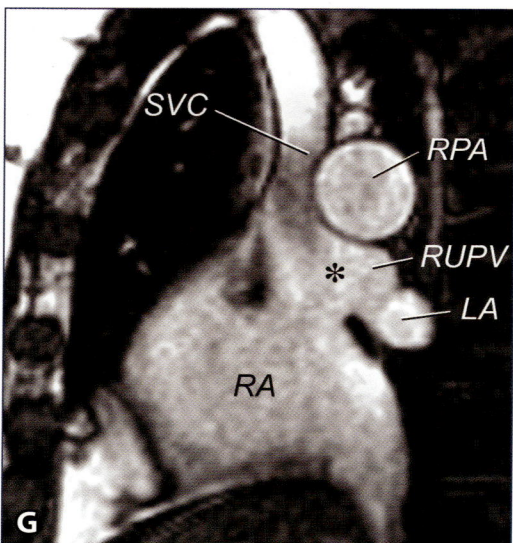

Figure 10-1. *(Continued)* **B,** Cine magnetic resonance image (MRI) in a four-chamber plane demonstrating the most common type of ASD—a secundum ASD (*arrow*). (*Adapted from* Valente and Powell [7]; with permission). **C,** Apical four-chamber echocardiogram image of a primum ASD (ASD 1°; *arrow*). Primum ASDs, a type of atrioventricular canal defect, are located near the crux of the heart and are usually associated with a cleft mitral valve. In one single-center experience of surgical correction of 33 adults with primum ASDs, 18% had perioperative complications, including heart block and 6% required reoperation within the first postoperative year due to residual defect and severe regurgitation [7]. **D,** Color Doppler echocardiogram image from an apical view demonstrating mild mitral regurgitation through the "cleft" of the mitral valve. **E,** Three-dimensional echocardiogram image demonstrating the cleft in the anterior leaflet of the mitral valve (*arrow*). **F** and **G,** Cine MRI images in axial (**F**) and sagittal (**G**) planes from a patient with a superior type sinus venosus septal defect. (*Adapted from* Valente and Powell [7]; with permission). Sinus venosus septal defects are not true defects in the atrial septum, but rather a deficiency of the posterior wall of the right atrium or the superior vena cava, and are associated with anomalous right pulmonary venous drainage. *Asterisk* indicates the defect in the wall that separates the superior vena cava (SVC) and the right upper pulmonary vein (RUPV). The *arrow* indicates the orifice of the RUPV through which blood can flow between the left atrium (LA) and the SVC. Ao—aorta; LV—left ventricle; RA—right atrium; RPA—right pulmonary artery; RPV—right pulmonary vein; RV—right ventricle.

Ventricular Septal Defect

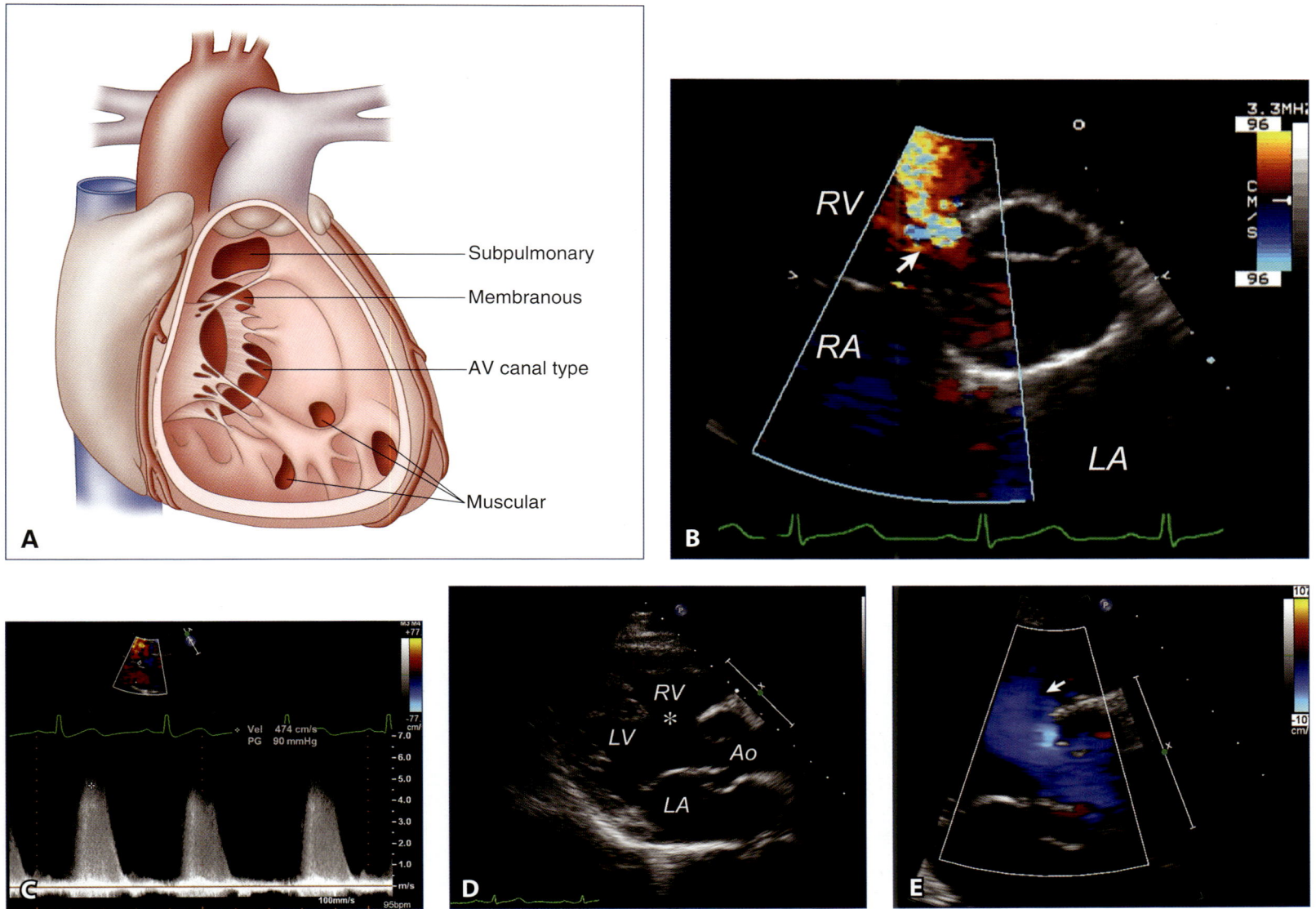

Figure 10-2. **A,** Diagrammatic representation of the location of the various types of ventricular septal defects (VSD). (*Adapted from Keane et al.* [8]; *with permission*). A VSD is a communication between the ventricles and is one of the most common congenital heart anomalies seen in children. VSDs may be isolated or associated with complex cardiac disease. Some VSDs, particularly those in the membranous and muscular septum, may become smaller over time and close spontaneously. The outcome for patients with small VSDs (without pulmonary hypertension or evidence of left ventricular volume overload) is generally excellent [9]. (*Adapted from an illustration provided by* Emily Flynn McIntosh.) **B,** Zoomed-in parasternal short-axis echocardiogram view of a small membranous VSD (*arrow*) with left-to-right flow by color Doppler. **C,** The peak instantaneous pressure gradient across the defect by continuous-wave Doppler is 90 mm Hg confirming that the defect is small enough to prevent equilibration of right and left ventricular pressures (*ie*, "restrictive" defect). **D,** Parasternal long-axis echocardiogram view of a large conoventricular septal defect (*asterisk*). Larger defects may lead to elevated pulmonary vascular resistance (Eisenmenger syndrome), which is associated with decreased long-term survival [10]. **E,** Color Doppler echocardiogram in the same patient demonstrating systolic right-to-left flow through the defect (*arrow*). Ao—aorta; AV—atrioventricular; LA—left atrium; LV—left ventricle; RA—right atrium; RV—right ventricle.

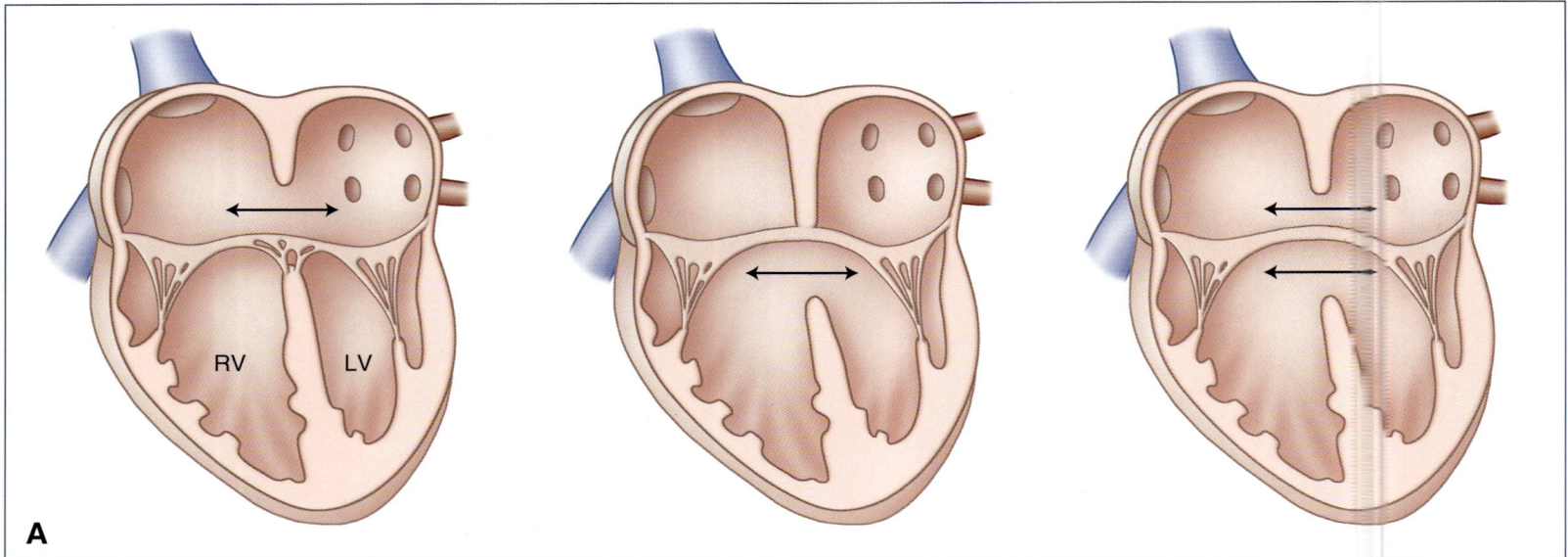

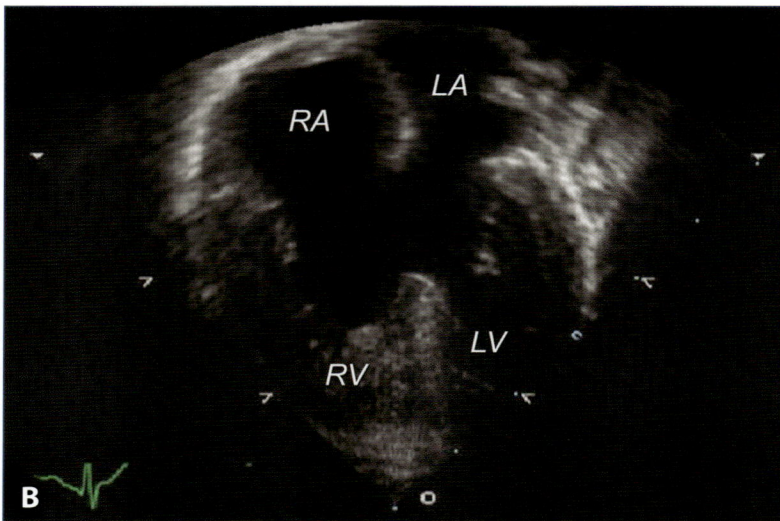

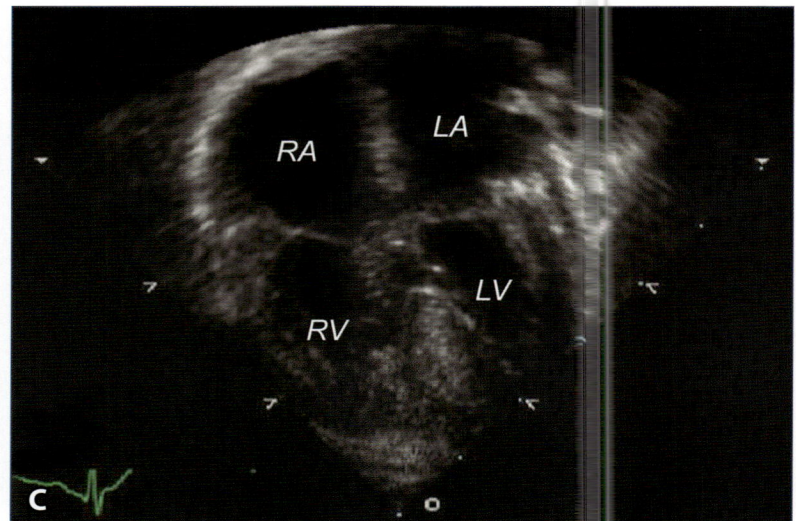

Figure 10-3. Atrioventricular canal defects (AVC) are present when the atrioventricular (AV) valves are partially or completely in common (*ie*, they are not separated by the septum of the AV canal). They are usually associated with a defect in the AV septum resulting in atrial or ventricular level shunts [11]. **A,** Diagrammatic representation of the various types of AVC defects. The *left diagram* illustrates an exclusively atrial level communication, with the common AV valve (AVV) densely attached to the ventricular septum. The type of AVC is termed a *primum atrial septal defect* (ASD). (*See* Fig. 10-1C.) The *middle diagram* has an exclusively ventricular communication. The common AVV valve is fused with the inferior limbic band of septum secundum, and thus there is no primum ASD. The *right diagram* has both atrial and ventricular defects and is termed a *complete common AVC defect*. (*Adapted from an illustration provided by* Emily Flynn McIntosh.) **B,** Echocardiographic four-chamber view in diastole showing a complete common AVC defect. Large atrial and ventricular communications are present. **C,** Systolic frame demonstrating closure of the common AVV. (**A** *adapted from* Keane *et al.* [6]; with permission.)

Continued on the next page

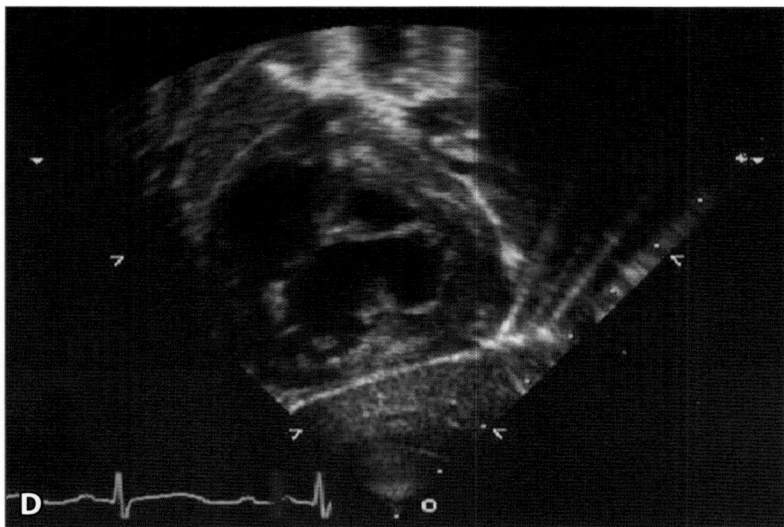

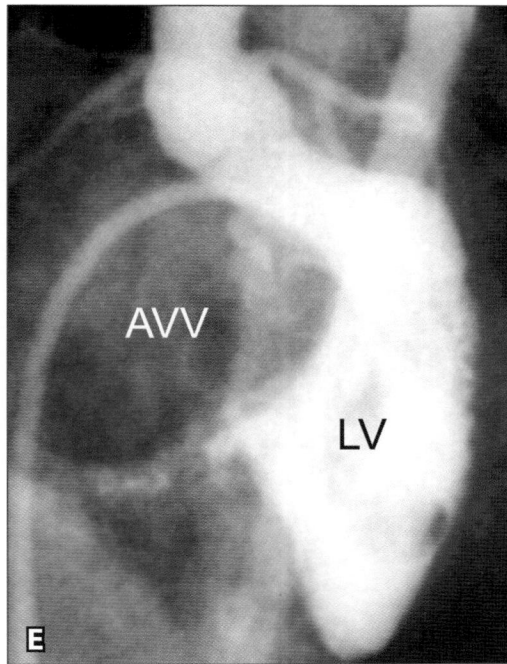

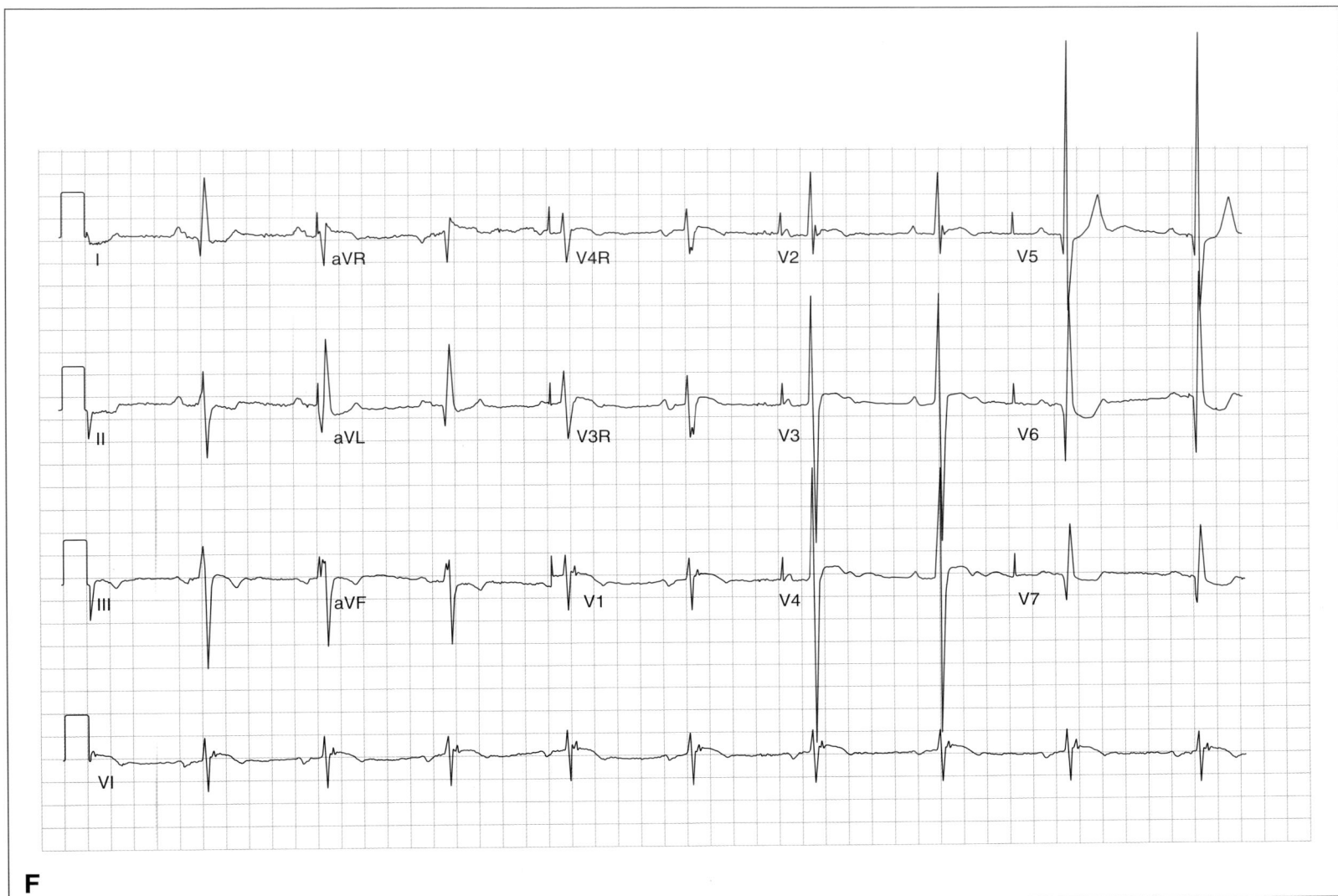

Figure 10-3. *(Continued)* **D,** Subxiphoid short-axis image demonstrating an en-face view of a common AV valve. **E,** Angiogram of the left ventricular outflow tract demonstrating the classic "gooseneck" deformity in a patient with a primum ASD. This appearance is the result of the inlet dimension of the left ventricle (LV) being shorter than the outlet dimension. *(Adapted from Lock et al.* [11]; with permission.) **F,** Twelve-lead electrocardiogram showing two common abnormalities frequently seen in patients with AVC defects: a superior QRS axis and first degree AV block. LA—left atrium; RA—right atrium; RV—right ventricle.

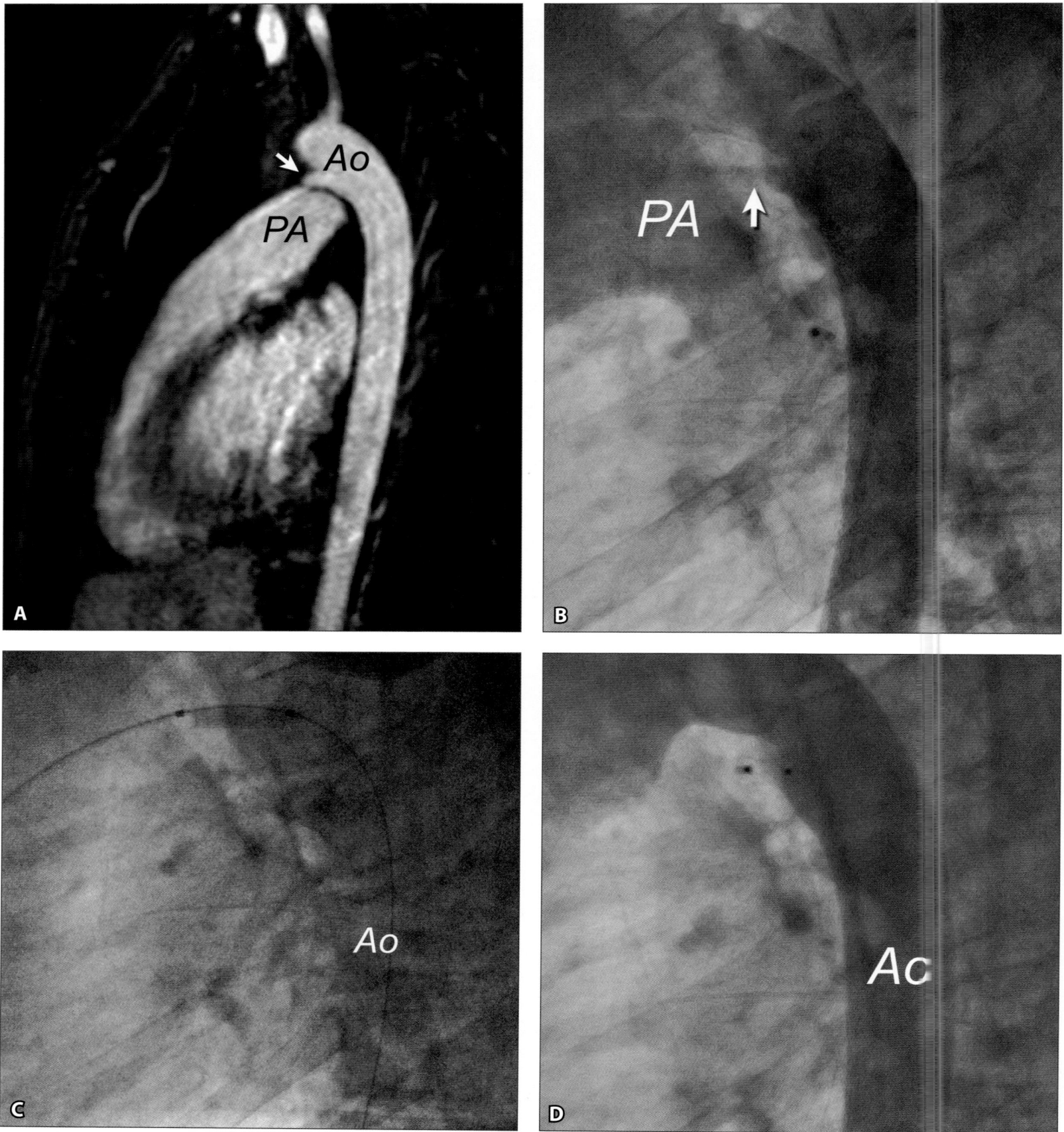

Figure 10-4. A patent ductus arteriosus (PDA) courses between the aortic isthmus and the origin of one of the branch pulmonary arteries (PA). Small PDAs may be associated with an increased risk of endocarditis [12]. Large PDAs over time may lead to left heart enlargement or chronically elevated pulmonary vascular resistance (ie, Eisenmenger syndrome). **A,** Gadolinium-enhanced three-dimensional magnetic resonance angiogram demonstrating a small PDA (*arrow*). **B,** Lateral angiographic projection of an aortogram revealing a small tubular PDA (*arrow*) with flow into the PA. **C,** A wire is placed retrograde in the descending aorta and balloon is inflated to size the PDA. **D,** Lateral angiogram demonstrating a ductal occlusion device (*black dots* at either end of implanted ductal occluder) in place which obliterates further aorta (Ao)–pulmonary arterial flow.

Pulmonary Stenosis

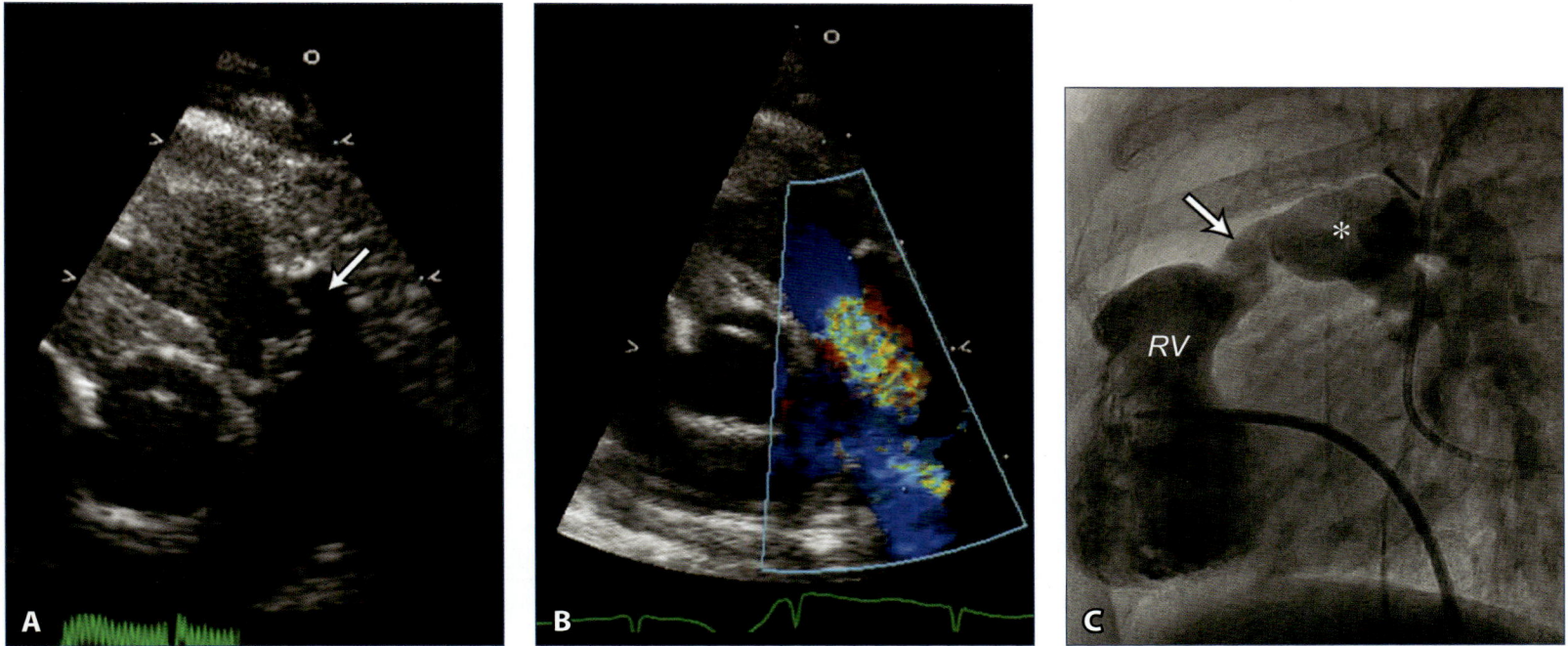

Figure 10-5. **A**, Parasternal short-axis echocardiogram view of pulmonary valve stenosis (*arrow*). **B**, Addition of color Doppler revealing increased flow velocity at the level of the pulmonary valve. **C**, Right ventricular (RV) radiograph angiogram demonstrating severe valvar pulmonary stenosis (PS) (*arrow*) and poststenotic dilation of the main pulmonary artery (*asterisk*). PS is one of the most common congenital heart defects, and it is associated with favorable long-term outcomes [13]. Mild PS (Doppler echocardiography peak instantaneous gradient < 30 mm Hg) [5] rarely progresses and does not warrant intervention. In the presence of symptoms, a peak instantaneous Doppler gradient greater than 50 mm Hg, and less than moderate pulmonary insufficiency, percutaneous balloon valvuloplasty is considered the therapeutic procedure of choice when the annulus is not hypoplastic [14]. A surgical commissurotomy is indicated for more complex lesions and valve replacement may be occasionally necessary if there is significant accompanying pulmonary insufficiency. Patients who have undergone surgical pulmonary valvotomy in childhood have excellent survival [15]. Patients who have undergone closed pulmonary valvotomy as the initial repair are more likely to require subsequent interventions, including pulmonary valve replacement for severe pulmonary regurgitation, and open valvotomy or pulmonary balloon valvuloplasty for residual pulmonary valve stenosis [16].

Double Chamber Right Ventricle

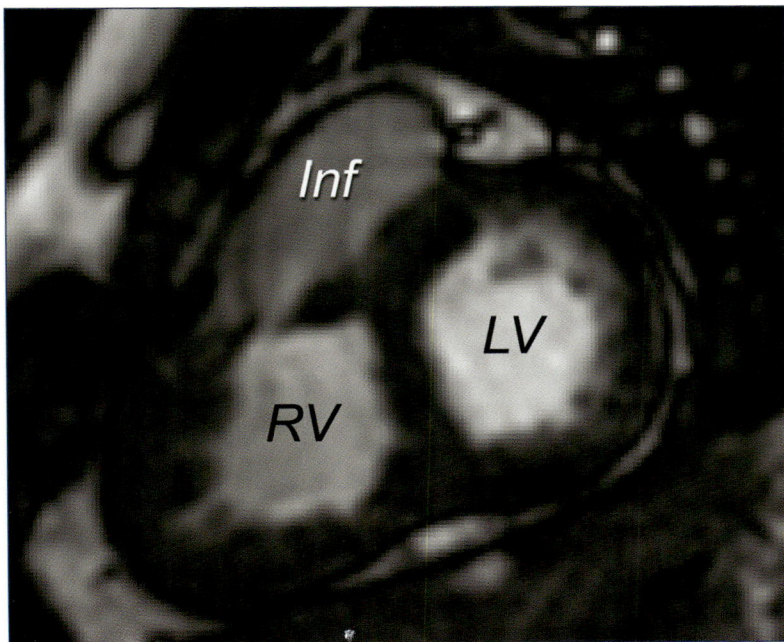

Figure 10-6. Cine magnetic resonance image in the short-axis plane demonstrating a double chamber right ventricle (RV). There is muscular narrowing at the proximal os infundibulum, which is the junction of the RV sinus and the infundibulum (Inf). The obstruction separates the RV into high and low pressure chambers and may be associated with a membranous ventricular septal defect. The long-term outcomes following surgical resection of the obstructing muscle in young patients are excellent [17]. LV—left ventricle.

Coarctation of the Aorta

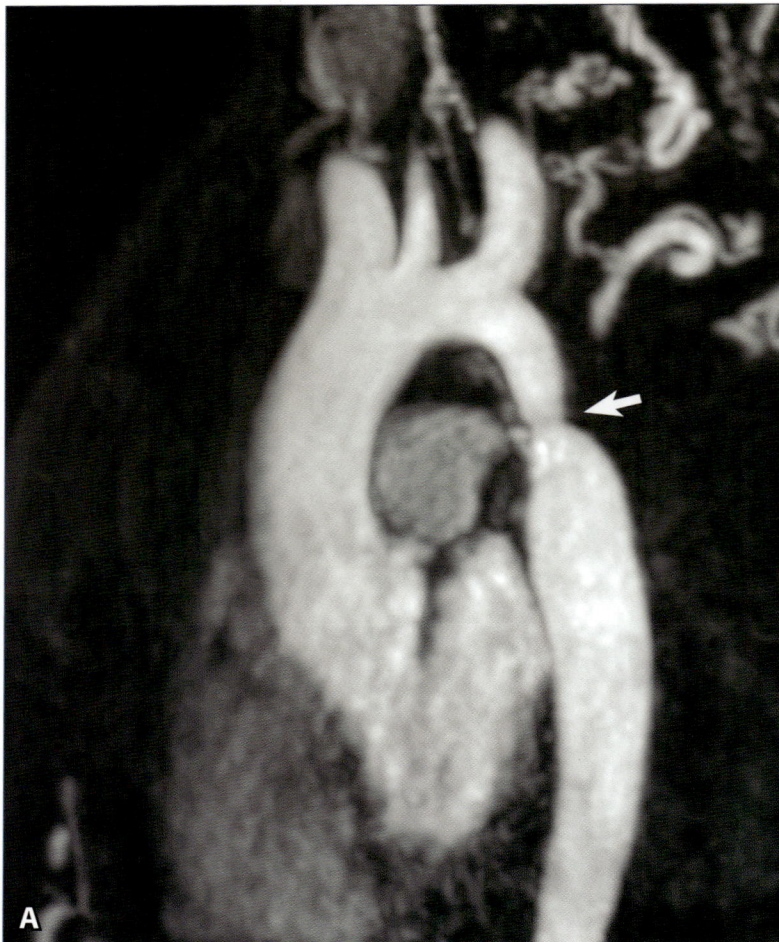

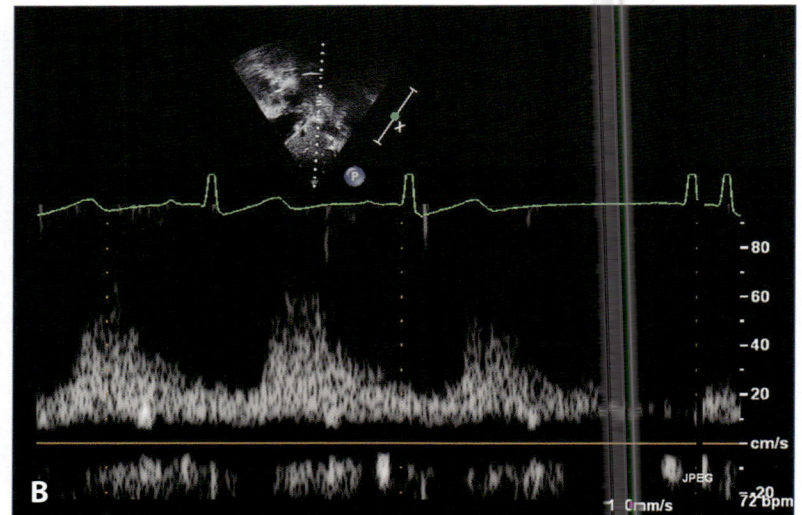

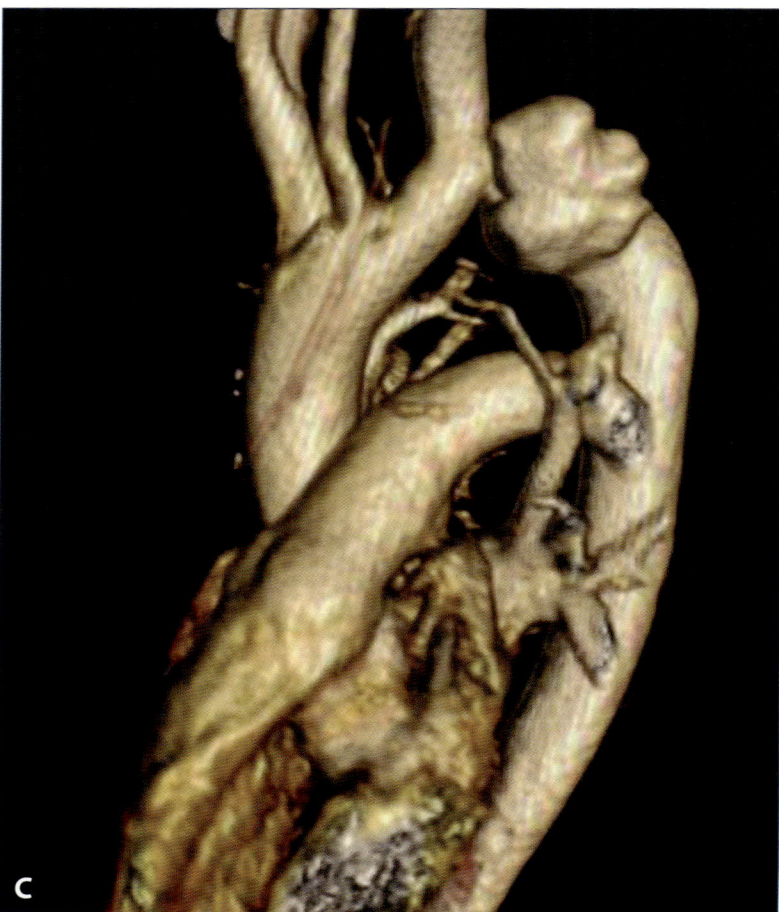

Figure 10-7. Vascular narrowing in coarctation of the aorta (CoA) most commonly involves the aortic isthmus, just distal to the left subclavian artery, but may also include the transverse arch and a portion of the descending aorta. A bicuspid aortic valve is a common association. The clinical presentation of the patient with CoA depends on several factors including age, associated lesions, and extent of collateral vessel formation. CoA is an important cause of secondary systemic arterial hypertension. Patients will typically have a higher blood pressure in the right arm (proximal to the obstruction) than in the lower extremities (distal to the obstruction). Patients with unrepaired CoA have a reported mortality as high as 75% by 46 years of age and median age of death of 31 years; the outcome with current hypertension and heart failure management is unknown [18]. Death is attributed to multiple factors including uncontrolled hypertension, congestive heart failure, infective endocarditis, aortic rupture or dissection, and cerebral hemorrhage. Patients who have undergone surgical repair have a 20-year survival rate greater than 80%; however they remain at risk for premature coronary artery disease and persistent hypertension, as well as aortic aneurysm, dissection, and recoarctation [19]. **A,** Magnetic resonance angiogram in an oblique sagittal projection demonstrating a CoA (*arrow*) at the aortic isthmus. **B,** Pulse-wave Doppler interrogation of the descending aorta in patients with CoA may show a blunted systolic velocity profile with persistent antero-grade flow into diastole. **C,** Volume rendering of a gadolinium-enhanced magnetic resonance angiogram demonstrating an aneurysm at the aortic isthmus following balloon angioplasty for CoA. (*Adapted from* Valente and Powell [7]; with permission.)

Physiologically Corrected Transposition of the Great Arteries

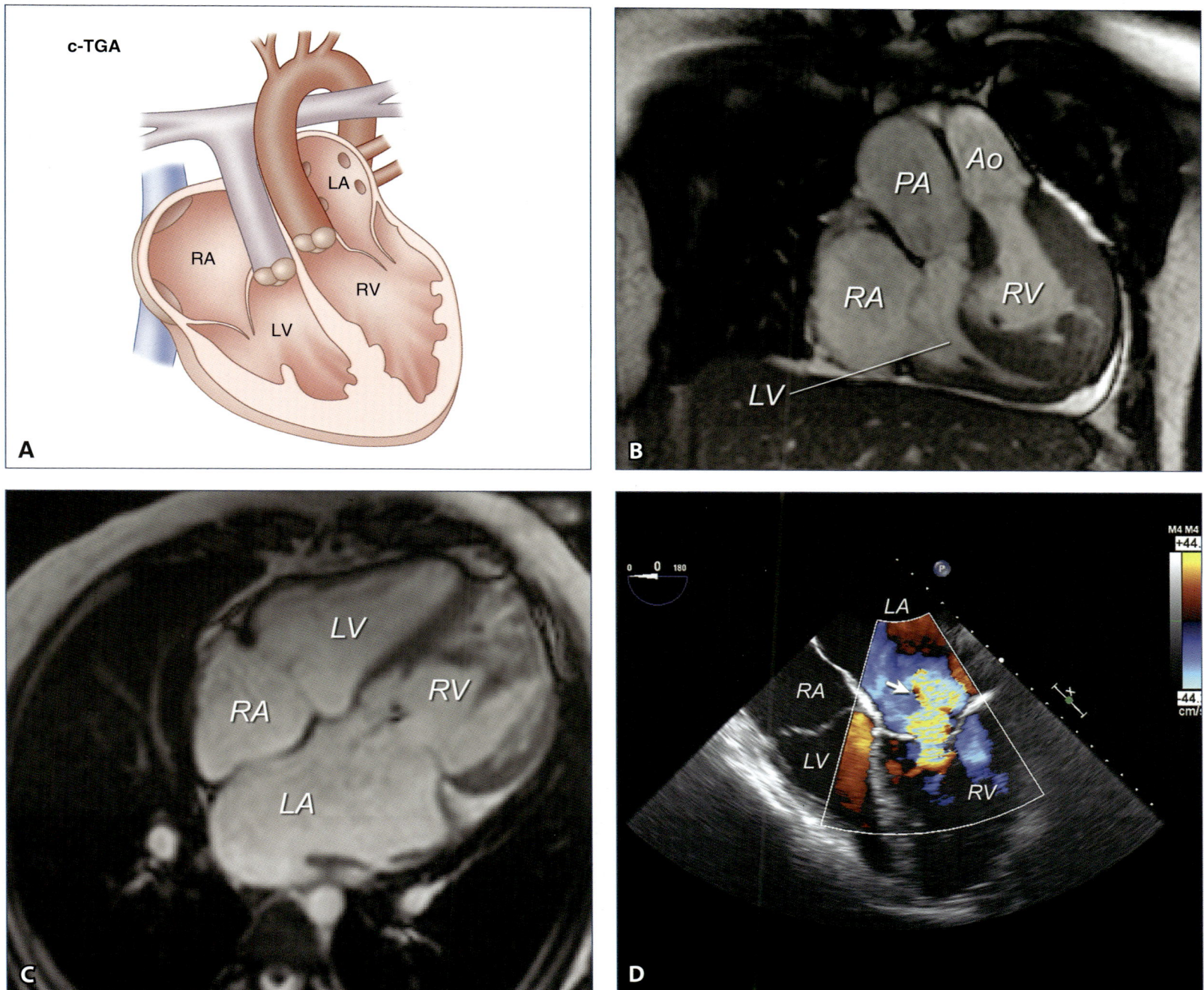

Figure 10-8. **A,** Diagrammatic representation of the most common form of physiologically corrected transposition of the great arteries (cTGA) with L-looping of the ventricles. cTGA is characterized by atrioventricular discordance and ventriculoarterial discordance. Systemic venous blood passes from the right atrium (RA) through the mitral valve into the morphologic left ventricle (LV) to the pulmonary artery (PA). Oxygenated blood then returns from the lungs to the left atrium (LA) through the tricuspid valve into the morphologic right ventricle (RV) and then out the aorta (Ao). RV outflow tract obstruction, ventricular septal defects, tricuspid valve abnormalities including Ebstein anomaly, complete heart block, and preexcitation may be associated with this lesion. Although some patients are asymptomatic, others develop congestive heart failure from right (systemic) ventricular failure and tricuspid valve (systemic atrioventricular valve) regurgitation [18]. Cine magnetic resonance image in the coronal (**B**) and four-chamber planes (**C**) demonstrating cTGA. **D,** Transesophageal echocardiogram demonstrating cTGA with dysplastic tricuspid valve and significant regurgitation (*arrow*).

Cyanotic Lesions

Transposition of the Great Arteries

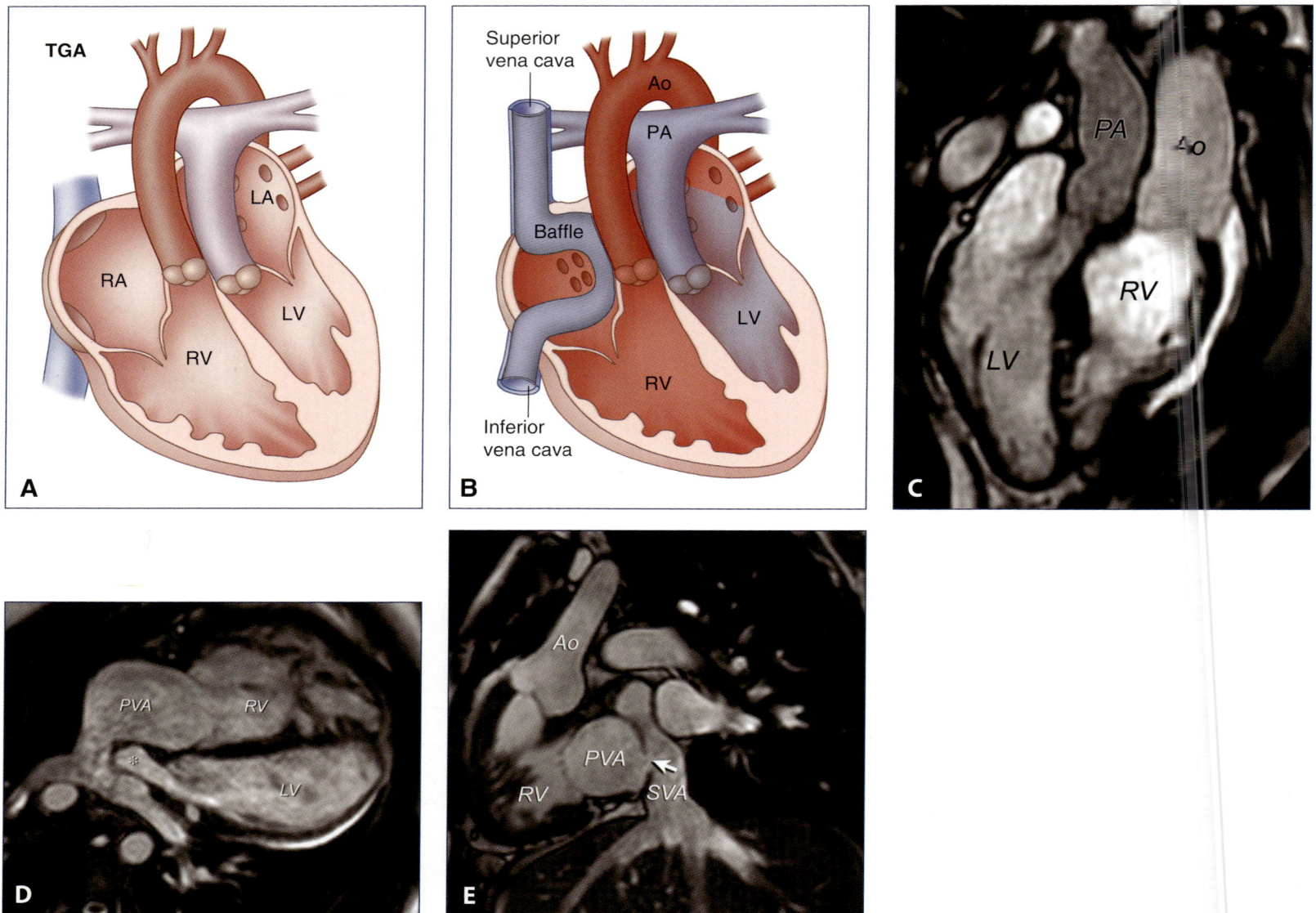

Figure 10-9. **A,** Diagrammatic representation of the most common form of transposition of the great arteries (TGA) with D-looping of the ventricles. In this condition, the aorta (Ao) arises from the right ventricle (RV) and the pulmonary artery (PA) from the left ventricle (LV). There is atrioventricular concordance and ventriculoarterial discordance. Low-oxygen systemic venous blood travels through the right heart, the aorta, the systemic circulation, and then back to the right heart. Oxygenated blood travels through the pulmonary veins, left heart, pulmonary arteries, and then back to the left heart. Thus, the systemic and pulmonary circulations run in parallel rather than in series. Survival depends on a communication between the two circuits (atrial septal defects, ventricular septal defects, or ductus arteriosus) to allow oxygenated blood to reach the body and low-oxygen blood to return to the lungs. In infancy, an emergent atrial septostomy may be performed to increase the mixing between the two circulations. Adult patients with TGA have usually undergone prior surgical repair. (*Adapted from an illustration provided by* Emily Flynn McIntosh.)

B, Diagram of the atrial switch repair (Senning or Mustard procedures), which was developed in the 1960s. With this surgery, systemic and pulmonary venous blood are redirected at the atrial level so that the systemic venous return (low-oxygen blood) flows to the LV and travels out the pulmonary artery, and the pulmonary venous blood (high-oxygen blood) flows to the RV and is ejected out the aorta. As a result, cyanosis is eliminated but the RV remains in the systemic position. The long-term morbidities of the atrial switch procedure are RV systolic dysfunction, atrial arrhythmias and defects, and obstruction in the venous pathways. (*Adapted from an illustration provided by* Emily Flynn McIntosh.) **C,** Cine magnetic resonance image (MRI) in the outflow tract plane. The Ao arises from the RV and the PA arises from the LV. (*Adapted from* Valente and Powell [7]; with permission.) **D,** Cine MRI in a four-chamber view demonstrating the pulmonary venous atrium (PVA) draining to the RV and the systemic venous atrium (SVA) (*asterisk*) draining to the LV. **E,** Cine MRI image in a sagittal plane demonstrating a baffle leak (*arrow*) in the atrial pathway.

Continued on the next page

F

G

H

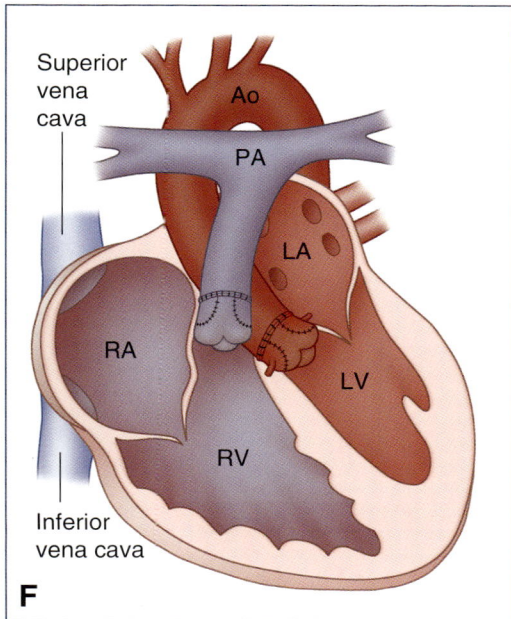

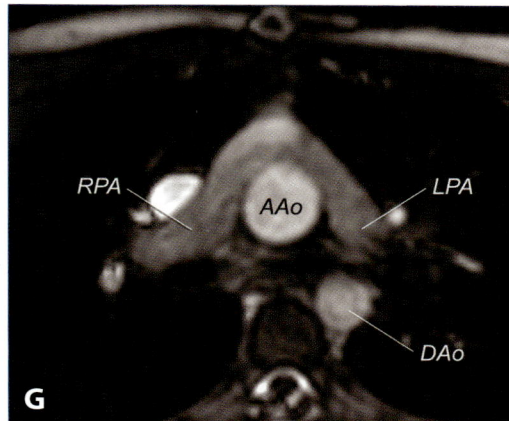

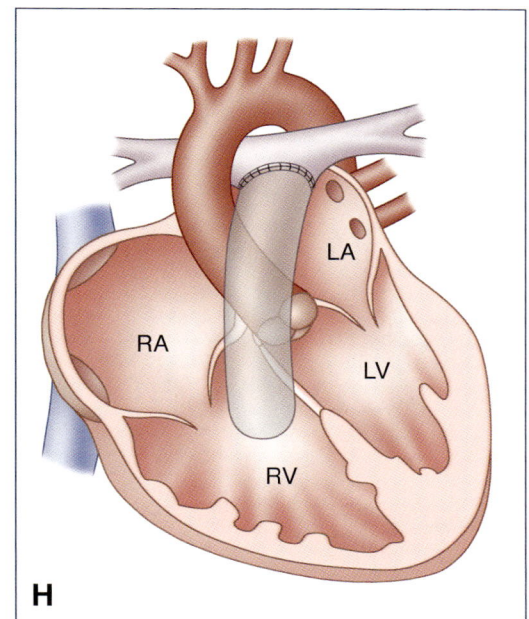

Figure 10-9. *(Continued)* **F,** Diagram of the arterial switch operation. In the 1980s, an alternative surgical treatment for TGA, the arterial switch operation, largely replaced the atrial switch operation. In this procedure, the ascending Ao and main pulmonary arteries are transected and then attached to the concordant ventricle, and the coronary arteries are detached and transferred to the new aortic root. To minimize kinking of the pulmonary arteries, the right pulmonary artery (RPA) is often positioned anterior to the ascending Ao (LeCompte maneuver). This surgery both eliminates cyanosis and establishes the LV as the systemic ventricle. Common sequelae from this surgery include PA stenosis, neoaortic root dilation, and neoaortic regurgitation [7]. *(Adapted from an illustration provided by* Emily Flynn McIntosh.) **G,** Cine MRI in the axial plane dem-onstrating the position of the pulmonary arteries and Ao following an arterial switch operation with a LeCompte maneuver. **H,** Patients with TGA, a ventricular septal defect, and significant pulmonary stenosis often undergo a Rastelli operation because an arterial switch operation would leave them with an obstructed LV outflow tract. A Rastelli operation involves patch closure of the ventricular septal defect to baffle LV blood to the Ao placement of an RV to PA conduit, and oversewing of the proximal main PA. Sequelae of this procedure include subaortic stenosis, conduit obstruction, ventricular septal defect patch leak, and heart block. *(Adapted from an illustration provided by* Emily Flynn McIntosh.) AAo—ascending aorta; DAo—descending aorta; LA—left atrium; LPA—left pulmonary artery; PVA—pulmonary venous atrium; RA—right atrium.

Tetralogy of Fallot

Figure 10-10. Tetralogy of Fallot (TOF) is the most common form of cyanotic congenital heart disease. The principal pathologic abnormality involves varying degrees of hypoplasia of the infundibulum (Inf) often with anterior, superior, and leftward deviation of the conal septum. As a result, TOF is characterized by right ventricular (RV) outflow tract obstruction, RV hypertrophy, a large conoventricular septal defect, and an aortic valve (AoV) that overrides the ventricular septum. Often the RV outflow tract obstruction is severe enough to cause right-to-left flow through the ventricular septal defect (VSD), which results in cyanosis. Patients with TOF born before the early 1970s were often palliated with systemic-to-pulmonary shunts to increase pulmonary blood flow. Definitive surgical repair is now often performed in infancy and typically involves patch closure of the VSD, and an infundibular or transannular RV outflow tract patch to relieve the obstruction. Relief of pulmonary valve (PV) stenosis can render the PV incompetent. Over time, pulmonary regurgitation may lead to RV dilation and dysfunction, exercise intolerance, and malignant ventricular

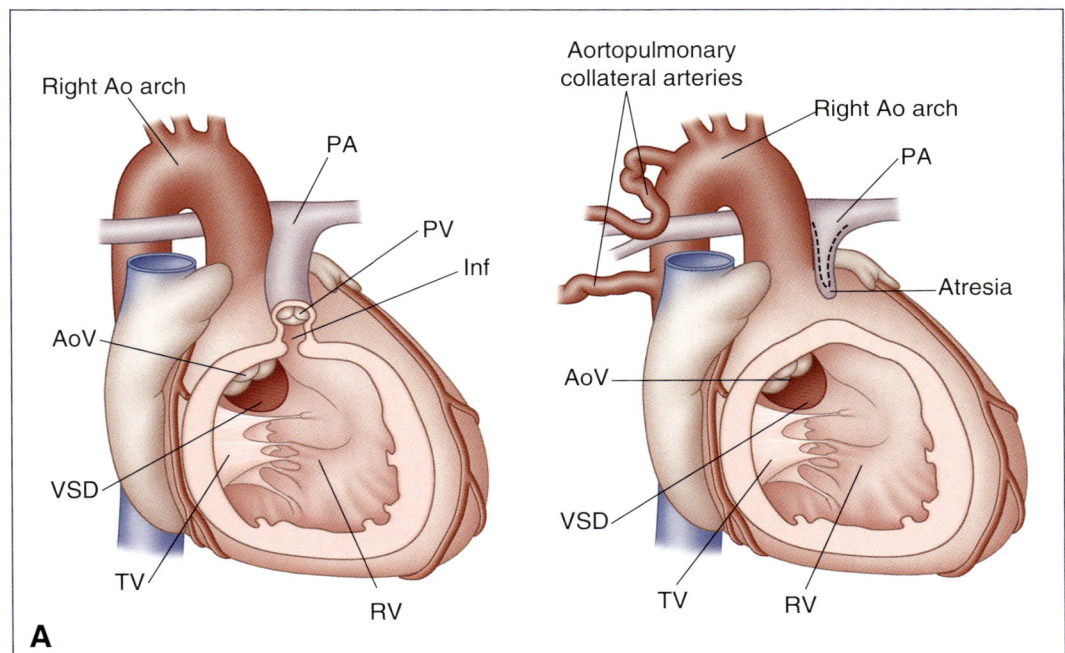

A

arrhythmias. **A,** Diagrammatic representations of two variations of TOF—the more common form with pulmonary stenosis and the more severe form with pulmonary atresia. *(Adapted from an illustration provided by* Emily Flynn McIntosh.)

Continued on the next page

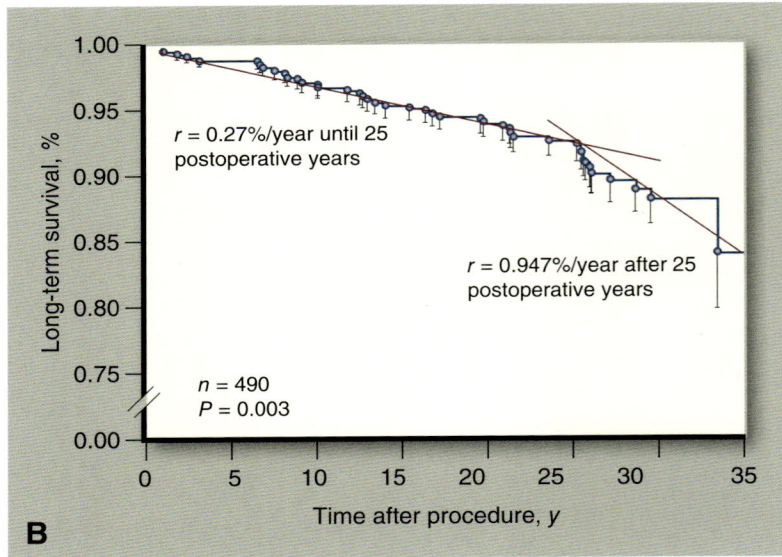

B

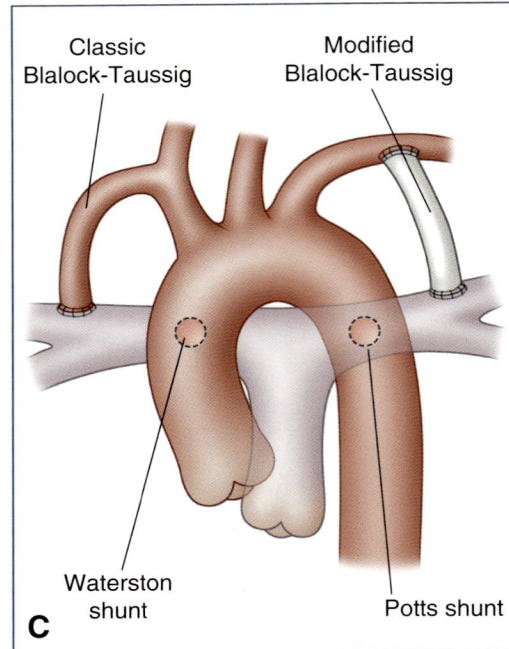

C

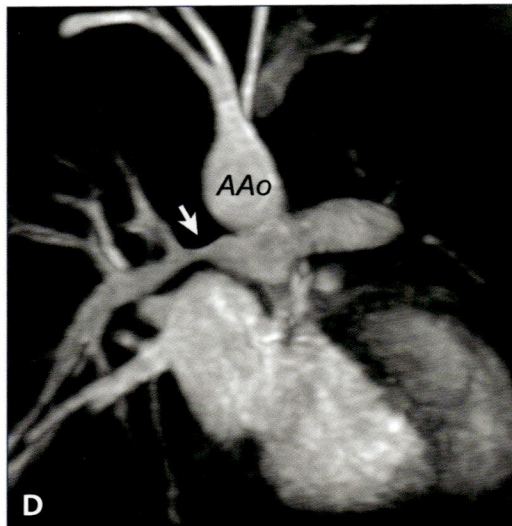

D

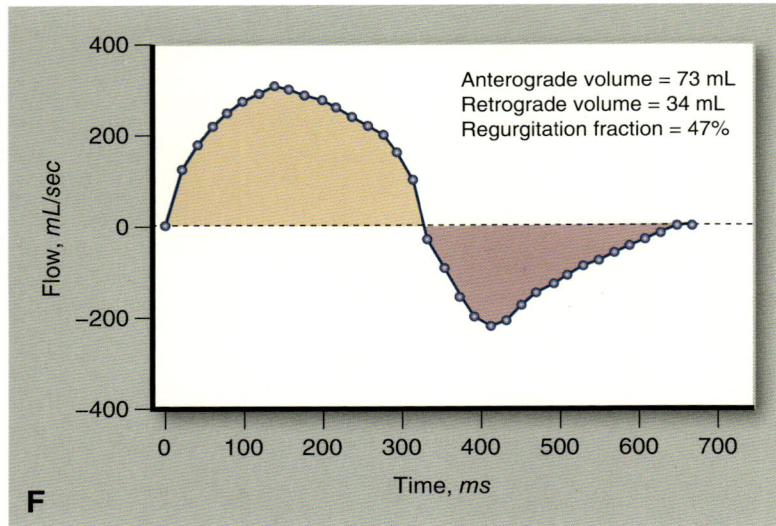

E

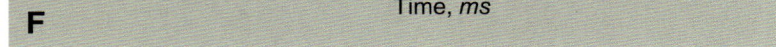

F

Figure 10-10. *(Continued)* **B,** Long-term survival curve after correction of TOF. Since the introduction of open-heart surgery for this condition, the 20-year survival rate has improved to nearly 90%. However, the risk of sudden cardiac death increases with time, and mortality approaches approximately 1% each postoperative (PO) year after 25 years. *(Adapted from* Nollert *et al.* 20 .) One risk factor that has been associated with worse outcomes is a QRS duration on a resting electrocardiogram greater than or equal to 180 ms, emphasizing the interrelationship between electrical and mechanical failure of the right-sided heart structures [21]. **C,** Diagrammatic representation of various types of systemic-to-pulmonary shunts. *(Adapted from an illustration provided by* Emily Flynn McIntosh.) **D,** Gadolinium-enhanced magnetic resonance angiogram in a coronal plane demonstrating a hypoplastic right pulmonary artery (PA) with focal narrowing *(arrow)* at the site of previous Waterston shunt. PA stenosis at the insertion site is a common complication of systemic-to-pulmonary shunts. **E,** Cine magnetic resonance image (MRI) in a ventricular short-axis plane demonstrating severe RV dilation (220 mL/m²) as a consequence of chronic PV regurgitation. **F,** Main PA flow curve generated by phase velocity MRI in a TOF patient with chronic pulmonary regurgitation. This technique allows precise quantitation of the severity of regurgitation. The area above the baseline is the anterograde flow volume and the area below the baseline is the regurgitant flow volume. The pulmonary regurgitation fraction is the ratio of the regurgitant and the anterograde flow volumes.

Continued on the next page

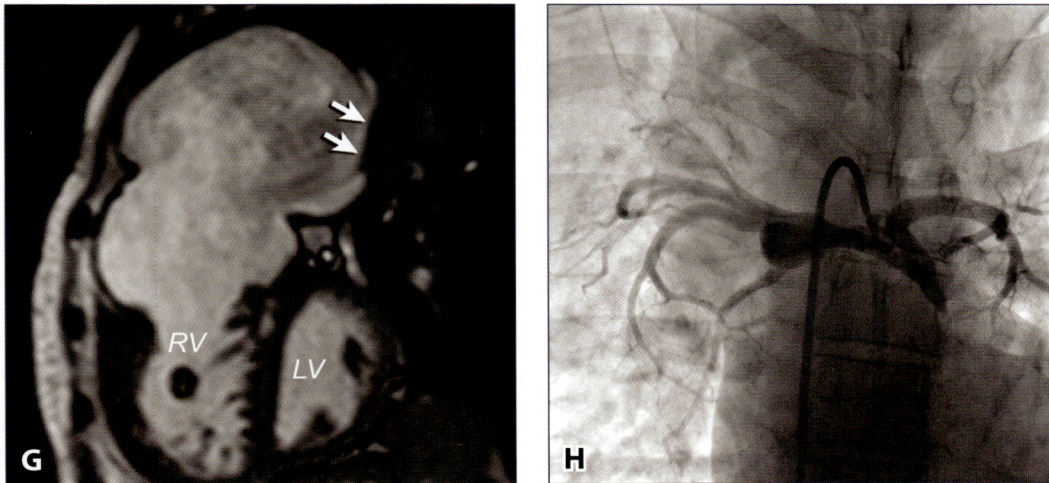

Figure 10-10. *(Continued)* **G,** Cine MRI in an oblique sagittal plane demonstrating a large RV outflow tract aneurysm with intravascular thrombus (*arrows*). RV outflow tract aneurysms occur in more than 15% of patients with repaired TOF and contribute to decreased RV systolic function [22]. **H,** Radiograph angiogram in an adult with unrepaired TOF with pulmonary atresia demonstrating the classically described "seagull" appearance of hypoplastic pulmonary arteries. In pulmonary atresia, the pulmonary blood supply may be from a patent ductus arteriosus or aorta-pulmonary collaterals. AAo—ascending aorta; LV—left ventricle; TV—tricuspid valve.

Single Ventricle Heart Disease

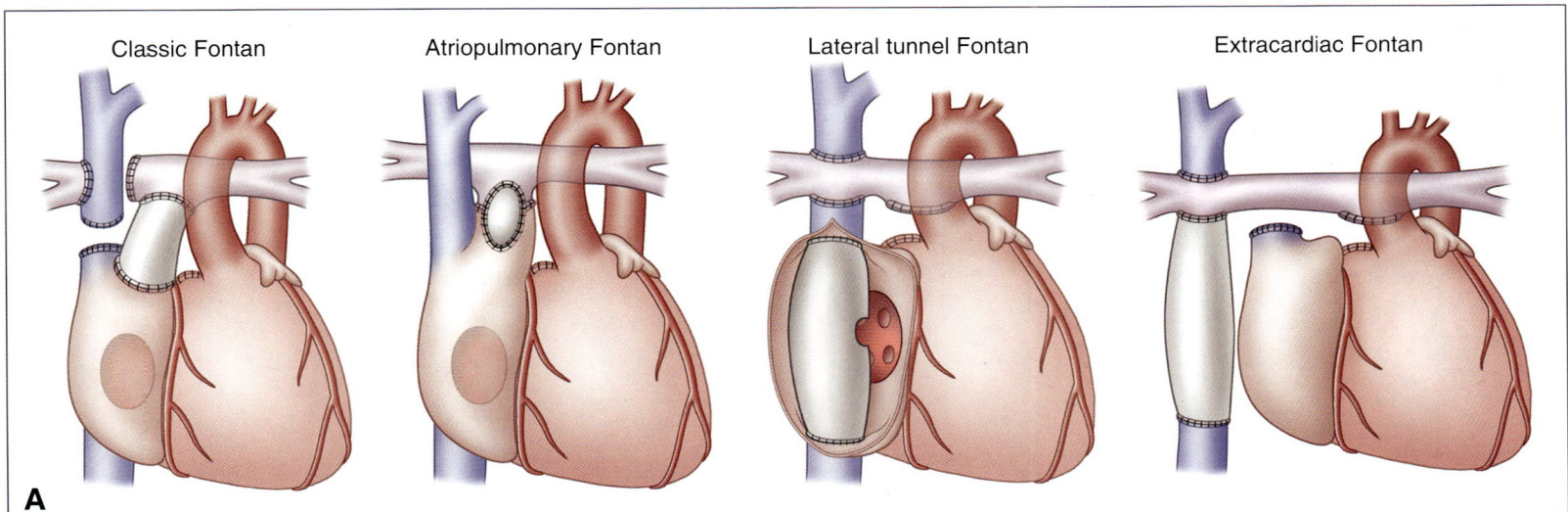

Figure 10-11. The term *single ventricle heart disease* is imprecise but useful in some settings. It generally refers to congenital heart lesions in which abnormalities of one ventricle or its valves preclude a biventricular circulation (*ie,* separate pulmonary and systemic circulations each supported by a ventricle). Common anatomic diagnoses in this category include tricuspid valve atresia, hypoplastic left heart syndrome, double inlet single left ventricle, and single right ventricle (RV). Most patients with single ventricle heart disease undergo a series of palliative surgeries culminating in a Fontan procedure. Since its initial application for tricuspid valve atresia in 1971, there have been many modifications to the Fontan procedure. In general, a Fontan procedure results in nearly complete separation of the pulmonary and systemic circulations with the "single ventricle" driving blood flow to the systemic circulation and "passive" venous return of blood flow to the lungs. Patients who have undergone a Fontan operation are predisposed to develop atrial arrhythmias, hepatic and renal dysfunction, thromboembolic events, and protein losing enteropathy [23]. **A,** Diagrammatic representation of the various types of Fontan surgeries. (*Adapted from an illustration provided by Emily Flynn McIntosh.*) **B,** Cine magnetic resonance image in the coronal plane in a patient with a classic Fontan operation demonstrating a dilated right atrium (*asterisk*) with sluggish blood flow.

Continued on the next page

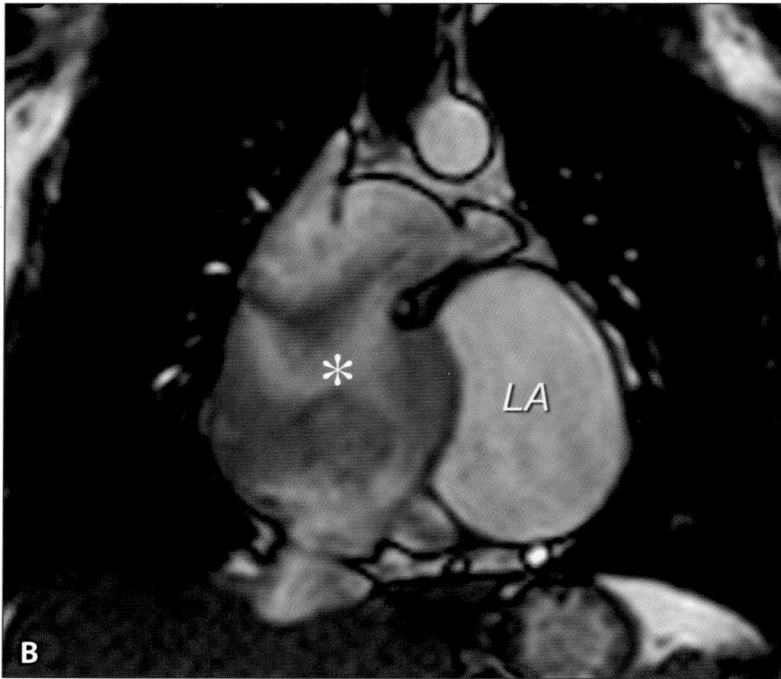

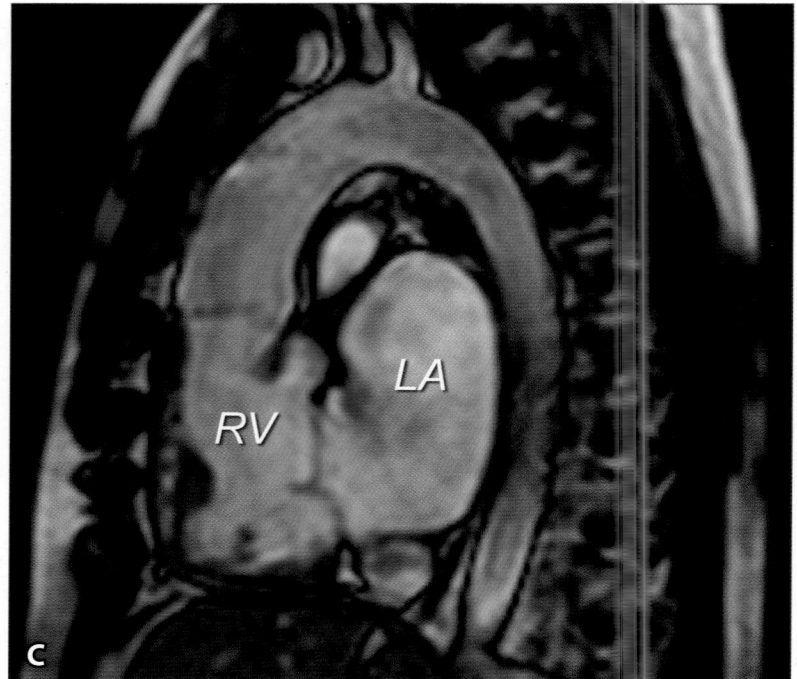

Figure 10-11. *(Continued)* **C,** Cine MRI image in a sagittal plane in the same patient. Oxygenated pulmonary venous blood drains to a left atrium (LA) and then into a single RV, which ejects blood into the aorta.

Ebstein Anomaly

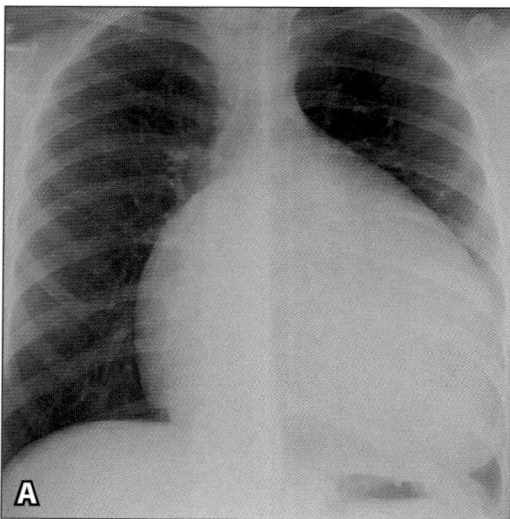

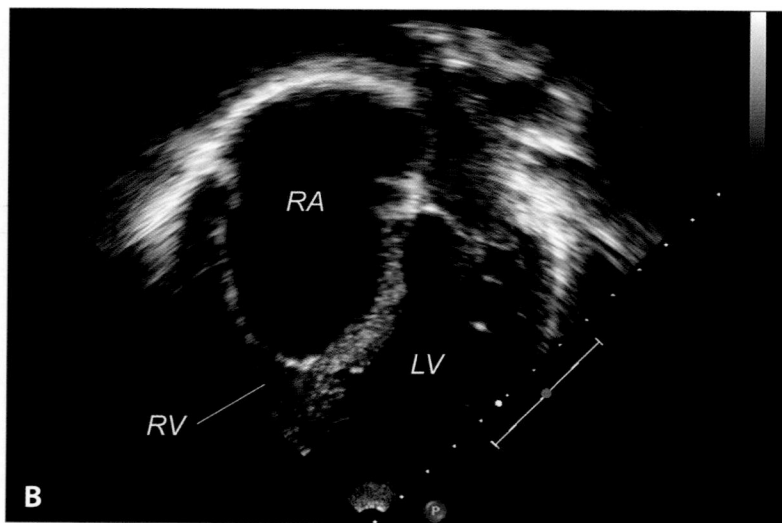

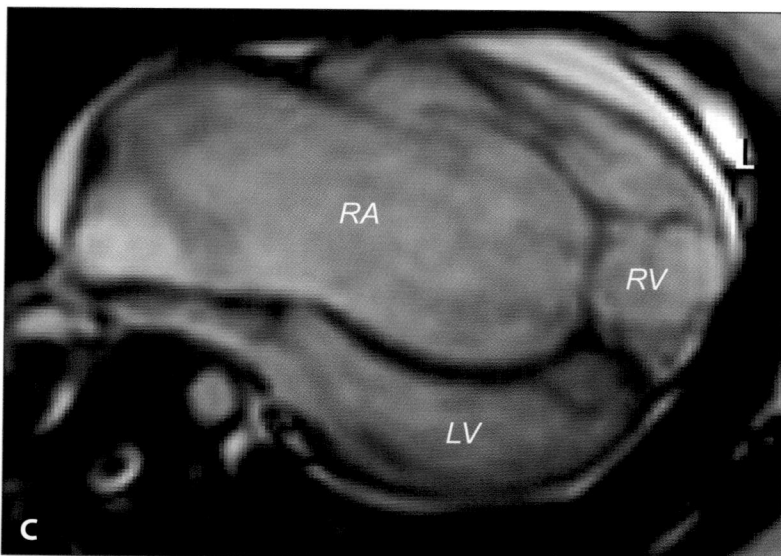

Figure 10-12. Ebstein anomaly is an abnormality of the tricuspid valve and right ventricular sinus. Failure of delamination of the septal leaflet of the tricuspid valve results in apical displacement of the tricuspid valve coaptation zone. Patients may be cyanotic from right-to-left shunting at the atrial level through an atrial septal defect or patent foramen ovale, which are commonly associated lesions. Progressive tricuspid regurgitation, right ventricular (RV) dilation and dysfunction, and atrial and ventricular arrhythmias may develop. Surgical treatment includes tricuspid valve repair or replacement, closure of any interatrial communications, and arrhythmia ablative procedures. Such interventions may improve systemic oxygen saturation, exercise tolerance, and functional class, and may reduce supraventricular and ventricular arrhythmias [24]. **A,** Chest radiograph demonstrating cardiomegaly and relatively oligemic lung fields typical of patients with severe Ebstein anomaly. Two-dimensional echocardiogram (**B**) and cine magnetic resonance images (**C**) in a four-chamber view. Failure of delamination of the tricuspid valve septal leaflet results in apical displacement of its hinge point.

Continued on the next page

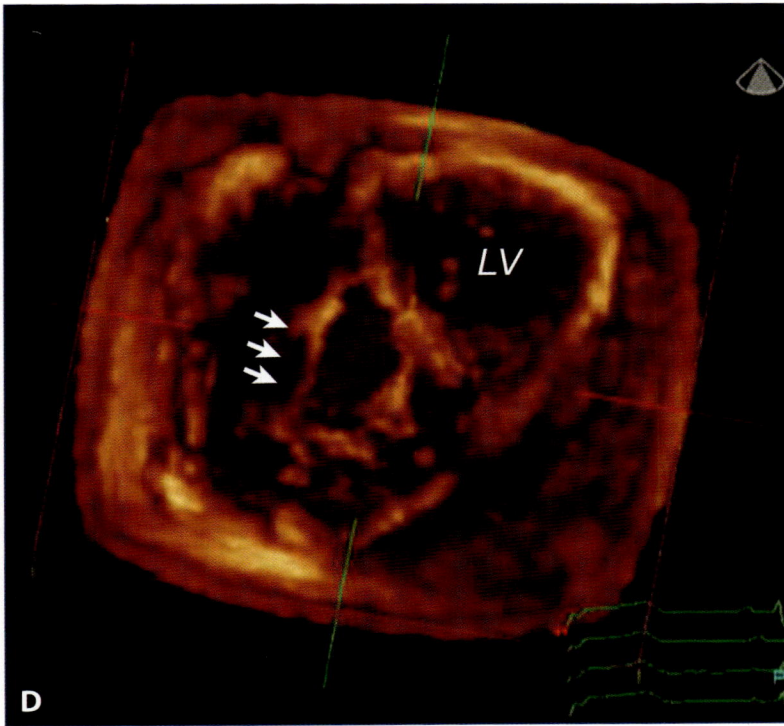

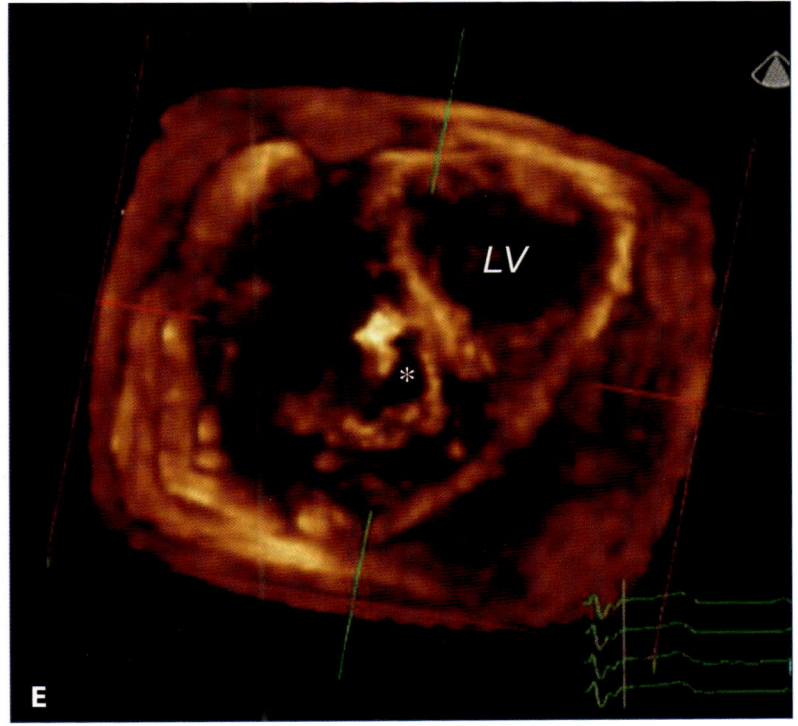

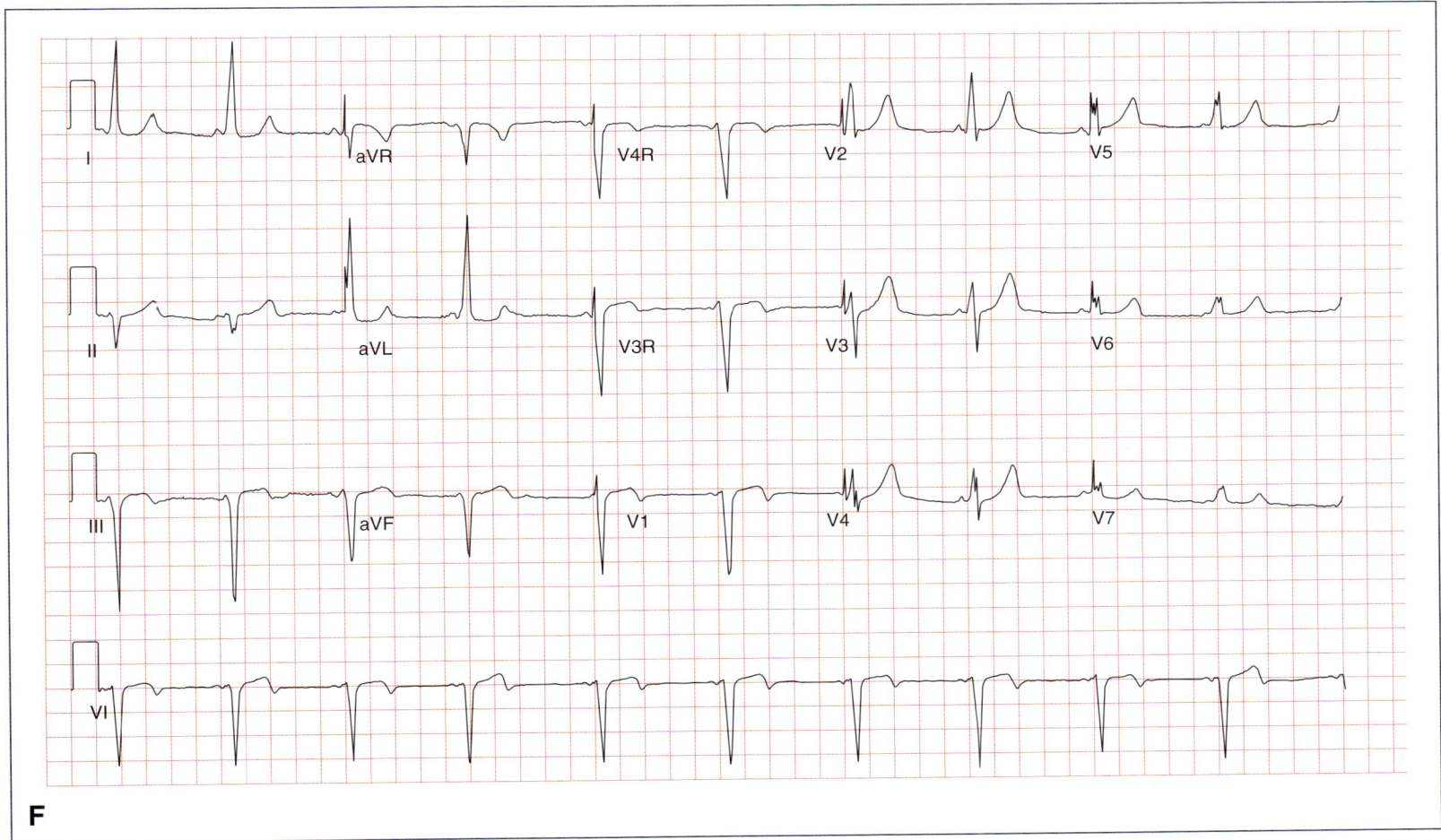

Figure 10-12. *(Continued)* **D,** Three-dimensional echocardiogram image in diastole demonstrating the redundant anterior leaflet of the tricuspid valve *(arrows)* with diminutive septal leaflet. **E,** Three-dimensional echocardiogram in systole illustrates failure of tricuspid valve coaptation *(asterisk).* **F,** Twelve-lead electrocardiogram in a patient with Ebstein anomaly demonstrating Wolff-Parkinson-White syndrome. Approximately 20% of patients with Ebstein anomaly have Wolff-Parkinson-White syndrome, and such accessory pathways are typically located along the posterior and septal aspects of the tricuspid valve ring [25,26]. LV—left ventricle; RA—right atrium.

References

1. Hoffman JI, Kaplan S: The incidence of congenital heart disease. *J Am Coll Cardiol* 2002, 39:1890–1900.

2. Warnes CA, Liberthson R, Danielson GK, *et al.*: Task force 1: the changing profile of congenital heart disease in adult life. *J Am Coll Cardiol* 2001, 37:1170–1175.

3. Niwa K, Perloff JK, Webb GD, *et al.*: Survey of specialized tertiary care facilities for adults with congenital heart disease. *Int J Cardiol* 2004, 96:211–216.

4. Hoffman JI, Kaplan S, Liberthson RR: Prevalence of congenital heart disease. *Am Heart J* 2004, 147:425–439.

5. Warnes CA, Williams RG, Bashore TM, *et al.*: ACC/AHA 2008 Guidelines for the management of adults with congenital heart disease. A report of the American College of Cardiology/American Heart Association task force for practice guidelines for the management of adults with congenital heart disease. *J Am Coll Cardiol* 2008, Nov 5 (epub ahead of print).

6. *NADAS' Pediatric Cardiology*, edn 2. Edited by Keane JF, Lock JF, Flyer DC. Philadelphia: WB Saunders; 2006:604.

7. Valente AM, Powell AJ: Clinical applications of cardiovascular magnetic resonance in congenital heart disease. *Cardiol Clin* 2007, 25:97–110.

8. *NADAS' Pediatric Cardiology*, edn 2. Edited by Keane JF, Lock JF, Flyer DC. Philadelphia: Elsevier; 2006:529.

9. Gabriel HM, Heger M, Innerhofer P, *et al.*: Long-term outcome of patients with ventricular septal defect considered not to require surgical closure during childhood. *J Am Coll Cardiol* 2002, 39:1066–1071.

10. Kidd L, Driscoll DJ, Gersony WM, *et al.*: Second natural history study of congenital heart defects. Results of treatment of patients with ventricular septal defects. *Circulation* 1993, 87:I38–I51.

11. Lock JE, Keane JF, Perry SB: *Diagnostic and Interventional Catheterization in Congenital Heart Disease*, edn 2. Norwell, MA: Kluwer Academic Publishers; 2000.

12. Sadiq M, Latif F, Ur-Rehman A: Analysis of infective endarteritis in patent ductus arteriosus. *Am J Cardiol* 2004, 93:513–515.

13. Hayes CJ, Hayes CJ, Driscoll DJ, *et al.*: Second natural history study of congenital heart defects. Results of treatment of patients with pulmonary valvar stenosis. *Circulation* 1993, 87:I28–I37.

14. Bonow RO, Carabello BA, Chatterjee K, *et al.*: ACC/AHA 2006 guidelines for the management of patients with valvular heart disease: a report of the American College of Cardiology/American Heart Association Task Force on Practice Guidelines (writing committee to revise the 1998 Guidelines for the Management of Patients With Valvular Heart Disease): developed in collaboration with the Society of Cardiovascular Anesthesiologists: endorsed by the Society for Cardiovascular Angiography and Interventions and the Society of Thoracic Surgeons. *Circulation* 2006, 48:e1–e148.

15. Reid JM, Coleman EN, Stevenson JG, *et al.*: Long-term results of surgical treatment for pulmonary valve stenosis. *Arch Dis Child* 1976, 51:79–81.

16. Earing MG, Connolly HM, Dearani JA, *et al.*: Long-term follow-up of patients after surgical treatment for isolated pulmonary valve stenosis. *Mayo Clin Proc* 2005, 80:871–876.

17. Hachiro Y, Takagi N, Koyanagi T, *et al.*: Repair of double-chambered right ventricle: surgical results and long-term follow-up. *Ann Thorac Surg* 2001, 72:1520–1522.

18. Campbell N: Natural history of coarctation of the aorta. *Br Heart* 1970, 62:633–640.

19. Oliver JM, Gallego P, Gonzalez A, *et al.*: Risk factors for aortic complications in adults with coarctation of the aorta. *J Am Coll Cardiol* 2004, 44:1641–1647.

20. Nollert G, Fischlein T, Bouterwek S, *et al.*: Long-term survival in patients with repair of tetralogy of Fallot: 36-year follow-up of 490 survivors of the first year after surgical repair. *J Am Coll Cardiol* 1997, 30:1374–1383.

21. Gatzoulis MA, Balaji S, Webber SA, *et al.*: Risk factors for arrhythmia and sudden cardiac death late after repair of tetralogy of Fallot: a multicentre study. *Lancet* 2000, 356:975–981.

22. Davlouros PA, Kilner PJ, Hornung TS, *et al.*: Right ventricular function in adults with repaired tetralogy of Fallot assessed with cardiovascular magnetic resonance imaging: detrimental role of right ventricular outflow aneurysms or akinesia and adverse right-to-left ventricular interaction. *J Am Coll Cardiol* 2002, 40:2044–2052.

23. Khairy P, Fernandes SM, Mayer JE Jr, *et al.*: Long-term survival, modes of death, and predictors of mortality in patients with Fontan surgery. *Circulation* 2008, 117:85–92.

24. Dearani JA, Danielson GK: Surgical management of Ebstein's anomaly in the adult. *Semin Thorac Cardiovasc Surg* 2005, 17:148–154.

25. Oh JK, Holmes DR Jr, Hayes DL, *et al.*: Cardiac arrhythmias in patients with surgical repair of Ebstein's anomaly. *J Am Coll Cardiol* 1985, 6:1351–1357.

26. Smith WM, Gallagher JJ, Kerr CR, *et al.*: The electrophysiologic basis and management of symptomatic recurrent tachycardia in patients with Ebstein's anomaly of the tricuspid valve. *Am J Cardiol* 1982, 49:1223–1234.

Deep Vein Thrombosis, Pulmonary Embolism, and Idiopathic Pulmonary Arterial Hypertension

11

Samuel Z. Goldhaber
Gregory Piazza

Venous thromboembolism, including deep vein thrombosis (DVT) and pulmonary embolism (PE), constitutes a major public health problem that requires the expertise of vascular medicine specialists. For patients with DVT alone, more than half will develop postthrombotic syndrome, with chronic leg swelling, abnormal skin pigmentation, and rarely, venous ulceration. PE causes complex pathophysiologic changes in cardiovascular hemodynamics and pulmonary gas exchange. The mortality rate from acute PE exceeds that from myocardial infarction. For survivors of PE, the possibility of developing disabling chronic thromboembolic pulmonary hypertension is 3% to 4%.

Although venous ultrasonography remains the test of choice for the diagnosis of DVT, improvements in computed tomography (CT) have made chest CT the dominant imaging modality for the evaluation of suspected PE. Contemporary diagnostic algorithms now focus on the combined use of a simplified clinical decision rule, D-dimer testing, and chest CT scanning [1].

Prognosis is best assessed with a combination of clinical evaluation, cardiac biomarkers, such as cardiac troponin, and imaging of the right ventricle (RV) [2]. RV enlargement on chest CT and RV dysfunction on echocardiography predict an elevated risk of adverse outcomes, even in the initial absence of hypotension or tachycardia. High-risk patients may be considered for primary therapies such as fibrinolysis, catheter or surgical embolectomy, or placement of an inferior vena cava filter. Options for immediate anticoagulation include unfractionated heparin, low-molecular weight heparin, and fondaparinux, whereas warfarin remains the mainstay of chronic anticoagulation. Patients with idiopathic DVT or PE continue to have a high risk of recurrence even after completing a standard course of anticoagulation and may benefit from indefinite anticoagulation.

Epidemiology and Risk Factors

Figure 11-1. Epidemiology of venous thromboembolism (VTE). VTE, which includes deep vein thrombosis (DVT) and pulmonary embolism (PE), is the third most common cardiovascular illness after acute coronary syndromes and stroke. In the Olmsted County population, the estimated annual incidence of VTE was 118 per 100,000 person-years [3]. The annual age-adjusted incidence of DVT has been estimated to be 61 per 100,000 [4]. DVT is a common condition among hospitalized inpatients, especially in the intensive care setting, and may often occur without symptoms [5,6]. An increasing number of patients with permanent pacemaker and implantable cardiac defibrillator leads, as well as chronic indwelling central venous

Epidemiology of Venous Thromboembolism

The annual incidence of VTE is estimated to be 118 per 100,000 person-years

The incidence of overall VTE rises dramatically for men and women after age 60, with PE accounting for the majority of the increase

The incidence of upper extremity DVT is rising as the number of patients with permanent pacemaker and implantable cardiac defibrillator leads as well as chronic indwelling central venous catheters increases

catheters, has resulted in a rise in the incidence of upper extremity DVT over the past decade [7].

The annual age-adjusted incidence of PE has been reported to be 88 per 100,000 [4]. The 90-day mortality rate for PE exceeds 15%, making it more life-threatening than acute myocardial infarction [8].

Figure 11-2. Major risk factors for venous thromboembolism (VTE). Clinicians should suspect inherited thrombophilias in patients with VTE at a young age, multiple family members with VTE, idiopathic or recurrent VTE, or a history of recurrent spontaneous abortions. Major inherited thrombophilias include factor V Leiden mutation resulting in activated protein C resistance, prothrombin gene mutation 20210, and deficiencies of antithrombin III, protein C, and protein S.

Other risk factors for VTE include advancing age, smoking, obesity, personal or family history of VTE, and recent surgery, trauma, or hospitalization. Acute infectious illnesses, such as urinary tract infections, have been associated with a transient increase in the risk of VTE in the community setting [9]. An increased incidence of pulmonary embolism has been observed in patients suffering from exacerbations of chronic obstructive pulmonary disease [10]. The presence of chronically indwelling central venous foreign bodies, such as pacemaker or implantable cardiac defibrillator leads, as well as venous catheters, significantly increases the risk of upper extremity deep vein thrombosis [7]. Recent studies suggest a pathophysiologic link between VTE and atherosclerotic disease, as well as atherothrombotic events [11,12].

Both active and occult malignancy have been associated with an elevated risk of VTE [13]. The increased risk of VTE is not restricted to adenocarcinomas and can also be observed in patients with myeloproliferative disorders, lymphoma, and leukemia [14].

Venous thromboembolism constitutes an important women's health concern. The correlation between pregnancy and an increased risk of VTE is well recognized. The use of oral contraceptive pills, especially those containing third-generation progestins, has been associated with an elevated risk of VTE [15]. In the Women's Health Initiative, women receiving

Major Risk Factors for Venous Thromboembolism

Factor V Leiden resulting in activated protein C resistance

Prothrombin gene mutation 20210

Antithrombin III deficiency

Protein C deficiency

Protein S deficiency

Advancing age

Smoking

Obesity

Personal or family history of venous thromboembolism

Recent surgery, trauma, or hospitalization

Acute infection

Chronic obstructive pulmonary disease

Long-haul air travel

Antiphospholipid antibody syndrome

Hyperhomocysteinemia (less commonly inherited secondary to a mutation in methylenetetrahydropholate reductase)

Pregnancy, oral contraceptive pills, or hormone replacement therapy

Atherosclerotic disease

Pacemaker or implantable cardiac defibrillator leads and indwelling venous catheters

estrogen plus progestin hormone replacement therapy had a twofold increase in the risk of VTE compared with those receiving placebo [16].

Long-haul air travel appears to increase risk by resulting in activation of coagulation in addition to physical immobility [17].

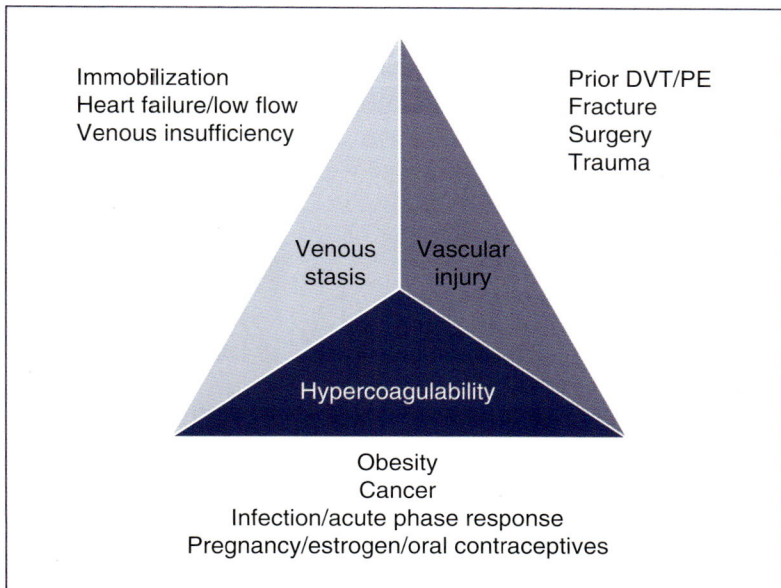

Figure 11-3. The 19th century German pathologist Rudolph Virchow posited three major factors that predispose to venous thrombosis. The acute phase response to infection or injury can cause hypercoagulability due to increased production of fibrinogen and the major endogenous inhibitor of fibrinolysis plasminogen activator inhibitor-1 (PAI-1). Estrogenic stimuli likewise increase fibrinogen and PAI-1. Vascular injury can be either due to direct trauma or biochemical or cellular stimuli such as activation of endothelial cells by proinflammatory cytokines or blood leukocytes. Obesity likewise causes inflammation that augments fibrinogen and PAI-1. Malignancies can produce a procoagulant state by producing tissue factor or inflammatory mediators. Venous stasis can arise from immobilization, such as prolonged travel, or from medical situations, such as hindered mobility due to postoperative state, trauma, or stroke. Low-flow states, such as heart failure, can also predispose to venous thrombosis. DVT—deep vein thrombosis; PE—pulmonary embolism.

Anatomy and Pathophysiology

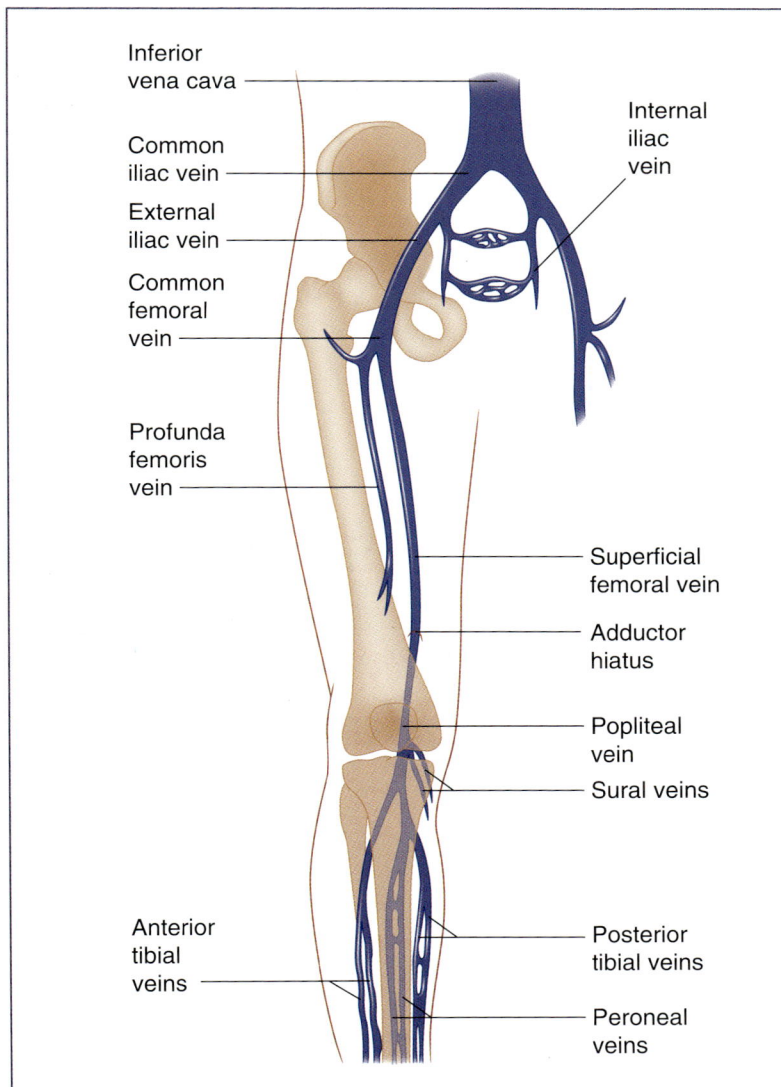

Figure 11-4. Venous anatomy of the lower extremities. The inferior vena cava is located to the right of the aorta and bifurcates into the common iliac veins. The left common iliac vein crosses below the right iliac artery or aorta, which may result in relative compression of the vein and is likely the cause of slower venous blood flow in the left leg compared with the right lower extremity. The common iliac vein bifurcates into external and internal iliac veins. The internal iliac vein tends to be smaller in diameter and connects with the contralateral internal iliac vein. As the external iliac vein descends through the pelvis, it becomes the common femoral vein as it crosses the inguinal ligament.

The common femoral vein then bifurcates into the profunda femoris (deep femoral) vein and the superficial femoral vein. The profunda femoris vein is responsible for venous drainage of the proximal two thirds of the thigh. The "superficial femoral vein" is actually a deep vein. The superficial femoral vein is responsible for the venous drainage of the distal third of the thigh.

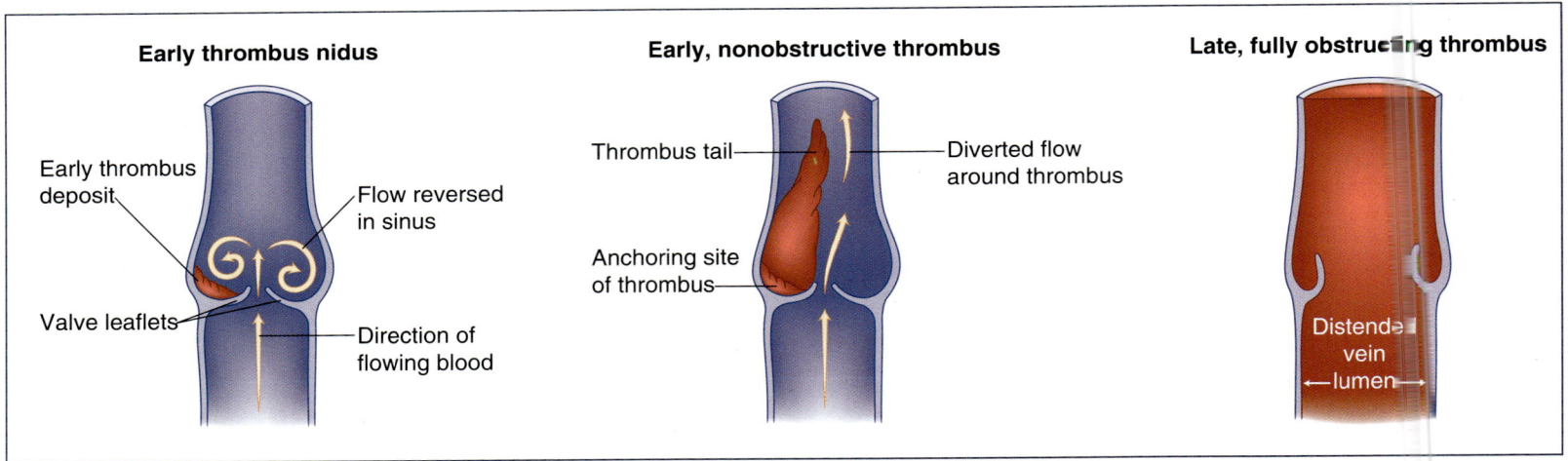

Figure 11-5. Pathophysiology of deep vein thrombosis. Early thrombi form in areas of stagnant blood flow (*left*), typically at the venous valve sinus where there is relative stasis of blood and reversal of blood flow. The inciting events for this early thrombus formation include traumatic injury to the endothelial lining of the vein, systemic or local alterations in coagulation, and stasis.

Aggregation of red blood cells and platelets within a fibrin mesh results in elongation of the thrombus from its anchoring point within the sinus of the vein valve (*middle*). The majority of thrombi never progress beyond this stage.

Under certain conditions, the thrombus can expand to fully occlude the lumen of the vein (*right*). Symptoms result from local distension and activation of pain receptors in the wall of the vein and surrounding tissues. Localized edema or inflammatory changes can further activate pain and stretch receptors in the contiguous tissues. Distal to the obstructing thrombus, impairment of venous return causes an increase in hydrostatic pressure, resulting in the extravasation of fluid into the extracellular space, which is manifested by edema on physical examination.

Figure 11-6. Pathophysiology of pulmonary embolism (PE). The hemodynamic impact of PE depends on the size of the embolus, the patient's underlying cardiopulmonary reserve, and the extent of compensatory neurohumoral adaptations [18]. Acute PE results in an increase in pulmonary vascular resistance (PVR) and right ventricular (RV) afterload through direct physical obstruction, hypoxemic vasoconstriction, and release of pulmonary artery vasoconstrictors [18]. The sudden increase in RV afterload can lead to RV dilatation and diminished systolic function, tricuspid regurgitation, and ultimately acute RV failure [18]. RV pressure overload can also result in flattening of the interventricular septum with deviation toward the left ventricle (LV) in diastole, thereby limiting LV filling [18]. This phenomenon of interventricular dependence can be observed as abnormal transmitral flow on Doppler echocardiography with left atrial contraction, represented by the A wave, making a greater contribution to LV diastole than passive filling, represented by the E wave [18]. RV pressure overload also increases wall stress and may induce ischemia by increasing myocardial oxygen demand while simultaneously limiting supply [1,18]. Evidence of RV injury secondary to acute RV pressure overload from PE may be observed in the form of elevated brain-type natriuretic peptide that results from RV shear stress and increases in cardiac troponins secondary to RV microinfarction [19].

Pulmonary embolism may also result in impaired gas exchange secondary to ventilation to perfusion mismatch, increases in total dead space, and right-to-left shunting [18]. While arterial hypoxemia and an increased

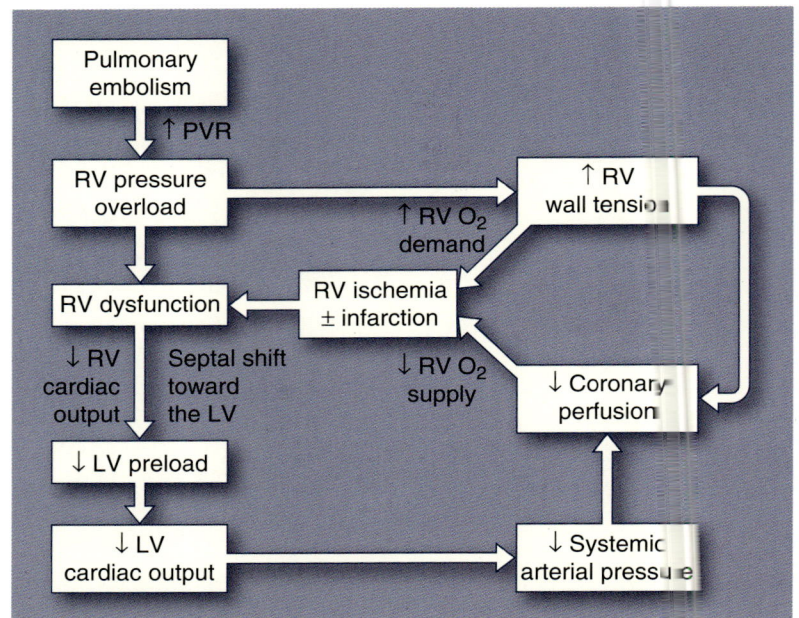

alveolar-arterial oxygen (O_2) gradient are the two most common abnormalities of gas exchange, patients may also present with hypocapnia and respiratory alkalosis due to hyperventilation [18]. Hypercapnia suggests massive PE with increased anatomic and physiologic dead space leading to impaired minute ventilation [18].

Diagnosis of Lower Extremity Deep Vein Thrombosis

Figure 11-7. Principal diagnostic studies for deep vein thrombosis (DVT). A nonspecific marker of ineffective endogenous fibrinolysis, D-dimer is elevated in venous thromboembolism (VTE), including DVT, as well as many other systemic conditions, such as pregnancy, surgery, and infection. Because many inpatients will have elevated levels secondary to other conditions, D-dimer is most useful in the evaluation of outpatients or emergency department patients with suspected VTE. D-dimer appears to offer the greatest accuracy in the evaluation of suspected DVT when coupled with a clinical assessment of probability [20]. While a negative D-dimer can exclude the diagnosis of proximal DVT without the need for further testing, such as ultrasonography in patients with low clinical probability, diagnostic imaging is warranted in patients with a higher clinical suspicion despite negative D-dimer results [20].

Venous ultrasonography remains the initial imaging test of choice in the evaluation of suspected lower and upper extremity DVT. Venous ultrasonography is superb for the diagnosis and exclusion of an initial episode of lower extremity DVT in both symptomatic and asymptomatic patients [21,22]. Duplex ultrasonography combines vein compression during B-mode imaging, and pulsed Doppler analysis with and without color. Failure to compress a vein is diagnostic of DVT.

Principal Diagnostic Studies for Deep Vein Thrombosis
D-dimer enzyme-linked immunosorbent assay
Duplex venous ultrasonography
CT venography
MR venography
Invasive contrast venography

Alternative imaging modalities, such as computed tomography (CT) venography, magnetic resonance (MR) venography, and invasive contrast venography, are used when the evaluation by duplex venous ultrasonography is inconclusive or inadequate. Anatomic constraints limit the ultrasonographic evaluation of the pelvic veins as well as the upper extremity veins proximal to the clavicle. CT and MR venography are preferred imaging modalities under these circumstances. CT, MR, or invasive contrast venography may also be useful if there is a high clinical suspicion of acute-on-chronic DVT.

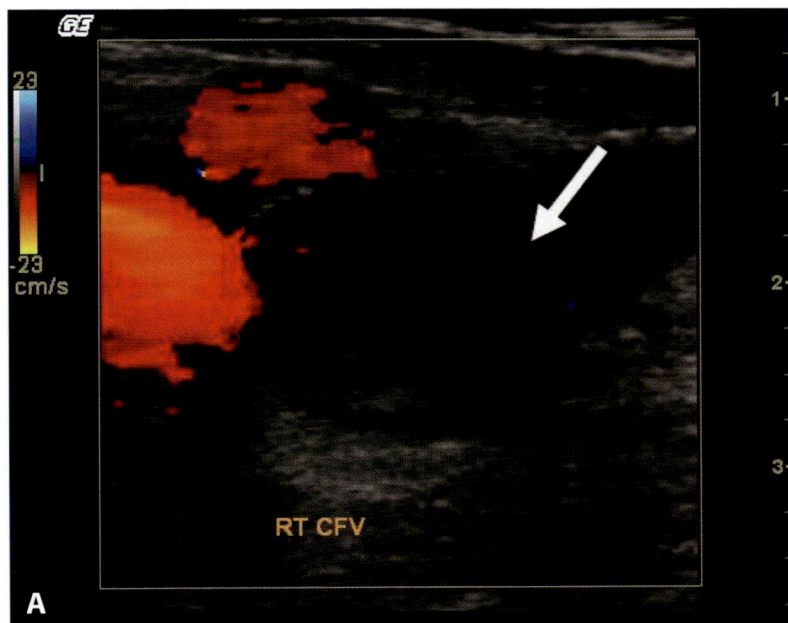

Figure 11-8. Duplex venous ultrasound of a patient with acute proximal deep vein thrombosis of the right leg. **A,** Color-assisted image of a thrombosed right common femoral vein (RT CFV) (*arrow*): the two larger, *red-filled areas* are the superficial and deep femoral arteries. **B,** Grayscale image of the femoral vein (FV) before and during compression. There is little change in lumen size of the FV (*arrows*) during compression because of the thrombus filling the vein. The other vessels labeled *A* are the superficial femoral artery and deep femoral artery. (*Courtesy of* Mark A. Creager, MD.)

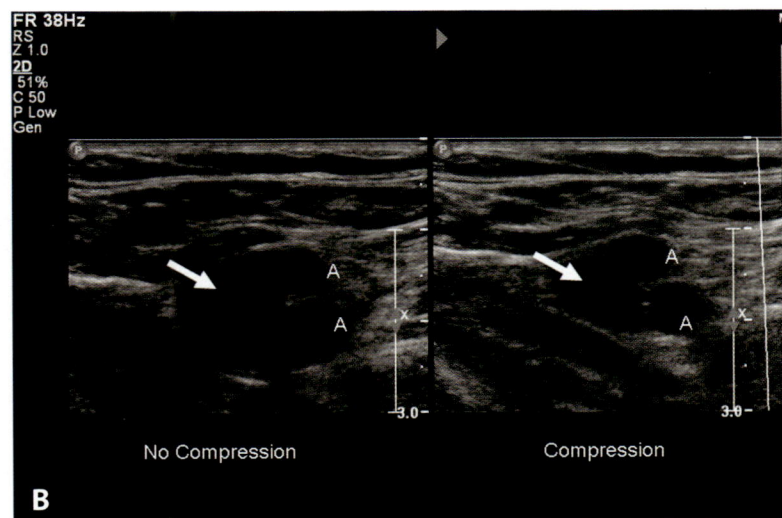

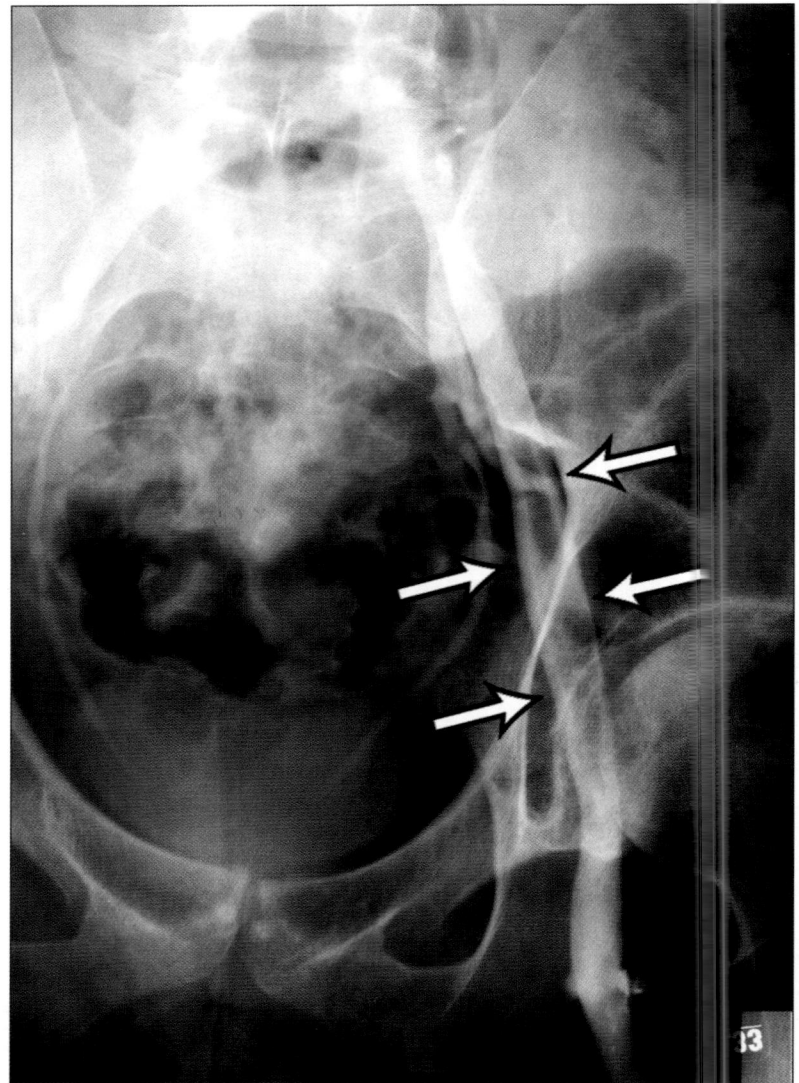

Figure 11-9. Contrast venography showing proximal and pelvic deep vein thrombosis. In this left lower extremity contrast venogram, a filling defect (*arrows*) present in the external iliac and common femoral veins is diagnostic for proximal lower extremity deep vein thrombosis extending into the pelvis. (*Courtesy of* Richard Baum, MD.)

Diagnosis of Pulmonary Embolism

Figure 11-10. A generally accepted clinical decision rule for the evaluation of patients with suspected pulmonary embolism (PE). The combination of a simplified clinical decision rule with further imaging when indicated by clinical suspicion and laboratory testing has been validated in major studies including the Christopher Study [23].

In the Christopher Study, the diagnosis of PE was established or excluded in no more than three steps: 1) a dichotomized clinical decision rule (ie, high clinical probability for PE versus non–high clinical probability for PE), 2) D-dimer testing, and 3) chest computed tomography (CT) [23]. These diagnostic tools were used to prospectively evaluate a cohort of patients with suspected acute PE. A modified version of the Wells clinical decision rule assigned 3 points for symptoms and signs of deep vein thrombosis (DVT), 3 points for an alternative diagnosis less likely than PE, 1.5 points for heart rate greater than 100 beats per minute, 1.5 points for recent immobilization or surgery, 1.5 points for previous venous thromboembolism (VTE), 1 point for hemoptysis, and 1 point for malignancy receiving therapy or palliative measures within the 6 months before presentation [23]. Patients were categorized as "PE unlikely" for scores of 4 or less and "PE likely" for scores greater than 4. Whereas patients in the "PE likely" category proceeded directly to chest CT, patients who were classified as "PE unlikely" underwent D-dimer testing and were referred to chest CT only if the result was positive. PE

Clinical Decisions for the Evaluation of Patients With Suspected Pulmonary Embolism	
Variable	**Points**
Clinical symptoms and signs of DVT	3
Alternative diagnosis less likely than PE	3
Heart rate > 100 beats per minute	1.5
Recent immobilization or surgery	1.5
Previous VTE	1.5
Hemoptysis	1
Malignancy receiving treatment or palliative care within the last 6 months	1
PE unlikely	≤ 4
PE likely	> 4

was considered to be excluded in patients classified as "PE unlikely" with negative D-dimer results and in patients with negative chest CT scans. The use of this simplified clinical algorithm permitted a management decision in 98% of patients with a low risk of VTE [23].

Figure 11-11. An integrated approach to diagnosis of pulmonary embolism (PE). A study of patients with suspected acute PE passing through a high-volume emergency department demonstrated that the D-dimer enzyme-linked immunosorbent assay (ELISA) had a sensitivity of 96.4% and a negative predictive value of 99.6% [24]. The high negative predictive value of the D-dimer ELISA allows clinicians to exclude the diagnosis of PE in outpatients with low to moderate clinical suspicion without the need for further costly imaging tests. Patients with a high pretest probability should proceed directly to an imaging study as the initial test for PE.

Multidetector CT scanners, with improved resolution, have markedly reduced the frequency of nondiagnostic studies. Chest CT has demonstrated negative predictive values of 99% for PE [25]. Chest CT for the diagnosis of acute PE is best utilized in combination with a clinical decision rule because its accuracy varies according to the pretest probability. In the Prospective Investigation of Pulmonary Embolism Diagnosis II (PIOPED II) trial, chest CT was shown to be accurate for the exclusion of PE in patients with low and intermediate clinical probability [26]. However, the results of PIOPED II suggest that further testing to confirm or exclude the diagnosis of PE is indicated when clinical suspicion and chest CT results are markedly discordant [26,27]. PIOPED II also demonstrated that the addition of venous phase imaging of the proximal lower extremity veins to chest CT only modestly increased the negative predictive value when compared with chest CT alone [26,27].

Other imaging modalities used to evaluate patients with suspected acute PE include ventilation-perfusion lung scanning, magnetic resonance angiography, and invasive contrast pulmonary angiography. Ventilation-perfusion lung scanning is currently reserved for patients with severe renal impairment, anaphylaxis to intravenous iodinated contrast, or pregnancy. Invasive contrast pulmonary angiography is reserved for the rare circumstance when other noninvasive imaging studies are nondiagnostic and a high clinical suspicion for PE remains.

Although insensitive for diagnosis, echocardiography may suggest the presence of PE by demonstrating evidence of right ventricular (RV) dysfunction. Transthoracic echocardiography is an excellent modality for the detection of RV dysfunction in the setting of RV pressure overload from PE.

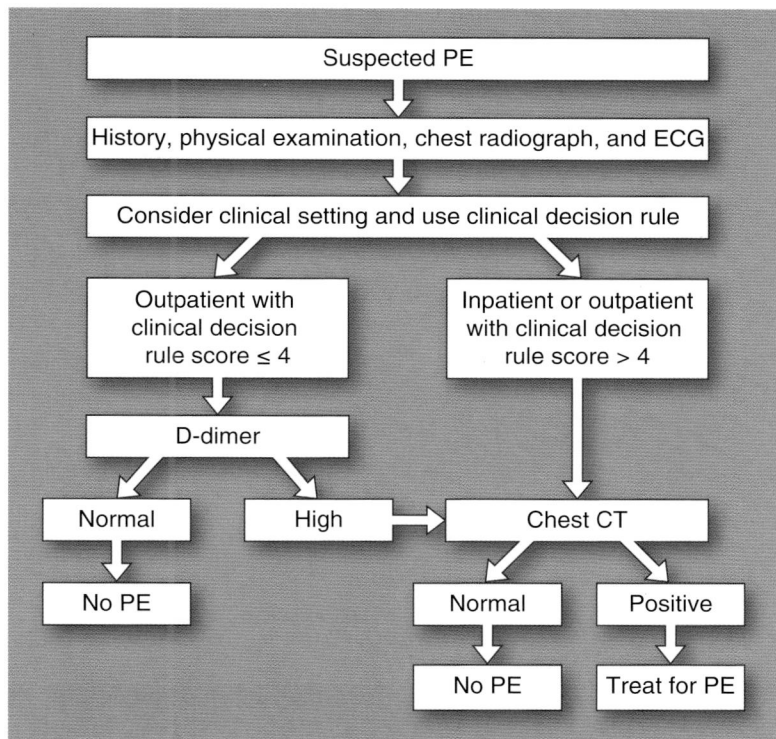

RV dilatation and hypokinesis, paradoxical interventricular septal motion toward the left ventricle, tricuspid regurgitation, and pulmonary hypertension as identified by a tricuspid regurgitant jet velocity greater than 2.6 m/sec are characteristic echocardiographic findings in patients with acute PE [28]. RV dysfunction in normotensive patients with acute PE is a clinically important finding because it is an independent risk predictor for early death [29]. In patients who have suffered cardiac arrest with a high suspicion of PE, who are not stable for travel to the CT scanner, or who may be referred to surgical embolectomy, transesophageal echocardiography may be used to establish the diagnosis of PE by direct visualization of the proximal pulmonary arteries [28]. ECG—electrocardiogram

Figure 11-12. Electrocardiogram of a 64-year-old woman who was hospitalized with "atypical chest pain" and subsequently diagnosed with pulmonary embolism (PE). This patient's electrocardiogram shows sinus tachycardia, incomplete right bundle branch block, an S wave in lead I, Q wave in lead III, and T-wave inversion in lead III. This so-called S1Q3T3 pattern along with the new incomplete right bundle branch block is indicative of right ventricular strain in the setting of pressure overload from PE. Other major findings in acute PE include right-axis deviation, complete right bundle branch block, T-wave inversions in V_1 through V_4, low voltage in the limb leads, and atrial fibrillation [1]. Of note, the electrocardiogram may be normal in young previously healthy patients.

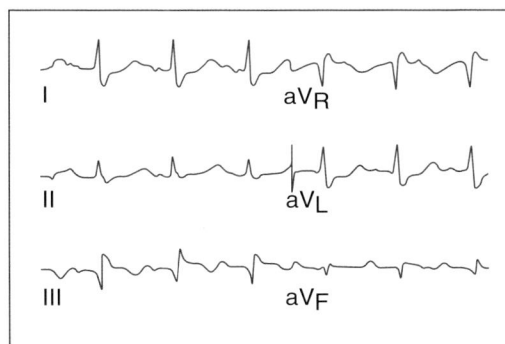

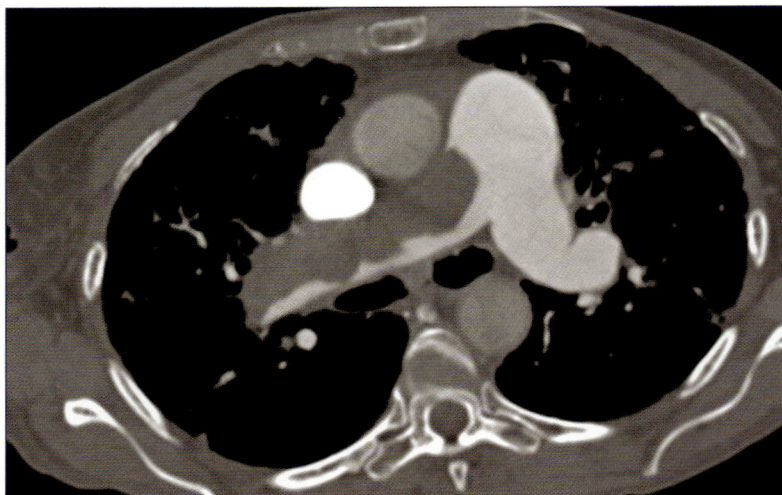

Figure 11-13. Diagnosis of acute pulmonary embolism (PE) by CT of the chest. This image is from a 59-year-old woman with advanced sarcoidosis who underwent chest CT as part of an evaluation before lung transplantation. The CT demonstrated a previously unsuspected PE indicated by the large filling defect in the right main pulmonary artery.

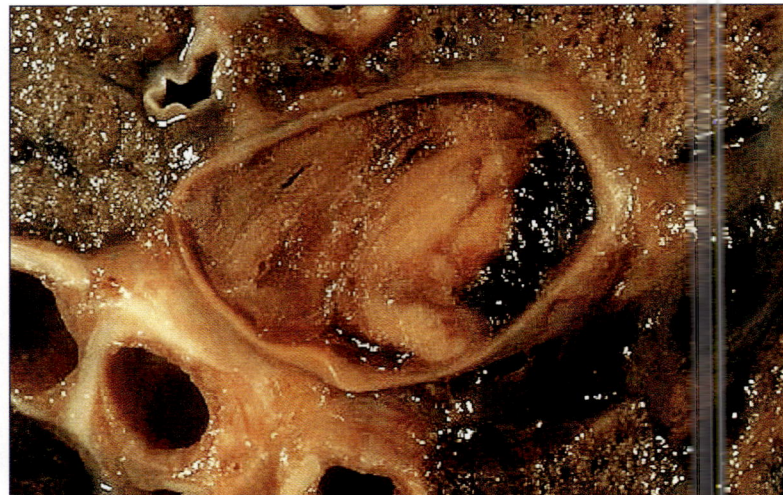

Figure 11-14. Autopsy specimen demonstrating pulmonary embolism. The patient in Figure 11-13 subsequently suffered a cardiac arrest and died 3 days later despite maximal resuscitative efforts. At autopsy, the right main pulmonary artery, seen in cross-section, was filled with thrombus of varying age.

Risk Stratification of Pulmonary Embolism

Figure 11-15. The spectrum of disease in acute pulmonary embolism (PE). Acute PE describes a spectrum of clinical syndromes. Patients with acute PE presenting with normal systemic arterial pressures and no evidence of right ventricular (RV) dysfunction have an excellent prognosis when treated with standard anticoagulation alone. Normotensive patients with PE and evidence of RV dysfunction are classified as having submassive PE and represent a population at increased risk for adverse events and early mortality [29]. Massive PE describes a subpopulation of patients presenting with syncope, systemic arterial hypotension, cardiogenic shock, or cardiac arrest. Patients with submassive and massive PE are candidates for primary therapy with fibrinolysis, embolectomy, or insertion of an inferior vena caval filter in addition to anticoagulation given their increased risk for adverse outcomes. Optimal management of submassive PE remains controversial.

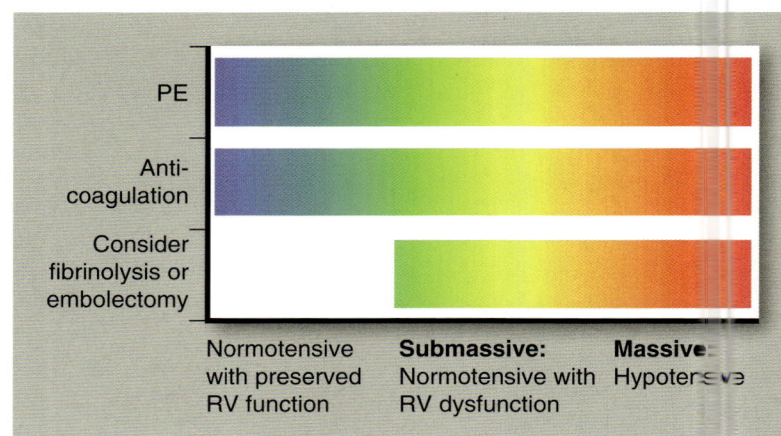

Figure 11-16. Tools for risk stratification of pulmonary embolism (PE). A subset of normotensive patients with PE will abruptly decompensate and experience systemic arterial hypotension, cardiogenic shock, and cardiac arrest despite standard anticoagulation. Risk stratification to identify such patients has become a critical step in the management of acute PE.

The history and physical examination can provide important clues for risk stratification of patients with PE. Congestive heart failure, chronic lung disease, cancer, systolic blood pressure 100 mm Hg or less, age greater than 70 years, and heart rate greater than 100 beats per minute have been shown to be significant predictors of increased mortality [29].

Cardiac biomarkers, such as troponin and brain-type natriuretic peptide (BNP) correlate with the presence of right ventricular (RV) dysfunction, which is a powerful independent predictor of early mortality in patients with acute PE [29]. Normal levels of cardiac troponin and BNP identify a low-risk subset of PE patients with negative predictive values for in-hospital death ranging from 97% to 100% [30].

In addition to its use for diagnosis of PE, chest CT can simultaneously assess for the presence of RV enlargement. RV enlargement, defined as a ratio of RV to left ventricular dimension of greater than 0.9, was found to be a significant independent predictor of 30-day mortality [31].

Echocardiography continues to be the imaging study of choice for risk stratification of patients with acute PE. The presence of RV hypokine-

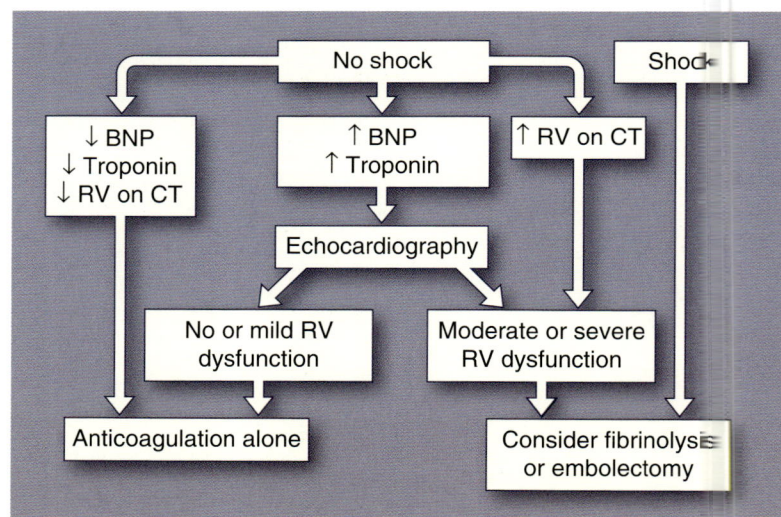

sis detects a subset of patients with acute PE and an increased risk of systemic arterial hypotension, cardiogenic shock, and death [28,29].

A risk stratification algorithm that incorporates clinical prognostic indicators, cardiac biomarkers such as troponin and BNP, and direct evidence of RV dysfunction on echocardiography or RV enlargement on chest CT is critical for detecting newly diagnosed acute PE patients with an increased likelihood of death or major nonfatal complications [2].

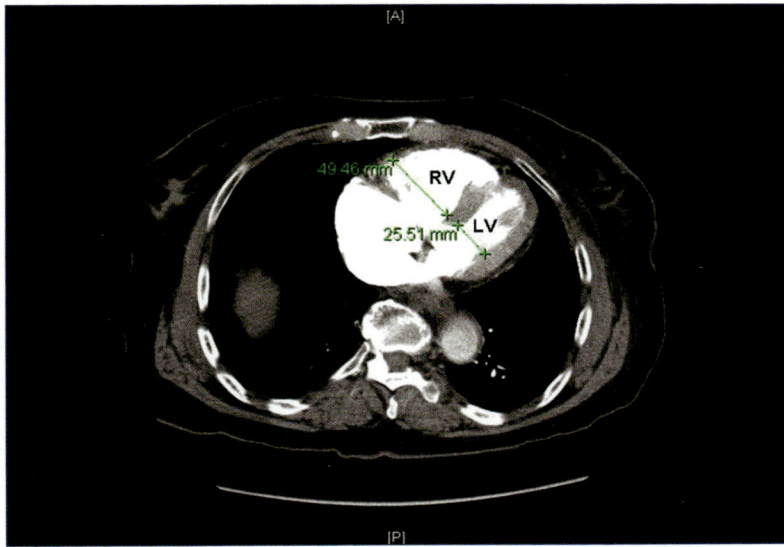

Figure 11-17. Chest computed tomography (CT) demonstrating right ventricular (RV) enlargement. This chest CT image demonstrates RV enlargement with a ratio of RV dimension to left ventricular (LV) dimension of 1.9. RV enlargement as defined by a ratio of RV dimension to LV dimension of greater than 0.9 has been shown to be a significant independent predictor of mortality at 30 days [31]. This patient was undergoing therapy for breast cancer and presented with acute onset dyspnea on exertion and hypotension. Chest CT demonstrated large bilateral pulmonary emboli (not shown) in addition to RV enlargement.

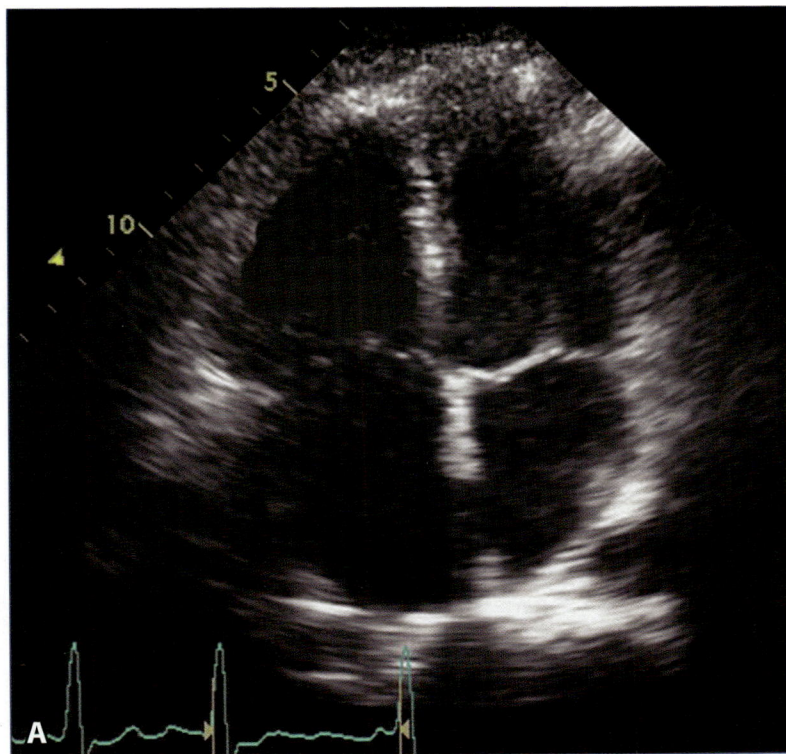

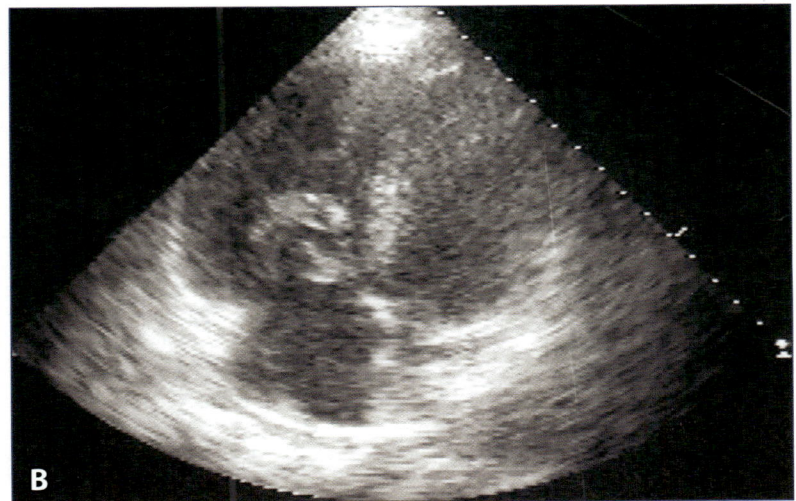

Figure 11-18. A, Transthoracic echocardiography demonstrating right ventricular (RV) dysfunction. In this transthoracic echocardiogram, the apical four-chamber view demonstrates an abnormally dilated RV. The RV appears larger than the left ventricle (LV), whereas it is normally no larger than 0.7 the size of the LV. (Courtesy of Mark A. Creager, MD.)

B, Transthoracic echocardiography demonstrating RV dysfunction. In this transthoracic echocardiogram of the patient in Figure 11-12, the api-

cal four-chamber view demonstrates an abnormally dilated RV. The RV appears larger than the LV, whereas it is normally no larger than 0.7 the size of the LV. In addition, a 3 × 4 cm globular mass is observed in the RV just underneath the tricuspid valve. This patient underwent emergency surgical embolectomy that revealed the mass to be a large curled-up thrombus, or "clot-in-transit." Additional thrombus was found in the pulmonary arteries.

Primary Therapy for Venous Thromboembolism

Figure 11-19. Options for primary therapy in deep vein thrombosis and pulmonary embolism (PE). Options for primary therapy in venous thromboembolism include fibrinolysis, embolectomy, and insertion of an inferior vena caval filter.

Fibrinolysis is generally accepted to be a life-saving intervention in patients presenting with massive PE [32]. The largest randomized trial of fibrinolysis in PE, the Management Strategies and Prognosis of Pulmonary Embolism-3 (MAPPET-3), evaluated the benefit of primary therapy with tissue plasminogen activator in patients with submassive PE [33]. Although a mortality benefit was not shown, the MAPPET-3 trial did demonstrate a reduction in the need for escalation of therapy among patients receiving tissue plasminogen activator [33]. All patients receiving fibrinolysis should be carefully screened for contraindications including risk factors for bleeding, especially intracranial hemorrhage.

Surgical thrombectomy is reserved for patients with massive or severely symptomatic deep vein thrombosis in whom fibrinolysis is contraindicated or has failed. Similarly, surgical embolectomy for PE may be considered in patients with massive or submassive PE in whom fibrinolysis is contraindicated or has been unsuccessful. At medical centers with experience in the management of such patients, surgical embolectomy is a safe and effective option for the treatment of massive and submassive PE [34].

Options for Primary Therapy in Deep Vein Thrombosis and Pulmonary Embolism

Deep vein thrombosis

Catheter-directed fibrinolysis

Surgical thrombectomy

Inferior vena cava filter

Pulmonary embolism

Fibrinolysis

Surgical embolectomy

Catheter-assisted embolectomy

Inferior vena cava filter

Catheter-assisted thrombectomy and embolectomy have been used in the primary therapy of deep vein thrombosis and PE, respectively. Catheter-assisted pulmonary embolectomy is an emerging technique for the primary therapy of massive and submassive PE.

Figure 11-20. Pulmonary angiography demonstrating successful fibrinolysis. This pulmonary angiogram (*left panel*) demonstrates a large thrombus (*arrow*) in the right main pulmonary artery. The patient was administered fibrinolytic therapy in the hope of achieving rapid and marked clot lysis, reversing right ventricular failure, and restoring systemic arterial perfusion. The US Food and Drug Administration approved 100 mg of tissue plasminogen activator as a continuous intravenous infusion over 2 hours for the fibrinolysis of acute pulmonary embolism. In contrast to fibrinolysis in acute ST-elevation myocardial infarction during which unfractionated heparin infusion is continued, anticoagulation is withheld during the administration of tissue plasminogen activator for venous thromboembolism and is not reinitiated until the activated partial thromboplastin time has fallen to less than twice the upper limit of normal. Pulmonary angiography immediately after fibrinolysis (*right panel*) demonstrates marked resolution of the thrombus.

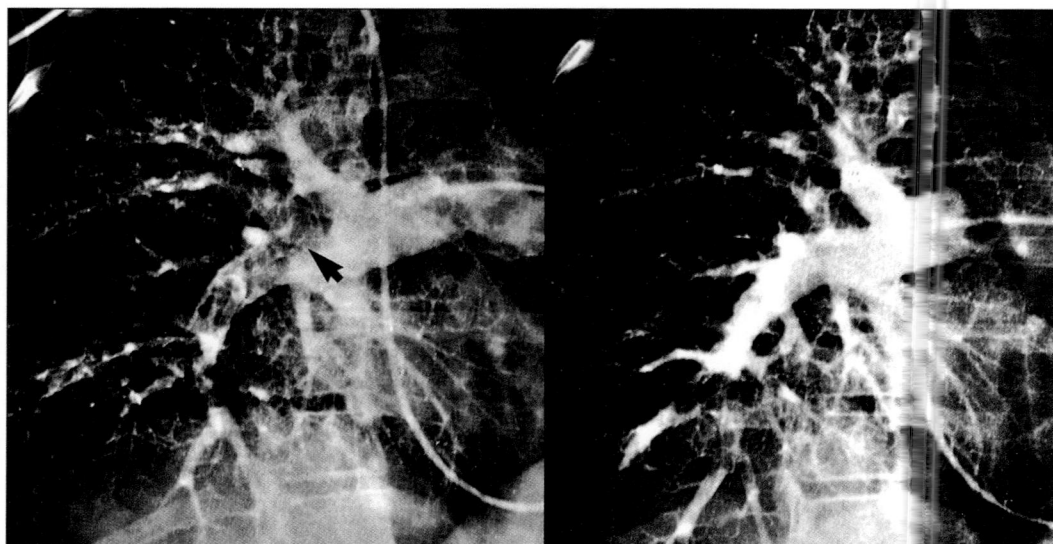

Figure 11-21. Successful fibrinolysis resulting in restoration of right ventricular function. Transthoracic echocardiography was performed in a patient who had presented with symptoms and signs of congestive heart failure. In the subcostal view (*left panel*), the right ventricle (RV) is markedly dilated, whereas the left ventricular (LV) diameter is markedly reduced. Because these findings were more suggestive of RV failure secondary to acute pulmonary embolism rather than LV failure, the patient underwent further evaluation including a contrast pulmonary angiogram, which ultimately revealed a large pulmonary embolism. After administration of fibrinolytic therapy, repeat echocardiography (*right panel*) revealed a marked decrease in RV diameter with a corresponding increase in LV size. PW—posterior wall; RA—right atrium; SEP—interventricular septum.

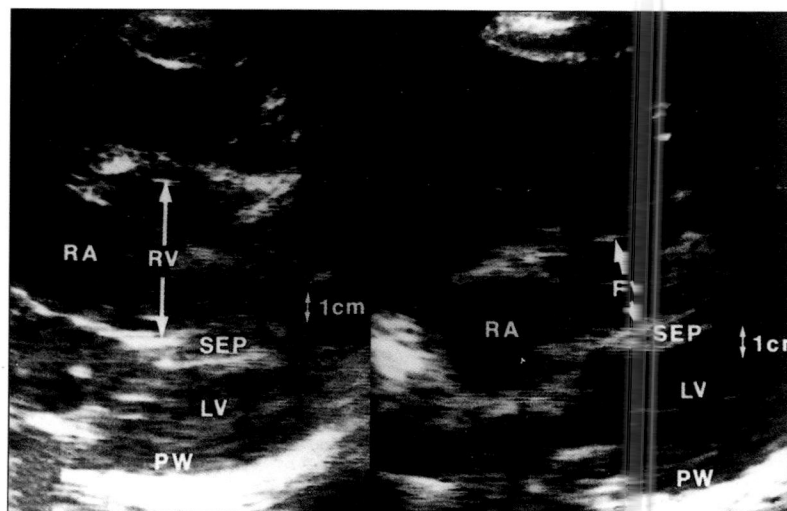

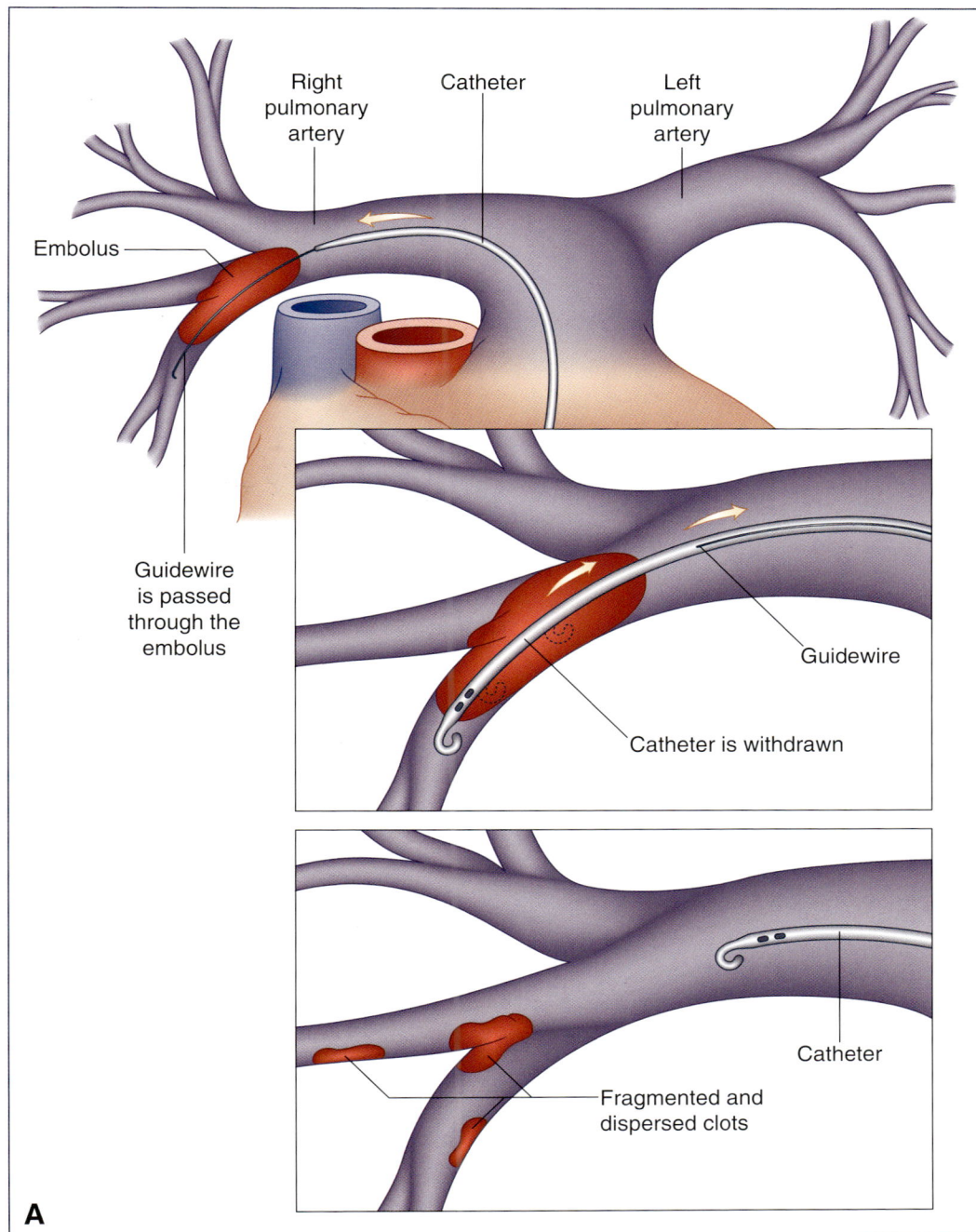

Figure 11-22. A, A technique for catheter-assisted embolectomy. In this schematic, a standard angiographic catheter is advanced over a J-tipped guidewire to the pulmonary artery trunk. The thrombus is first pushed forward by advancing the catheter and guidewire together. The guidewire is then passed through the thrombus, and, subsequently, the catheter is advanced over the guidewire. The guidewire is withdrawn, allowing the catheter tip to return to its normal curled conformation (*inset, upper panel*). The catheter is then withdrawn, resulting in fragmentation of the large thrombus into smaller ones that disperse into the distal branches of the pulmonary arterial tree (*inset, lower panel*).

B, Surgical embolectomy specimen from the patient in Figures 11-12 and 11-18B. The patient was referred for emergency surgical embolectomy and was subsequently found to have massive thrombus burden in the pulmonary arterial tree. As had been demonstrated on transthoracic echocardiography before embolectomy, a large thrombus was found in the right side of the heart. The patient responded well to surgical embolectomy and had an uncomplicated postoperative course.

Figure 11-23. **A**, Angiography of the right pulmonary arterial vasculature demonstrating evidence of chronic pulmonary thromboembolic disease. Single and recurrent episodes of pulmonary embolism may result in pulmonary hypertension. Pulmonary hypertension secondary to chronic thromboembolic disease is more common than previously thought. This pulmonary angiogram image demonstrates abrupt narrowing of the right descending pulmonary artery and absence of middle and lower lobe vascularity typical of pulmonary hypertension secondary to chronic pulmonary thromboembolic disease.

B, Angiography of the left pulmonary arterial vasculature demonstrating evidence of chronic pulmonary thromboembolic disease. This pulmonary angiogram image from the patient in **A** demonstrates diminished flow to the left lower lobe pulmonary artery and lingula.

C, Pulmonary thromboendarterectomy specimens. Pulmonary hypertension secondary to chronic pulmonary thromboembolic disease is an often debilitating condition that may be amenable to surgical intervention. Depending on the extent and location of the thromboembolic obstruction, surgical thromboendarterectomy may reduce and even cure pulmonary hypertension [35]. Chronic thromboemboli obtained from the patient in **A** and **B** at the time of pulmonary thromboendarterectomy are shown here. When pulmonary thromboendarterectomy is not possible, balloon pulmonary angioplasty may be an alternative strategy.

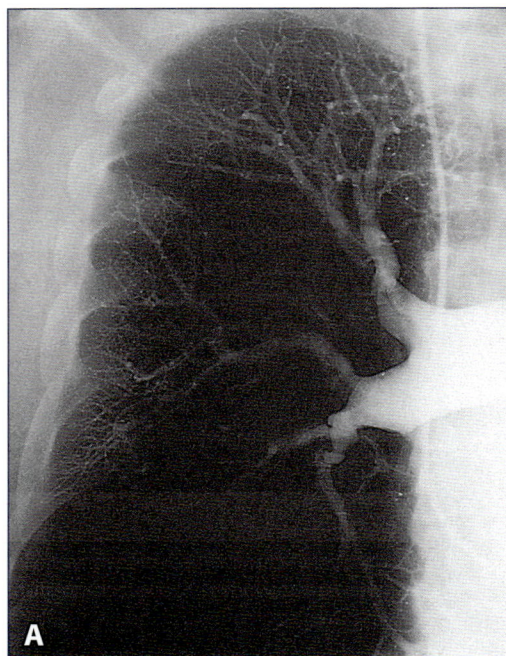

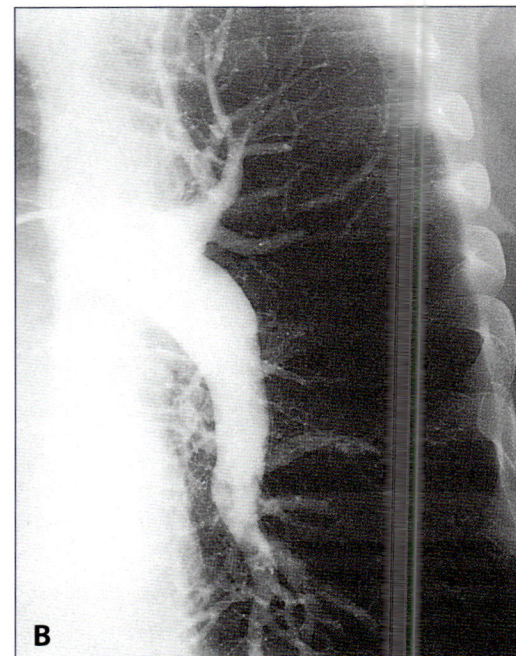

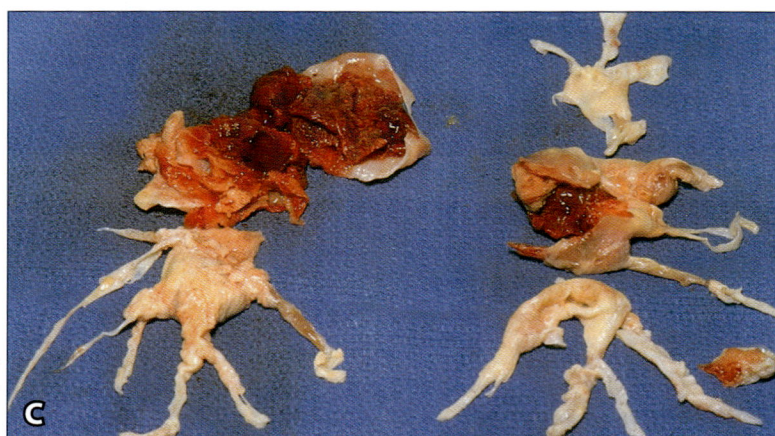

Tips for the Supportive Care of Massive Pulmonary Embolism

High-dose intravenous unfractionated heparin should be administered as soon as massive PE is suspected and should be continued while primary therapy is being considered

Higher doses of unfractionated heparin are often needed because standard weight-based dosing protocols often fail to achieve adequate therapeutic anticoagulation in patients with massive PE

Avoid excessive volume resuscitation in patients with massive PE, as the increased preload may worsen right ventricular failure

While an initial trial of volume may be successful in patients without signs of increased right-sided preload, administration of vasopressors and inotropes should be the first step in the hemodynamic support of patients with an estimated or measured central venous pressure of > 12 to 15 mm Hg

Norepinephrine, epinephrine, and dopamine are reasonable agents for the initial vasopressor support of patients with massive PE

If an inotrope with vasodilator properties, such as dobutamine, is required, the addition of a vasopressor may be necessary

In patients with massive PE and sinus tachycardia or atrial fibrillation with rapid ventricular rates, a strict vasopressor such as phenylephrine may be most appropriate to avoid accelerating the heart rate further and thereby impairing diastolic function

Figure 11-24. Tips for the supportive care of massive pulmonary embolism (PE). High-dose intravenous unfractionated heparin should be administered as soon as massive PE is suspected [32]. The initial reaction to hemodynamic instability is often to administer boluses of crystalloid to augment right ventricular (RV) preload. However, many patients with massive PE have markedly elevated right-sided filling pressures that may predispose to sudden RV failure in the setting of excessive volume resuscitation [32]. In patients without signs of increased right-sided preload such as those with an estimated or measured central venous pressure of less than 12 to 15 mm Hg, an initial trial of 500 mL of volume is reasonable [19,32]. However, in patients with signs of increased right-sided preload such as those with a central venous pressure of greater than 12 to 15 mm Hg, volume loading should be avoided and administration of a vasopressor or inotrope should be the initial step to improve hemodynamic support [19].

Ideal drugs for the support of massive PE should aim to improve RV contractility through positive inotropic effects while maintaining systemic arterial perfusion [19]. This usually requires empiric trial and error. Norepinephrine, epinephrine, and dopamine act both as inotropes and vasopressors and therefore may be favorable initial choices for the hemodynamic support of patients with massive PE [19]. Dobutamine may be necessary to improve RV contractility and cardiac output but carries the risk of systemic arterial hypotension because of its vasodilator properties [19].

Anticoagulation

Figure 11-25. Options for immediate anticoagulation in venous thromboembolism. Agents for immediate anticoagulation as a bridge to therapeutic oral anticoagulation with warfarin include unfractionated heparin, low molecular weight heparin (LMWH), and fondaparinux.

Intravenous unfractionated heparin is preferred in patients undergoing fibrinolysis, surgery, or catheter-assisted intervention for venous thromboembolism because it can be easily discontinued and rapidly reversed.

LMWHs have several advantages over unfractionated heparin, including a longer half-life, more consistent bioavailability, and a more predictable dose response. Among patients with deep vein thrombosis, a large meta-analysis documented a 30% reduction in mortality and a 40% lower risk of major bleeding associated with LWMH use [36]. Clinical trials have also demonstrated that LMWHs are as safe and effective as unfractionated heparin in the prevention of recurrent venous thromboembolism among patients with acute pulmonary embolism (PE).

Options for Immediate Anticoagulation in Venous Thromboembolism	
Agent	**Advantages**
Intravenous unfractionated heparin	Can be easily discontinued and rapidly reversed
	Preferred in patients undergoing fibrinolysis, surgery, or catheter-assisted intervention
	Can be used in severe renal insufficiency
Low molecular weight heparin	Longer half-life
	Consistent bioavailability
	More predictable dose response
	Does not require dose adjustment or laboratory monitoring under usual circumstances
	Lower risk of heparin-induced thrombocytopenia
	May be preferred in patients with active cancer
Fondaparinux	Longer half-life
	Consistent bioavailability
	More predictable dose response
	Does not require dose adjustment or laboratory monitoring under usual circumstances
	Does not cause heparin-induced thrombocytopenia

LMWH as monotherapy without transition to oral anticoagulation is a promising alternative that may be preferred for patients with active malignancy [37,38]. Although unfractionated heparin is largely eliminated by the liver, LMWHs are cleared renally.

Approved by the US Food and Drug Administration for treatment of deep vein thrombosis and PE, the synthetic pentasaccharide fondaparinux has been shown to be at least as safe and effective as LMWH in treatment of deep vein thrombosis and intravenous unfractionated heparin in treatment of acute PE [39,40]. Fondaparinux is administered subcutaneously in fixed once-daily doses of 5 mg for body weight less than 50 kg, 7.5 mg for body weight between 50 and 100 kg, and 10 mg for body weight greater than 100 kg. Fondaparinux does not require monitoring or dose adjustment based on laboratory coagulation tests. Cleared by the kidneys, fondaparinux is contraindicated in patients with severe renal impairment. In contrast to unfractionated heparin and LMWH, fondaparinux is not associated with heparin-induced thrombocytopenia.

Figure 11-26. Pathogenesis of heparin-induced thrombocytopenia. Heparin-induced thrombocytopenia is caused by heparin-dependent IgG antibodies directed against the heparin-platelet factor 4 (PF4) complex [41]. Platelets release PF4 when activated by agonists such as thrombin, collagen, and heparin. Heparin, PF4, and antiheparin-PF4 antibodies form immune complexes that can interact with platelet Fc receptors and trigger platelet activation, aggregation, and thrombin generation. This cascade of events can result in devastating arterial and, more commonly, venous thromboembolic complications. Although the risk is lower with low molecular weight heparin (LMWH), unfractionated heparin and LMWH can result in heparin-induced thrombocytopenia. A decrease in platelet count of greater than 50% from baseline or a new thromboembolic event while administering any heparin product, including heparin flushes, should raise concern for heparin-induced thrombocytopenia and prompt the discontinuation of all heparin-containing products.

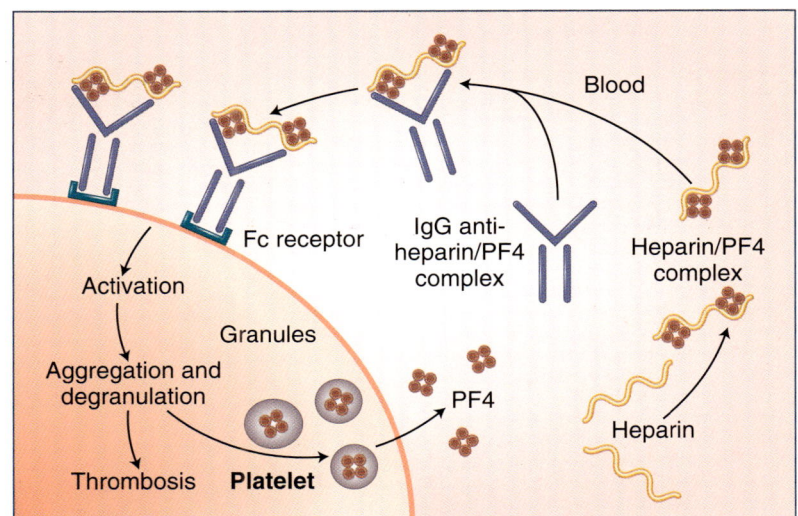

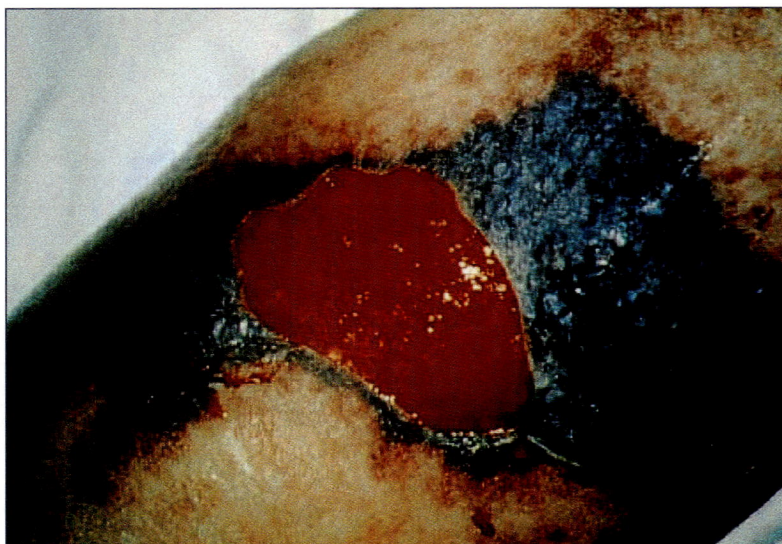

Figure 11-27. Gangrene caused by heparin-induced thrombocytopenia. Heparin-induced thrombocytopenia may result in severe and even limb-threatening gangrene.

Tips for Management of Heparin-Induced Thrombocytopenia

When heparin-induced thrombocytopenia is confirmed or even suspected, a direct thrombin inhibitor such as argatroban, bivalirudin, or lepirudin should be administered

Warfarin as monotherapy should not be used for anticoagulation because it may worsen the procoagulant state and result in gangrene or limb-threatening ischemia

Platelet transfusions "add more fuel to the fire" and may precipitate massive arterial or venous thromboembolism

Low molecular weight heparin may cross react with heparin-platelet factor 4 antibodies once heparin-induced thrombocytopenia has developed and may result in worsening thrombocytopenia and life-threatening thromboembolic events

Figure 11-28. Tips for management of heparin-induced thrombocytopenia (HIT). The management of HIT can present a challenge because of many potential pitfalls. When HIT is confirmed or even suspected, a direct thrombin inhibitor such as argatroban, bivalirudin, or lepirudin should be initiated to prevent arterial and venous thromboembolism. Of note, lepirudin and bivalirudin require dose adjustment for renal impairment. Argatroban is hepatically cleared and should be used with caution in patients with impaired liver function. Warfarin as monotherapy for anticoagulation should be avoided as it may worsen the procoagulant state and lead to possible limb-threatening gangrene. Similarly, platelet transfusions can perpetuate the tendency toward thromboembolism by "adding more fuel to the fire." Inferior vena cava filters should not be placed in lieu of anticoagulation because they may serve as a nidus for massive caval, pelvic, and lower extremity vein thrombosis. While less likely to initiate HIT, low molecular weight heparin may occasionally cross react with heparin-platelet factor 4 antibodies, resulting in worsening thrombocytopenia and thrombosis.

Tips for Management of Oral Anticoagulation

Clearly designate who will manage the patient's anticoagulation

Insist on detailed and explicit communication between all of the patient's health care providers

Clearly explain to the patient and family the rationale for anticoagulation and the major risks of supertherapeutic levels (hemorrhage) and subtherapeutic levels (thromboembolism)

Define the relationship between important terms such as prothrombin time, international normalized ratio (INR), and dose adjustment of the anticoagulant

Consider using a software-supported electronic surveillance and data management system that will keep track of prior anticoagulation levels, complications, and laboratory results that are expected but have not been reported

Consider the use of centralized anticoagulation clinics

Avoid warfarin dose adjustments of > 20% of the previous dose

Changes in the INR are most reflective of warfarin dose adjustments made 3 to 5 days previously

Figure 11-29. Tips for management of oral anticoagulation. Initial warfarin doses of 5 or 10 mg daily appear to be safe and effective for the majority of patients with venous thromboembolism [42]. Management of anticoagulation with warfarin can often be quite challenging because of many drug-food, drug-alcohol, and drug-drug interactions. Recently described mutations in cytochrome P450 2C9 and the gene encoding vitamin K epoxide reductase complex 1 (VKORC1) help to explain the wide variation in warfarin dosing requirements encountered from one patient to the next [43,44].

The optimal duration of warfarin therapy depends on the individual patient's risk of recurrent venous thromboembolism. The risk of recurrence persists after completion of standard anticoagulation in patients with idiopathic deep vein thrombosis or pulmonary embolism. Several studies have validated the safety and efficacy of indefinite duration anticoagulation for patients with idiopathic venous thromboembolism [45–47].

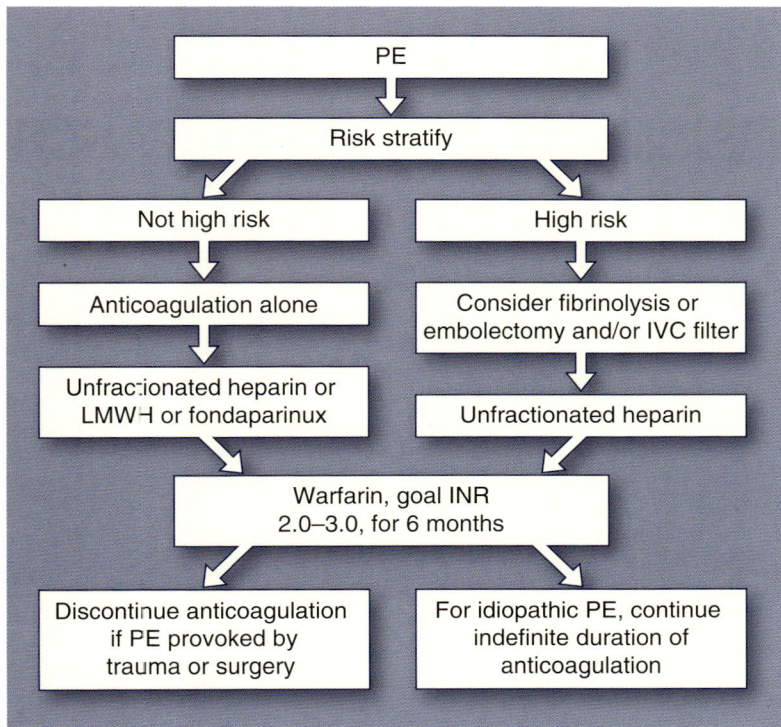

Figure 11-30. An integrated approach to pulmonary embolism (PE). Overall management of PE should consider primary therapy for high-risk patients and indefinite anticoagulation for patients with idiopathic venous thromboembolism [2]. INR—international normalized ratio; IVC—inferior vena cava; LMWH—low molecular weight heparin.

Inferior Vena Cava Filters

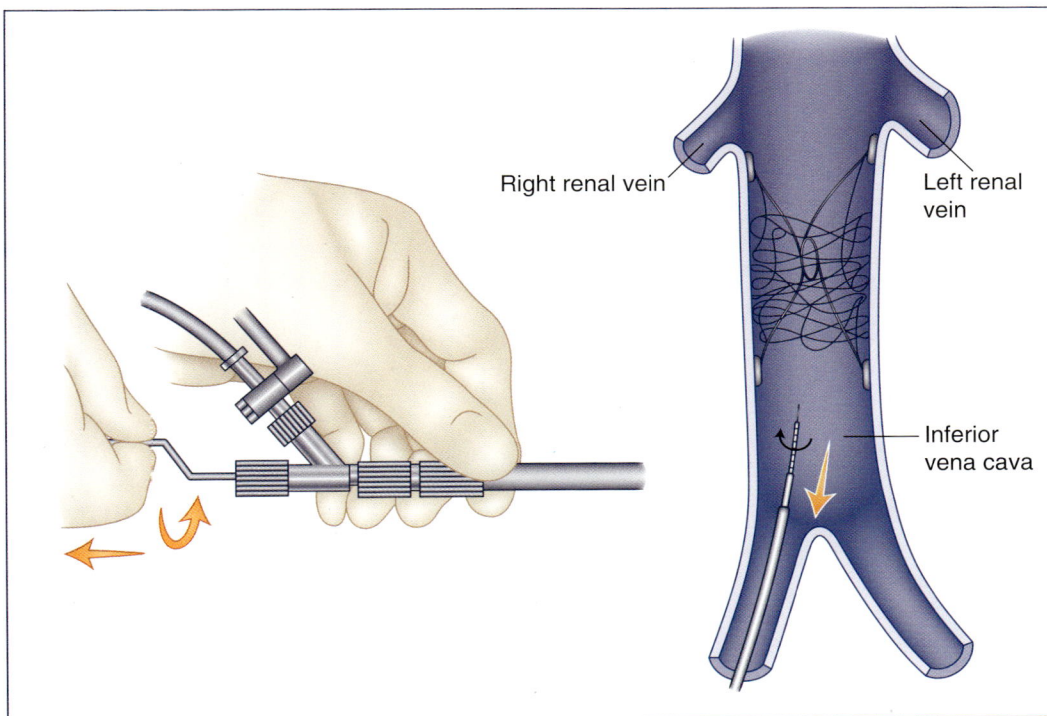

Figure 11-31. Insertion of an inferior vena cava (IVC) filter. The goal of IVC filter placement is to prevent potentially life-threatening pulmonary embolism (PE) in patients who have contraindications to anticoagulation, suffer recurrent PE despite adequate anticoagulation, or are undergoing surgical embolectomy. Although effective in the prevention of PE, IVC filters have been shown to increase the incidence of deep vein thrombosis [48]. A review of the International Cooperative Pulmonary Embolism Registry (ICOPER) data noted a significant reduction in 90-day mortality associated with the placement of IVC filters [49]. Further prospective stud-ies are warranted to corroborate this finding. Retrievable IVC filters are safe and effective alternatives for patients with transient contraindications to anticoagulation.

This image demonstrates deployment of the Bird's Nest filter (Cook Inc., Bloomington, IN). The right-angled handle of the wire guide pusher is rotated counterclockwise for 10 to 15 turns in order to disengage the filter. Then the wire guide pusher is removed, followed by the empty filter catheter. The introducing sheath is temporarily left in place to allow for a postprocedure cavogram to be performed.

Prevention

Figure 11-32. Options for venous thromboembolism (VTE) prophylaxis. VTE prophylaxis continues to be underutilized even in high-risk hospitalized patients. Mechanical prophylaxis devices, such as graduated compression stockings and intermittent pneumatic compression boots, reduce venous stasis and may enhance endogenous fibrinolysis-resulting in reductions in VTE [50]. Pharmacologic options for VTE prevention include subcutaneously administered unfractionated heparin, low molecular weight heparin, fondaparinux, and warfarin. Certain high-risk populations such as neurosurgical, thoracic surgery, and medical intensive care patients may benefit from combinations of mechanical and pharmacologic modalities.

Despite an improved understanding of the risk factors for venous thromboembolism, the utilization of VTE prophylaxis among inpatients continues to be low [6]. Computerized provider order entry programs offer a unique opportunity to improve implementation of VTE prevention by alerting health care providers to patients with an increased risk of VTE who are not receiving prophylaxis. A computer alert program at Brigham and Women's Hospital improved physician utilization of VTE prophylaxis and resulted in a 41% reduction in the incidence of symptomatic deep vein thrombosis and pulmonary embolism [51].

Options for Venous Thromboembolism Prophylaxis
Mechanical modalities
Graduated compression stockings
Intermittent pneumatic compression devices
Pharmacologic modalities
Subcutaneously administered unfractionated heparin
Low molecular weight heparin
Fondaparinux
Warfarin

In addition to consistent utilization, the proper duration of prophylaxis must be prescribed to protect patients from potentially life-threatening VTE. A significant number of patients, especially those who have had surgery, experience deep vein thrombosis or pulmonary embolism while at a rehabilitation center or even at home, demonstrating that the risk of VTE persists well after discharge from the acute care hospital. Multiple studies have validated the use of extended-duration prophylaxis for up to 4 to 6 weeks in high-risk patients, such as those who have undergone orthopedic or oncologic surgery [52–54].

Regimens for Venous Thromboembolism Prevention

Patient Population	Prophylaxis
General surgery	Unfractionated heparin, 5000 U SC TID or
	Enoxaparin 40 mg SC QD or
	Dalteparin 2500 or 5000 U SC QD
Orthopedic surgery	Warfarin (target INR 2.0–3.0) or
	Enoxaparin 30 mg SC BID or
	Enoxaparin 40 mg SC QD or
	Dalteparin 2500 or 5000 U SC QD or
	Fondaparinux 2.5 mg SC QD
Neurosurgery	Unfractionated heparin, 5000 U SC TID or
	Enoxaparin 40 mg SC QD and
	Graduated compression stockings/intermittent pneumatic compression
	Consider surveillance lower extremity ultrasonography
Oncologic surgery	Enoxaparin 40 mg SC QD
Thoracic surgery	Unfractionated heparin, 5000 U SC TID and
	Graduated compression stockings/intermittent pneumatic compression
Medical patients	Unfractionated heparin 5000 U SC TID or
	Enoxaparin 40 mg SC QD or
	Dalteparin 5000 U SC QD or
	Fondaparinux 2.5 mg SC QD (not FDA approved) or
	Graduated compression stockings/intermittent pneumatic compression for patients with contraindications to anticoagulation
	Consider combination pharmacologic and mechanical prophylaxis for very high-risk patients such as intensive care patients
	Consider surveillance lower extremity ultrasonography for intensive care patients

Figure 11-33. Regimens for venous thromboembolism (VTE) prevention. Prophylactic regimens must consider the patient population as well as the individual patient's risk factors for VTE. Certain high-risk populations may warrant a combination of mechanical and pharmacologic modalities as well as surveillance lower extremity ultrasonography.

Continue on the next page

Figure 11-33. *(Continued)* Hospitalized medical patients are a particularly vulnerable patient population with a high incidence of VTE risk factors and frequent under-utilization of VTE prophylaxis [6]. Various regimens have been validated for the prevention of VTE among hospitalized medical patients. The low molecular weight heparins (LMWHs) enoxaparin and dalteparin have been shown to safely and effectively reduce the risk of VTE in patients with acute medical illness [55,56]. Fondaparinux, 2.5 mg of administered subcutaneously once daily, nearly halved the incidence of VTE among medical patients [57].

Orthopedic patients represent another patient population at a particularly high risk for VTE after discharge from the hospital. Extended out-of-hospital prophylaxis with either warfarin or LMWH has been shown to be safe and effective in the prevention of VTE in orthopedic patients [53,54]. In addition, fondaparinux (2.5 mg subcutaneously once daily) has been shown to be a safe and effective alternative in patients undergoing major orthopedic surgery [58].

Patients undergoing abdominal or pelvic surgery for malignancy, such as ovarian cancer, have a significantly elevated risk for postoperative VTE. The Enoxaparin and Cancer (ENOXACAN) II study demonstrated that extended-duration enoxaparin significantly reduced the risk of VTE in this high-risk patient population [54]. BID—twice daily; INR—international normalized ratio; QD—daily; SC—subcutaneous; TID—three times daily.

Idiopathic Pulmonary Arterial Hypertension

Clinical Features of Idiopathic Pulmonary Arterial Hypertension

Idiopathic pulmonary arterial hypertension is defined by resting mean pulmonary artery pressure greater than 25 mm Hg in the absence of a secondary cause such as parenchymal lung disease, chronic thromboembolic disease, left-sided valvular disease, left ventricular systolic or diastolic dysfunction, congenital heart disease, or a systemic connective tissue disorder

While the vast majority of cases are sporadic, idiopathic pulmonary arterial hypertension may be rarely inherited secondary to an autosomal dominant mutation in the *PPH1* gene, which encodes bone morphogenetic protein receptor 2

Among patients with sporadic idiopathic pulmonary arterial hypertension, risk factors include mutations in bone morphogenetic protein receptor 2, portal hypertension, HIV infection, human herpesvirus-8 infection, anoretic drug use, and use of cocaine or amphetamines

Presenting symptoms and signs include exertional dyspnea, syncope, chest discomfort, and findings of right-sided heart failure such as jugular venous distension, tricuspid regurgitation, hepatomegaly, and lower extremity edema

Figure 11-34. Clinical features of idiopathic pulmonary arterial hypertension. Idiopathic pulmonary arterial hypertension (IPAH), formerly known as primary pulmonary hypertension, is defined by a mean pulmonary artery pressure greater than 25 mm Hg at rest and 30 mm Hg during exercise in the absence of secondary causes. IPAH appears to be more common among women and tends to present in the fourth decade of life.

Although the vast majority of cases are sporadic, IPAH may be rarely inherited secondary to an autosomal dominant mutation in the *PPH1* gene, which encodes bone morphogenetic protein receptor 2 [59]. Risk factors for noninherited IPAH include sporadic mutations in bone morphogenetic protein receptor 2, portal hypertension, HIV, human herpesvirus-8 infection, anorectic drug use, and use of cocaine or amphetamines.

Patients with IPAH may present with initial complaints of exertional dyspnea, lightheadedness, syncope, chest discomfort, and lower extremity swelling. Physical examination may reveal signs of right-sided heart failure, such as distended jugular veins, tricuspid regurgitation, hepatomegaly, and lower extremity edema.

The diagnosis of IPAH is suggested by a compatible clinical presentation, documentation of pulmonary hypertension on Doppler echocardiography or cardiac catheterization, and exclusion of secondary causes of pulmonary hypertension.

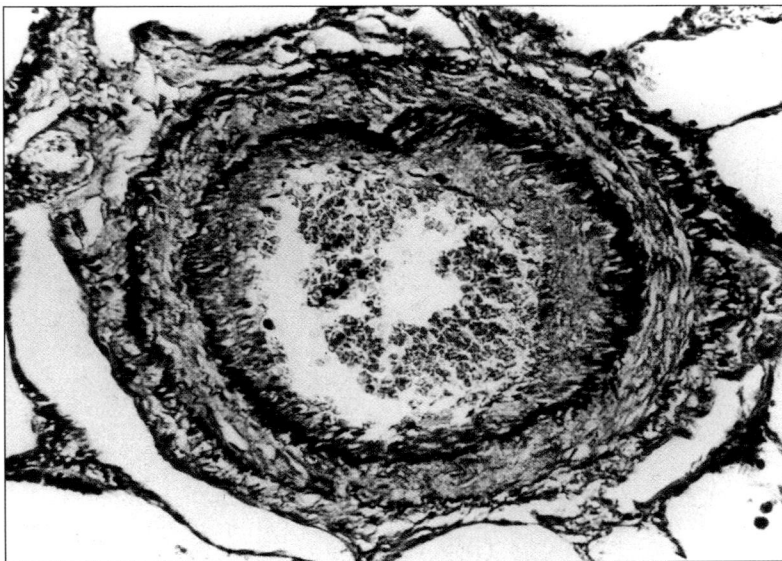

Medial hypertrophy

Figure 11-35. Vascular pathologic findings in idiopathic pulmonary arterial hypertension. Pathologic findings in idiopathic pulmonary arterial hypertension include medial hypertrophy, intimal hypertrophy and fibrosis, plexogenic arteriopathy, and thrombotic arteriopathy. This image demonstrates prominent medial hypertrophy in a specimen from a patient with idiopathic pulmonary arterial hypertension.

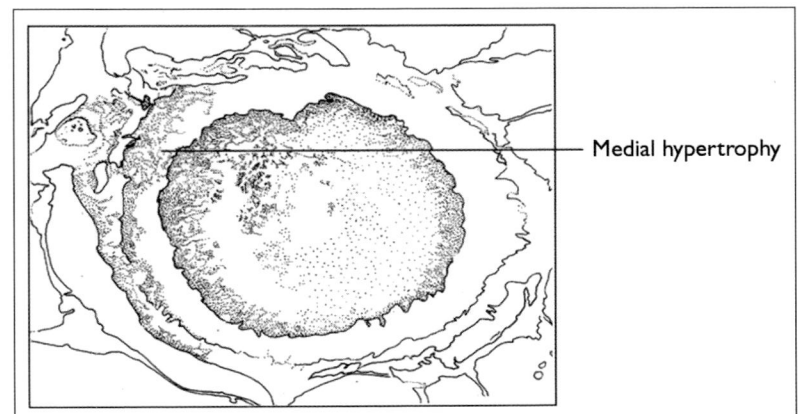

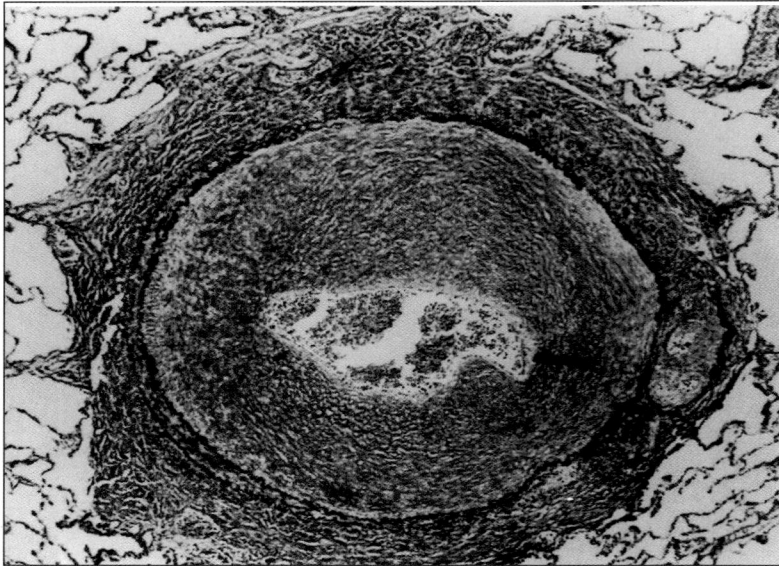

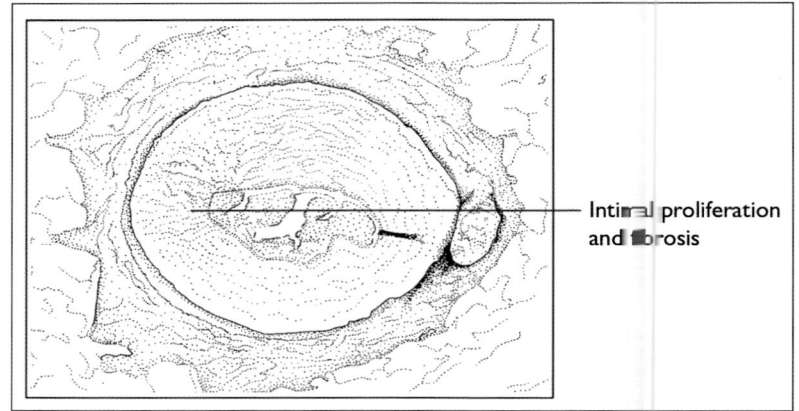

Figure 11-36. Marked intimal proliferation and fibrosis in a pathologic specimen from a patient with idiopathic pulmonary arterial hypertension.

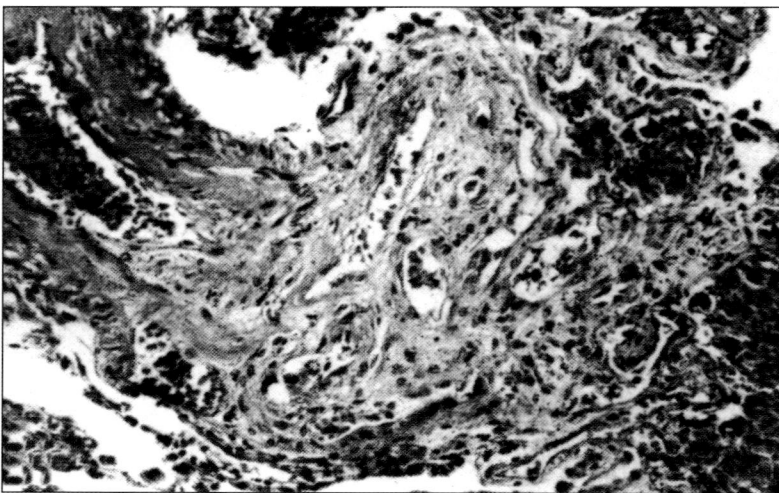

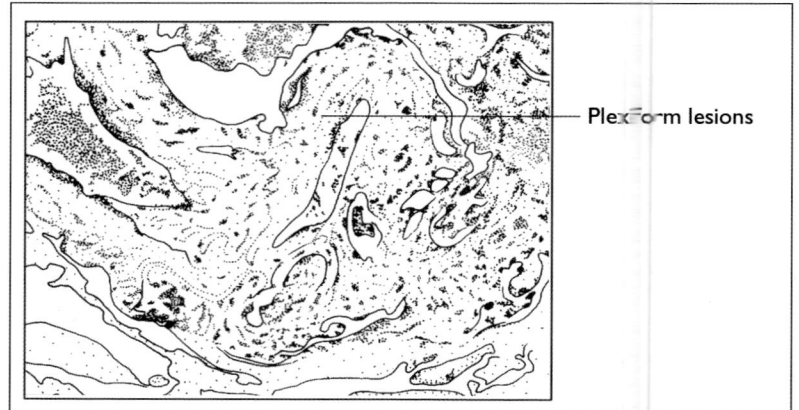

Figure 11-37. Plexogenic arteriopathy in a pathologic specimen from a patient with idiopathic pulmonary arterial hypertension. Pathologic specimens from patients with idiopathic pulmonary arterial hyper- tension may show disorganized proliferation of capillary-like vessels called plexogenic arteriopathy.

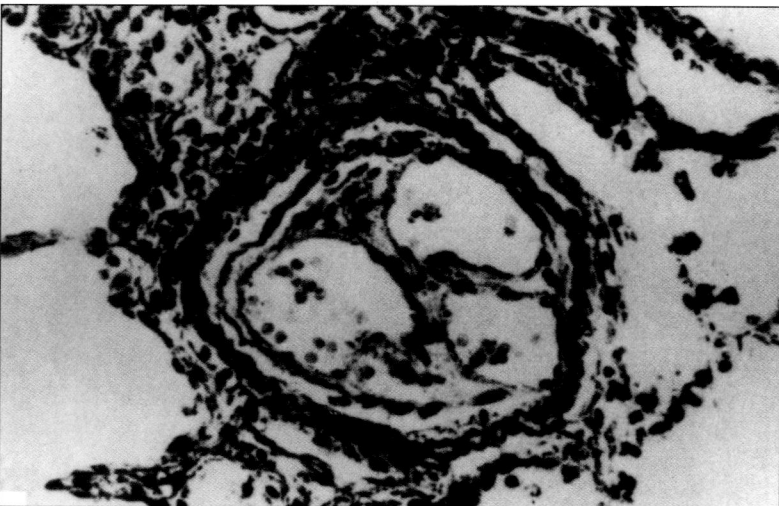

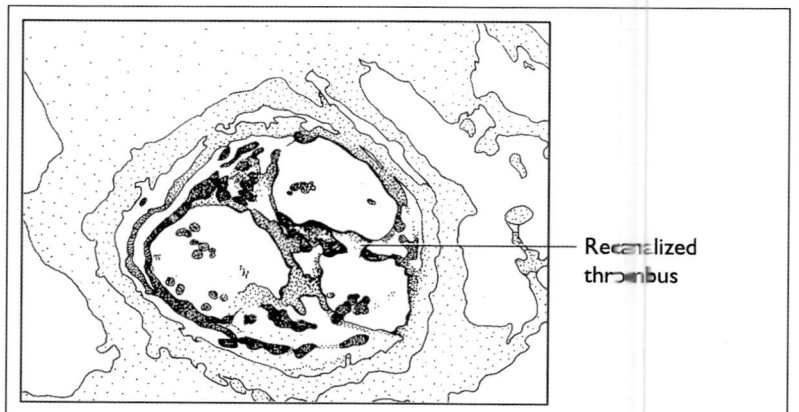

Figure 11-38. Thrombotic arteriopathy in a pathologic specimen from a patient with idiopathic pulmonary arterial hypertension. Evidence of thrombosis with recanalization can be observed in pathologic specimens from patients with idiopathic pulmonary arterial hypertension.

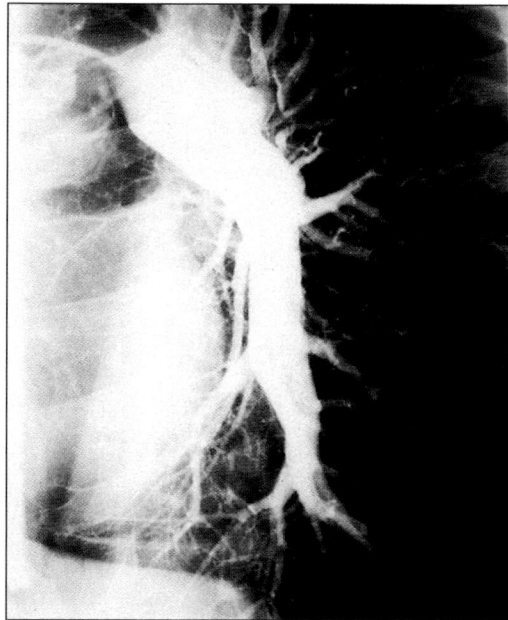

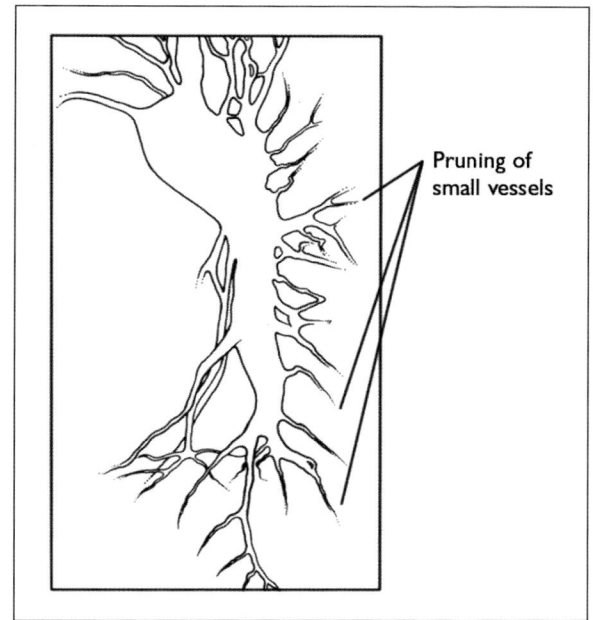

Figure 11-39. Contrast pulmonary angiography in a patient with diopathic pulmonary arterial hypertension. In this image, marked "pruning" of the small vessels and nearly absent peripheral flow characterize the classic findings in idiopathic pulmonary arterial hypertension. No segmental or larger vascular abnormalities are noted.

Figure 11-40. Therapies for idiopathic pulmonary arterial hypertension (IPAH). Without treatment, the median survival after diagnosis of IPAH is approximately 3 years. Until recently, patients with IPAH had very limited options that focused primarily on supportive care and surgical interventions, such as lung transplantation. However, advances in vasodilator therapy have dramatically increased the number of therapeutic options available to patients with IPAH [60].

Supportive care still constitutes a major focus in management of patients with IPAH. Oral anticoagulation with warfarin has been shown to improve survival in patients with IPAH [61]. Diuretics may be helpful in managing right ventricular overload, although overly aggressive volume reduction may result in hypotension and renal failure. Supplemental oxygen used to maintain an oxygen saturation of greater than 90% should be administered to overcome the vasoconstrictor effect of hypoxemia.

Patients with IPAH who demonstrate a hemodynamic response to vasodilators have several options. Prolonged therapy with calcium channel blockers has been shown to improve survival in patients with IPAH who have a documented response to short-acting vasodilators [61]. However, calcium channel blockers have fallen out of favor and are rarely prescribed. In patients with IPAH, continuous intravenous infusion of prostacyclin via a chronically indwelling central venous catheter improves hemodynamics, exercise capacity, and survival [62]. Other prostanoids such as treprostinil and iloprost have been shown to improve hemodynamics and functional capacity. Bosentan, an oral endothelin-receptor antagonist, improves hemodynamics, exercise capacity, and New York Heart Association functional class while also alleviating symptoms and reducing the frequency of clinical deterioration [63]. Primarily used to treat erectile dysfunction, the oral phosphodi-

Therapies for Idiopathic Pulmonary Arterial Hypertension
Supportive
Anticoagulation
Diuretics for right ventricular volume overload
Supplemental oxygen to maintain an oxygen saturation > 90%
Vasodilators
Calcium channel blockers
Continuous intravenous infusion of prostacyclin
Subcutaneously administered treprostinil
Inhaled iloprost
Oral endothelin-receptor antagonist (bosentan)
Oral phosphodiesterase-5 inhibitors (sildenafil, starting dose of 20 mg orally three times daily)
Surgery
Atrial septostomy
Lung transplantation

esterase-5 inhibitor sildenafil has been shown to improve hemodynamics, exercise capacity, and functional class in patients with IPAH [64].

Surgical interventions are generally reserved for patients with IPAH in whom vasodilator therapy has been unsuccessful. Atrial septostomy involves the creation of a right-to-left shunt that decompresses the failing right ventricle and increases left-sided preload in an effort to augment overall cardiac output and oxygen delivery. For patients with IPAH unresponsive to medical therapy, bilateral lung transplantation can be considered.

References

1. Piazza G, Goldhaber SZ: Acute pulmonary embolism, part I: epidemiology and diagnosis. *Circulation* 2006, 114:e28–e32.

2. Piazza G, Goldhaber SZ: Acute pulmonary embolism, part II: treatment and prophylaxis. *Circulation* 2006, 114:e42–e47.

3. Heit JA: The epidemiology of venous thromboembolism in the community: implications for prevention and management. *J Thromb Thrombolysis* 2006, 21:23–29.

4. Silverstein MD, Heit JA, Mohr DN, *et al.*: Trends in the incidence of deep vein thrombosis and pulmonary embolism: a 25-year population-based study. *Arch Intern Med* 1998, 158:585–593.

5. Stein PD, Beemath A, Olson RE: Trends in the incidence of pulmonary embolism and deep venous thrombosis in hospitalized patients. *Am J Cardiol* 2005, 95:1525–1526.

6. Goldhaber SZ, Tapson VF: A prospective registry of 5,451 patients with ultrasound-confirmed deep vein thrombosis. *Am J Cardiol* 2004, 93:259–262.

7. Joffe HV, Kucher N, Tapson VF, Goldhaber SZ: Upper-extremity deep vein thrombosis: a prospective registry of 592 patients. *Circulation* 2004, 110:1605–1611.

8. Goldhaber SZ, Visani L, De Rosa M: Acute pulmonary embolism: clinical outcomes in the International Cooperative Pulmonary Embolism Registry (ICOPER). *Lancet* 1999, 353:1386–1389.

9. Smeeth L, Cook C, Thomas S, *et al.*: Risk of deep vein thrombosis and pulmonary embolism after acute infection in a community setting. *Lancet* 2006, 367:1075–1079.

10. Tillie-Leblond I, Marquette CH, Perez T, *et al.*: Pulmonary embolism in patients with unexplained exacerbation of chronic obstructive pulmonary disease: prevalence and risk factors. *Ann Intern Med* 2006, 144:390–396.

11. Prandoni P, Bilora F, Marchiori A, *et al.*: An association between atherosclerosis and venous thrombosis. *N Engl J Med* 2003, 348:1435–1441.

12. Bova C, Marchiori A, Noto A, *et al.*: Incidence of arterial cardiovascular events in patients with idiopathic venous thromboembolism. A retrospective cohort study. *Thromb Haemost* 2006, 96:132–136.

13. Schulman S, Lindmarker P: Incidence of cancer after prophylaxis with warfarin against recurrent venous thromboembolism: duration of anticoagulation trial. *N Engl J Med* 2000, 342:1953–1958.

14. Stein PD, Beemath A, Meyers FA, *et al.*: Incidence of venous thromboembolism in patients hospitalized with cancer. *Am J Med* 2006, 119:60–68.

15. Vandenbroucke JP, Rosing J, Bloemenkamp KW, *et al.*: Oral contraceptives and the risk of venous thrombosis. *N Engl J Med* 2001, 344:1527–1535.

16. Rossouw JE, Anderson GL, Prentice RL, *et al.*: Risks and benefits of estrogen plus progestin in healthy postmenopausal women: principal results from the Women's Health Initiative randomized controlled trial. *JAMA* 2002, 288:321–333.

17. Schreijer AJ, Cannegieter SC, Meijers JC, *et al.*: Activation of coagulation system during air travel: a crossover study. *Lancet* 2006, 367:832–838.

18. Goldhaber SZ, Elliott CG: Acute pulmonary embolism: part I: epidemiology, pathophysiology, and diagnosis. *Circulation* 2003, 108:2726–2729.

19. Piazza G, Goldhaber SZ: The acutely decompensated right ventricle: pathways for diagnosis and management. *Chest* 2005, 128:1836–1852.

20. Wells PS, Owen C, Doucette S, *et al.*: Does this patient have deep vein thrombosis? *JAMA* 2006, 295:199–207.

21. Kearon C, Ginsberg JS, Hirsh J: The role of venous ultrasonography in the diagnosis of suspected deep venous thrombosis and pulmonary embolism. *Ann Intern Med* 1998, 129:1044–1049.

22. Bressollette L, Nonent M, Oger E, *et al.*: Diagnostic accuracy of compression ultrasonography for the detection of asymptomatic deep venous thrombosis in medical patients: the TADEUS project. *Thromb Haemost* 2001, 86:529–533.

23. van Belle A, Buller HR, Huisman MV, *et al.*: Effectiveness of managing suspected pulmonary embolism using an algorithm combining clinical probability, D-dimer testing, and computed tomography. *JAMA* 2006, 295:172–179.

24. Dunn KL, Wolf JP, Dorfman DM, *et al.*: Normal D-dimer levels in emergency department patients suspected of acute pulmonary embolism. *J Am Coll Cardiol* 2002, 40:1475–1478.

25. Quiroz R, Kucher N, Zou KH, *et al.*: Clinical validity of a negative computed tomography scan in patients with suspected pulmonary embolism: a systematic review. *JAMA* 2005, 293:2012–2017.

26. Stein PD, Fowler SE, Goodman LR, *et al.*: Multidetector computed tomography for acute pulmonary embolism. *N Engl J Med* 2006, 354:2317–2327.

27. Perrier A, Bounameaux H: Accuracy or outcome in suspected pulmonary embolism. *N Engl J Med* 2006, 354:2383–2385.

28. Goldhaber SZ: Echocardiography in the management of pulmonary embolism. *Ann Intern Med* 2002, 136:691–700.

29. Kucher N, Rossi E, De Rosa M, Goldhaber SZ: Prognostic role of echocardiography among patients with acute pulmonary embolism and a systolic arterial pressure of 90 mm Hg or higher. *Arch Intern Med* 2005, 165:1777–1781.

30. Kucher N, Goldhaber SZ: Cardiac biomarkers for risk stratification of patients with acute pulmonary embolism. *Circulation* 2003, 108:2191–2194.

31. Schoepf UJ, Kucher N, Kipfmueller F, *et al.*: Right ventricular enlargement on chest computed tomography: a predictor of early death in acute pulmonary embolism. *Circulation* 2004, 110:3276–3280.

32. Kucher N, Goldhaber SZ: Management of massive pulmonary embolism. *Circulation* 2005, 112:e28–e32.

33. Konstantinides S, Geibel A, Heusel G, *et al.*: Heparin plus alteplase compared with heparin alone in patients with submassive pulmonary embolism. *N Engl J Med* 2002, 347:1143–1150.

34. Leacche M, Unic D, Goldhaber SZ, *et al.*: Modern surgical treatment of massive pulmonary embolism: results in 47 consecutive patients after rapid diagnosis and aggressive surgical approach. *J Thorac Cardiovasc Surg* 2005, 129:1018–1023.

35. Jamieson SW, Kapelanski DP, Sakakibara N, *et al.*: Pulmonary endarterectomy: experience and lessons learned in 1,500 cases. *Ann Thorac Surg* 2003, 76:1457–1462; discussion 1462–1454.

36. Gould MK, Dembitzer AD, Doyle RL, *et al.*: Low-molecular-weight heparins compared with unfractionated heparin for treatment of acute deep venous thrombosis: a meta-analysis of randomized, controlled trials. *Ann Intern Med* 1999, 130:800–809.

37. Lee AY, Levine MN, Baker RI, *et al.*: Low-molecular-weight heparin versus a coumarin for the prevention of recurrent venous thromboembolism in patients with cancer. *N Engl J Med* 2003, 349:146–153.

38. Kucher N, Quiroz R, McKean S, *et al.*: Extended enoxaparin monotherapy for acute symptomatic pulmonary embolism. *Vasc Med* 2005, 10:251–256.

39. Buller HR, Davidson BL, Decousus H, *et al.*: Subcutaneous fondaparinux versus intravenous unfractionated heparin in the initial treatment of pulmonary embolism. *N Engl J Med* 2003, 349:1695–1702.

40. Buller HR, Davidson BL, Decousus H, *et al.*: Fondaparinux or enoxaparin for the initial treatment of symptomatic deep venous thrombosis: a randomized trial. *Ann Intern Med* 2004, 140:867–873.

41. Arepally GM, Ortel TL: Clinical practice: heparin-induced thrombocytopenia. *N Engl J Med* 2006, 355:809–817.

42. Quiroz R, Gerhard-Herman M, Kosowsky JM, *et al.*: Comparison of a single end point to determine optimal initial warfarin dosing (5 mg versus 10 mg) for venous thromboembolism. *Am J Cardiol* 2006, 98:535–537.

43. Rieder MJ, Reiner AP, Gage BF, *et al.*: Effect of VKORC1 haplotypes on transcriptional regulation and warfarin dose. *N Engl J Med* 2005, 352:2285–2293.

44. Joffe HV, Xu R, Johnson FB, *et al.*: Warfarin dosing and cytochrome P450 2C9 polymorphisms. *Thromb Haemost* 2004, 91:1123–1128.

45. Schulman S, Wahlander K, Lundstrom T, *et al.*: Secondary prevention of venous thromboembolism with the oral direct thrombin inhibitor ximelagatran. *N Engl J Med* 2003, 349:1713–1721.

46. Ridker PM, Goldhaber SZ, Danielson E, *et al.*: Long-term, low-intensity warfarin therapy for the prevention of recurrent venous thromboembolism. *N Engl J Med* 2003, 348:1425–1434.

47. Kearon C, Ginsberg JS, Kovacs MJ, *et al.*: Comparison of low-intensity warfarin therapy with conventional-intensity warfarin therapy for long-term prevention of recurrent venous thromboembolism. *N Engl J Med* 2003, 349:631–639.

48. Eight-year follow-up of patients with permanent vena cava filters in the prevention of pulmonary embolism: the PREPIC (Prevention du Risque d'Embolie Pulmonaire par Interruption Cave) randomized study. *Circulation* 2005, 112:416–422.

49. Kucher N, Rossi E, De Rosa M, Goldhaber SZ: Massive pulmonary embolism. *Circulation* 2006, 113:577–582.

50. Urbankova J, Quiroz R, Kucher N, Goldhaber SZ: Intermittent pneumatic compression and deep vein thrombosis prevention: a meta-analysis in postoperative patients. *Thromb Haemost* 2005, 94:1181–1185.

51. Kucher N, Koo S, Quiroz R, *et al.*: Electronic alerts to prevent venous thromboembolism among hospitalized patients. *N Engl J Med* 2005, 352:969–977.

52. Hull RD, Pineo GF, Stein PD, *et al.*: Extended out-of-hospital low-molecular-weight heparin prophylaxis against deep venous thrombosis in patients after elective hip arthroplasty: a systematic review. *Ann Intern Med* 2001, 135:858–869.

53. Eikelboom JW, Quinlan DJ, Douketis JD: Extended-duration prophylaxis against venous thromboembolism after total hip or knee replacement: a meta-analysis of the randomised trials. *Lancet* 2001, 358:9–15.

54. Bergqvist D, Agnelli G, Cohen AT, *et al.*: Duration of prophylaxis against venous thromboembolism with enoxaparin after surgery for cancer. *N Engl J Med* 2002, 346:975–980.

55. Samama MM, Cohen AT, Darmon JY, *et al.*: A comparison of enoxaparin with placebo for the prevention of venous thromboembolism in acutely ill medical patients. Prophylaxis in Medical Patients with Enoxaparin Study Group. *N Engl J Med* 1999, 341:793–800.

56. Leizorovicz A, Cohen AT, Turpie AG, *et al.*: Randomized, placebo-controlled trial of dalteparin for the prevention of venous thromboembolism in acutely ill medical patients. *Circulation* 2004, 110:874–879.

57. Cohen AT, Davidson BL, Gallus AS, *et al.*: Efficacy and safety of fondaparinux for the prevention of venous thromboembolism in older acute medical patients: randomised placebo controlled trial. *BMJ* 2006, 332:325–329.

58. Turpie AG, Bauer KA, Eriksson BI, Lassen MR: Fondaparinux vs enoxaparin for the prevention of venous thromboembolism in major orthopedic surgery: a meta-analysis of 4 randomized double-blind studies. *Arch Intern Med* 2002, 162:1833–1840.

59. Lane KB, Machado RD, Pauciulo MW, *et al.*: Heterozygous germline mutations in BMPR2, encoding a TGF-beta receptor, cause familial primary pulmonary hypertension. The International PPH Consortium. *Nat Genet* 2000, 26:81–84.

60. Ghofrani HA, Wilkens MW, Rich S: Uncertainties in the diagnosis and treatment of pulmonary artery hypertension. *Circulation* 2008, 118:1195–1201.

61. Rich S, Kaufmann E, Levy PS: The effect of high doses of calcium-channel blockers on survival in primary pulmonary hypertension. *N Engl J Med* 1992, 327:76–81.

62. Barst RJ, Rubin LJ, Long WA, *et al.*: A comparison of continuous intravenous epoprostenol (prostacyclin) with conventional therapy for primary pulmonary hypertension. The Primary Pulmonary Hypertension Study Group. *N Engl J Med* 1996, 334:296–302.

63. Rubin LJ, Badesch DB, Barst RJ, *et al.*: Bosentan therapy for pulmonary arterial hypertension. *N Engl J Med* 2002, 346:896–903.

64. Galie N, Ghofrani HA, Torbicki A, *et al.*: Sildenafil citrate therapy for pulmonary arterial hypertension. *N Engl J Med* 2005, 353:2148–2157.

Interventional Cardiology

12

Pinak B. Shah, Jean-Francois Dorval, Marc Z. Krichavsky, and Frederic S. Resnic

Interventional cardiovascular medicine has undergone explosive growth since 1977, when Dr. Andreas Grüntzig performed the first coronary balloon angioplasty in an awake human. The first 15 years of the field were marked by improvements in balloon technology, as well as the development of atherectomy devices for plaque removal and ablation. The early 1990s saw the development of coronary stents that improved long-term outcomes of coronary interventional procedures over balloon angioplasty. However, both modalities were limited by unacceptably high restenosis rates, resulting in the need for repeat intervention. Drug-eluting stents are now the mainstay of therapy for the percutaneous treatment of coronary artery disease.

With the development of interventional therapies for the treatment of coronary artery disease, innovations were also made in the treatment of peripheral vascular disease. Interventions to relieve symptomatic obstructive disease of the carotid, subclavian, renal, and lower extremity vascular beds are now mainstay procedures in catheterization laboratories (see Ch. 4).

Interventional cardiologists have also expanded their expertise to treat a variety of structural heart conditions. With advancements in intraprocedural echocardiography and closure device technology, interventional cardiologists now routinely perform valvular interventions, including aortic and mitral valvuloplasty. Further, advancements are being made in the percutaneous repair of valvular disorders. Congenital heart disease (eg, patent foramen ovale and atrial septal defect) is also routinely treated in catheterization laboratories. This chapter provides an atlas of important images in the fields of coronary, peripheral vascular, and structural heart disease intervention.

Coronary Intervention

Coronary Arterial Response to Injury

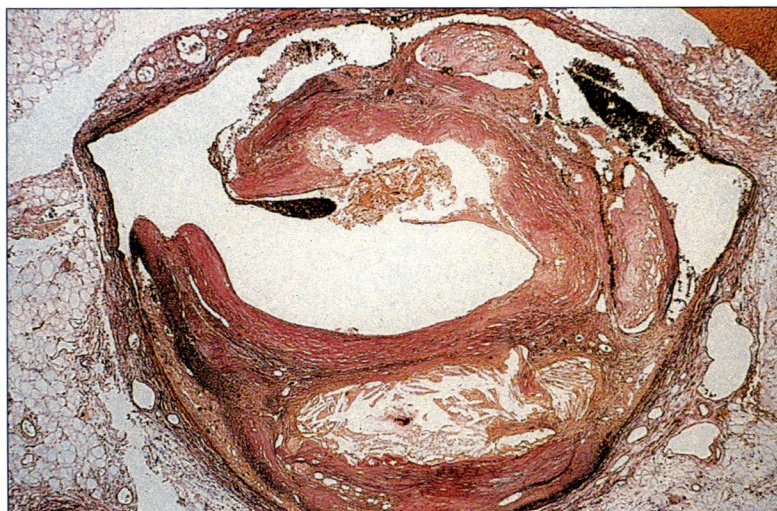

Figure 12-1. Acute pathology specimen of a patient who underwent balloon coronary angioplasty. Percutaneous coronary intervention necessarily injures the coronary artery vessel wall. The arterial response to this injury, which is a critical determinant to the long-term success or failure of such procedures [1], results in neointimal hyperplasia and adventitial thickening (the latter may manifest as negative remodeling). The primary mechanism of lumen improvement after balloon angioplasty appears to be fracture of the atheromatous plaque or the media itself. In this figure, note the dissection across the superior border of the artery and laceration of the vessel at the plaque site. (Hematoxylin and eosin stain.)

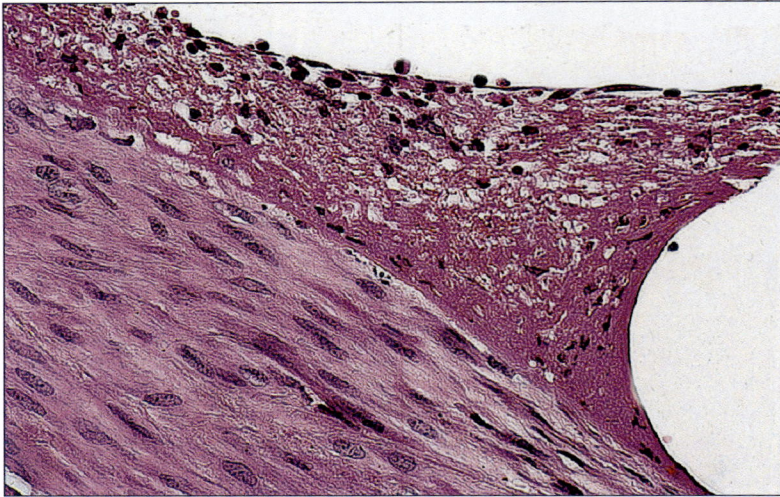

Figure 12-2. Normal pig artery 4 days after stent placement. Placement of a stent prevents negative vessel remodeling after coronary intervention. Therefore, neointimal hyperplasia is the prime determinant of in-stent restenosis. Accumulation of mural thrombus along the stent strut is apparent. Macrophages and lymphocytes are colonizing the thrombus at this early stage; an inflammatory response is much more common when the stent strut has been embedded in a lipid core or injured media rather than in fibrous plaque. Endothelialization is present at this early stage in this injured coronary pig model; in general, by 30 days after implantation in humans, stent endothelialization is present, although not necessarily complete.

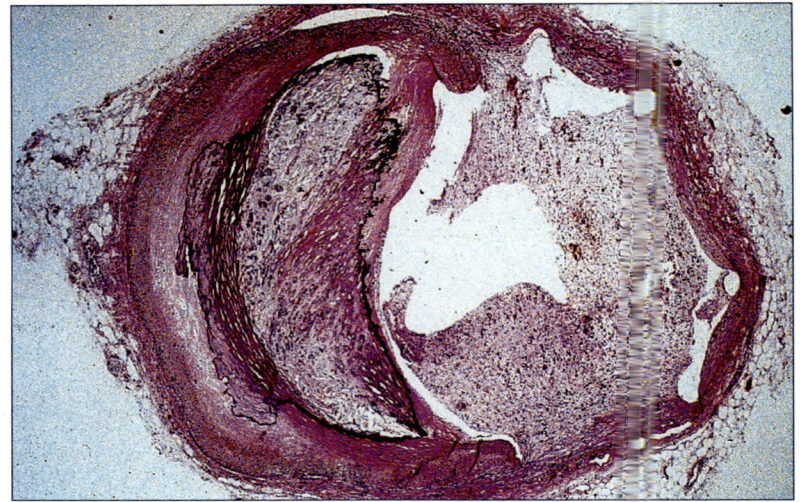

Figure 12-3. Pathology specimen of a coronary artery 30 days after stent placement. Inflammation is the source of neointimal thickening. In this pathologic specimen of a coronary artery 30 days after stent implantation, densely cellular neointimal expansion has caused restenosis. In summary, coronary revascularization results in vessel injury (ie, disruption of the vascular endothelium and exposure of deep tissue components to blood). Potential repair mechanisms that are basic to survival of the species are triggered by these occurrences, which result in thrombus formation and acute inflammation with subsequent neointima formation. A better understanding of these processes enables the development of more effective anti-restenosis strategies, including the continuing evolution of drug-eluting stents.

Invasive Lesion Assessment: Beyond Coronary Angiography

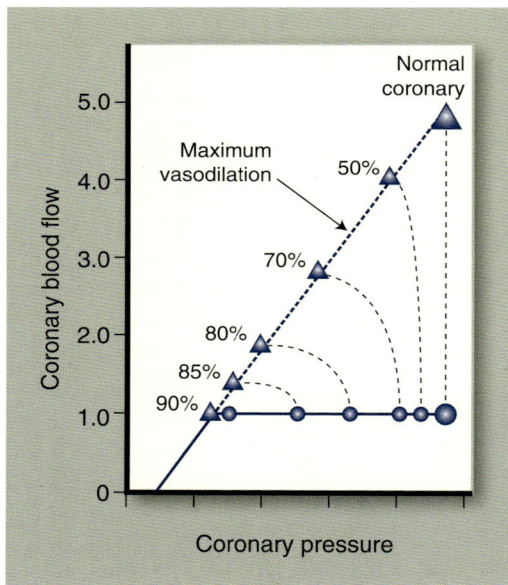

Figure 12-4. Coronary pressure-flow relationship at rest and during hyperemia. Coronary guidewires with distal pressure sensors can assess the functional significance of coronary stenoses that are of indeterminate severity using coronary angiography. Appreciation of coronary physiology can aid in the application of these techniques to clinical practice. At rest, coronary blood flow (CBF) is maintained at near constant levels over a range of perfusion pressures by the process of autoregulation. In the presence of an obstructive coronary stenosis in the epicardial vessel, the distal coronary pressure falls and the microcirculation undergoes compensatory vasodilation. With increasingly severe stenoses (indicated by the percentage values, triangles, and circles connected to the corresponding triangles by the dashed lines), the translesional pressure drop increases and autoregulation is overcome as the resistance vessels become unable to further dilate. This figure demonstrates that, even with relatively high-grade stenoses and variable coronary perfusion pressure, coronary blood flow remains constant under resting conditions (*circles*). However, with increased demand during stress or maximal hyperemia induced in the catheterization laboratory, the ability to increase CBF becomes diminished with increasingly severe epicardial stenoses.

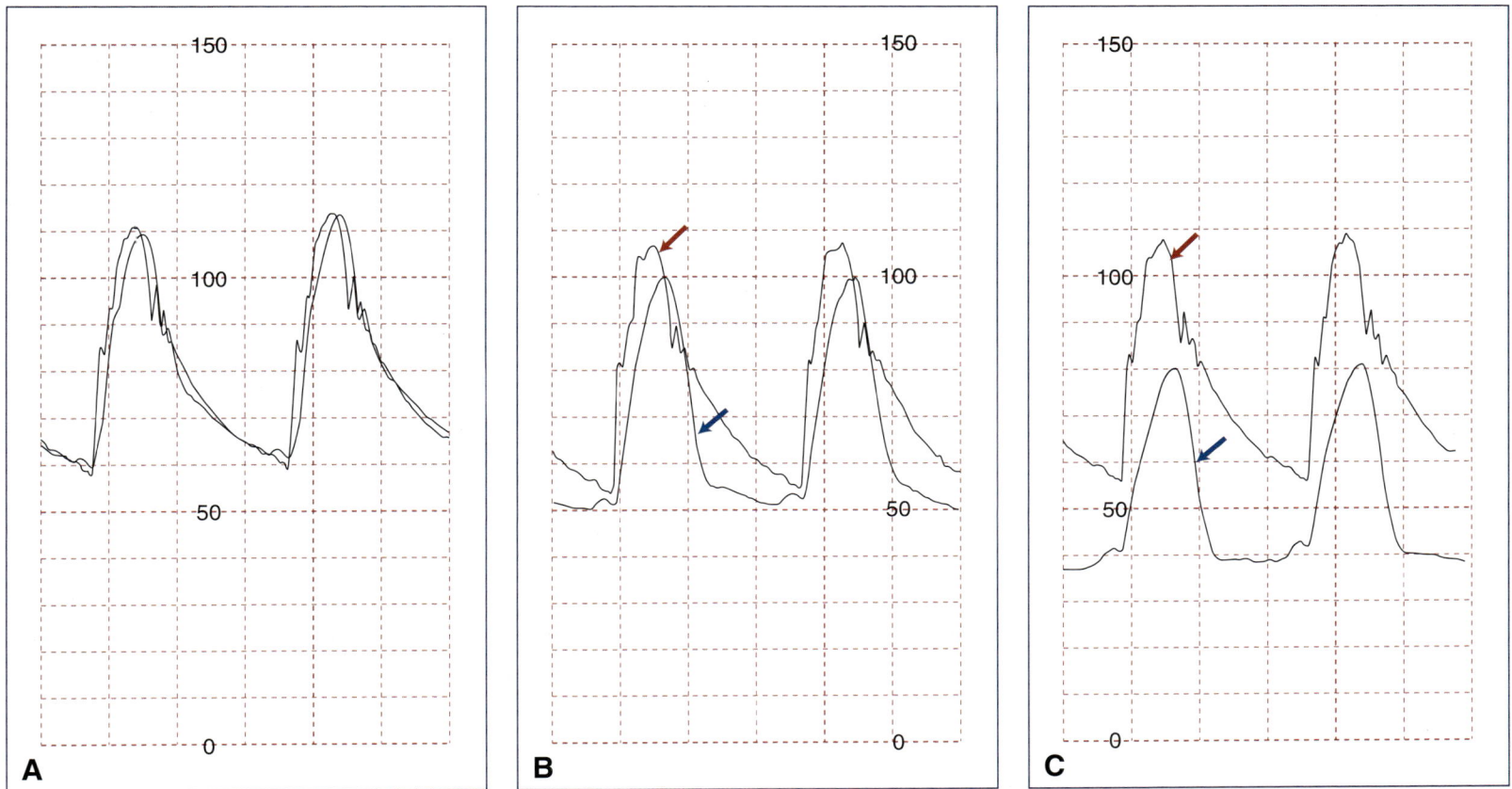

Figure 12-5. Measurement of fractional flow reserve (FFR). To measure FFR, a coronary guidewire with a pressure sensor located near the wire tip is advanced to the ostium of the guiding catheter. The pressures measured by the guide catheter and wire are equalized (**A**). The guidewire is advanced distal to the epicardial stenosis. The pressure gradient across the stenosis is measured in resting (**B**) and then maximum hyperemic conditions (**C**). *Red arrow* indicates pressure proximal to the lesion; *blue arrow* indicates pressure distal to the lesion. Coronary hyperemia is induced with adenosine by either intracoronary bolus (20–60 mcg) or intravenous infusion (140–180 mcg/kg/min). The FFR is defined as the ratio of distal pressure (Pd)/proximal pressure (Pa) at maximal hyperemic conditions. Several studies have shown that an FFR less than 0.75 correlates with an abnormal noninvasive stress test for ischemia and is generally thought to be consistent with a hemodynamically significant lesion [2,3]. Careful attention to technical and theoretical limitations—including signal drift, guide catheter-induced pressure dampening, ostial stenoses, tandem lesions, diffuse disease, and microvascular disease—is required when interpreting the data.

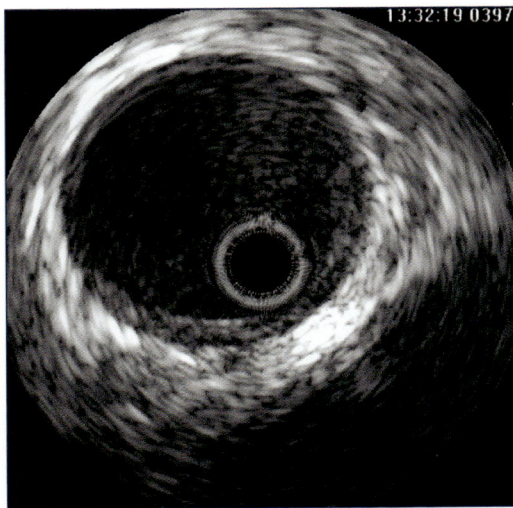

Figure 12-6. Intravascular ultrasound (IVUS) image of a normal coronary artery. IVUS provides detailed tomographic cross-sectional images of the lumen, vessel wall, and adjacent structures. Using automated pullback devices and associated computer software, these images can be converted into longitudinal and three-dimensional reconstructed images of the vessel. This figure depicts a normal left main coronary artery. The IVUS catheter and coronary guidewire are seen in the vessel lumen. The three layers of the vessel wall can often be identified with an innermost echodense intima, an echolucent media, and an outermost echodense adventitia. Quantitative measurements, including cross-sectional area (CSA), minimum, and maximum luminal diameters, can be calculated.

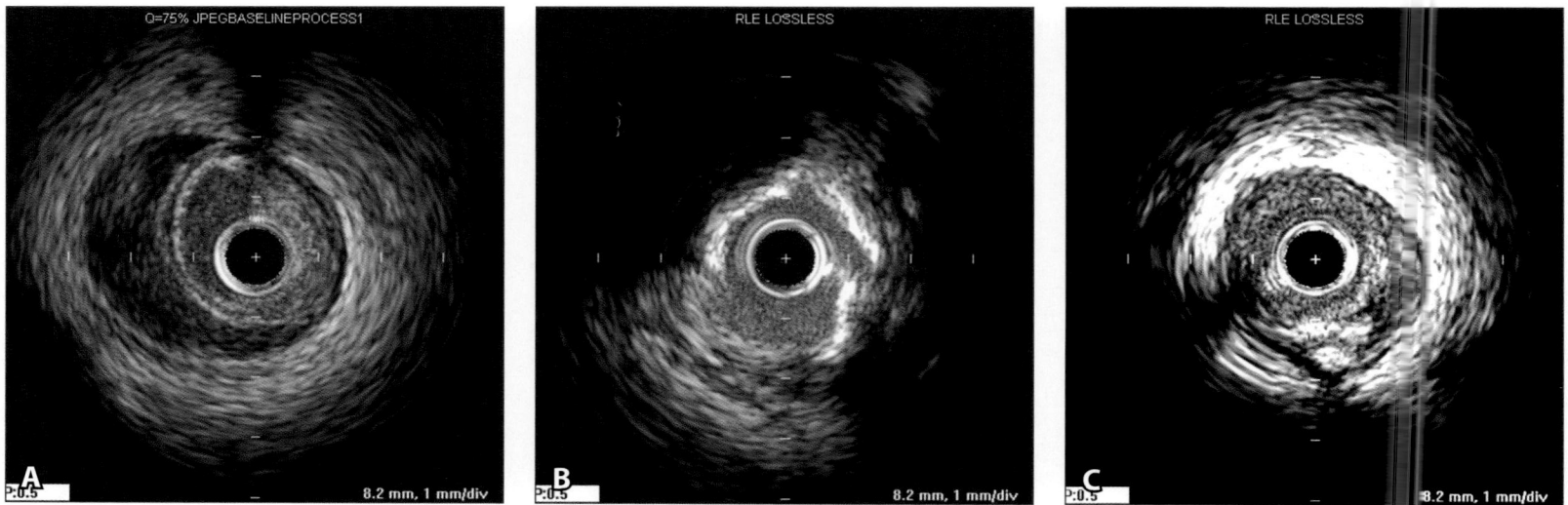

Figure 12-7. Coronary pathology identified with intravascular ultrasound (IVUS). IVUS imaging provides additional diagnostic information beyond coronary angiography. **A,** Dissection of left anterior descending artery. The dissection flap and crescent-shaped false lumen are appreciated from 4 to 12 o'clock. **B,** Stenosis of the left main artery associated with heavy calcification. Characteristic acoustic shadowing can be seen behind the echodense calcium from 9 to 5 o'clock. **C,** IVUS can distinguish calcified stenoses from eccentric stenoses associated with echolucent lipid laden plaque (4 o'clock). Both types of lesions may have a "hazy" appearance on coronary angiography.

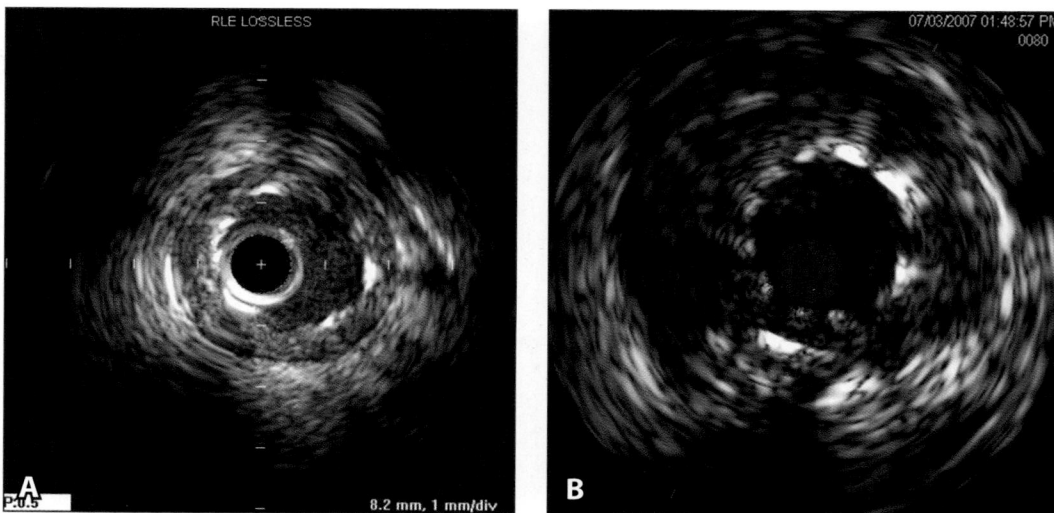

Figure 12-8. Placement and assessment of coronary stents with intravascular ultrasound (IVUS). IVUS can provide accurate measurements of vessel diameter and length of stenosis to guide in appropriate stent selection. Apposition of the stent with the vessel wall is best assessed with IVUS. Underdeployment is an important risk factor for stent thrombosis. In cases of stent thrombosis, IVUS can help assess the cause, including malapposition due to an underdeployed stent indicated by the gap between the echodense struts and the echolucent medial stripe (**A**) or acquired coronary aneurysm (echolucent) following drug-eluting stent placement, which is identified by the circle of echodense struts (**B**).

Stent Designs

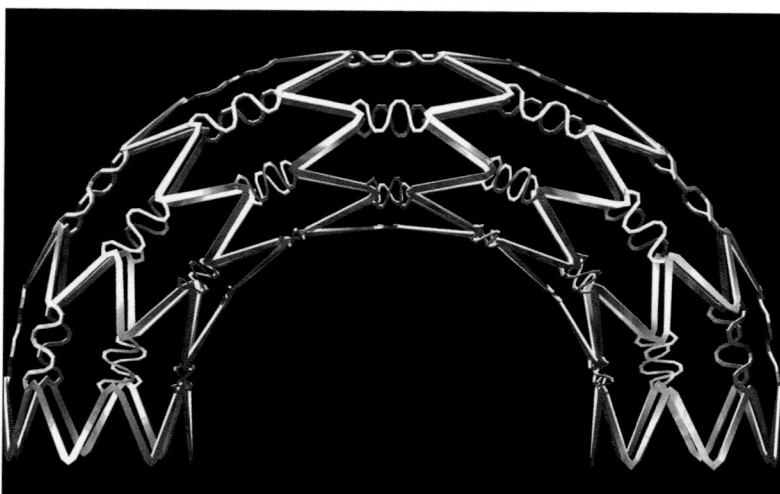

Figure 12-9. The Cypher stent (Cordis, Miami Lakes FL). Contemporary coronary stents are primarily balloon expandable and can be classified according to their basic design (slotted tube versus open cell) and their composition (stainless steel, cobalt-alloy, or nitinol). An ideal coronary stent would have the attributes of flexibility, ability to maneuver stent to distal vessel locations ("trackability"), adequate surface coverage, visibility, radial strength, side branch access, and low crossing profile. Each stent design has relative advantages and disadvantages in each of these categories; therefore, stent selection needs to account for angiographic and procedural issues for a specific case. This figure shows the Cordis Cypher stent, which is the rapamycin-eluting version of the BX Velocity stent (Cordis). The BX Velocity stent is laser cut from a single tube of stainless steel. It uses a closed-cell design to maintain flexibility while trying to preserve vessel coverage. Rapamycin is a cytostatic drug that blocks the cell cycle by blocking growth-factor induced cellular proliferation. (*Courtesy of* Cordis.)

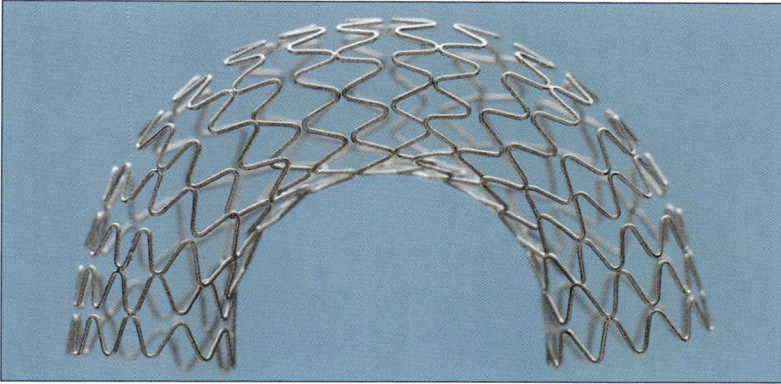

Figure 12-10. The Medtronic Driver coronary stent (Medtronic, Santa Rosa, CA). The Driver stent is based on a single sinusoidal element configured in a series of interconnected crowns and struts. Although the early generation of this stent focused on deliverability, the more recent generations have evolved to emphasize radial strength and vessel scaffolding with radio-opacity. The Driver is the most recent version of Medtronic's bare metal coronary stent designs and is a cobalt alloy open-cell system. The Medtronic Endeavor drug-eluting stent is based on the Driver bare metal stent design coated with a phosphorylcholine biocompatible polymer carrying Zotarolimus as the antiproliferative drug. (*Courtesy of* Medtronic.)

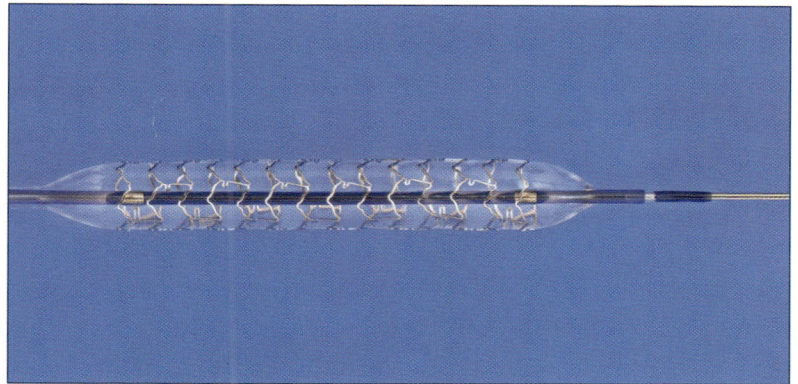

Figure 12-11. The Abbott Vascular Xience stent (Abbott Laboratories, Abbott Park, IL). The Xience stent is a drug-eluting stent based on the Multi-Link Vision bare-metal-stent platform. The Vision coronary stent is a cobalt chromium alloy with extremely thin struts (0.0032"). The Multi-Link stents were originally based on a slotted tube design composed of multiple rings connected by small bridging elements. The Vision stent represents the seventh generation of this stent design. The Xience drug-eluting stent (Abbott Laboratories) and the Promus stent (Boston Scientific, Natick, MA) is coated with a biocompatible polymer carrying Everolimus as the anti-proliferative agent. (*Courtesy of* Abbott Laboratories).

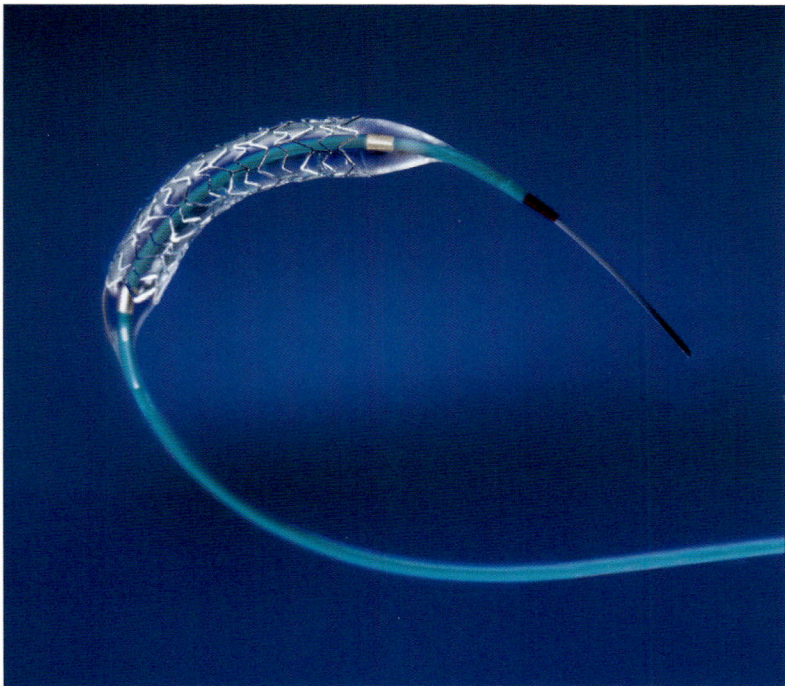

Figure 12-12. Express² bare metal stent (Boston Scientific, Natick, MA). The Express² stent is a closed-cell design that serves as the platform for the TAXUS Express drug eluting stent. The TAXUS stent utilizes paclitaxel, an antiproliferative agent that stabilizes intracellular microtubules, thereby preventing smooth muscle cell proliferation and in-stent restenosis. (*Courtesy of* Boston Scientific, Natick, MA.)

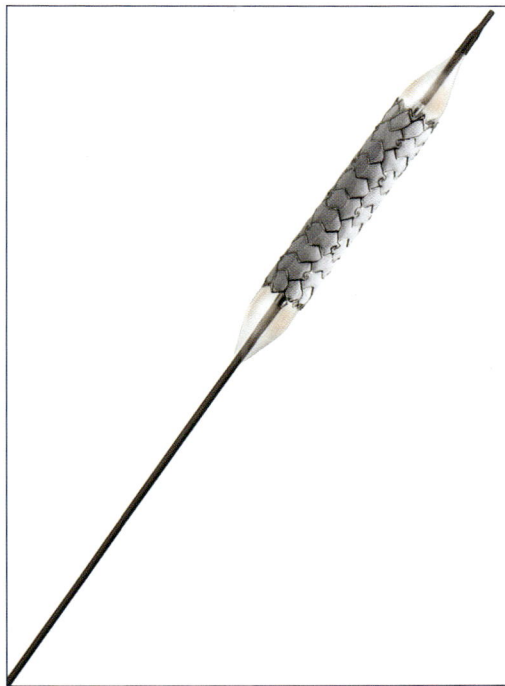

Figure 12-13. The Abbott Vascular JoStent Graftmaster covered stent (Abbott Vascular, Abbott Park, IL). The Graftmaster is a unique stent design approved for the treatment of coronary perforation in the United States. The Graftmaster possesses a thin polytetrafluoroethylene (PTFE) layer sandwiched between two stainless steel stents that serve to secure the membrane but impairs the deliverability of the system. However, this stent design is effective for the treatment of coronary perforations that are not responsive to conventional measures of prolonged balloon inflation and reversal of anticoagulation, and it can eliminate the need for emergent surgery in many patients experiencing this unusual life-threatening complication of coronary intervention. The Graftmaster is currently available in the United States only under Human Device Exemption. (*Courtesy of* Abbott Vascular, Abbott Park, IL.)

Drug-Eluting Stents

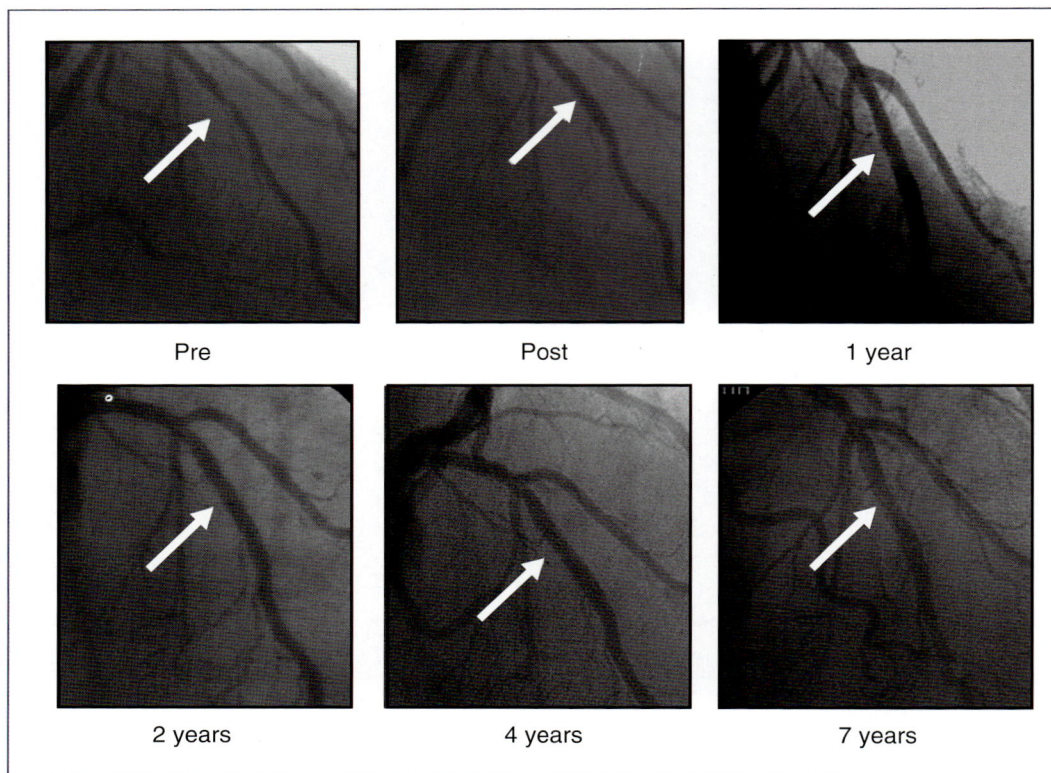

Pre　　　Post　　　1 year

2 years　　　4 years　　　7 years

Figure 12-14. Reduction of in-stent restenosis with drug-eluting stents. The initial studies of the Sirolimus-eluting Cypher stent (Cordis, Miami Lakes, FL) showed dramatic reduction in the rates of in-stent restenosis in patients treated with the drug-eluting stent. This figure shows the preintervention, postintervention, and serial follow-up angiograms to 7 years of the left anterior descending artery of the first patient treated with the Cypher stent, demonstrating no late lumen loss or evidence of restenosis at the treated vessel segment. (*Courtesy of* Cordis). Similarly dramatic results have been demonstrated for the other US Food and Drug Administration–approved drug-eluting stents, including Taxus (Boston Scientific, Natick, MA), Endeavor (Medtronic, Santa Rosa, CA), and Xience (Abbott Laboratories, Abbott Park, IL).

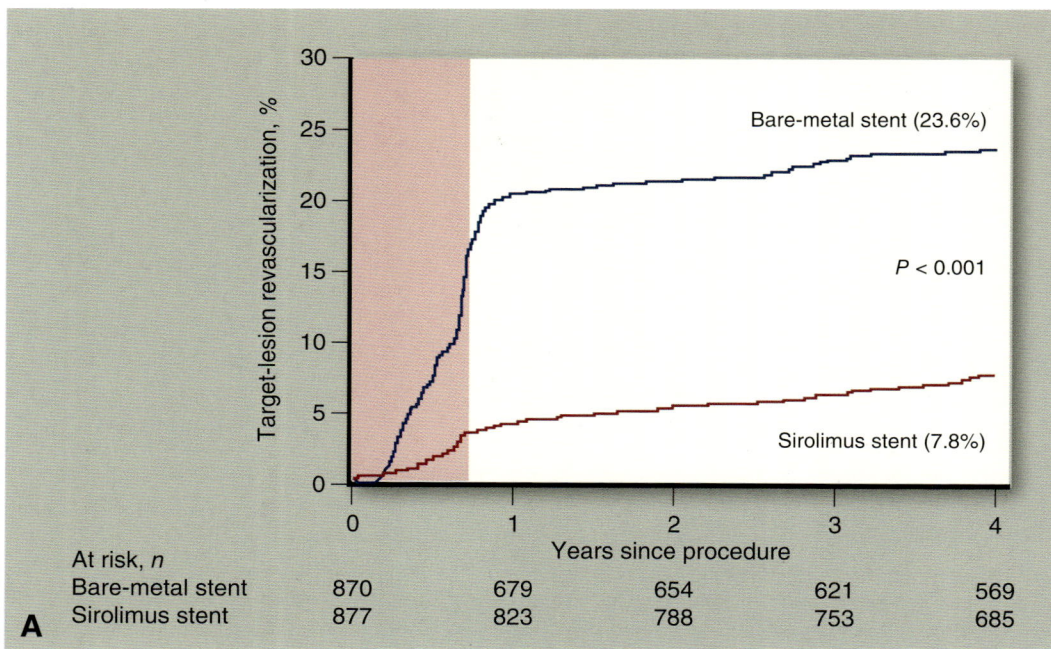

At risk, *n*				
Bare-metal stent	870	679	654	621	569
Sirolimus stent	877	823	788	753	685

A

Figure 12-15. Efficacy of drug-eluting stents. **A,** The sustained reduction in restenosis for the Cypher (Cordis, Miami Lakes, FL) Sirolimus-eluting stent compared with the bare metal stent counterpart in the four randomized prospective trials assessing the Cypher stent. Revascularization at the target lesion was reduced by 67% at 4 years. (*Courtesy of* Massachusetts Medical Society).

Continued on the next page

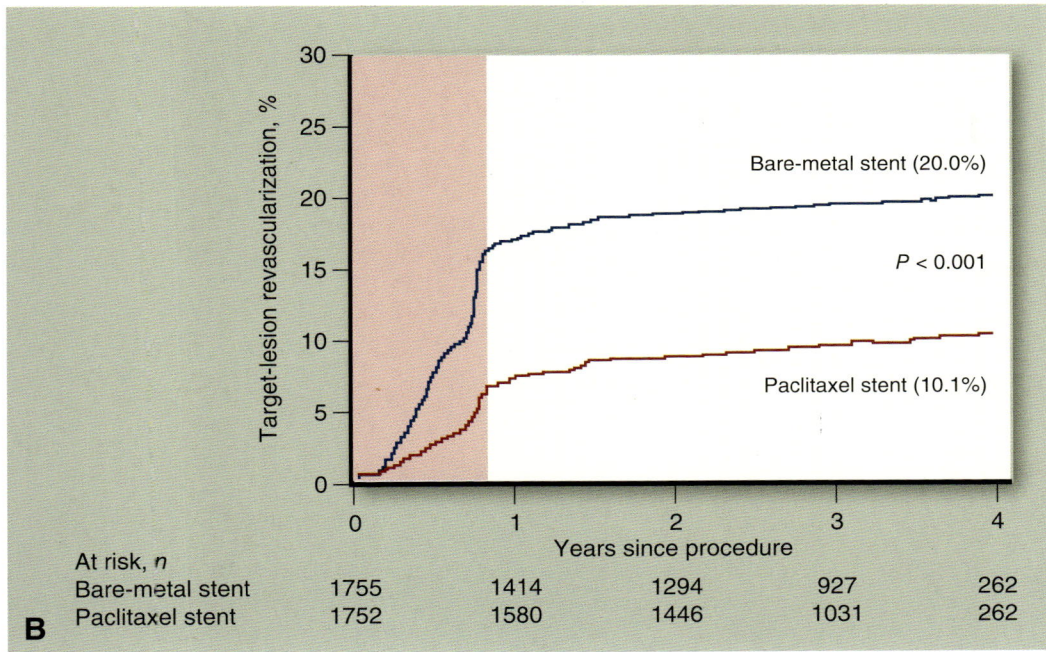

B

At risk, n

Bare-metal stent	1755	1414	1294	927	262
Paclitaxel stent	1752	1580	1446	1031	262

Figure 12-15. *(Continued)* **B,** The sustained efficacy of the paclitaxel-eluting Taxus stent (Boston Scientific, Natick, MA), demonstrating 50% reduction in the need for target lesion revascularization out to 4 years of follow-up. In both drug-eluting stents, nearly all of the benefit occurs in the first 8 months of the studies, consistent with the known time-course for the development of coronary in-stent restenosis *(pink-shaded area).* *(Courtesy of* Massachusetts Medical Society.) [4].

Drug-Eluting Stents Approved for Use in the United States

	Cypher	TAXUS	Endeavor	Xience
Manufacturer	Cordis (Miami Lakes, FL)	Boston Scientific (Natick, MA)	Medtronic (Santa Rosa, CA)	Abbott Vascular (Abbott Park, IL)
Stent design	Closed cell stainless stell	Closed cell stainless steel	Open cell cobalt alloy	Closed cell chromium cobalt
Active agent	Sirolimus	Paclitaxel	Zotarolimus	Everolimus
Polymer	Ekastomeric polymer	Proprietary translute polymer	Phosphorocholine based	Fluoroploymer
US pivotal trial	Sirius ($n = 1058$)	Taxus IV ($n = 1314$)	Endeavor IV ($n = 1548$)	Spirit III ($n = 1002$)
US approval	2003	2004	2008	2008

Figure 12-16. Drug-eluting stents (DES) approved for use in the United States. The chart lists the stents approved for use in the United States as of September 1, 2008.

Complications of Stents: In-Stent Restenosis

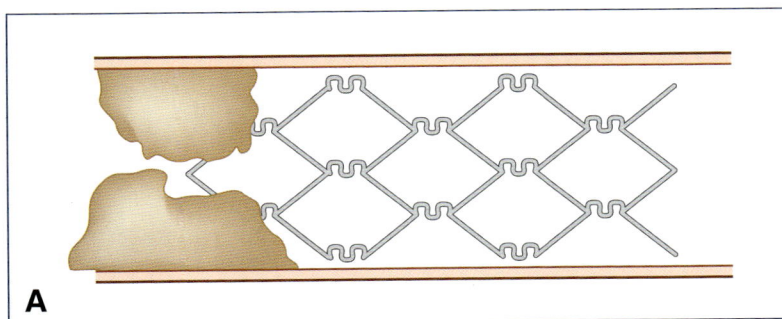

A

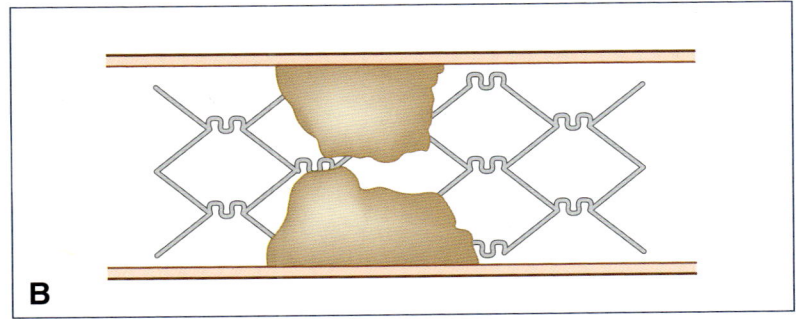

B

Figure 12-17. Classification of in-stent restenosis. Bare metal stenting is associated with less restenosis compared with conventional balloon angioplasty. However, bare metal stenting is still limited by target lesion revascularization rates exceeding 20%. In-stent restenosis can be divided into two broad categories: focal and diffuse. Focal lesions are less than or equal to 10 mm in length and may occur within the body of the stent, the proximal or distal margin, or a combination of these. **A**, **B**, and **C** represent proximal edge restenosis, focal body restenosis, and multifocal restenosis diffusely, respectively.

Continued on the next page

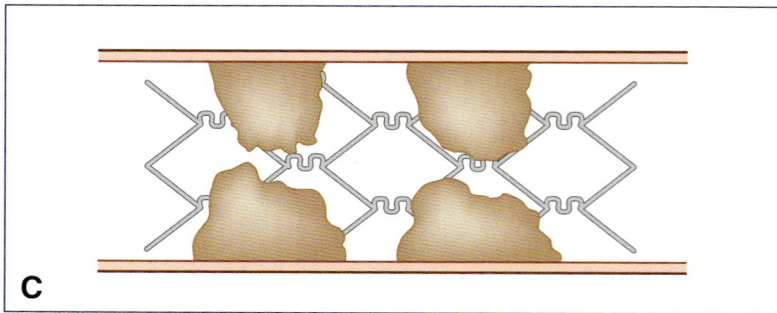

C

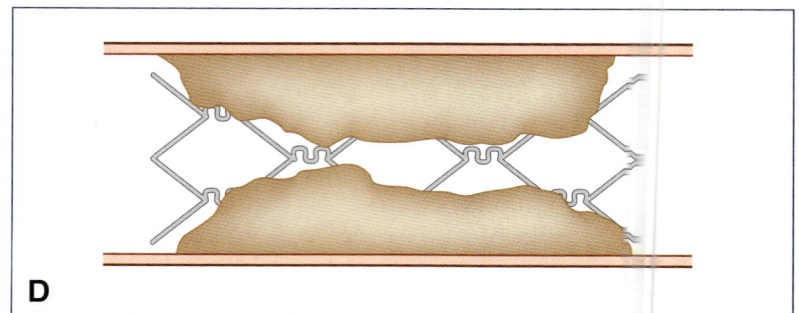

D

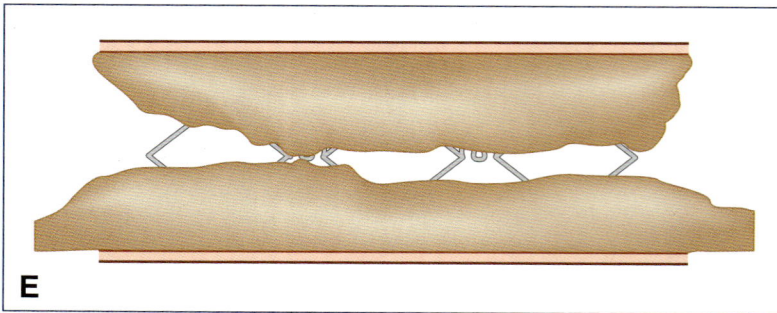

E

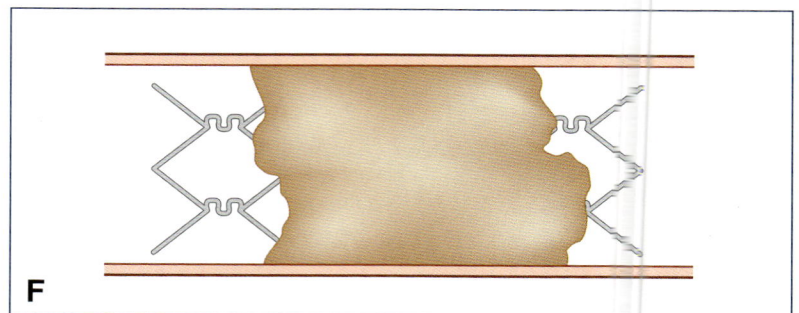

F

Figure 12-17. *(Continued)* **D** represents diffuse (> 10 mm in length) restenosis. **E** represents diffuse proliferative restenosis, extending beyond the margins of the stent. Very aggressive restenosis may totally occlude the stent as demonstrated in **F** [5,6].

Drug-eluting stents (DES) have reduced target lesion revascularization rates in clinical trials to 5% to 7%. As a result, in-stent restenosis is encountered less frequently in the modern era of percutaneous coronary intervention. When in-stent restenosis is encountered, it is generally focal and treated with balloon angioplasty or repeat stenting with drug-eluting stents.

Complications of Stents: Stent Thrombosis

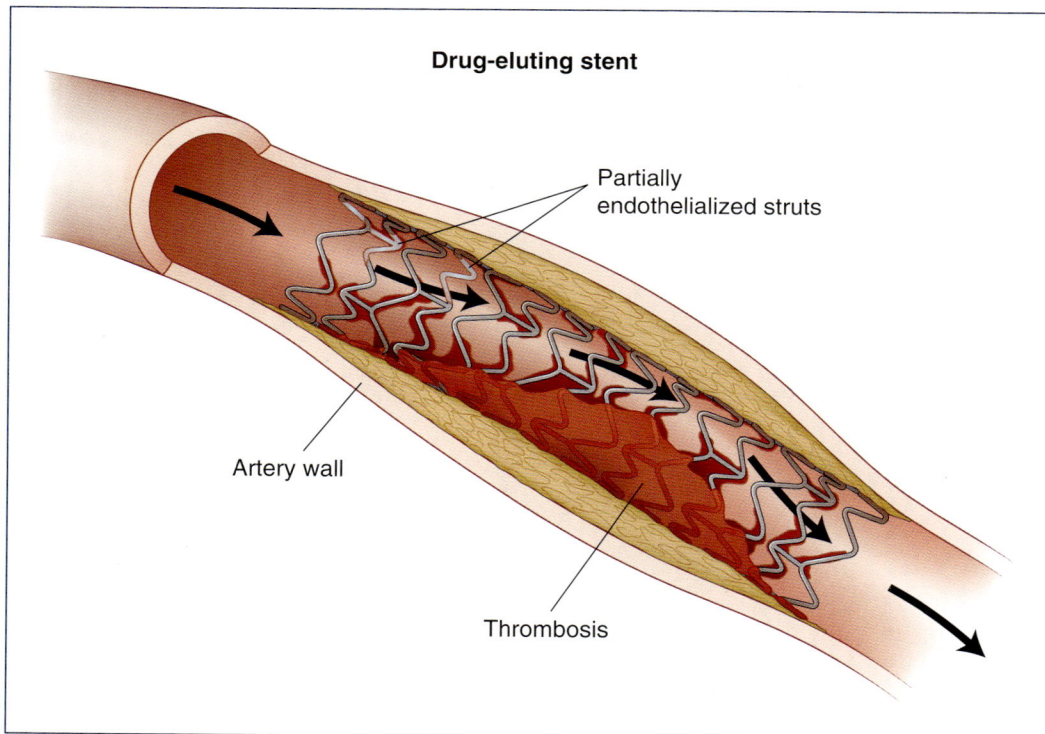

Drug-eluting stent

Partially endothelialized struts

Artery wall

Thrombosis

Figure 12-18. Stent thrombosis. Acute occlusion of a coronary stent typically occurs when thrombus forms within the stent as a result of a mechanical complication of stent implantation, such as an untreated edge dissection at the margin of the stent or unrecognized underdilation of the stent struts (*see* Fig 12-8A). Thrombus may occlude the entire lumen precipitating an ST segment myocardial infarction, which is associated with very high rates of morbidity and mortality, even with prompt treatment. The rates of stent thrombosis declined substantially with the evolution of coronary stent implantation technique, including high pressure postdilation of coronary stents and recognition of the importance of treatment with dual antiplatelet therapy, including aspirin and a thienopyridine, such as clopidogrel. Stent thrombosis is described by classifying the time between stent implantation to the development of the thrombosis: early stent thrombosis (0–30 days following implantation), late stent thrombosis (31–365 days), and very late stent thrombosis (more than 1 year following stent implant) [7]. (*Courtesy of* Massachusetts Medical Society.)

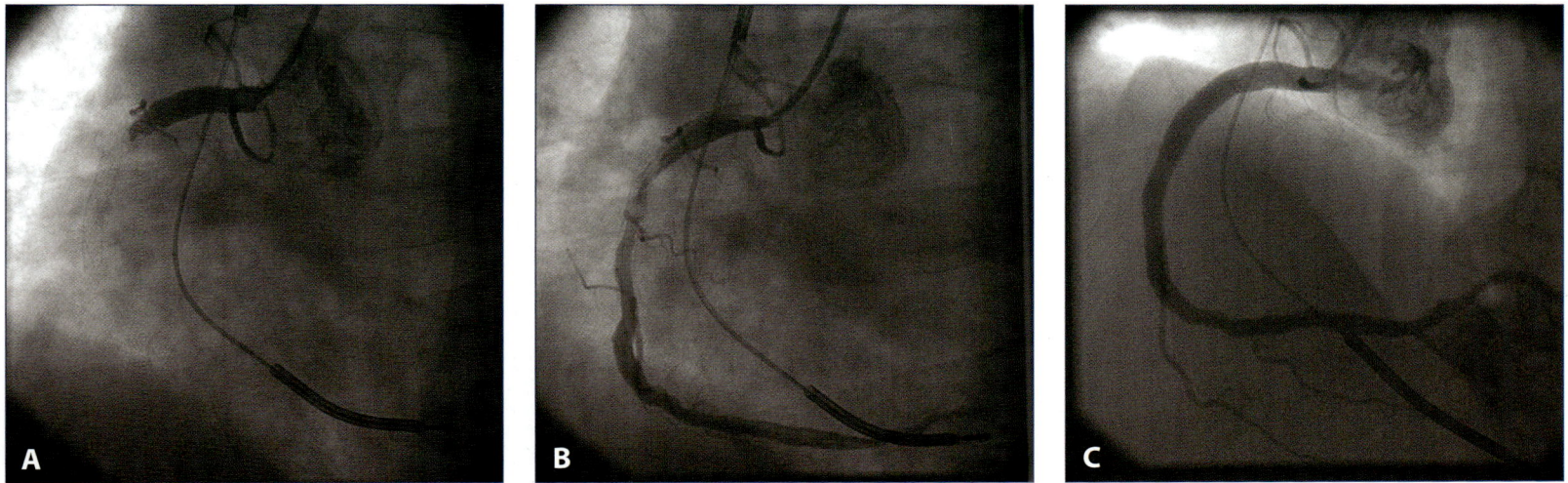

Figure 12-19. Very late stent thrombosis (VLST) in a bare metal stent. This figure illustrates very late stent thrombosis in a patient who had undergone bare metal stenting of the proximal right coronary artery for unstable angina. He had been compliant with his dual antiplatelet therapy through 30 days following stent implantation and continued taking aspirin as prescribed. The patient developed severe substernal chest pain 18 months after his initial procedure without prodromal symptoms, and was evaluated emergently where an electrocardiogram demonstrated acute ST segment elevation in the inferior leads. He was promptly taken for coronary angiography, which demonstrated complete occlusion of the proximal right coronary artery in the mid portion of the previously placed stent (**A**). Note that the thrombosis extends through the length of the stent. After initial balloon dilation, Thrombosis in Myocardial Infarction Trial grade 3 (TIMI-3) flow was restored, but with evidence of extensive filling defect consistent with a large thrombus burden (**B**). Glycoprotein IIb-IIIa inhibitor was administered and thrombectomy and repeat stenting was performed of the right coronary artery, with the result shown in **C**.

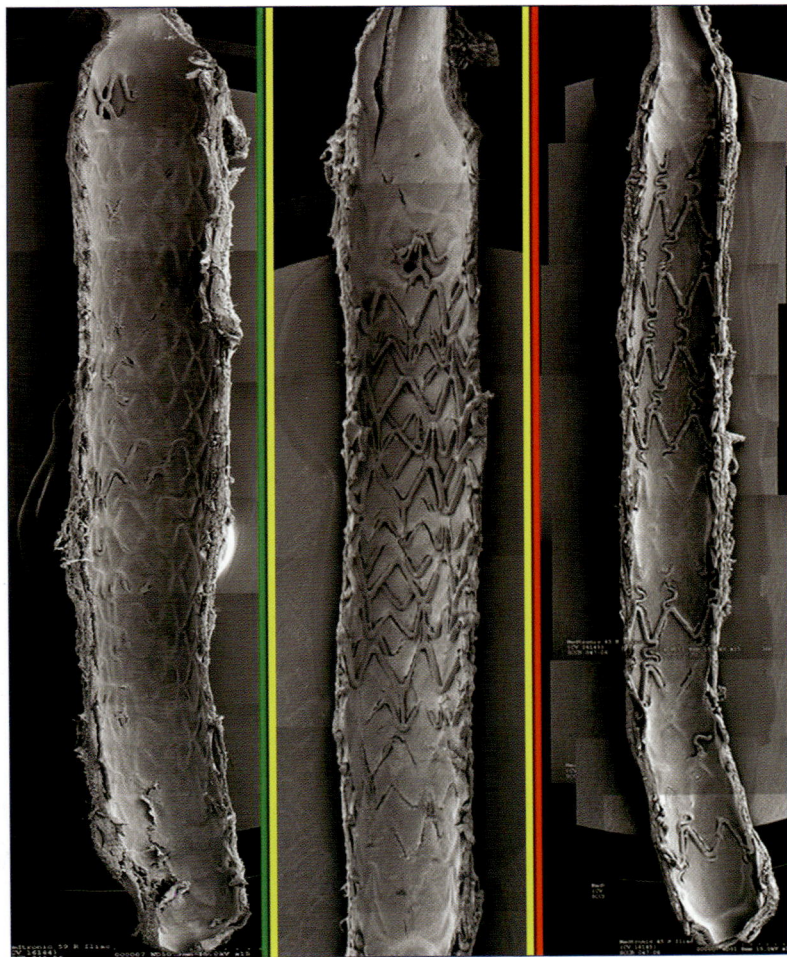

Figure 12-20. Delayed vessel wall healing following drug-eluting stent implantation [8]. A common feature of the vascular response to implantation of current drug-eluting stents is the delayed healing of the vessel wall. As shown in the electron micrographs in the figure, drug-eluting stents variably inhibit the completeness of vessel wall healing demonstrated by uncovered stent struts 21 days after implantation into an animal arterial injury model. In the left panel, the Medtronic Endeavor drug-eluting stent (Medtronic, Santa Rosa, CA) demonstrates 75% stent strut coverage 21 days after implantation, while 50% of the Boston Scientific Taxus stent (Boston Scientific, Natick, MA) is covered by a cellular layer (*center panel*) and 30% of the Cordis Cypher stent (Cordis, Miami Lakes, FL) demonstrates strut coverage (*right panel*). The delayed vessel wall healing is posited as one possible explanation for a potential increased risk of delayed stent thrombosis for drug-eluting stents compared with bare metal stents. The pathologic observation of delayed endothelialization and vessel wall healing supports the recommendation of prolonged dual antiplatelet therapy as compared with bare metal stents. Importantly, other factors, including compliance with dual antiplatelet therapy, malapposition of stent struts to the vascular wall, and the treatment of complex lesions (*eg*, bifurcations with multiple stents) may also contribute to the observe rates of stent thrombosis for both drug-eluting and bare metal coronary stents. (*From* Medtronic; with permission).

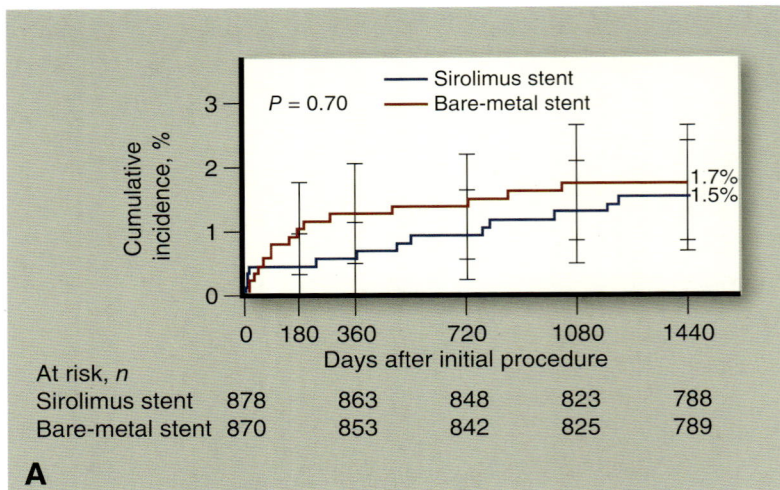

A

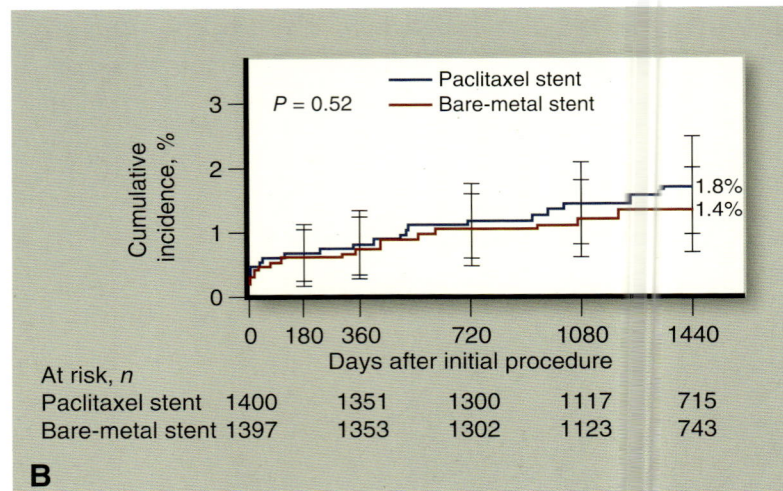

B

Figure 12-21. Stent thrombosis in drug-eluting stents. Although there have been concerns raised regarding the potential for increased rates of stent thrombosis after implantation of drug-eluting stents, clinical trial data have not supported this hypothesis. **A,** The rates of stent thrombosis from the pooled randomized trial results for the Cypher stent versus the Cordis Velocity bare metal stent (Cordis, Miami Lakes, FL), demonstrated no difference in the rates of thrombosis over the 4 years of follow-up when using uni-form definitions for stent thrombosis (*Courtesy of* Massachusetts Medical Society).

B, Similarly, there was no significant difference in the long-term rates of stent thrombosis for the paclitaxel-eluting Taxus stent compared with the Express[2] bare metal stent (Boston Scientific, Natick, MA). Both drug-eluting stents and bare metal stents appear to have a constant rate of late stent thrombosis of approximately 0.4% per year [9]. (*Courtesy of* Massachusetts Medical Society.)

Lesion Subsets

Ostial Lesions

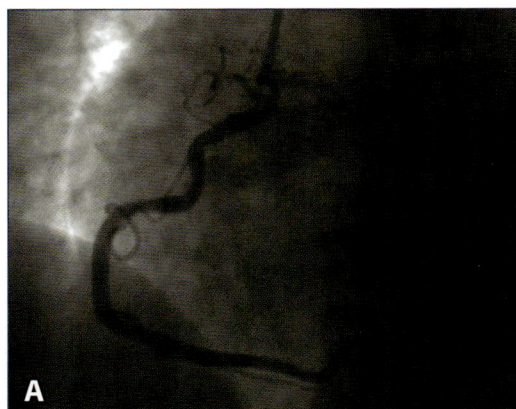

A

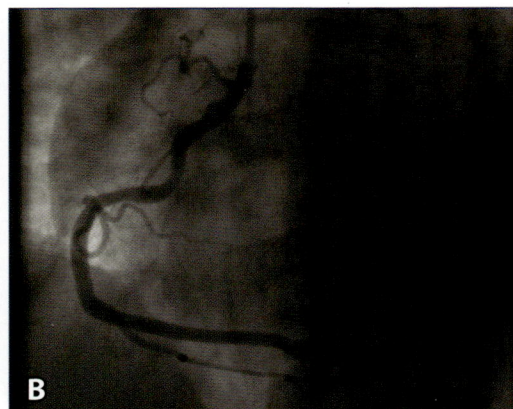

B

Figure 12-22. Aorto-ostial right coronary artery lesions are a challenging lesion subset to treat as these lesions are often heavily calcified and stent placement can be difficult. It is critical that the stent fully cover the ostium of the vessel with no more than 2 mm of stent extending into the aorta. **A,** Aorto-ostial lesion of the right coronary artery. **B,** Final angiographic result after predilatation and drug-eluting stent placement.

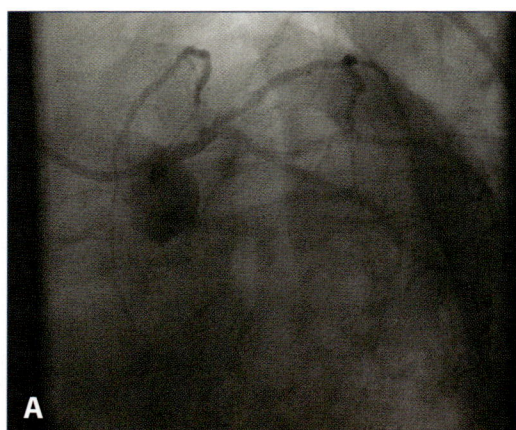

A

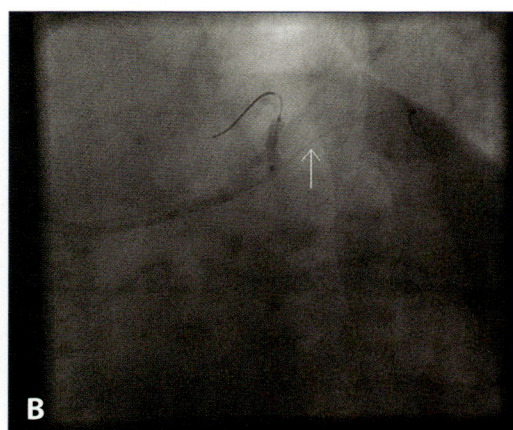

B

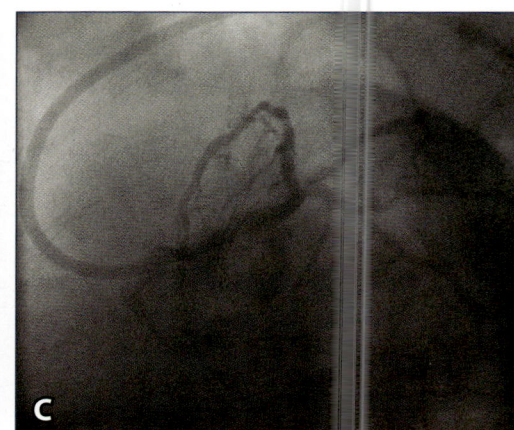

C

Figure 12-23. Ostial lesions of the left anterior descending artery and left circumflex arteries pose a significant challenge because of the tendency of plaque in the diseased vessel to be pushed into the other vessel resulting in lumen compromise of the second vessel. Patients are often referred for coronary artery bypass grafting for ostial left anterior descending or ostial left circumflex coronary artery if coronary intervention is not felt to be safe or feasible. **A,** Ostial lesion of the left anterior descending artery. **B,** Stent deployment following balloon predilatation. Note second coronary guidewire (*arrow*) placed in the large ramus medianus for protection from plaque shift. **C,** Final angiographic result.

Bifurcation Lesions

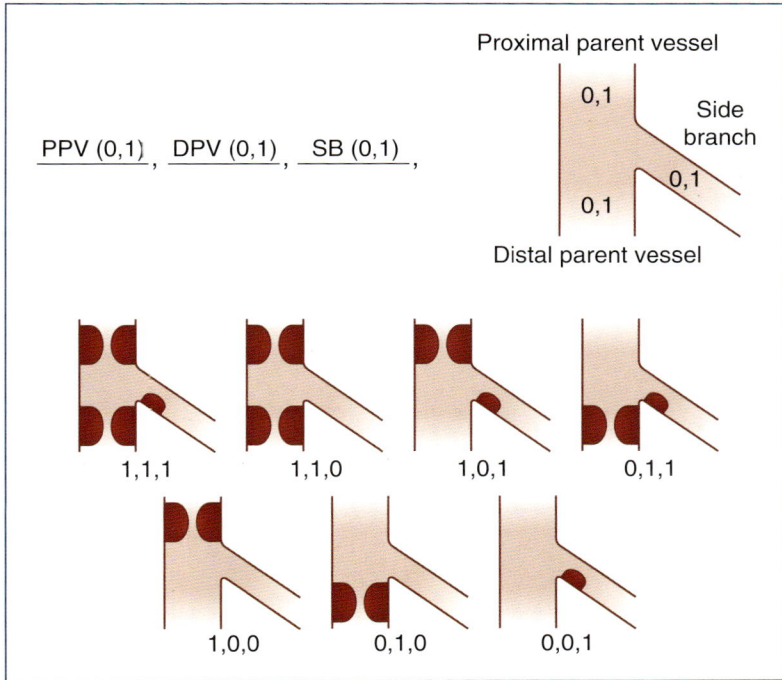

Figure 12-24. The Medina classification of bifurcation lesions [10]. Numerous classifications for bifurcation lesions have been proposed; however, the Medina classification is the simplest to understand. Significant obstruction is noted by *1* and no obstruction is noted by *0*. The lesion is then classified with a three-number system, with the first number representing the proximal parent vessel, the second number representing the distal parent vessel, and the third number representing the side branch.

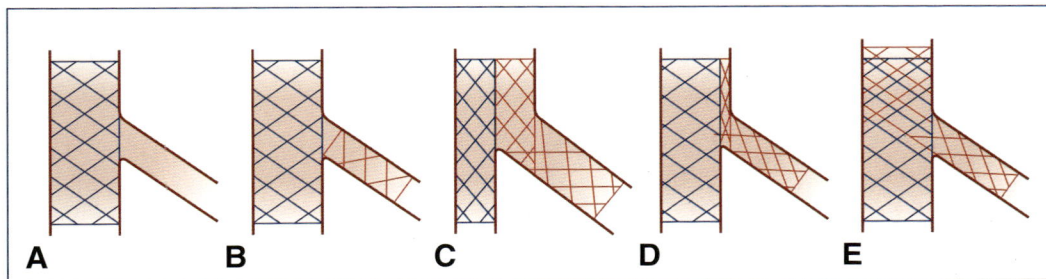

Figure 12-25. Stenting techniques for bifurcation lesions. **A,** Stenting of the main branch with balloon only of the side branch. This is the most common method of bifurcation stenting. **B,** T-stenting. The side branch is first stented, then the parent vessel. Although technically simple, T-stenting can result in incomplete coverage of the ostium of the side branch. **C,** Simultaneous kissing stent. Two stents are simultaneously deployed in a side-by-side fashion. **D,** Crush technique. The side-branch stent is first deployed with the proximal portion of the stent crushed by the deployment of the parent vessel stent. **E,** Culotte technique. The side branch is stented first with the stent originating in the parent vessel. Through the side branch stent, the parent vessel stent is deployed. For all techniques, a final kissing balloon inflation is performed after stent deployment.

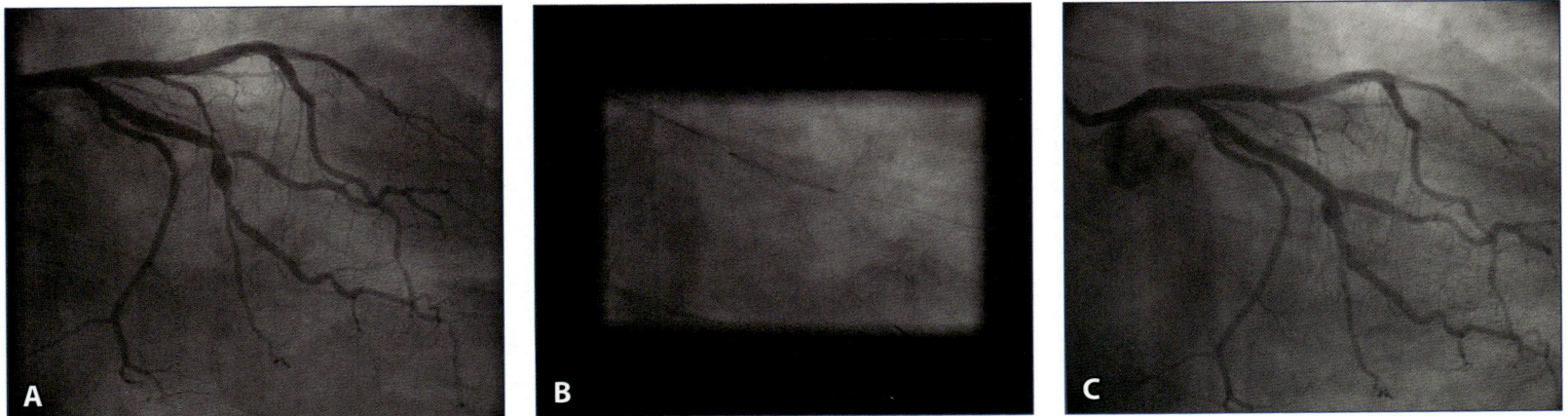

Figure 12-26. Example of the culotte bifurcation stent technique. **A,** Bifurcation lesion with significant disease in the parent vessel and side-branch with planned culotte stenting approach. **B,** Stent positioning of the side branch stent after placement of the parent vessel stent. **C,** Final angiographic result.

Total Occlusion

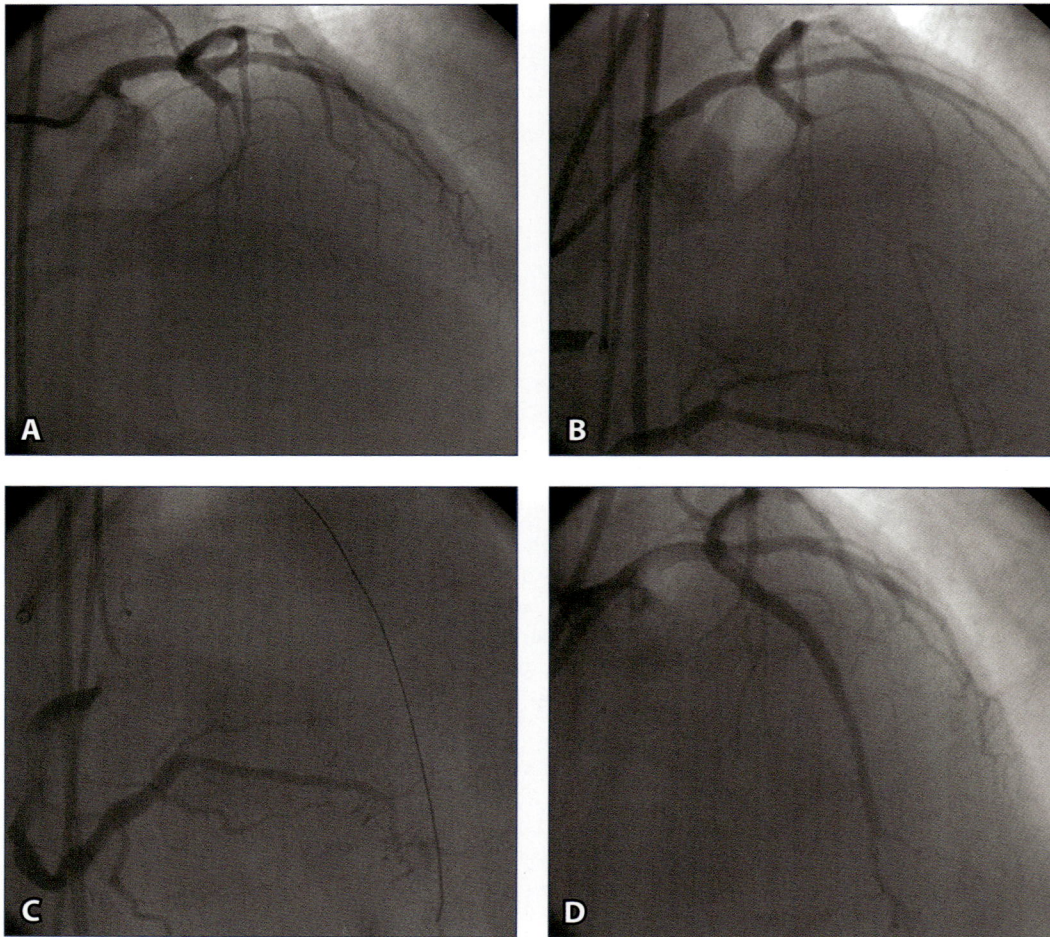

Figure 12-27. Chronic total occlusion. Chronic total occlusions remain the most technically challenging lesion subset to treat with percutaneous coronary intervention. There have been recent advancements in guidewire technology as well as novel techniques that have enhanced the outcomes of total occlusion intervention. **A,** Total occlusion of the left anterior descending artery. **B,** Simultaneous injection of the left coronary and right coronary artery to better delineate the length of occlusion. **C,** Use of contralateral injection to ensure intraluminal position of guidewire. **D,** Final result.

Thrombus-Containing Lesions

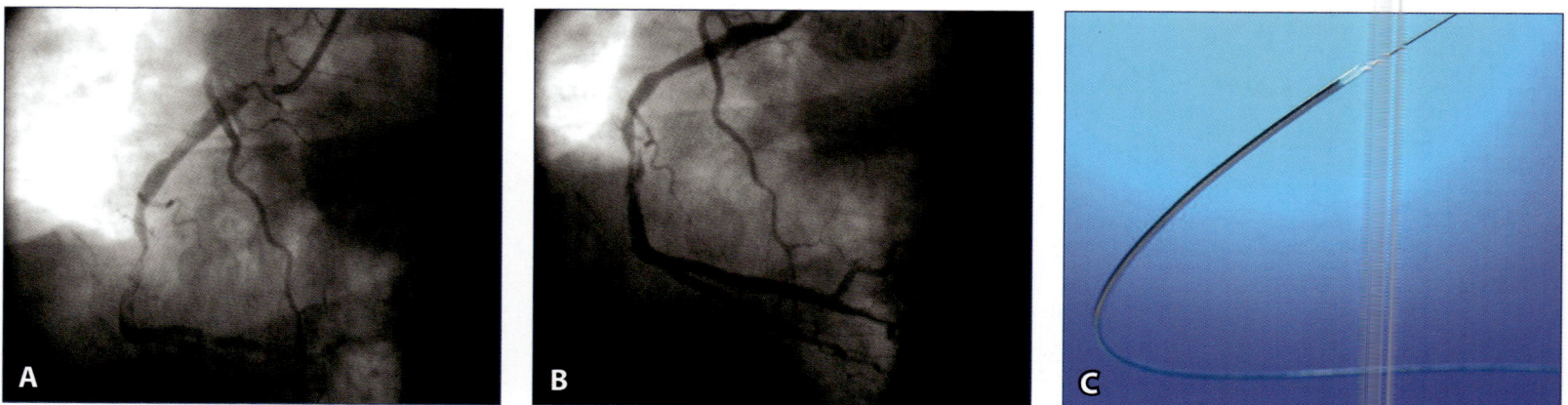

Figure 12-28. Thrombus-containing lesions. Thrombus-containing lesions are common particularly in acute coronary syndromes such as ST-segment elevation myocardial infarction. Recent studies have suggested an improvement in outcomes with thrombus removal using a thrombectomy catheter during percutaneous treatment of ST-segment elevation myocardial infarction [11]. **A,** Right coronary with thrombus in a young man presenting with ST-segment elevation myocardial infarction. **B,** Result after thrombectomy with the Export catheter (*Courtesy of* Medtronic, Santa Rosa, CA). **C,** Export catheter (*Courtesy of* Medtronic). This device consists of a suction catheter attached to a syringe at negative pressure. Once the catheter is in place, the syringe is opened to the catheter resulting in aspiration of vessel contents.

Continued on the next page

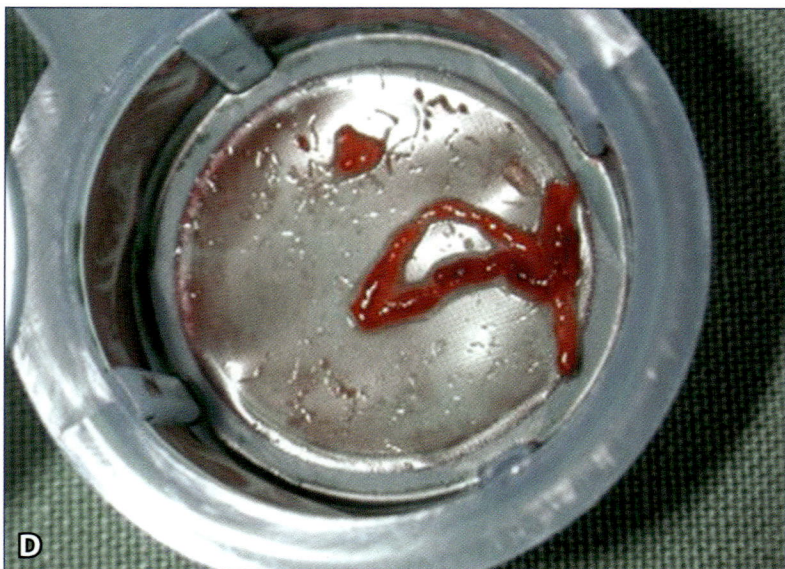

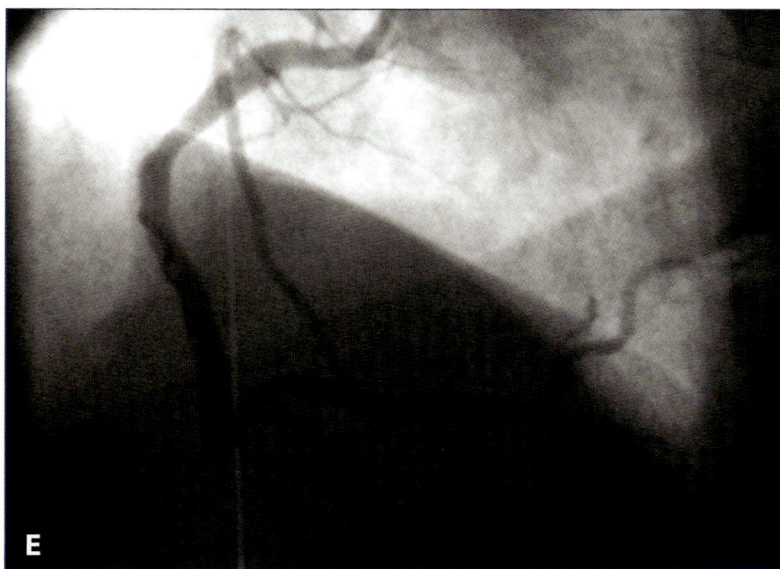

Figure 12-28. *(Continued)* **D,** Thrombus removed after Export thrombectomy. **E,** Final result after stenting.

Calcified Lesions

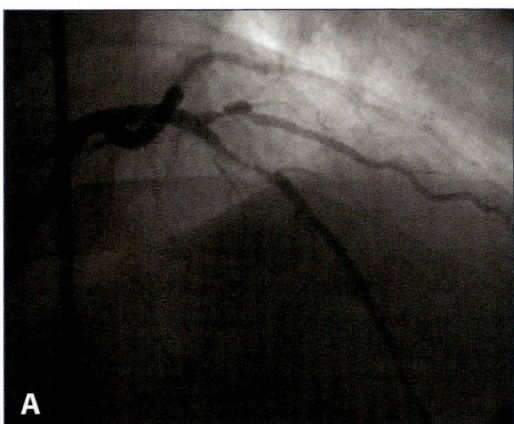

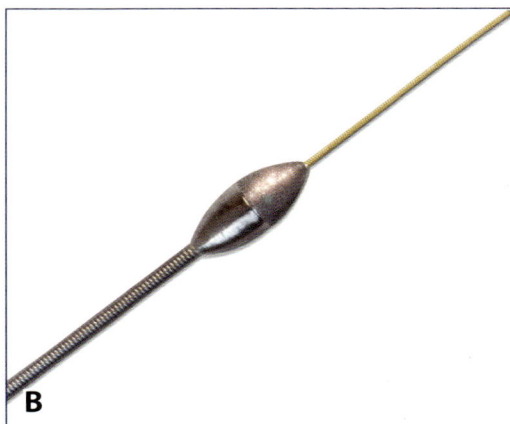

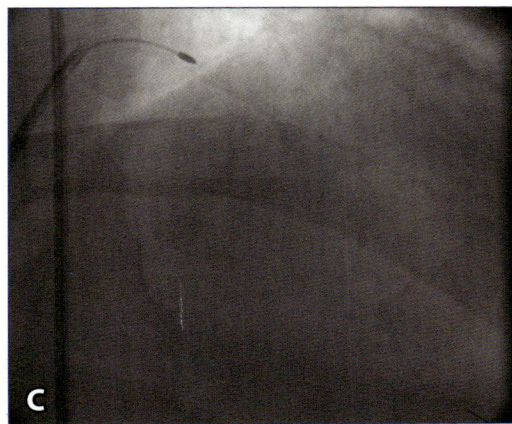

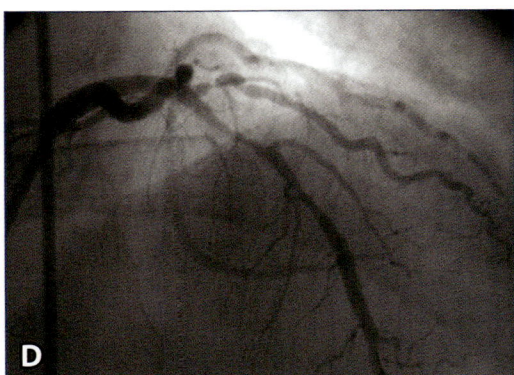

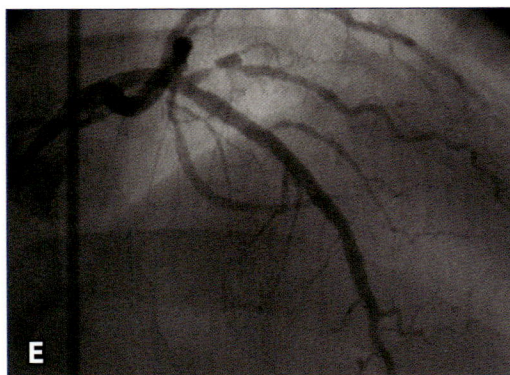

Figure 12-29. Treatment of calcified lesions. **A,** Heavily calcified left anterior descending artery lesion in a patient with exertional angina and stress test showing anterior ischemia. Calcification of the artery was evident on fluoroscopy before injection of contrast. Heavily calcified lesions pose a unique challenge to percutaneous intervention as device advancement and lesion dilatation can be difficult if not impossible. Often, rotational atherectomy is used to debulk the calcification before predilatation and stent deployment. In this case, a 1.5 mm balloon could not be advanced for predilatation. **B,** Rotational atherectomy burr. Rotational atherectomy is a niche device and used mostly to treat calcified, undilatable lesions. The burrs are available in diameters ranging from 1.25 mm to 2.25 mm. The distal half of the burr is covered with diamond chips. The burr rotates at 150,000 to 180,000 RPM and ablates inelastic (*ie,* calcified) plaque without injuring healthy elastic tissue. Clinical trials of rotational atherectomy have failed to show a clear benefit of rotational atherectomy in terms of reduction of restenosis; however, it remains an important device in coronary interventional practice for the treatment of heavily calcified lesions. (*Courtesy of* Boston Scientific, Natick, MA.) **C,** Treatment of a heavily calcified lesion in *A,* with a 1.5 mm rotational atherectomy burr delivered proximal to the lesion. **D,** Result post-atherectomy with a 1.5 mm burr. **E,** Result following successful balloon delivery, lesion predilatation, and stenting.

Left Main Disease

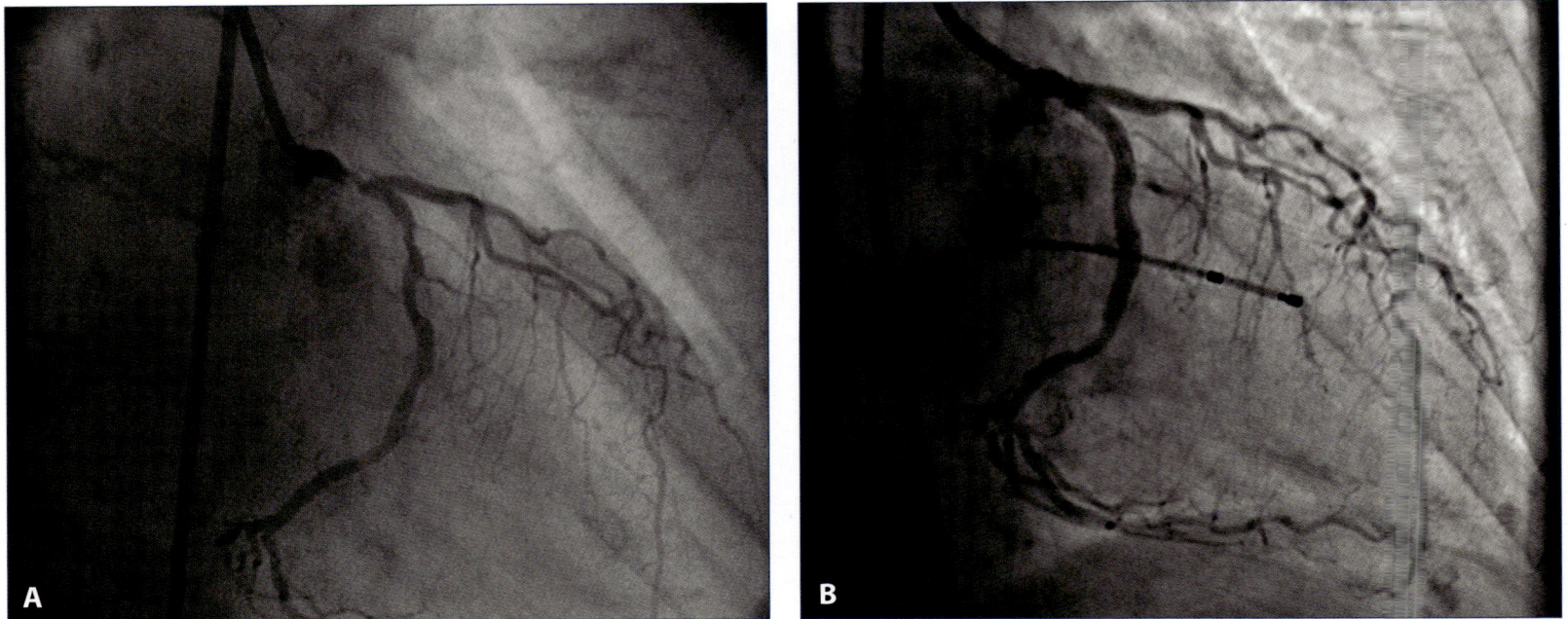

Figure 12-30. Coronary artery bypass grafting is still the revascularization strategy of choice for most patients with left main coronary artery disease. Numerous observational studies have shown excellent outcomes with left main stenting in the drug-eluting stent era, particularly in patients with ostial and midshaft left main disease. The results of percutaneous coronary intervention (PCI) for distal left main disease are not as favorable. Two randomized trials of PCI with drug-eluting stents versus coronary artery bypass grafting are under way (SYNTAX and FREEDOM) to determine the role of PCI for this challenging patient subset. **A,** Critical mid-to-distal left main stenosis in an elderly woman with exertional angina. This patient refused surgery and wished to proceed with PCI. **B,** Excellent angiographic result after culotte stenting with two drug-eluting stents.

In-Stent Restenosis

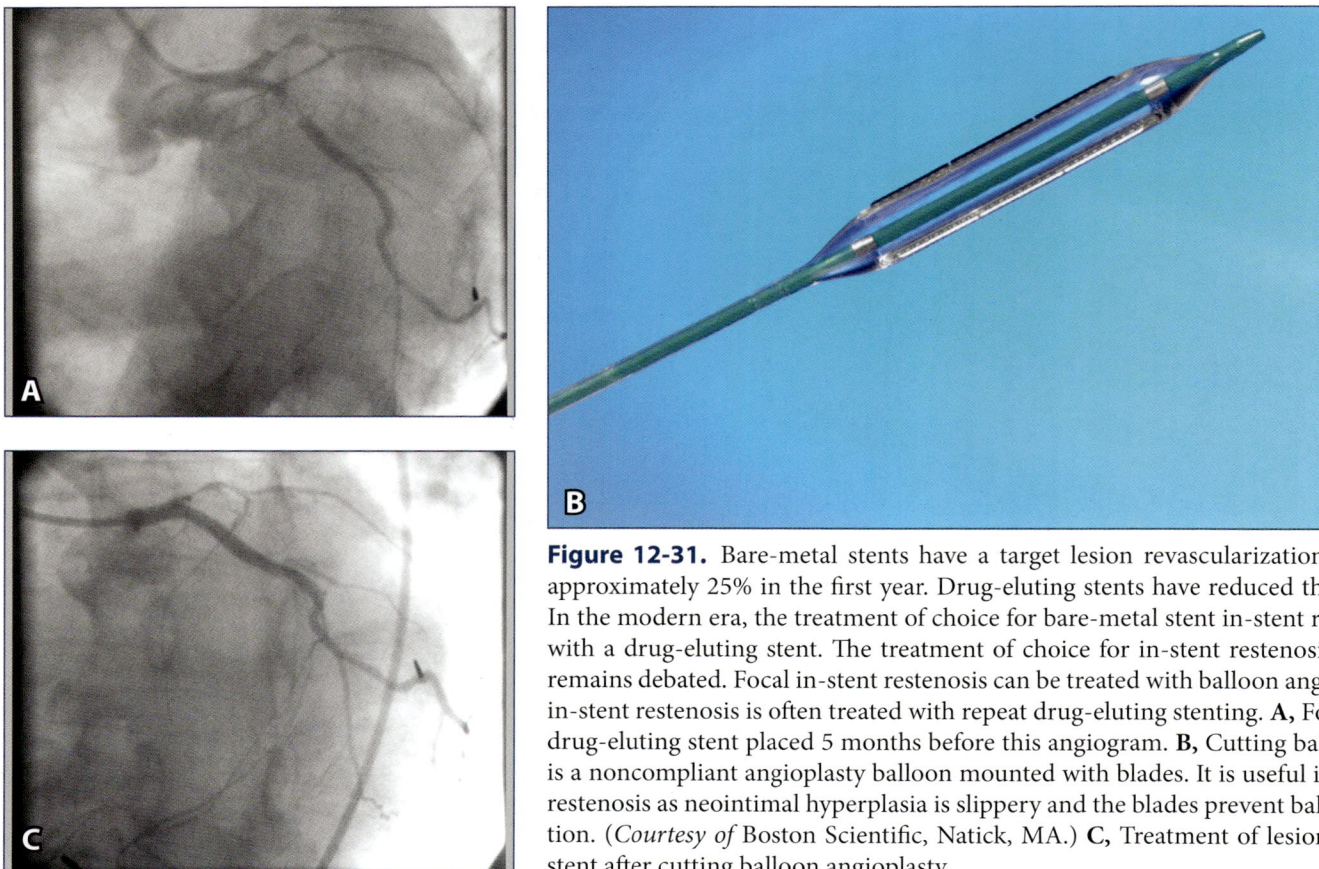

Figure 12-31. Bare-metal stents have a target lesion revascularization rate due to restenosis of approximately 25% in the first year. Drug-eluting stents have reduced this rate to about 5% to 7%. In the modern era, the treatment of choice for bare-metal stent in-stent restenosis is repeat stenting with a drug-eluting stent. The treatment of choice for in-stent restenosis with drug-eluting stents remains debated. Focal in-stent restenosis can be treated with balloon angioplasty only. More diffuse in-stent restenosis is often treated with repeat drug-eluting stenting. **A,** Focal in-stent restenosis in a drug-eluting stent placed 5 months before this angiogram. **B,** Cutting balloon. The Cutting balloon is a noncompliant angioplasty balloon mounted with blades. It is useful in the treatment of in-stent restenosis as neointimal hyperplasia is slippery and the blades prevent balloon slipping during inflation. (*Courtesy of* Boston Scientific, Natick, MA.) **C,** Treatment of lesion with repeat drug-eluting stent after cutting balloon angioplasty.

Saphenous Vein Grafts

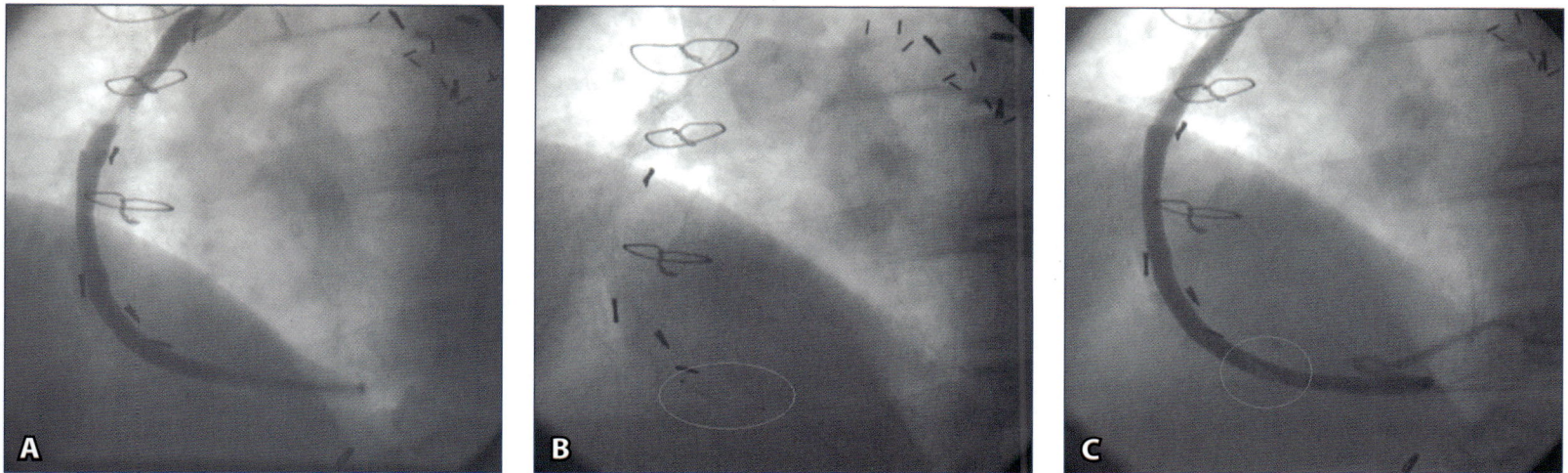

Figure 12-32. Intervention on saphenous vein grafts is associated with a significant risk of ischemic complications including no-reflow and periprocedural myocardial infarction. The SAFER (Saphenous Vein Graft Angioplasty Free of Emboli Randomized) trial showed a nearly 50% reduction in such complications with use of the GuardWire embolic protection device [12]. These devices are now considered standard of care for use in saphenous vein graft intervention. **A,** Bulky lesion in a saphenous vein graft to the distal right coronary artery. **B,** Spider FX (ev3, Plymouth, MN) embolic protection filter seen in vein graft before stent placement (*oval*). **C,** Result after stent deployment with embolic material seen in the distal filter (*oval*).

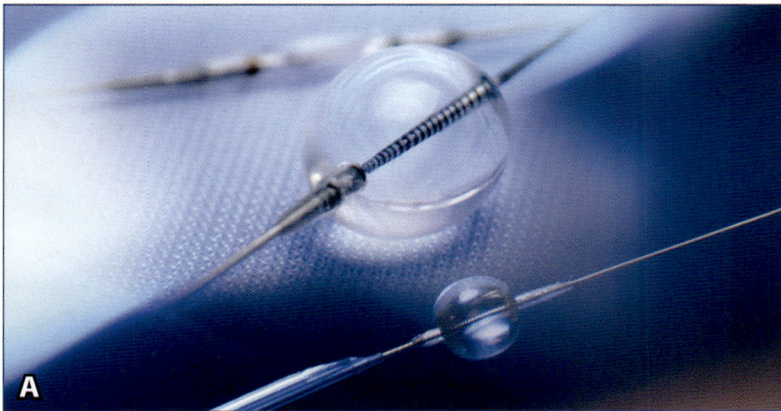

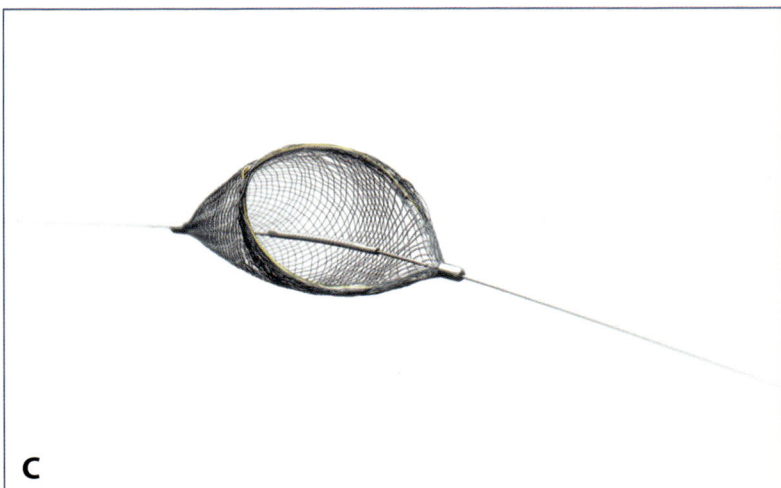

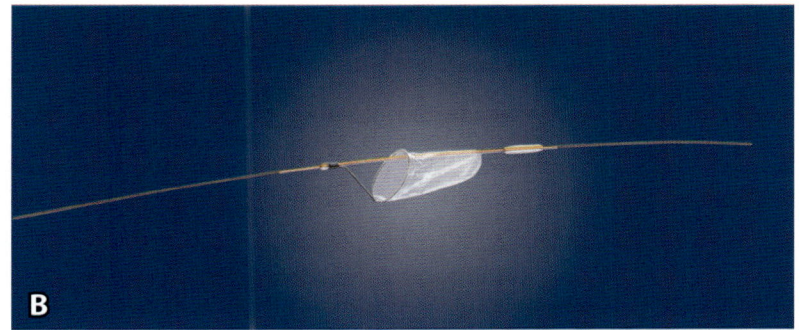

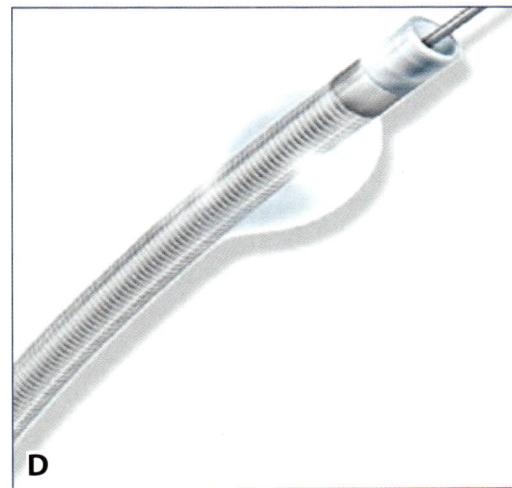

Figure 12-33. Approved embolic protection devices for saphenous vein graft intervention. **A,** GuardWire (Medtronic, Santa Rosa, CA). The GuardWire is a 0.014" coronary guidewire mounted with balloon that occludes the graft during intervention. The embolic material is then aspirated with an Export catheter (Medtronic) before deflating the balloon. (*Courtesy of* Medtronic.) **B,** FilterWire EZ (Boston Scientific, Natick, MA). A membrane filter is mounted on a coronary guidewire and delivered distal to the lesion before intervention and retrieved after intervention. (*Courtesy of* Boston Scientific.) **C,** Spider FX (ev3, Plymouth, MN). A nitinol based filter delivered distal to the lesion before intervention. (*Courtesy of* ev3.) **D,** Proxis (St. Jude Medical, St. Paul, MN). A proximal balloon is inflated, stopping anterograde flow while intervention is performed. Embolic material is then aspirated before deflation of the balloon. (*Courtesy of* St. Jude Medical.)

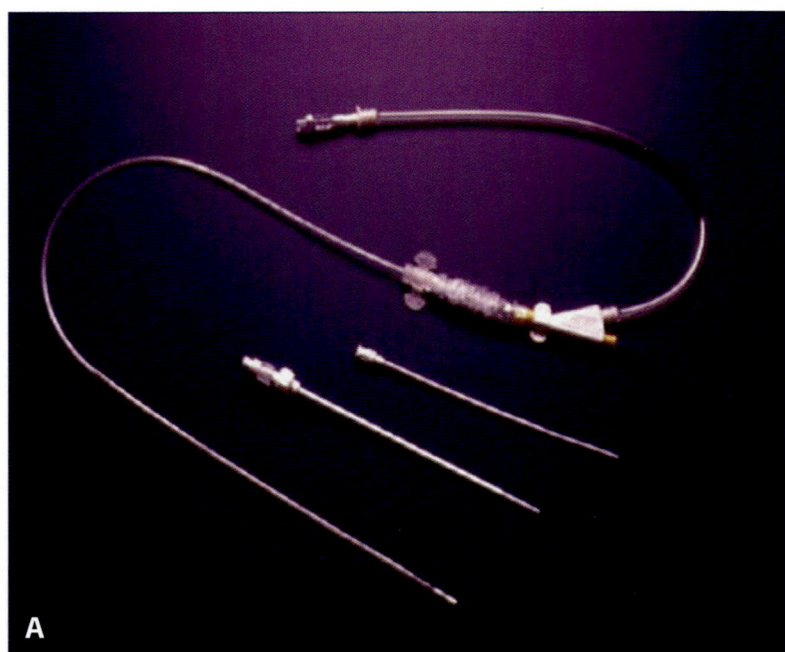

A

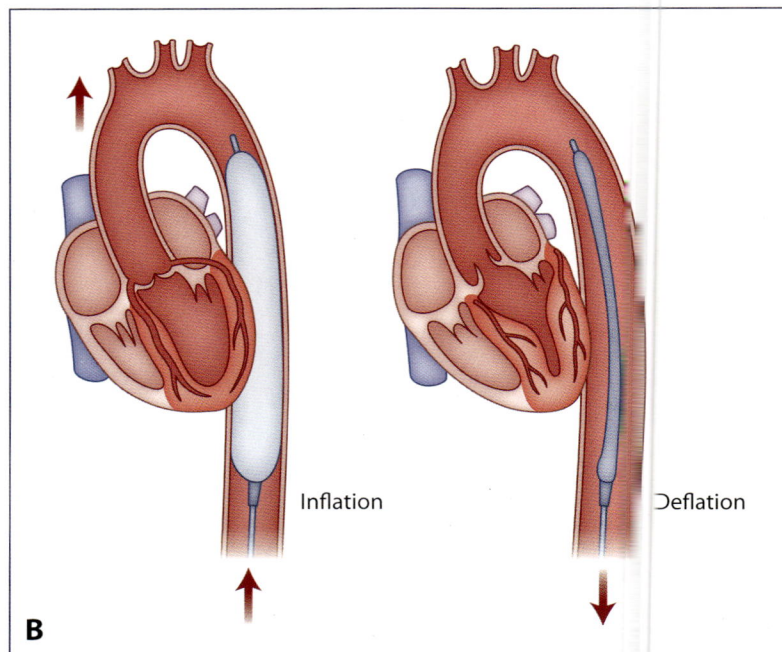

Inflation   Deflation

B

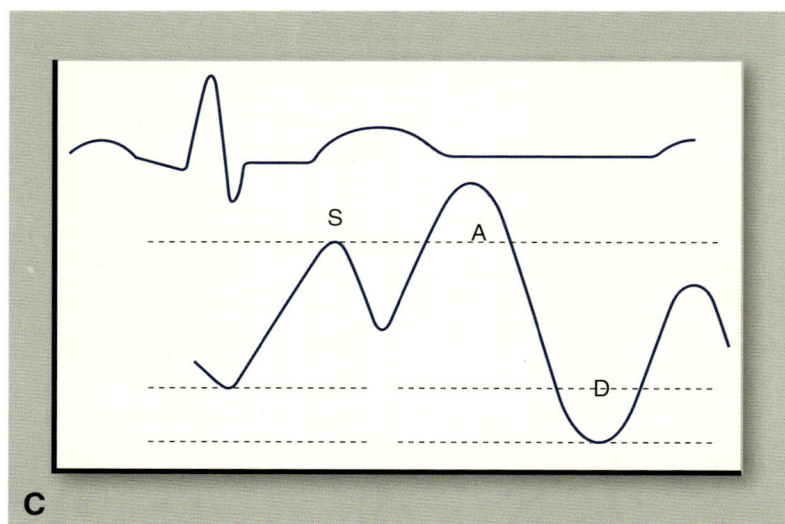

C

Figure 12-34. The intra-aortic balloon pump is the first-line hemodynamic assist device for the treatment of cardiogenic shock. **A,** Intra-aortic balloon pump catheter. **B,** The catheter inflates at the onset of diastole thereby enhancing coronary and systemic perfusion. Just before systole, the balloon deflates creating a maximally reduced afterload state thereby enhancing stroke volume. **C,** The patient's systolic pressure is noted by S. The pressure is augmented with balloon inflation noted by A and should be higher than the patient's systolic pressure. The diastolic pressure, enhanced by balloon deflation, is noted at D. (*Courtesy of* Datascope, Montvale, NJ.)

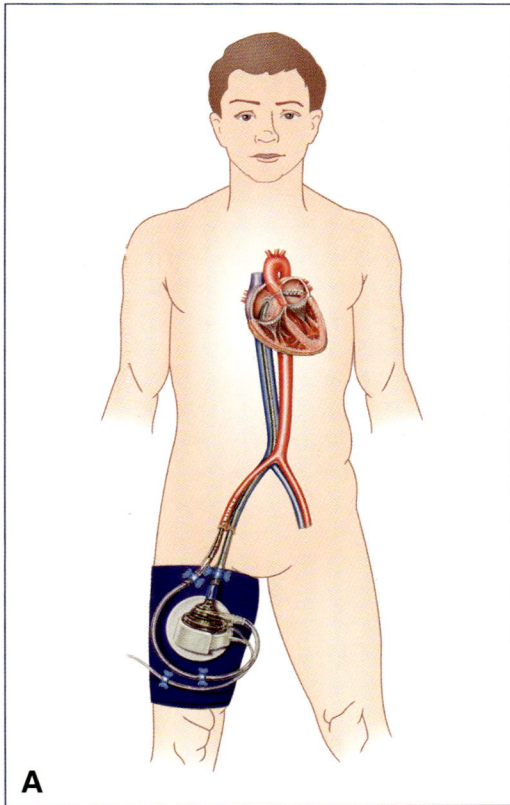

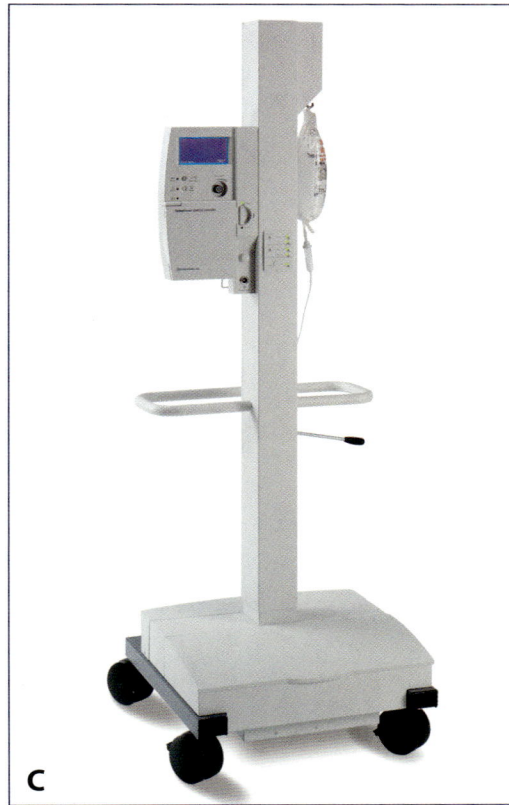

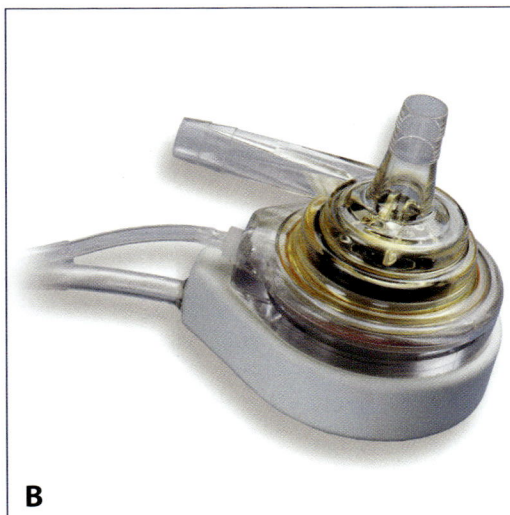

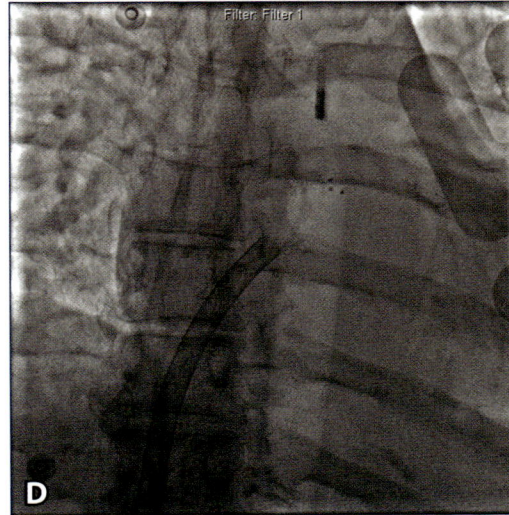

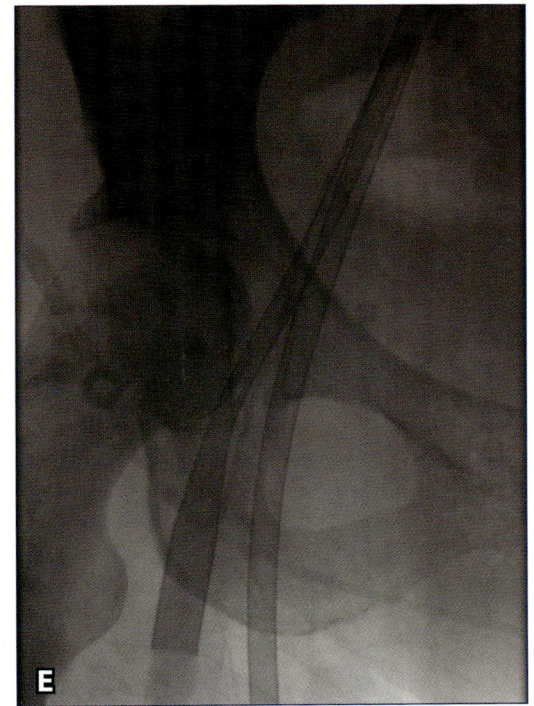

Figure 12-35. The Tandem Heart percutaneous ventricular assist device (Cardiac Assist, Pittsburgh, PA). This device provides continuous flow for the hemodynamic support of cardiogenic shock. **A,** Schematic of the Tandem Heart device. A 21 Fr venous cannula is inserted into the right common femoral vein and advanced transseptally into the left atrium and serves as the inflow cannula to the external pump attached to the patient's right lower extremity. A 17 Fr arterial cannula is inserted into the right common femoral artery and serves as the outflow cannula from the pump. Oxygenated blood is taken from the left atrium via the inflow cannula and pumped to the systemic circulation via the outflow cannula. **B,** The centrifugal pump is supported by a hydrodynamic fluid bearing and provides flow rates of up to 5 L/min. Flow rates are adjusted by the pump controller (**C**). (*Courtesy of* Cardiac Assist.) **D,** Fluoroscopic image of the chest showing the inflow cannula across the intra-atrial septum in the left atrium. **E,** Fluoroscopic image of the 17 Fr outflow cannula in the right common femoral artery.

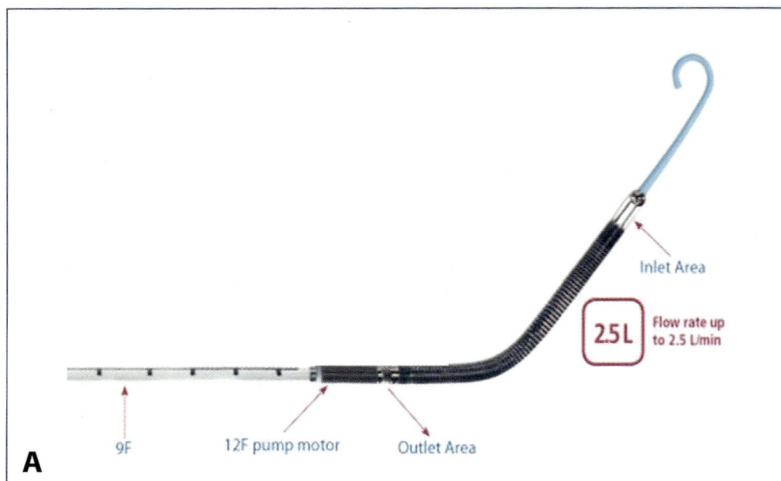

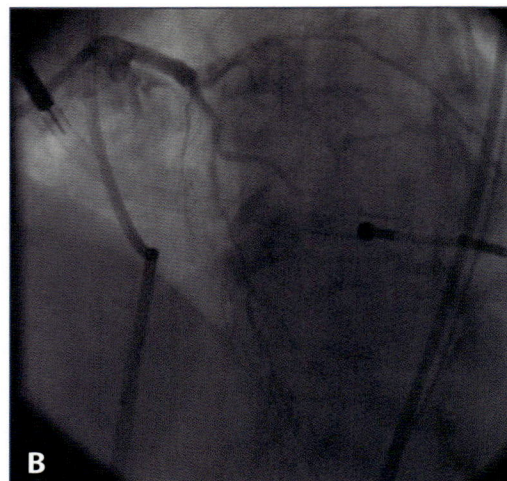

Figure 12-36. The Impella percutaneous ventricular assist device (Abiomed, Danvers, MA). **A,** The Impella device is a 9 Fr pigtail catheter that is advanced across the aortic valve into the left ventricle. A 12 Fr motor is housed at the angle of the pigtail. Using a screw mechanism, blood is removed from the left ventricle at the inlet area and pumped into the aorta at the outlet area. Flow rates of 2.5 L/min can be achieved. The device now has 510(k) approval by the US Food and Drug Administration for use. **B,** Fluoroscopic image of the chest showing the Impella device in the left ventricle during high-risk coronary intervention. (*Courtesy of* Abiomed.)

Peripheral Vascular Interventions

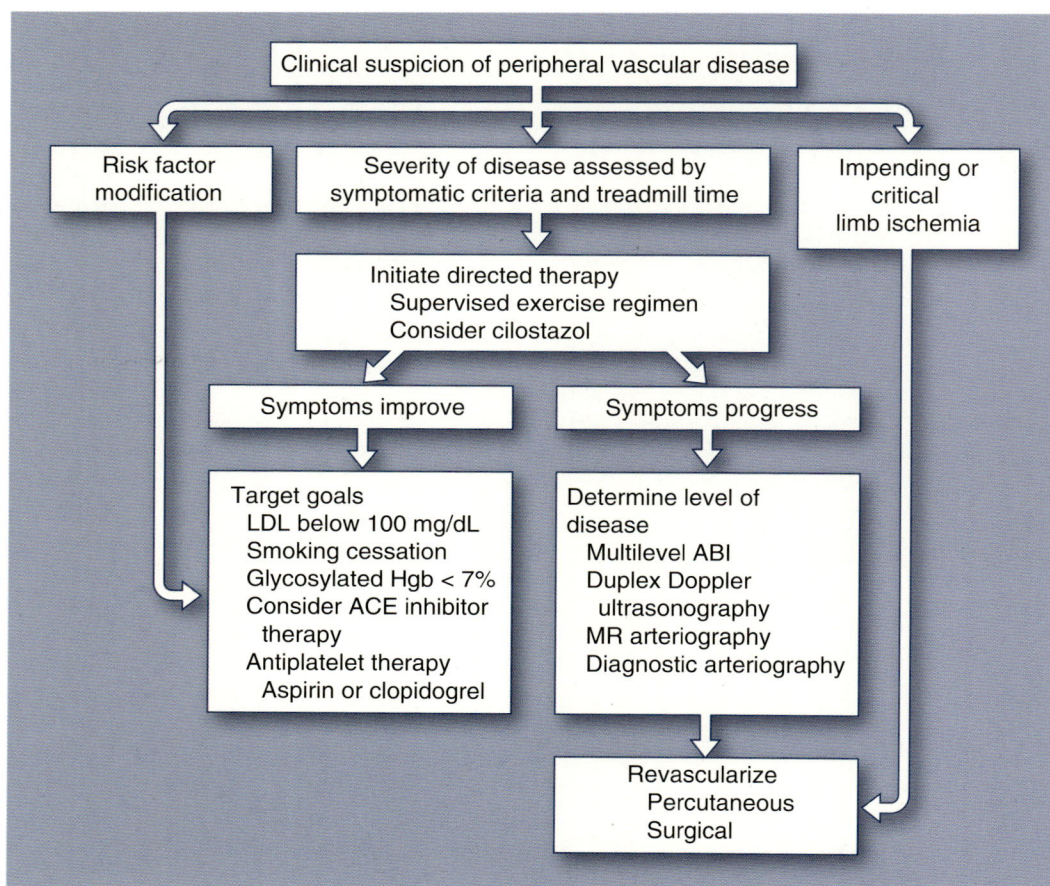

Figure 12-37. Clinical approach to and management of patients with suspected peripheral vascular disease. The incidence of peripheral arterial disease is increasing as the patient population becomes older. Some data suggest that peripheral arterial disease is often present but not diagnosed. This may relate to the fact that symptoms can be misinterpreted, the patient is not severely symptomatic, or there is limited expertise in examining the peripheral vascular tree. The clinical approach and management of patients with suspected peripheral arterial disease requires a heightened clinical suspicion of its presence. ABI—ankle brachial index; ACE—angiotensin-converting enzyme; Hgb—hemoglobin; LDL—low-density lipoprotein. (*Adapted from* Hiat [13].)

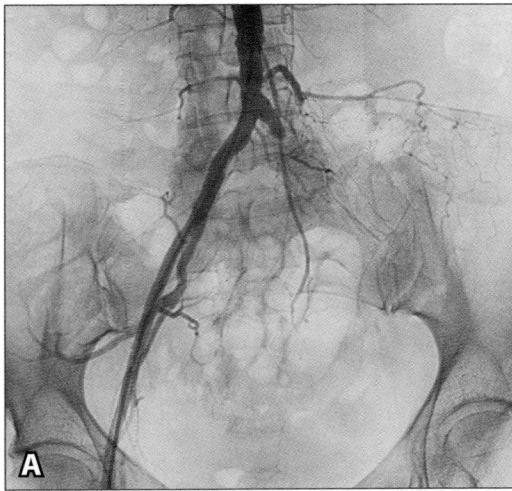

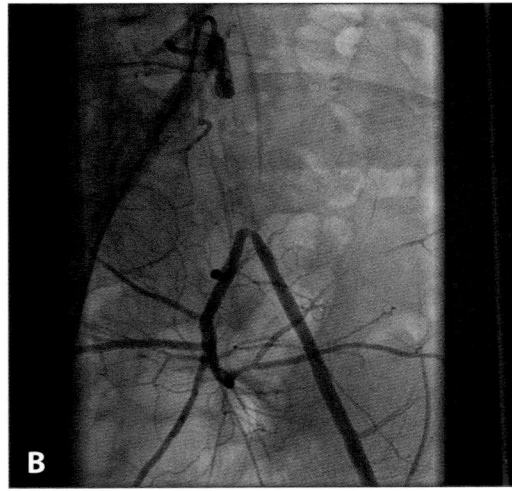

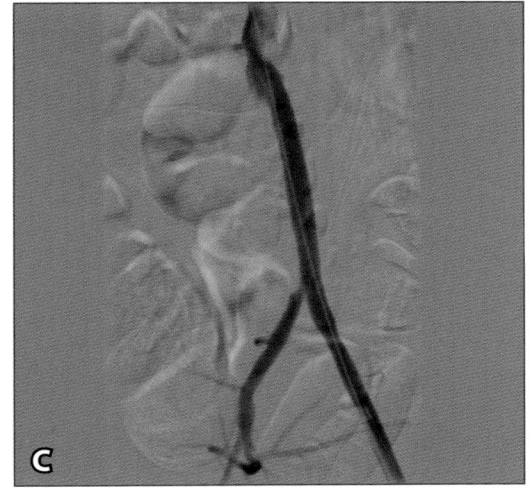

Figure 12-38. Iliac artery stenosis. Atherosclerotic disease of the iliac artery is effectively treated with percutaneous endovascular techniques. Proximal "in flow" disease frequently presents with lifestyle-limiting claudication. Resting ankle brachial index (ABI) can appear falsely normal and sometimes requires postexercise ABI assessment for accurate diagnosis. Diagnostic angiography in a patient with limiting left buttock and calf claudication depicts a proximally occluded left common iliac that reconstitutes at the bifurcation of the internal and external iliac arteries (**A** and **B**). Following balloon dilation and stent placement, final angiography demonstrates an excellent result (**C**).

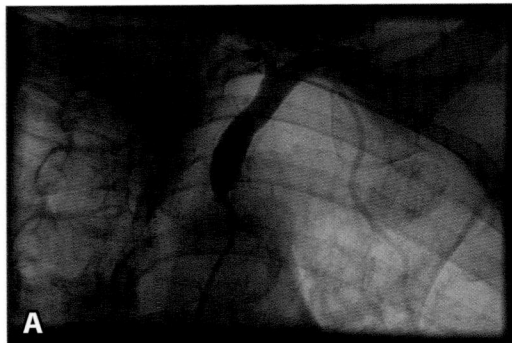

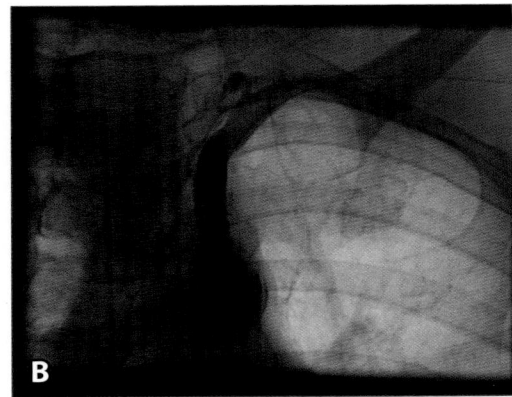

Figure 12-39. Subclavian stenosis. Subclavian artery stenosis can present as upper extremity claudication or angina in patients who have undergone coronary artery bypass grafting (CABG) with an internal mammary artery (IMA) graft. This patient presented with angina and anterior ischemia on stress testing following CABG. Diagnostic angiography demonstrates a severe ostial stenosis of the left subclavian artery (**A**) with no significant disease in the left IMA. Final angiography following balloon angioplasty and placement of a self expanding stent shows an excellent angiographic result (**B**).

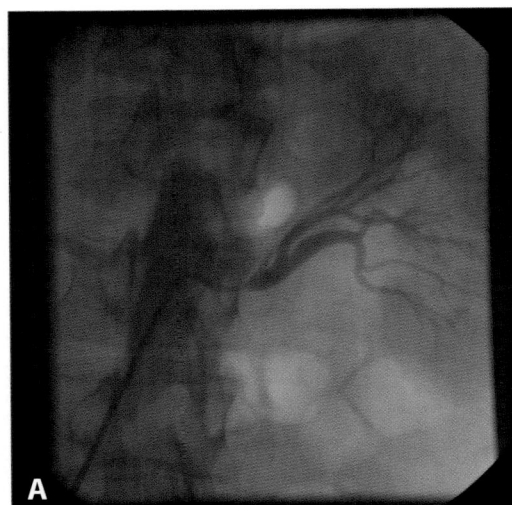

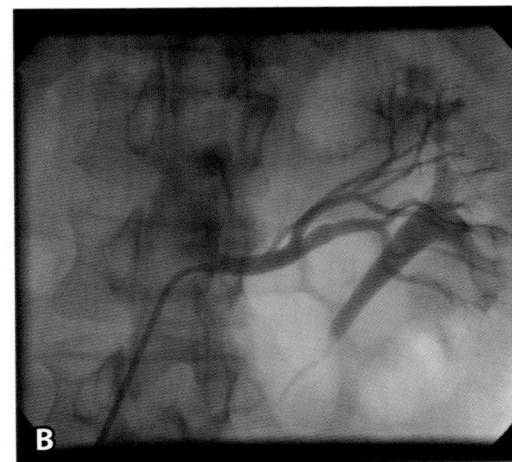

Figure 12-40. Renal artery stenosis. Renal artery stenosis frequently presents with hypertension refractory to multiple anti-hypertensive medications and renal insufficiency. Endovascular revascularization can provide improvement in blood pressure though rarely are patients able to discontinue all anti-hypertensive medications. Distal embolic protection devices may help preserve maximal renal function. Selective angiography of the left renal artery demonstrates a severe ostial stenosis (**A**). Due to the bifurcation of the renal artery in close proximity to the stenosis, distal protection was not used in this case. Following stent placement, final angiography demonstrated an excellent angiographic result (**B**).

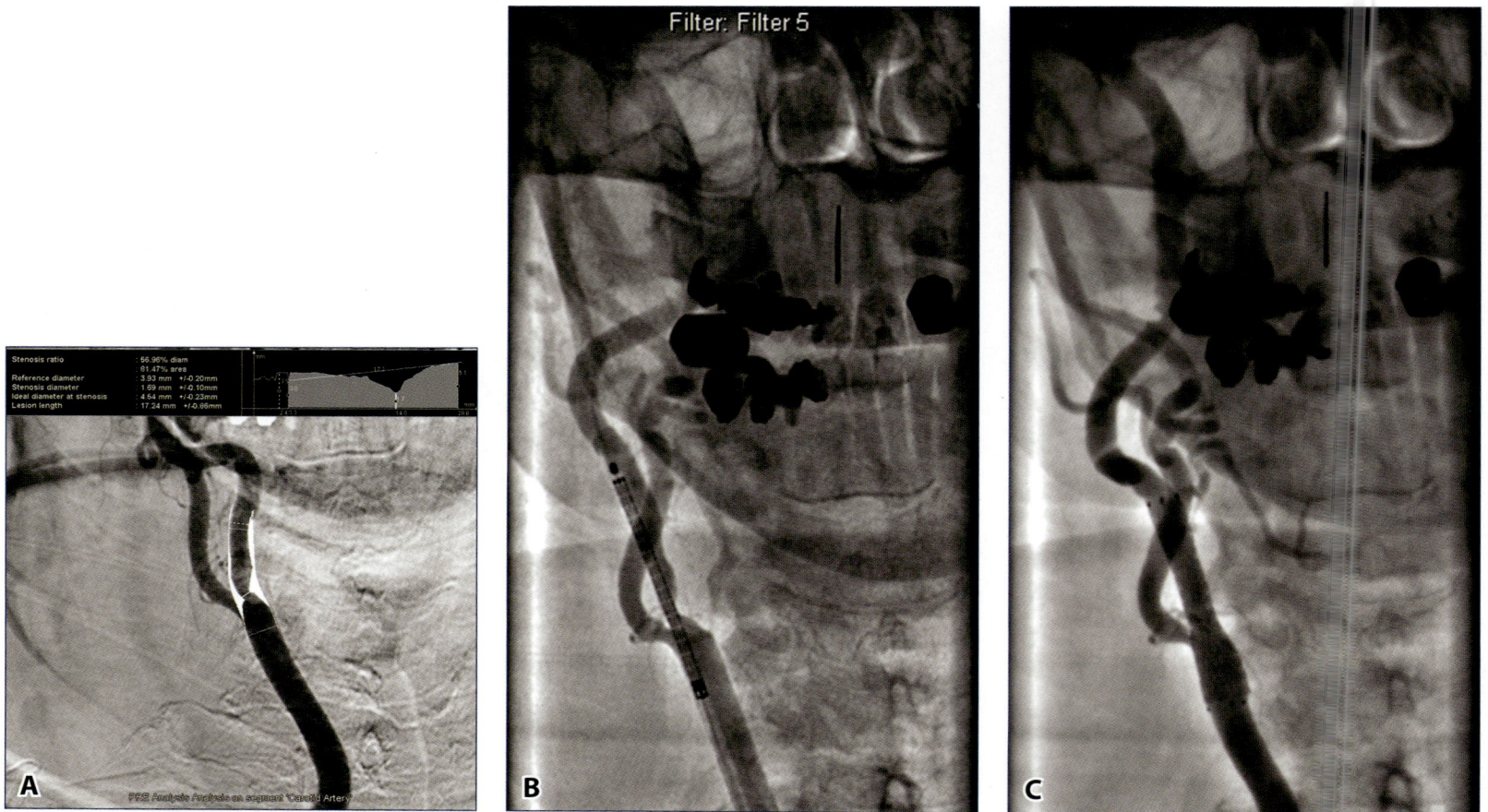

Figure 12-41. Carotid artery stenosis. Carotid artery stenting has emerged as an alternative to surgical carotid endarterectomy (CEA), particularly in patients who are at higher risk for surgical complications due to age, comorbidities, prior CEA with restenosis, neck irradiation, or difficult surgical access to the stenosis. Distal embolic protection is routinely used during carotid stenting to reduce the risk of periprocedural neurologic complications. This elderly patient with severe chronic obstructive pulmonary disease and coronary artery disease presented with a right hemispheric transient ischemic attack (TIA). A noninvasive carotid ultrasound demonstrated a greater than 50% stenosis of the right internal carotid artery (RICA). Angiography with quantitative measurements confirmed a greater than 50% stenosis of the RICA (**A**). After placement of a distal embolic protection device (**B**), balloon angioplasty and stenting were performed using a self-expanding stent. Final angiography (**C**) revealed an excellent angiographic result with only mild recoil and a residual stenosis of less than 20%.

Interventions for Structural Heart Disease

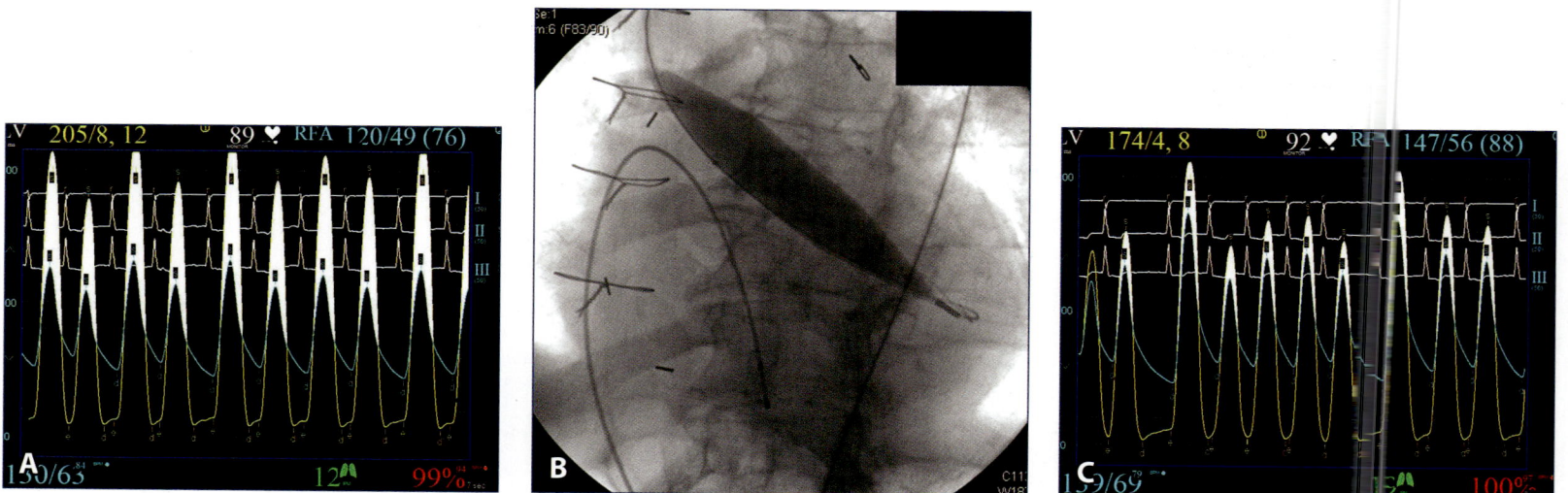

Figure 12-42. Aortic valvuloplasty. Balloon aortic valvuloplasty can be used as a bridge to aortic valve replacement surgery in unstable patients with intercurrent illnesses, or as palliative therapy for patients who are nonoperative candidates. **A,** Hemodynamic profile showing the gradient (*white*) between the left ventricular pressure (*yellow*) and the femoral arterial pressure (*blue*) before the procedure. **B,** The stenotic aortic valve is dilated with a 20 mm × 4 cm × 120 cm Atlas balloon (Bard Peripheral Vascular, Tempe, AZ) at high pressure. **C,** The gradient is dramatically lowered following balloon inflation. Unfortunately, recurrence of aortic stenosis usually occurs with time following aortic valvuloplasty.

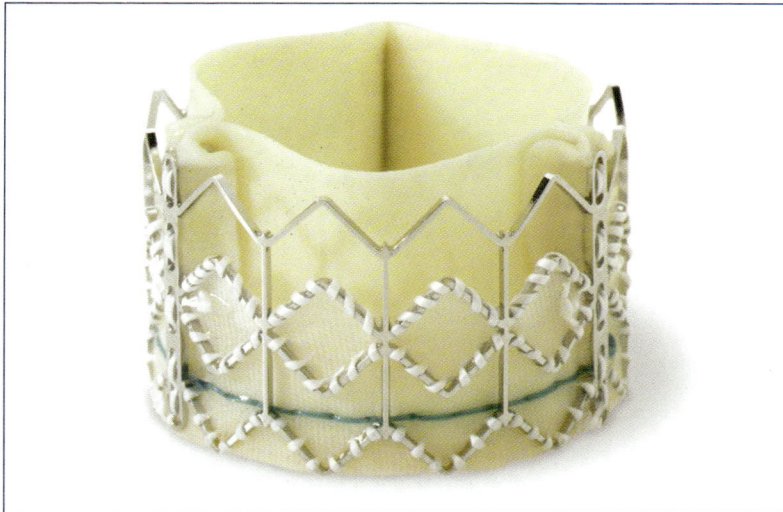

Figure 12-43. Percutaneous valve replacement. Percutaneous aortic valve technology is presently being evaluated in clinical trials as an alternative to surgical aortic valve replacement. This image shows the Edwards Sapien Transcatheter Heart Valve (Edwards LifeSciences, Irvine, CA). The valve is a porcine valve mounted on a balloon-expandable stainless steel stent. The device is mounted on a balloon, delivered across the aortic valve, and deployed with a balloon inflation. (*Courtesy of* Edwards LifeSciences.)

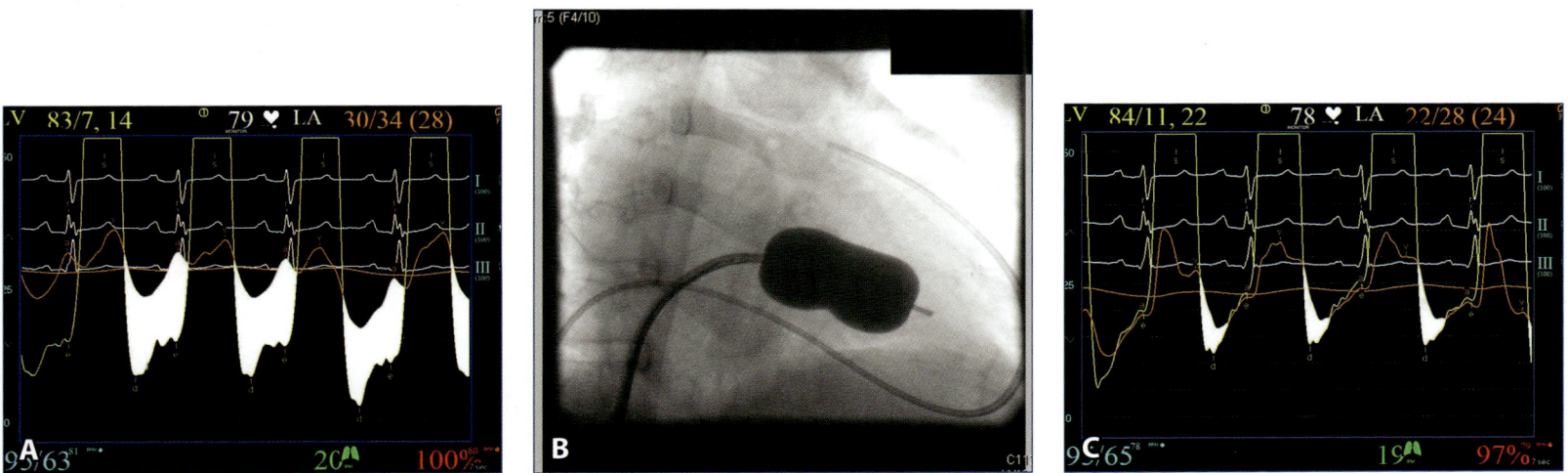

Figure 12-44. Mitral valvuloplasty. Balloon mitral valvuloplasty is the treatment of choice for symptomatic rheumatic mitral stenosis. **A,** Hemodynamic profile showing a significant transmitral gradient (*white*) between the left ventricular pressure (*yellow*) and the left atrial pressure (*orange*) in a patient with rheumatic mitral stenosis. **B,** A 28 mm Inoue balloon (Toray Industries, Tokyo, Japan) is inflated across the mitral valve. The "waist" in the balloon is positioned at the level of the mitral valve. **C,** Hemodynamic profile showing significant reduction of gradient after balloon inflation.

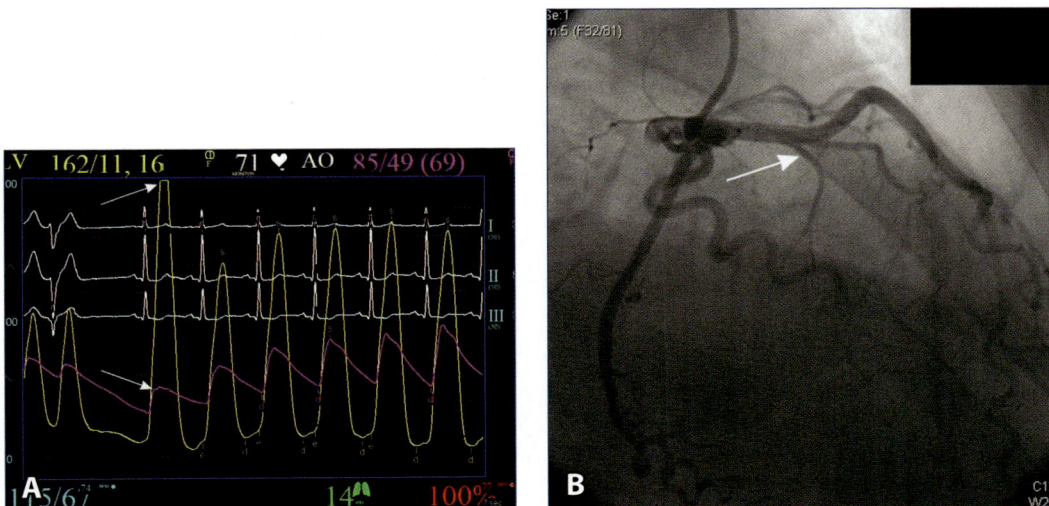

Figure 12-45. Alcohol septal ablation for hypertrophic cardiomyopathy. Alcohol septal ablation is used as an alternative to surgical myomectomy for left ventricular outflow tract reduction in patients with hypertrophic cardiomyopathy and symptomatic elevation of outflow tract gradient. **A,** Hemodynamic profile showing a significant gradient between the left ventricle (*yellow*) and the aorta (*pink*). Note the increased systolic left ventricular pressure and decreased systemic arterial pressure following a premature ventricular contraction (Braunwald-Brockenbrough sign). **B,** Angiogram of the left coronary circulation in the same patient. The most proximal septal branch of the left anterior descending artery (*arrow*) is chosen for alcohol injection as it corresponds to the greatest level of septal hypertrophy on echocardiography.

Continued on the next page

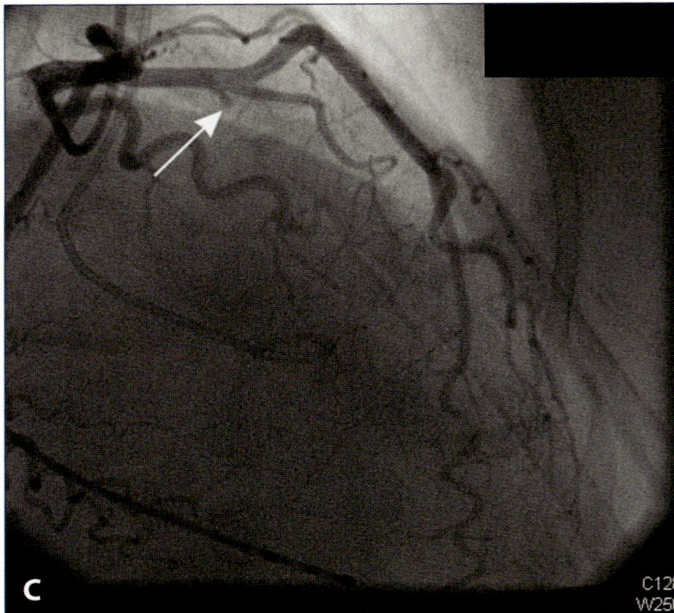

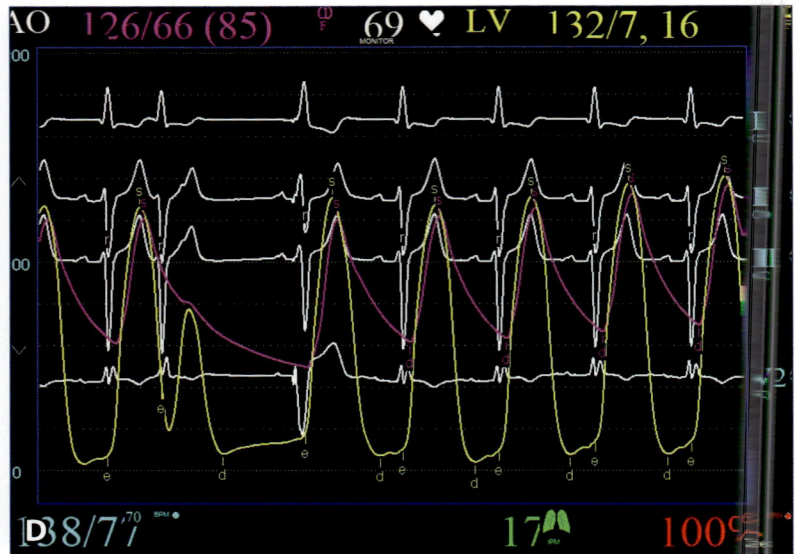

Figure 12-45. *(Continued)* **C,** After alcohol injection into the septal branch, the septal branch shows no flow correlating with the localized myocardial infarct induced by the alcohol. **D,** Postprocedure hemo-dynamics showing significant reduction in gradient and elimination of the Braunwald-Brockenbrough sign.

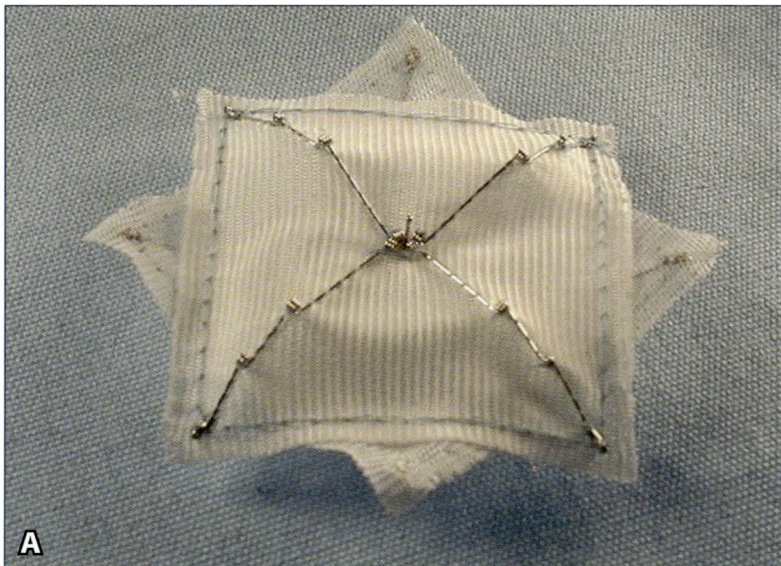

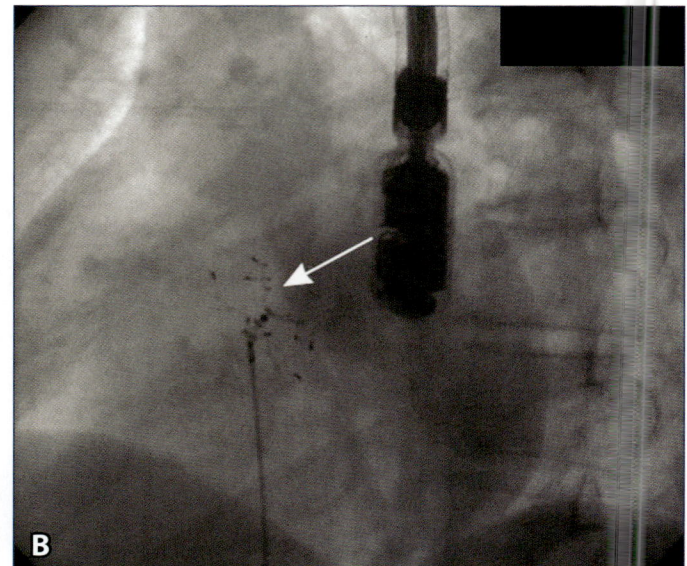

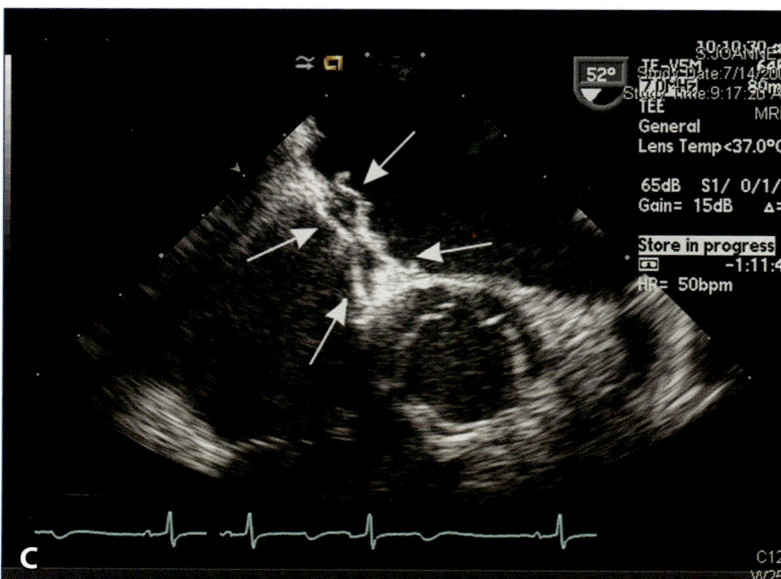

Figure 12-46. Patent foramen ovale closure. Several atrial septal closure devices can be used for closure of patient foramen ovale in patients with cryptogenic stroke. These devices are not presently approved for this indication and are being evaluated in clinical trials. **A,** The CardioSeal device (NMT Medical, Boston, MA) consists of two fabric "umbrellas" held open by nitinol arms. The device sits across the patent foramen ovale with one side on the left atrial side of the septum and the other side on the right atrial side. **B,** Fluoroscopic image of a 28 mm CardioSeal device placed across a patent foramen ovale. **C,** Echocardiogram showing the device in place (*arrows*) and sealing the foramen ovale.

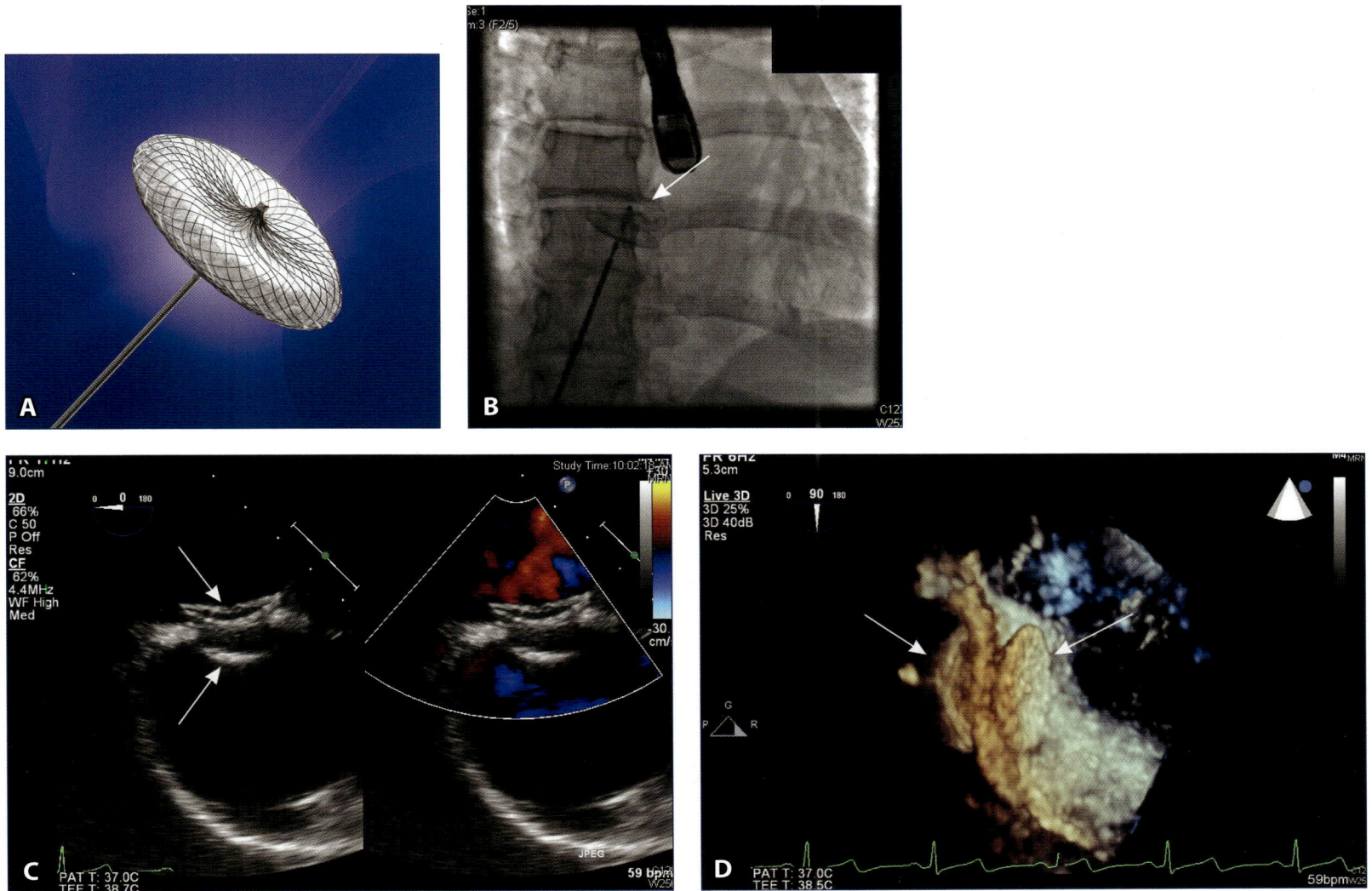

Figure 12-47. Atrial septal defect closure. Ostium secundum atrial septal defects can be closed percutaneously in selected patients with an approved atrial septal occluder device. **A,** The Amplatzer device (AGA Medical, Minneapolis, MN) is presently approved for secundum atrial septal defect closure and consists of two nitinol discs that sit on either side of the intra-atrial septum. Within each disc is a fabric membrane that enhances endothelialization of the device. (*Courtesy of* AGA Medical, Minneapolis, MN). **B,** Fluoroscopic image of an Amplatzer deployed across a secundum atrial septal defect. **C,** Intraprocedural transesophageal echocardiographic image showing an Amplatzer device successfully placed across a secundum atrial septal defect. **D,** Three-dimensional echocardiograph image demonstrating the Amplatzer device successfully placed across a secundum atrial septal defect.

References

1. Schwartz RS, Murphy JG, Edwards WD, *et al.*: Restenosis occurs with internal elastic lamina laceration and is proportional to severity of vessel injury in a porcine coronary artery model [abstract]. *Circulation* 1990, 82:III–656.

2. Pijls NH, De Bruyne B, Peels K, *et al.*: Measurement of fractional flow reserve to assess the functional severity of coronary-artery stenoses. *N Engl J Med* 1996, 334:1703–1708.

3. De Bruyne B, Bartunek J, Sys SU, Heyndrickx GR: Relation between myocardial fractional flow reserve calculated from coronary pressure measurements and exercise-induced myocardial ischemia. *Circulation* 1995, 92:39–46.

4. Stone GW, Moses JW, Ellis SG, *et al.*: Safety and efficacy of sirolimus- and paclitaxel-eluting coronary stents. *N Engl J Med* 2007, 356:998–1008.

5. Kimura T, Tamura T, Yokoi H, *et al.*: Long-term clinical and angiographic follow-up after placement of Palmaz-Schatz coronary stent: a single center experience. *J Intervent Cardiol* 1994, 7:129–139.

6. Mehran R, Dangas G, Abizaid AS, *et al.*: Angiographic patterns of in-stent restenosis: classification and implications for long-term outcome. *Circulation* 1999, 100:1872–1878.

7. Curfman GD, Morrisey S, Jarcho JA, *et al.*: Drug-eluting stents: promise and uncertainty. *N Engl J Med* 2007, 356:1059–1060.

8. Sudhir K: Abbott Vascular Drug Eluting Stent Program. FDA Presentation SE2925108A. December 8, 2006. Available at http://www.fda.gov/ohrms/dockets/ac/06/slides/2006-4253oph2_18_Sudhir.pdf.

9. Mauri L, Hsieh W, Massaro JM, *et al.*: Stent thrombosis in randomized clinical trials of drug-eluting stents. *N Engl J Med* 2007, 356:1020–1029.

10. Medina A, Suarez de Lezo J, Pan M: A new classification of coronary bifurcation lesions [in Spanish]. *Rev Esp Cardiol* 2006, 59:183.

11. Svilaas T, Vlaar PJ, van der Horst I, *et al.*: Thrombus aspiration during primary percutaneous coronary intervention. *N Engl J Med* 2008, 358:557–567.

12. Baim DS, Wahr D, George B, *et al.*: Randomized trial of distal embolic protection device during percutaneous intervention of saphenous vein aorto-coronary bypass grafts. *Circulation* 2002, 105:1285–1290.

13. Hiat R: Medical treatment of peripheral arterial disease and claudication. *N Engl J Med* 2001, 344:1608–1621.

Echocardiography

13

Judy Mangion and Scott D. Solomon

Echocardiography remains the most common imaging modality in cardiovascular medicine. An echocardiographic study requires no patient exposure to radiation, and uses ultrasound and Doppler technology to seamlessly combine anatomy and physiology to provide clinicians with real-time information about cardiac chamber size and morphology, ventricular systolic and diastolic function, and valvular morphology and function—more combined information than available with any other imaging modality. The technology continues to advance with frequent improvements in image quality, portability, and morphologic and quantitative modalities—such as three-dimensional echocardiography—that offer more sophisticated ways to visualize the heart. Indeed, echocardiographic studies can be performed in a laboratory, at bedside in the most advanced hospitals, and even in remote locations.

Echocardiography is by nature a visual specialty, and the images in this chapter illustrate the basic principles of echocardiography, emphasizing the use of this technology in the care of patients with heart disease, and highlighting some of the newer technologies that continue to maintain echocardiography on the cutting edge of cardiovascular imaging.

Principles of Echocardiography

Figure 13-1. Physical principles of echocardiography. Ultrasound waves are high-frequency sound waves that have a general range of more than a million cycles per second. In contrast, sound that is audible to humans falls within the 20 to 20,000 Hz range. The oscillatory nature of sound waves is caused by the compression and rarefaction of particles. The properties of ultrasound (as is the case in all waves) include 1) frequency (f): the number of cycles occurring per second; 2) wavelength (λ): the length of the wave—one cycle; and 3) velocity (c): propagation speed or velocity. These properties are related by the equation $c = f\lambda$ (*top panel*).

Amplitude represents the "height" or power of the wave. The intensity represents the power in watts divided by the area in square centimeters. Ultrasound waves are subject to attenuation—the decrease in amplitude relative to the distance traveled as sound waves weaken as they travel through a medium.

Ultrasound waves are primarily reflected from the boundaries between tissues of different acoustic impedance (*bottom panel*). This type of reflection is referred to as a "specular" reflection. Although part of the ultrasound is reflected as the echo, a percentage is transmitted (transmission) through the reflector. Ultrasound waves can interact with tissue in the following ways: 1) Refraction is a change in the direction of a non–perpendicular incident ultrasound beam without a change in frequency. This results in the bending of a portion of the incident ultrasound waves away from the main beam axis. 2) Scattering is a combination of reflection and refraction of incident ultrasound waves within tissues, which diverts them in multiple directions. Interaction with tissues and tissue boundaries produces a pattern of echoes that are characteristic of the tissues imaged, which gives them their signature appearance. Hyperechoic structures produce greater amplitude of reflections and appear white. Hypoechoic tissues produce echoes with smaller amplitudes and appear as various shades of gray. Anechoic or echolucent structures appear echo-free because they completely absorb all the incident ultrasound waves. 3) Attenuation refers to the loss of amplitude or beam intensity with distance traveled within the imaged tissue due to absorption and scattering. 4) Absorption is the transmission of ultrasound waves with complete loss of acoustic energy and with no reflected echoes. A fraction of the acoustic energy is lost as heat.

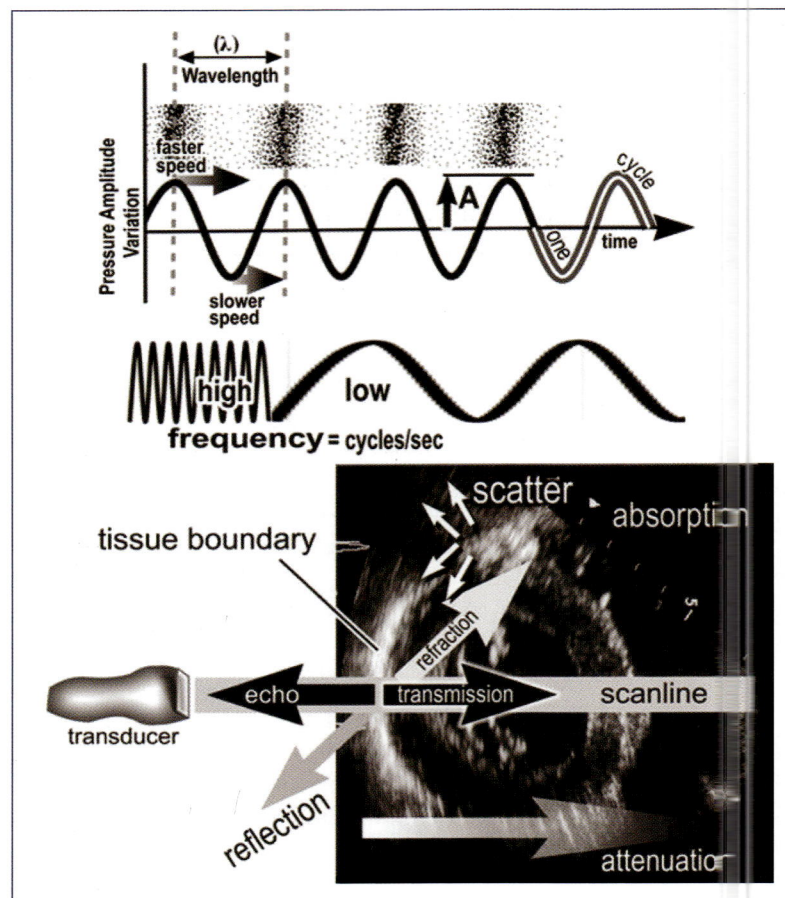

Figure 13-2. Color flow Doppler echocardiography. One advance in cardiac ultrasound has been the development of color flow Doppler (CFD) imaging. It has dramatically improved the assessment of cardiovascular hemodynamics, and complements the cross-sectional and spectral Doppler examination. CFD is a pulse wave (PW)–based modality that, unlike PW, uses multiple gates (*ie,* multiple sample volumes) simultaneously instead of a single gate and provides spatial display of real-time color-coded velocities superimposed upon real-time two-dimensional (2D) imaging. CFD thus provides information on flow velocity and direction. CFD imaging is subject to the same physical principles as PW Doppler and is thus subject to aliasing when velocities are high enough that the Doppler shift is greater than half the pulse repetition frequency.

Schema of apical view showing CFD sector scan superimposed upon real-time 2D grayscale image (*left panel*). The active color scan sector employs multiple gates (trains or ensemble) that are color-coded velocities. Apical view showing color Doppler superimposed on B-mode 2D imaging

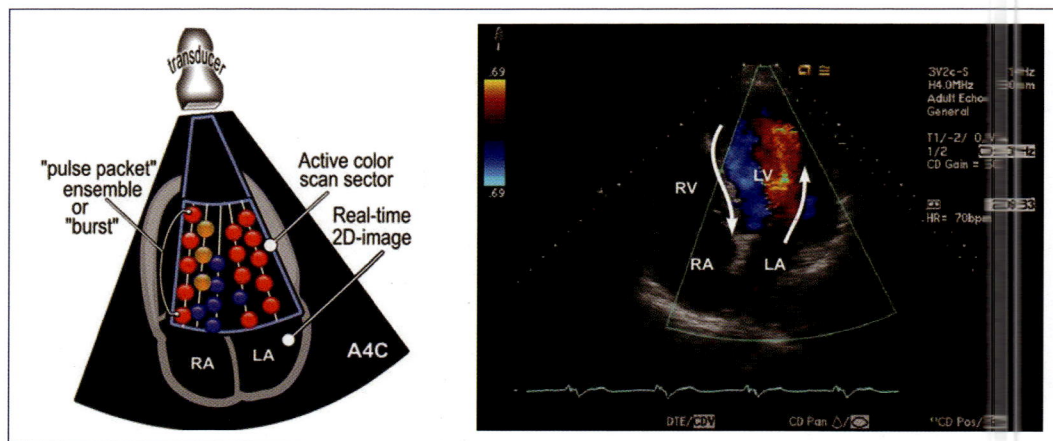

(*right panel*). Flow direction during early systole reveals blue flow along the left ventricular (LV) outflow tract. Red flow indicating flow momentum from left atrium (LA) into LV is also visualized.

CFD provides an intuitive assessment of cardiovascular hemodynamics because it permits an "angiographic" view of the flow, and is therefore more intuitive than spectral Doppler. It allows for rapid qualitative assessment of abnormal flow patterns. It is an important guide to PW and continuous wave Doppler position and alignment. PZE—piezoelectric crystal.

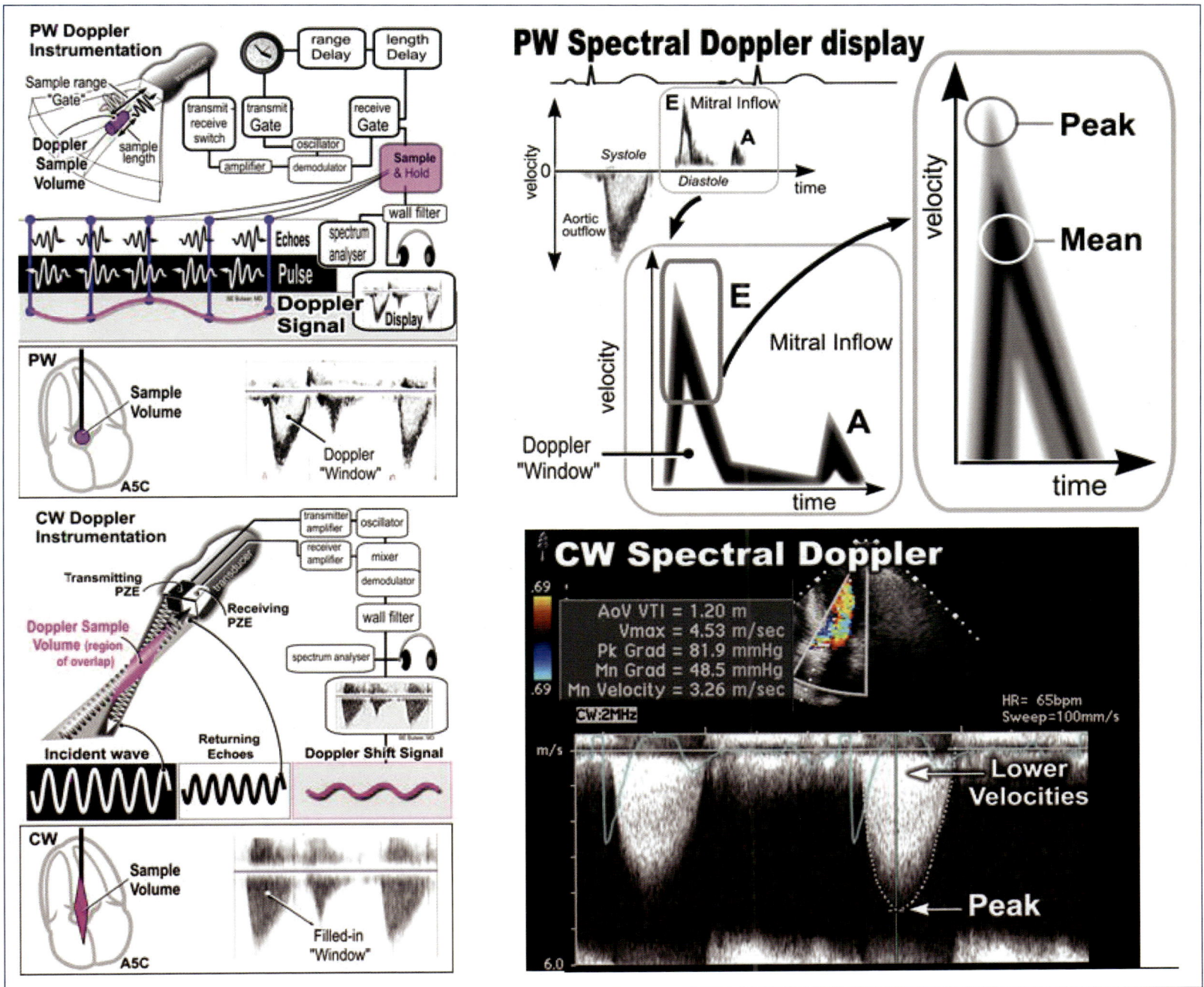

Figure 13-3. Doppler echocardiography. In pulsed-wave Doppler (*upper left panel*), the ultrasound signal is emitted repeatedly from the transducer and the return signal is "listened for" by the transducer. Sending out Doppler in pulses allows the equipment to interrogate velocities at particular depths by gating, or only "listening" at a certain time after the pulse is emitted. By focusing on a particular scan line, a region of interest (sample volume) can be defined by both the "depth" using time gating and the lateral location. Because pulsed Doppler is sent out and received in "pulses," the Doppler velocities are essentially being "sampled" at the pulse repetition frequency and are therefore subject to sampling issues, which can limit the velocity of the blood flow that can be interrogated. All spectral Doppler signals (*upper right panel*) show time on the X-axis and velocity on the Y-axis. When the pulsed-wave Doppler signal appears hollow (Doppler "window"), it is indicative of laminar flow where the majority of red blood cells are traveling within a narrow range of velocities.

With continuous wave (CW) Doppler (*lower left panel*) the Doppler signal is emitted continuously (similar to a continuous tone) and continuously listened for. For this reason, CW Doppler can be used to identify peak velocities, but cannot localize velocities to particular depths. Note the filled in appearance of the CW spectral Doppler display in the (*lower right panel*). This reflects the wide spectrum of velocities detected within the much larger sample volume.

Assessment of Cardiac Function

Transthoracic Echocardiography: Windows, Imaging Planes, and Views

① **Transducer Position or "Window"**

Each view is described using three (3) components:
- 1. **Transducer Position or "Window"**, *e.g. Parasternal, Apical, or Subcostal*
- 2. **Echocardiographic Imaging Plane**, *e.g. LAX, SAX, or 4C*
- 3. **Region or Structures visualized**, *e.g. Aortic valve (AV) level, Two-Chamber*

P: Parasternal
A: Apical
SC: Subcostal
SSN: Suprastenal Notch

② **Echocardiographic Imaging Planes**
- LAX; SAX; 4C

③ **Region or Structures Visualized**

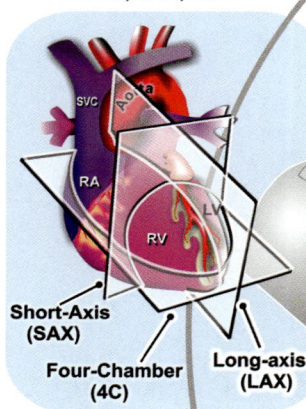
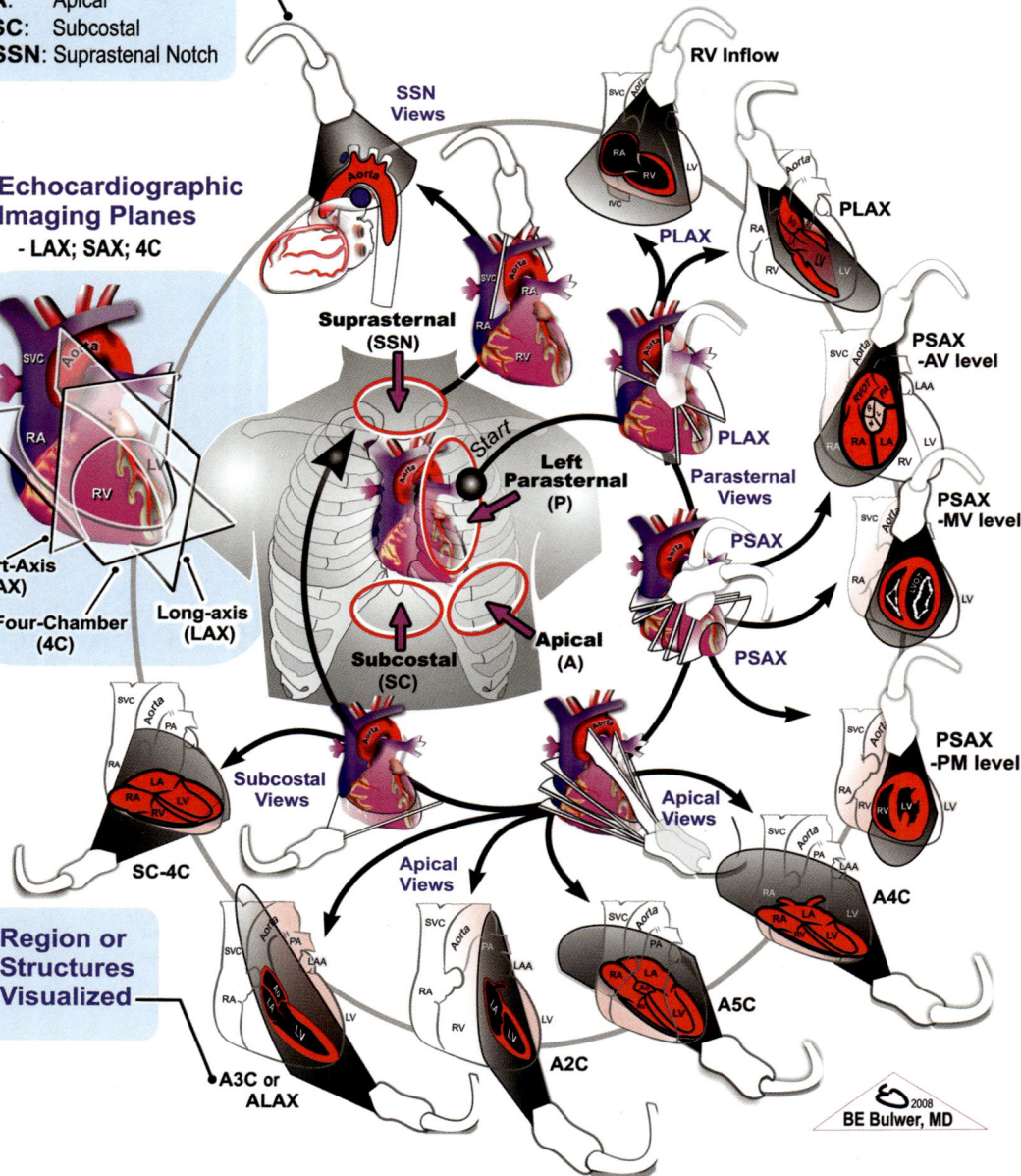

Comprehensive Transthoracic Two-Dimensional Echocardiographic Examination Protocol

Left Pararasternal Views (P) ⟶ **Apical Views (A)** ⟶ **Subcostal Views (SC)**

Left Pararasternal Views (P)	Apical Views (A)	Subcostal Views (SC)
PLAX: Parasternal Long-Axis (LV Inflow/Ouflow)	A4C: Apical Four-Chamber	SC-4C: Subcostal Four-Chamber View
PLAX: RV inflow +/- RV Outflow	A5C: Apical Five-Chamber	SC-SAX and SC-LAX Views *(optional)*
PSAX: Parasternal Short-Axis (Aortic Valve level)	A2C: Apical Two-Chamber	Inferior Vena Cava and Hepatic Veins
PSAX: Parasternal Short-Axis (Mitral Valve level)	A3C: Apical Three-Chamber	Abdominal Aorta
PSAX: Parasternal Short-Axis (Papillary Muscle level)		
PSAX: Parasternal Short-Axis (Apical LV level)		

⟶ **Suprasternal Notch Views (SSN)**
SSN Aortic Arch Long-Axis Views
SSB Aortic Arch Short-Axis Views *(optional)*

Figure 13-4. Transthoracic echocardiography imaging planes, windows, and views. Transthoracic two-dimensional echocardiography: imaging planes, transducer positions, and standard views. A2C—apical two-chamber view; A3C—apical three-chamber view; A4C—apical four-chamber view; A5C—apical five-chamber view; PLAX—parasternal long-axis view; PSAX—parasternal short-axis view; PSAX-AV—parasternal short-axis view-aortic valve level; PSAX-MV—parasternal short-axis view-mitral valve level; PSAX-PM—parasternal short-axis view papillary muscle level; SC-4C—subcostal view (four-chamber).

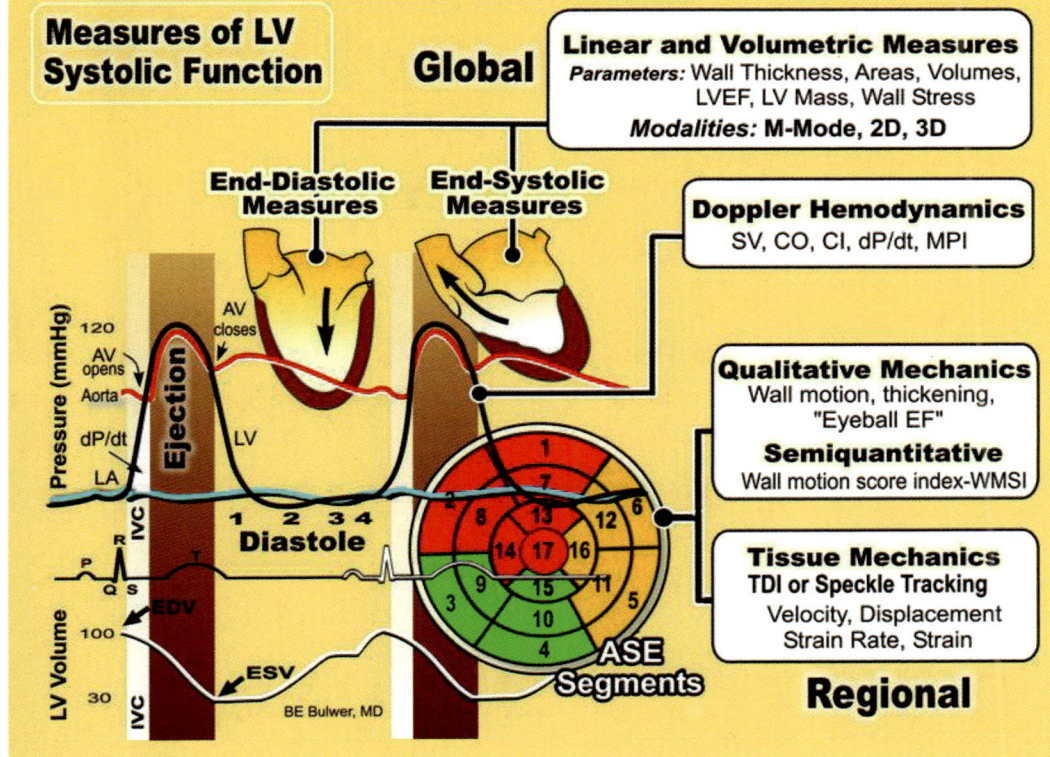

Summary of Measures of LV Systolic Function

Measures of LV Systolic Function

Global

Linear and Volumetric Measures
Parameters: Wall Thickness, Areas, Volumes, LVEF, LV Mass, Wall Stress
Modalities: M-Mode, 2D, 3D

End-Diastolic Measures

End-Systolic Measures

Doppler Hemodynamics
SV, CO, CI, dP/dt, MPI

Qualitative Mechanics
Wall motion, thickening, "Eyeball EF"

Semiquantitative
Wall motion score index-WMSI

Tissue Mechanics
TDI or Speckle Tracking
Velocity, Displacement
Strain Rate, Strain

ASE Segments

Regional

BE Bulwer, MD

Figure 13-5. Assessment of systolic function. Echocardiographic assessment of ventricular systolic function includes measures of both global and regional systolic function [1,2]. The primary measures of systolic function include 1) measurement of ventricular dimensions (*eg,* distances between opposite walls, ventricular areas, and volumes), in which ejection fraction can be easily calculated from ventricular volumes; 2) Doppler hemodynamic measures of stroke volumes and cardiac output (the myocardial performance index [MPI]); and 3) measures of regional systolic function based on the ASE (American Society of Echocardiography) 17 segment model are performed by qualitative "eyeball" assessment, as well as promising new semiquantitative automated techniques. CI—cardiac index; CO—cardiac output; dP/dt—rate of change of pressure during ejection; LVEF—left ventricular ejection fraction; SV—stroke volume; TDI—tissue Doppler imaging; WMSI—wall motion score index.

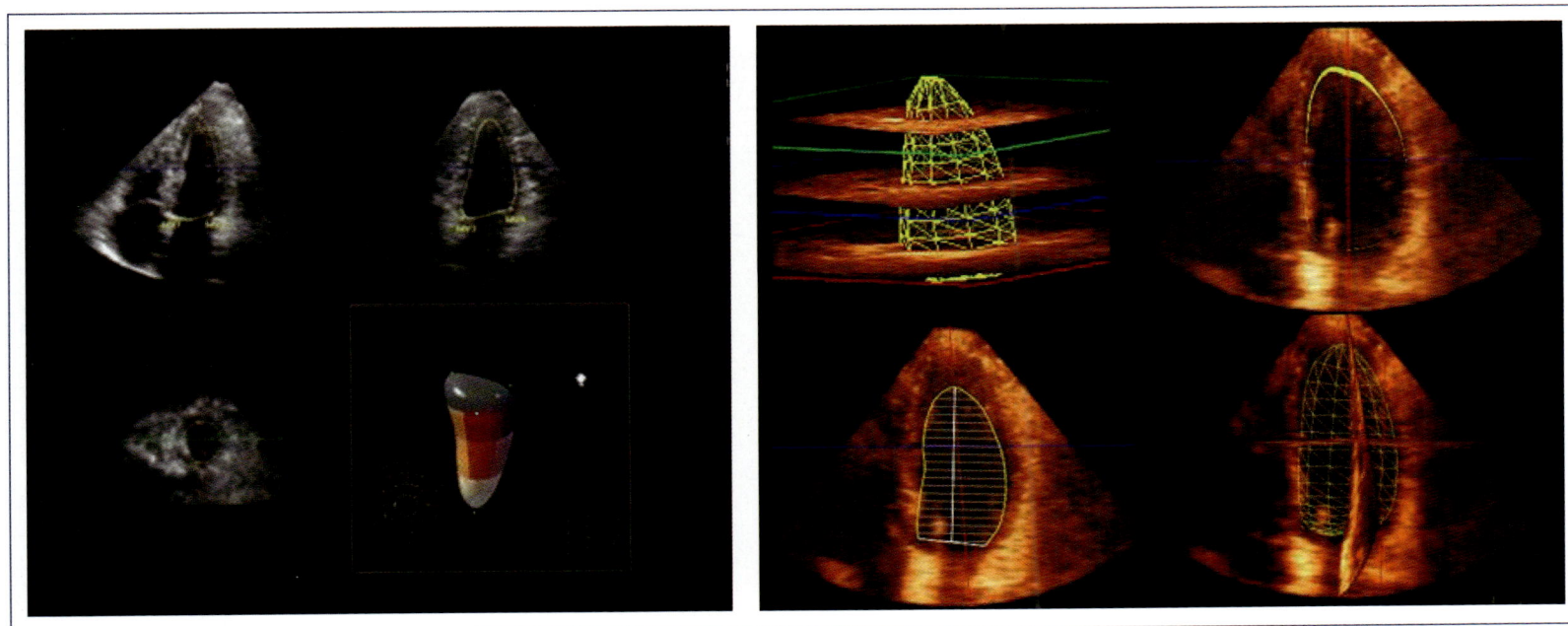

Figure 13-6. Assessment of systolic function with real-time three-dimensional echocardiography. Volumetric three-dimensional echocardiography can potentially give the most accurate assessment of ventricular volumes and function because these methods do not rely on geometric assumptions about the ventricle (*left panel*) [3,4]. Semiautomatic border detection with multiplanar reconstruction in three-dimensional echocardiography is also shown (*right panel*).

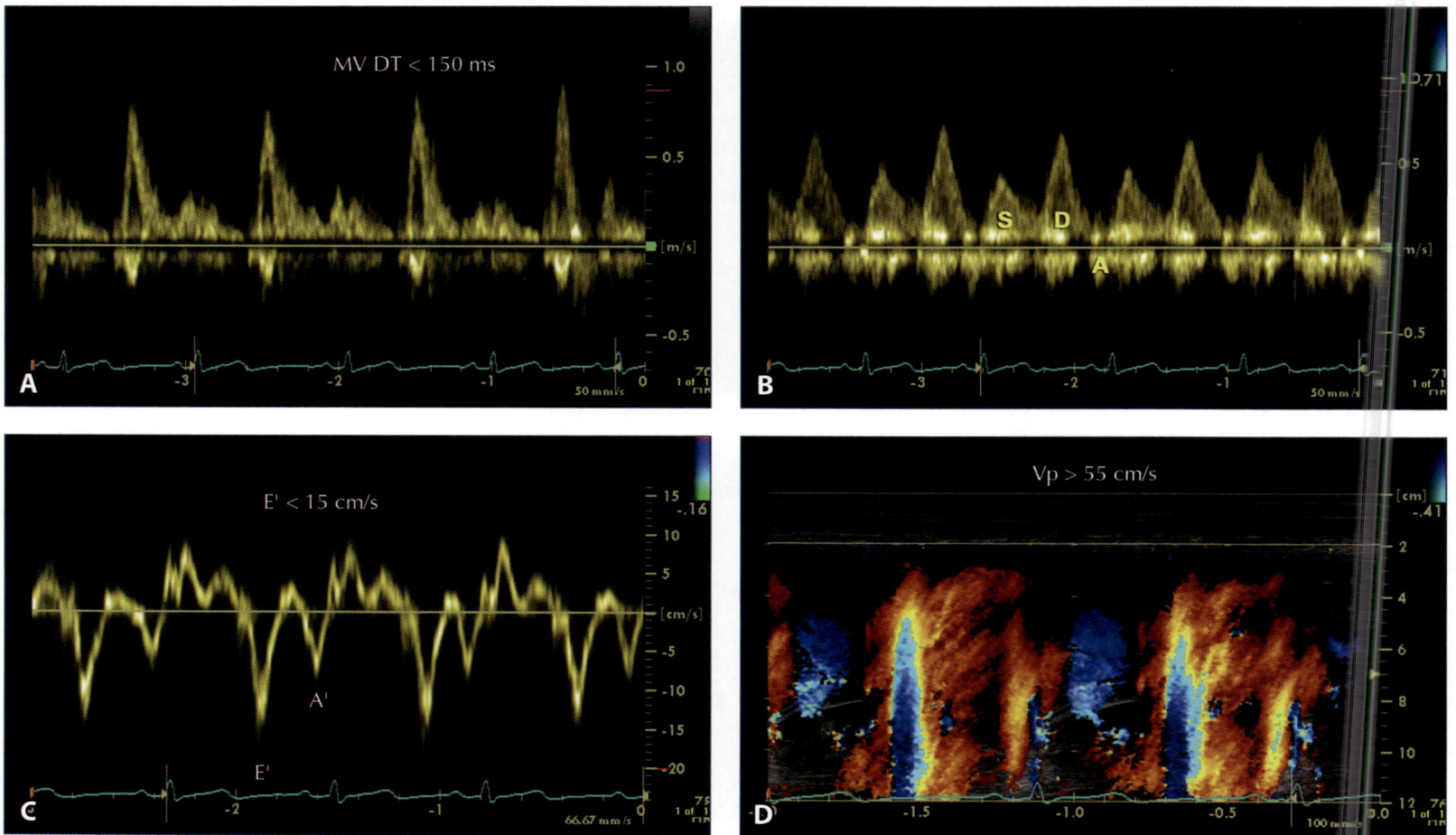

Figure 13-7. Assessment of diastolic function. The assessment of diastolic function with echocardiography is made by careful analysis of pulsed wave Doppler throughout the mitral valve and pulmonary veins, with tissue Doppler recordings of mitral annular velocities, and color M-mode recordings of blood flow from the base to the apex of the left ventricle. This figure demonstrates mitral inflow from a normal 15-year-old boy with a rapid deceleration time, reflecting vigorous relaxation with a compliant ventricle. **A,** Mitral inflow with a normal E wave velocity and a deceleration time, which is less than 150 ms. **B,** The pulmo-nary vein flows demonstrate dominant flow in diastole with blunting in systole. Interpreting the pulmonary vein flow in isolation would lead to an incorrect diagnosis of diastolic dysfunction. **C,** The tissue annular velocities are normal, reflecting normal relaxation. **D,** The flow propagation velocities are normal, once again reinforcing normal relaxation. The constellation of findings indicate normal diastolic function in this young adult. A′—late mitral annular relaxation velocity; E′—early mitral annular relaxation velocity; MV DT—mitral valve deceleration time; Vp—propagation velocity.

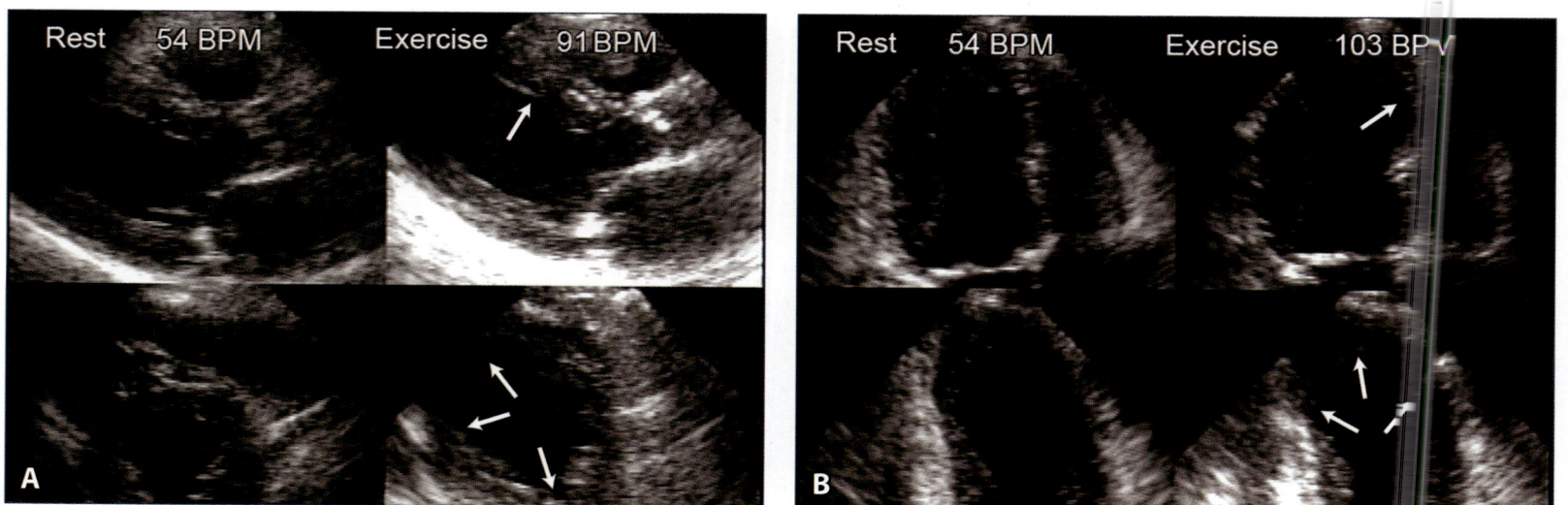

Figure 13-8. Assessment of ischemic heart disease: stress echocardiography. Marked ischemia with exercise in a patient with a normal exercise electrocardiogram. In this patient who presented with exertional dyspnea, left ventricular systolic function appeared normal at rest, but there was marked worsening of function with exercise. This is shown in both the parasternal (**A**) and apical (**B**) views. Heart rate response to exercise was attenuated because of β-blocker therapy for hypertension. Regions of akinesis or dyskinesis (*arrows*) are shown in all four views and are manifested in end-systolic images as bulging. This patient had multivessel coronary artery disease. This illustrates the incremental value of exercise echocardiography. The test provides information beyond that available from clinical, rest echocardiographic, or exercise electrocardiogram predictors of prognosis [5].

Valvular Heart Disease

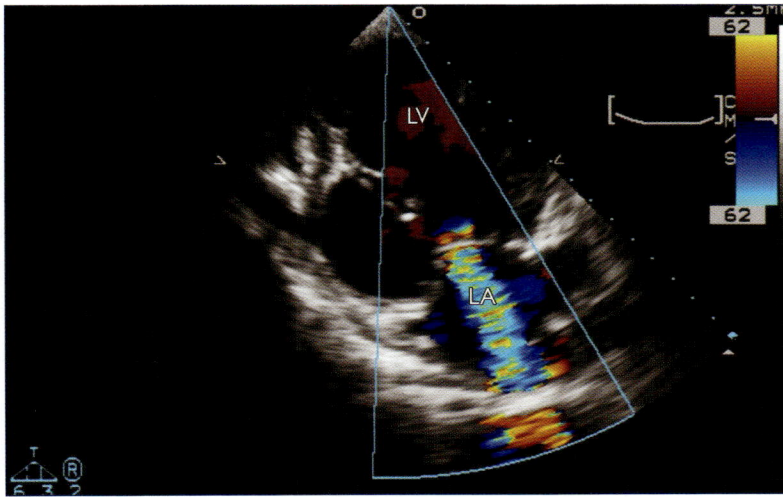

Figure 13-9. Assessment of mitral regurgitation. Moderate to severe mitral regurgitation that has developed from tethering of the mitral leaflets is shown. LA—left atrium; LV—left ventricle.

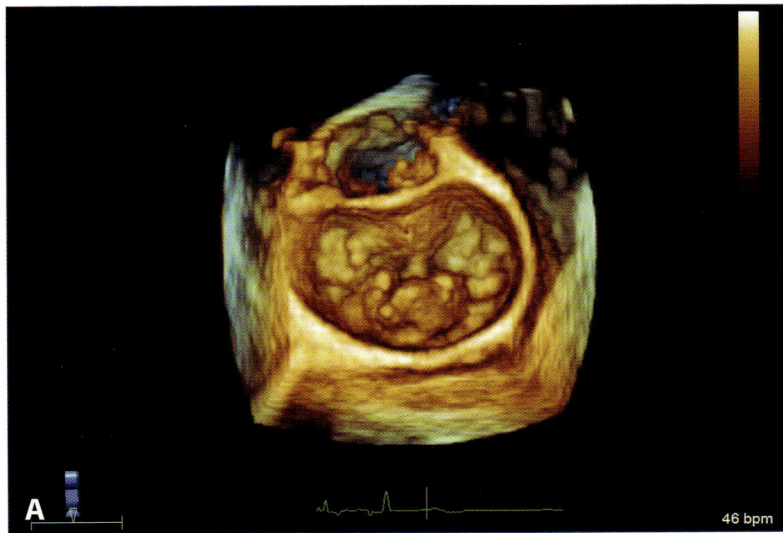

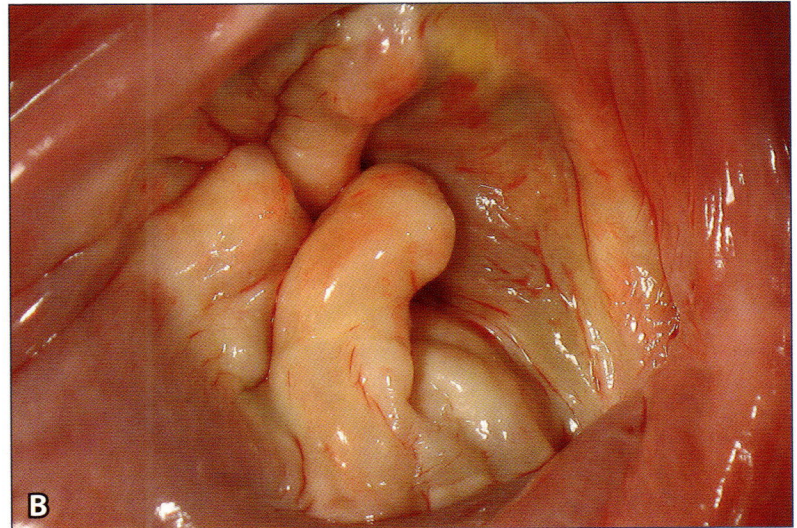

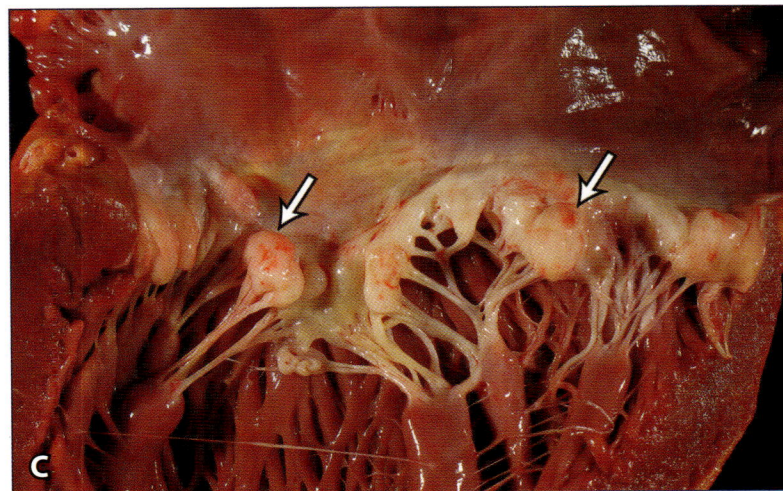

Figure 13-10. Mitral valve morphology and prolapse. Myxomatous thickening and prolapse of the mitral valve can occur in isolation in 2% to 3% of the general population [6], or may be associated with heritable collagen vascular disorders and aortic root dilatation, such as Marfan syndrome [7]. Myxomatous degeneration of the valve predisposes to severe regurgitation and chordal rupture and is a frequent indication for mitral valve repair or replacement [8]. Prolapse can affect only one or both leaflets to varying degrees. **A,** Three-dimensional transesophageal echocardiogram showing a myxomatous mitral valve from the left atrial *en face* aspect. There is billowing and prolapse of the entire middle scallop of the posterior leaflet (*courtesy of* Douglas C. Shook, Brigham and Women's Hospital, Boston, MA). **B,** The posterior leaflet of the mitral valve demonstrates marked prolapse and hooding in all segments and severe redundancy in this photograph taken from the vantage point of the left atrium. **C,** Opening the left side of the heart reveals prominent mitral leaflet hooding (*arrows*). The chordae are focally thickened but are not fused, which would be the case in rheumatic valve disease.

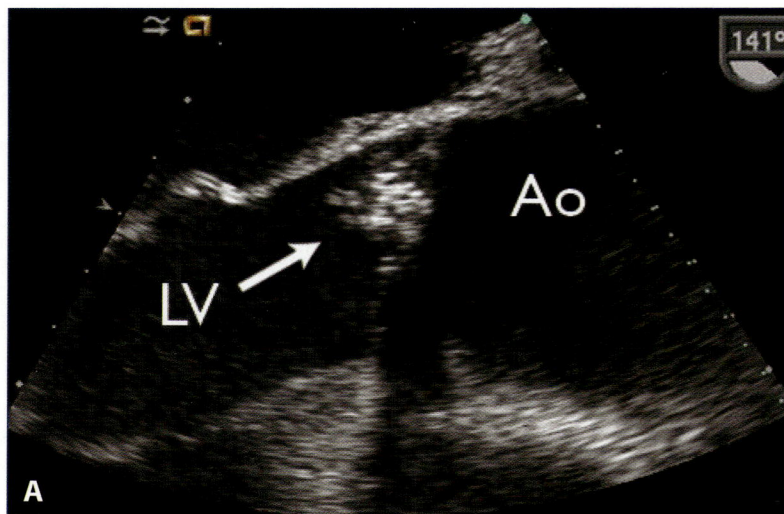

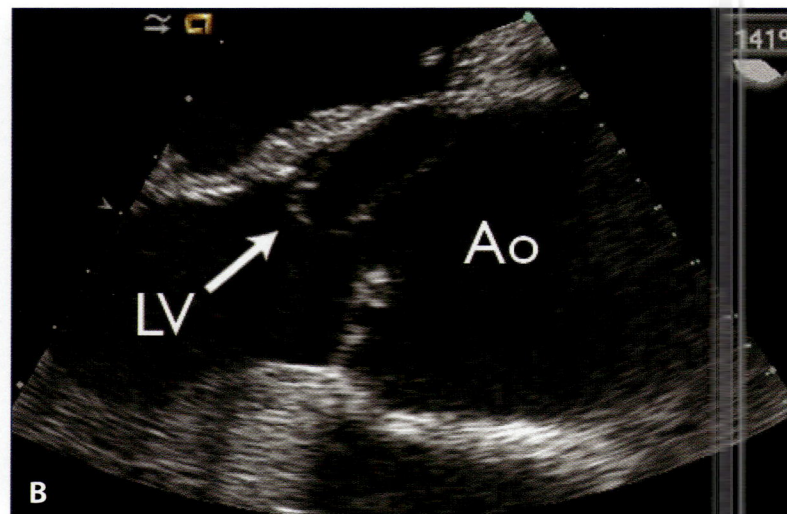

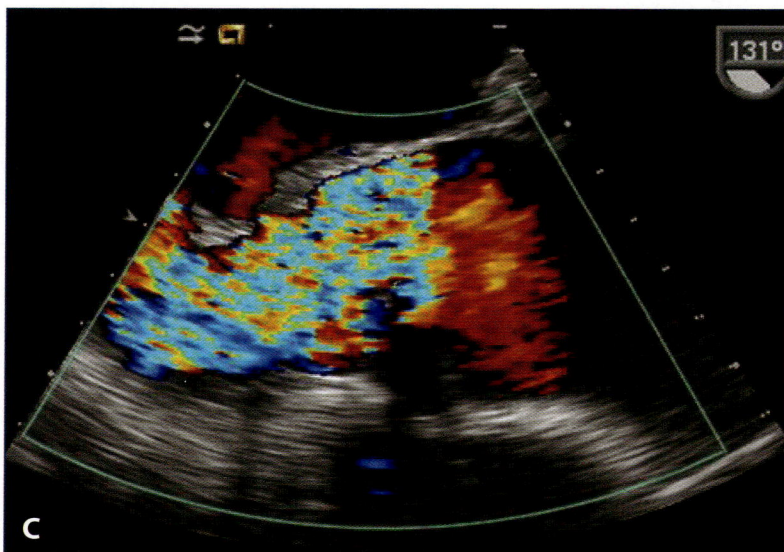

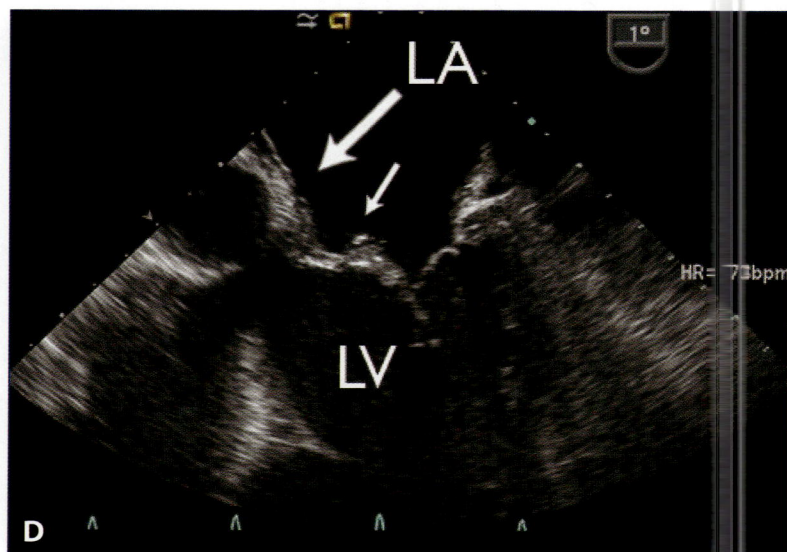

Figure 13-11. Transesophageal assessment of endocarditis. Native aortic valve endocarditis with subaortic complications. Multiple studies have demonstrated the superiority of transesophageal echocardiography (TEE) compared with transthoracic echocardiography (TTE) in identifying left-sided valvular vegetations [9,10]. A recent study comparing TTE with harmonic imaging to TEE demonstrated the continuing superiority of TEE. In this case-control study of 50 patients with valvular vegetations identified by TEE, TTE had a sensitivity of only 55%. The sensitivity of TTE was slightly greater for mitral valve vegetations (62%) versus aortic valve vegetations (50%). TEE is especially more sensitive than TTE in diagnosing subaortic complications of aortic valve endocarditis, as seen in these images. Midesophageal long-axis view of the aortic valve (**A**) demonstrates a vegeta- tion on the ventricular aspect of the aortic valve. This was a bicuspid aortic valve. This infection also caused leaflet aneurysm with prolapse (**B** arrow) just adjacent to the vegetation. Aortic valve leaflet perforation was present in this same location (**C**) with severe associated aortic insufficiency. In the midesophageal five-chamber view, abnormal thickening of the interval- vular fibrosa consistent with abscess is present (**D**, *long arrow*). This view also demonstrates abnormal thickening of the anterior mitral valve leaflet with a small vegetation present on its atrial aspect (**D**, *short arrow*). This patient also had evidence of an anterior mitral leaflet aneurysm with leaf- let perforation. Compared with TEE, the sensitivity of TTE in diagnosing intervalvular fibrosa abscess, aneurysm, or perforation is reported as low as 21% [11]. Ao—aorta; LA—left atrium; LV—left ventricle.

Doppler Assessment of Stenotic Lesions: Aortic Stenosis

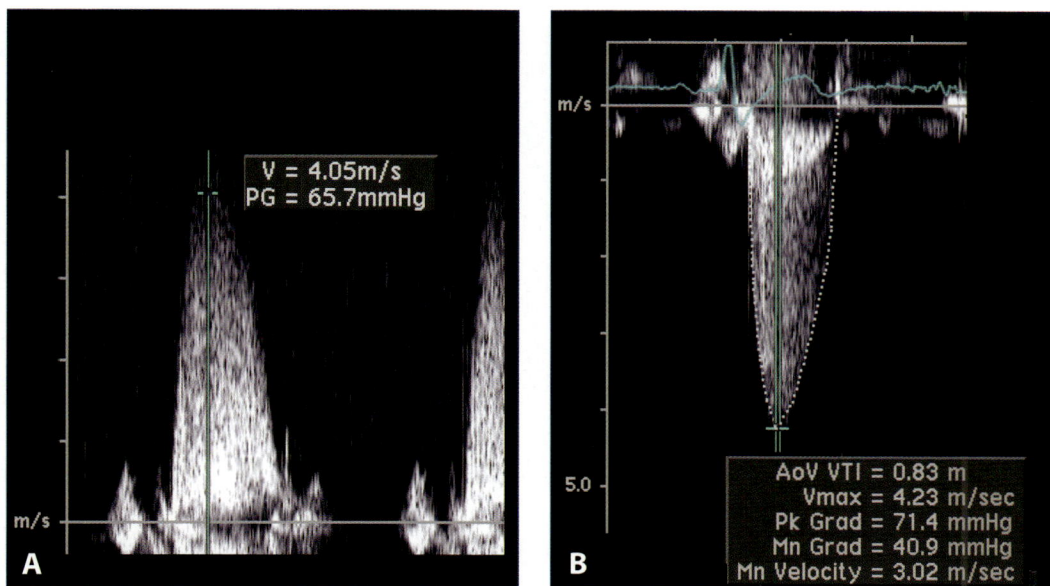

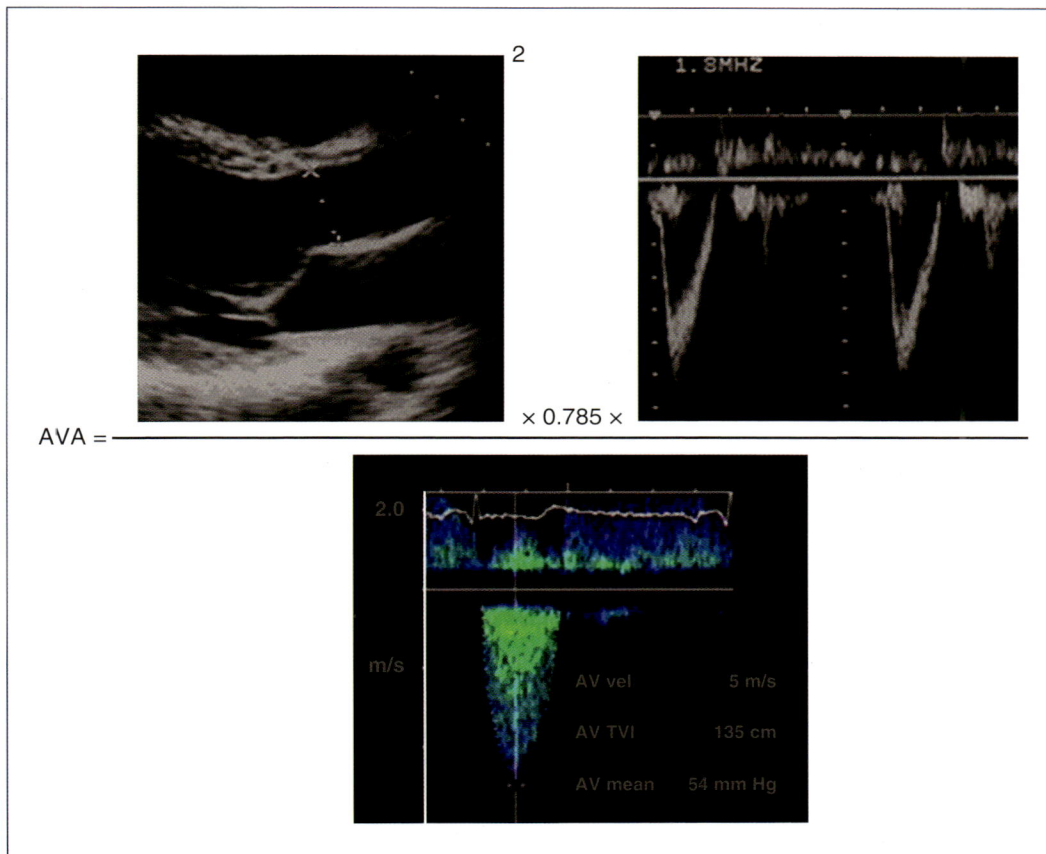

Figure 13-12. A clinical example of severe aortic stenosis with continuous wave Doppler flow directed toward the transducer (**A**) (from a suprasternal notch window) and flow directed away from the transducer (**B**) (from an apical window). The highest velocity (V) obtained from all views should be used in pressure calculations as this corresponds to the gradient when ultrasound beam alignment is most parallel with flow. In this case, the highest peak velocity was obtained from the apical position (4.23 m/sec). Peak transaortic pressure gradient (PG) is calculated using the simplified Bernoulli equation. Note inset (*upper right*) showing location of Doppler cursor.

Figure 13-13. Assessment of valve area by the "continuity" or conservation of mass principle. In a noncompressible fluid system, such as blood, flow is the same at any point. Thus, $area_1 \times$ time velocity integral $(TVI)_1 = area_2 \times TVI_2$. This is the "continuity equation." Flow $(cm^3) =$ area $(cm^2) \times$ length traveled by the volume per beat (cm). The length traveled by the volume per beat is the TVI, obtained by integration of the area under the curve of the Doppler spectral envelope. Area $= \pi r^2 = \pi \times (diameter/2)^2 = diameter^2 \times \pi/4 = diameter^2 \times 0.785$. The diagram shows how to calculate the aortic valve area (AVA) by multiplying the square of the left ventricular outflow tract (LVOT) diameter obtained in the parasternal long-axis view by 0.785 and then by the TVI calculated by integrating the area under the curve (black-white interface) of the LVOT pulsed-wave spectral Doppler on the apical three-chamber view. This is then divided by the TVI of the continuous spectral Doppler signal through the aortic valve. Care must be taken when placing the pulse-wave sample volume near the aortic valve to avoid the high velocity flow convergence laminar flow area that precedes the aortic valve. This would cause overestimation of the AVA (underestimation of the severity of stenosis). This is achieved by placing the sample volume 0.5 to 1 cm before the aortic valve [12].

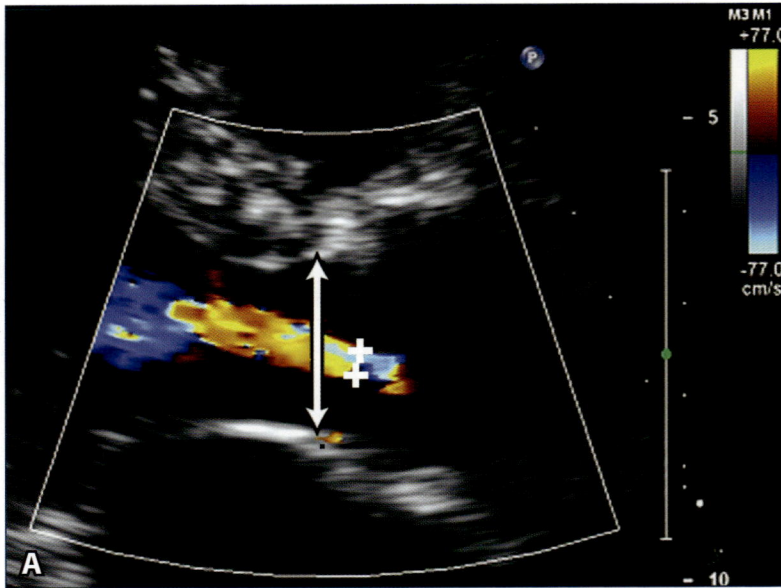

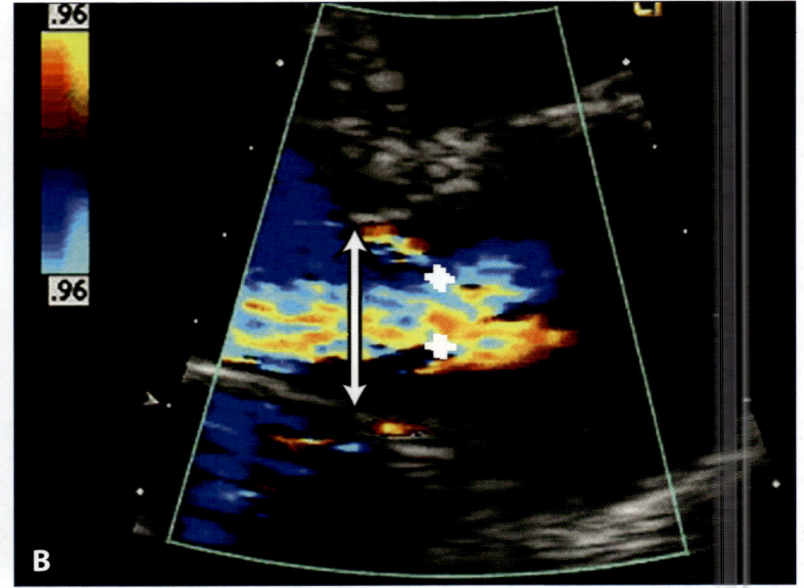

Aortic Regurgitation Severity

Type of echocardiographic information	Mild	Moderate		Severe
Specific and supportive signs	Vena contracta < 0.3 cm	Intermediate values		Vena contracta > 0.6 cm
	Central jet width < 25% of LVOT			Central jet width > 65% of LVOT
	No or brief early diastolic flow reversal in descending aorta			Prominent holodiastolic flow reversal in descending aorta
	Pressure half time > 500 ms			Pressure half time < 200 ms
	Normal LV size			LV enlargement
Quantitative parameters	Mild	Moderate	Moderate–Severe	Severe
ERO, cm²	< 0.1	0.1–0.19	0.20–0.29	≥ 0.30
	< 30	30–44	45–59	≥ 60

C

Figure 13-14. Assessment of regurgitation severity in aortic valve disease. Vena contracta and jet width/left ventricular outflow tract (LVOT) width. Shown are parasternal long-axis transthoracic echo images of a patient with mild aortic regurgitation (**A**) and severe regurgitation (**B**). The vena contracta is 0.3–0.7 cm (**A** and **B**), respectively (**C**). Note that the central jet width is less than or equal to 25% of the LVOT width (**A**, *two-headed arrow*) and greater than or equal to 65% of the LVOT width (**B**, *two-headed arrow*). The quantification of aortic regurgitation can be a challenging task for the echocardiographer. It is not recommended to rely on one or two measure- ments, but to combine multiple measurements in a comprehensive manner. A simple reliable method is measurement of the vena contracta; the small- est width of the regurgitant flow at the orifice immediately beyond the flow convergence region (**A** and **B**, *calipers*) and before expansion of the turbulent regurgitant jet, which is a surrogate measure of the effective regurgitant ori- fice (ERO) [13]. Measurement of vena contracta is carried out in the para- sternal long-axis with a zoomed view and optimized color Doppler settings at early to mid diastole [14]. Vena contracta has been shown to be superior to the jet/LVOT ratio for quantification of aortic regurgitation.

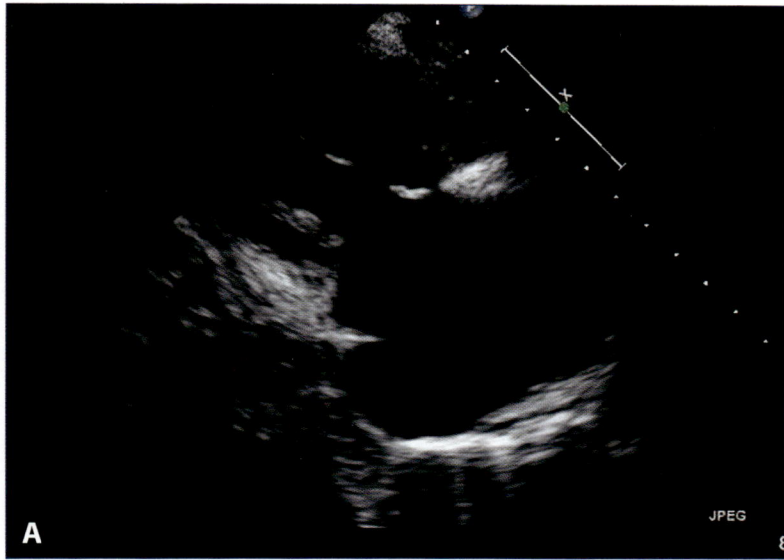

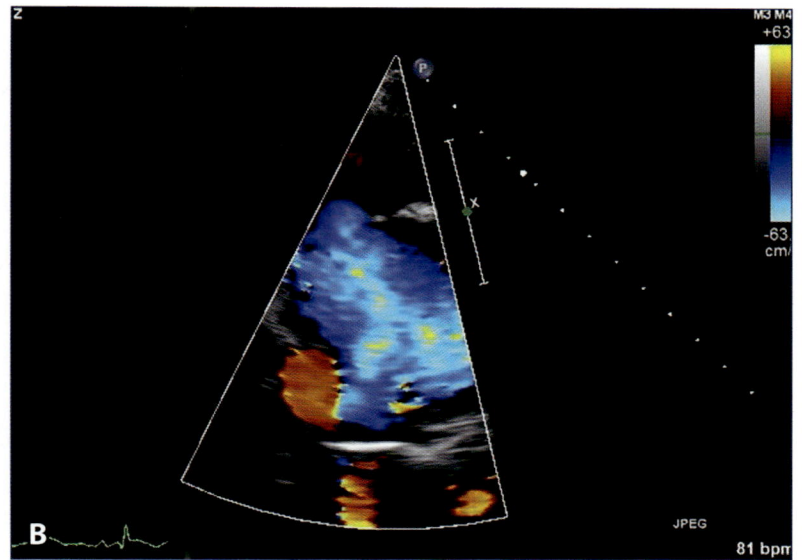

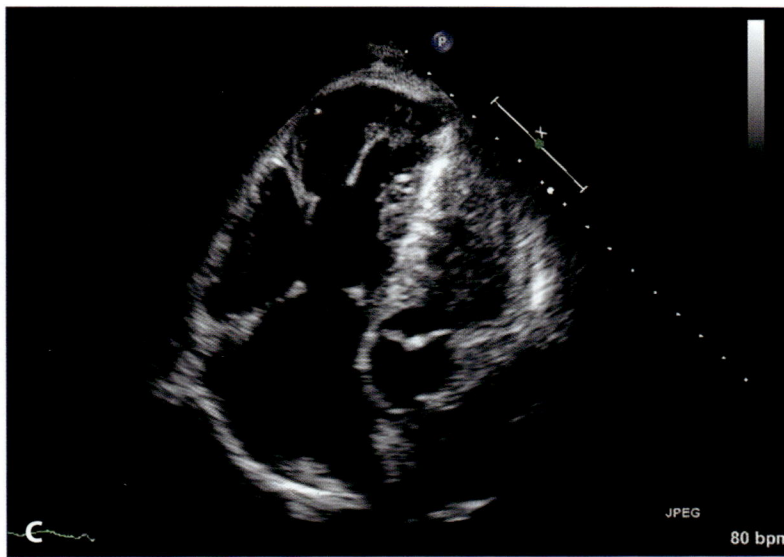

Figure 13-15. Carcinoid heart disease involving the tricuspid valve. Right ventricular inflow tract views (**A** and **B**) demonstrate the typical features of carcinoid heart disease. The leaflets are thickened, retracted, and immobilized, creating a large regurgitant orifice. As a result, there is unrestricted tricuspid regurgitation, and the color regurgitant jet may appear relatively monochromic. In the apical five-chamber view of the same patient (**C**), the classic "drum stick" appearance of the leaflets is evident. The vulvopathy occurs when serotonin and its metabolite 5-hydroxytryptophan secreted by carcinoid tumors causes an inflammatory reaction in the valves. Because the active metabolite is inactivated in the lungs, left-sided involvement occurs only when there is an intracardiac shunt or pulmonary metastases.

Pulmonic Valve Morphology

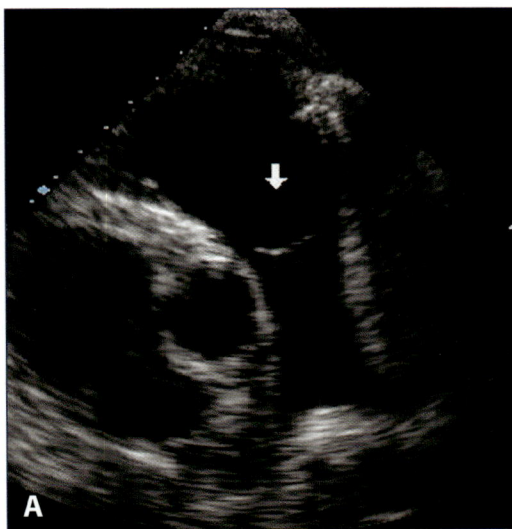

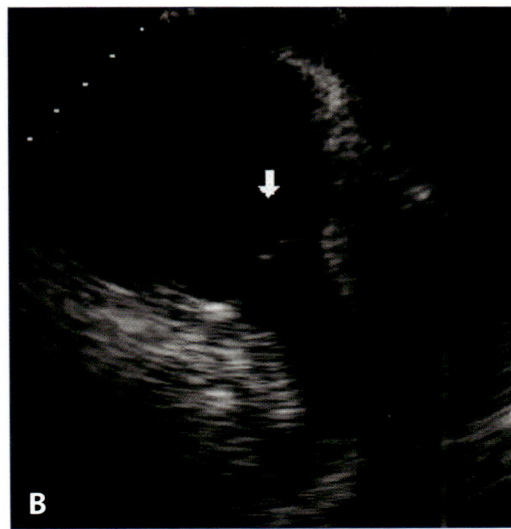

Figure 13-16. Pulmonic valve morphology. Although the pulmonic valve has three cusps (right, left, and anterior), it is rare to see all three in a single, short, two-dimensional echocardiographic image. Long-axis images of the valve (*arrowhead*) may be obtained transthoracically using basal parasternal (**A**), steeply anteriorly angulated apical (**B**) with the valve indicated (*arrowhead*), and subcostal (**C**) windows.

Continued on the next page

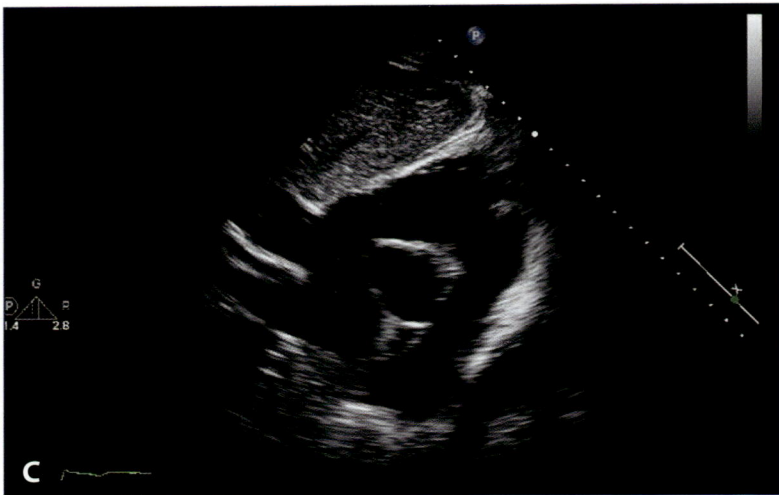

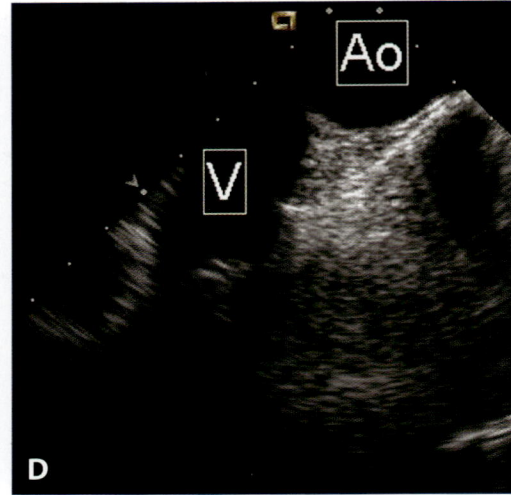

Figure 13-16. *(Continued)* Comparable views may be obtained with transesophageal echocardiography (TEE). TEE offers a unique view of the valve using a high esophageal window rotated slightly from that used to image the aortic arch (**D**). Ao—aorta; V—valve.

Echocardiography in Myocardial Diseases and Miscellaneous Diseases

Myocardial Infarction

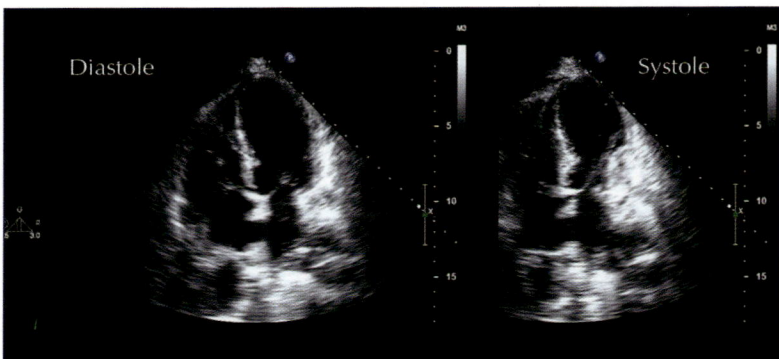

Figure 13-17. Regional left ventricle (LV) wall motion abnormality on echocardiography is the hallmark of coronary artery disease and myocardial infarction. It is one of the earliest signs of myocardial ischemia and infarction and serves as a key component in the latest definition of both acute and prior myocardial infarction [15]. During ischemia and infarction, there is decreased thickening of the myocardium and reduced inward motion of the endocardial wall. Shown here is a transthoracic echocardiographic apical four-chamber view with regional wall motion abnormality during anterior myocardial infarction (diastole and systole). The extent of dysfunction involves the apical portion of the LV.

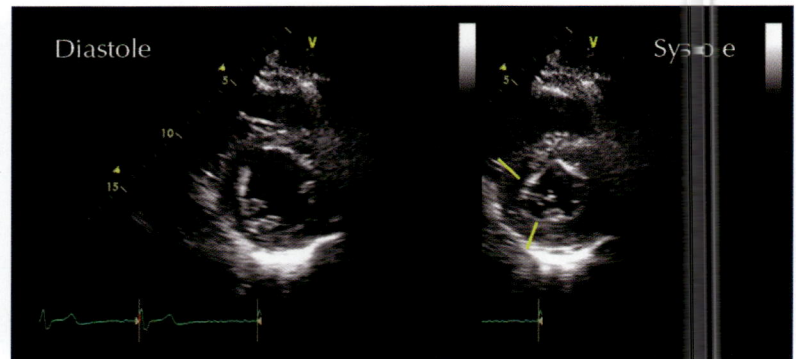

Figure 13-18. Diastolic and systolic frames from a transthoracic echocardiographic parasternal short axis view at mid–left ventricle level demonstrate the circumferential extent of regional wall motion abnormality during inferior myocardial infarction (*between yellow lines*). The inferior septum and inferior wall are involved.

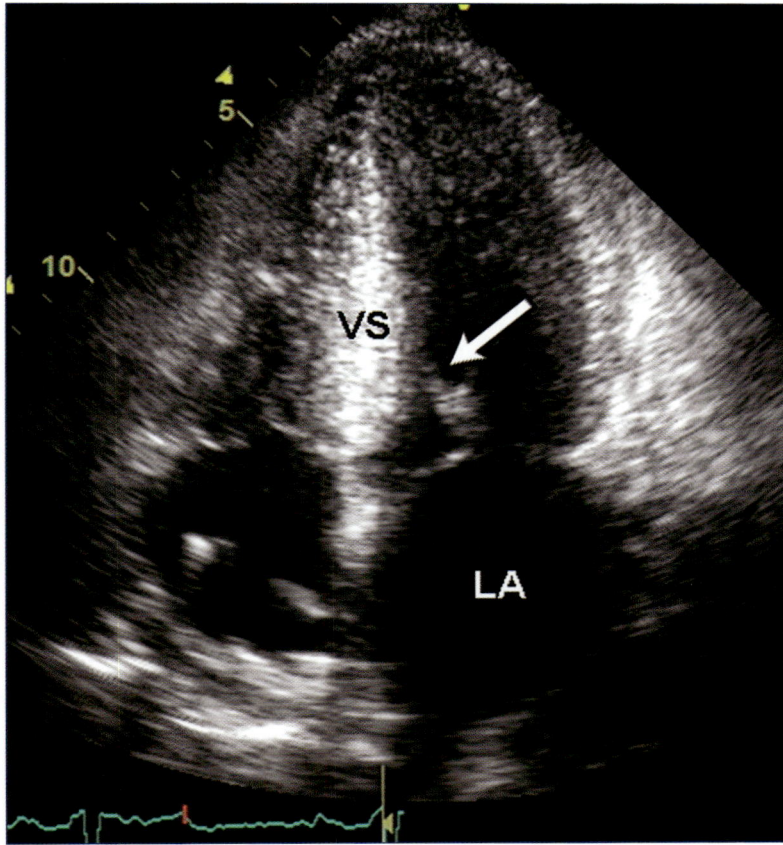

Figure 13-19. Hypertrophic cardiomyopathy with systolic anterior motion of the mitral calve. Proposed mechanisms for systolic anterior motion (SAM) include Venturi effect or drag forces (the more likely of the two). The Venturi effect theory proposes that the hypertrophied basal septum creates a local low pressure region in the outflow tract that acts to pull the mitral valve anteriorly. The drag effect theory emphasizes the importance of anterior displacement of the mitral apparatus, which exposes more leaflet surface area to blood flow in the left ventricular (LV) outflow tract. The hypertrophied proximal septum redirects blood flow posteriorly and laterally, creating a pressure gradient between the LV cavity and outflow tract, which pushes the underside of the mitral leaflets toward the septum and creates a self-amplifying loop where longer durations of SAM septal contact lead to further increases in the gradient [16]. LA—left atrium; VS—ventricular septum.

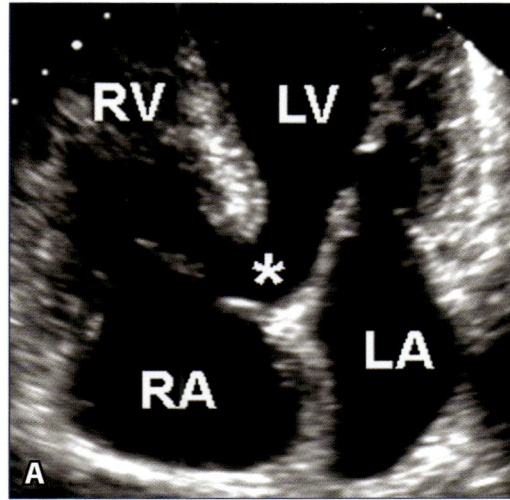

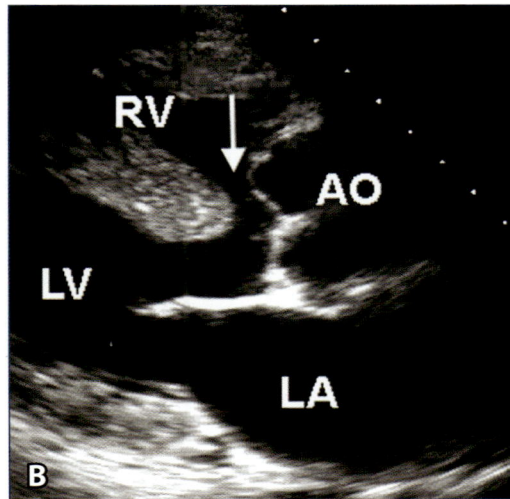

Figure 13-20. Adult congenital heart disease: tetralogy of Fallot. Tetralogy of Fallot is the most common conotruncal defect seen in the adult population with congenital heart disease. **A,** An apical four-chamber view of a patient with tetralogy of Fallot shows a normal left ventricle (LV), a nonrestrictive perimembranous malalignment ventricular septal defect (*asterisk*), right ventricular (RV) hypertrophy, and an enlarged aorta (not shown) overriding the ventricular septum. **B,** Parasternal long-axis view of tetralogy of Fallot shows a large unrestrictive malalignment-type ventricular septal defect (*arrow*) and an enlarged aorta (AO) overriding the outlet septum. The anterior RV is hypertrophied. (*See also* Fig. 10-10.) LA—left atrium; RA—right atrium.

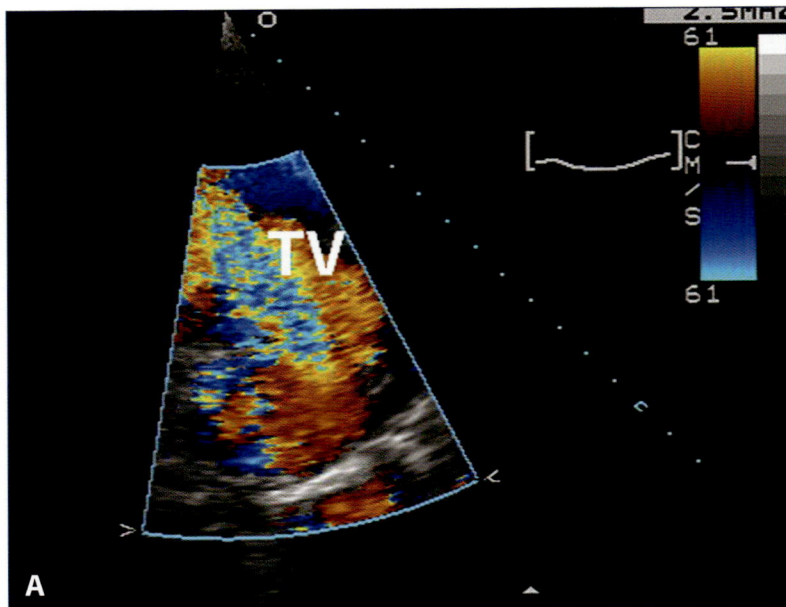

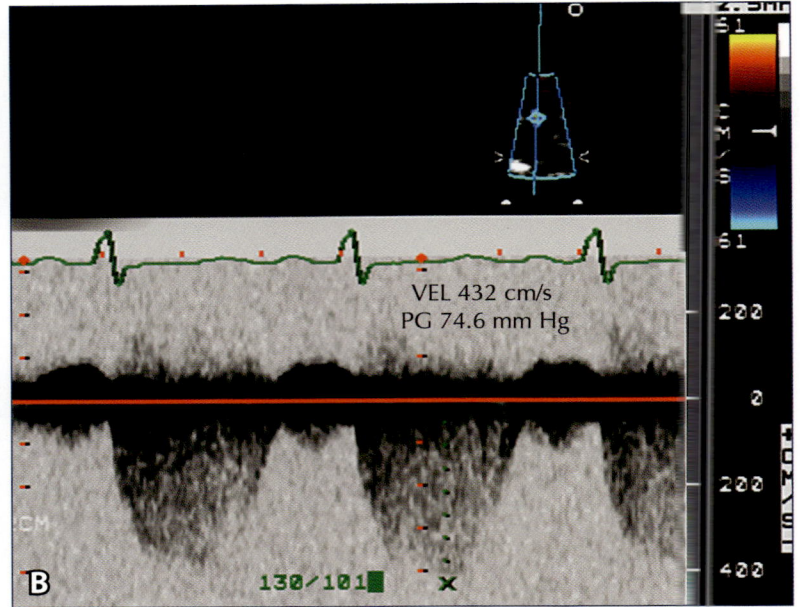

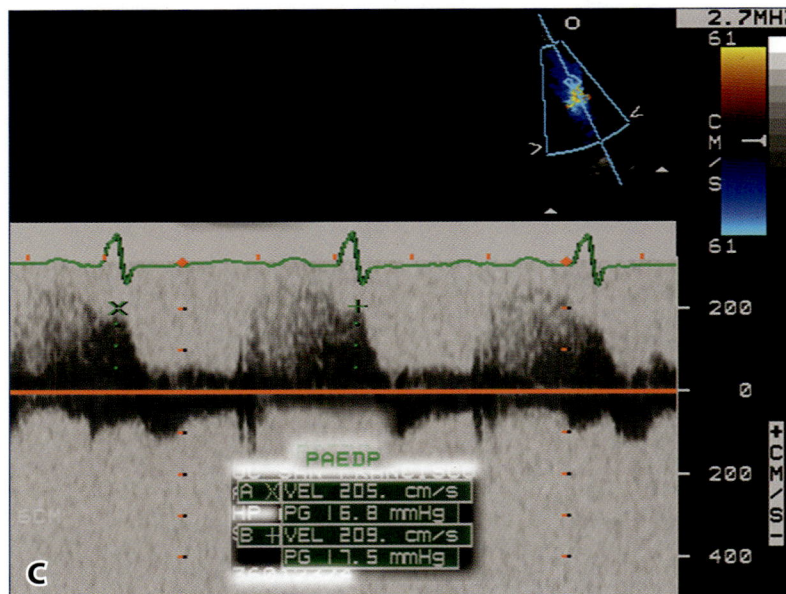

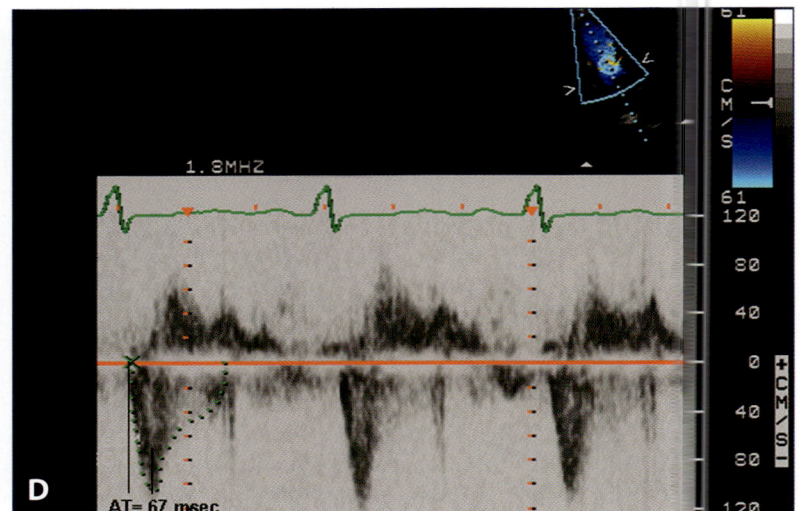

Figure 13-21. Severe pulmonary hypertension in patients with sickle cell disease. Doppler echocardiography shows severe pulmonary hypertension in a patient with sickle cell disease. **A,** Color Doppler of the tricuspid valve (TV) shows severe tricuspid regurgitation. **B,** Continuous wave Doppler echocardiography across the TV is indicative of a markedly elevated pulmonary artery systolic pressure of 85 mm Hg, with a right atrial pressure esti- mated to be 10 mm Hg in this patient. **C,** Continuous wave Doppler suggests a significantly elevated pulmonary artery end-diastolic pressure of 27 mm Hg in the same patient. **D,** Pulsed wave Doppler of the right ventricular out- flow tract flow shows an abnormal flow pattern with a shortened accelera- tion time (time interval between onset of the flow to its peak velocity (VEL), suggestive of severe pulmonary hypertension). PG—peak gradient.

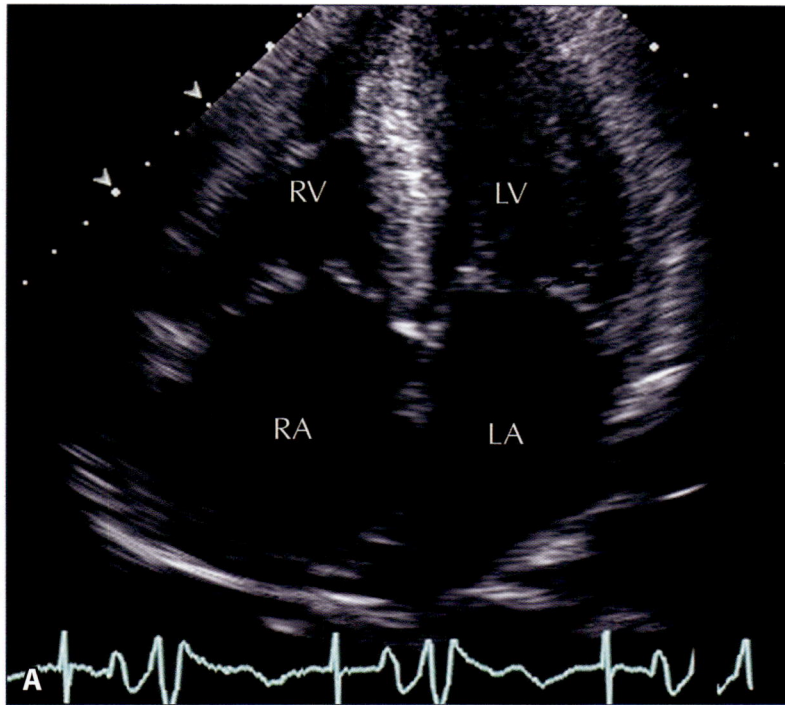

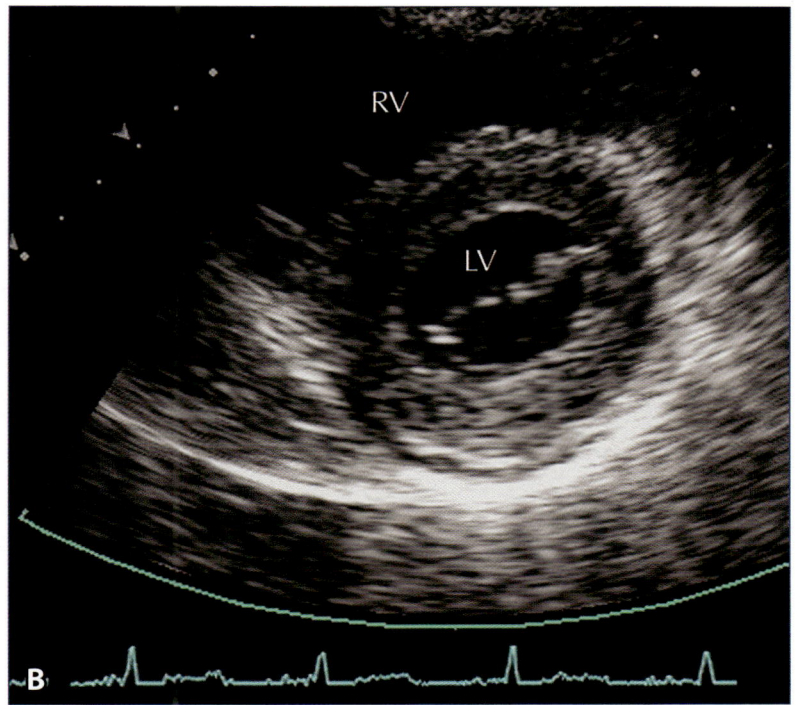

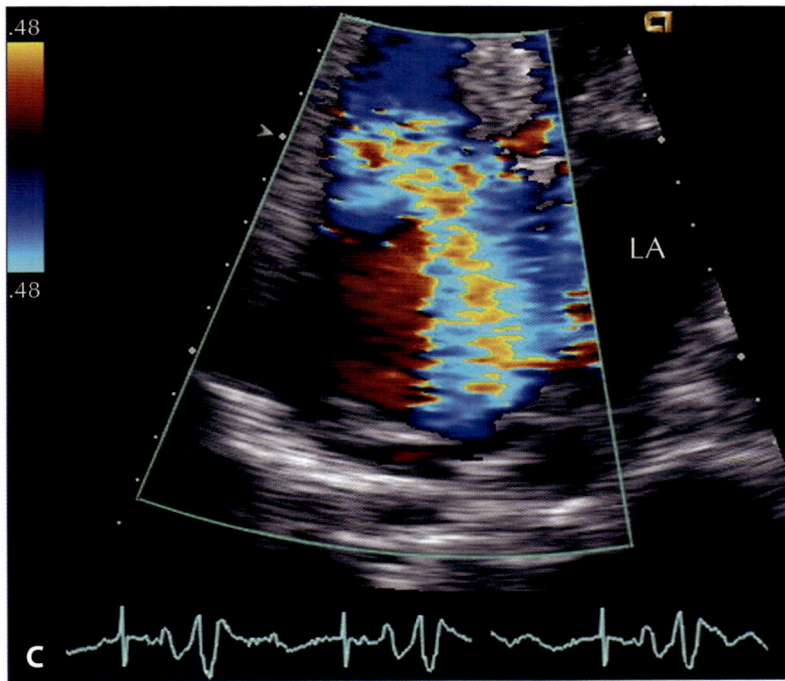

Figure 13-22. Amyloid heart disease. Two-dimensional echocardiography shows restrictive cardiomyopathy in a patient with cardiac amyloidosis. **A,** Apical four-chamber view shows left ventricular (LV) hypertrophy, small left ventricle size, and bi-atrial enlargement. LV ejection fraction was estimated to be 55% in this patient. LV systolic function is usually preserved initially without dilatation of the ventricular chamber, and as the disease progresses, the systolic function can gradually deteriorate. **B,** Short-axis view of the left ventricle in the same patient shows concentric LV hypertrophy and thickening of the mitral valve. Amyloid deposits can also occur diffusely in the heart valves, resulting in thickening of the heart valves, which can lead to significant valvular insufficiency. **C,** Severe mitral insufficiency due to involvement of the mitral valve in cardiac amyloidosis is shown. LA—left atrium; RA—right atrium.

Echocardiographic Emergencies

Figure 13-23. Pulmonary embolism. Apical four-chamber view, demonstrating right ventricular (RV) dilatation, hypokinesis, as well as McConnell's sign (*arrow*), which are markers of acute pulmonary embolism. Echocardiography is an outstanding clinical tool in selecting patients with pulmonary embolism who may have a poor prognosis, with RV systolic dysfunction being the most powerful predictor of in-hospital death (six-fold increase). McConnell's sign refers to the presence of RV free wall segmental hypokinesis with sparing of the RV apex, resulting in a "hinge" appearance of RV contraction, which is most apparent in real-time. This sign may be a helpful screening tool to distinguish acute pulmonary embolism from other etiologies of RV systolic dysfunction, and it has been estimated to have a sensitivity of 77%, specificity of 94%, and negative predictive value of 96%.

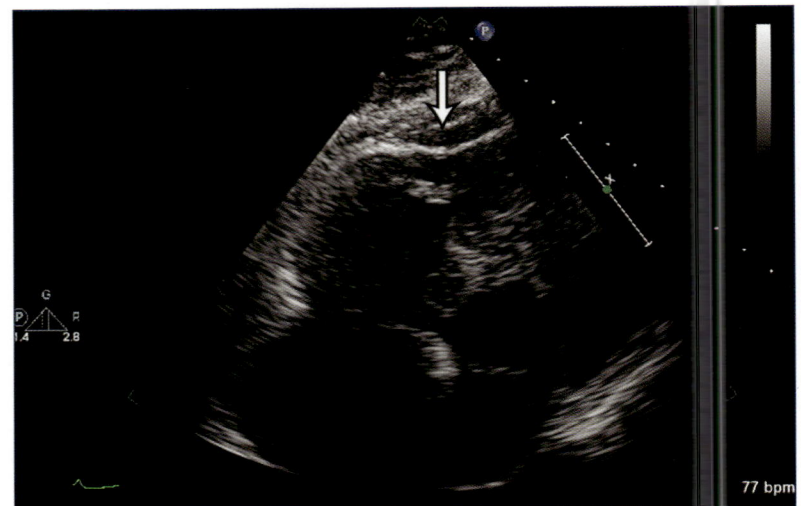

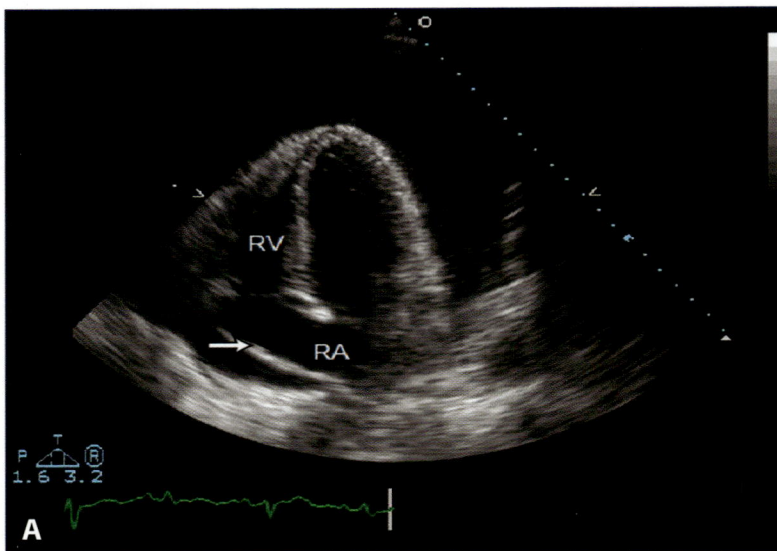

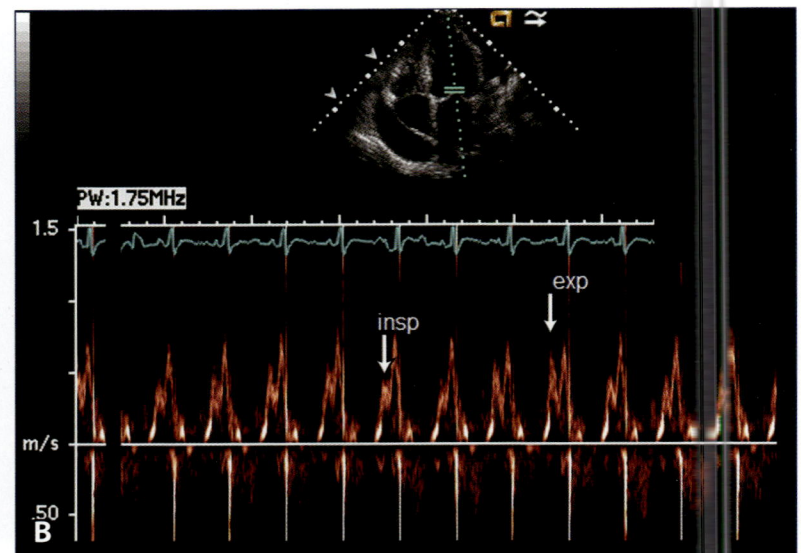

Figure 13-24. Cardiac tamponade. **A,** Physiology of cardiac tamponade, right atrial inversion. The urgent need to use echocardiography in assessing pericardial effusions always involves determining the presence or absence of tamponade physiology. Cardiac tamponade physiology occurs when the pressure in the pericardium exceeds the pressure in the cardiac chambers, resulting in impaired cardiac filling. The compressive effect of the pericardium is seen most clearly in the phase of the cardiac cycle when the pressure is lowest in that chamber. Hence, one of the earliest manifestations of tamponade is late diastolic early systolic collapse of the right atrium (RA), as is present in this apical four-chamber image (*arrow*) of a patient with massive circumferential pericardial effusion. RV—right ventricle.

B, Respiratory variation in transmitral E wave with pulsed Doppler, apical four-chamber view. This image demonstrates an inspiratory decrease in transmitral E wave velocities of greater than 25% (*arrows*), which is highly suggestive of cardiac tamponade. Intrapericardial and intrathoracic pressures normally decrease to the same degree with inspiration (insp). In tamponade, intrapericardial pressures fall substantially with inspiration as opposed to intrathoracic pressures, and as a consequence there is decreased left atrial filling pressure, which results in a decrease in E wave peak velocity. The diagnosis of pericardial tamponade always includes both clinical hemodynamic parameters and the echocardiographic findings. exp—expiration.

C, Respiratory variation in transaortic spectral Doppler, apical five-chamber view. This image demonstrates an inspiratory decrease in trans-

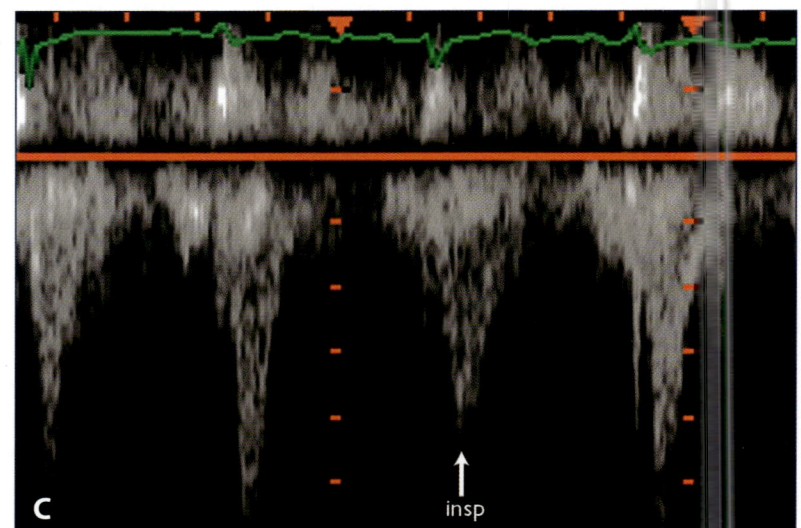

aortic spectral Doppler velocities of greater than 25%, which is highly suggestive of cardiac tamponade (*arrow*). In cardiac tamponade, the increased venous return to the RV with inspiration causes a shift of septal motion toward the left ventricle, which in turn leads to decreased left ventricular filling and resultant pulsus paradoxus or inspiratory decrease in transaortic spectral Doppler velocities.

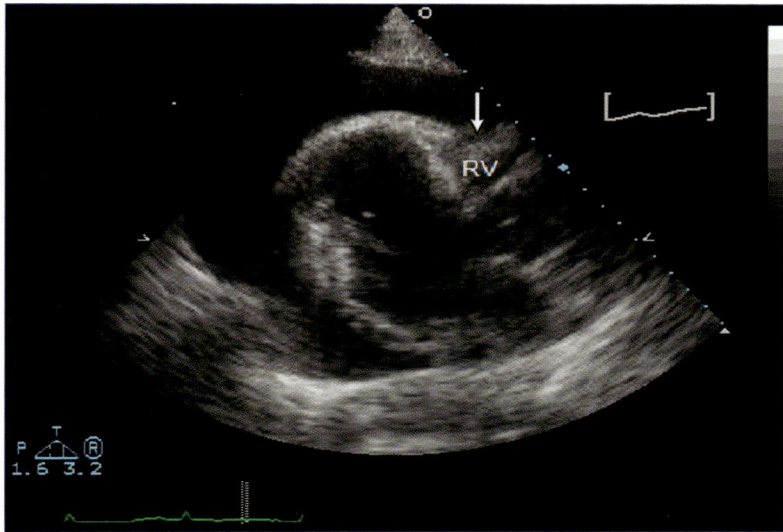

Figure 13-25. Right ventricular indentation in cardiac tamponade. Physiology of cardiac tamponade, right ventricular (RV) diastolic collapse (*arrow*), parasternal long-axis view. When intrapericardial pressure exceeds RV diastolic pressure, collapse of the free wall of the right ventricle occurs. This is a less sensitive, but more specific finding, consistent with cardiac tamponade.

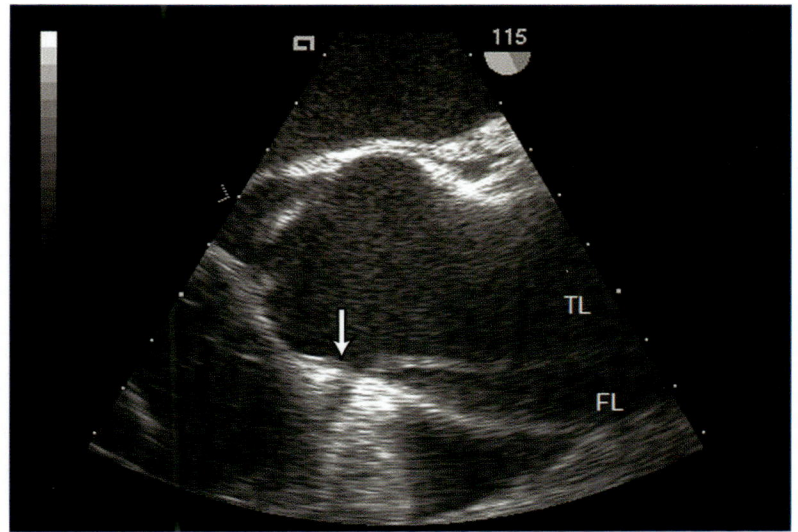

Figure 13-26. Acute aortic dissection. Transesophageal echocardiogram, longitudinal view of the aorta, demonstrating a Debakey type I aortic dissection. A mobile linear dissection flap originates just distal to the right coronary artery (*arrow*). According to the Debakey classification, type I dissection starts in the ascending aorta and extends to the arch and often beyond. These are surgical emergencies. FL—false lumen; TL—true lumen.

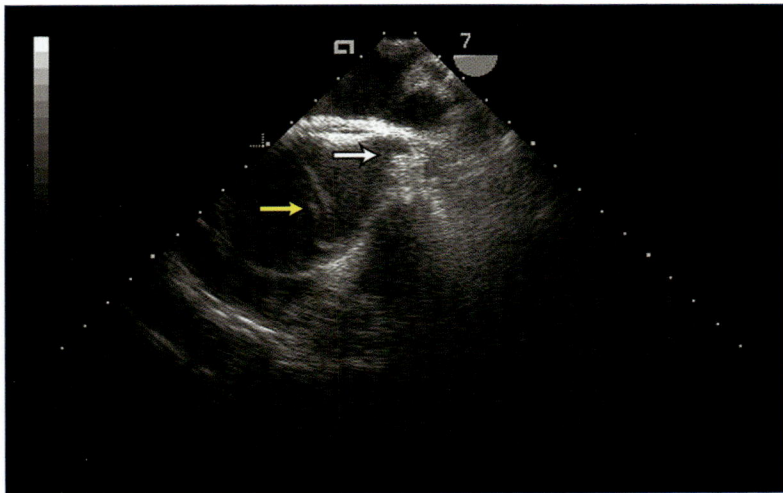

Figure 13-27. Type I aortic dissection, same patient as in Fig. 13-26. Transesophageal transverse view of the aortic root and ascending aorta, demonstrating no left coronary artery involvement (*white arrow*) by the dissection flap (*yellow arrow*). It is important to carefully examine the left and right coronary artery ostia in all patients with dissection involving the ascending aorta, as flaps can often dissect into the coronary artery, causing myocardial infarction. The identification of coronary artery involvement would warrant coronary artery bypass grafting at the time of surgical repair.

New Technologies in Echocardiography

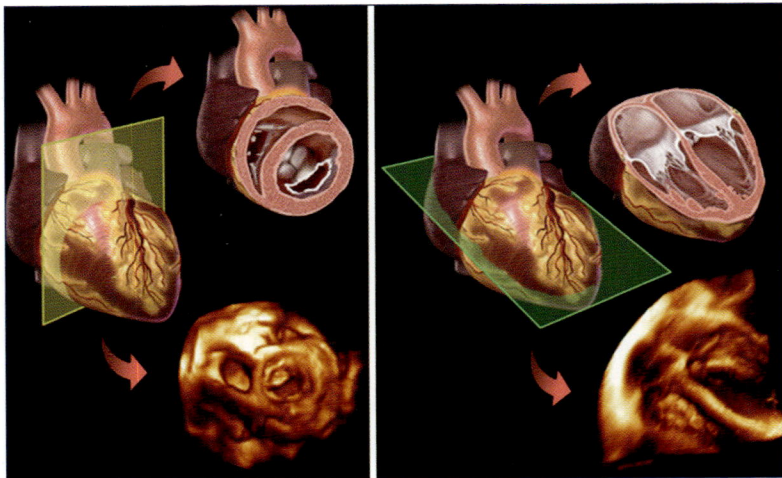

Figure 13-28. Three-dimensional echocardiography. Schematic representation of how different cut planes of the heart can be extracted from a pyramidal three-dimensional dataset. The basal short-axis view of the left ventricle depicts the mitral and tricuspid valves (*left panel, yellow cut plane*). The apical four-chamber view depicts the inferoseptal, inferior, and inferolateral walls (*right panel, green plane*). (*From* Nanda *et al.* [17]; with permission.)

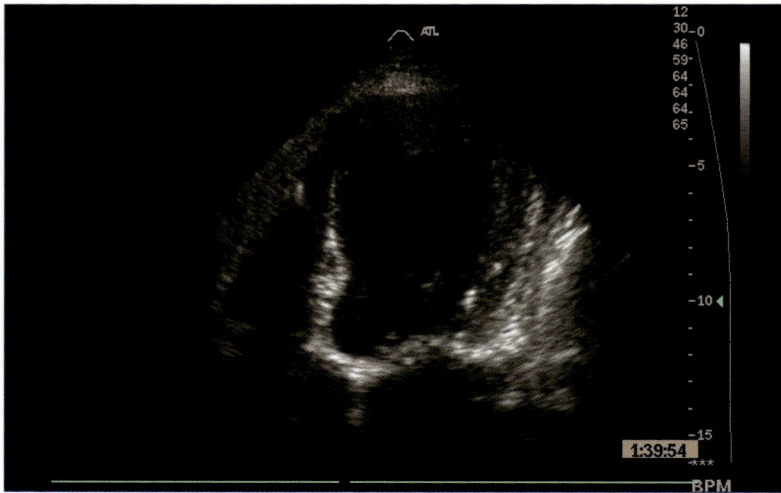

Figure 13-29. Tissue harmonic imaging in a patient with dilated cardio-myopathy and a vague echo density in the left ventricular (LV) apex is suggestive of an apical LV thrombus.

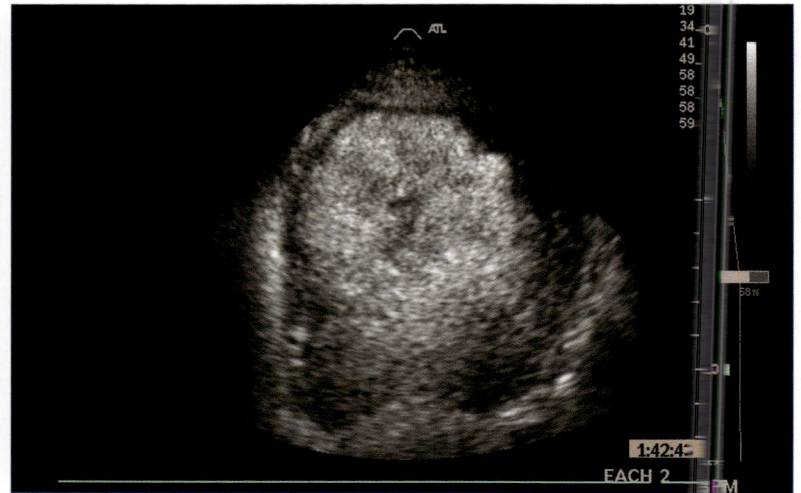

Figure 13-30. Apical four-chamber view. Image enhancement with intra-venous contrast demonstrates left ventricular (LV) opacification and out-lines the normal smooth endocardial border. The apical image artifact is eliminated, thus excluding an LV thrombus.

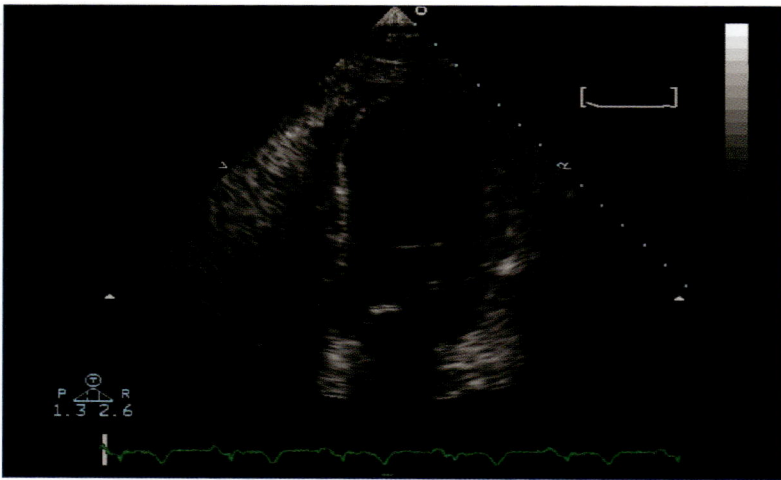

Figure 13-31. Apical four-chamber view. Tissue harmonic imaging in a patient with recent anteroseptal acute myocardial infarction demonstrates suboptimal endocardial borders. A vague echo density at the apex suggests an apical thrombus.

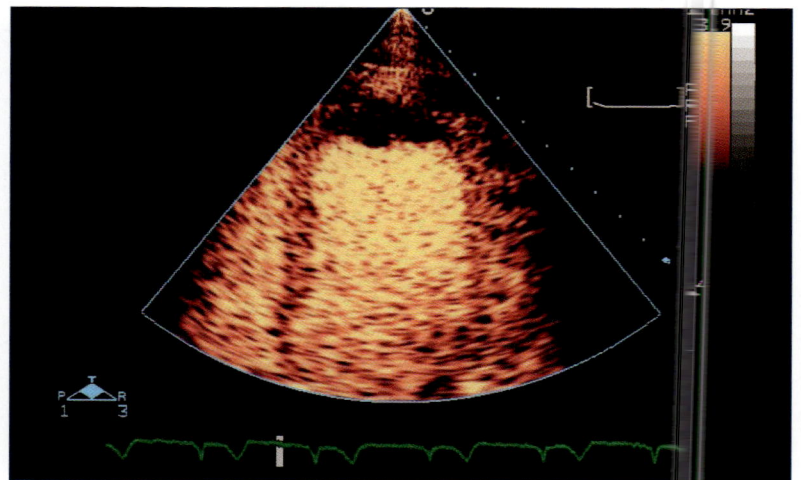

Figure 13-32. Apical four-chamber view. After contrast enhancement, a distinct filling defect is noted in the apex consistent with left ventricular apical thrombus.

Essential Features of a Hand-Carried Ultrasound Device

	Traditional echocardiography platform	HCU
Controls	Complex	Simple
Power supply	A/C	Battery
Weight	+++++	+
Price	+++++	++
A		

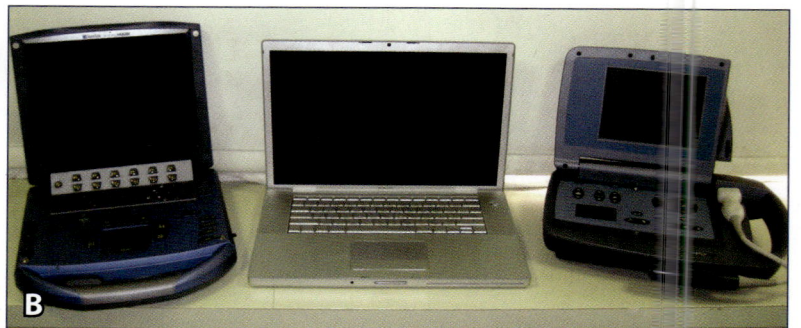

Figure 13-33. Hand-carried echocardiography. Although devices of 10 to 20 lbs can be "carried" (**A**), most would only consider using hand-carried echocardiography (HCU) device instruments that can be easily carried from patient room to patient room; this would typically mean platforms lighter than 6 to 7 lbs. More recent devices weighing less than 3 lbs are currently available. The other key features are battery power, simplicity of operation, and relatively low cost. Typical hand-carried devices (**B**, *left and right*) are shown with a laptop computer (**B**, *middle*) for scale.

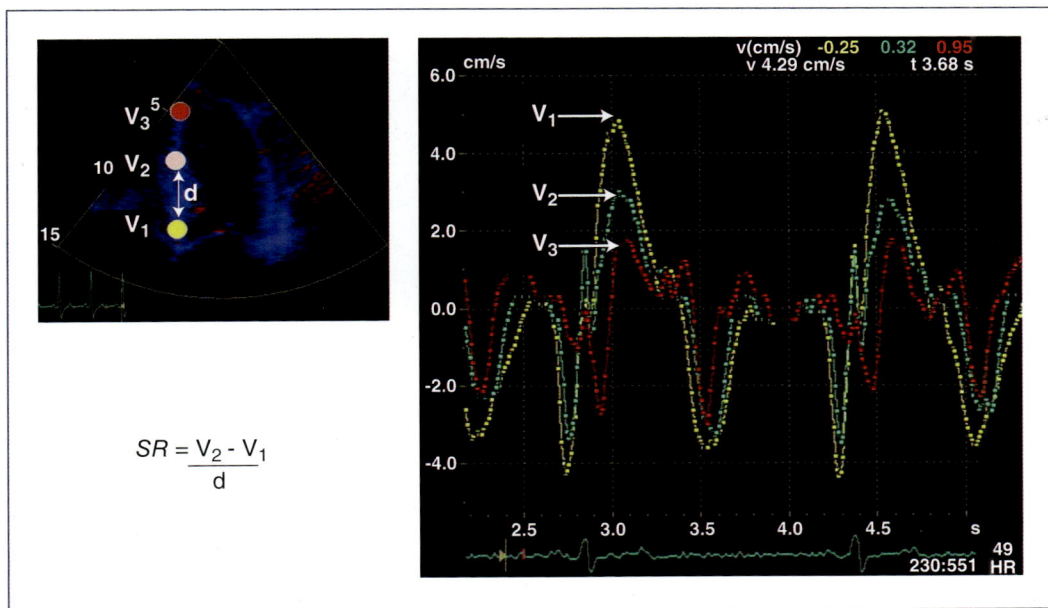

Figure 13-34. Assessment of myocardial strain with Doppler techniques. In the longitudinal orientation, normal heart motion is such that the base moves toward the apex, which moves very little or not at all. Thus, tissue velocity is maximal at the base (V_1), lower in the middle (V_2), and least at the apex (V_3). This gradient in velocities is used to calculate strain rates (SR). SR is calculated (using tissue Doppler) as the difference between two tissue velocities along the ultrasound beam (V_2–V_1) normalized to the intervening distance (d) between these two velocities. Colored circles indicate the positions of the region of interest in the myocardium (*left panel*) for the corresponding tissue velocity traces (*right panel*). (*From* Abraham *et al.* [18]; with permission.)

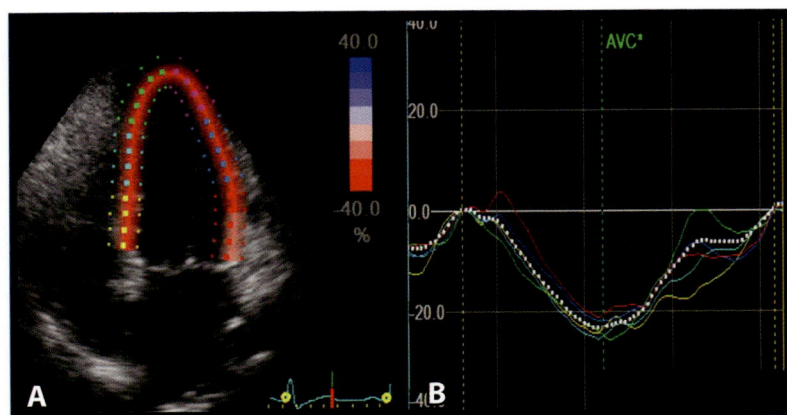

$$SR = \frac{V_2 - V_1}{d}$$

Figure 13-35. Assessment of myocardial strain using two-dimensional speckle tracking. In this representative figure of two-dimensional speckle tracking strain measurement of longitudinal strain, the color overlay indicates peak systolic strain along the longitudinal direction per the color scale in the right upper corner (**A**). Absolute values of strain per segment (*individual traces in solid line*) and global strain (*dotted white line*) are shown (**B**). AVC—aortic valve closure.

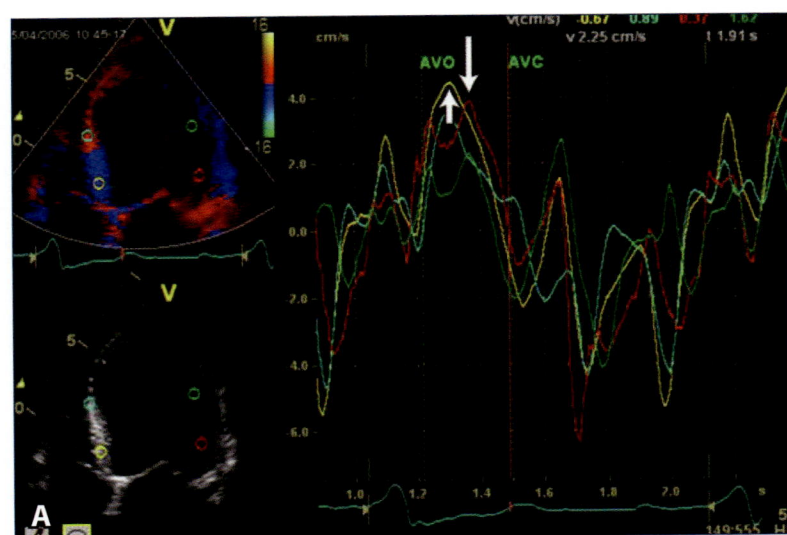

Figure 13-36. Assessment of cardiac dyssynchrony with echocardiography. Tissue Doppler imaging (TDI) is often used to determine which patients may benefit from cardiac resynchronization therapy (CRT), using biventricular pacing, as illustrated. Yu *et al.* [19] proposed measuring the standard deviation of the time-to-peak systolic velocity among 12 left ventricular (LV) segments (six basal, six mid) on apical two-, three-, and four-chamber images to calculate the dyssynchrony index (Ts-SD). Examples of color-coded TDI at apical four-chamber (**A** and **B**), apical two-chamber (**C** and **D**), and three-chamber (**E** and **F**) views before (**A, C,** and **E**) and after (**B, D,** and **F**) CRT are shown.

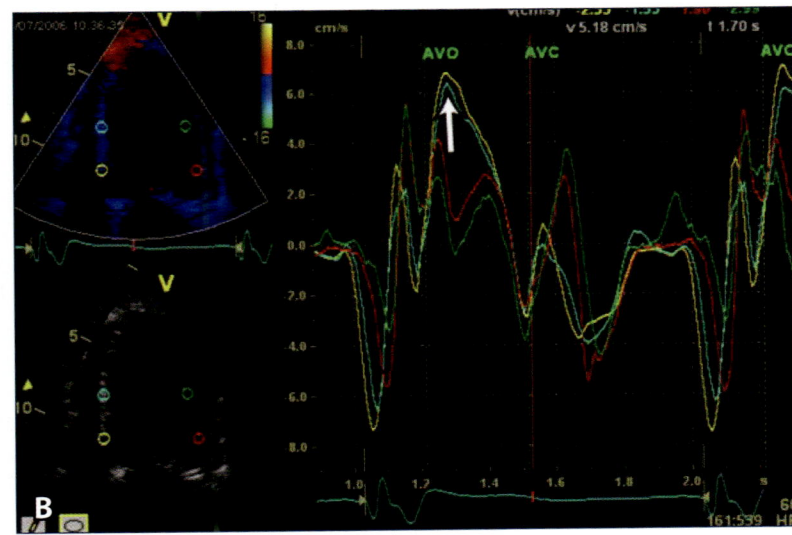

Continued on the next page

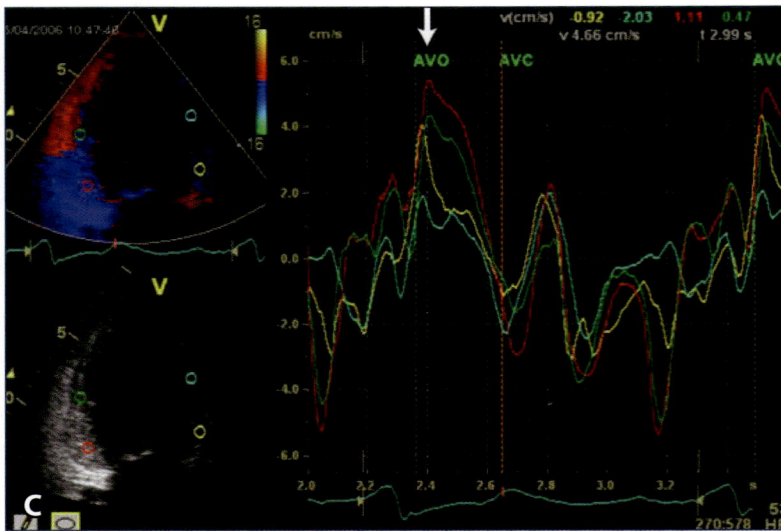

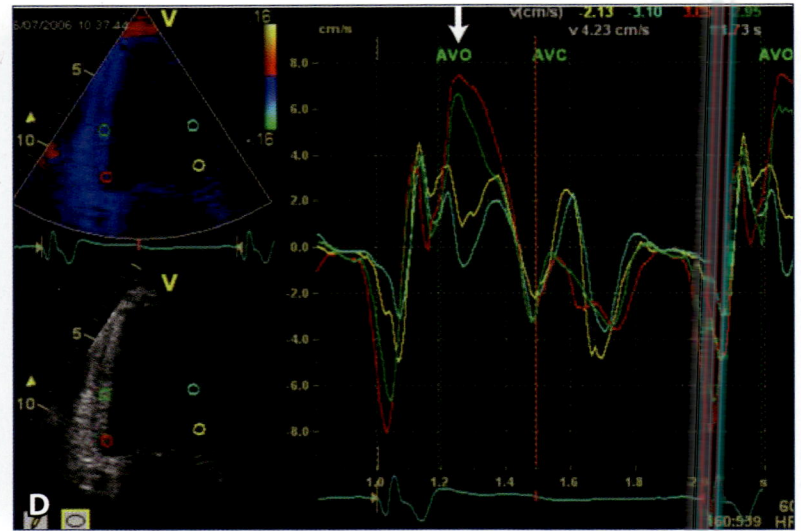

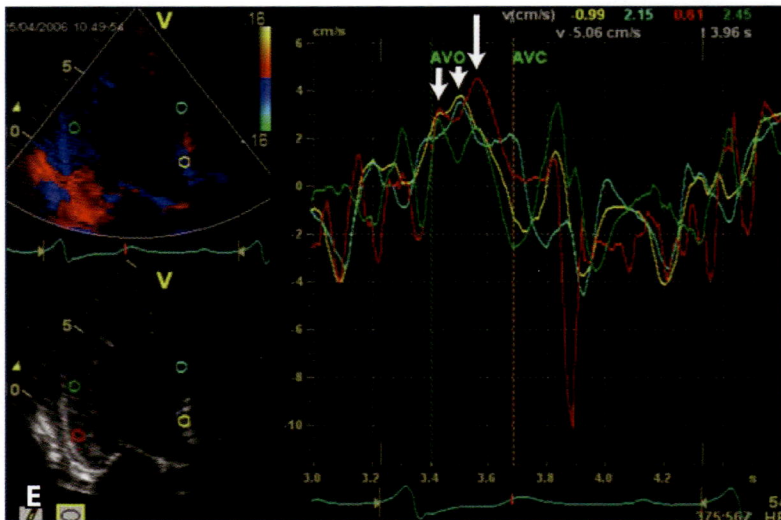

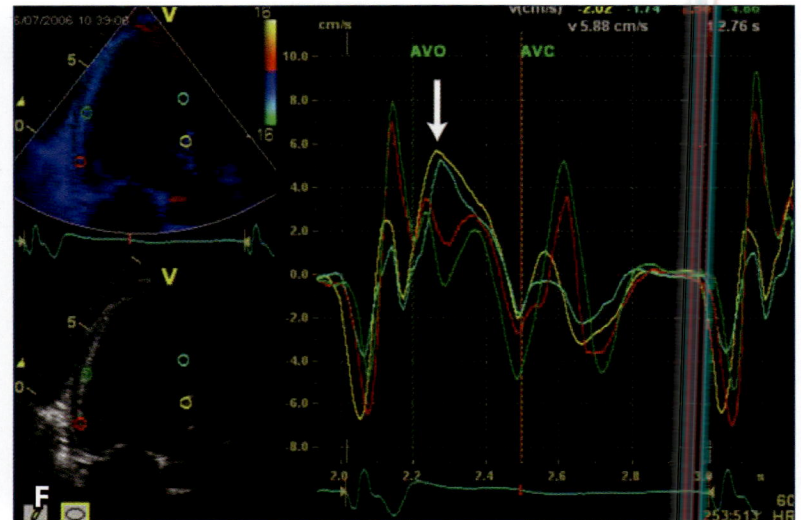

Figure 13-36. *(Continued)* The use of three apical views can establish the six-basal and six-midsegmental LV model for assessing LV dyssynchrony. Delay in the time-to-peak systolic velocity is evident in the lateral (**A**) and posterior walls (**C**) at baseline. Peak systolic velocities are shown (**A** and **C**, *arrows*). After CRT, there is a realignment of the systolic velocities, in particular in the ejection phase where the peak systolic velocities occur almost at the same time. Peak systolic velocities are shown (*all panels, arrows*). The Ts-SD can be calculated from the standard deviation of time-to-peak systolic velocity in the ejection phase of the 12 LV segments, which is decreased from 51 ms before CRT to 20 ms after the therapy. The cut-off value of Ts-SD for substantial LV dyssynchrony is 33 ms [19]. AVC—aortic valve closure; AVO—aortic valve opening.

References

1. Thomas JD, Popovic ZB: Assessment of left ventricular function by cardiac ultrasound. *J Am Coll Cardiol* 2006, 48:2012–2025.

2. Kirkpatrick JN, Vannan MA, Narula J, Lang RM: Echocardiography in heart failure: applications, utility, and new horizons. *J Am Coll Cardiol* 2007, 50:381–396.

3. Sugeng L, Mor-Avi V, Weinert L, *et al.*: Quantitative assessment of left ventricular size and function: side-by-side comparison of real-time three-dimensional echocardiography and computed tomography with magnetic resonance reference. *Circulation* 2006, 114:654–661.

4. Kirkpatrick JN, Vannan MA, Narula J, Lang RM: Echocardiography in heart failure: applications, utility, and new horizons. *J Am Coll Cardiol* 2007, 50:381–396.

5. Arruda-Olson AM, Juracan EM, Mahoney DW, *et al.*: Prognostic value of exercise echocardiography in 5798 patients: is there a gender difference? *J Am Coll Cardiol* 2002, 39:625–631.

6. Freed LA, Levy D, Levine RA, *et al.*: Prevalence and clinical outcome of mitral-valve prolapse. *N Engl J Med* 1999, 341:1–7.

7. Weyman AE, Scherrer-Crosbie M: Marfan syndrome and mitral valve prolapse. *J Clin Invest* 2004, 114:1543–1546.

8. Wilcken DE, Hickey AJ: Lifetime risk for patients with mitral valve prolapse of developing severe valve regurgitation requiring surgery. *Circulation* 1988, 78:10–14.

9. Erbel R, Rohmann S, Drexler M, *et al.*: Improved diagnostic value of echocardiography in patients with infective endocarditis by transoesophageal approach: a prospective study. *Eur Heart J* 1988, 9:43–53.

10. Mugge A, Daniel WG, Frank G, Lichtlen PR: Echocardiography in infective endocarditis: reassessment of prognostic implications of vegetation size determined by the transthoracic and the transesophageal approach. *J Am Coll Cardiol* 1989, 14:631–638.

11. Karalis DG, Bansal RC, Hauck AJ, *et al.*: Transesophageal echocardiographic recognition of subaortic complications in aortic valve endocarditis: clinical and surgical implications. Clinical and surgical implications. *Circulation* 1992, 86:353–362.

12. Quinones MA, Otto, CM, Stoddard M, *et al.*: American Society of Echocardiography Recommendations for Quantification of Doppler Echocardiography: A Report from the Doppler Quantification Task Force of the Nomenclature and Standards Committee of the American Society of Echocardiography. Accessible at asecho.org. Accessed March 24, 2008.

13. Enriquez-Sarano M, Tajik AJ: Clinical practice. Aortic regurgitation. *N Engl J Med* 2004, 351:1539–1546.

14. Tribouilloy CM, Enriquez-Sarano M, Bailey KR, *et al.*: Assessment of severity of aortic regurgitation using the width of the vena contracta: a clinical color Doppler imaging study. *Circulation* 2000, 102:558–564.

15. Thygesen K, Alpert JS, White HD: Universal definition of myocardial infarction. *Eur Heart J* 2007, 28:2525–2538.

16. Sherrid MV, Gunsburg DZ, Moldenhauer S, Pearle G: Systolic anterior motion begins at low left ventricular outflow tract velocity in obstructive hypertrophic cardiomyopathy. *J Am Coll Cardiol* 2000, 36:1344–1354.

17. Nanda NC, Kisslo J, Lang R, *et al.*: Examination protocol for three-dimensional echocardiography. *Echocardiography* 2004, 21:763–768.

18. Abraham TP, Dimaano VL, Liang HY: Role of tissue Doppler and strain echocardiography in current clinical practice. *Circulation* 2007, 116:2597–2609.

19. Yu CM, Chau E, Sanderson JE, *et al.*: Tissue Doppler echocardiographic evidence of reverse remodeling and improved synchronicity by simultaneously delaying regional contraction after biventricular pacing therapy in heart failure. *Circulation* 2002, 105:438–445.

Nuclear Cardiology

14

Vasken Dilsizian, Marcelo F. Di Carli, and Jagat Narula

R adionuclide-based imaging offers a diverse range of approaches to evaluate cardiovascular physiology and pathophysiology, including assessment of myocardial perfusion, metabolism, neuronal function, cardiac function, and more recently, molecularly targeted imaging. The regional
distribution of radionuclides in the heart can be imaged tomographically using single-photon emission computed tomography (SPECT) or positron emission tomography (PET). These approaches offer
high sensitivity and quantitative results, which is another key strength of nuclear cardiology–based
imaging. These technologies are now being integrated with computed tomography (CT) and possibly
magnetic resonance imaging (MRI) (eg, SPECT/CT, PET/CT, PET/MRI) with the hope of exploiting
the unique strengths of each component to allow improved diagnosis of disease and better patient
care. In addition, the miniaturization of SPECT and PET scanners with dramatic increases in sensitivity and spatial resolution, coupled with the development of quantitative targeted imaging approaches
for evaluating physiology and pathophysiology at the cellular and molecular level provide a promising
platform for a new era in diagnostic imaging. Myocardial perfusion and metabolism imaging using
both SPECT and PET play a critical role in diagnosis and risk assessment of patients with known or
suspected coronary artery disease, and are widely used for guiding patient management. This chapter
reviews the essentials of radionuclide imaging and its current clinical applications with a focus on
coronary artery disease. It also provides a glimpse to the future, especially in areas currently being
tested in clinical trials, including imaging of myocardial metabolism to assess ischemic memory and
neuronal imaging to identify patients at risk of sudden cardiac death.

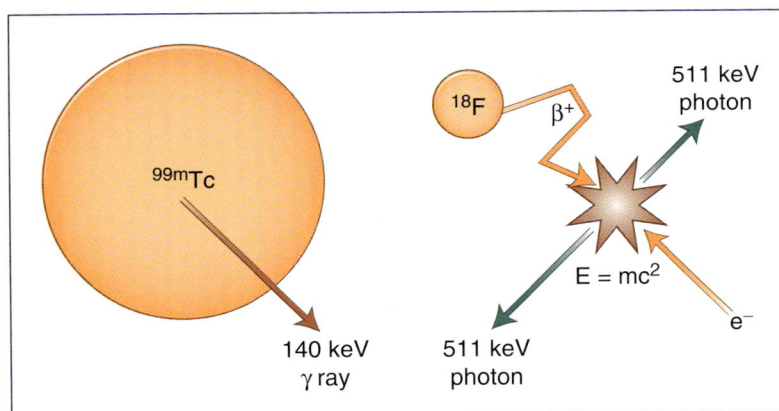

Figure 14-1. Single-photon emission computed tomography (SPECT) versus positron emission tomography
(PET) radionuclides. The figure shows two very different types of radionuclides, technetium-99m (^{99m}Tc) and fluo-
rine-18 (^{18}F). ^{99m}Tc is a large radionuclide that emits a single photon or γ-ray per radioactive decay that is used in
SPECT to create images. The energy of the emitted photon is 140 keV. The *m* in ^{99m}Tc means that the nucleus is
meta-stable (almost stable but really unstable). ^{18}F is a much smaller radionuclide that emits a positron (β+) antiparticle. This ionized antiparticle travels through a medium interacting with it, losing energy and slowing down
until it interacts with an electron, usually from some atom. Because the electron and the positron are antiparticles
of each other, *ie*, same mass but opposite charge, they undergo a phenomenon called pair annihilation. In pair
annihilation, the mass of both particles disintegrates and is converted into energy as explained by Einstein's famous
equation, $E = mc^2$, where *E* is the emitted energy, *m* is the mass of the two particles, and *c* is the speed of light in a
vacuum. Because of the nature of the interaction, most of the time the energy is emitted in the form of two photons
traveling in exactly opposite directions from each other and each having the same energy, 511 keV, which is the
energy equivalent to the rest mass of an electron. It is these two photons that are used to create images in PET.

Properties of SPECT Flow Tracers

Tracer	Mechanism of Myocyte Uptake	Usual Dose, *mCi*
^{201}Tl	Na-K ATPase—sarcolemma	3.0–4.5
^{99m}Tc sestamibi	Negative transmembrane potential—mitochondria	8–40
^{99m}Tc tetrofosmin	Negative transmembrane potential—mitochondria	8–40

A

Properties of PET Flow Tracers

Tracer	Mechanism of Myocyte Uptake	Usual Dose, *mCi*
^{82}Rb	Na-K ATPase—sarcolemma	30–60
^{13}N ammonia	Trapped as ^{13}N glutamine (mediated by ATP)—cytoplasm	10–20

B

C

D

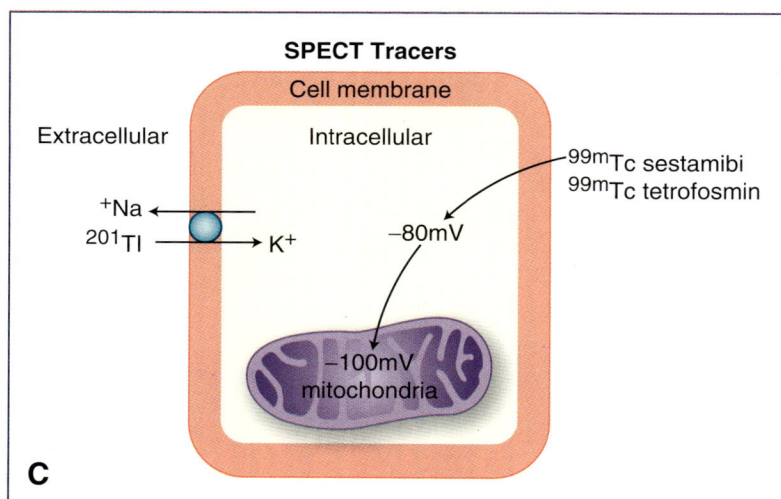

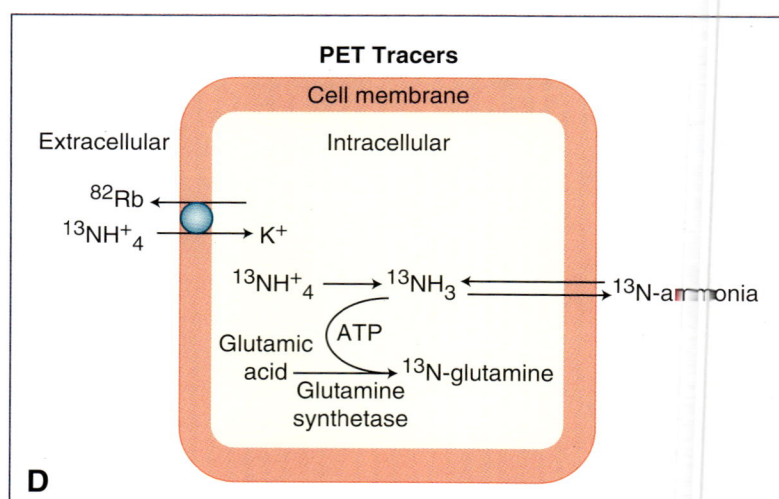

Figure 14-2. **A,** Properties of single-photon emission computed tomography (SPECT) and positron emission tomography (PET) flow tracers (**B**). To reflect regional myocardial perfusion, radiotracers commonly used with SPECT and PET must have high extraction by the heart and rapid clearance from the blood. Clinically available radiopharmaceuticals that meet these criteria are ^{201}Tl and ^{99m}Tc-labeled sestamibi and tetrofosmin with SPECT (**C**), and ^{82}Rb and ^{13}N ammonia with PET (**D**). Radiotracers that are not highly extracted (< 50%), or if the residence time in the blood is prolonged (clearance half-time of > 5 minutes), cannot be used to assess regional perfusion.

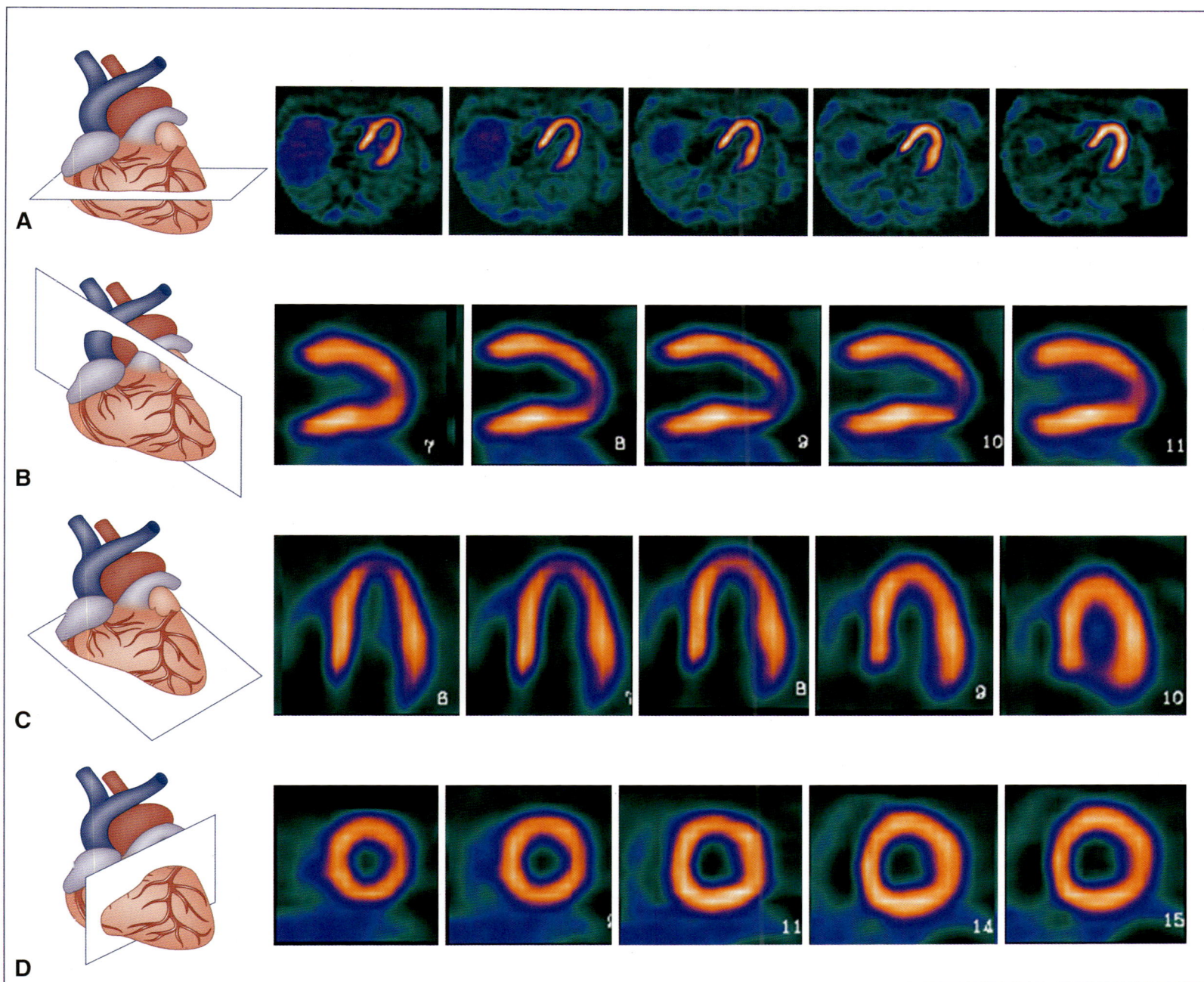

Figure 14-3. Oblique angle reorientation. *Transaxial images:* The natural products of rotational tomography are images that represent cross-sectional slices of the body, perpendicular to the imaging table (or long axis of the body). These images are called transverse or transaxial slices. An example of transaxial slices can be seen in **A**.

Oblique images: We are not restricted to the natural x, y, and z directions, however, for the display of images. The computer may be used to extract images at any orientation, and these images are called oblique images. Because of the variation in the heart orientation of different patients, it is important that oblique slices are adjusted to try to match the same anatomy from patient to patient. The important oblique sections used for viewing cardiac images are defined thusly: *Vertical long-axis slices:* The three-dimensional set of transaxial sections, some of which are shown in **A**, is resliced parallel to the long axis and perpendicular through the transaxial slices. Each of the resulting oblique images is called a vertical long-axis slice, as shown in **B**. They are displayed with the base of the left ventricle toward the left side of the image and the apex toward the right. Serial slices are displayed from medial (septal) to lateral, left to right. *Horizontal long-axis slices:* The three-dimensional block of vertical long-axis slices is recut parallel to the denoted long axis and perpendicular to the stack. The resulting oblique cuts are called horizontal long-axis slices, as seen in **C**. They contain the left ventricle with its base toward the bottom of the image and its apex toward the top. The right ventricle appears on the left side of the image. Serial horizontal long-axis slices are displayed from inferior to anterior, from left to right. *Short-axis slices:* Slices perpendicular to the denoted long axis and perpendicular to the vertical long-axis slices are also cut from the stack. These are termed short-axis slices; they contain the left ventricle with its anterior wall toward the top, its inferior wall toward the bottom, and its septal wall toward the left. Serial short-axis slices are displayed from apex to base, from left to right, in **D**.

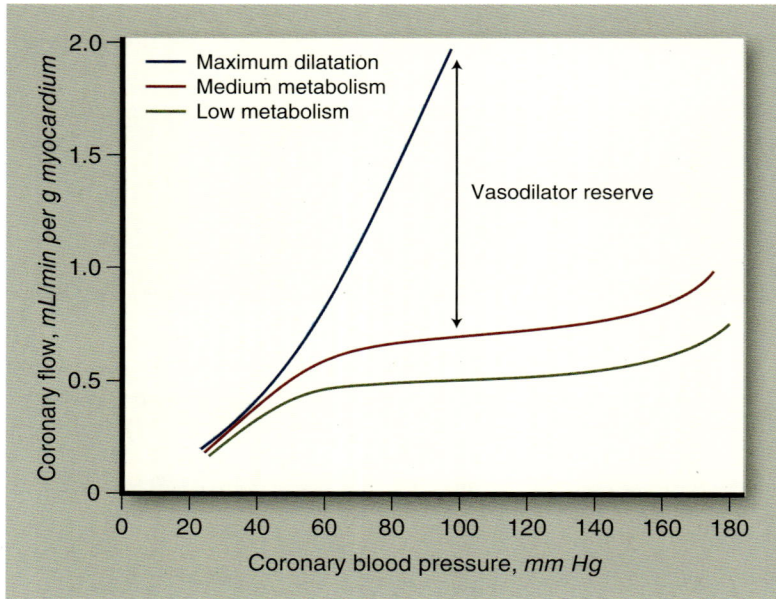

Figure 14-4. Autoregulation of coronary blood flow. The coronary circulation underlies an active autoregulation [1] that keeps coronary blood flow relatively constant despite changes in coronary driving pressure. Autoregulation of coronary blood flow depends on myocardial oxygen requirements [2] so that coronary flow changes in proportion to changes in oxygen demand and consumption. Mechanisms responsible for the active changes in coronary vascular resistance relate to both myogenic control and local metabolic needs. Myogenic control implies that pressure distention of the vessel due to increases in coronary perfusion pressure lead to active vasoconstriction that increases vascular resistance and maintains flow relatively constant. In contrast, local metabolic feedback control entails intrinsic local mechanisms that adjust coronary blood flow to changes in oxygen consumption. An increase in oxygen consumption, for example due to increases in contractile state or heart rate and thus in myocardial work, is associated with a decrease in myocardial oxygen tension that leads to release or activation of local vasodilator substances such as adenosine, K^+ adenosine triphosphate channels, and/or nitric oxide, which in turn increase coronary blood flow and oxygen supply.

The vasodilator capacity represents the increase in flow from rest to hyperemia either during exercise or pharmacologically induced vasodilation. However, the autoregulation is lost at coronary driving pressures less than 60 mm Hg. Further, during maximum vasodilation as induced by vascular smooth muscle relaxing agents, coronary flow becomes dependent on coronary driving pressure.

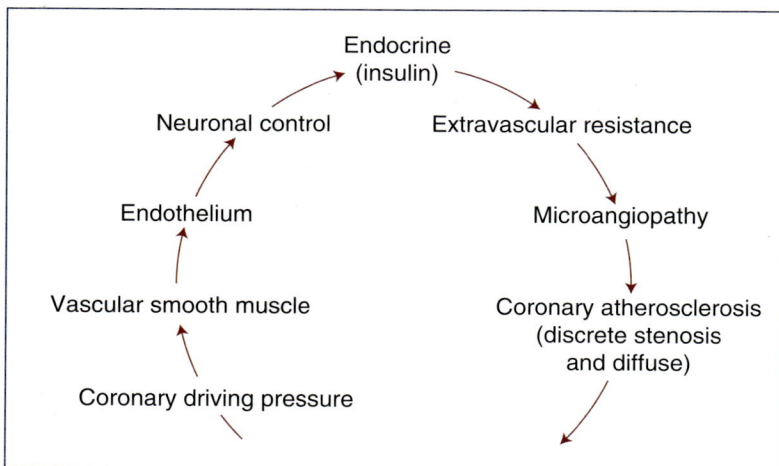

Figure 14-5. Determinants of vasodilator-induced hyperemic myocardial blood flows.

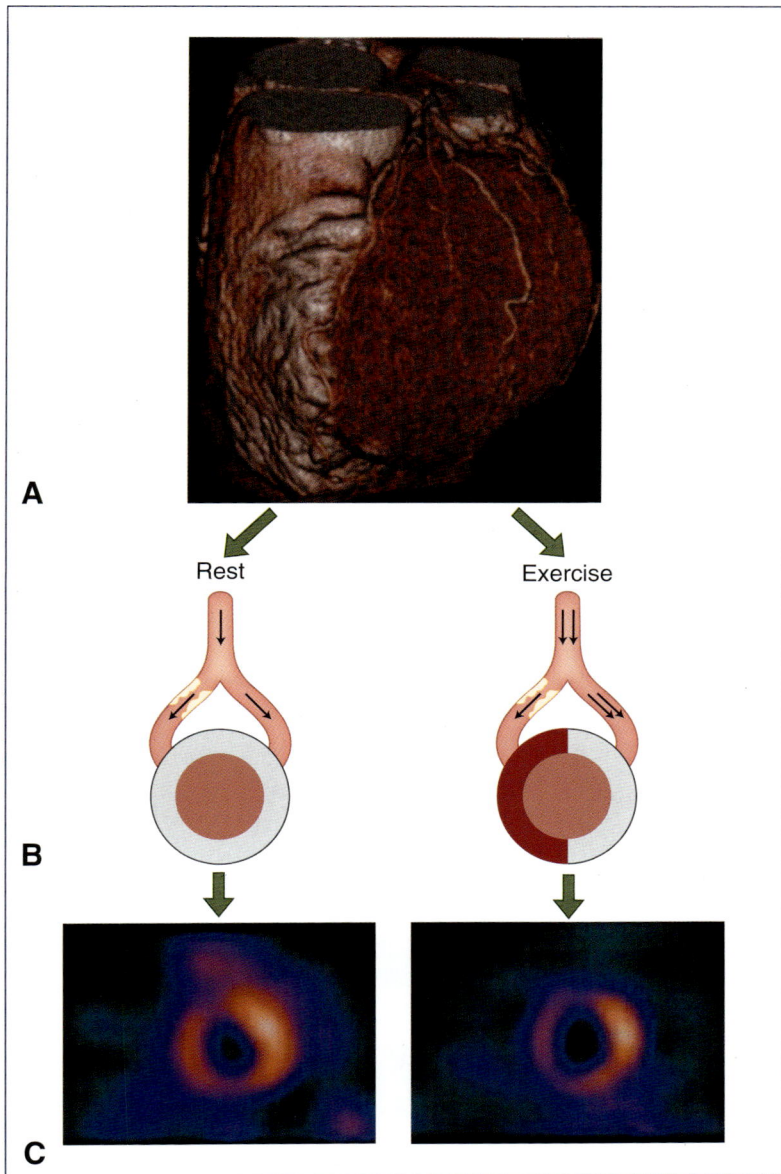

Figure 14-6. Myocardial blood flow and coronary anatomy: disparate yet complementary information. Regional myocardial blood flow is critically dependent on the driving pressure gradient and the resistance of the vascular bed. Advanced degrees of coronary artery disease may exist at rest (**A**) without myocardial ischemia due to compensatory dilatation of the resistance vessels. As illustrated in **B** and **C**, at rest, regional myocardial blood flow is preserved in both patent and stenosed coronary artery branches. Such disparity between myocardial blood flow and coronary anatomy attests to the complementary information that physiologic study such as myocardial perfusion single photon emission computed tomography (SPECT) or positron emission tomography (PET) provides to that of coronary angiography with CT or diagnostic catheterization. In dogs, more than 80% occlusion of the coronary artery was necessary before ischemia was observed under basal state. Because the pressure drop across a stenosis varies directly with the length of the stenosis and inversely with the fourth power of the radius (Bernoulli's theorem), resistance almost triples as the severity of coronary artery stenosis increases from 80% to 90%. Consequently, during exercise or pharmacologic stress testing, when the resistance to the distal bed and the pressure distending the stenotic coronary artery declines, myocardial ischemia ensues (**B** and **C**).

Coronary blood flow in myocardial regions without coronary artery stenosis may increase about two- to threefold during vigorous aerobic exercise. However, in the setting of moderate-to-severe coronary artery stenosis, the degree of coronary flow increase may be attenuated when compared to myocardial regions without coronary artery stenosis (**B**). The insufficient coronary blood flow increase during stress results in impaired perfusion and myocardial ischemia (**C**). In patients with coronary artery disease, an inverse relationship has been shown between the increase in myocardial blood flow and the percentage of coronary artery stenosis once the lumen is narrowed by approximately 40% to 50%. Thus, when a radiotracer such as thallium is injected at peak exercise, the relative differences in regional myocardial blood flow will be reflected in disproportionate concentrations of regional thallium activity on the stress images. Myocardial perfusion imaging, therefore, identifies subcritical coronary artery stenosis when performed in conjunction with exercise or pharmacologic stress, but not at rest.

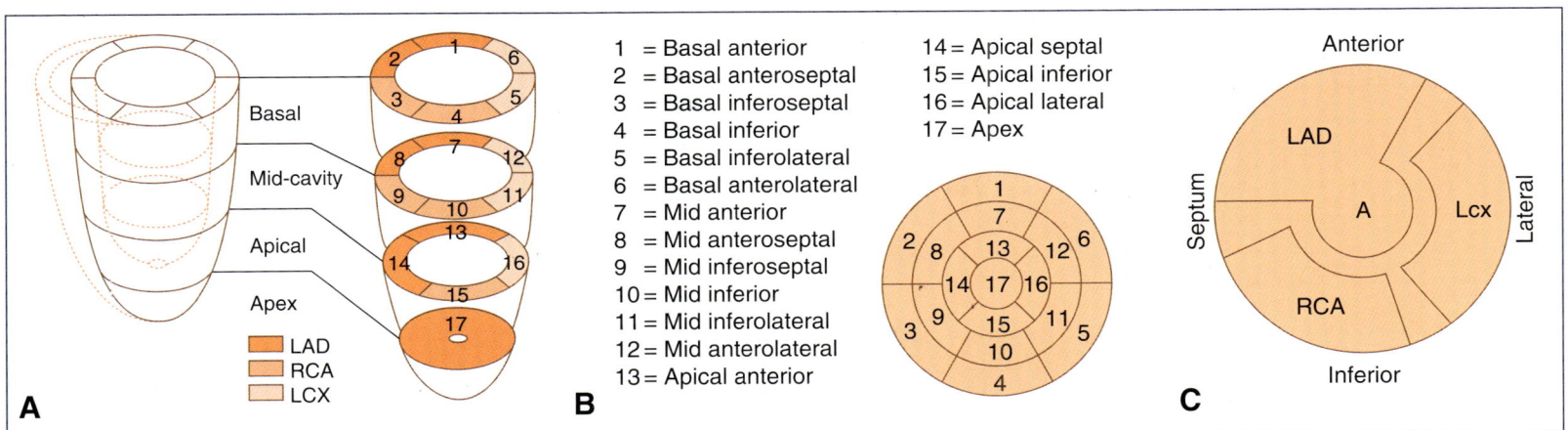

Figure 14-7. Myocardial segmentation, standard nomenclature and vascular territories. Single photon emission computed tomography (SPECT) myocardial perfusion images are interpreted on the basis of the presence, location, extent, and severity of perfusion defects using a standard 17-segment model [3] and visual scoring. **A,** Standard segmentation model divides the left ventricle into three major short-axis slices: apical, mid-cavity, and basal. The apical short-axis slice is divided into four segments, whereas the mid-cavity and basal slices are divided into six segments. The apex is analyzed separately, usually from a vertical long-axis slice. Although the anatomy of coronary arteries may vary in individual patients, the anterior, septal, and apical segments are usually ascribed to the left anterior descending (LAD) coronary artery, the inferior and basal septal segments to the right coronary artery (RCA), and the lateral segments to the left circumflex (LCX) coronary artery. The apex can also be supplied by the RCA and LCX artery. **B,** Data from the individual short-axis tomograms can be combined to create a bull's-eye polar plot, representing a two-dimensional compilation of all the three-dimensional short-axis perfusion data. Standard nomenclature for the 17 segments is outlined. **C,** The two-dimensional compilation of perfusion data can then easily be assigned to specific vascular territories.

A　　　　　　　**B**　　　　　　　**C**

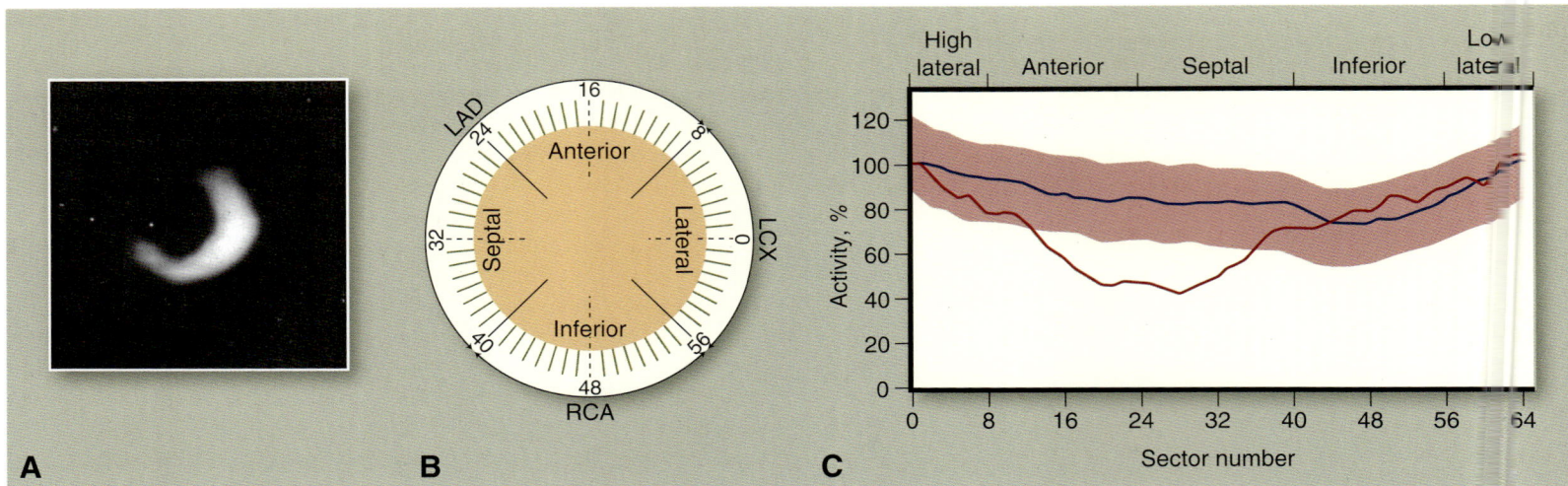

Figure 14-8. Quantitative analysis. Because radionuclide images are intrinsically digital images, true quantification of tracer uptake in myocardial regions is feasible [4]. The methodology of semiautomatic quantitative circumferential-profile analysis applied to a short-axis ^{201}Tl tomogram obtained after exercise in a patient with coronary artery disease is shown in **A**. The left ventricular myocardium is divided into 64 sectors, representing four myocardial regions (**B**). **C** shows the patient's thallium uptake during stress imaging in each section (*red line*) and the normal range (mean ± 2 SD for normal subjects; *shaded area with blue,*

centered line). The patient's count profile displays the distribution of counts in the tomogram relative to maximal counts counter-clockwise, starting at 0, representing the high lateral region that is designated the value of 100% (maximal count density). Whenever a region of the circumferential profile falls below the lower limit of normal, that region of the patient's myocardium is considered to have a perfusion defect. In this patient, thallium perfusion defects are apparent in the anterior and septal regions. LAD—left anterior descending; LCX—left circumflex; RCA—right coronary artery.

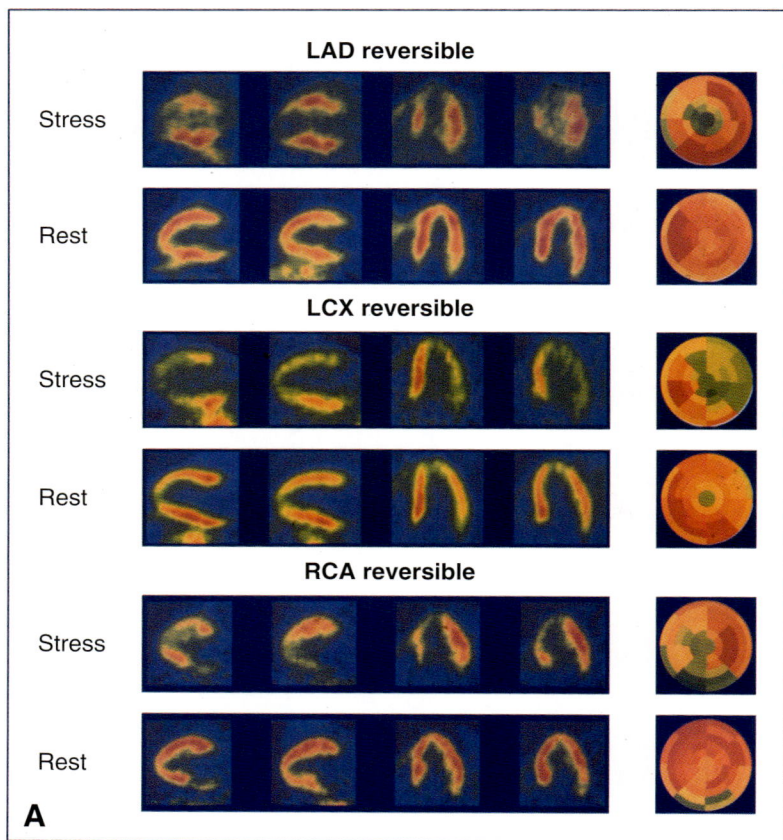

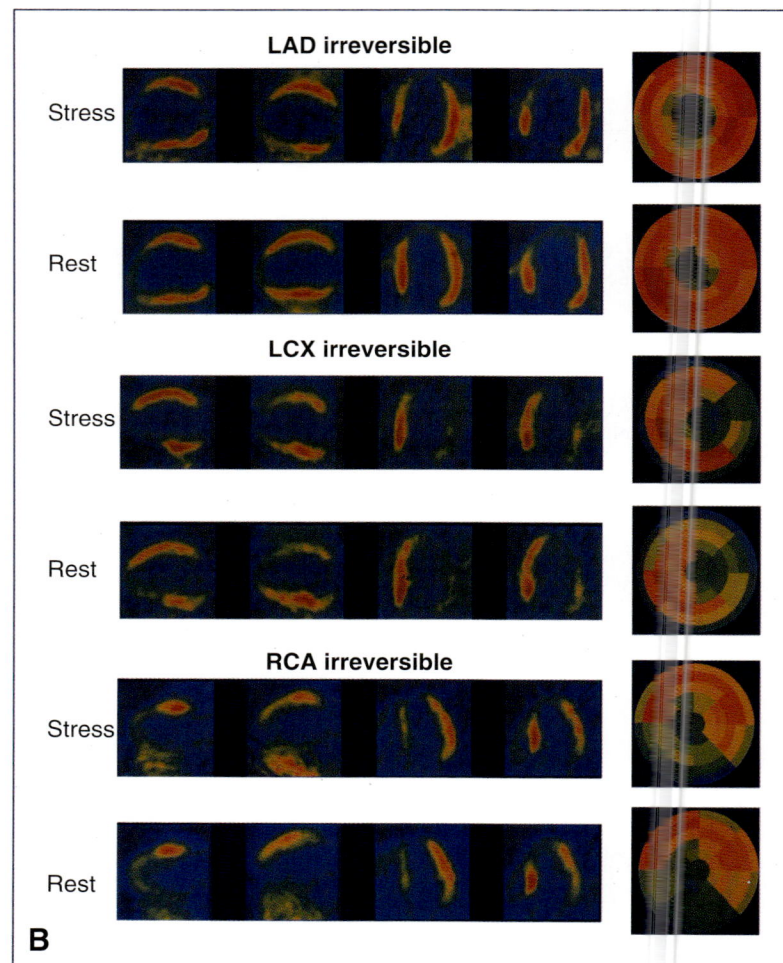

A　　　　　　　**B**

Figure 14-9. Reversible and irreversible perfusion defects: myocardial ischemia and infarction. Imbalance between oxygen supply (usually due to reduced myocardial perfusion) and oxygen demand (determined primarily by the rate and force of myocardial contraction) is termed *ischemic myocardium*. Clinical presentation of such imbalance may be symptomatic (angina pectoris) or asymptomatic (silent ischemia). If the oxygen supply-

demand imbalance is transient (ie, triggered by exertion) it represents reversible ischemia. The scintigraphic hallmark of reversible ischemia is a reversible perfusion defect. **A,** Examples of patients with reversible perfusion defects in the 1) left anterior descending (LAD), 2) left circumflex (LCX), and 3) right coronary artery (RCA) territories are shown.

Continued on the next page

Figure 14-9. (Continued) However, if regional oxygen supply-demand imbalance is prolonged (ie, during myocardial infarction), high-energy phosphates will be depleted, regional contractile function will progressively deteriorate, and cell membrane rupture with cell death will follow (myocardial infarction).

The scintigraphic hallmark of myocardial infarction is a fixed or irreversible perfusion defect. **B**, Examples of patients with irreversible (fixed) perfusion defects in the 1) LAD, 2) LCX, and 3) RCA territories are shown.

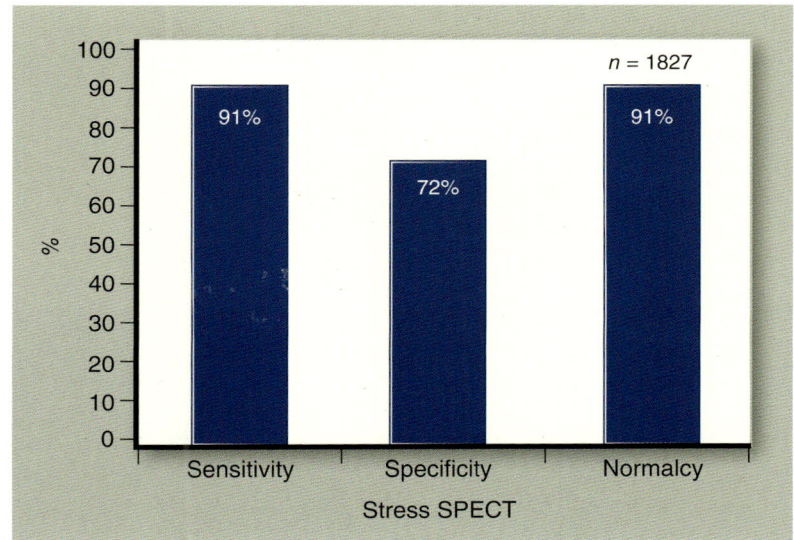

Figure 14-10. Detection of angiographic coronary artery disease with radiotracers. Extensive literature exists on the diagnostic yield of stress single photon emission computed tomography (SPECT) myocardial perfusion imaging [5–16]. Among 1827 patients referred for evaluation of chest discomfort (pooled data from 12 studies performed between 1989 and 1999), the overall sensitivity of myocardial perfusion SPECT for the detection of angiographic coronary artery disease was 91%, the specificity was 72%, and the normalcy rate (in subjects with low likelihood for coronary artery disease who did not undergo coronary angiography) was 91%.

Figure 14-11. High- and low-risk single-photon emission computed tomography (SPECT) images. SPECT images should not be interpreted as either normal or abnormal. The prognosis of a patient is related to the degree of myocardial perfusion abnormality. Quantification or semiquantification provides that important prognostic information. High-risk SPECT images are characterized by large perfusion defects on the stress images that involve multiple coronary artery territories (if two or more coronary territories are involved, the study should be considered high risk). Large stress-induced reversible defects represent extensive myocardial ischemia, which may be associated with increased lung uptake, transient ischemic left ventricular (LV) cavity dilation, and transient increased right ventricular (RV) myocardial visualization.

One of the strongest features of stress myocardial perfusion SPECT imaging is its ability to identify low-risk patients. Patients with unequivocal normal exercise or pharmacologic stress myocardial perfusion SPECT images exhibit less than a 1% future cardiac event rate, the same as the general population. For those undergoing an exercise study, this presumes that the patient achieved greater than 85% predicted maximum heart rate for a man or woman of their age. Similarly, presuming that adequate exercise was performed, patients with small myocardial perfusion defects on stress and small regions of defect reversibility have low risk for future cardiac events.

High- and Low-Risk SPECT Images

High-risk

Large perfusion defect on stress imaging

Multiple coronary artery territories

Large reversibility

Increased lung uptake

Transient LV dilation

Low-lisk

Normal stress images

Small stress defect

Small reversibility

These patients should be treated aggressively with medical therapy because of the presence of coronary artery disease. It is important to emphasize that stress myocardial perfusion SPECT images should always be interpreted in conjunction with clinical and electrocardiographic data. For example, a rare patient may have a markedly abnormal exercise portion of the test but normal or near-normal SPECT images. It is the responsibility of the nuclear cardiologist to determine the significance of such disparate data.

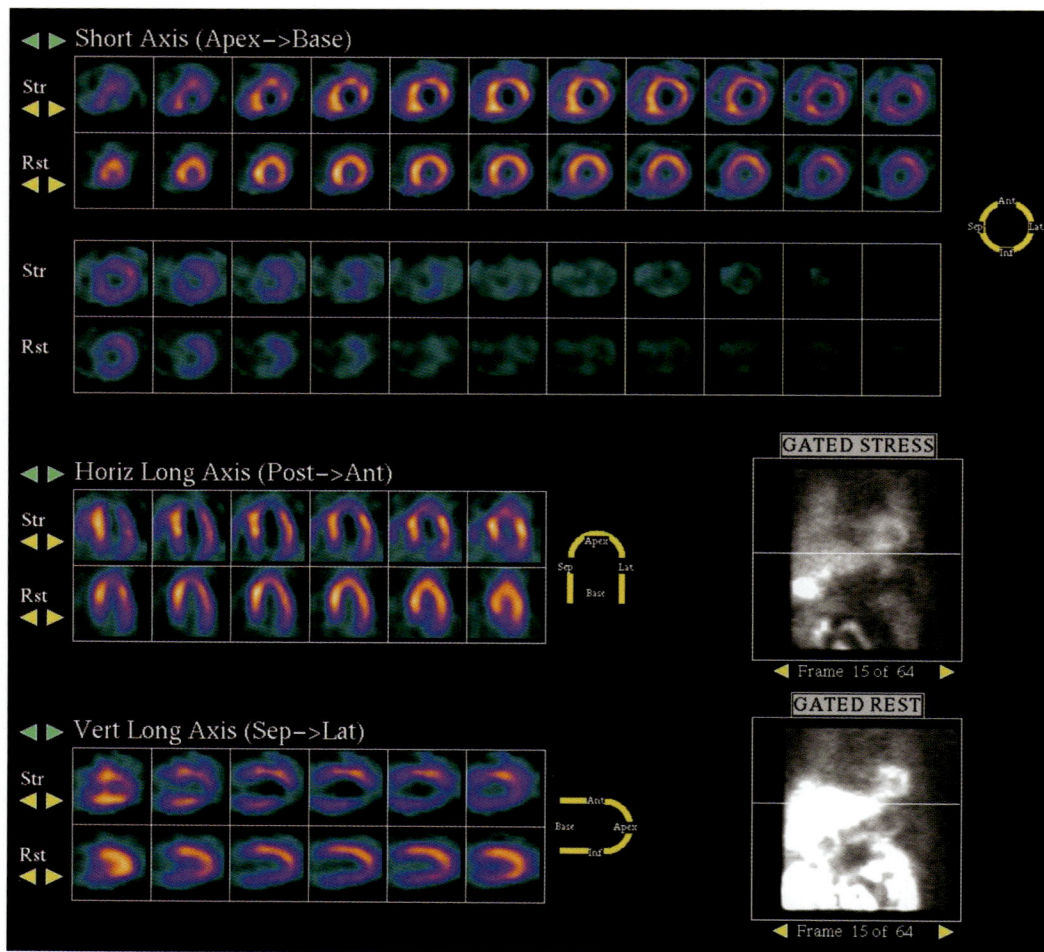

Figure 14-12. Example of a patient with severe and extensive stress-induced perfusion abnormalities. A 51-year-old man with atypical chest pain who had diabetes and a family history of premature coronary artery disease as risk factors and repolarization abnormalities on resting electrocardiography (ECG), exercised for 5 minutes and 20 seconds to a heart rate of 160 beats per minute (88% of maximal predicted). The patient developed chest discomfort and had an ischemic ECG response to stress. There was no exercise hypotension. Exercise rest-stress ^{99m}Tc-sestamibi images are interlaced in the alternate rows, which show short-axis images (*top four rows*) horizontal long-axis images (*middle two rows*), and vertical long-axis images (*bottom two rows*). The raw (projection) images of the stress (*top*) and rest (*bottom*) ^{99m}Tc-sestamibi images displaying the pulmonary distribution of the radionuclide are shown in the lower right corner. The myocardial perfusion single photon emission computed tomography (SPECT) images reveal severe perfusion defects throughout the distribution of the mid left anterior descending and left circumflex coronary arteries. The summed stress score is very high at 21, the summed rest score is low at 3, and the summed difference score is 18. Severe and extensive ischemia is confirmed by evidence of transient ischemic dilation of the left ventricle, measured at 1.33, and increased pulmonary uptake during stress.

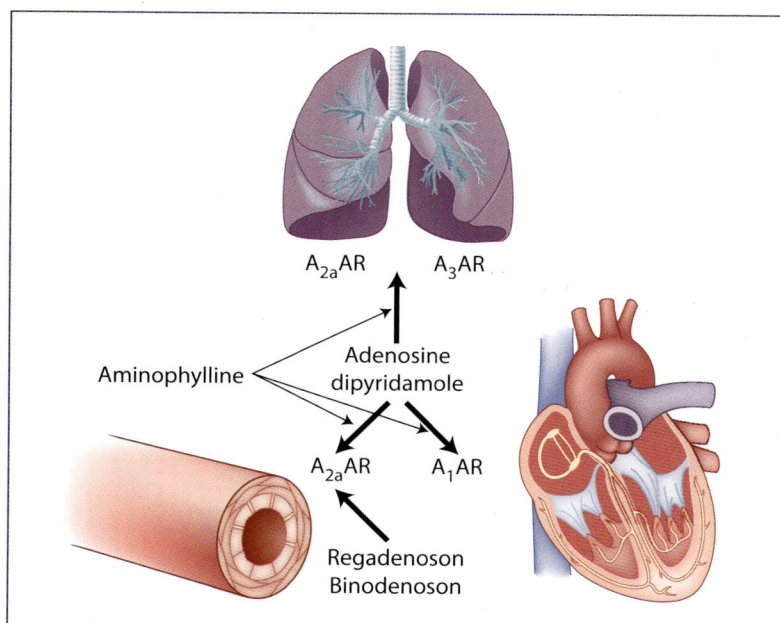

Figure 14-13. Schematic of the direct and indirect action of adenosine and dipyridamole on vascular (A_{2a} receptors [A_{2a}AR]) and bronchial (A_{2b} [A_{2a}AR] and A_3 [A_3AR] receptors) smooth muscle cells, and on cardiac conduction cells (A_1 receptors [A_1AR]). Also shown is a new class of specific adenosine 2a receptor agonists (regadenoson and binodenoson). The latter are associated with a lower incidence of adverse effects and considered safer, especially for patients with chronic lung disease or heart block [17–20]. The "antidote" that reverses the effects of dipyridamole, adenosine, and the new A_{2a} agonists is aminophylline. Patient preparation for pharmacologic stress testing is similar to that for 12–24 hours for exercise stress, although all methylxanthines must be withheld before adenosine or dipyridamole testing. β-Blockers should be withheld for 24 hours before dobutamine stress testing. With vasodilator single photon emission computed tomography (SPECT) imaging, the increased splanchnic activity mandates a delay in image acquisition for 30 to 60 minutes following the injection of a ^{99m}Tc agent.

Adenosine is a small, heterocyclic, endogenous compound produced by the endothelial cell. It is a non-specific agonist of adenosine receptors (A_1, A_{2a}, A_{2b}, and A_3). It causes vasodilatation via the production of adenyl cyclase and the subsequent local increase in cyclic adenosine monophosphate. Theophylline and other methylxanthines, including caffeine, are competitive antagonists of adenosine and dipyridamole. Adenosine enters endothelial and red blood cells by a facilitated transport mechanism. Intracellular adenosine is then deaminated or converted to other inactive metabolites.

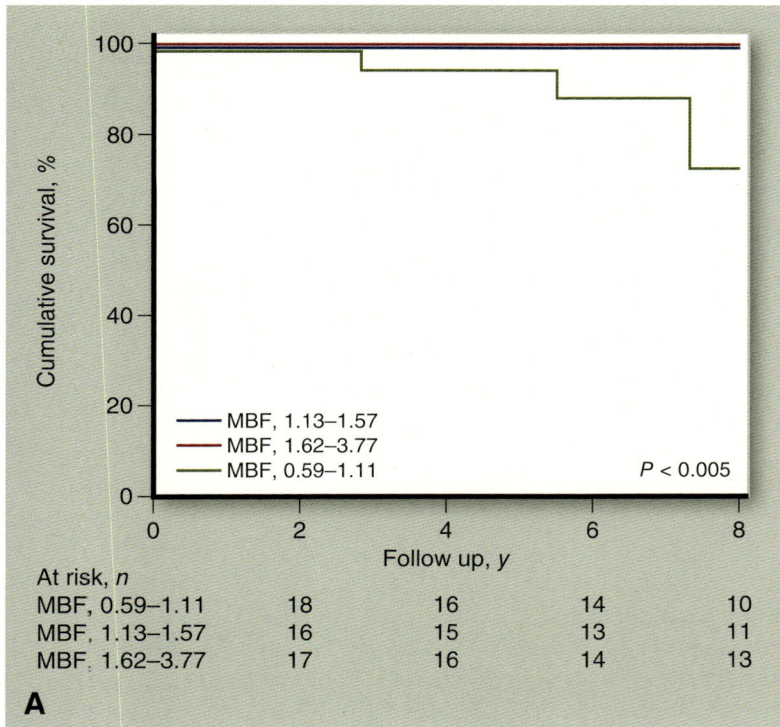

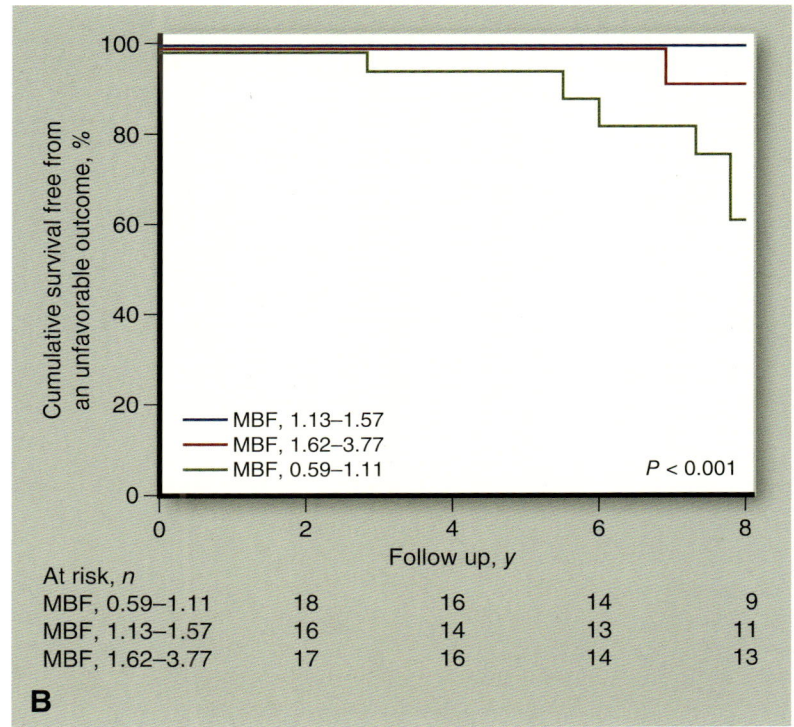

Figure 14-14. Prognostic value of diminished vasodilator responses in patients with hypertrophic cardiomyopathy. Fifty-one patients with hypertrophic cardiomyopathy were submitted positron emission tomography (PET) measurements of myocardial blood flow (MBF) at rest and during pharmacologic vasodilation and were observed for an average of 8.1 ± 2.1 years [21]. Sixteen patients had cardiovascular events, including cardiovascular death, worsening of congestive heart failure symptoms, or implantation of cardioverter/defibrillator for sustained ventricular arrhythmias. **A** and **B**, Patients were grouped into three approximately equal groups according to the PET estimates of hyperemic MBFs. The overall accu- mulative survival (**A**) and cumulative survival free from an unfavorable outcome (**B**) were strongly associated with the level of hyperemic MBFs achieved during dipyridamole vasodilation. The degree of microvascular dysfunction related to functional or structural abnormalities of the coronary microcirculation and as reflected by the diminished total vasodilator capacity on PET was predictive of future cardiovascular outcome. The observation made in this study with PET is consistent with earlier observations in patients with and without coronary artery disease and in which the coronary vasodilator capacity was assessed with highly invasive quantitative angiographic and flow velocity measurement approaches [22,23].

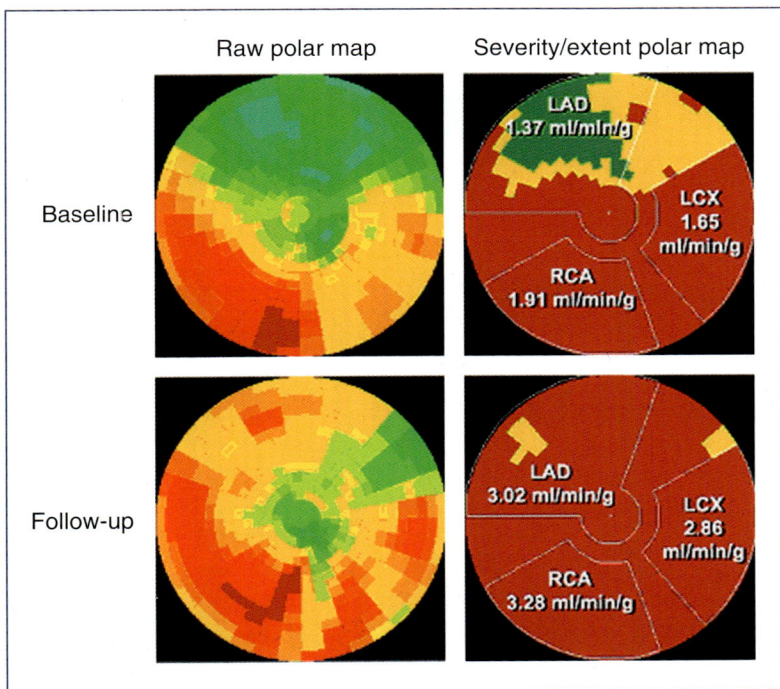

Figure 14-15. Statin treatment and regional myocardial blood flow. Polar maps of the distribution of myocardial blood flow during adenosine-stimulated hyperemia in a patient with a coronary artery disease at baseline and after 1 year of treatment with pravastatin. The extent of the stress-induced defect declined from 51% of the left anterior descending (LAD) territory to only 3%. Myocardial blood flow in each of the three coronary artery territories (as listed in the figure) increased and importantly normalized in the region with a prior stress induced defect. Only measurements of myocardial blood flow, but not the evaluation of the relative distribution of the radiotracer uptake in the myocardium, demonstrates the improvement in the flow reserve in remote or normally appearing myocardium. LCX—left circumflex; RCA—right coronary artery.

Figure 14-16. Gated myocardial perfusion single-photon emission CT (SPECT): acquisition. It is estimated that over 90% of myocardial perfusion SPECT studies performed in the United States in 2004 used electrocardiographic (ECG) gating, which makes it possible to provide both perfusion and function information with a single radiopharmaceutical injection and a single acquisition sequence. A gated cardiac SPECT acquisition proceeds almost exactly like an ungated one: the camera detector(s) rotate around the patient, collecting projection images at equally spaced angles along a 180° or 360° arc, and these projections are then filtered and reconstructed into tomographic short- and long-axis images [24,25]. Gated SPECT imaging's distinguishing feature is that at each angle, not one but several (eight, 16, or even 32) projection images are acquired, each corresponding to a specific phase of the cardiac cycle. Reconstruction of all same-phase projections produces a three-dimensional "snapshot" of the patient's heart, frozen in time at that particular phase, and doing so for all phases results in four-dimensional image volumes (x, y, z, and time) from which cardiac function can be readily assessed.

In our laboratory, we do not increase the injected dose or the acquisition time when gating a myocardial SPECT study: typical parameters used are low-energy high-resolution (LEHR) collimator(s), patient weight–based injection of 25 to 40 mCi of ^{99m}Tc-sestamibi/tetrofosmin or 3 to 4.5 mCi of ^{201}Tl, 3° spacing between adjacent projections, and 25 seconds (^{99m}Tc) or 35 seconds (^{201}Tl) acquisition time per projection [26]. The resulting total acquisition time can be as short as 12.5 minutes (^{99m}Tc) or 17.5 minutes (^{201}Tl), if a dual-detector camera with the detectors at a 90° angle is used. (*Adapted from* Germano and Berman [26].)

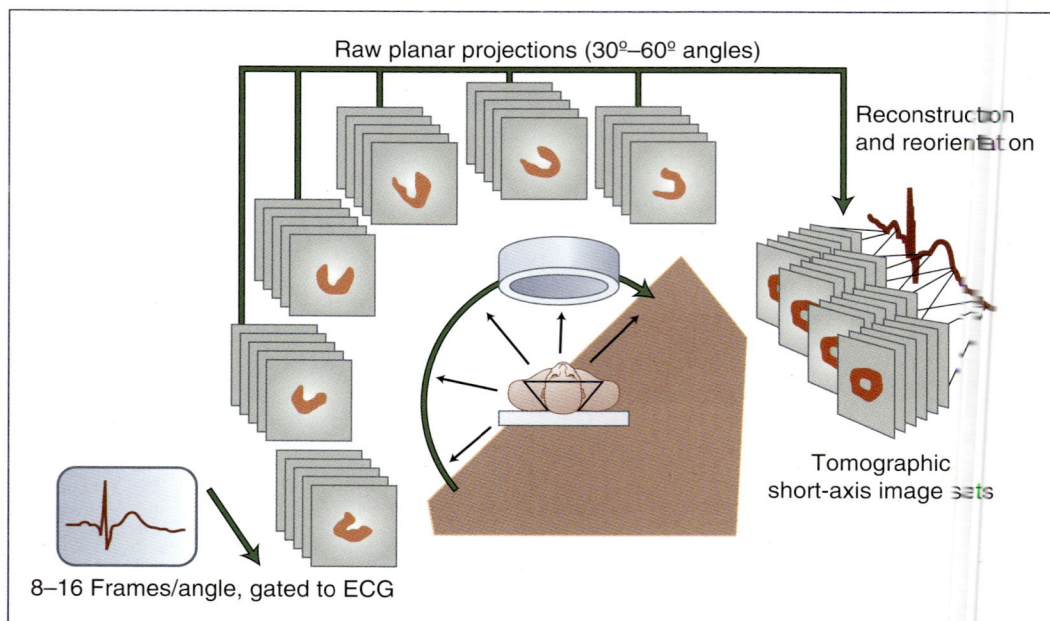

Figure 14-17. A and B, The time-volume curve, eight- versus 16-frame gating, and diastolic function. The time-volume curve graphs the value of the left ventricular cavity volume as a function of the gated single-photon emission CT (SPECT) interval. In addition to identifying the intervals corresponding to end diastole and end systole (maximum and minimum volume, respectively), the time-volume curve represents an important tool for the quality control of the gating process; ideally, in an eight-frame gated acquisition, the first interval ought to correspond to end diastole (because the inception of gating is triggered by the electrocardiographic QRS complex) whereas end systole ought to occur at interval 3 or 4. Moreover, the curve would be expected to follow a relatively smooth "U" pattern.

It should be noted that using eight-frame instead of 16-frame gated SPECT data causes a slight undersampling of the time-volume curve from which the left ventricular ejection fraction (LVEF) is derived, resulting in underestimation of the LVEF by about four ejection fraction (EF) percentage points; this underestimation is remarkably uniform over a wide range of ejection fractions [27–32]. We recommend 16-frame acquisition as the technique of choice for gated SPECT, particularly because this approach allows for meaningful measurement of diastolic function and has been reported to yield excellent agreement with the multigated radionuclide angiography standard [29,30,33–36]. Measurable parameters include the peak filling ratio (PFR), denoting the maximum value of the derivative of the time-volume curve; the time to peak filling ratio (TPFR), or the time interval between the lowest point of the time-volume curve and the time at which PFR occurs; and the one-third mean filling rate (1/3 MFR), expressing the value of the derivative of the time-volume curve at one third the global filling time. HR—heart rate; RR—time between successive R waves. (*Adapted from* Nakajima *et al.* [34].)

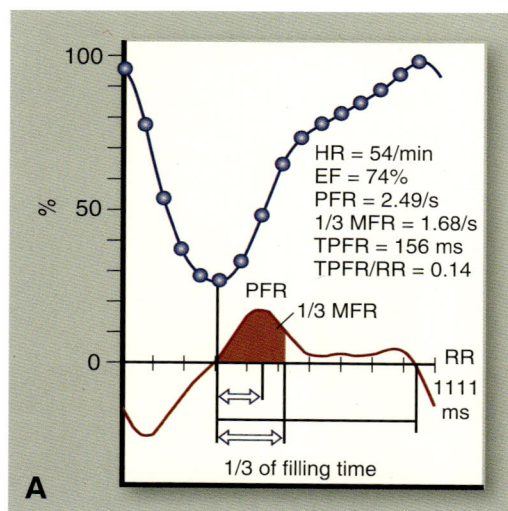

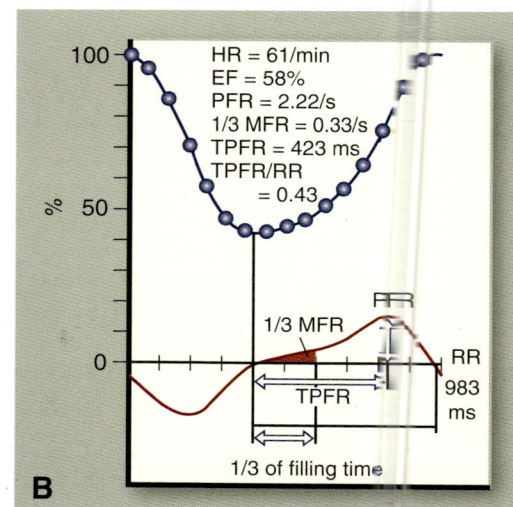

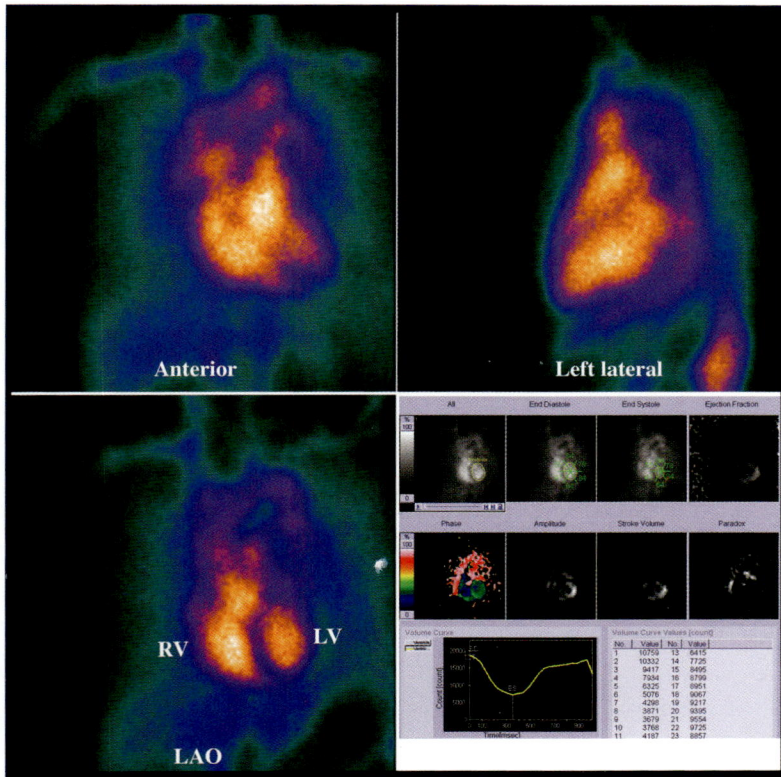

Figure 14-18. Example of a gated radionuclide blood pool study performed to evaluate right and left ventricular function in a patient with cancer before undergoing chemotherapy. Planar images are displayed in anterior, lateral, and oblique projections for optimal visualization of the right and left ventricles and calculation of ejection fraction.

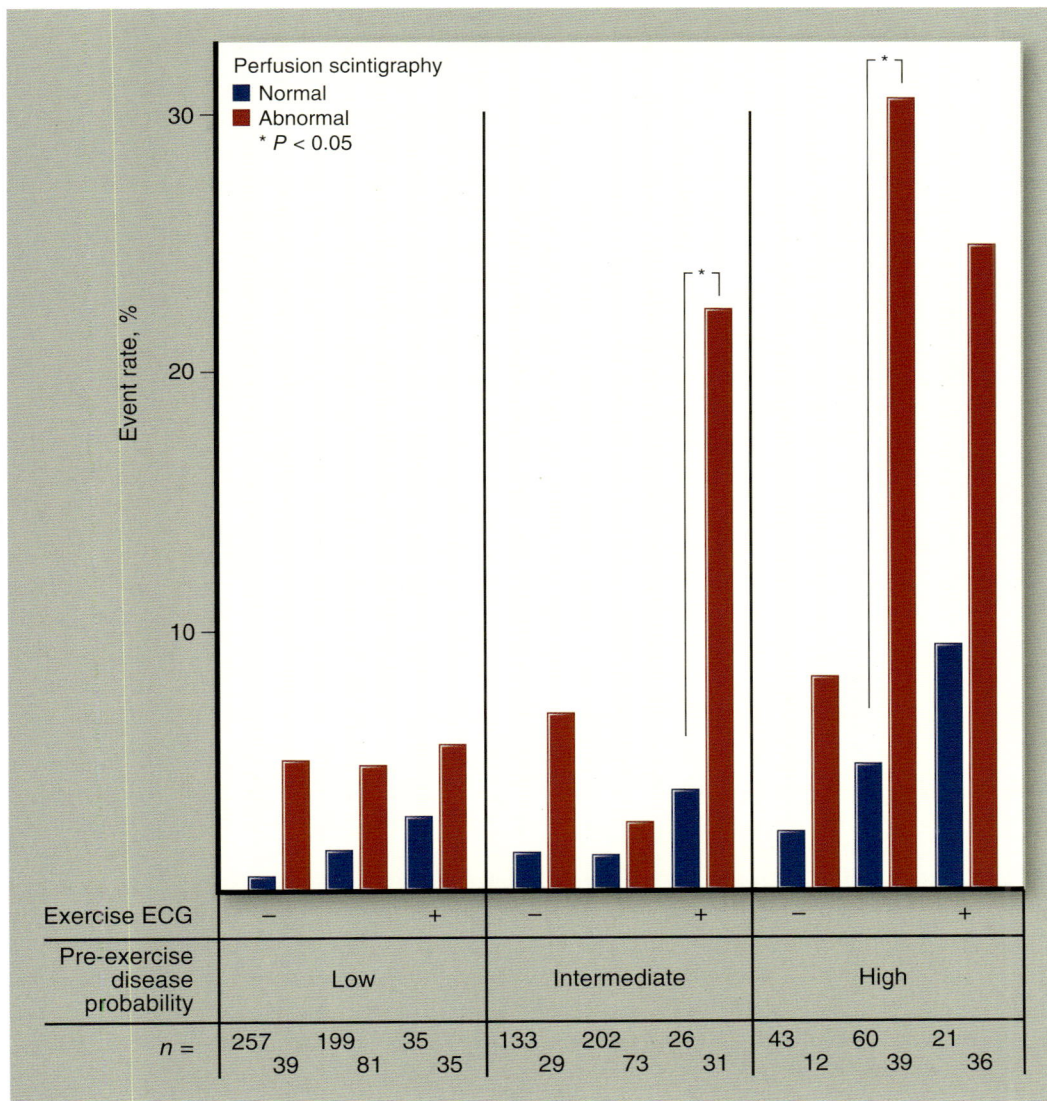

Figure 14-19. Incremental prognostic value of myocardial perfusion scintigraphy in a large series of patients without known coronary artery disease (CAD). Patients were categorized by their pre-exercise probability of CAD, by their response to stress testing, and then by their response on planar myocardial perfusion scintigraphy [37]. In the nine categories illustrated, an abnormal ^{201}Tl scan was associated with a higher risk than a normal scan. However, marked differences in event rates were noted only in categories in patients with an intermediate likelihood of CAD and an abnormal stress test response, and patients with a high likelihood of CAD. Until the time of this study, the use of ^{201}Tl imaging was confined predominantly to patients with an intermediate likelihood of having CAD, because prior research had shown that testing with nuclear studies in this patient population was highly effective for diagnostic purposes. The results of this study demonstrated that for prognostic purposes, patients with a high likelihood of CAD either before or after treadmill ECG are the patients in whom the greatest incremental benefit of myocardial perfusion scintigraphy is noted. (*Adapted from* Ladenheim *et al.* [37].)

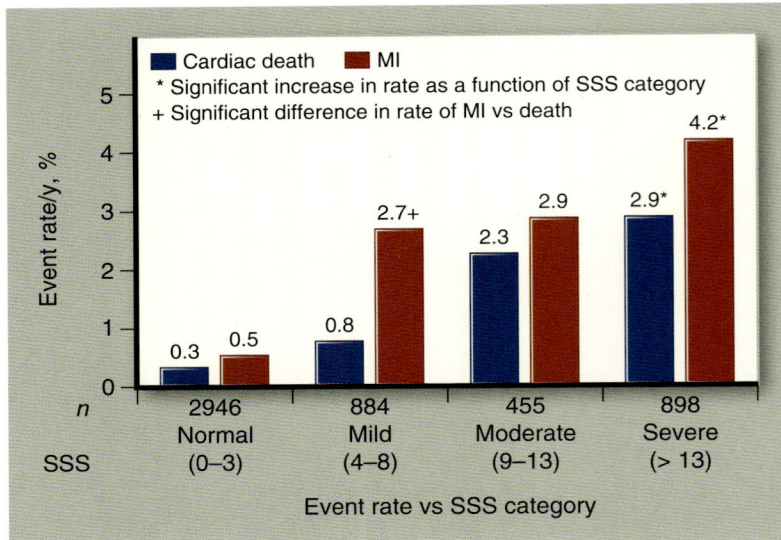

Figure 14-20. Prediction of myocardial infarction (MI) versus cardiac death by myocardial perfusion single photon emission computed tomography (SPECT). The extent of abnormality of the myocardial perfusion SPECT provides important additional information regarding risk. The annualized cardiac death and MI rates of a large group of patients undergoing stress myocardial perfusion SPECT is shown. The extent of stress perfusion defect as measured by the summed stress score (SSS) is plotted horizontally. The progressive increase in the cardiac death rate as a function of the SSS is shown. The rate of nonfatal MI is low when the scans are normal but increases abruptly even when mild myocardial perfusion in defect is noted. (*Adapted from* Hachamovitch *et al.* [38].)

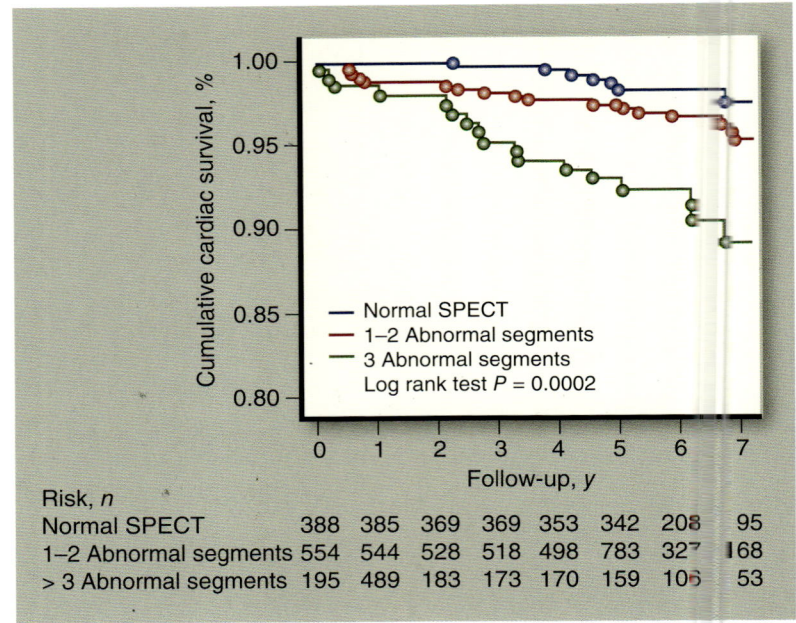

Figure 14-21. Long-term prognostic value of ^{201}Tl single photon emission computed tomography (SPECT). Vanzetto *et al.* [39] reported the results of a large series of patients who were followed for long-term cardiac events. In the presence of a normal ^{201}Tl SPECT study, the event-free survival was excellent. A progressive worsening of event-free survival was noted as a function of the number of abnormal segments on stress myocardial perfusion SPECT studies. (*Adapted from* Vanzetto *et al.* [39].)

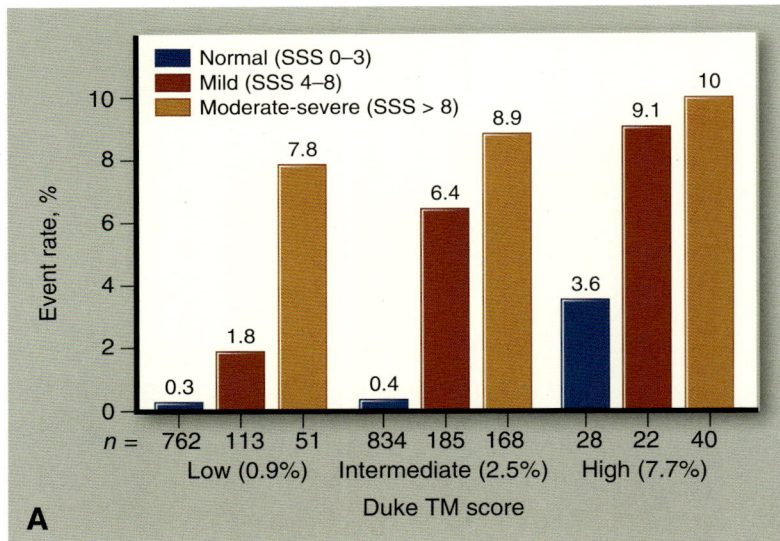

Figure 14-22. Hard event rate as a function of summed stress score (SSS) and Duke University treadmill score (TM). In patients with interpretable stress electrocardiographs (ECGs), it has been demonstrated that the Duke TM score can separate patients into groups with low, intermediate, and high risk of cardiac events. Thus, current guidelines suggest beginning with a stress ECG in these patients [40]. However, nuclear testing is useful in the patients with intermediate- or high-risk Duke TM scores. **A,** Stress myocardial perfusion single photon emission computed tomography (SPECT) studies further risk-stratify patients within each of these Duke TM score categories [41]. All patients examined had no known coronary artery disease (patients with prior catheterization, myocardial infarction [MI], or revascularization were excluded). The hard event (cardiac death or MI) rate as a function of the Duke treadmill score category and the nuclear scan results are illustrated. The normal, mild, and severe SSS categories are based on the subgroups of SSS abnormality. Due to small patient numbers, for purposes of this study those patients with moderate to severe SSS were categorized as severe. Overall, patients with a low-risk Duke TM score had such a low rate of cardiac events that it would not be cost effective to study them for prognostic purposes. Additionally, since patients with a high-risk Duke TM score usually undergo catheterization, these patients are generally not sent for further nuclear testing. However, 55% of the population had the intermediate risk Duke TM score with a cardiac event rate of 2.5%. Thus, myocardial perfusion SPECT provided excellent stratification of these patients with respect to risk of hard event [41].

Continued on the next page

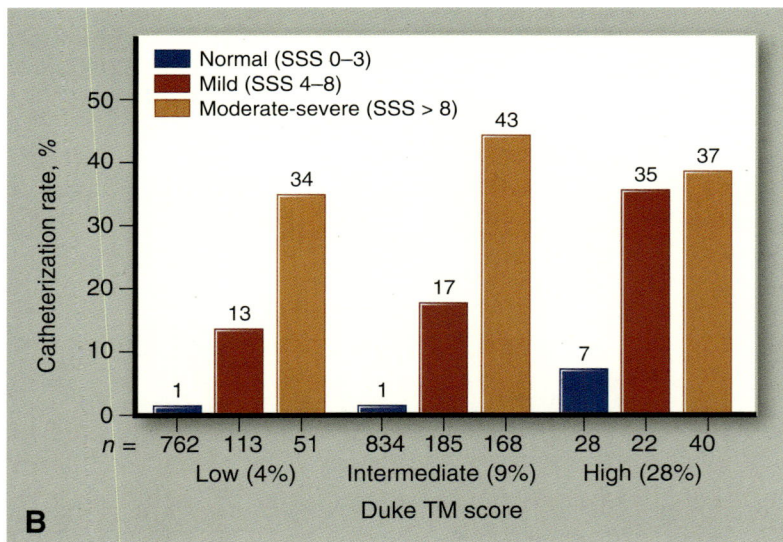

B

Figure 14-22. (*Continued*) **B**, Catheterization rate as a function of SSS and the Duke TM score. The catheterization rates are seen to follow the event rates in panel A. Note that of the patients in the intermediate Duke TM score group, only 1% of the patients found to have a normal myocardial perfusion SPECT study underwent subsequent early catheterization. Similarly, in the patients in the high Duke TM score group, only 7% of the patients found to have a normal myocardial perfusion SPECT study underwent subsequent early catheterization. (*Adapted from* Hachamovitch *et al.* [41].)

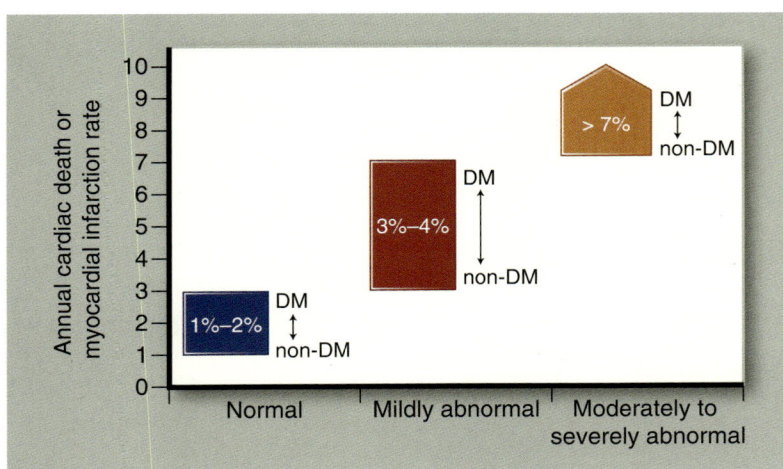

Figure 14-23. Cardiac event rates in diabetic versus nondiabetic patients. Diabetic patients have a life expectancy that is estimated to be approximately one decade less than that of their nondiabetic counterparts, and for our purposes, their ensuing risk associated with any single-photon emission computed tomography (SPECT) abnormality will be exacerbated. The benefit of screening diabetics is that because of the frequent occurrence of neuropathy, silent ischemia and infarction are more prevalent. Thus, an imaging strategy, such as that utilizing SPECT, is valuable in order to discern the extent and severity of provocative ischemia. As microvascular and macrovascular complications occur at the onset of hyperglycemia, on initial diagnosis, some assessment of cardiac risk should be performed. From a recent meta-analysis, annual cardiac death or myocardial infarction rates were 1.9% for diabetics and 0.6% for nondiabetics with a normal stress perfusion scan [42]. For a severely abnormal SPECT study, the annual rates increased to 5.8% for nondiabetics and were as high as 9.6% for diabetics. These results reveal that diabetics have a higher than expected cardiac event rate when compared with nondiabetic patients [43]. So for the nuclear cardiologist, one could expect that concurrent with their higher baseline risk, all predicted event rates will be elevated and adjusted accordingly for diabetic patients. As noted in the recent report by Kang *et al.* [43], we can expect that any risk associated with a given severity of SPECT abnormalities is higher for diabetics than nondiabetics. This statement is probably also true for patients with the metabolic syndrome, particularly those with four or five risk factors for the metabolic syndrome (defined as insulin resistance [with or without glucose intolerance], low high-density lipoprotein cholesterol, increased triglycerides, hypertension, and abdominal obesity). DM—diabetes mellitus. (*Adapted from* Kang *et al.* [43].)

Figure 14-24. Risk stratification in pharmacologic versus exercise stress testing. It is expected that by 2030, nearly 20% of the US population will be 65 years of age or older [44]. As elderly patients have more frequent chronic diseases, including coronary artery disease, prevalence rates approach one in three patients for those older than 70 years. Comorbid conditions are also prevalent, including hypertension, vascular diseases, and osteoarthritis [44]. Elderly patients also have frequent physical disability, with recent estimates from the Centers for Disease Control and Prevention reporting that from one to three in 10 elderly individuals require assistance or are unable to perform activities of daily living including self-care and household cleaning [44]. For a single-photon emission computed tomography (SPECT) imaging laboratory, this would translate into an estimated physical work capacity of less than four metabolic equivalent units (METs) and an increased need for the use of pharmacologic stress imaging [44,45]. Experientially, we have observed the representation of patients referred to pharmacologic stress grow from approximately 20% to 40% of any laboratory's patient population. Approximately 15 years ago, the majority of referrals to pharmacologic stress were for patients with significant orthopedic limitations or for preoperative risk stratification in which exercise testing was not advisable (eg, in aortic aneurysm).

Physiologically, peak maximal oxygen consumption values decline with age. Based on a recent report, the average peak MET value for patients older than 74 years is less than five METs [46]. Thus, one can envision that the vast majority of elderly patients would require the use of pharmacologic stress SPECT. Consequent to this, it is essential to note whether risk stratification is equally accurate for exercise and pharmacologic stress. From a recent meta-analysis, a similarly marked separation in expected cardiac event rates is seen for patients undergoing exercise and pharmaco-

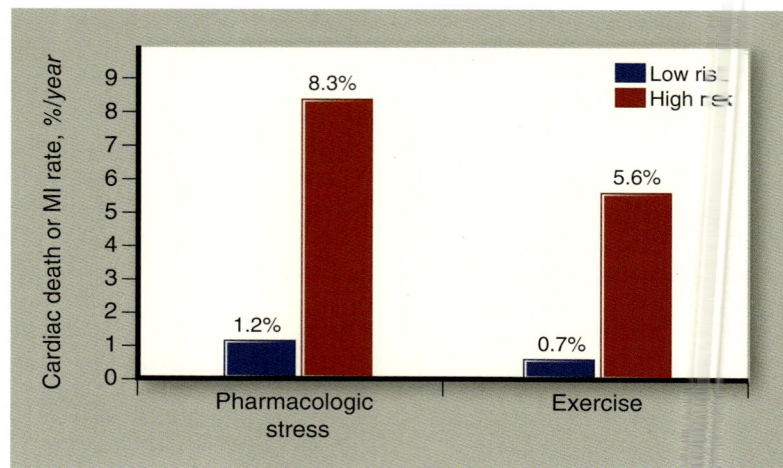

logic stress (ie, the death or myocardial infarction rates are low for patients with normal stress perfusion SPECT results and increase dramatically for those with abnormal stress myocardial perfusion findings). However, as the degree of comorbidity drives the expected event rate and pharmacologic stress patients are frequently encumbered with multiple chronic conditions, there is a necessary escalation in expected event rates for low-risk to severely abnormal findings. As can be seen from this recent meta-analysis, low-risk pharmacologic stress SPECT is associated with an annual rate of cardiac death or nonfatal myocardial infarction of approximately 1.2%, as compared with 0.7% for exercise stress with normal perfusion [42]. A similarly greater event rate is noted for pharmacologic versus exercise stress in patients with abnormal myocardial perfusion results.

Cardiac Stress Myocardial Perfusion Single-Photon Emission Computed Tomography (SPECT) in Patients Able to Exercise

Recommendations for diagnosis of patients with an intermediate likelihood of coronary artery disease (CAD) and/or risk stratification of patients with an intermediate or high likelihood of CAD who are able to exercise (to at least 85% maximum predicated heart rate)

Class I

1. Exercise myocardial perfusion SPECT to identify the extent, severity, and location of ischemia in patients who do not have left bundle branch block or an electronically paced ventricular rhythm but do have a baseline electrocardiograph (ECG) abnormality that interferes with the interpretation of exercise-induced ST segment changes (ventricular pre-excitation, left ventricular hypertrophy, digoxin therapy, or more than 1 mm ST depression). (Level of evidence: B)

2. Adenosine or dipyridamole myocardial perfusion SPECT in patients with LBBB or electronically paced ventricular rhythm. (Level of evidence: B)

3. Exercise myocardial perfusion SPECT to assess the functional significance of intermediate (25%–75%) coronary lesions. (Level of evidence: B)

4. Exercise myocardial perfusion SPECT in patients with intermediate DUKE treadmill score. (Level of evidence: B)

5. Repeat exercise myocardial perfusion imaging after initial perfusion imaging in patients whose symptoms have changed to redefine the risk of cardiac event. (Level of evidence: C)

Class IIa

1. Exercise myocardial perfusion SPECT at 3–5 years after revascularization (either percutaneous coronary intervention or coronary artery bypass graft) in selected, high-risk asymptomatic patients. (Level of evidence: B)

2. Exercise myocardial perfusion SPECT as the initial test in patients who are considered to be at high risk (patients with diabetes or patients otherwise defined as having more than 20% 10-year risk of a coronary heart disease event). (Level of evidence: B)

Class IIb

1. Repeat exercise myocardial perfusion SPECT 1–3 years after initial perfusion imaging in patients with a known or high likelihood of CAD, stable symptoms, and a predicted mortality or more than 1%, to redefine the risk of a cardiac event. (Level of evidence: C)

2. Repeat exercise myocardial perfusion SPECT on cardiac active medications after initial abnormal perfusion imaging to asses the efficacy of medical therapy. (Level of evidence: C)

3. Exercise myocardial perfusion SPECT in symptomatic or asymptomatic patients who have severe coronary calcification (CT CCS more than 75th percentile for age and sex) in the presence on the resting ECG of pre-excitation (Wolff-Parkinson-White) syndrome or more than 1 mm ST segment depression. (Level of evidence: B)

4. Exercise myocardial perfusion SPECT in asymptomatic patients who have a high-risk occupation. (Level of evidence: B)

A

Figure 14-25. A, **B**, and **C**, American College of Cardiology (ACC)/ American Heart Association (AHA)/American Society of Nuclear Cardiology (ASNC) guideline recommendations for radionuclide imaging in patients with suspected or known coronary artery disease [47].

Continued on the next page

Cardiac Stress Myocardial Perfusion Single-Photon Emission Computed Tomography (SPECT) in Patients Unable to Exercise

Recommendations for diagnosis of patients with an intermediate likelihood of coronary artery disease (CAD) and/or risk stratification of patients with an intermediate or high likelihood of CAD who are unable to exercise.

Class I

1. Adenosine or dipyridamole myocardial perfusion SPECT to identify the extent, severity, and location of ischemia

2. Adenosine or dipyridamole myocardial perfusion SPECT to asses the functional significance of intermediate (25%–75%) coronary lesions. (Level of evidence: B)

3. Adenosine or dipyridamole myocardial perfusion SPECT after initial perfusion imaging in patients whose symptoms have changed to redefine the risk for cardiac event. (Level of evidence: C)

Class IIa

1. Adenosine or dipyridamole myocardial perfusion SPECT at 3–5 years after revascularization (either percutaneous coronary intervention or coronary artery bypass graft) in selected, high-risk asymptomatic patients. (Level of evidence: B)

2. Adenosine or dipyridamole myocardial perfusion SPECT as the initial test in patients who are considered to be at high risk (patients with diabetes or patients otherwise defined as having a more than 20% 10-year risk of a coronary heart disease event). (Level of evidence: B)

3. Dobutamine myocardial perfusion SPECT in patients who have a contraindication to adenosine or dipyridamole. (Level of evidence: C)

Class IIb

1. Repeat adenosine or dipyridamole myocardial perfusion imaging in patients with known or a high likelihood of CAD, stable symptoms, and a predicted annual mortality of more than 1% to redefine the risk of a cardiac event. (Level of evidence: C)

2. Repeat adenosine or dipyridamole myocardial perfusion SPECT on cardiac active medications after initial abnormal perfusion imaging to assess the efficacy of medical therapy. (Level of evidence: C)

3. Adenosine or dipyridamole myocardial perfusion SPECT in symptomatic or asymptomatic patients who have severe coronary calcification (CT coronary calcium score more than 75th percentile for age and sex) in the presence on the rest electrocardiograph (ECG) of left bundle branch block or an electronically paced ventricular rhythm. (Level of evidence: B)

4. Adenosine or dipyridamole myocardial perfusion SPECT in asymptomatic patients who have a high-risk occupation. (Level of evidence: C)

B

Cardiac Stress Myocardial Perfusion Positron Emission Tomography (PET)

Recommendations for diagnosis of patients with an intermediate likelihood of coronary artery disease (CAD) and/or risk stratification of patients with an intermediate or high likelihood of CAD.

Class I

Adenosine or dipyridamole myocardial perfusion PET in patients in whom an appropriately indicated myocardial perfusion single photon emission computed tomography (SPECT) study has been found to be equivocal for diagnostic or risk-stratification purposes. (Level of evidence: B)

Class IIa

1. Adenosine or dipyridamole myocardial perfusion PET to identify the extent, severity, and location of ischemia as the initial diagnostic test in patients who are unable to exercise. (Level of evidence: B)

2. Adenosine or dipyridamole myocardial perfusion PET to identify the extent, severity, and location of ischemia as the initial diagnostic test in patients who are able to exercise but have left bundle branch block or an electronically paced rhythm. (Level of evidence: B)

C

Figure 14-25. *(Continued)*

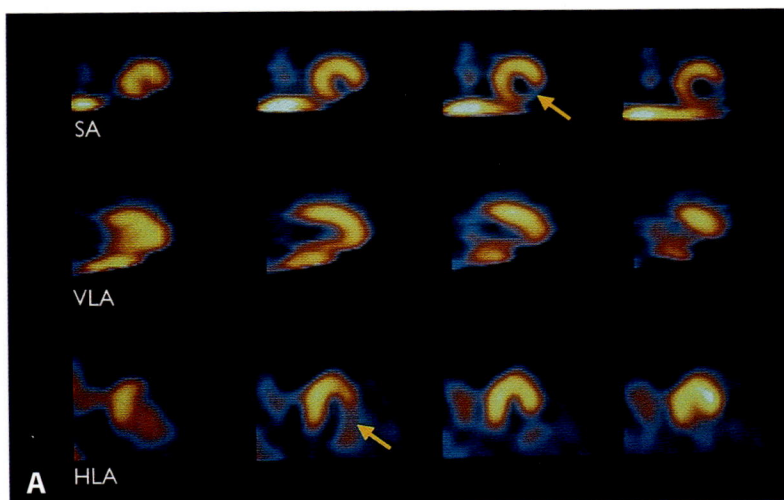

Figure 14-26. Significant myocardial perfusion abnormalities in patients with chest pain but nondiagnostic electrocardiographic alterations. **A,** Short-axis (SA), vertical long-axis (VLA), and horizontal long-axis (HLA) resting single-photon emission computed tomography (SPECT) myocardial perfusion images (MPIs) of a 39-year-old-man who presented to the emergency room (ER) with chest pain atypical for angina and a normal initial ECG. He was injected with ^{99m}Tc-sestamibi at rest in the ER and underwent SPECT imaging soon thereafter. The images show a dense inferolateral resting perfusion defect (*arrows*), which in the setting of ongoing symptoms was most suggestive of resting ischemia and acute coronary syndrome (ACS). He was immediately triaged to the catheterization laboratory.

Continued on the next page

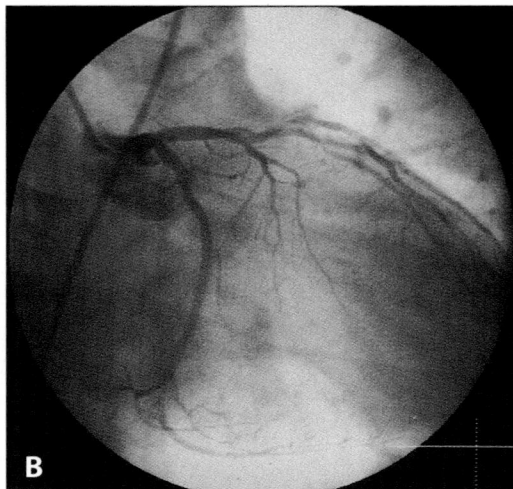

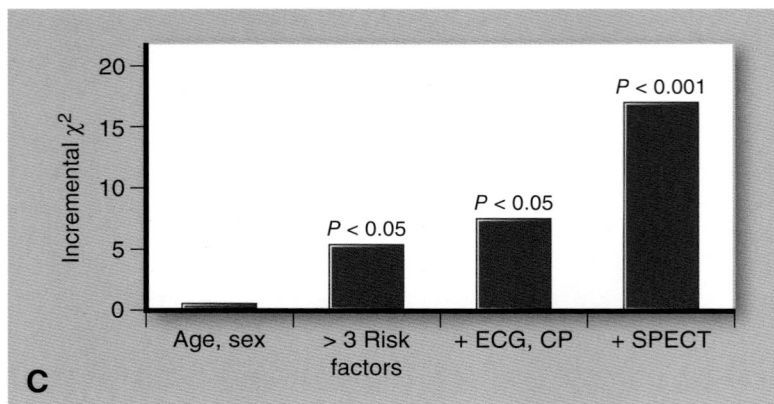

Figure 14-26. *(Continued)* **B,** Right anterior oblique view of the left coronary artery injection showing an acutely occluded left circumflex artery in the patient in *panel A*. Left circumflex occlusions are not always well seen on the standard 12-lead ECG. The patient subsequently underwent successful percutaneous coronary intervention of the left circumflex artery, with an excellent anatomic result. Had MPI not been performed, he may have been admitted for observation, and serial enzyme analysis may have been positive for a myocardial infarction. The use of MPI likely allowed significantly earlier intervention in this case.

C, Analysis of the incremental value of resting MPI data to predict cardiac events in patients presenting to the ER with suspected ischemia. The incremental x^2 value measures the strength of the association between individual factors added to a clinician's knowledge base in incremental fashion and unfavorable cardiac events. Addition of resting SPECT MPI data (+ SPECT) in the ER setting adds highly statistically significant value on detection of ACS and events even given knowledge of age, sex, multiple (> 3) risk factors for coronary artery disease, and ECG changes and the presence or absence of chest pain (CP). (*Panel C adapted from* Heller *et al.* [48].)

ACC/AHA/ASNC Guideline Recommendations for Radionuclide Imaging in Patients With Suspected ACS Presenting to the Emergency Department

Patient Subgroup	Imaging Modality	Recommendation/Evidence Level
Assessment of risk in suspected ACS with nondiagnostic initial ECG	Rest MPI	I, A
Diagnosis of CAD in suspected ACS with nondiagnostic ECG and negative biomarkers or normal rest MPI	Stress/rest MPI	I, B

A

ACC/AHA/ASNC Guideline Recommendations for Radionuclide Imaging in Diagnosis, Risk Assessment, Prognosis, and Assessment of Therapy After Acute ST-Segment Elevation MI

Patient Subgroup/Indication	Imaging Modality	Recommendation/Evidence Level
Assessment of LV function (all patients)	Rest RNA or gated SPECT	I, B
Detection of inducible ischemia and myocardium at risk in patients after thrombolytic therapy who do not undergo catheterization	Stress MPI or gated SPECT	I, B
Assessment of infarct size and myocardial viability post-MI	Rest and/or MPI with gated SPECT	I, B
Assessment of RV function in suspected RV MI	Rest RNA or FP RNA	IIa, B

B

Figure 14-27. A, American College of Cardiology (ACC)/American Heart Association (AHA)/American Society of Nuclear Cardiology (ASNC) guideline recommendations for radionuclide imaging in patients with suspected acute coronary syndrome (ACS) presenting to the emergency department. Based on the growing literature regarding imaging in patients with suspected ACS, recent guidelines have recommended the use of perfusion imaging, with a class I recommendation for specific situations. First, in patients who present with symptoms consistent with ACS but with a nondiagnostic initial electrocardiography, rest perfusion imaging will supply substantial risk stratification information to inform clinical decisions regarding triage (*ie*, whether the patient needs to be admitted or is safe to discharge home). Second, among patients who have been observed and have negative serial biomarkers, stress/rest perfusion imaging may be strongly recommended for detection of coronary artery disease (CAD) as well as for risk stratification. MPI—myocardial perfusion imaging.

B, American College of Cardiology (ACC)/American Heart Association (AHA)/American Society of Nuclear Cardiology (ASNC) guideline recommendations for radionuclide imaging in diagnosis, risk assessment, prognosis, and assessment of therapy after acute ST-segment elevation myocardial infarction (MI). Based on the totality of data that have been published over the years, recent guidelines have summarized recommendations for the use of radionuclide imaging in patients with acute ST-segment elevation MI. Radionuclide assessment of left ventricular (LV) function (by resting radionuclide angiography [RNA] or gated single proton emission CT [SPECT]) is recommended at a class I level and is particularly useful when quantitative assessment is indicated.

Continued on the next page

ACC/AHA/ASNC Guideline Recommendations for Radionuclide Imaging in Risk Assessment/Prognosis in Patients With Non–ST-Segment Elevation MI and Unstable Angina

Patient subgroup/Indication	Imaging modality	Recommendation/Evidence level
Identification of inducible ischemia in patients with low or intermediate clinical risk	Stress MPI with gated SPECT	I, B
Identification of inducible ischemia in patients whose angina has been stabilized medically	Stress MPI with gated SPECT	I, A
Identification of hemodynamic significance of a coronary stenosis after angiography	Stress MPI with gated SPECT	I, B
Assessment of LV function	Rest RNA or gated SPECT	I. B
Identification of the severity/extent of ischemia/CAD in patients with ongoing suspected ischemia symptoms when ECG changes are nondiagnostic	Rest MPI	IIa, B

C

Figure 14-27. *(Continued)* Risk stratification by stress/rest myocardial perfusion imaging (MPI) gated SPECT in stable patients in the aftermath of acute ST-segment elevation MI who receive thrombolytic reperfusion therapy and who are not routinely undergoing angiography provides information on two of the most important parameters defining risk: the extent and severity of inducible ischemia and the status of LV function. Imaging after rest injection with single-photon agents now has substantial literature supporting its use for quantitation of infarct size as well as for defining regional viability in the setting of regional dysfunction. Finally, in the appropriate setting, assessment of right ventricular (RV) function, by first-pass (FP) or equilibrium RNA, is given a class IIa recommendation (ie, is indicated in most circumstances).

C, ACC/AHA/ASNC guideline recommendations for radionuclide imaging in risk assessment/prognosis in patients with non–ST-segment elevation MI and unstable angina. Current guidelines recommend radionuclide assessment of perfusion and/or function in various situations for patients with non–ST-segment elevation MI or unstable angina. Most commonly, imaging is used, and is supported by randomized trials of strategies, in patients with "medically stabilized" acute coronary syndromes in whom the clinical signs or laboratory tests (such as troponin levels) do not suggest clear benefit from an "invasive" strategy (direct to catheterization with revascularization as appropriate). Stress/rest gated SPECT MPI can provide information on the extent and severity of inducible ischemia (which directly relates to subsequent natural history risk), as well as the status of LV function. This information can guide decisions on the potential benefit of revascularization, or whether a "conservative" strategy (no catheterization with aggressive risk factor control) is appropriate. Among patients who are catheterized and have lesions identified of unclear significance, stress/rest imaging is recommended to assess the impact of the stenosis on coronary flow reserve.

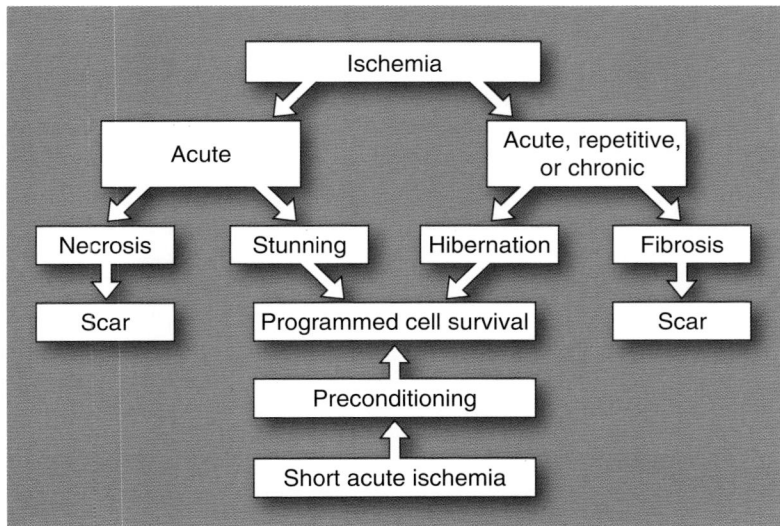

Figure 14-28. Imbalance between oxygen supply, usually due to reduced myocardial perfusion, and oxygen demand, determined primarily by the rate and force of myocardial contraction, is termed *ischemic myocardium*. If the oxygen supply-demand imbalance is transient (ie, triggered by exertion), it represents reversible ischemia. However, if regional oxygen supply-demand imbalance is prolonged, high-energy phosphates will be depleted, regional contractile function will progressively deteriorate, and cell membrane rupture with cell death will follow (myocardial necrosis and fibrosis). The phenomena of stunning, hibernation, and ischemic preconditioning represent different mechanisms of acute and chronic adaptation to a temporary or sustained reduction in coronary blood flow. Such modulated responses to ischemia are regulated to preserve sufficient energy to protect the structural and functional integrity of the cardiac myocyte. In contrast to programmed cell death, or apoptosis, Taegtmeyer [49] has coined the term *programmed cell survival* to describe the commonality between myocardial stunning, hibernation, and ischemic preconditioning independent from their disparate myocardial responses to acute and chronic ischemia. (*Adapted from* Taegtmeyer [49].)

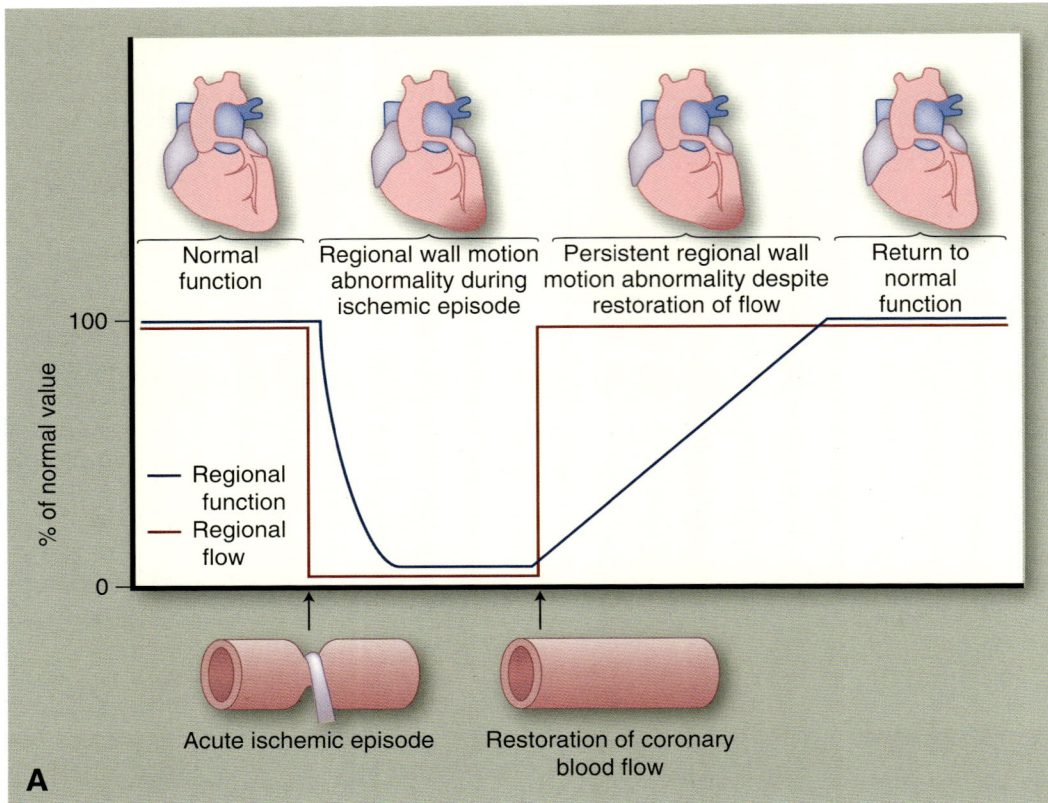

A

Acute ischemic episode   Restoration of coronary blood flow

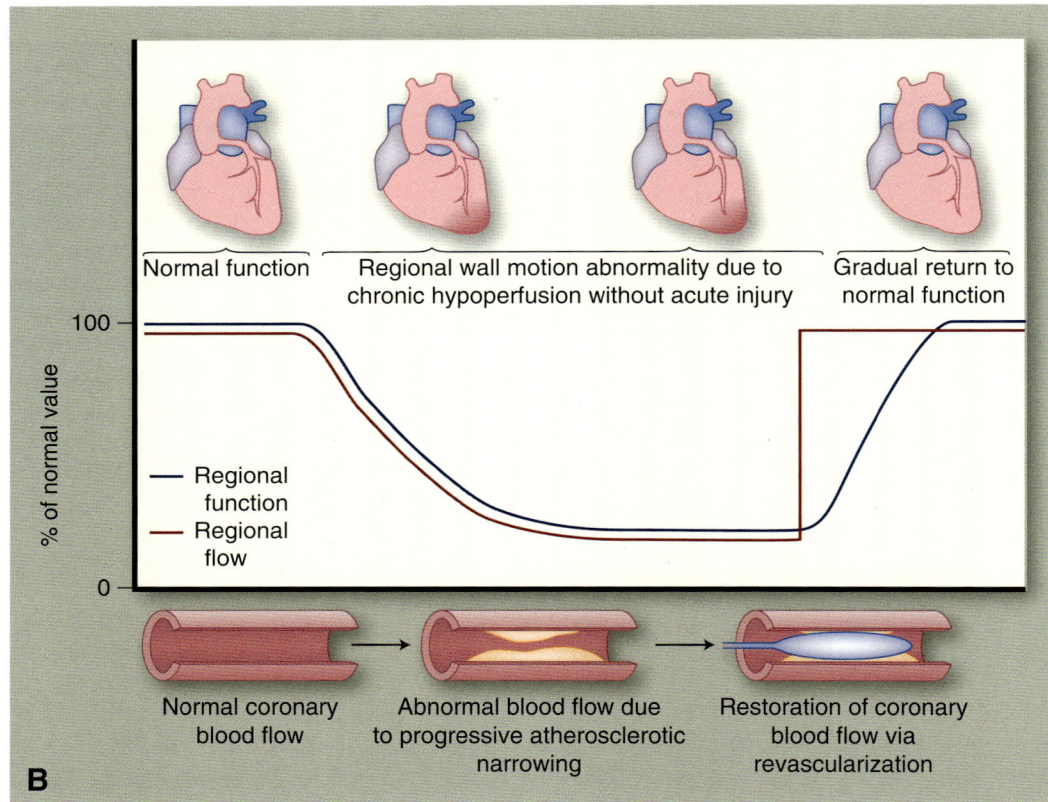

B

Normal coronary blood flow → Abnormal blood flow due to progressive atherosclerotic narrowing → Restoration of coronary blood flow via revascularization

Figure 14-29. Pathophysiologic paradigms concerning the relationship between myocardial perfusion and left ventricular function in stunned and hibernating myocardium. **A,** Stunned myocardium refers to the state of delayed recovery of regional left ventricular dysfunction after a transient period of ischemia that has been followed by reperfusion [50]. The ischemic episodes that ultimately lead to myocardial stunning can be single or multiple, brief or prolonged but never severe enough to result in myocardial necrosis. **B,** Hibernating myocardium refers to an adaptive rather than injurious response of the myocardium, in which viable but dysfunctional myocardium arises from prolonged myocardial hypoperfusion at rest in the absence of clinically evident ischemia [51]. In stunning interventions aimed at decreasing the frequency, severity, or duration of ischemic episodes would result in improved contractile function. In hibernation, interventions that favorably alter the supply/demand relationship of the myocardium, either improvement in blood flow or reduction in demand, would be expected to improve contractile function. It is very likely, however, that in patients with chronic coronary artery disease, the adaptive responses of hibernation and injurious responses of stunning coexist.

Figure 14-30. Post-revascularization functional outcome of asynergic regions in relation to prerevascularization ^{201}Tl patterns of normal, reversible, partially reversible, mild to moderate irreversible, and severe irreversible defects using stress-redistribution-reinjection ^{201}Tl protocol. The probabilities of functional recovery after revascularization were over 90% in normal or completely reversible defects, 63% in partially reversible defects, 30% in mild to moderate irreversible defects, and 0% in severe irreversible defects. Asynergic regions with reversible defects (complete or partial) on the prerevascularization ^{201}Tl study were shown more likely to improve function after revascularization when compared with asynergic regions with mild-to-moderate irreversible defects (79% vs 30%, respectively; $P < 0.001$). Even at a similar mass of viable myocardial tissue (as reflected by the final ^{201}Tl content), the presence of inducible ischemia (reversible defect) was associated with an increased likelihood of functional recovery. (*Adapted from* Kitsiou *et al.* [52].)

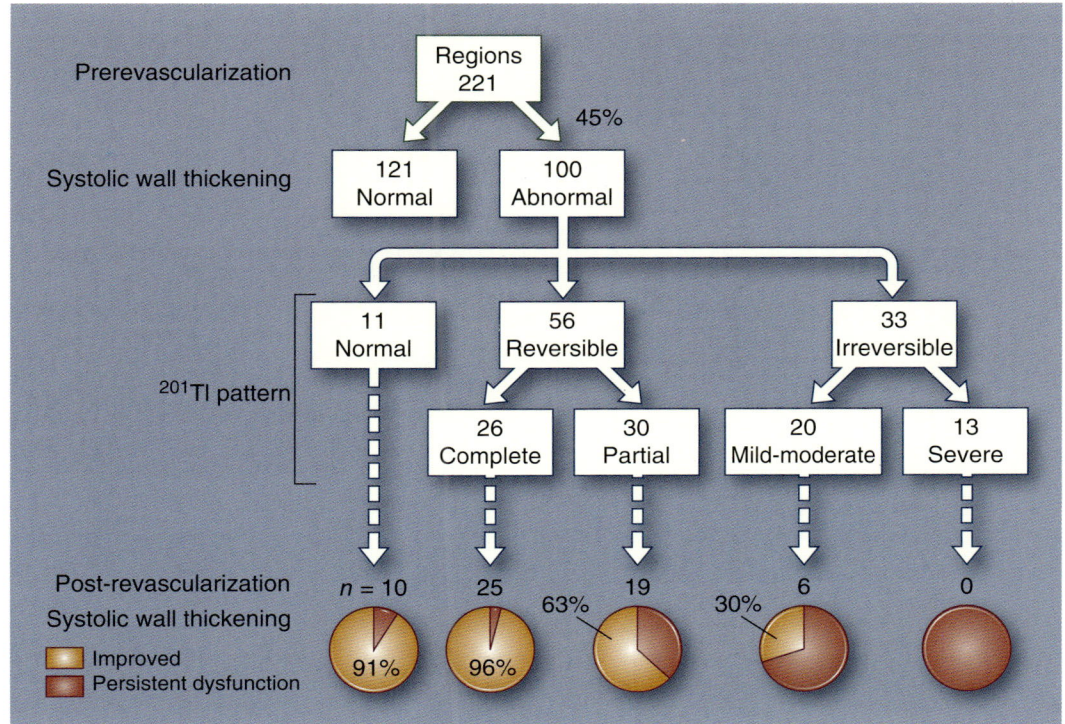

Figure 14-31. Major metabolic pathways and regulatory steps of a myocyte. Breakdown of fatty acids in the mitochondria via β-oxidation is exquisitely sensitive to oxygen deprivation. Therefore, in the setting of reduced oxygen supply, the myocytes compensate for the loss of oxidative potential by shifting toward greater utilization of glucose to generate high-energy phosphates. Glycolysis occurs in the cytoplasm under anaerobic conditions and leads to the formation of pyruvate. For every mol of glucose metabolized through glycolysis, 2 mol adenosine triphosphate (ATP) are generated (anaerobic condition), and 36 mol ATP are generated from pyruvate entering the citric acid cycle in the mitochondria (aerobic oxidative phosphorylation). Because glycolysis can generate ATP under anaerobic conditions, glycolysis becomes an attractive alternate metabolic pathway for ATP generation in hypoperfused myocardium with a limited supply of oxygen. Although the amount of energy produced by glycolysis may be adequate to maintain myocyte viability and preserve the electrochemical gradient across the cell membrane, it may not be sufficient to sustain contractile function. In hibernation, the adaptive response of the myocardium in the setting of prolonged resting hypoperfusion (reduced oxygen supply) is a reduction in myocardial contractile function (reduced oxygen demand), thereby preserving myocardial viability in the absence of clinically evident ischemia. FDG—[18F]-fluorodeoxyglucose. ADP—adenosine diphosphate. (*Adapted from* Dilsizian [53].)

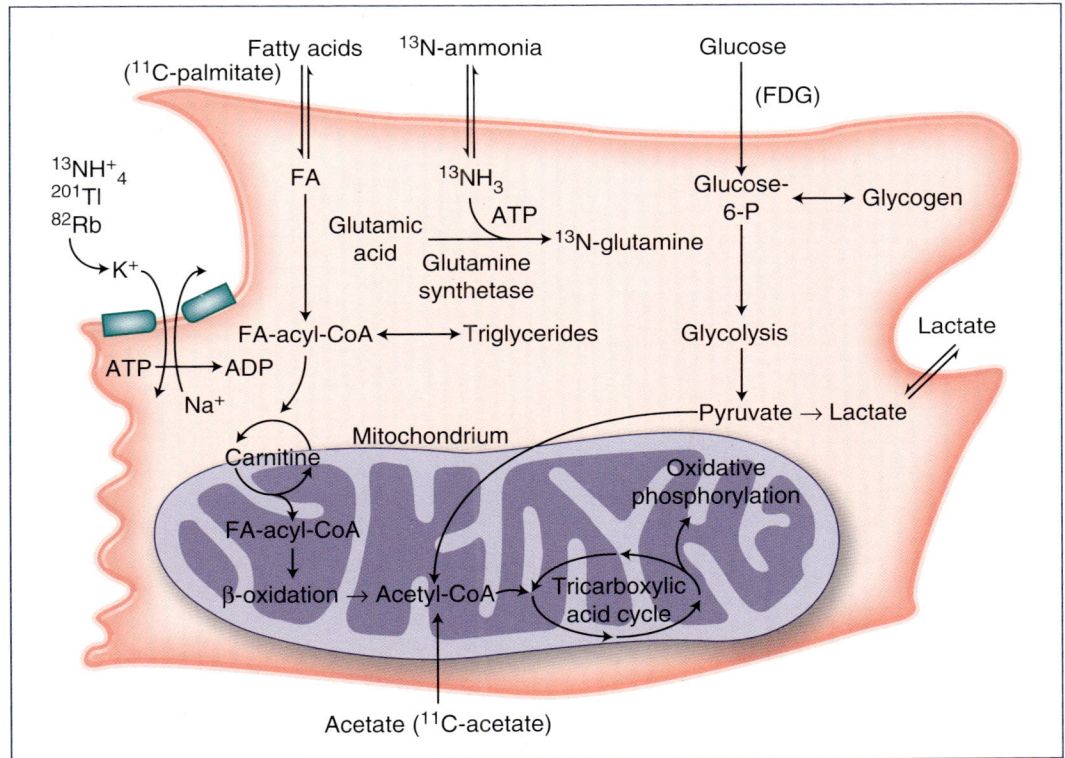

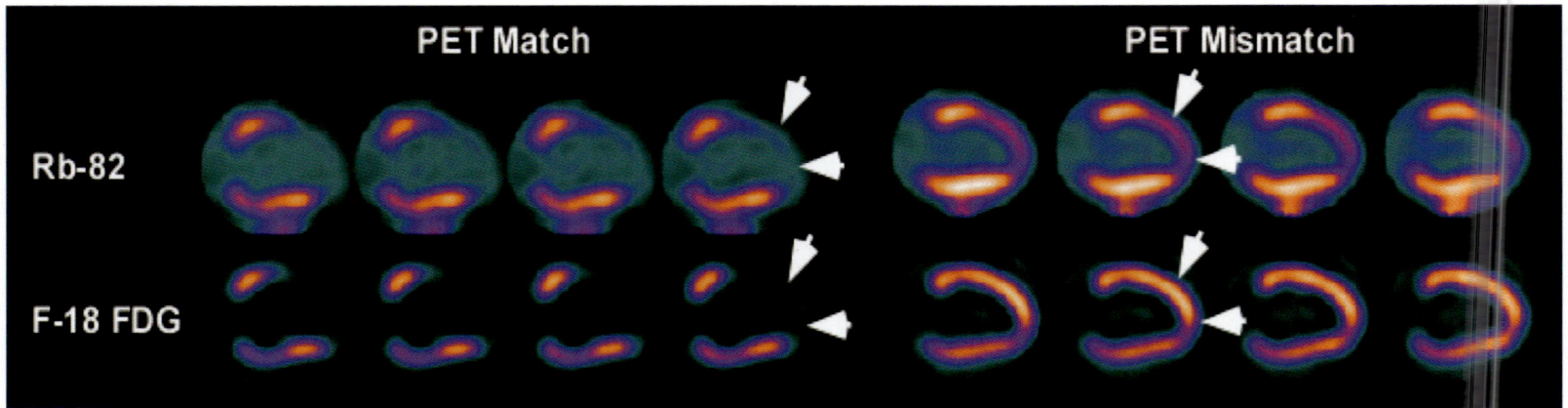

Figure 14-32. Positron emission tomographic patterns of myocardial viability in patients with chronic ischemic left ventricular (LV) dysfunction and heart failure symptoms. The so-called perfusion-metabolism mismatch (reduced blood flow with preserved or enhanced [18F]-fluorodeoxyglucose [FDG] uptake) identifies patients with residual myocardial viability and potentially reversible LV dysfunction following revascularization. In contrast, the perfusion-metabolism match pattern (concordantly reduced blood flow FDG uptake) identifies patients with predominantly scarred myocardium and irreversible LV dysfunction following revascularization. The principle of using a metabolic tracer, such as FDG, is based on the concept that viable myocytes in hypoperfused and dysfunctional regions are metabolically active, while scarred or fibrotic tissue is metabolically inactive. Although fatty acids are the primary source of myocardial energy production in the fasting state, in the setting of reduced oxygen supply (a consequence of hypoperfusion at rest), the myocytes compensate for the loss of oxidative potential by shifting toward greater glucose utilization to generate high-energy phosphates. Thus, in chronic ischemia, aerobic metabolism is slowed while the anaerobic metabolism is accelerated, a reversal of the well-known Pasteur effect. Such increased FDG uptake (anaerobic metabolism) in asynergic myocardial regions with reduced blood flow at rest has become a scintigraphic marker of hibernation.

Left panel, vertical long-axis ^{82}Rubidium scan (*top row*) demonstrating a large anterior and apical perfusion defects at rest. The corresponding [18F]-fluorodeoxyglucose (FDG) scan (*bottom row*) shows a concordant reduction in glucose uptake consistent with non-viable myocardium. **Right panel,** vertical long-axis ^{82}Rubidium scan (*top row*) demonstrating a large anterior and apical perfusion defects at rest. The corresponding FDG scan (*bottom row*) shows a preserved glucose uptake consistent with viable but hibernating myocardium. PET—positron emission tomography. (*Reproduced with permission from Di Carli and Hachamovitch [54].*)

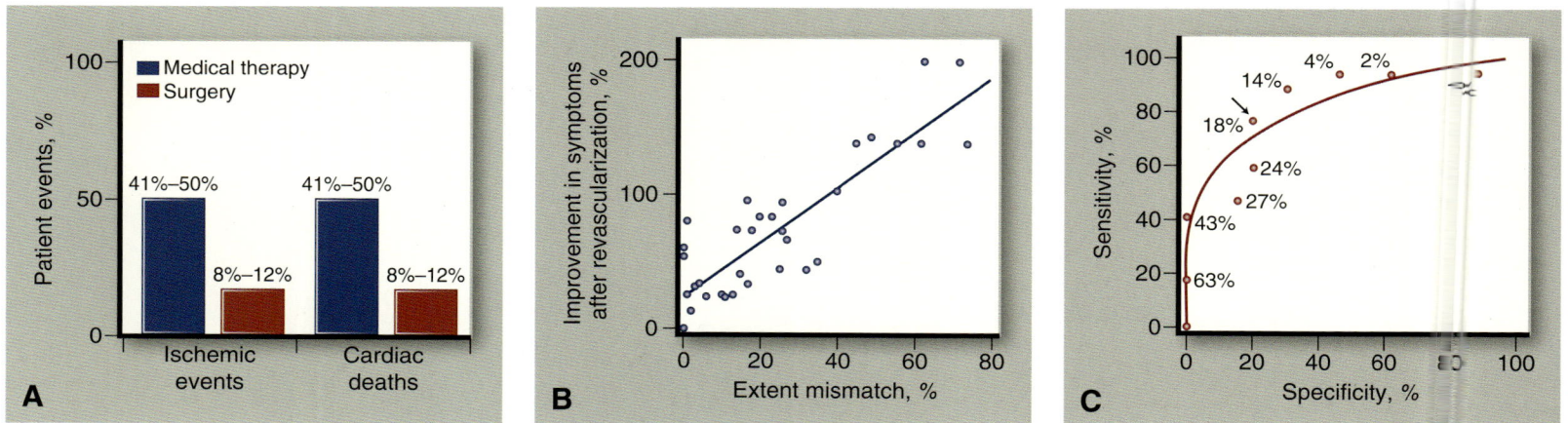

Figure 14-33. Positron emission tomography (PET) mismatch and prognosis. The prognostic significance of perfusion-metabolism mismatch pattern in ischemic cardiomyopathy has been shown in a number of non-randomized, retrospective studies with PET [55,56]. **A,** Patients with perfusion-metabolism mismatch pattern who were treated surgically had lower ischemic event rates and fewer deaths when compared with those treated with medical therapy. In contrast, patients with perfusion-metabolism match pattern displayed no such difference in outcomes between surgical and medical management. Moreover, the patients with myocardial viability (mismatch pattern) who underwent revascularization manifested a significant improvement in heart failure symptoms and exercise tolerance [57,58]. **B,** The relation between the anatomic extent of perfusion. Metabolism PET mismatch pattern (expressed as percent of the left ventricle) and the change in functional status after revascularization (expressed as percent improvement from baseline) is shown. The scatterplot shows that the greatest improvement in heart failure symptoms occurs in patients with the largest mismatch defects on quantitative analysis of PET images. **C,** Receiver-operating characteristic curve for different anatomic extent of perfusion-metabolism mismatch to predict a change (at least one grade) in functional status after revascularization is shown. When the extent of PET mismatch involves 18% or more of the left ventricular mass, the sensitivity for predicting a change in functional status after revascularization is 76% and the specificity is 78% (area under the fitted curve = 0.82). (**A,** adapted from Eitzman et al. [55] and Di Carli et al. [56]; **B** and **C,** adapted from Di Carli et al. [57].)

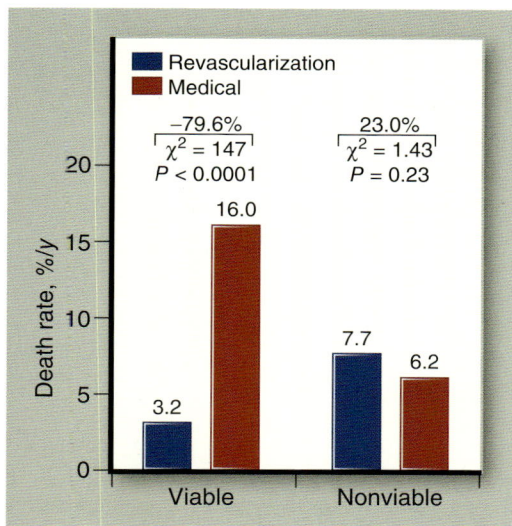

Figure 14-34. Prognostic implications of myocardial viability testing in patients with coronary artery disease and left ventricular dysfunction. Data from meta-analysis of 3088 patients (mean left ventricular ejection fraction, 32%, followed for 25 ± 10 months) demonstrates that in patients with preserved myocardial viability, the annual mortality rate was significantly lower in those who were treated with revascularization (3.2%) compared with those treated with medical therapy alone (16%). This represents a 79.6% decrease in annual mortality for patients with viability treated with revascularization ($P < 0.0001$). Moreover, there was a direct relationship between severity of left ventricular dysfunction and magnitude of benefit from revascularization among patients with myocardial viability ($P < 0.001$). In contrast, among patients without evidence of viable myocardium, there was no incremental benefit of revascularization over medical therapy. These data, along with other papers presented in this chapter, support the role of myocardial viability testing for the management of patients with chronic left ventricular dysfunction and in guiding therapeutic decisions for revascularization. (Adapted from Allman et al. [59].)

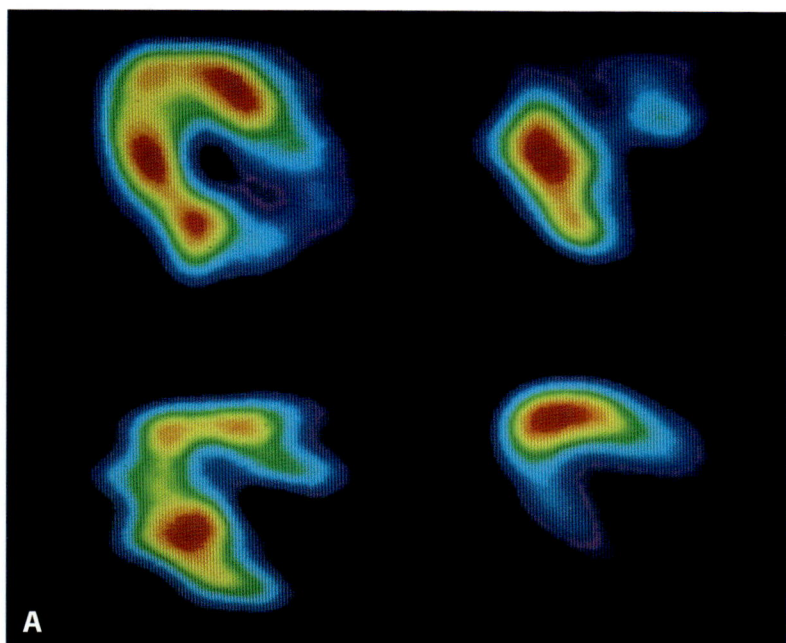

A

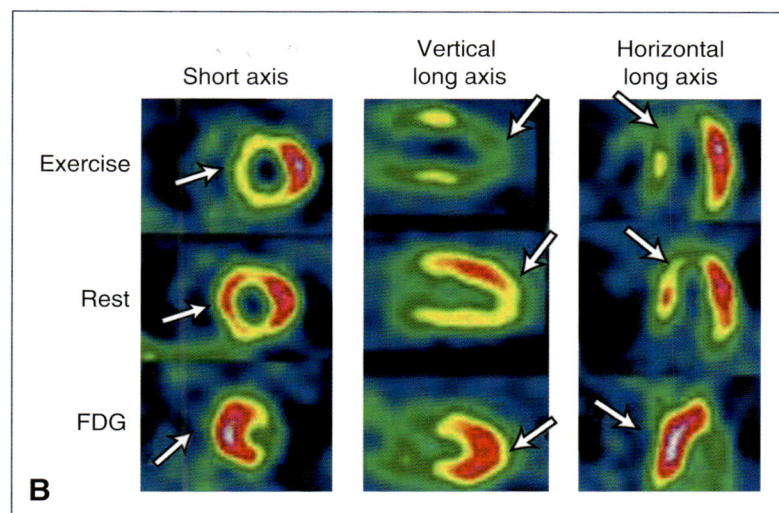

B

Figure 14-35. Metabolic alterations in postischemic myocardium in patients with angina. Physical exercise is probably the most common precipitating factor responsible for myocardial ischemia in patients with coronary artery disease, manifested as angina and, most importantly, left ventricular dysfunction. Although recovery of such stress-induced left ventricular dysfunction is thought to occur within minutes after the termination of exercise, persistent contractile dysfunction has been observed in some patients up to 90 minutes after the termination of exercise, which has been attributed to stunned myocardium. A, Transaxial rubidium-82 (^{82}Rb) positron emission tomography images reflecting myocardial blood flow at rest, during exercise, and after exercise are shown along with [18F]-fluorodeoxyglucose (FDG) images after exercise. At rest (top left), the distribution of myocardial blood flow is homogeneous in all myocardial regions. During exercise (top right), there are extensive blood flow abnormalities in the apical and anteroseptal regions that improve on the postexercise images (bottom left) and are comparable to the ^{82}Rb rest image (top left). FDG

was injected 8 minutes after the termination of exercise. The FDG image recorded 60 minutes after tracer injection (bottom right) shows metabolic alterations in the previously ischemic regions. (From Camici et al. [60]; with permission.)

B, Simultaneous myocardial perfusion and metabolism imaging after dual intravenous injection of Tc-99m sestamibi and FDG at peak exercise. Dual isotope simultaneous acquisition (DISA) was carried out 40–60 minutes after the exercise study was completed. Rest Tc-99m sestamibi imaging was carried out separately. In this patient with angina and no prior myocardial infarction, there is evidence for extensive reversible perfusion defect in the anterior, septal, and apical regions. The coronary angiogram showed 90% stenosis of the left anterior descending and 60% stenosis of the left circumflex coronary arteries. The corresponding FDG image shows intense uptake in the regions with reversible sestamibi defects reflecting the metabolic correlate of exercise-induced myocardial ischemia. (Adapted from He et al. [61].)

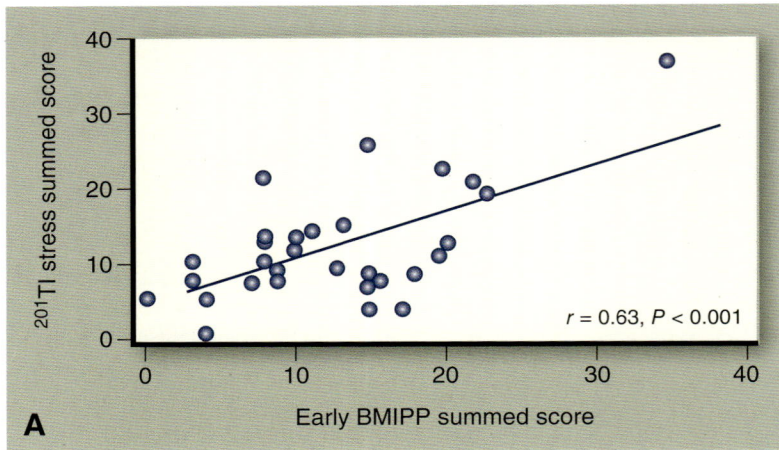

A

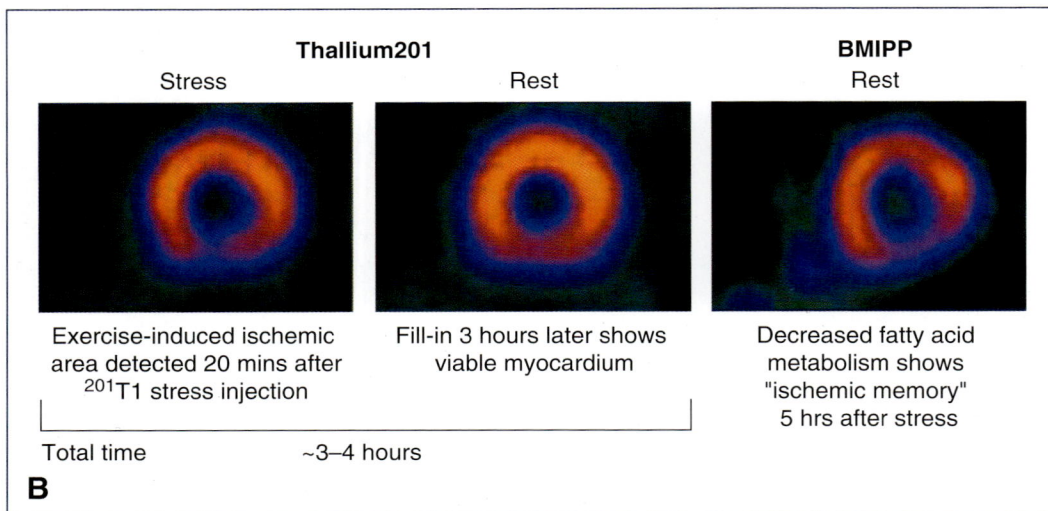

Thallium201

Stress

Exercise-induced ischemic
area detected 20 mins after
201T1 stress injection

Rest

Fill-in 3 hours later shows
viable myocardium

BMIPP

Rest

Decreased fatty acid
metabolism shows
"ischemic memory"
5 hrs after stress

Total time   ~3–4 hours

B

Figure 14-36. A and **B,** Evidence for metabolic imprint of a stress-induced ischemic episode, also known as *ischemic memory*. Recovery of regional perfusion is a prerequisite for recovery of regional function and metabolism. While delayed recovery of regional function after reperfusion is well documented in the clinical setting as stunned myocardium, delayed recovery of regional fatty acid metabolism, termed metabolic stunning, was only recently recognized in the clinical setting [62]. In patients with exercise-induced ischemia on ^{201}TI single-photon emission computed tomography (SPECT), β-methly-p-[123I]-iodophenyl-pentadecanoic acid (BMIPP) was injected at rest (within 30 hours of treadmill ischemia) and BMIPP SPECT images were acquired approximately 10 minutes thereafter. Agreement between BMIPP and ^{201}TI data for the presence of an abnormality, on a patient basis, was 91%. Agreement between BMIPP and ^{201}TI was 95% among patient studies on the same day, mean 6.2 ± 1.4 hours after exercise-induced ischemia and 91% among patients studied on the same day, mean 24.9 ± 2.6 hours after ischemia (P = NS). Moreover, the magnitude of resting BMIPP metabolic defect by semiquantitative visual analysis was correlated to the magnitude of exercise-induced ^{201}TI perfusion defect (r = 0.63, $P <$ 0.001) (**A**). Example of similar extent and severity of rest metabolic BMIPP defect compared with exercise-induced ^{201}TI perfusion defect is shown (**B**). Representative stress (*left*) and rest reinjection (*middle*) short-axis ^{201}TI tomograms demonstrate a reversible inferior defect consistent with exercise-induced myocardial ischemia. BMIPP tomogram (*right*) injected and acquired at rest 5 hours after exercise-induced ischemia show persistent metabolic abnormality in the inferior region despite complete recovery of regional perfusion at rest, as evidenced by ^{201}TI reinjection image. (*Adapted from* Dilsizian *et al.* [62].)

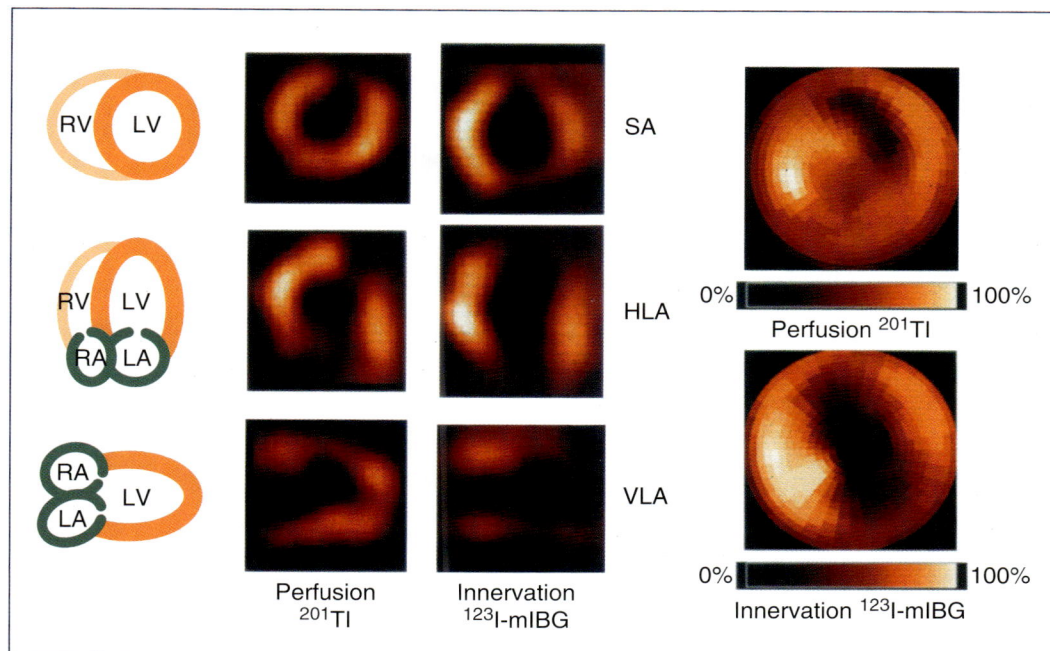

Figure 14-37. Assessment of neuronal function in the infarct zone. Single-photon emission computed tomography (SPECT) images were obtained in a patient within 14 days of an anterior myocardial infarction. The tomographic slices are displayed in short-axis (SA), horizontal long-axis (HLA), and vertical long-axis views (VLA). Regional retention of 10 mCi I-123 metaiodobenzylguanidine (^{123}I-mIBG) after 4 hours was compared with the myocardial perfusion as assessed from images acquired 20 minutes after injection of 2 mCi of [201]Tl. There is a perfusion abnormality in the ^{201}Tl images involving the anterolateral wall of the left ventricle. The images obtained after ^{123}I-mIBG injection reveal a markedly larger area of reduced ^{123}I-mIBG retention involving the anterolateral wall as well as the distal inferior wall. Polar maps display the disparity of perfusion and neuronal abnormality, reflecting the infarct size and area of denervation. This mismatch between perfusion and ^{123}I-mIBG retention indicates denervation of areas that survived the ischemic event. The mismatch between infarct size and denervation is present in almost 80% of patients after acute myocardial infarction. Although there is no clear correlation between extent and severity of myocardial denervation following myocardial infarction and clinical outcome, this disparity between denervation and infarct size has been linked to perioperative complications.

Several studies have investigated the incidence of reinnervation following myocardial infarction [63–65]. The results are controversial because some studies show no reinnervation for up to 6 months, while others show that reinnervation takes place within a few months after the acute event. About 40% of infarcted segments show some degree of reinnervation, most likely reflecting a different degree of neuronal injury [66]. LA—left atrium; LV—left ventricle; RA—right atrium; RV—right ventricle.

Figure 14-38. Neuronal damage in ischemic myocardium. ^{99m}Tc-sestamibi and ^{123}I-metaiodobenzylguanidine (^{123}I-mIBG) images were acquired in a 78-year-old man with anterior myocardial infarction, and polar maps were plotted to evaluate the area of risk, area of infarct, and neuronal integrity. After injection of the first sestamibi dose in the emergency room, the patient was transferred to the cardiac catheterization laboratory and percutaneous intervention of the left anterior descending artery was performed. Several hours after the intervention, single-photon emission computed tomography (SPECT) images were taken. Using a 50% threshold of regional ^{99m}Tc-sestamibi activity, the area of risk was determined to be 58% of the left ventricle (left). The SPECT imaging was repeated at rest 14 days after the acute event. Based on the relative retention of ^{99m}Tc-sestamibi, the final infarct size was calculated again using a 50% threshold. The final infarct size was determined to be 15% of the left ventricle, documenting considerable salvage of myocardium following reperfusion therapy (center). The ^{123}I-mIBG images obtained on the 15th day following myocardial infarction display a large area of denervation within the left ventricle (59.3% of the left ventricle) comparable to the area at ischemic risk (right).

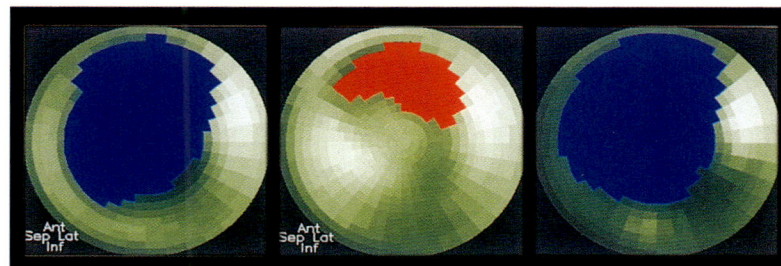

These data indicate that the area of denervation, as determined by ^{123}I-mIBG images of tracer retention in the myocardium, is considerably larger than the infarct size, suggesting a mismatch between denervation and final infarct size. Interestingly, the area of denervation accurately matches the area of risk determined early during the ischemic event. This example confirms animal data, which indicate the higher sensitivity of neuronal activities to myocardial ischemia. Therefore, the ^{123}I-mIBG images obtained at 14 days after the ischemic event still reflect the area of risk as evidence of the extent and severity of the initial ischemic area [67–70].

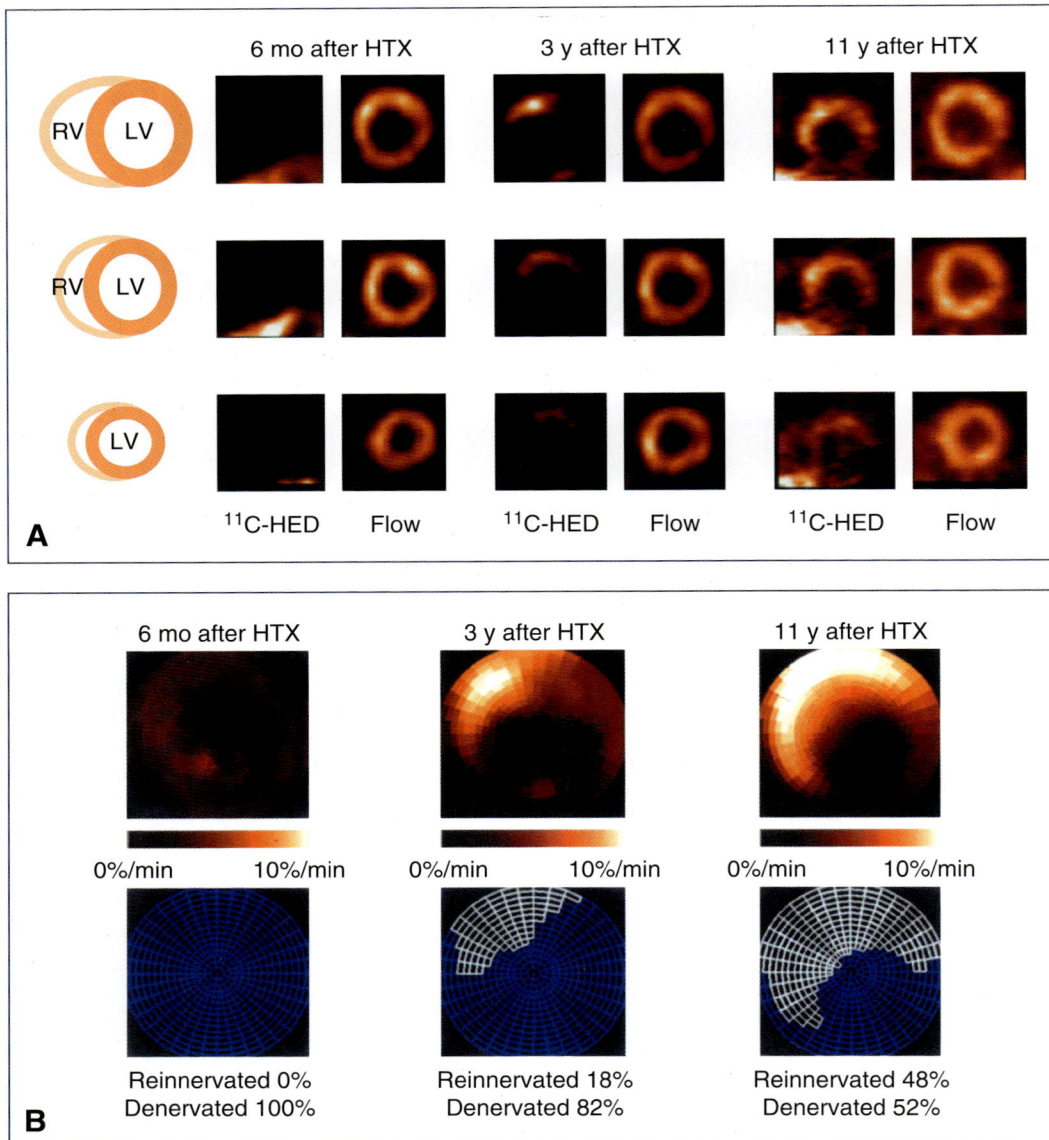

Figure 14-39. Reinnervation of cardiac allograft. Cardiac transplantation (HTX) represents the best model of cardiac denervation because the neuronal fibers are cut during the transplantation surgery. However, as time after cardiac transplantation passes, there is evidence for regional reinnervation [71]. Uptake of radiolabeled catecholamines in the anterior wall, septum, and base of the left ventricle indicates the reappearance of functioning sympathetic nerve terminals. The pharmacologic integrity of these nerve terminals has been demonstrated by studies of neurotransmitter released following the intracoronary injection of tyramine [72].

A study linking regional tracer uptake with exercise capacity indicates that the reinnervation process is beneficial for the exercise performance of patients following heart transplantation [73]. **A,** Neuronal imaging with C-11 hydroxyephedrine (^{11}C-HED) obtained 6 months after transplantation shows little retention of the tracer in the myocardium 40 minutes after tracer injection in comparison to the myocardial perfusion assessed with ^{13}N-ammonia. In a patient studied 3 years after heart transplantation, myocardial perfusion is homogeneous throughout the left ventricle (LV), but the ^{11}C-HED images obtained 40 minutes after injection reveal reappearance of regional ^{11}C-HED retention in the anteroseptal area of the LV. The area of reinnervation appears larger in a patient studied 11

years after transplantation, but regional denervation remains detectable in the inferior aspects of the LV that display normal perfusion. These examples of PET images at different time points after transplantation depict the reinnervation process occurring in about 40% to 50% of the patients. The reinnervation process does not result in complete reinnervation, but shows regional reappearance of sympathetic nerve terminals. Functional studies have shown that patients with reinnervation show greater heart rate variability, better exercise tolerance, and improved LV function with exercise [73].

B, PET–^{11}C-HED polar maps of cardiac transplantation patients at various time points after surgery. Early after transplantation, the retention index is reduced throughout the entire left ventricular myocardium. Using a threshold of 7%/min retention index, no reinnervated area can be detected. At 3 years after transplantation, the anteroseptal areas show reinnervated territories (about 18% of the left ventricle). The PET images obtained 11 years after transplantation show a reinnervated area of 48% of the left ventricle, illustrating the progress of the reinnervation process in the anterior septal wall towards the apex. However, the inferior inferolateral wall remains denervated as seen in most of the patients undergoing neuronal imaging late after cardiac transplantation [73–75].

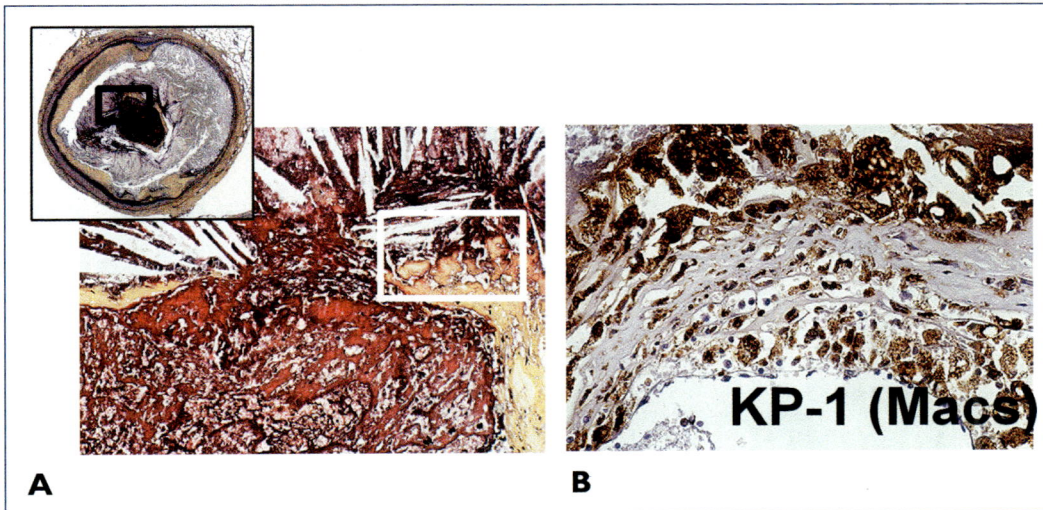

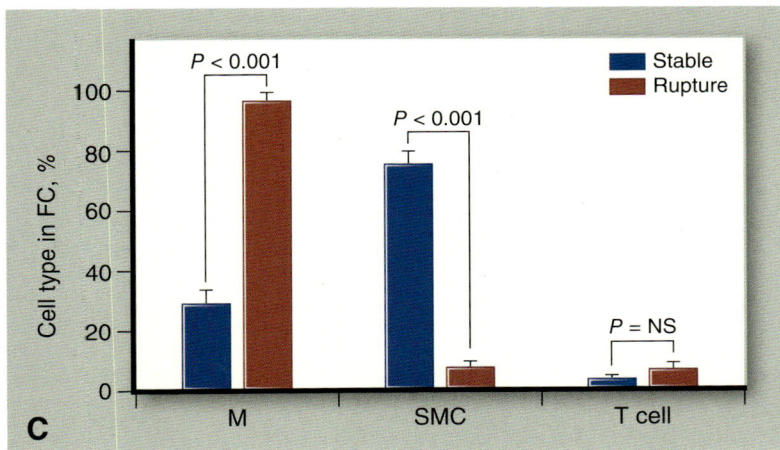

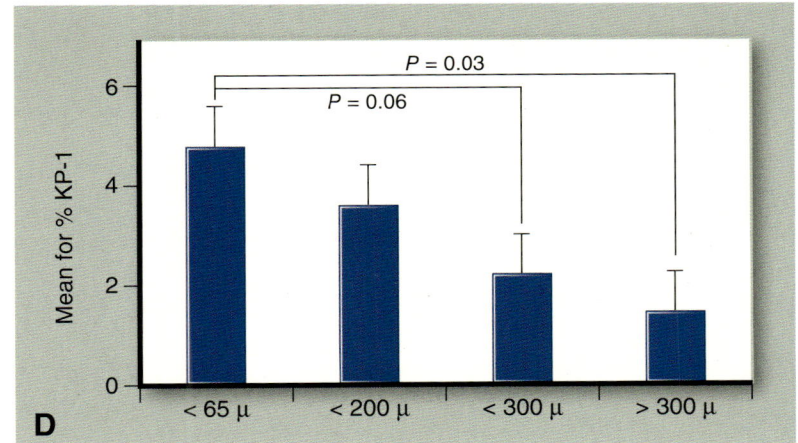

Figure 14-40. Imaging of inflammatory process. Inflammation is a common pathologic manifestation or substrate of numerous cardiovascular diseases. Myocardial inflammation has been commonly imaged with gallium-67 imaging that targets the monocyte-macrophage population or by radiclabeled autologous white blood cells. However, since myocardial inflammation is almost invariably accompanied by myocardial injury, imaging of necrosis or apoptosis have been commonly employed for the clinical detection of myocarditis and transplant rejection. Inflammation in atherosclerotic lesions determines susceptibility of atherosclerotic plaques to acute coronary events [76,77]. This figure demonstrates the culprit coronary lesion from a patient with sudden death (**A,** *inset*). The larger magnification (**A**) highlights the area of rupture characterized by thin disrupted fibrous cap that allows interaction of the thrombogenic neointima necrotic core (with numerous cholesterol crystals) and the luminal thrombus (Movat's pentachrome × 40). Further magnification of the area of cap rupture and its immunohistochemical characterization reveals intense infiltration of the cap by macrophages (staining with KP-1 or antimacrophage antibody × 40) (**B**). Predominant cell population in fibrous caps of ruptured and vulnerable plaques comprises macrophages (M), whereas smooth muscle cells (SMC) are more commonly seen in stable plaques (**C**). In fact, the larger the number of macrophages the more attenuated becomes the fibrous cap (FC) (**D**). It is therefore conceivable that the imaging of the macrophage infiltration in atherosclerotic lesions will allow identification of plaques prone to rupture. Nuclear imaging of macrophages has been performed by targeting of neoexpression of receptors for various chemotactic peptides or adhesion molecules. Radiolabeled monocyte chemoattractant peptide (MCP-1) has been employed in experimental atherosclerotic lesions. In addition, from oncology imaging experience it is well established that the cells with high respiratory burst preferentially accumulate glucose. (*Courtesy of* Renu Virmani, MD, Washington, DC.)

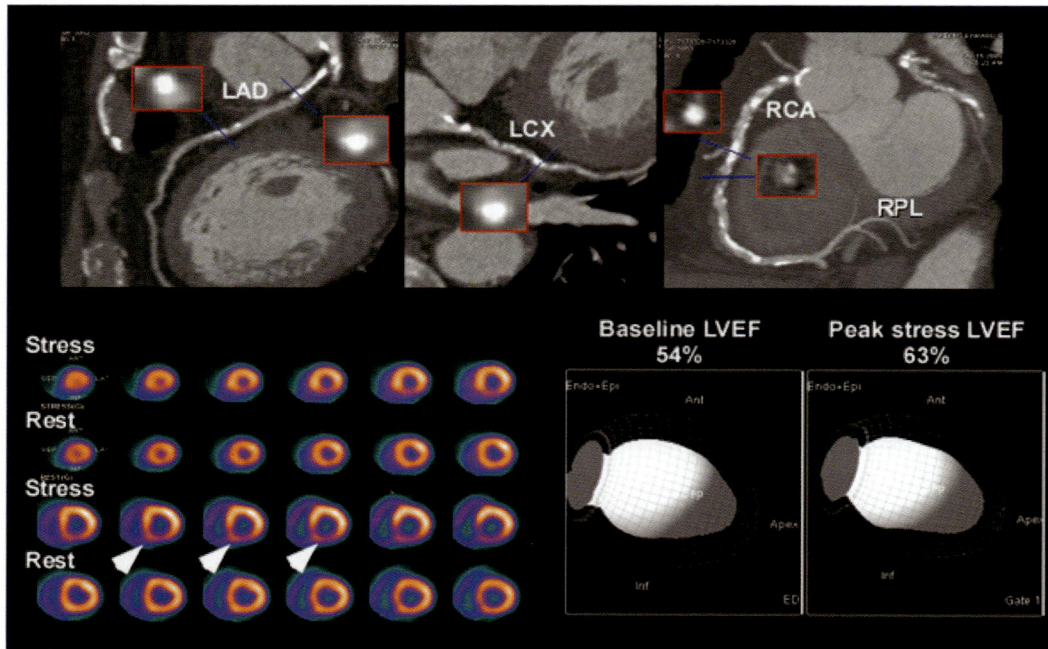

Figure 14-41. Integrated positron emission tomography (PET)/computed tomography angiogram study. There is extensive calcified plaque burden throughout the coronary arteries. The left anterior descending and circumflex coronary arteries show severe calcified plaque in their proximal and mid segments. The dominant right coronary artery shows multiple calcified plaques, with a severe, predominantly noncalcified plaque in its mid segment. However, the rest and peak adenosine stress myocardial perfusion PET study (*lower left panel*) demonstrates only moderate ischemia in the inferior wall (*arrows*). In addition, left ventricular ejection fraction was normal at rest and demonstrated a normal rise during peak stress, effectively excluding the presence of flow-limiting three-vessel CAD (*Reproduced from* Di Carli and Hachamovitch [54].)

References

1. Mosher P, Ross J Jr, McFate PA, Shaw RF: Control of coronary blood flow by an autoregulatory mechanism. *Circ Res* 1964, 14:250–259.

2. Feigl E, Schaper W: Physiology of coronary circulation. In *Cardiology*. Edited by Crawford M, DiMarco J. London: Mosby; 2001:1.1–1.9.

3. Cerqueira MD, Weissman NJ, Dilsizian V, *et al.*: Standardized myocardial segmentation and nomenclature for tomographic imaging of the heart. AHA Writing Group on Myocardial Segmentation and Registration for Cardiac Imaging. *Circulation* 2002, 105:539–542.

4. Dilsizian V, Rocco TP, Freedman NM, *et al.*: Enhanced detection of ischemic but viable myocardium by the reinjection of thallium after stress-redistribution imaging. *N Engl J Med* 1990, 323:141–146.

5. Maddahi J, Van Train K, Prigent F, *et al.*: Quantitative single photon emission computed thallium-201 tomography for detection and localization of coronary artery disease: optimization and prospective validation of a new technique. *J Am Coll Cardiol* 1989, 14:1689–1699.

6. Fintel DJ, Links JM, Brinker JA, *et al.*: Improved diagnostic performance of exercise thallium-201 single photon emission computed tomography over planar imaging in the diagnosis of coronary artery disease: A receiver operating characteristic analysis. *J Am Coll Cardiol* 1989, 13:600–612.

7. Iskandrian AS, Heo J, Kong B, *et al.*: Effect of exercise level on the ability of thallium-201 tomographic imaging in detecting coronary artery disease: analysis of 461 patients. *J Am Coll Cardiol* 1989, 14:1477–1486.

8. Go RT, Marwick TH, MacIntyre WJ, *et al.*: A prospective comparison of rubidium-82 PET and thallium-201 SPECT myocardial perfusion imaging utilizing a single dipyridamole stress in the diagnosis of coronary artery disease. *J Nucl Med* 1990, 31:1899–1905.

9. Mahmarian JJ, Boyce, Goldberg RK, *et al.*: Quantitative exercise thallium-201 single photo emission computed tomography for the enhanced diagnosis of ischemic heart disease. *J Am Coll Cardiol* 1990, 15:318–329.

10. Van Train KF, Maddahi J, Berman DS, *et al.*: Quantitative analysis of tomographic stress thallium-201 myocardial scintigrams: a multicenter trial. *J Nucl Med* 1990, 31:1168–1179.

11. Kiat H, Maddahi J, Roy L, *et al.*: Comparison of technetium 99m methoxy isobutyl isonitrile and thallium-201 for evaluation of coronary artery disease by planar and tomographic methods. *Am Heart J* 1989, 117:1–11.

12. Iskandrian AS, Heo J, Long B, *et al.*: Use of technetium-99m isonitrile (RP-30A) in assessing left ventricular perfusion and function at rest and during exercise in coronary artery disease, and comparison with coronary arteriography and exercise thallium-201 SPECT imaging. *Am J Cardiol* 1989, 64:270–275.

13. Kahn JK, McGhie I, Akers MS, *et al.*: Quantitative rotational tomography 201Tl and 99mTc 2-methoxly-isobutyl-isonitrile. *Circulation* 1989, 79:1282–1293.

14. Solot G, Hermans J, Merlo P, *et al.*: Correlation of 99Tcm-sestamibi SPECT with coronary angiography in general hospital practice. *Nucl Med Commun* 1993, 14:23–29.

15. Van Train KF, Garcia EV, Maddahi J, *et al.*: Multicenter trial validation for quantitative analysis of same-day rest-stress technetium-99m-sestamibi myocardial tomograms. *J Nucl Med* 1994, 35:609–618.

16. Azzarelli S, Galassi AR, Foti R, *et al.*: Accuracy of 99m-tetrofosmin myocardial tomography in the evaluation of coronary artery disease. *J Nucl Cardiol* 1999, 6: 8–189.

17. Udelson JE, Heller GV, Wackers FJ, *et al.*: Randomized, controlled dose-ranging study of the selective adenosine A2A receptor agonist binodenoson for pharmacological stress as an adjunct to myocardial perfusion imaging. *Circulation* 2004, 109:457–464.

18. Iskandrian AE, Bateman TM, Belardinelli L, *et al.*: Adenosine versus regadenoson comparative evaluation in myocardial perfusion imaging: results of the ADVANCE phase 3 multicenter international trial. *J Nucl Cardiol* 2007,14:645–658

19. Leaker BR, O'Connor B, Hansel TT, *et al.*: Safety of regadenoson, an adenosine A2A receptor agonist for myocardial perfusion imaging, in mild asthma and moderate asthma patients: a randomized, double-blind, placebo-controlled trial. J Nucl Cardiol 2008, 15:329–336.

20. Thomas GS, Tammelin BR, Schiffman GL, *et al.*: Safety of regadenoson, a selective adenosine A2A agonist, in patients with chronic obstructive pulmonary disease: a randomized, double-blind, placebo-controlled trial (RegCOPD trial). *J Nucl Cardiol* 2008, 5:319–328.

21. Cecchi F, Olivotto I, Gistri R, *et al.*: Coronary microvascular dysfunction and prognosis in hypertrophic cardiomyopathy. *N Engl J Med* 2003, 349: 27–1035.

22. Schachinger V, Britten MB, Zeiher AM: Prognostic impact of coronary vasodilator dysfunction on adverse long-term outcome of coronary heart disease. *Circulation* 2000, 101:1899–1906.

23. Britten MB, Zeiher AM, Schachinger V: Microvascular dysfunction in angiographically normal or mildly diseased coronary arteries predicts adverse cardiovascular long-term outcome. *Coron Artery Dis* 2004, 15:259–264.

24. Germano G: Technical aspects of myocardial SPECT imaging. *J Nucl Med* 2001, 42:1499–1507.

25. The Cardiovascular Imaging Committee, American College of Cardiology; The Committee on Advanced Cardiac Imaging and Technology, Council on Clinical Cardiology, American Heart Association; and Board of Directors, Cardiovascular Council, Society of Nuclear Medicine: Standardization of cardiac tomographic imaging. *J Am Coll Cardiol* 1992, 20:255–256.

26. Germano G, Berman D: Acquisition and processing for gated perfusion SPECT: technical aspects. In *Clinical Gated Cardiac SPECT*. Edited by Germano G, Berman D. Armonk, NY: Futura Publishing Company; 1999:93–113.

27. Germano G, Kiat H, Kavanagh PB, *et al.*: Automatic quantification of ejection fraction from gated myocardial perfusion SPECT. *J Nucl Med* 1995, 36:2138–2147.

28. Manrique A, Koning R, Cribier A, Véra P: Effect of temporal sampling on evaluation of left ventricular ejection fraction by means of thallium-201 gated SPECT: comparison of 16- and 8-interval gating, with reference to equilibrium radionuclide angiography. *Eur J Nucl Med* 2000, 27:694–699.

29. Kikkawa M, Nakamura T, Sakamoto K, *et al.*: Assessment of left ventricular diastolic function from quantitative electrocardiographic-gated (99)mTc-tetrofosmin myocardial SPECT. *Eur J Nucl Med* 2001, 28:593–601. [Published erratum appears in *Eur J Nucl Med* 2001, 28:1579.]

30. Kumita S, Cho K, Nakajo H, *et al.*: Assessment of left ventricular diastolic function with electrocardiography-gated myocardial perfusion SPECT: comparison with multigated equilibrium radionuclide angiography. *J Nucl Cardiol* 2001, 8:568–574.

31. Roelants V, Gerber B, Vanoverschelde J: Comparison between 16- and 8-interval gating for the evaluation of LV function with G-SPECT in patients with history of myocardial infarction and severe ischemic cardiomyopathy: a comparison to MRI [abstract]. *J Nucl Cardiol* 2003, 10:S6.

32. Navare SM, Wackers FJT, Liu YH: Comparison of 16-frame and 8-frame gated SPECT imaging for determination of left ventricular volumes and ejection fraction. *Eur J Nucl Med Mol Imaging* 2003, 30:1330–1337.

33. Higuchi T, Nakajima K, Taki J, *et al.*: Assessment of left ventricular systolic and diastolic function based on the edge detection method with myocardial ECG-gated SPECT. *Eur J Nucl Med* 2001, 28:1512–1516.

34. Nakajima K, Taki J, Kawano M, *et al.*: Diastolic dysfunction in patients with systemic sclerosis detected by gated myocardial perfusion SPECT: an early sign of cardiac involvement. *J Nucl Med* 2001, 42:183–188.

35. Higuchi T, Nakajima K, Taki J, *et al.*: The accuracy of left-ventricular time volume curve derived from ECG-gated myocardial perfusion SPECT [abstract]. *J Nucl Cardiol* 2001, 8:S18.

36. Akincioglu C, Abidov A, Nishina H, *et al.*: Determination and prospective validation of normal values of diastolic parameters in 16-frame Tc-99m MIBI gated myocardial perfusion SPECT [abstract]. *J Nucl Cardiol* 2004, 11:S3–S4.

37. Ladenheim ML, Kotler TS, Pollock BH, *et al.*: Incremental prognostic power of clinical history, exercise electrocardiography and myocardial perfusion scintigraphy in suspected coronary artery disease. *Am J Cardiol* 1987, 59:270–277.

38. Hachamovitch R, Berman DS, Shaw LJ, *et al.*: Incremental prognostic value of myocardial perfusion single photon emission computed tomography for the prediction of cardiac death: differential stratification for risk of cardiac death and myocardial infarction. *Circulation* 1998, 97:535–543.

39. Vanzetto G, Ormezzano O, Fagret D, *et al.*: Long-term additive prognostic value of thallium-201 myocardial perfusion imaging over clinical and exercise stress test in low to intermediate risk patients: study in 1137 patients with 6-year follow-up. *Circulation* 1999, 100:1521–1527.

40. Gibbons RJ, Chatterjee K, Daley J, *et al.*: ACC/AHA/ACP-ASIM guidelines for the management of patients with chronic stable angina: a report of the American College of Cardiology/American Heart Association Task Force on Practice Guidelines (Committee on Management of Patients With Chronic Stable Angina) [published correction appears in *J Am Coll Cardiol* 1999, 34:314]. *J Am Coll Cardiol* 1999, 33:2092–2197.

41. Hachamovitch R, Berman DS, Kiat H, *et al.*: Exercise myocardial perfusion SPECT in patients without known coronary artery disease: incremental prognostic value and use in risk stratification. *Circulation* 1996, 93:905–914.

42. Shaw LJ, Iskandrian AE: Prognostic value of stress gated SPECT in patients with known or suspected coronary artery disease. *J Nucl Cardiol* 2004, 11:171–185.

43. Kang X, Berman DS, Lewin HC, *et al.*: Incremental prognostic value of myocardial perfusion single photon emission computed tomography in patients with diabetes mellitus. *Am Heart J* 1999, 138:1025–1032.

44. National Center for Health Statistics: Health, United States 1999: health and aging chart book. Accessible at http://www.cdc.gov/nchs/data/hus/hus99cht.pdf. Accessed August 22, 2008.

45. Gibbons RJ, Balady GJ, Bricker JT, *et al.*: American College of Cardiology/American Heart Association Task Force on Practice Guidelines. Committee to Update the 1997 Exercise Testing Guidelines: ACC/AHA 2002 guideline update for exercise testing: summary article. A report of the American College of Cardiology/American Heart Association Task Force on Practice Guidelines (Committee to Update the 1997 Exercise Testing Guidelines). *J Am Coll Cardiol* 2002, 40:1531–1540.]

46. Gulati M, Black HR, Shaw LJ, *et al.*: The prognostic value of exercise capacity in women: nomogram for the female population. *N Engl J Med* 2005, 353:468–475.

47. Klocke FJ, Baird MG, Lorell BH, *et al.*: ACC/AHA/ASNC guidelines for the clinical use of cardiac radionuclide imaging—executive summary: a report of the American College of Cardiology/American Heart Association Task Force on Practice Guidelines (ACC/AHA/ASNC Committee to Revise the 1995 Guidelines for the Clinical Use of Cardiac Radionuclide Imaging). *J Am Coll Cardiol* 2003, 42:1318–1333.

48. Heller GV, Stowers SA, Hendel RC, *et al.*: Clinical value of acute rest technetium-99m tetrofosmin tomographic myocardial perfusion imaging in patients with acute chest pain and nondiagnostic electrocardiograms. *J Am Coll Cardiol* 1998, 31:1011–1017.

49. Taegtmeyer H: Modulation of responses to myocardial ischemia: metabolic features of myocardial stunning, hibernation, and ischemic preconditioning. In *Myocardial Viability: A Clinical and Scientific Treatise*. Edited by Dilsizian VA. New York: Futura; 2000:25–36.

50. Braunwald E, Kloner RA: The stunned myocardium: prolonged, postischemic ventricular dysfunction. *Circulation* 1982, 66:1146–1149.

51. Rahimtoola SH: A perspective on the three large multicenter randomized clinical trials of coronary bypass surgery for chronic stable angina. *Circulation* 1985, 72(suppl V):V123–V135.

52. Kitsiou AN, Srinivasan G, Quyyumi AA, *et al.*: Stress-induced reversible and mild-to-moderate irreversible thallium defects: Are they equally accurate for predicting recovery of regional left ventricular function after revascularization? *Circulation* 1998, 98:501–508.

53. Dilsizian V: Perspectives on the study of human myocardium: viability. In *Myocardial Viability: A Clinical and Scientific Treatise*. Edited by Dilsizian V. Armonk, New York: Futura; 2000:3–22.

54. Di Carli MF, Hachamovitch R: New technology for noninvasive evaluation of coronary artery disease. *Circulation* 2007, 115:1464–1480.

55. Eitzman D, Al-Aouar Z, Kanter HL, *et al.*: Clinical outcome of patients with advanced coronary artery disease after viability studies with positron emission tomography. *J Am Coll Cardiol* 1992, 20:559–565.

56. Di Carli MF, Davidson M, Little R, *et al.*: Value of metabolic imaging with positron emission tomography for evaluating prognosis in patients with coronary artery disease and left ventricular dysfunction. *Am J Cardiol* 1994, 73:527–533.

57. Di Carli MF, Asgarzadie F, Schelbert HR, *et al.*: Quantitative relation between myocardial viability and improvement in heart failure symptoms after revascularization in patients with ischemic cardiomyopathy. *Circulation* 1995, 92:3436–3444.

58. Haas F, Haehnel CJ, Picker W, *et al.*: Preoperative positron emission tomography viability assessment and perioperative and postoperative risk in patients with advanced ischemic heart disease. *J Am Coll Cardiol* 1997, 30:1693–1670.

59. Allman KC, Shaw LJ, Hachamovitch R, Udelson JE: Myocardial viability testing and impact of revascularization on prognosis in patients with coronary artery disease and left ventricular dysfunction: a meta-analysis. *J Am Coll Cardiol* 2002, 39:1151–1158.

60. Camici P, Araujo LI, Spinks T, *et al.*: Increased uptake of 18F-fluorodeoxyglucose in postischemic myocardium of patients with exercise-induced angina. *Circulation* 1986, 74:81–88.

61. He ZX, Shi RF, Wu YJ, *et al.*: Direct imaging of exercise-induced myocardial ischemia with fluorine-18-labeled deoxyglucose and Tc-99m-sestamibi in coronary artery disease. *Circulation* 2003, 108:1208–1213.

62. Dilsizian V, Bateman TM, Bergmann SR, *et al.*: Metabolic imaging with β-methly-p-[123I]-iodophenyl-pentadecanoic acid (BMIPP) identifies ischemic memory following demand ischemia. *Circulation* 2005, 112:2169–2174.

63. Allman KC, Wieland DM, Muzik O, *et al.*: Carbon-11 hydroxyephedrine with positron emission tomography for serial assessment of cardiac adrenergic neuronal function after acute myocardial infarction in humans. *J Am Coll Cardiol* 1993, 22:368–375.

64. Fallen EL, Coates G, Nahmias C, *et al.*: Recovery rates of regional sympathetic reinnervation and myocardial blood flow after acute myocardial infarction. *Am Heart J* 1999, 137:863–869.

65. Simula S, Lakka T, Kuikka J, *et al.*: Cardiac adrenergic innervation within the first 3 months after acute myocardial infarction. *Clin Physiol* 2000, 20:366–373.

66. Patel A, Iskandrian A: MIBG imaging. *J Nucl Cardiol* 2002, 9:75–94.

67. Matsunari I, Schricke U, Bengel FM, *et al.*: Extent of cardiac sympathetic neuronal damage is determined by the area of ischemia in patients with acute coronary syndromes. *Circulation* 2000, 101:2579–2585.

68. Schwaiger M, Guiborg H, Rosenspire K, *et al.*: Effect of regional myocardial ischemia on sympathetic nervous system as assessed by fluorine-18-metaraminol. *J Nucl Med* 1990, 31:1352–1357.

69. Schwaiblmair M, von Scheidt W, Uberfuhr P, *et al.*: Functional significance of cardiac reinnervation in heart transplant recipients. *J Heart Lung Transplant* 1999, 18:838–845.

70. Wolpers H, Nguyen N, Rosenspire K, *et al.*: C-11 hydroxyephedrine as marker for neuronal catecholamine retention in reperfused canine myocardium. *Coronary Artery Disease* 1991, 2:923–929.

71. Schwaiger M, Hutchins GD, Kalff V, *et al.*: Evidence for regional catecholamine uptake and storage sites in the transplanted human heart by positron emission tomography. *J Clin Invest* 1991, 87:1681–1690.

72. Odaka K, von Scheidt W, Ziegler SI, *et al.*: Reappearance of cardiac presynaptic sympathetic nerve terminals in the transplanted heart: correlation between PET using (11)C-hydroxyephedrine and invasively measured norepinephrine release. *J Nucl Med* 2001, 42:1011–1016.

73. Bengel FM, Ueberfuhr P, Schiepel N, *et al.*: Effect of sympathetic reinnervation on cardiac performance after heart transplantation. *N Engl J Med* 2001, 345:731–738.

74. De Marco T, Dae M, Yuen-Green MS, *et al.*: Iodine-123 metaiodobenzylguanidine scintigraphic assessment of the transplanted human heart: evidence for late reinnervation. *J Am Coll Cardiol* 1995, 25:927–931.

75. Estorch M, Camprecios M, Flotats A, *et al.*: Sympathetic reinnervation of cardiac allografts evaluated by 123I-MIBG imaging. *J Nucl Med* 1999, 40:911–916.

76. Narula J, Virmani R, Iskandrian AE: Strategic targeting of atherosclerotic lesions. *J Nucl Cardiol* 1999, 6:81–90.

77. Narula J, Finn AV, Demaria AN: Picking plaques that pop . . . *J Am Coll Cardiol* 2005, 45:1970–1973.

Cardiac Computed Tomography

15

Matthew J. Budoff and Marcelo F. Di Carli

ardiac computed tomography (CT) is emerging as a powerful noninvasive imaging tool for the evaluation of atherosclerosis in patients with known or suspected coronary artery disease (CAD). Although it was initially introduced as a sensitive means of assessing the extent and severity of coronary artery calcifications, advances in imaging technology with fast scanners capable of 'freezing' cardiac motion and sub-millimeter resolution are making noninvasive assessments of the coronary arteries possible. Unlike invasive coronary angiography, CT coronary angiography (CTA) not only assesses disease within the coronary lumen but it can also provide direct qualitative and quantitative information about nonobstructive atherosclerotic plaque burden within the vessel wall. Thus, it is possible that CTA-based patient evaluation may provide more clinically relevant information on which to base risk assessments when compared to conventional "luminography." New generations of fast scanners are also paving the way for the evaluation of the aorta and peripheral circulation with high accuracy. This chapter reviews the strengths and weaknesses of cardiac CT and its expanding clinical role in areas such as coronary atherosclerosis, peripheral arterial disease, and electrophysiology.

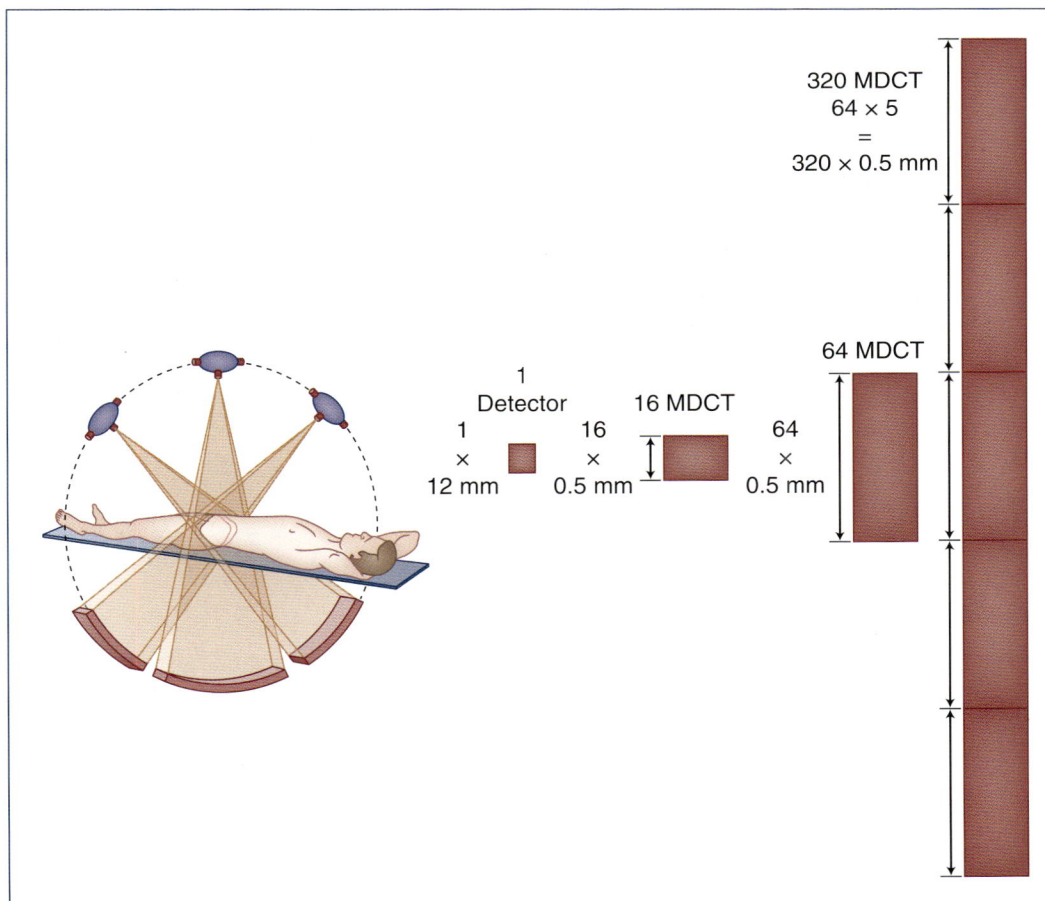

Figure 15-1. Schematic of computed tomography (CT) imaging and detector configuration for multislice CT scanners. The words "computed tomography" refer to a method of tomographic imaging in which a cross-sectional slice is imaged with the aid of computer processing to obtain an exact representation of the anatomic structures within each slice.

Continued on the next page

Figure 15-1. (Continued) With modern multislice CT scanners, images are collected as the radiograph tube rotates around the patient's body and the table moves through the gantry (so-called "helical acquisition;" *left panel*). The radiograph projections at each angle are recorded and subsequently reconstructed to generate tomographic images. Multislice CT scanners can have different detector configurations, with state-of-the-art scanners for cardiac imaging having 64 slices or higher. The number of slices dictates the width of the axial field of view or anatomic coverage during each rotation of the radiograph tube, which in turn defines the length of the scan. The higher the number of slices the shorter the scan acquisition. Newer volume CT scanners with 320 slices (16 cm field of view) acquire an entire scan of the heart in a single rotation of the radiograph tube (< 0.5 sec). MDCT—multidetector computed tomography.

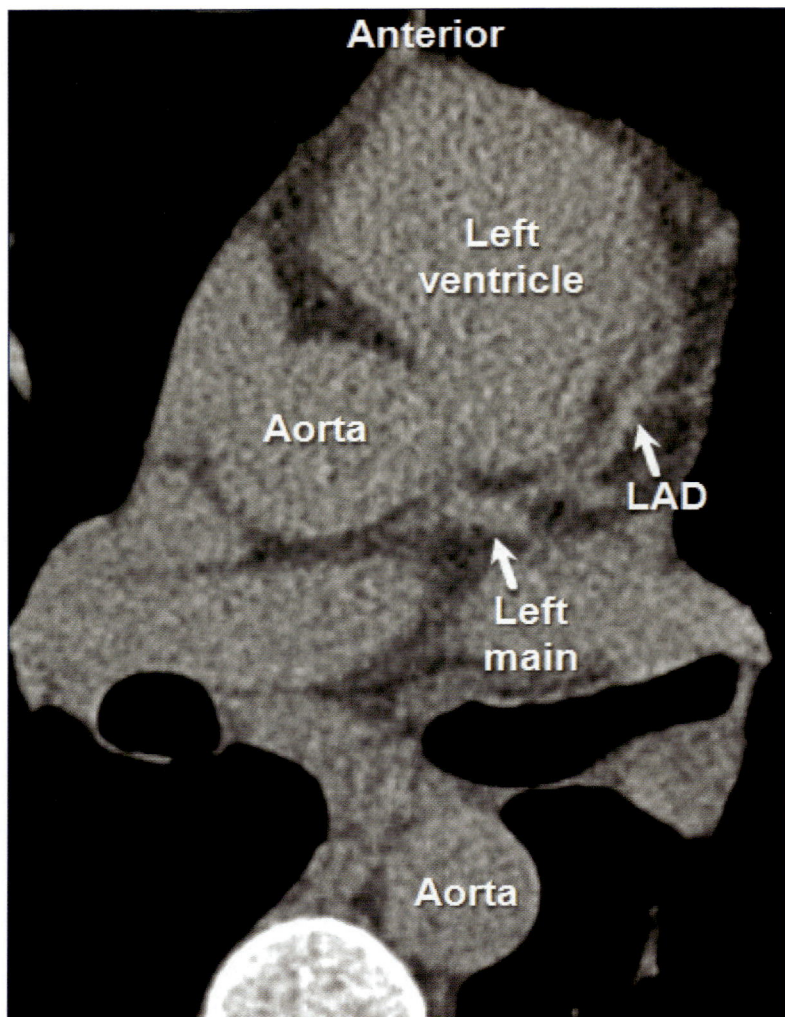

Figure 15-2. A 53-year-old male with moderate hypercholesterolemia who underwent coronary artery calcium scanning. The selected cross-sectional image demonstrates absence of coronary artery calcification. Based on multiple large prospective trials, a coronary artery calcium score of zero in an asymptomatic individual is associated with a less than 0.1% annual event rate [1]. LAD—left anterior descending artery.

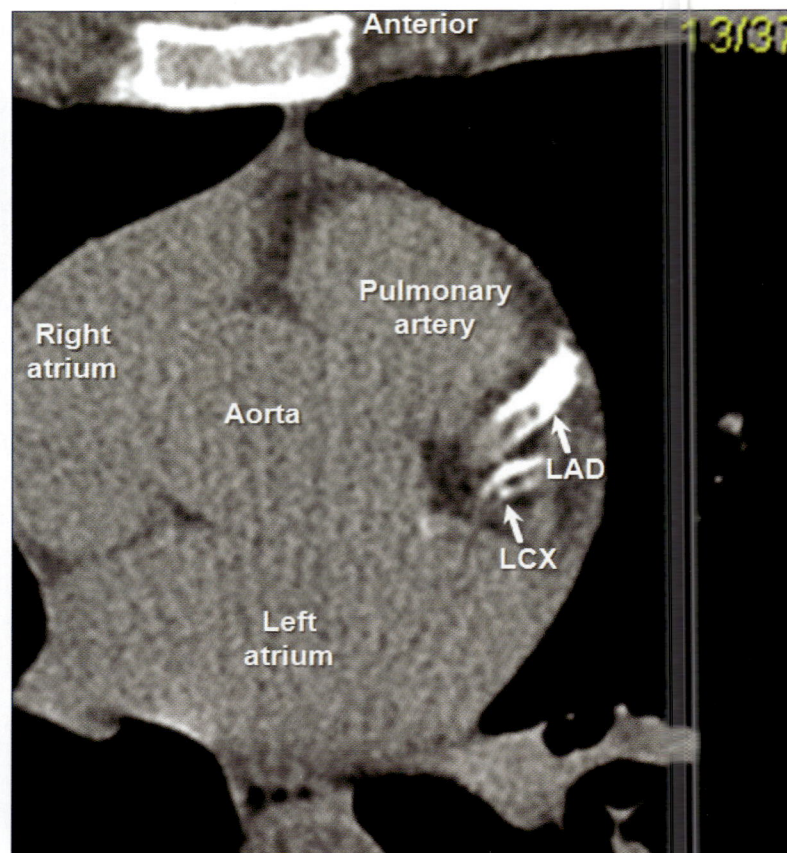

Figure 15-3. A 56-year-old postmenopausal woman, initially assessed at low risk based on age, gender, and risk factors (4% Framingham 10-year risk) underwent coronary artery calcium (CAC) testing. The selected cross-sectional image demonstrates dense coronary artery calcification in the left anterior descending (LAD) and left circumflex (LCX) arteries. A CAC score greater than 100 is associated with a 10-fold risk of cardiovascular events over the next 3 to 5 years, based on a large population study, the Multi-Ethnic Study of Atherosclerosis [1].

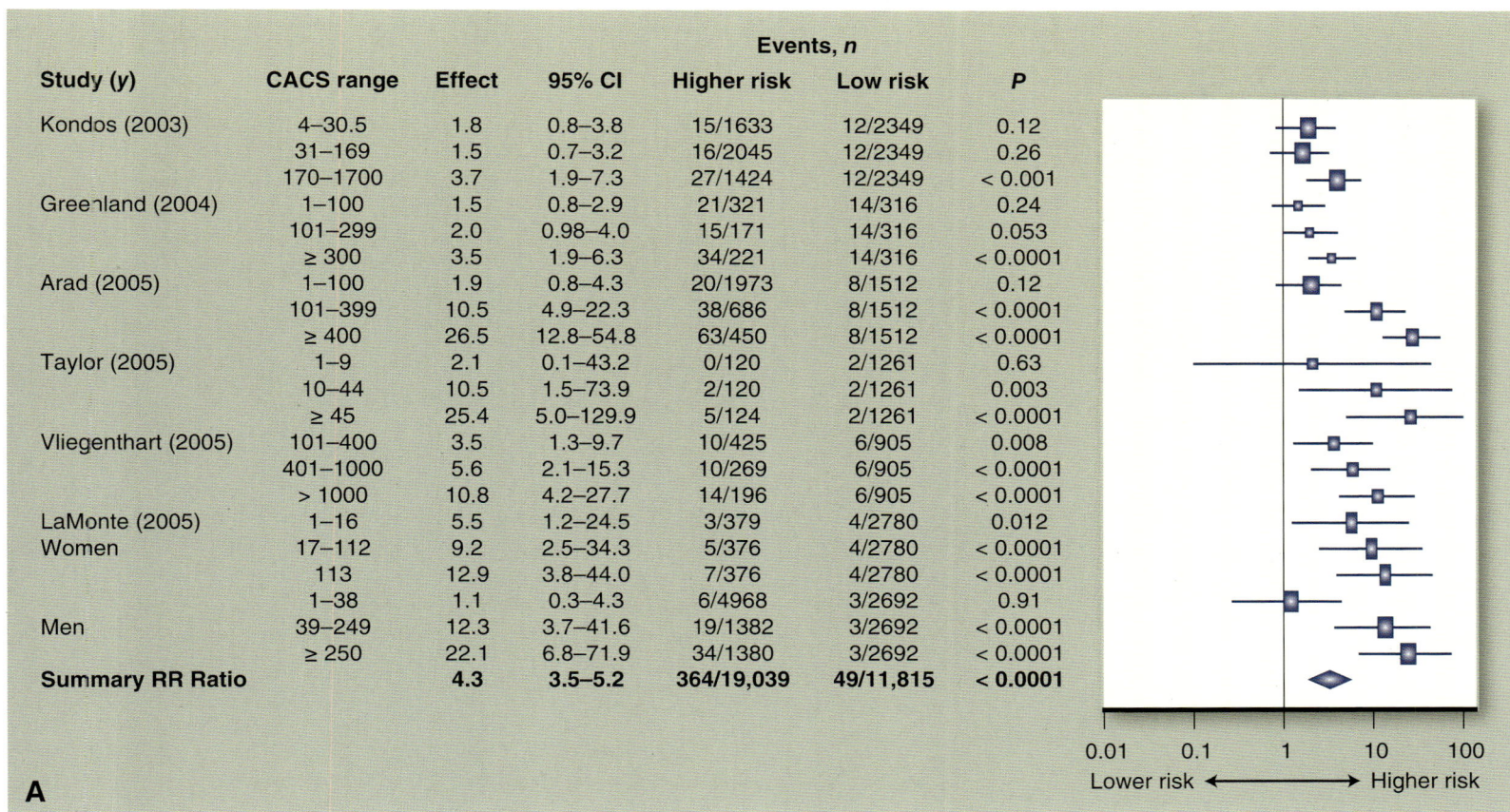

Study (y)	CACS range	Effect	95% CI	Events, n Higher risk	Events, n Low risk	P
Kondos (2003)	4–30.5	1.8	0.8–3.8	15/1633	12/2349	0.12
	31–169	1.5	0.7–3.2	16/2045	12/2349	0.26
	170–1700	3.7	1.9–7.3	27/1424	12/2349	< 0.001
Greenland (2004)	1–100	1.5	0.8–2.9	21/321	14/316	0.24
	101–299	2.0	0.98–4.0	15/171	14/316	0.053
	≥ 300	3.5	1.9–6.3	34/221	14/316	< 0.0001
Arad (2005)	1–100	1.9	0.8–4.3	20/1973	8/1512	0.12
	101–399	10.5	4.9–22.3	38/686	8/1512	< 0.0001
	≥ 400	26.5	12.8–54.8	63/450	8/1512	< 0.0001
Taylor (2005)	1–9	2.1	0.1–43.2	0/120	2/1261	0.63
	10–44	10.5	1.5–73.9	2/120	2/1261	0.003
	≥ 45	25.4	5.0–129.9	5/124	2/1261	< 0.0001
Vliegenthart (2005)	101–400	3.5	1.3–9.7	10/425	6/905	0.008
	401–1000	5.6	2.1–15.3	10/269	6/905	< 0.0001
	> 1000	10.8	4.2–27.7	14/196	6/905	< 0.0001
LaMonte (2005)	1–16	5.5	1.2–24.5	3/379	4/2780	0.012
Women	17–112	9.2	2.5–34.3	5/376	4/2780	< 0.0001
	113	12.9	3.8–44.0	7/376	4/2780	< 0.0001
	1–38	1.1	0.3–4.3	6/4968	3/2692	0.91
Men	39–249	12.3	3.7–41.6	19/1382	3/2692	< 0.0001
	≥ 250	22.1	6.8–71.9	34/1380	3/2692	< 0.0001
Summary RR Ratio		**4.3**	**3.5–5.2**	**364/19,039**	**49/11,815**	**< 0.0001**

A

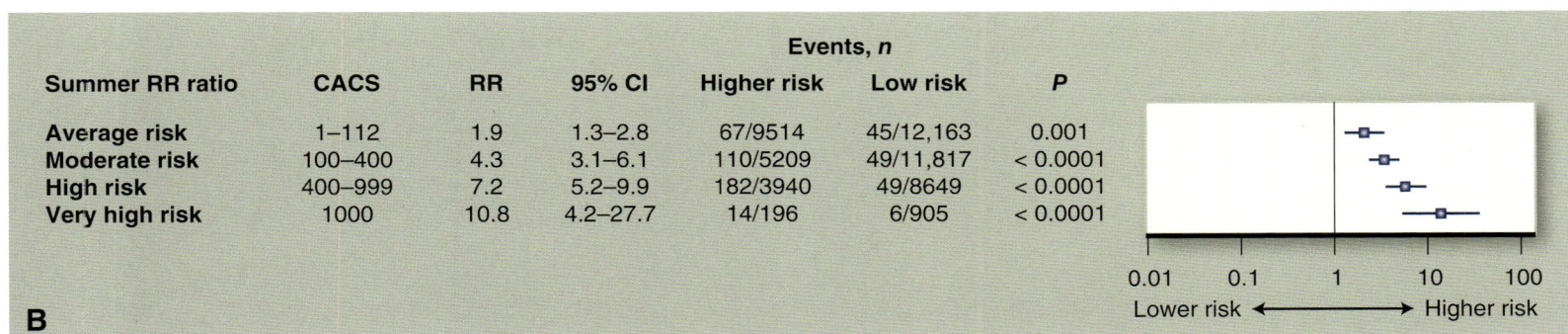

Summer RR ratio	CACS	RR	95% CI	Events, n Higher risk	Events, n Low risk	P
Average risk	1–112	1.9	1.3–2.8	67/9514	45/12,163	0.001
Moderate risk	100–400	4.3	3.1–6.1	110/5209	49/11,817	< 0.0001
High risk	400–999	7.2	5.2–9.9	182/3940	49/8649	< 0.0001
Very high risk	1000	10.8	4.2–27.7	14/196	6/905	< 0.0001

B

Figure 15-4. **A** depicts the results of a meta-analysis on the prognostic value of coronary artery calcium scoring, whereas **B** shows relative risk ratios according to level of risk for coronary artery calcium scores, from average risk to very high risk. CACS—coronary artery calcium score. (*Adapted from* Greenland *et al.* [1].)

ACC/AHA Expert Consensus Interpretation and Recommendations for CT Heart Scanning and Coronary Artery Calcium Scoring

1. A negative test (score 0) makes the presence of atherosclerotic plaque, including unstable or vulnerable plaque, highly unlikely

2. A negative test (score 0) makes the presence of significant luminal obstructive disease highly unlikely (negative predictive power by EBCT on the order of 95%–99%)

3. A negative test is consistent with a low risk (0%–1% per year) of a cardiovascular event in the next 2 to 5 years

4. A positive test (CACS 0) confirms the presence of a coronary atherosclerotic plaque

5. The greater the amount of coronary calcium correlates best with the total amount of atherosclerotic plaque, although the true "atherosclerotic burden" is underestimated

7. A high calcium score (an Agatston score 100) is consistent with a high risk of a cardiac event within the next 2 to 5 years (2% annual risk)

8. Coronary artery calcium measurement can improve risk prediction in conventional intermediate-risk patients, and CACP scanning should be considered in individuals at intermediate risk for a coronary event (1.0% per year to 2.0% per year) for clinical decision-making with regard to refinement of risk assessment

9. Decisions for further testing (such as stress testing or cardiac catheterization) beyond assistance in risk stratification in patients with a positive CAC score cannot be made on the basis of coronary calcium scores alone, as calcium score correlates poorly with stenosis severity in a given individual and should be based on clinical history and other conventional clinical criteria

Figure 15-5. American College of Cardiology/American Heart Association expert consensus interpretation and recommendations for computed tomography (CT) heart scanning and coronary artery calcium scoring. (*Adapted from* Budoff *et al.* [2].) CACP—coronary artery calcified plaque; CACS—coronary artery calcium score; CI—confidence interval; EBCT—electron beam computed tomography; RR—relative risk.

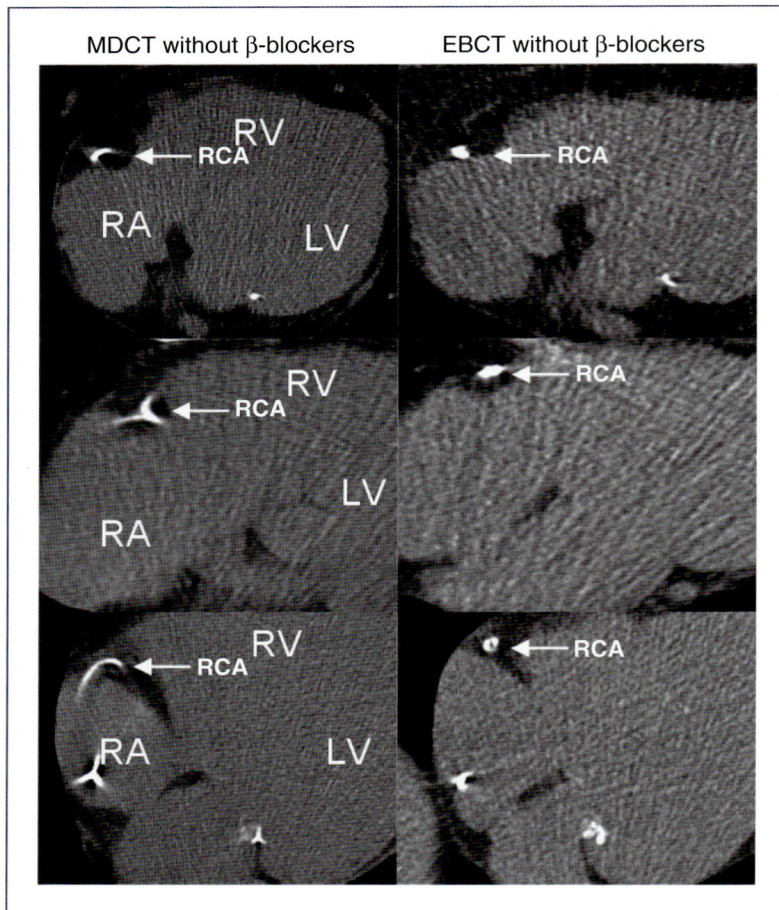

MDCT without β-blockers   EBCT without β-blockers

Figure 15-6. Due to the somewhat limited temporal resolution of computed tomography (CT) scanners, cardiac imaging with CT requires careful consideration of the potential need for heart rate control to minimize motion artifacts. Images on the left panel reflect a coronary artery calcium (CAC) scan done with multidetector computed tomography (MDCT) without use of β-blockers on a patient with a relatively fast heart rate (> 70 beats per minute). The images on the right panel show the CAC scan on the same patient acquired with electron beam CT (EBCT), which allows faster imaging with lower motion artifacts. The images on the left illustrate a typical artifact in the right coronary artery (RCA; *arrow*) depicted as a line streak rather than the normal circular shape shown on the right, which is caused by cardiac motion. Motion artifacts also apply to coronary CT angiography imaging. This example illustrates the need for heart rate control with β-adrenergic blocking agents in patients referred for cardiac CT. With adequate heart rate control, calcium score results from MDCT and EBCT are very similar [3]. LV—left ventricle; RA—right atrium; RV—right ventricle.

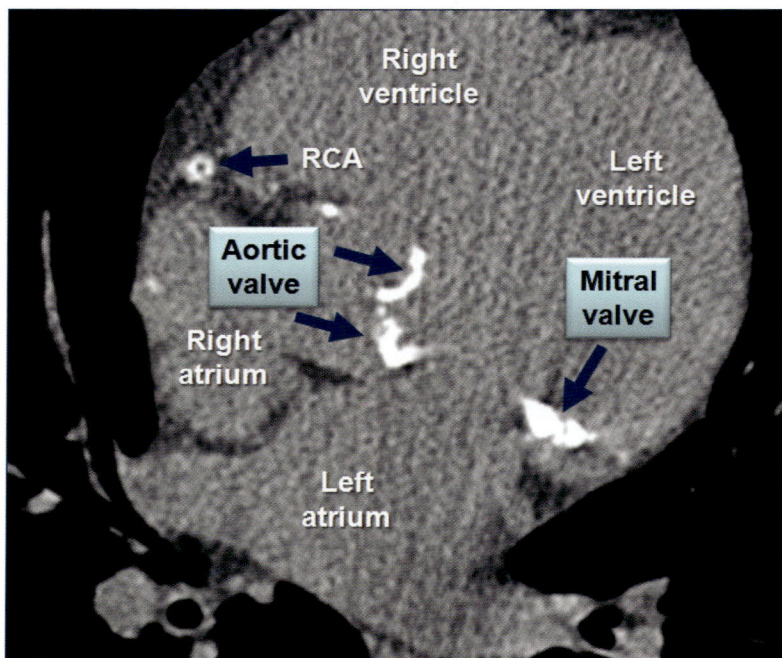

Figure 15-7. Patient with aortic valve calcification and mitral annular calcification (*arrows*). Cardiac computed tomography (CT) is quite robust at visualizing and quantifying calcifications of valves, coronary arteries, and the aorta. Evidence is accumulating that these measures may add independently prognostic information to the results of the coronary arteries. RCA—right coronary artery.

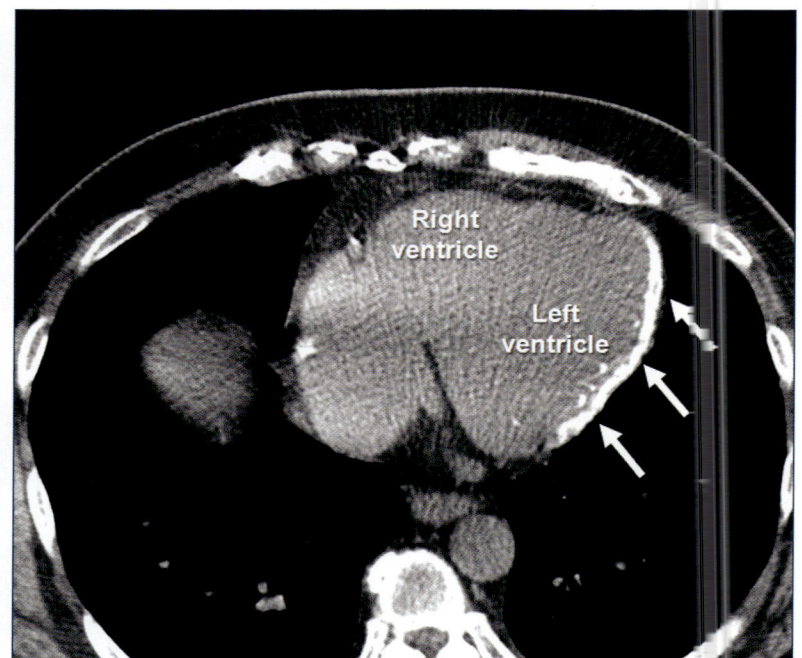

Figure 15-8. A patient with severe calcifications of the lateral pericardium (*arrows*). Calcifications are easy to detect on computed tomography (CT). However, quantification of pericardial physiology or assessment of constrictive pericarditis is not possible with CT.

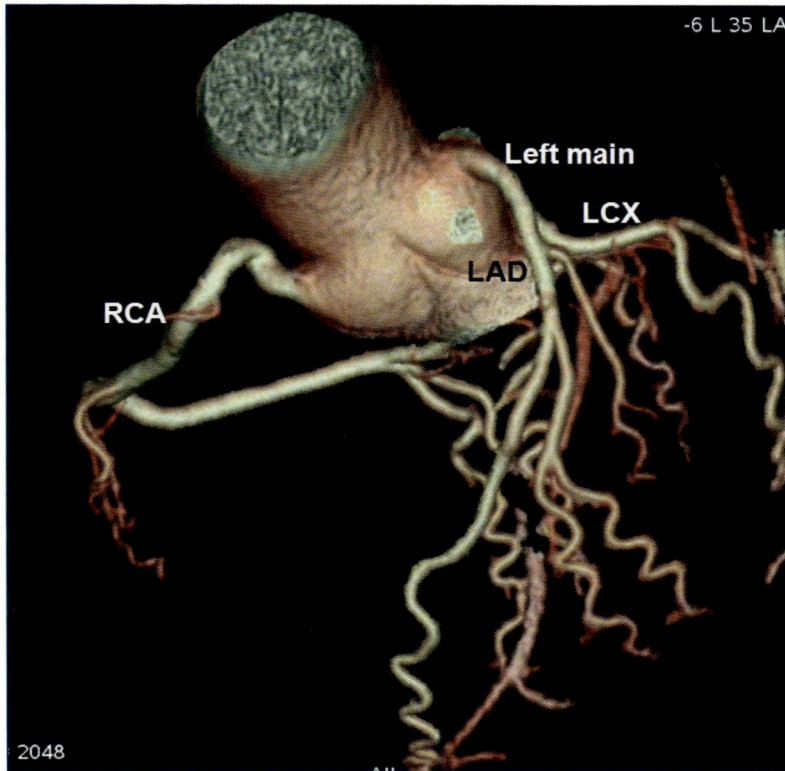

Figure 15-9. A volume-rendered computed tomography (CT) angiographic image of the coronary arteries of a 72-year-old woman who presented with hypertension and atypical chest pain. This study reveals tortuous coronary arteries but no stenosis. Multidetector computed tomography (MDCT) coronary angiography remains a very sensitive method for detecting atherosclerosis with a consistently high negative predictive value. In contrast, specificity and positive predictive value remain moderate in patients with high prevalence of coronary artery disease [4–6]. LAD—left anterior descending artery; LCX—left circumflex; RCA—right coronary artery.

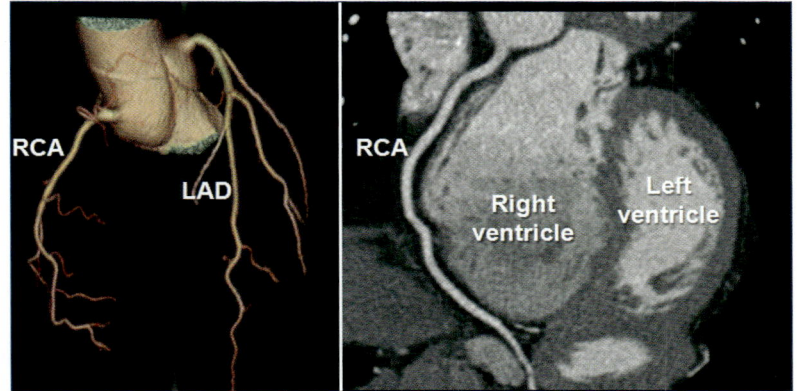

Figure 15-10. A volume-rendered computed tomography angiogram (CTA) image (*left*) and curved multiplanar image of the right coronary artery (RCA), revealing normal coronary arteries. Multiple different protocols can be used on the dataset to allow for comprehensive examination of the studies. Most readers use two to three reconstruction techniques, starting with axial data, progressing to different reconstruction techniques. Each imaging method has strengths and weaknesses. For example, curved multiplanar images allow the entire vessel to be seen on one image, but normal anatomic landmarks are lost. LAD—left anterior descending artery; RCA—right coronary artery.

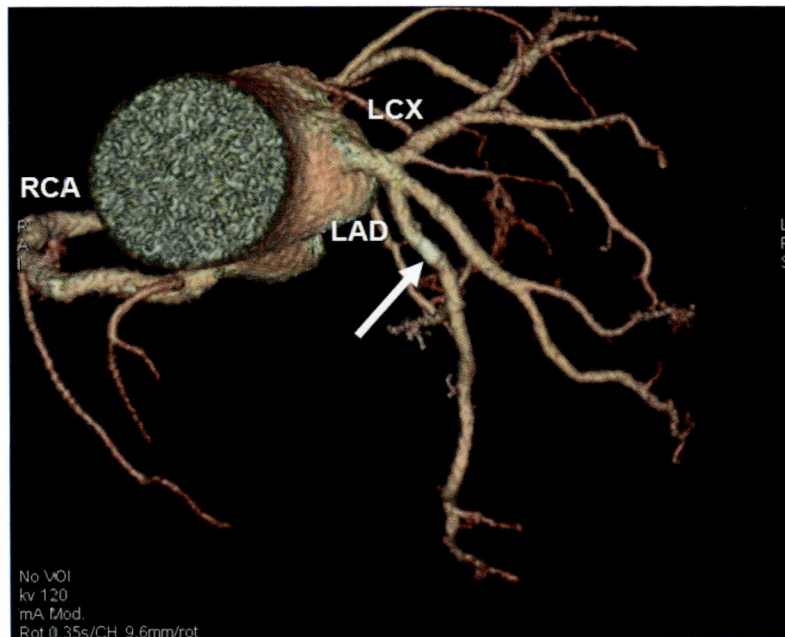

Figure 15-11. Volume rendering of a computed tomography coronary angiogram showing a densely calcified plaque in the left anterior descending artery (LAD). Volume rendering is less useful in the setting of stents or coronary calcium, as the lumen is obscured. LCX—left circumflex artery; RCA—right coronary artery.

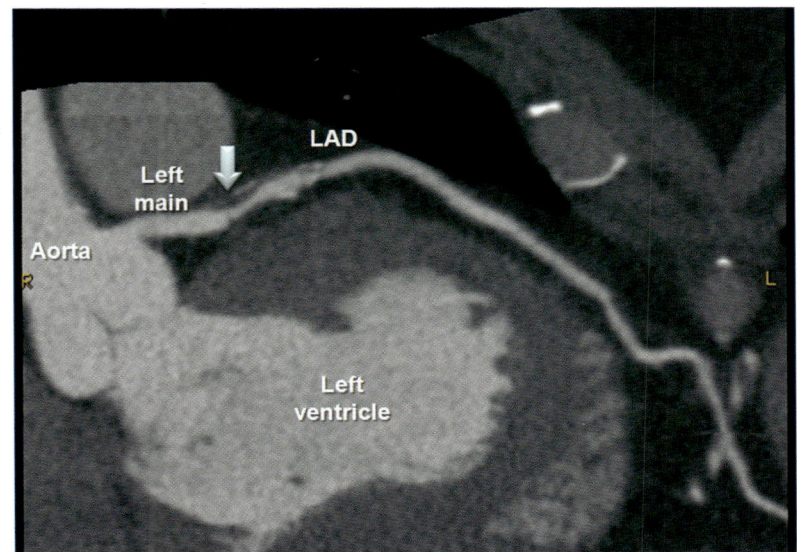

Figure 15-12. A curved multiplanar reformat computed tomography angiographic (CTA) view of a left anterior descending (LAD) artery with significant (> 50%), noncalcified stenosis in its proximal segment. Several studies comparing CTA and intravascular ultrasound (IVUS) have shown that CTA can delineate calcified and noncalcified plaque with high accuracy, but has difficulty in discerning fibrous from lipid-laden plaque [7].

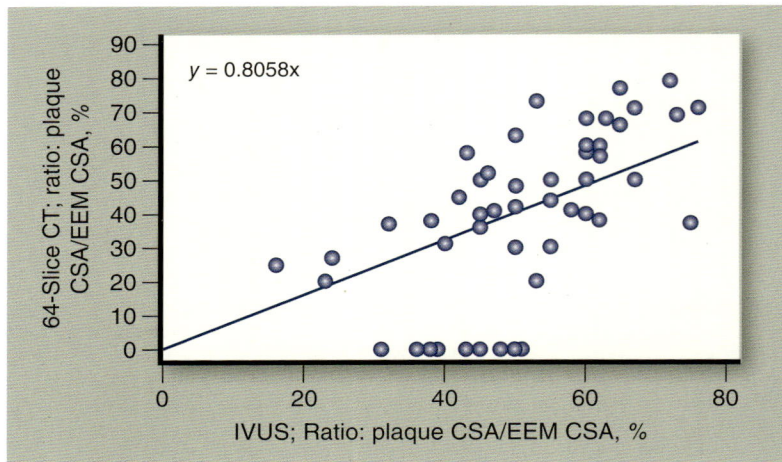

Figure 15-13. Correlation between 64-slice computed tomography angiogram measurements of plaque volume and intravascular ultrasound (IVUS) in diseased coronary artery segments. CSA—cross-sectional area; EEM—external elastic membrane. (*Adapted from* Leber *et al.* [7].)

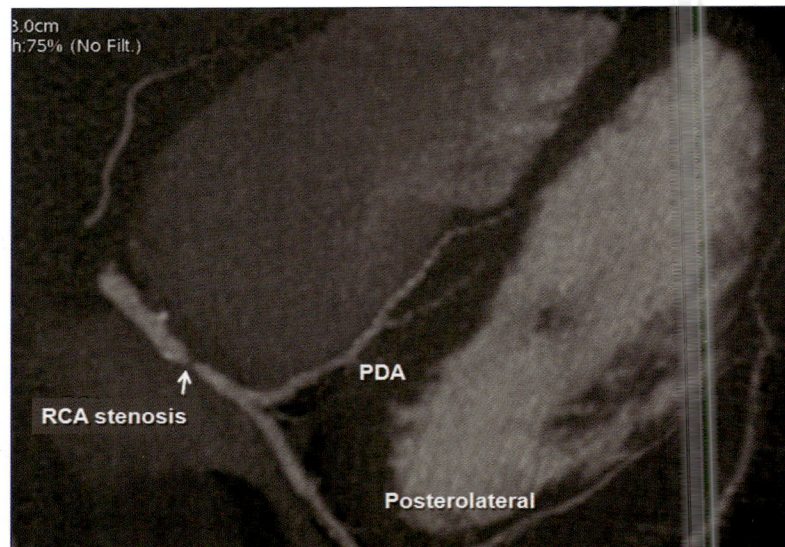

Figure 15-14. A maximum intensity projection CT angiographic view of the distal right coronary (RCA), posterior descending (PDA) arteries, and a posterolateral branch. The distal right coronary artery shows severe stenosis. The patient subsequently had angiography and stenting of the vessel.

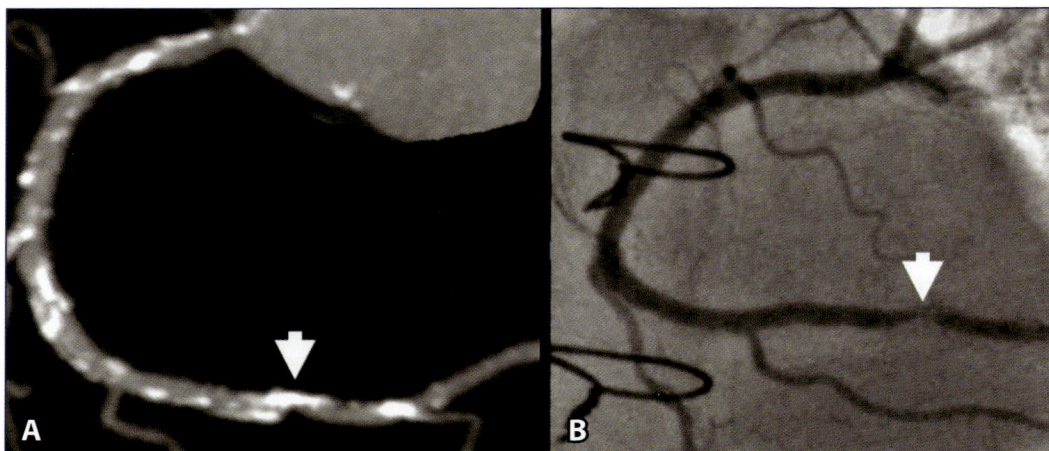

Figure 15-15. A multiplanar computed tomography angiographic (CTA) view of the right coronary artery (**A**), demonstrating severe and diffuse calcifications throughout the vessel. The distal stenosis (seen on invasive angiography in **B**) is not well visualized on the CTA, as the calcium "blooming" obscures the visualization of the lumen (*arrows*). Future directions of cardiac computed tomography are evaluating dual energy (*ie*, scanning patients with both 120 kilovolts [kVp] and 80 kilovolts) to evaluate whether this technique can differentiate better calcification from contrast.

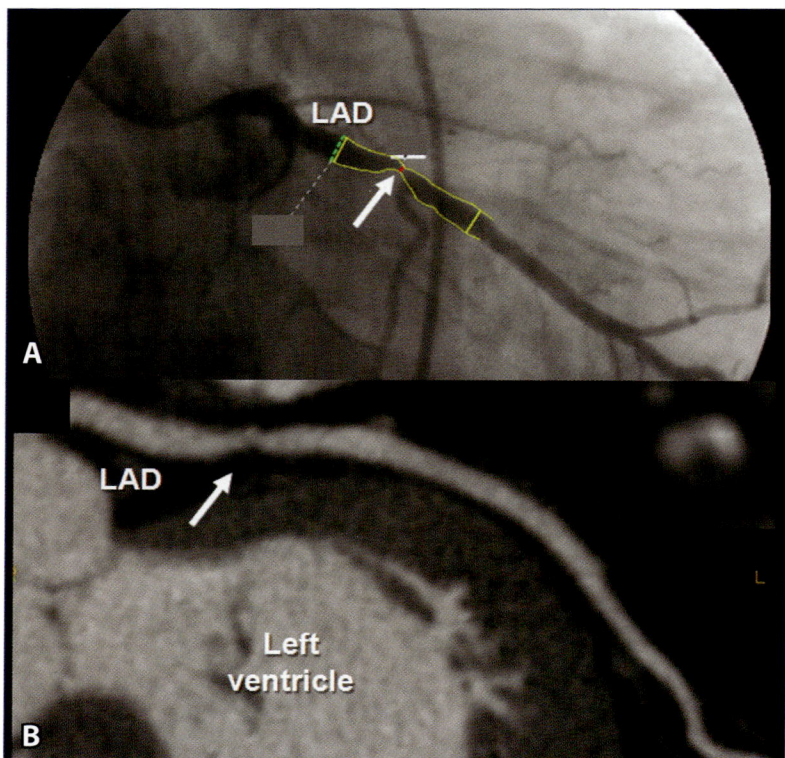

Figure 15-16. A patient with angina who underwent computed tomography (CT) coronary angiography (**B**) and then subsequent invasive angiography (**A**). The left anterior descending artery (LAD) has a significant stenosis, assessed similarly by both modalities. The lack of coronary calcium in that segment and motion artifacts facilitates the interpretation of CT angiography.

Overall diagnostic accuracy of 64 detector CT angiography compared with cardiac catheterization, defined by the first prospective multicenter trial (Assessment by Coronary Computed Tomographic Angiography of Individuals Undergoing Invasive Coronary Angiography [ACCURACY] study). This study enrolled 230 patients with chest pain who were referred for invasive coronary angiography. By quantitative coronary angiography, disease prevalence was 25%. On a per patient basis, sensitivity was 94% to 95% depending on the cut-point chosen to represent a positive invasive coronary angiogram and specificity was 83%. Post-test probabilities for a negative test (negative predictive value) was 99% for both stenosis greater than 50% and greater than 70% [8].

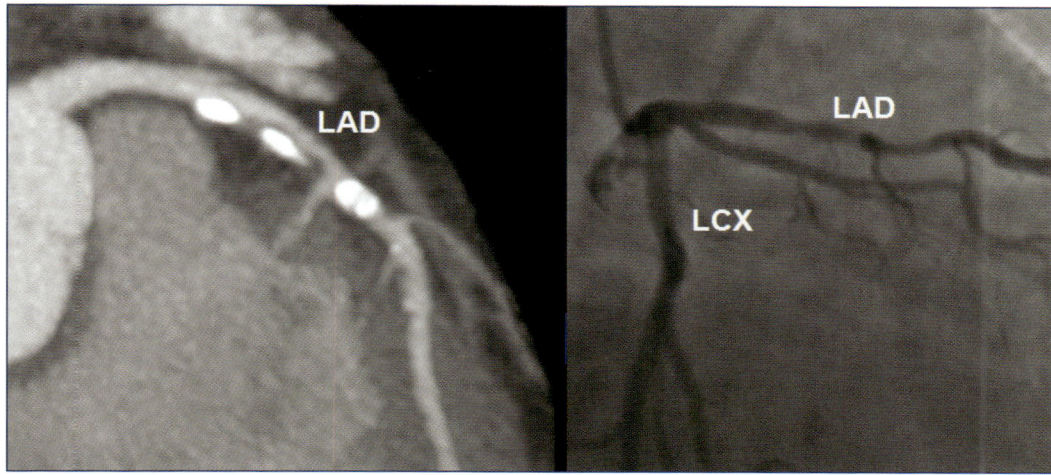

Figure 15-17. Patient with a normal stress nuclear myocardial perfusion study. The computed tomography (CT) angiogram (*left*) revealed a high-grade stenosis in the mid left anterior descending artery (LAD). However, the invasive angiogram (*right*) demonstrated only a moderate stenosis in the mid LAD. The patient ultimately underwent intravascular ultrasound that revealed a 60% stenosis, which in the absence of objective evidence of ischemia on stress imaging was interpreted as non–flow-limiting and the patient was treated medically. CT angiography has a tendency to "over-call" the stenosis severity. LCX—left circumflex artery, (*Courtesy of* Dr. Karlsberg, Cardiovascular Medical Group, Beverly Hills, CA.)

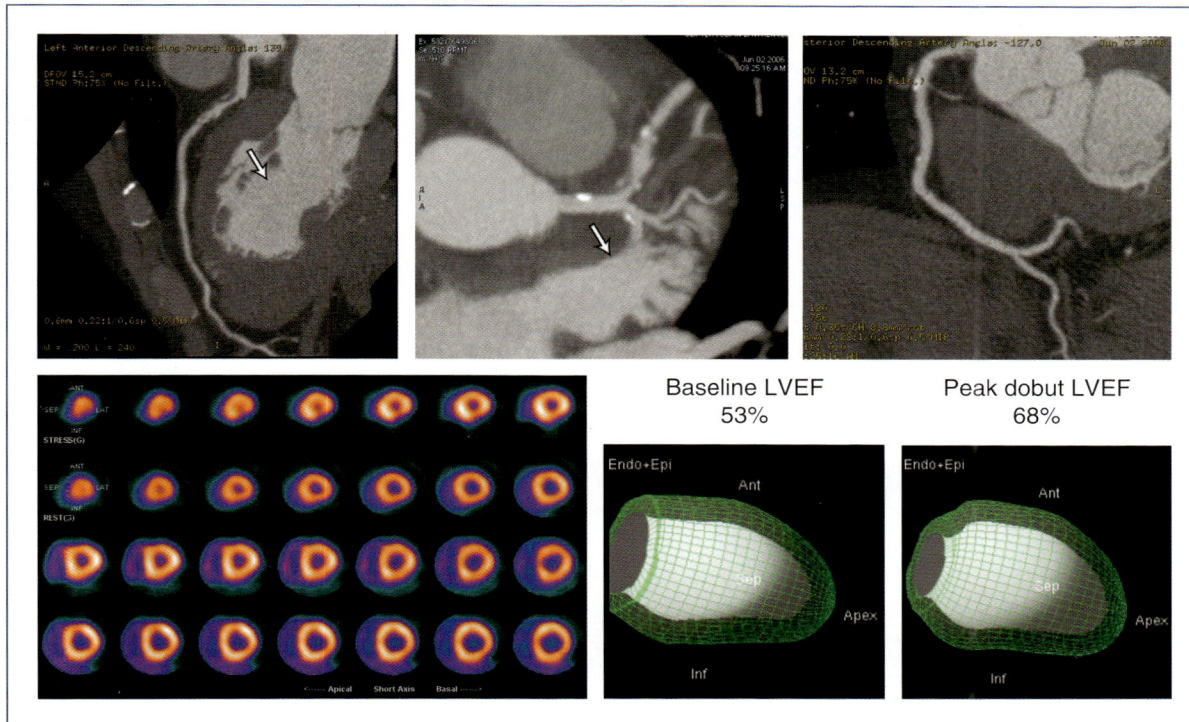

Figure 15-18. Integrated positron emission tomography (PET)/computed tomography angiogram (CTA) study. The CTA images demonstrate a noncalcified plaque (*arrow*) in the proximal left anterior descending artery with 50% to 70% stenosis. However, the rest and peak dobutamine stress myocardial perfusion PET study (*lower left*) demonstrates only minimal inferoapical ischemia. In addition, left ventricular ejection fraction (LVEF) was normal at rest and demonstrated a normal rise during peak dobutamine stress, suggesting only mild ischemia. The patients was treated medically. (*Adapted from* Di Carli and Hachamovitch [6].)

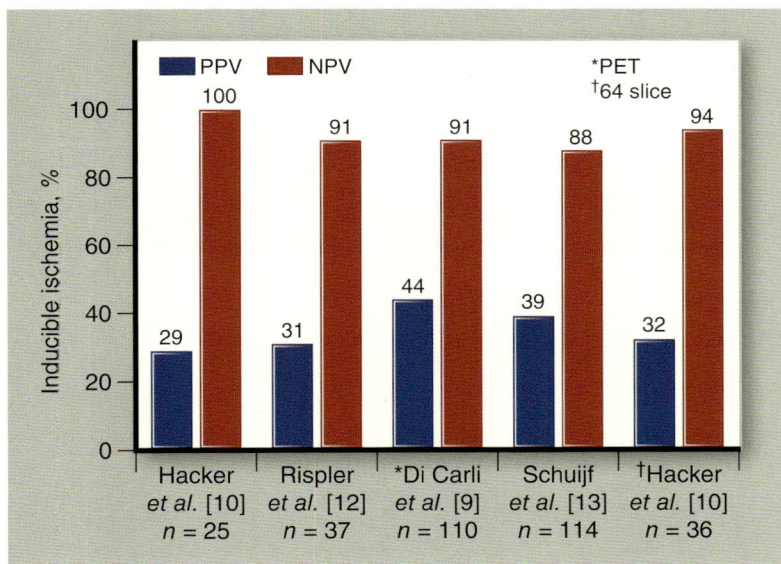

Figure 15-19. Frequency of inducible ischemia by myocardial perfusion imaging in territories supplied by stenosis greater than 50% on CT coronary angiography. Although these data confirm the excellent negative predictive value (NPV) of CT coronary angiography to exclude significant coronary artery disease, the low positive predictive value (PPV) emphasizes the limited value of CTA to identify flow-limiting coronary stenoses and, thus, the potential need for revascularization. PET—positron emission tomography. (*From* Di Carli *et al.* [9], Hacker *et al.* [10,11], Rispler *et al.* [12], and Schuijf *et al.* [13].)

Study	Slices	Vendor	Method	Mean effective dose estimates, mSv					
				CTCA			Calcium scoring		
				Without ECTCM	Mixed	With ECTCM	Without ECTCM	With ECTCM	Prospective Gating
Hunold et al. [22]	4	Siemens*	TLD-ARP (low)	6.7 (M), 8.1 (F)	–	–	3.0 (M), 3.6 (F)	–	1.5 (M), 1.8 (F)
	4	Siemens	TLD-ARP (high)	10.9 (M), 13.0 (F)	–	–	5.2 (M), 6.2 (F)	–	–
McCollough [23]	4	NS (1st)	Multiple	9	–	–	2.5	–	0.9
	4	NS (2nd)	Multiple	12	–	–	4.5	–	1
Poll et al. [24]	4	Siemens	DLP	8.3 (M), 11.0 (F)	–	4.0 (M), 5.4 (F)	1.9 (M), 2.5 (F)	1.2 (M), 1.6 (F)	–
	4	Siemens	TLD-ARP	10.3 (M), 12.7 (F)	–	4.6 (M), 5.6 (F)	2.4 (M), 2.9 (F)	1.5 (M), 1.8 (F)	–
Hacker et al. [25]	12	Siemens	–	–	–	4.3	–	–	–
Coles et al. [26]	12	Siemens	CTDosimetry.xls	14.2	–	–	4.1	2.6	–
	16	Siemens	CTDosimetry.xls	15.3	–	–	–	–	–
Flohr et al. [27]	16	Siemens	WinDose	7.1 (M), 10.5 (F)	–	4.3 (M), 6.4 (F)	2.2 (M), 3.1 (F)	–	0.45 (M), 0.65 (F)
Garcia et al. [28]	16	Phillips[†]	DLP	–	8	–	–	–	–
Gerber et al. [29]	16	Siemens	Modified DLP	11.3	–	8.1	–	–	–
Hoffmann et al. [30]	16	Phillips	–	4.9	–	8.1	–	–	–
Nawfel and Yoshizumi [31]	16	General Electric[‡]	MOSFET-CIRS	20.6	–	–	–	–	–
Sato et al. [32]	4	Siemens	–	4–5	–	–	–	–	–
	16	Toshiba[¶]	–	7–8	–	–	–	–	–
Trabold et al. [33]	16	Siemens	TLD-ARP	8.1 (M), 10.9 (F)	–	4.3 (M), 5.6 (F)	2.9 (M), 3.6 (F)	1.6 (M), 2.0 (F)	–
Gaspar et al. [34]	40	Phillips	Modified DLP	9.9	–	–	–	–	–
Caussin et al. [35]	64	Siemens	–	–	8.4	–	–	–	–
Hausleiter et al. [36]	16	Siemens	DLP	10.6	–	6.4	–	–	–
	64	Siemens	DLP	14.8	–	9.4	–	–	–
Ghostine et al. [37]	64	Siemens	DLP	–	–	7	–	–	–
Leber et al. [38]	64	Siemens	–	–	–	10–14	–	–	–
Mollet et al. [39]	64	Siemens	WinDose	15.2 (M), 21.4 (F)	–	–	–	1.3 (M), 1.7 (F)	–
Muhlenbruch et al. [40]	64	Siemens	–	13.6 (M), 17.2 (F)	–	–	–	–	–
Nikolaou et al. [41]	64	Siemens	WinDose	8–10	–	–	–	–	–
Pugliese et al. [42]	64	Siemens	–	15 (M), 20 (F)	–	–	–	–	–
Raff et al. [43]	64	Siemens	–	13 (M), 18 (F)	–	–	–	–	–

*New York, NY.

[†]Amesterdam, The Netherlands.

[‡]Fairfield, CT.

[¶]Tokyo, Japan.

CIRS—Computerized Imaging Reference Systems (Norfolk, VA); DLP—Derived from dose-length product on scanner console; F—female; M—male; MOSFET-CIRS—metal oxide semiconductor field effect transistors in a CIRS phantom; NS—not specified; TLD-ARP—thermoluminescent dosimeteres in an Alderson-Rando phantom.

Figure 15-20. Total body mean effective doses from computed tomography coronary angiography (CTCA). Reported radiation doses are quite variable and highly dependent on the available technology. The reported mean effective dose for calcium scoring using prospective gating ranges from 0.5 to 1.8 mSv. The reported mean effective dose for coronary CTCA ranges from 4.0 to 21.4 mSv. It is generally accepted that using state-of-the-art CT technology (64 slices or higher combined with electrocardiogram-controlled dose modulation or prospective gating) and careful patient selection, radiation dose from CTCA can be reduced substantially to levels equal or below those from cardiac catheterization ($\leq$ 7 mSv). ECTCM—electrocardiographically controlled tube current modulation. (*Adapted from* Einstein et al. [14].)

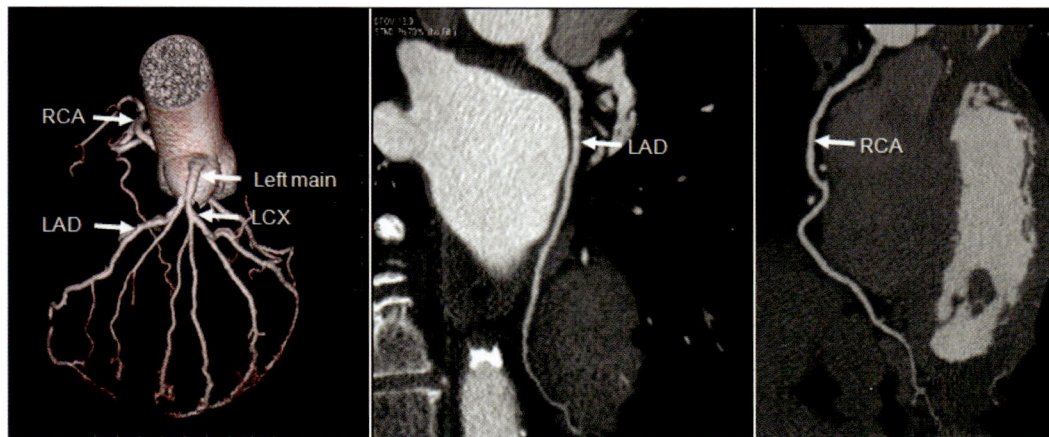

Figure 15-21. Radiation doses have been of increasing concern with cardiac computed tomography, given the rapid growth of this modality. Prospective imaging (using a "step-and-shoot" acquisition protocol, whereby the radiograph tube is only turned on during a short phase of the cardiac cycle, typically end-diastole) allows doses to be reduced by 70% to 80% [15]. The volume rendered computed tomography angiography of the coronary arterial tree (*left*), curved multiplanar views of the left anterior descending (LAD; *middle*), and the right coronary artery (RCA; *right*) demonstrate a high-quality study without evidence of obstructive coronary artery disease. This example used 100 kVp to reduce radiation by up to 40% to 50% and prospective triggering (similar to calcium score protocols). This study was performed with a total dose of 0.95 mSv, and was highly diagnostic, revealing only mild calcifications/stenosis of the left anterior descending artery. LCX—left circumflex artery. (*Courtesy of* Dr. Jay Earls, Fairfax, VA.)

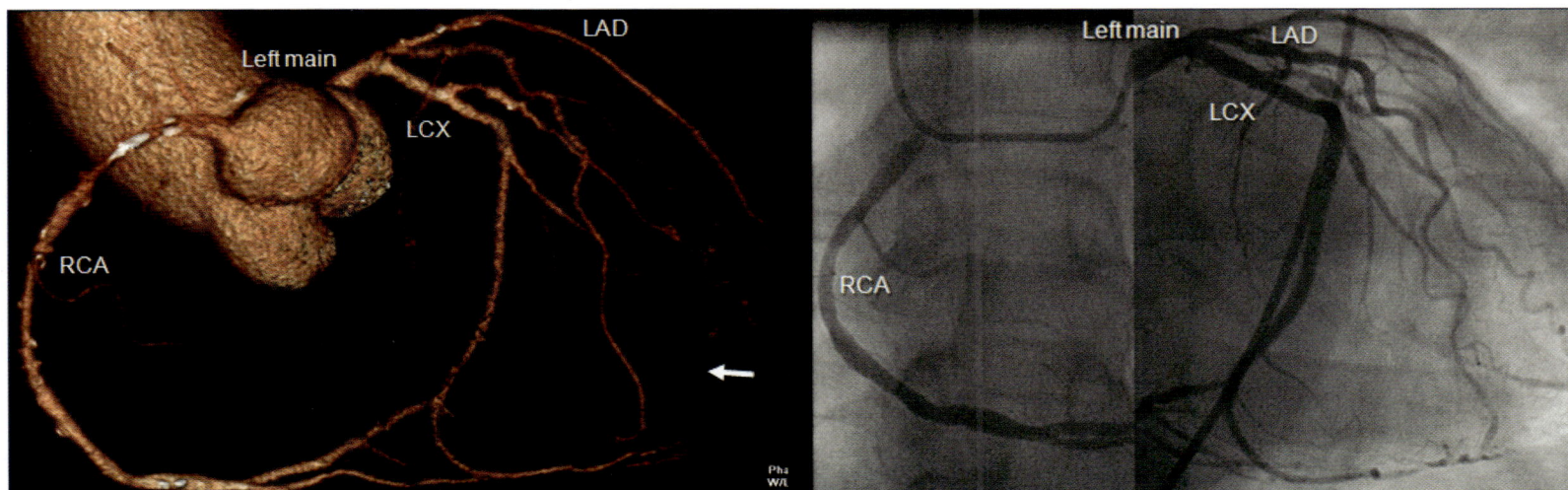

Figure 15-22. Prospective gated computed tomography (CT) coronary angiography study (*left*) from a volumetric 320-slice scanner and corresponding images from invasive coronary angiography (*right*) on a patient with atypical chest pain. The study delivered an effective dose of 3 mSv [16]. State-of-the-art cardiac CT scanners now offer 64 slices or higher. As explained in the legend to Fig. 15-1, the more slices, the shorter the scan acquisition, which allows for consistently high image quality and importantly reduction of radiation dose. In the future, advanced CT scanners may permit first-pass myocardial perfusion imaging in addition to the contrast CT angiogram. RCA—right coronary artery; LAD—left anterior descending artery; LCX—left circumflex artery. (*Images courtesy of* Dr. Frank Rybicki, Brigham and Women's Hospital, Boston, MA.)

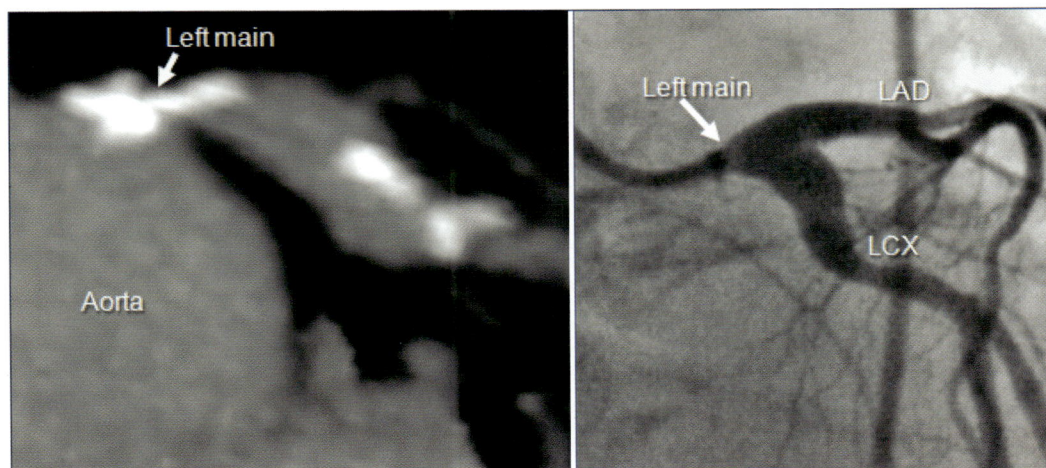

Figure 15-23. A patient with a normal nuclear stress test who underwent CT angiography and was found to have high grade stenosis at the ostium of left main coronary artery (*left*), confirmed on invasive angiography (*right*). Nuclear imaging may underestimate the severity and/or extent of underlying coronary artery disease in cases of balanced flow reduction. This situation reduces the sensitivity of stress perfusion imaging [17]. (*Courtesy of* Dr. Karlsberg, Cardiovascular Medical Group, Beverly Hills, CA.) LAD—left anterior descending artery; LCX—left circumflex artery

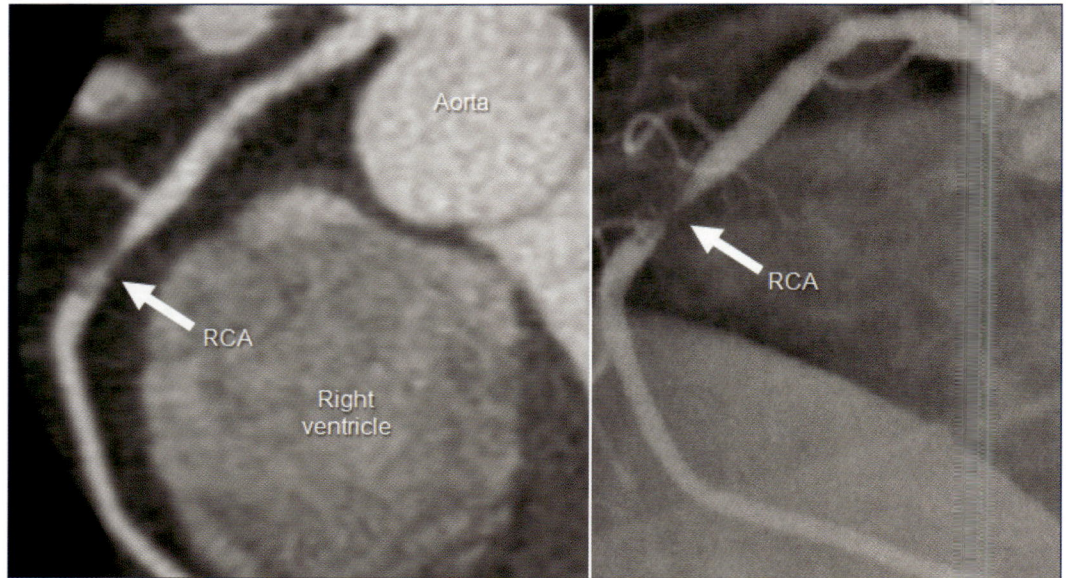

Figure 15-24. CT angiogram (curved multi-planar image; *left*) demonstrating a high-grade stenosis of the mid right coronary artery (RCA), with invasive angiography confirmation (*right*). This is a noncalcified plaque, which is more prevalent in patients with acute coronary syndromes. (*Courtesy of* Dr. Karlsberg, Cardiovascular Medical Group, Beverly Hills, CA.)

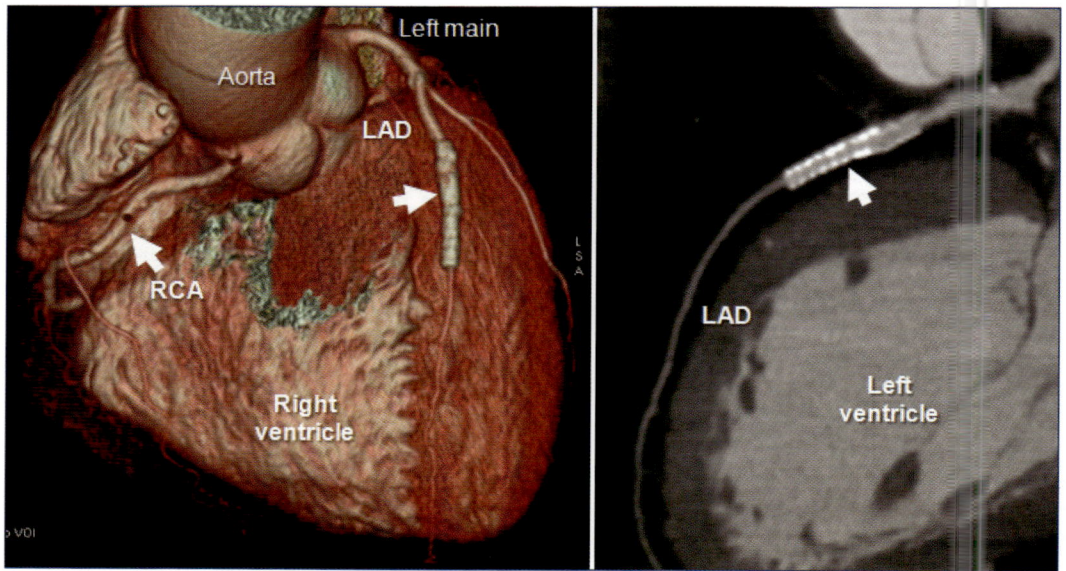

Figure 15-25. Patient with a patent stent (*arrow*) in the left anterior descending artery (LAD) on volume rendering (left) and curved multiplanar CT view (right). Volume rendering is not adequate for imaging within a calcified or stented segment.

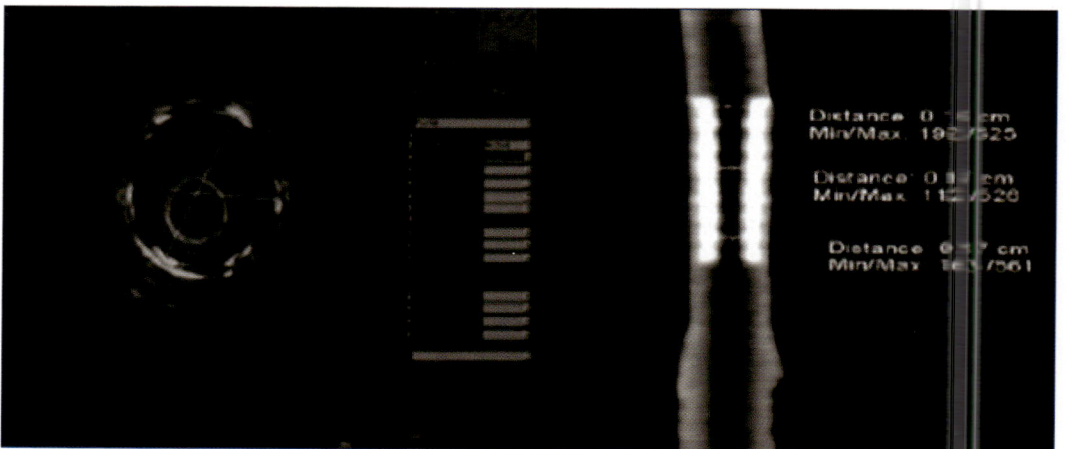

Figure 15-26. This phantom study illustrates intravascular ultrasound (IVUS) (*left*) and the blooming effect of metallic stents when imaged with multidetector computed tomography (MDCT) (*right*). The blooming artifact caused by metal, generally underestimates the coronary lumen compared with IVUS. In this phantom experiment, computed tomography angiography (CTA) systematically underestimated the lumen within the stent area used, regardless of the number of CT slices. To date, a limited number of studies assessing the value of CTA to detect in-stent restenosis have been published. However, they all show a consistently low sensitivity to identify in-stent restenosis [6]. The limited spatial resolution of CT, type of stent, and, especially, stent diameter (< 3 mm being associated with the highest number of partial lumen visualization and nondiagnostic scans) contribute to limited clinical results. (*Adapted from* Beohar *et al.* [18].)

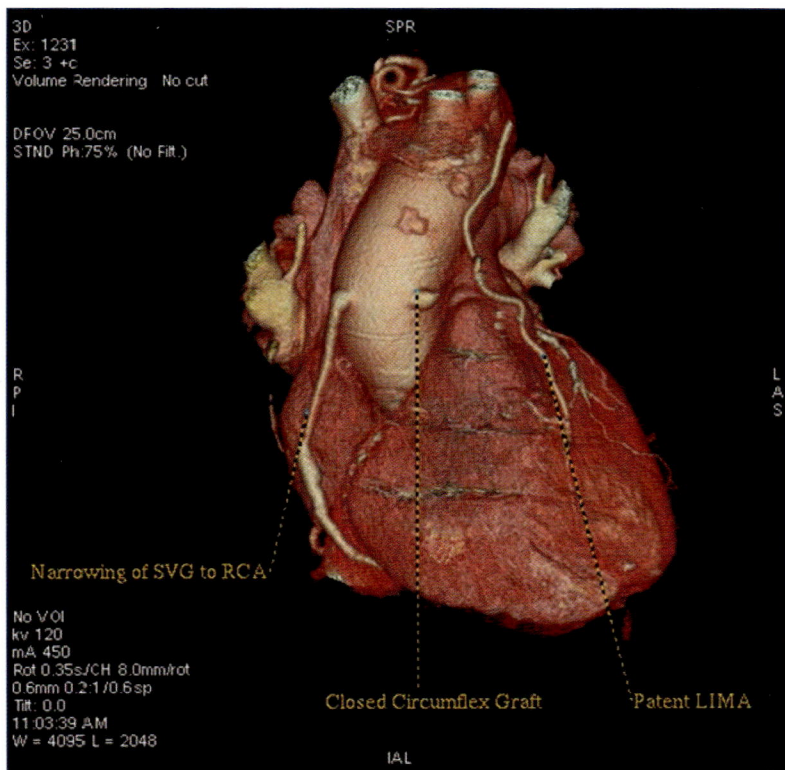

Figure 15-27. Bypass graft evaluation with computed tomography (CT) volume rendering is quite robust. This study demonstrates a closed saphenous vein graft (SVG) to the circumflex, patent left internal mammary graft to the left anterior descending and mildly (< 30% stenosis) diseased segment of the graft to the right coronary artery. Assessing patency and progression of coronary artery disease (CAD) in bypass grafts is less challenging than the native coronary arteries, as they are generally larger and less subject to motion. Occasionally, evaluation of internal mammary grafts can be difficult due to blooming artifact from metal clips. On a per graft basis, the average sensitivity for detecting at least one graft with more than 50% stenosis or total occlusion is 99% (range, 96%–100%), whereas the average specificity is 93% (range, 68%–100%). The corresponding average positive and negative predictive values are 83% (range, 37%–98%) and 99% (range, 98%–100%) respectively, and the overall diagnostic accuracy is 97% (range, 95% to 99%) [6]. Importantly, there is no appreciable difference in the reported diagnostic accuracies for the detection of stenosis or total occlusions between arterial and vein grafts. In general, false-positive findings are related to difficulties in evaluating distal anastomosis. Despite the high degree of accuracy to detect occlusions and stenosis within grafts, computed tomography angiography has limited value in the evaluation of the patient with recurrent chest pain after coronary artery bypass graft because this also requires an assessment of the native coronary arteries, which tend to be more challenging because they are usually very small and heavily calcified.

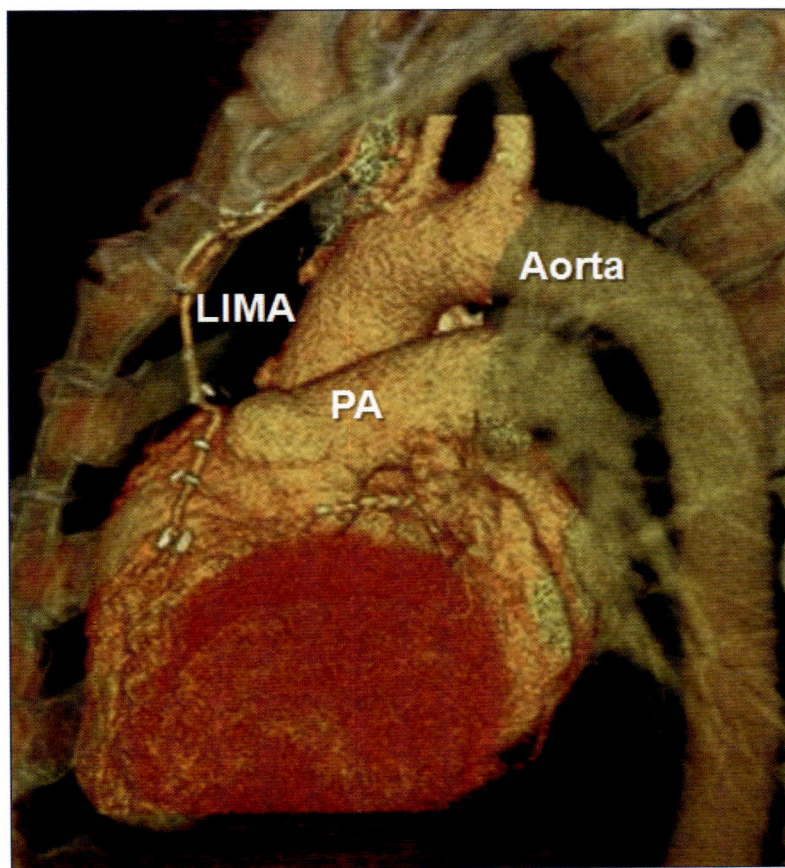

Figure 15-28. Volume rendered computed tomography angiography (CTA) images of a patient with a prior history of coronary artery bypass graft (CABG) obtained before undergoing repeat CABG for coronary artery disease progression. CTA delineates the precise location of the grafts, especially the left internal mammary artery (LIMA), in relation to the site of sternotomy and is very useful for surgical planning. PA—pulmonary artery. (*Adapted from* Gasparovic *et al.* [19].)

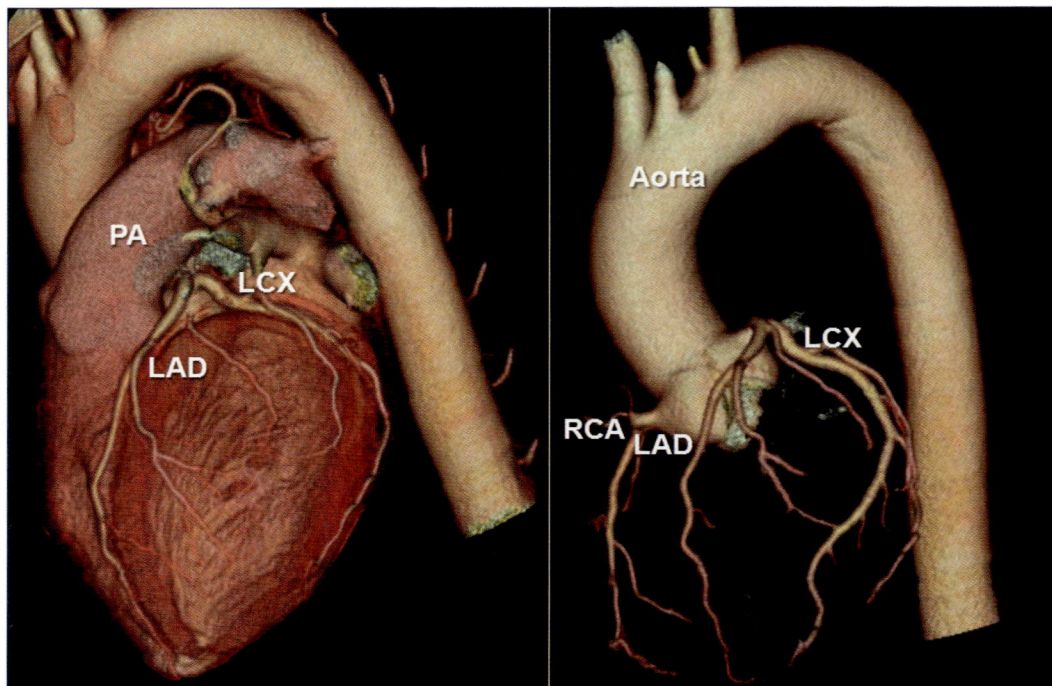

Figure 15-29. A patient presenting to an emergency room with atypical chest pain, underwent computed tomography angiography (CTA) imaging to evaluate coronary artery stenosis, aortic dissection, and pulmonary embolism. This patient was found to have a normal study, and was subsequently discharged. Preliminary data using CTA in the emergency room setting suggest that, in selected patients, CTA may save cost and time compared with nuclear imaging [20]. LAD—left anterior descending artery; LCX—left circumflex artery; PA—pulmonary artery; RCA—right coronary artery.

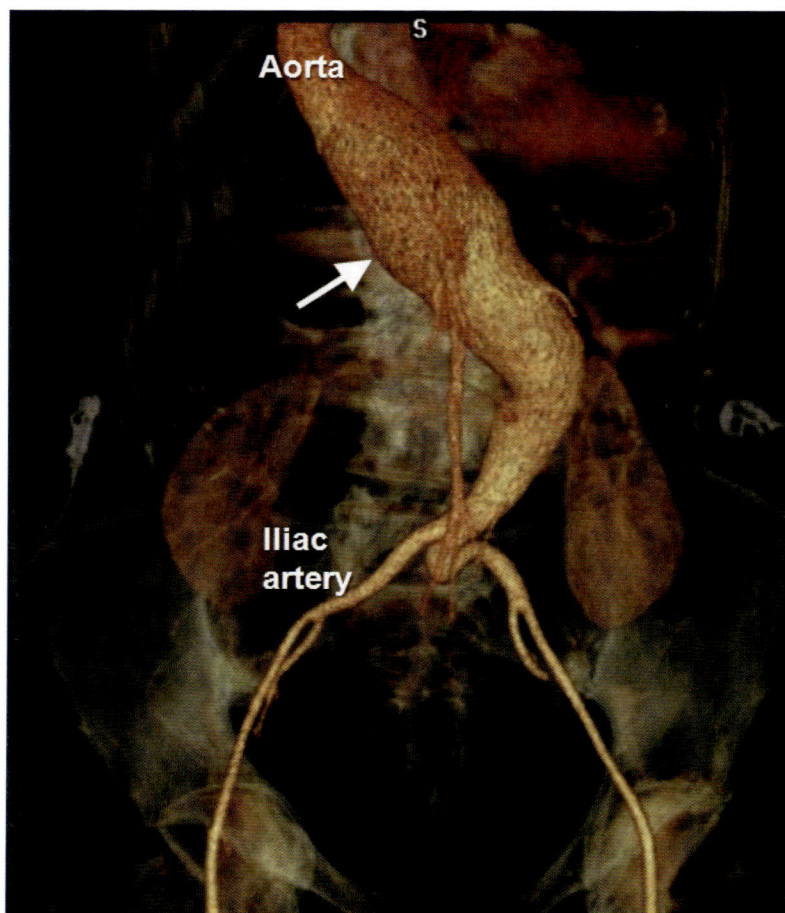

Figure 15-30. Multidetector computed tomography angiography (CTA) in a patient with a saccular abdominal aortic aneurysm (arrow). CTA is very helpful in the evaluation of patients with acute or chronic aortic pathology. (Courtesy of Dr. Michael Steigner, Brigham and Women's Hospital, Boston, MA.)

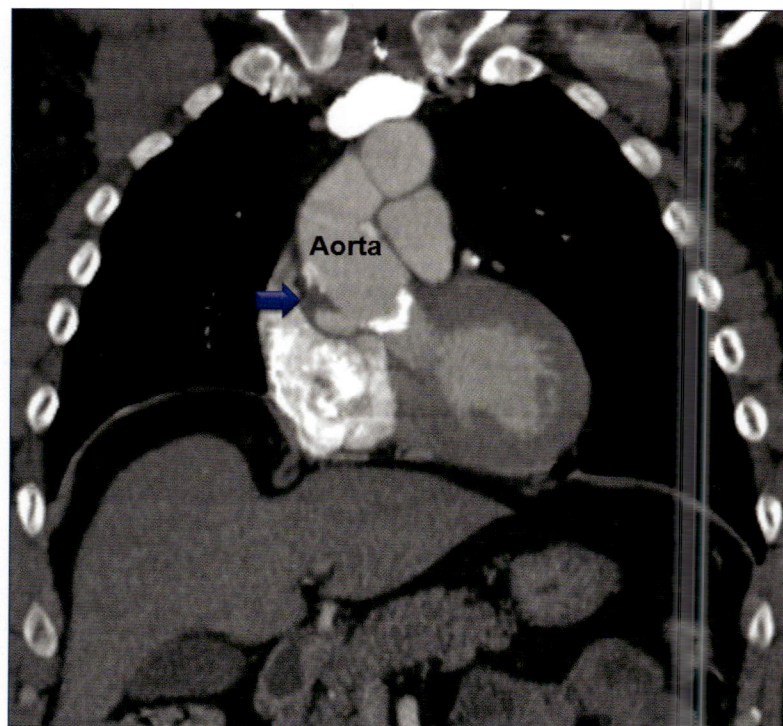

Figure 15-31. Multidetector computed tomography angiography (MDCT) in a patient with a history of aortic valve replacement, demonstrating a pseudoaneurysm of the ascending aorta (arrow). (Courtesy of Dr. Michael Steigner, Brigham and Women's Hospital, Boston, MA.)

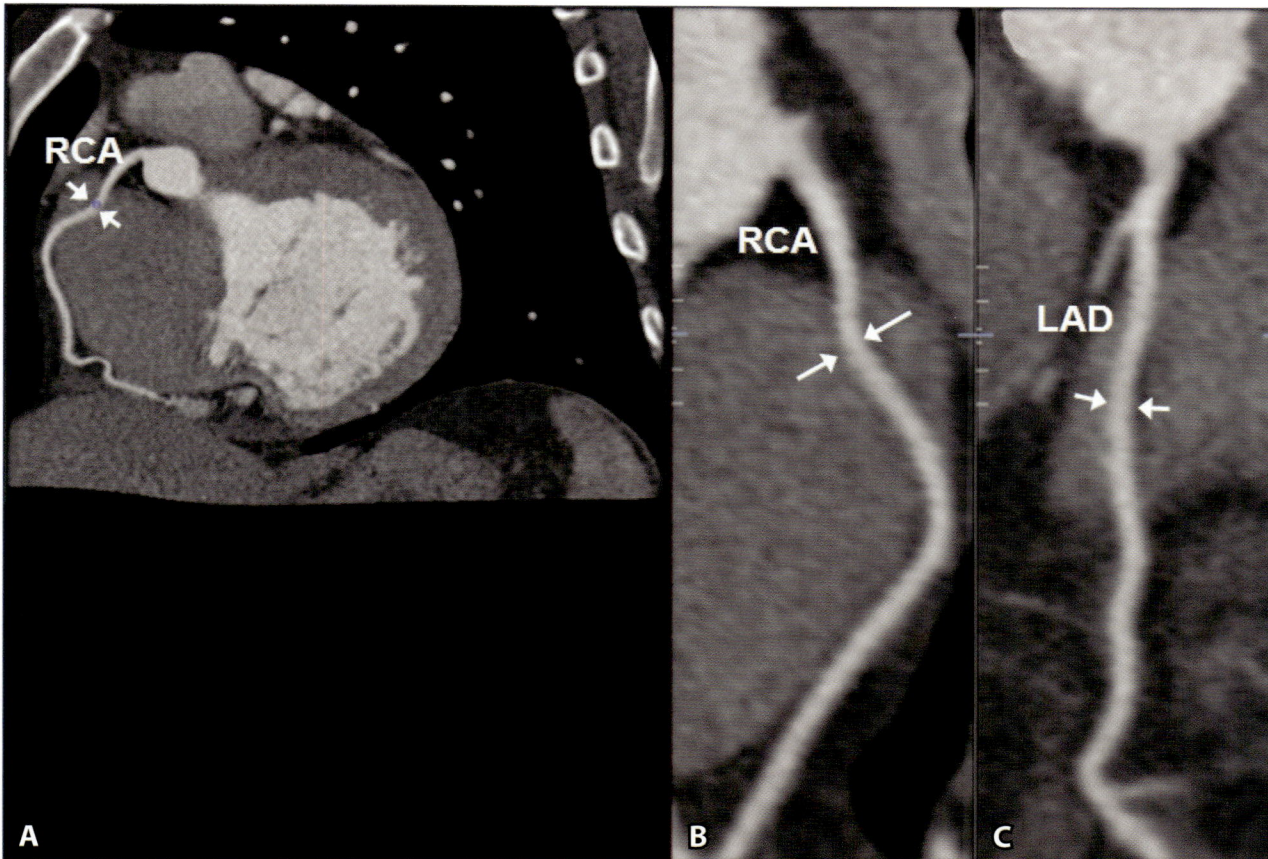

Figure 15-32. Multiplanar computed tomography (CT) angiographic views demonstrating muscle bridges along the proximal right coronary artery (RCA) (**A** and **B**) and left anterior descending (LAD) (**C**) coronary arteries. In this example, the RCA and LAD coronary arteries traverse between layers of muscle encasing the vessel (*arrows*) and sometimes leading to dynamic compression of the lumen. Myocardial bridges are frequent findings on CT. (*Courtesy of* Dr. Michael Steigner, Brigham and Women's Hospital, Boston, MA.)

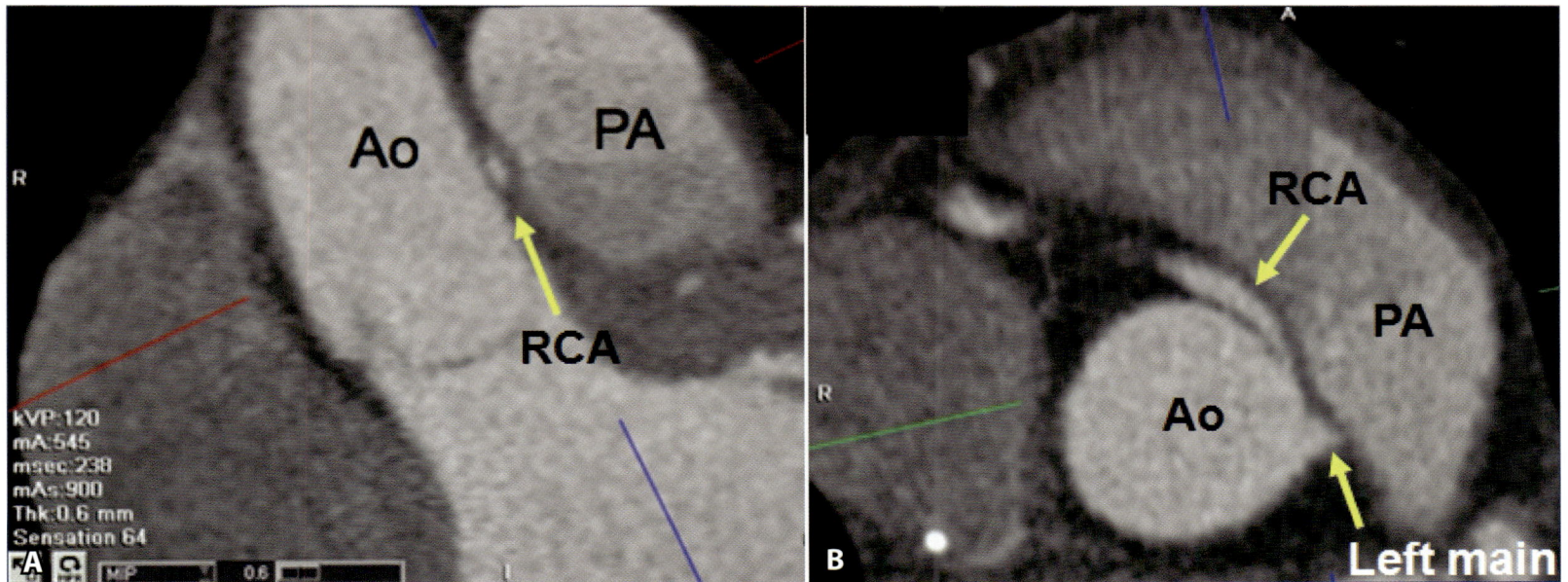

Figure 15-33. A, Coronary computed tomography angiography (CTA) study in a patient with atypical chest pain, demonstrating an anomalous right coronary artery (RCA) arising from the left coronary ostium (**B**), near the origin of the left main. The RCA traverses between the pulmonary artery (PA) and the aorta (Ao; *arrows*). Occasionally, there is dynamic compression of the RCA, especially during exercise, which may lead to ischemia. (*Courtesy of* Dr. Michael Steigner, Brigham and Women's Hospital, Boston, MA.)

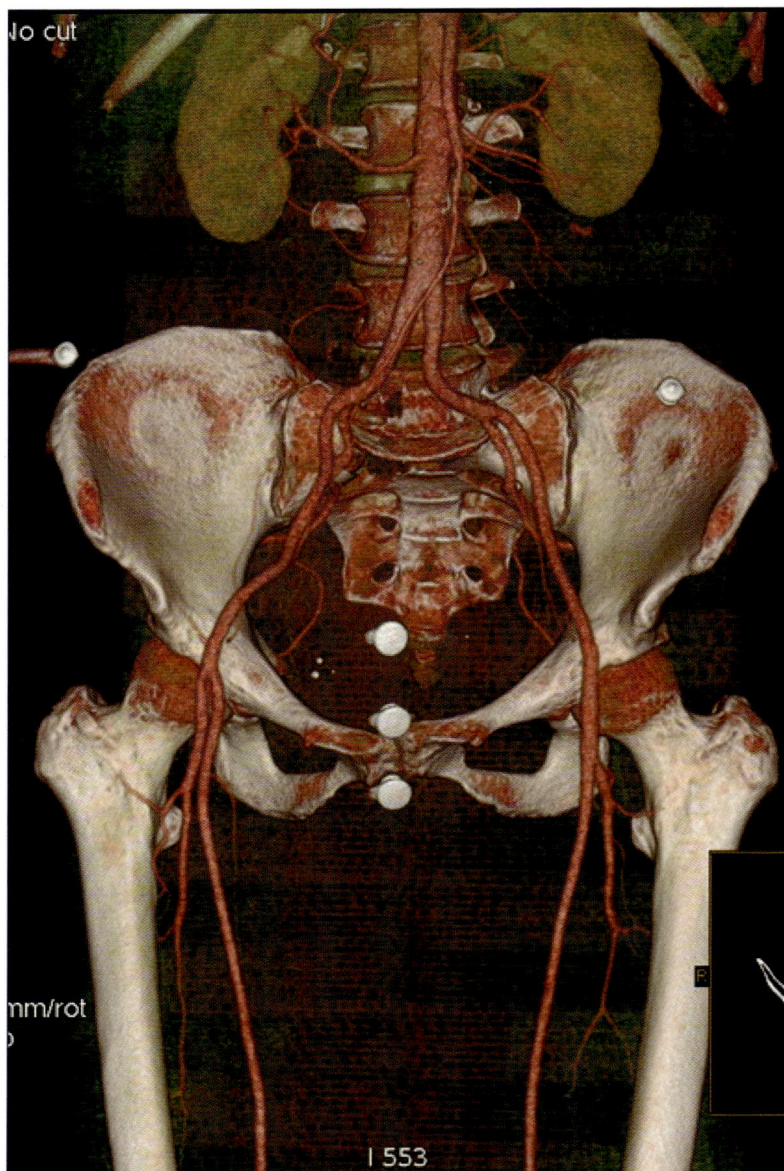

Figure 15-34. This image shows a three-dimensional reconstruction of a normal aorta, iliac, and femoral arteries of a patient. Images of peripheral arteries can be obtained with less contrast (approximately 30–40 mL), less radiation (approximately 4–6 mSev) and with higher accuracy (sensitivities and specificities > 95%) than coronary computed tomography angiography [21]. This advantage results in part from the larger vessel size, as well as lack of motion artifacts in non-cardiac imaging.

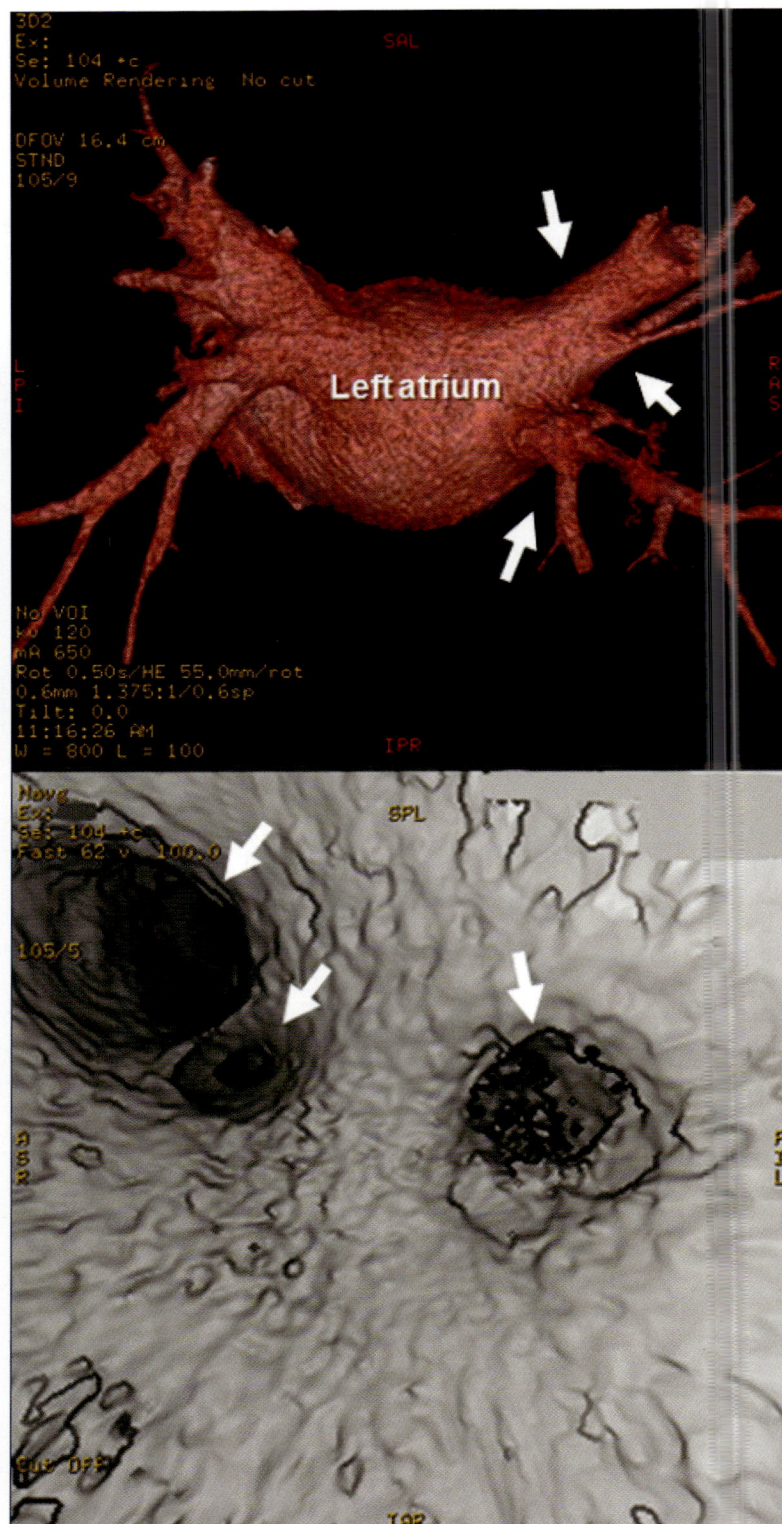

Figure 15-35. A three-dimensional reconstruction of the left atrium and associated pulmonary veins (*top*). *Arrows* depict the three pulmonary veins entering the left atrium from the right. An endoscopic view of the same patient, with visualization of the three pulmonary veins entering the left atrium from the right (*bottom*). Distances, diameters, and locations can be ascertained, and the figure can be merged with fluoroscopic data in invasive suite and are useful for planning complex interventions, such as radiofrequency ablations, in the electrophysiology laboratory.

References

1. Greenland P, Bonow RO, Brundage BH, *et al.*: ACCF/AHA 2007 clinical expert consensus document on coronary artery calcium scoring by computed tomography in global cardiovascular risk assessment and in evaluation of patients with chest pain: a report of the American College of Cardiology Foundation Clinical Expert Consensus Task Force (ACCF/AHA Writing Committee to Update the 2000 Expert Consensus Document on Electron Beam Computed Tomography) developed in collaboration with the Society of Atherosclerosis Imaging and Prevention and the Society of Cardiovascular Computed Tomography. *J Am Coll Cardiol* 2007, 49:378–402.

2. Budoff MJ, Achenbach S, Blumenthal RS, *et al.*: Assessment of coronary artery disease by cardiac computed tomography: a scientific statement from the American Heart Association Committee on Cardiovascular Imaging and Intervention, Council on Cardiovascular Radiology and Intervention, and Committee on Cardiac Imaging, Council on Clinical Cardiology. *Circulation* 2006, 114:1761–1791.

3. Mao SS, Pal RS, McKay CS, *et al.*: Comparison of Coronary Artery Calcium Scores Between Electron Beam Computed Tomography and 64-Multidetector Computed Tomographic Scanner. *J Comput Assist Tomogr* 2008, In press.

4. Hamon M, Biondi-Zoccai GG, Malagutti P, *et al.*: Diagnostic performance of multislice spiral computed tomography of coronary arteries as compared with conventional invasive coronary angiography: a meta-analysis. *J Am Coll Cardiol* 2006, 48:1896–1910.

5. Hamon M, Biondi-Zoccai GG, Malagutti P, *et al.*: Diagnostic performance of multislice spiral computed tomography of coronary arteries as compared with conventional invasive coronary angiography: a meta-analysis. *J Am Coll Cardiol* 2006, 48:1896–1910.

6. Di Carli MF, Hachamovitch R: New technology for noninvasive evaluation of coronary artery disease. *Circulation* 2007, 115:1464–1480.

7. Leber AW, Knez A, von Ziegler F, *et al.*: Quantification of obstructive and nonobstructive coronary lesions by 64-slice computed tomography: a comparative study with quantitative coronary angiography and intravascular ultrasound. *J Am Coll Cardiol* 2005, 46:147–154.

8. Budoff MJ, Dowe D, Jollis JG, *et al.*: Diagnostic performance of 64-detector row coronary computed tomographic angiography of individuals undergoing invasive coronary prospective multicenter ACCURACY (Assessment by Coronary Computed Individuals Without Known Coronary Artery Disease: Results From the Tomographic Angiography for Evaluation of Coronary Artery Stenosis in Angiography) trial. *J Am Coll Cardiol* 2008, 52:1724–1732.

9. Di Carli MF, Dorbala S, Curillova Z, *et al.*: Relationship between CT coronary angiography and stress perfusion imaging in patients with suspected ischemic heart disease assessed by integrated PET-CT imaging. *J Nucl Cardiol* 2007, 14:799–809.

10. Hacker M, Jakobs T, Hack N, *et al.*: Sixty-four slice spiral CT angiography does not predict the functional relevance of coronary artery stenoses in patients with stable angina. *Eur J Nucl Med Mol Imaging* 2007, 34:4–10.

11. Hacker M, Jakobs T, Matthiesen F, *et al.*: Comparison of spiral multidetector CT angiography and myocardial perfusion imaging in the noninvasive detection of functionally relevant coronary artery lesions: first clinical experiences. *J Nucl Med* 2005, 46:1294–1300.

12. Rispler S, Roguin A, Keidar Z, *et al.*: Integrated SPECT/CT for the assessment of hemodynamically significant coronary artery lesions. *J Am Coll Cardiol* 2006, 47:115A.

13. Schuijf JD, Wijns W, Jukema JW, *et al.*: Relationship between noninvasive coronary angiography with multi-slice computed tomography and myocardial perfusion imaging. *J Am Coll Cardiol* 2006, 48:2508–2514.

14. Einstein AJ, Moser KW, Thompson RC, *et al.*: Radiation dose to patients from cardiac diagnostic imaging. *Circulation* 2007, 116:1290–1305.

15. Earls JP, Berman EL, Urban BA, *et al.*: Prospectively gated transverse coronary CT angiography versus retrospectively gated helical technique: improved image quality and reduced radiation dose. *Radiology* 2008, 246:742–753.

16. Steigner ML, Otero HJ, Cai T, *et al.*: Narrowing the phase window width in prospectively ECG-gated single heart beat 320-detector row coronary CT angiography. *Int J Cardiovasc Imaging* 2009, 25:85–90.

17. Berman DS, Kang X, Slomka PJ, *et al.*: Underestimation of extent of ischemia by gated SPECT myocardial perfusion imaging in patients with left main coronary artery disease. *J Nucl Cardiol* 2007, 14:521–528.

18. Beohar N, Robbins JD, Cavanaugh BJ, *et al.*: Quantitative assessment of in-stent dimensions: a comparison of 64 and 16 detector multislice computed tomography to intravascular ultrasound. *Catheter Cardiovasc Interv* 2006, 68:8–10.

19. Gasparovic H, Rybicki FJ, Millstine J, *et al.*: Three dimensional computed tomographic imaging in planning the surgical approach for redo cardiac surgery after coronary revascularization. *Eur J Cardiothorac Surg* 2005, 28:244–249.

20. Goldstein JA, Gallagher MJ, O'Neill WW, *et al.*: A randomized controlled trial of multi-slice coronary computed tomography for evaluation of acute chest pain. *J Am Coll Cardiol* 2007, 49:863–871.

21. Nasir K, Budoff MJ: Peripheral angiography. In *Cardiac CT Imaging: Diagnosis of Cardiovascular Disease*, edn 1. London, UK: Springer; 2006.

22. Hunold P, Vogt FM, Schmermund A, *et al.*: Radiation exposure during cardiac CT: effective doses at multi-detector row CT and electron-beam CT. *Radiology* 2003, 226:145–152.

23. McCollough CH: Patient dose in cardiac computed tomography. *Herz* 2003, 28:1–6.

24. Poll LW, Cohnen M, Brachten S, *et al.*: Dose reduction in multi-slice CT of the heart by use of ECG-controlled tube current modulation ("ECG pulsing"): phantom measurements. *Rofo* 2002, 174:1500–1505.

25. Hacker M, Jakobs T, Matthiesen F, *et al.*: Comparison of spiral multidetector CT angiography and myocardial perfusion imaging in the noninvasive detection of functionally relevant coronary artery lesions: first clinical experiences. *J Nucl Med* 2005, 46:1294–1300.

26. Coles DR, Smail MA, Negus IS, *et al.*: Comparison of radiation doses from multislice computed tomography coronary angiography and conventional diagnostic angiography. *J Am Coll Cardiol* 2006, 47:1840–1845.

27. Flohr TG, Schoepf UJ, Kuettner A, *et al.*: Advances in cardiac imaging with 16-section CT systems. *Acad Radiol* 2003, 10:386–401.

28. Garcia MJ, Lessick J, Hoffmann MH, CATSCAN Study Investigators: Accuracy of 16-row multidetector computed tomography for the assessment of coronary artery stenosis. *JAMA* 2006, 296:403–411.

29. Gerber TC, Stratmann BP, Kuzo RS, *et al.*: Effect of acquisition technique on radiation dose and image quality in multidetector row computed tomography coronary angiography with submillimeter collimation. *Invest Radiol* 2005, 40:556–563.

30. Hoffmann MH, Shi H, Schmitz BL, *et al.*: Noninvasive coronary angiography with multislice computed tomography. *JAMA* 2005, 293:2471–2478.

31. Nawfel R, Yoshizumi T: Update on radiation dose in CT. *Am Assoc Physicists Med Newsletter* 2005, 30:12–13.

32. Sato Y, Matsumoto N, Ichikawa M, *et al.*: Efficacy of multislice computed tomography for the detection of acute coronary syndrome in the emergency department. *Circ J* 2005, 69:1047–1051.

33. Trabold T, Buchgeister M, Kuttner A, *et al.*: Estimation of radiation exposure in 16-detector row computed tomography of the heart with retrospective ECG-gating. *Rofo* 2003, 175:1051–1055.

34. Gaspar T, Halon DA, Lewis BS, *et al.*: Diagnosis of coronary in-stent restenosis with multidetector row spiral computed tomography. *J Am Coll Cardiol* 2005, 46:1573–1579.

35. Caussin C, Larchez C, Ghostine S, *et al.*: Comparison of coronary minimal lumen area quantification by sixty-four-slice computed tomography versus intravascular ultrasound for intermediate stenosis. *Am J Cardiol* 2006, 98:871–876.

36. Hausleiter J, Meyer T, Hadamitzky M, *et al.*: Radiation dose estimates from cardiac multislice computed tomography in daily practice: impact of different scanning protocols on effective dose estimates. *Circulation* 2006, 113:1305–1310.

37. Ghostine S, Caussin C, Daoud B, *et al.*: Noninvasive detection of coronary artery disease in patients with left bundle branch block using 64-slice computed tomography. *J Am Coll Cardiol* 2006, 48:1929–1934.

38. Leber AW, Knez A, von Ziegler F, *et al.*: Quantification of obstructive and nonobstructive coronary lesions by 64-slice computed tomography: a comparative study with quantitative coronary angiography and intravascular ultrasound. *J Am Coll Cardiol* 2005, 46:147–154.

39. Mollet NR, Cademartiri F, van Mieghem CA, *et al.*: High-resolution spiral computed tomography coronary angiography in patients referred for diagnostic conventional coronary angiography. *Circulation* 2005,112:2318–2323.

40. Muhlenbruch G, Seyfarth T, Soo CS, *et al.*: Diagnostic value of 64-slice multi-detector row cardiac CTA in symptomatic patients. *Eur Radiol* 2007, 17:603–609.

41. Nikolaou K, Knez A, Rist C, *et al.*: Accuracy of 64-MDCT in the diagnosis of ischemic heart disease. *AJR Am J Roentgenol* 2006, 187:111–117.

42. Pugliese F, Mollet NR, Runza G, *et al.*: Diagnostic accuracy of non-invasive 64-slice CT coronary angiography in patients with stable angina pectoris. *Eur Radiol* 2006, 16:575–582.

43. Raff GL, Gallagher MJ, O'Neill WW, Goldstein JA: Diagnostic accuracy of noninvasive coronary angiography using 64-slice spiral computed tomography. *J Am Coll Cardiol* 2005, 46:552–557.

Cardiac Magnetic Resonance Imaging

16

Raymond Y. Kwong

ardiac magnetic resonance (CMR) is currently the most complex imaging technology of the heart, but its versatile capabilities within a single examination have ensured it an increasing role in clinical cardiology. With the advent of imaging hardware and post-processing techniques, a CMR examination that can quantitatively assess a multitude of structural or physiologic problems can be achieved in less than 1 hour. This chapter presents some of these imaging applications by CMR based on case examples.

Cardiac Magnetic Resonance Imaging in Coronary Artery Disease

Imaging of Myocardial Infarction and Viability

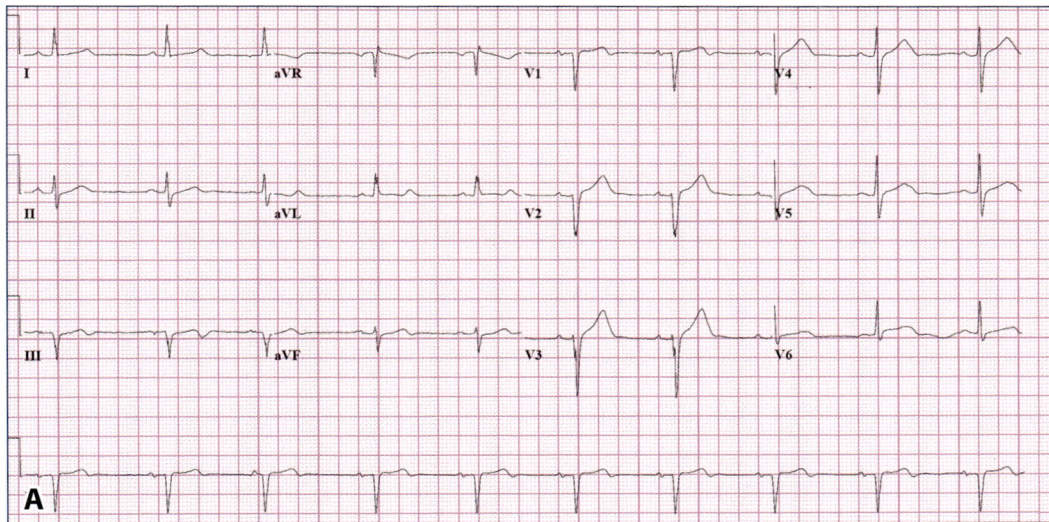

Figure 16-1. A number of pulse sequence techniques in cardiac magnetic resonance (CMR) have clinical applications in assessing coronary artery disease (CAD). Cine steady-state free precession gradient-echo imaging has been the standard technique at 1.5 Tesla, in volumetrically quantifying left (LV) and right ventricular (RV) sizes, global and regional functions, and myocardial mass. Excellent spatial (1.5–2 mm in-plane) and temporal resolution (30 ms) can be achieved without the need for contrast use. Tissue contrast between normal and infarcted myocardium can be brought out by gadolinium-based contrast agent.

In this example, a 39-year-old construction worker developed acute chest pain after use of cocaine. The patient presented 2 days after the initial chest pain and was found to have a three-fold elevation of serum creatine kinase MB. **A,** Serial echocardiogram (ECG) on admission was unremarkable for acute ischemia and there was not definite pathologic Q waves.

Continued on the next page

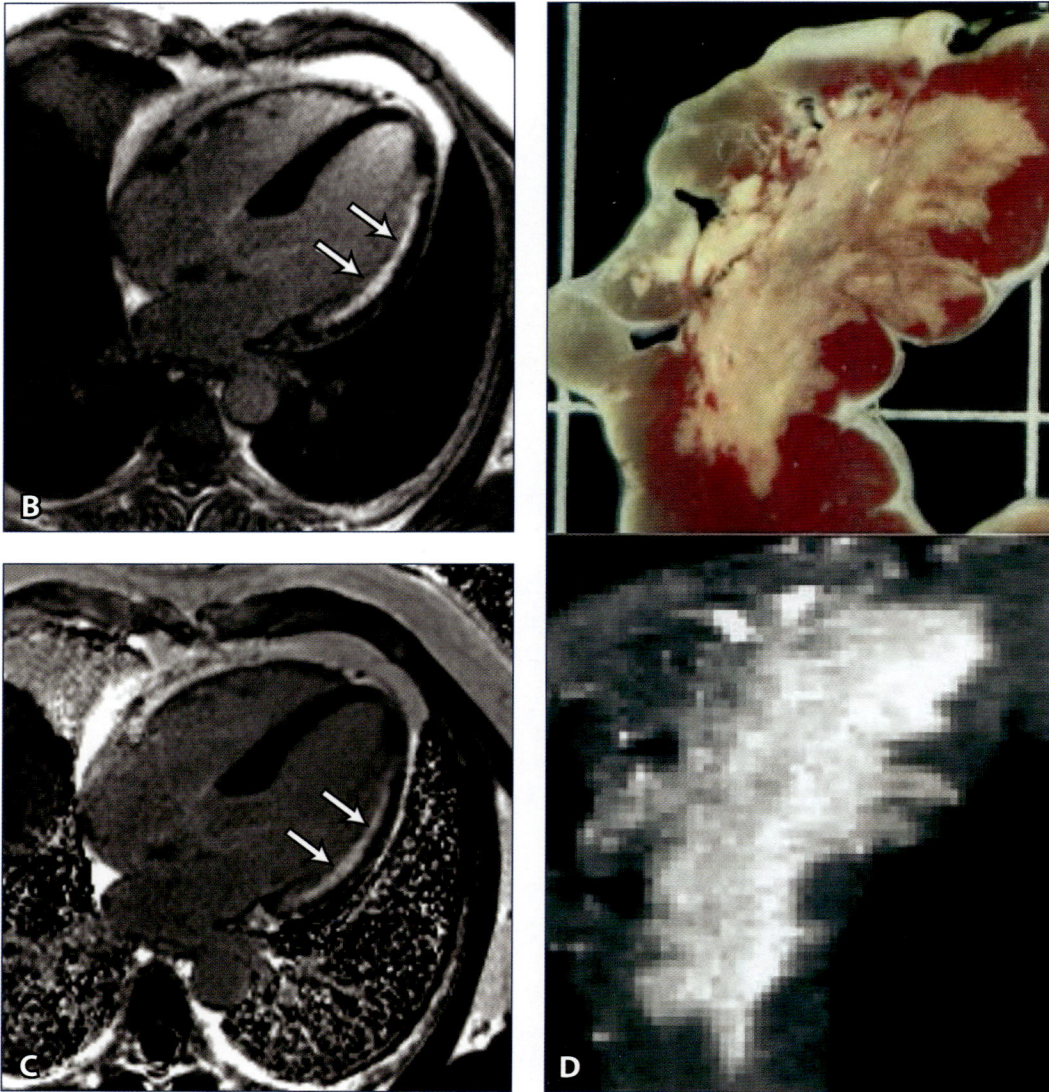

Figure 16-1. *(Continued)* **B,** By contrast-enhanced CMR, late gadolinium enhancement (LGE) imaging, there is subendocardial myocardial damage of the basal and mid-anterolateral wall. Coronary angiography showed a severe stenosis in the proximal diagonal branch of the left anterior descending artery and an occluded obtuse marginal branch of the circumflex artery (*arrows*). However, his LV ejection fraction (LVEF) was preserved at 60%. High contrast noise ratio, spatial resolution, and tomographic approach of contrast-enhanced CMR can detect myocardial damage from myocardial infarction (MI) missed by ECG and in some cases serum biomarkers. In this case, myocardial damage in the lateral wall may have been electrically "silent" and was not detected by ECG. **C,** This image represents LGE imaging where phase-sensitive reconstruction of the imaging data was applied to enhance the contrast between normal and infarcted myocardium [1,2]. **D,** The myocardial extent of infarction by LGE imaging has extensive validation against animal model of MI by triphenyltetrazolium chloride staining. (*From* Kim *et al.* [3]; with permission.)

Assessment for Presence of Myocardial Infarction

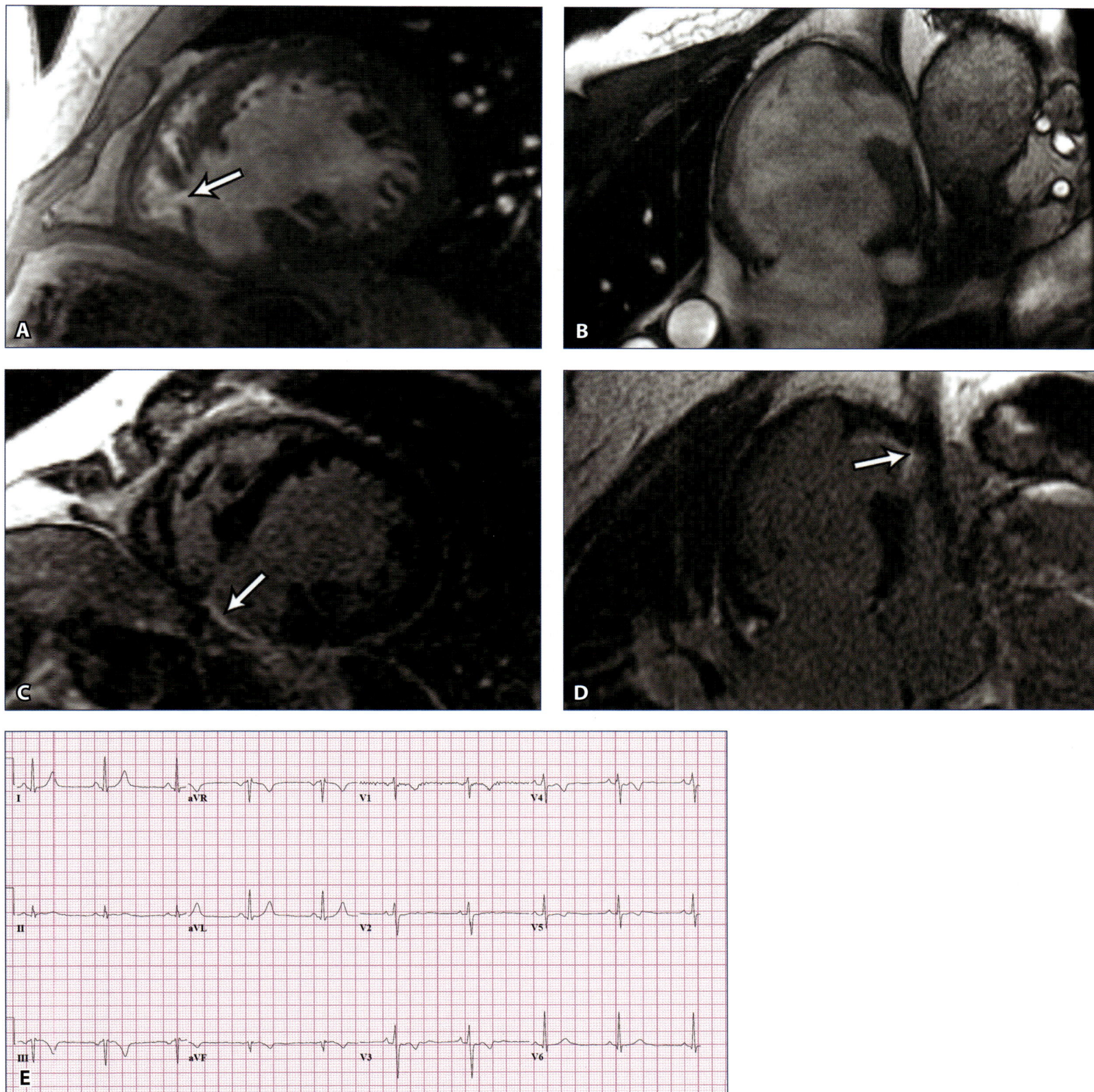

Figure 16-2. A 52-year-old executive without any prior history of coronary artery disease presented with a 2-week history of dyspnea and was found to have a ventricular septal defect (VSD) on echocardiography. Cardiac magnetic resonance (CMR) was referred to assess the size of the VSD to assist in planning of closure of the septal defect by percutaneous versus surgical approach. **A,** This figure demonstrates a small slit-like VSD with left-to-right shunting during systole (*arrow*). However, precontrast cine imaging (**A** and **B**) revealed akinesis of the inferior and inferoseptal walls with myocardial thinning. **C** and **D,** Contrast-enhanced late gadolinium enhancement imaging of these matching views demonstrate thinned myocardial scarring consistent with myocardial infarction of the inferior and inferoseptal walls (*arrows*). Upon further questioning, the patient recalled having an episode of prolonged chest pain while traveling abroad on a business trip 4 weeks before presentation. He did not seek medical attention at the time. Interestingly, the admission echocardiogram did not show any evidence of inferior infarction or abnormality from the presence of a VSD (**E**). This patient was subsequently found to have severe coronary stenoses in the left anterior descending and right coronary arteries, both of which were successfully treated with percutaneous revascularization. The VSD was closed by implantation of a percutaneous closure device and the patient has been doing well 2 years after his initial presentation.

Cardiac Magnetic Resonance Is the Most Sensitive Current Technique for Subendocardial Infarction

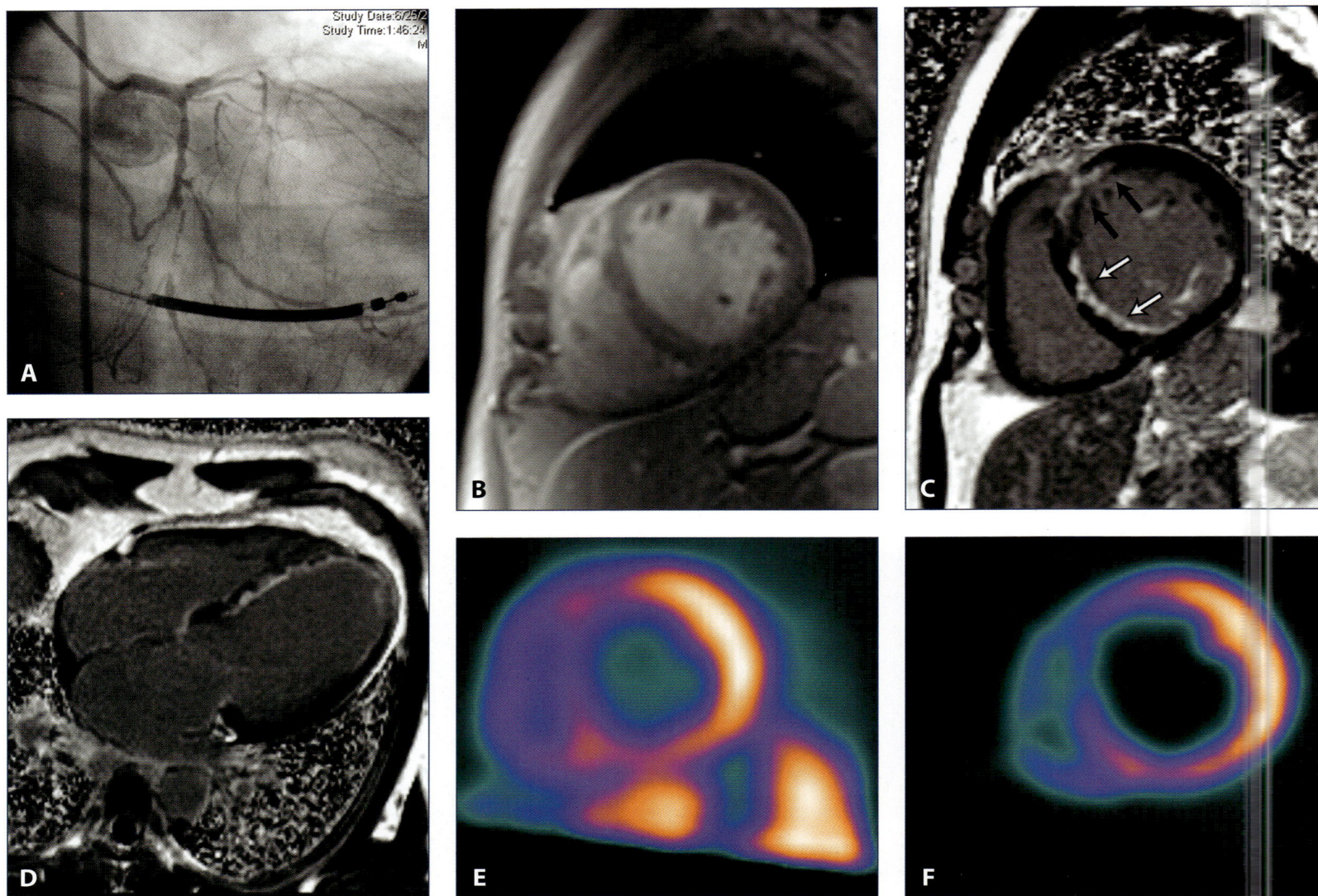

Figure 16-3. A 56-year-old male with a remote history of myocardial infarction and congestive heart failure was admitted with several weeks' history of progressive dyspnea. He was noted to have severe global systolic left ventricular (LV) dysfunction with a left ventricular ejection fraction (LVEF) of 15% by echocardiography. **A,** Cardiac catheterization revealed diffuse three-vessel coronary artery disease. He was referred for cardiac magnetic resonance (CMR) to assess myocardial viability in each coronary territory. **B,** This figure showed a dilated left ventricle with marked global systolic dysfunction. Quantitative LVEF by cine CMR was 19%. There is a medium-sized infarction (with > 75% transmural extent) in the left anterior descending territory involving the basal to mid-anteroseptal wall, distal septum, and the true LV apex (**C** and **D**). On positron emission tomography (PET) imaging, these myocardial segments demonstrated reduced perfusion tracer (rubidium-82) uptake (**E**) matched by reduced fluorodeoxyglucose F-18 uptake (**F**) indicative of infarction. **C,**

There is another region of late gadolinium enhancement (LGE) involving the subendocardium of the inferior and inferoseptal walls (*white arrows*). This subendocardial infarction was not easily recognized by the corresponding views by PET (**E** and **F**). In this case, the identification of the inferior and inferoseptal infarction was important because the patient was considered for LV reconstructive surgery (Dor Procedure), and the coexistence of inferior infarction made reconstruction of the anterior wall alone less likely to benefit the patient.

Current LGE technique by CMR can achieve an in-plane spatial resolution of 1.5 × 1.5 mm while maintaining a high contrast-noise ratio of 20. Applying this technical advantage, the transmural extent of infarction as quantified by LGE can accurately predict the likelihood of recovery of segmental contractile function from successful coronary revascularization. Subendocardial infarction detected by CMR LGE is often undetected by imaging of regional wall thickening or by nuclear scintigraphy.

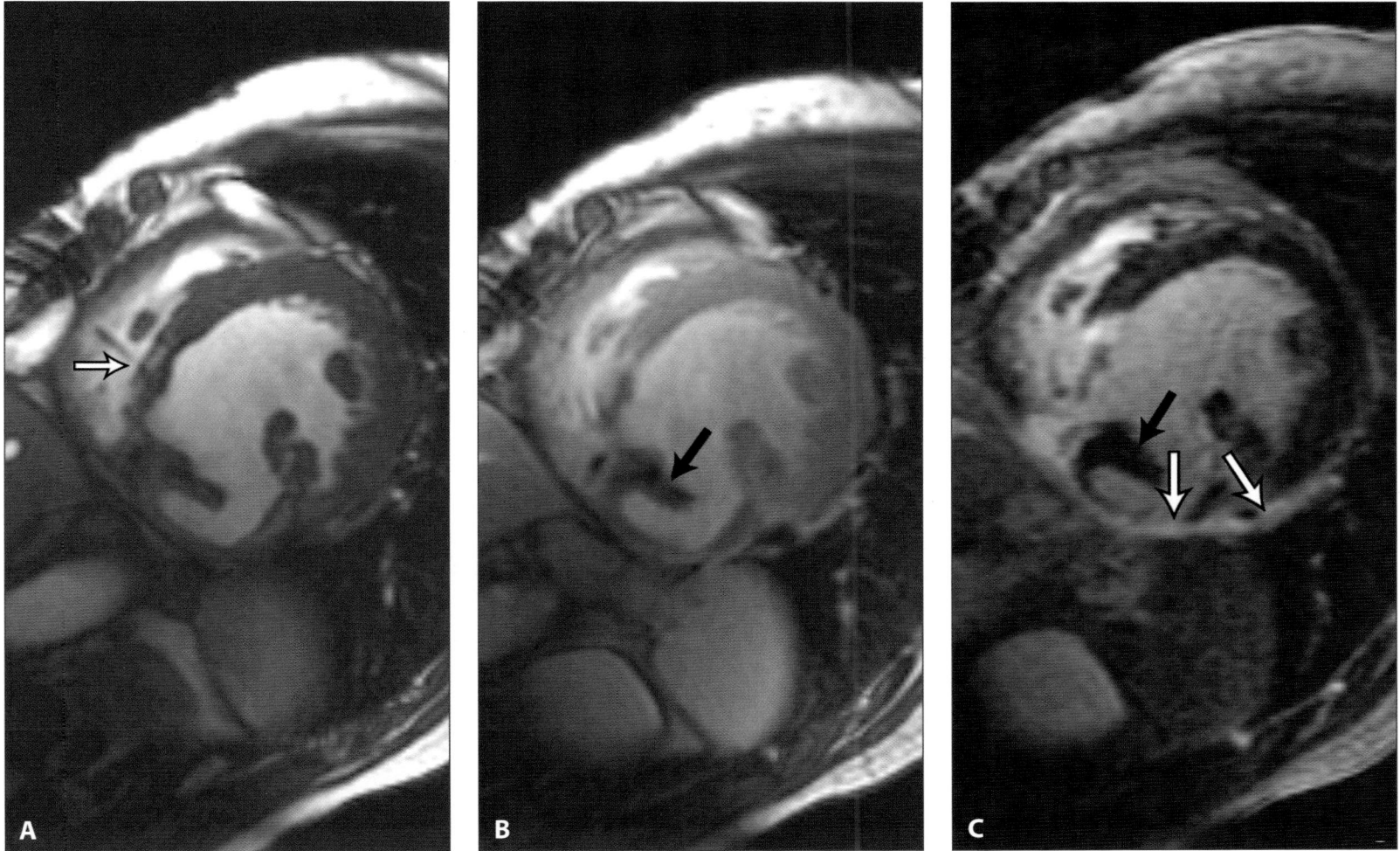

Figure 16-4. A 78-year-old female experienced an ST-elevation myocardial infarction (MI) and presented late to the hospital. Despite percutaneous revascularization of the infarct-related coronary artery, the post-MI course was complicated by heart failure with a left ventricular ejection fraction (LVEF) of 35% at hospital discharge. Due to a large region of inferior akinesis, the patient was treated with anticoagulation and with afterload-reducing medications in an attempt to reduce any adverse ventricular remodeling. Three months later, the patient presented to the hospital again with signs and symptoms of severe congestive heart failure and was referred to undergo cardiac magnetic resonance (CMR) to assess her cardiac status. **A,** Systolic frame of a short-axis cine image demonstrating a severe dilated and distorted left ventricle (LV) with a dyskinetic and thinned inferior and inferoseptal walls. **B** and **C,** Matching postcontrast images. LVEF quantified by CMR cine steady-state free precession yields an LVEF of 20%. Matching postcontrast late gadolinium enhancement (LGE) imaging (**C**) demonstrates full thickness infarction (*white arrows*) of the segments matching the extent of the dyskinesis. A large mural thrombus is seen with markedly suppressed signal intensity in the postcontrast LGE imaging (*black arrows*). In addition, the post-MI status of this patient was complicated by a small ventricular septal perforation at the edge of the infarction (*arrow* on **A**, indicating the presence of a left-to-right flow jet through the ventricular septal defect (VSD). This patient underwent urgent repair of the VSD and surgical reconstruction of the LV.

Matching tomographic scan planes, high spatial resolution, and tissue characterization can provide diagnostic information complementary to imaging of cardiac structure by echocardiography. In this case, myocardial extent of the infarcted myocardium and formation of mural thrombus was readily detected by gadolinium-enhanced CMR. Klem *et al.* [4] recently studied 784 consecutive patients with systolic dysfunction, demonstrating that tissue characterization by LGE, rather than anatomical appearance, was the strongest imaging marker to detect intracavitary thrombus or embolic events within the subsequent 6 months after CMR.

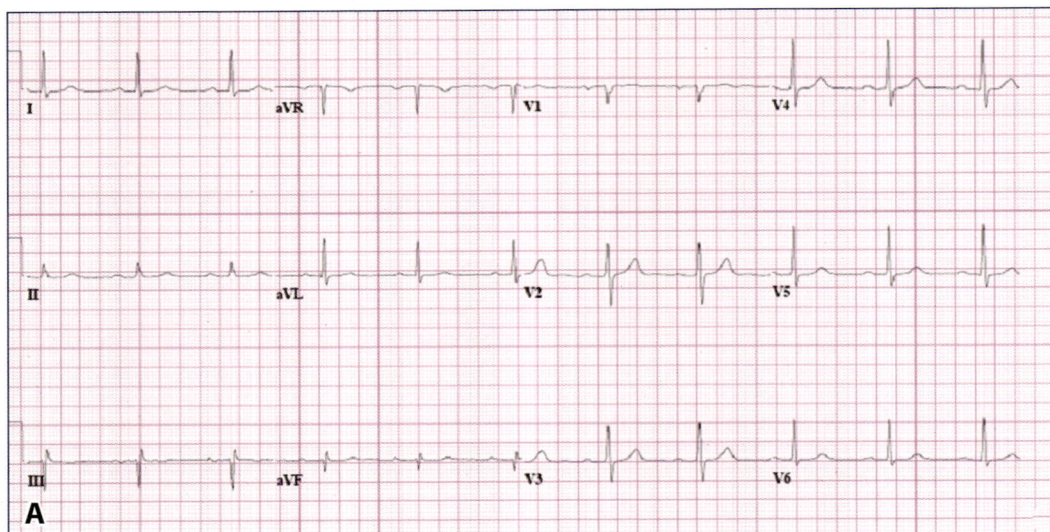

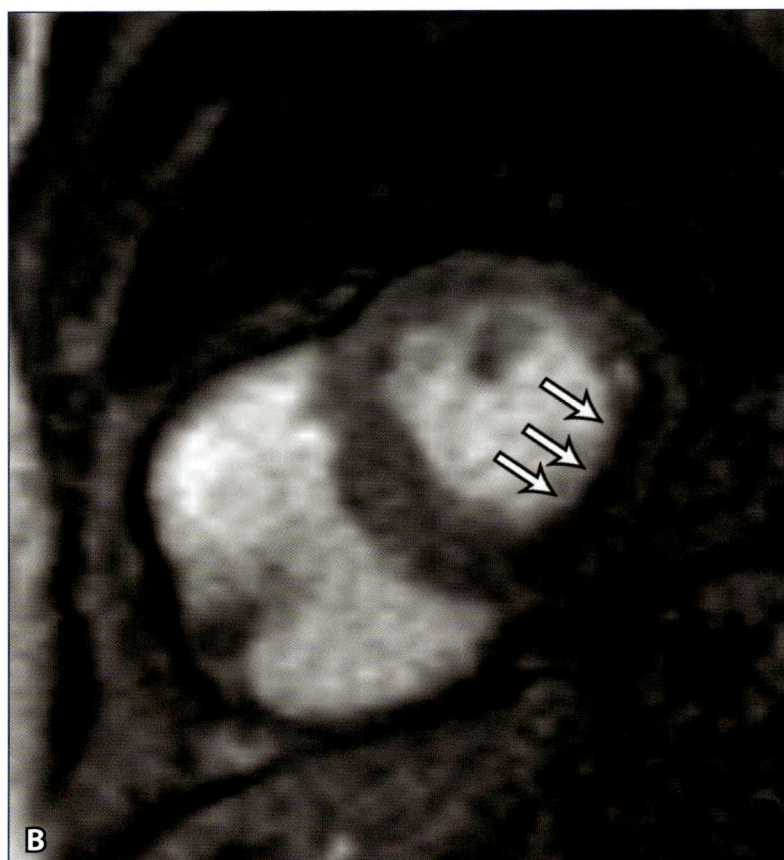

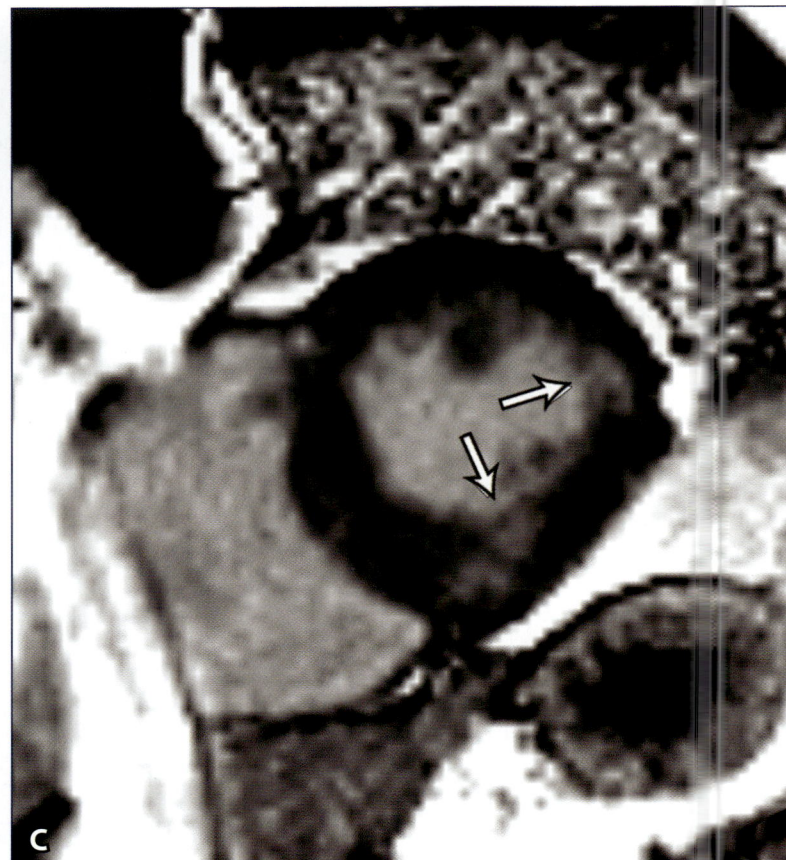

Figure 16-5. A 60-year-old male with history of chronic hypertension but no prior cardiac disease presented with a 3-month history of bilateral ankle swelling and atypical chest discomfort. **A,** Resting echocardiography did not reveal any abnormality to suggest significant coronary artery disease (CAD). Cardiac magnetic resonance (CMR) first-pass perfusion is demonstrated during adenosine vasodilatation (**B**) and late enhancement imaging (**C**) in a matching short-axis location. **C,** There are two foci of late gadolinium enhancement (LGE) in the inferior wall and the inferolateral wall. During adenosine vasodilatation, there is a moderate-sized first-pass perfusion defect (in **B**, *arrows*) that is larger in extent than the LGE areas.

This patient was found to have two-vessel severe coronary stenoses of the right coronary and circumflex arteries amendable by coronary stenting.

This case demonstrates that CMR can detect clinically unrecognized myocardial infarction (MI) and first-pass CMR perfusion imaging can complement by assessing for evidence of significant flow-limiting coronary stenosis. LGE imaging by CMR is currently the most sensitive technique for detecting small subendocardial MI [5–7], which can portend adverse cardiac outcomes [8]. Numerous single-center studies and a recent multicenter study have consistently reported excellent sensitivities and high specificities in detecting angiographically significant CAD [9–11].

Continued on the next page

At risk, n

Normal DSMR	353	316	228	96	20	0
Abnormal DSMR	108	79	50	21	3	0

D

At risk, n

Normal MR perfusion	302	272	205	84	16	0
Abnormal MR perfusion	159	123	73	33	7	0

E

F

G

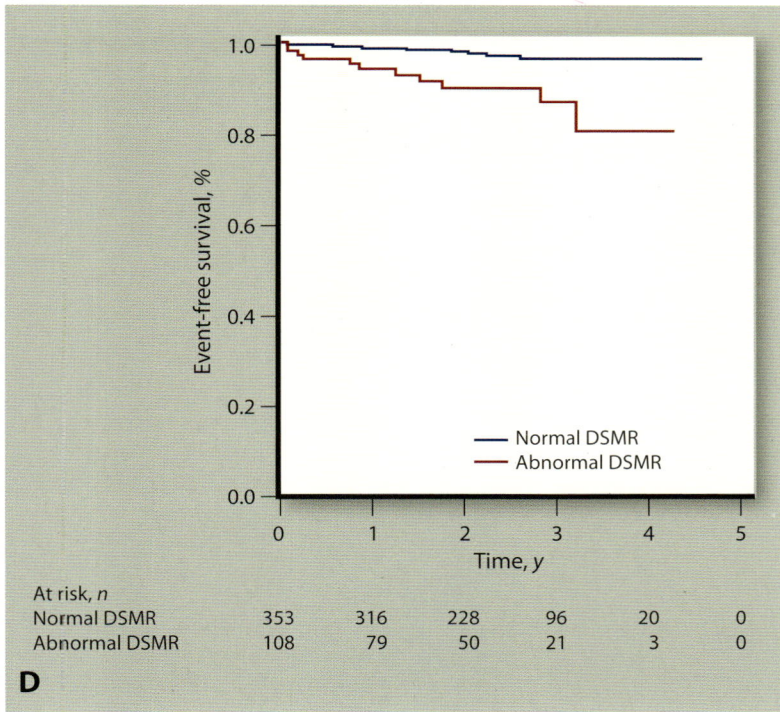

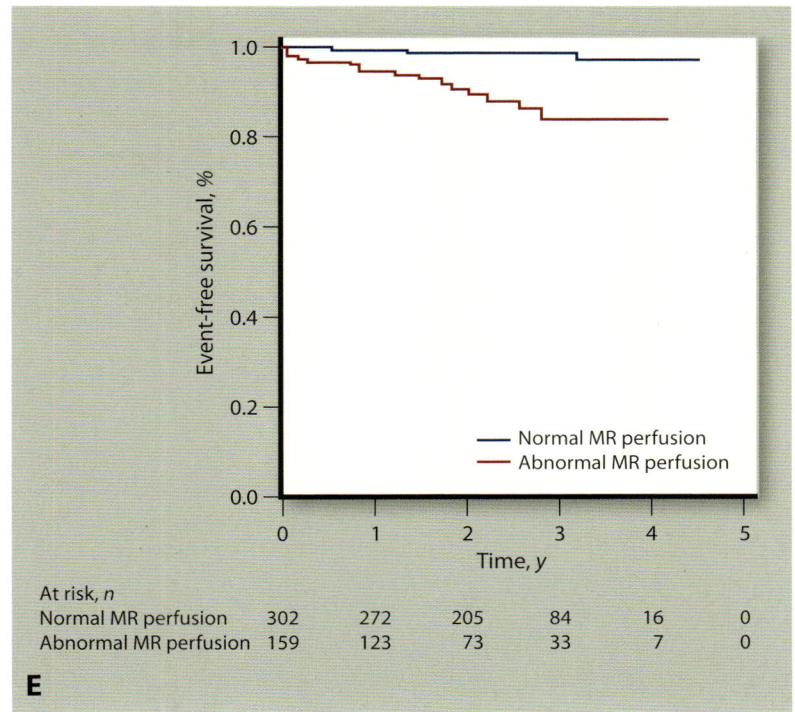

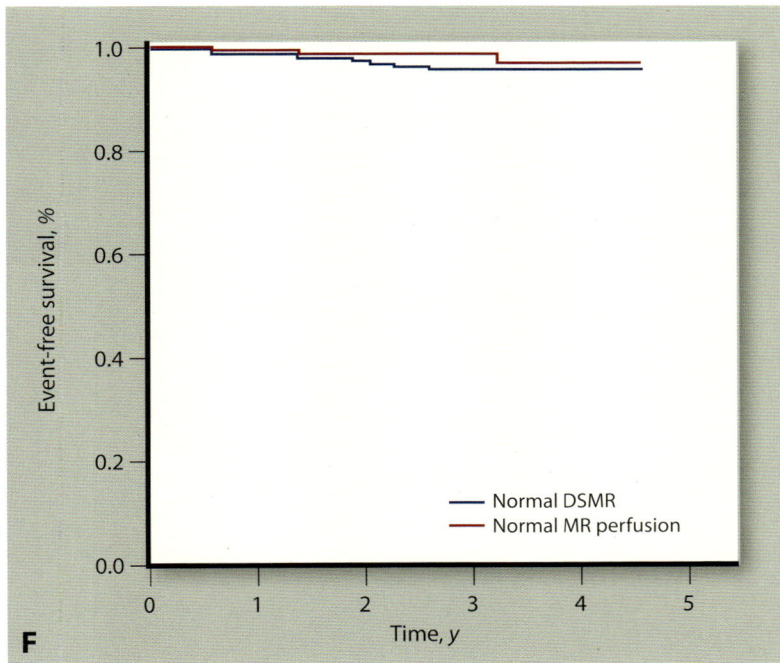

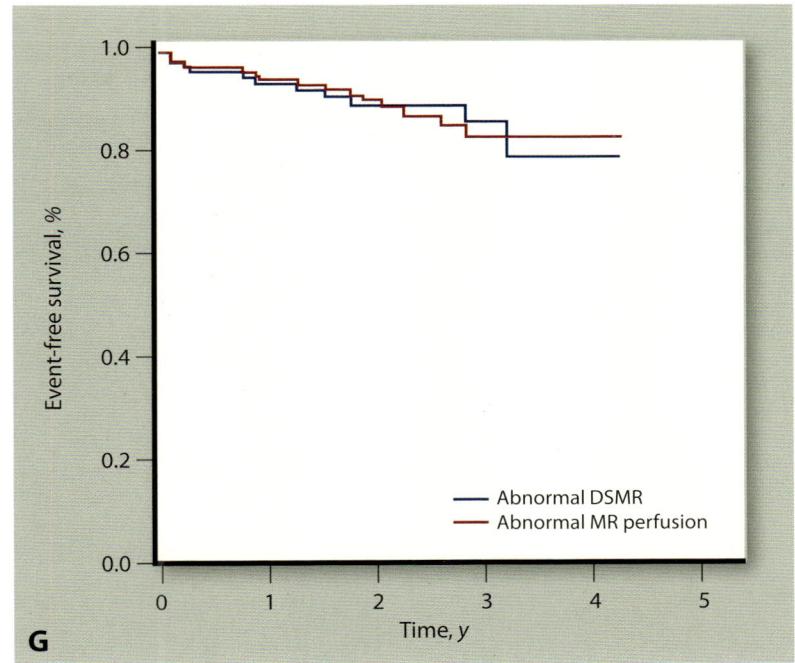

Figure 16-5. *(Continued)* **D, E, F,** and **G,** In addition, recent studies have reported strong prognostic implication of CMR first-pass perfusion imaging in assessing patients with chest pain syndromes [12–15]. Jahnke *et al.* [15] studied 513 chest pain patients with intermediate pre-test likelihood of CAD with first-pass CMR adenosine stress perfusion imaging. Patients who had a negative CMR stress study experienced a 3-year event-free survival of 99.2%. DSMR—dobutamine stress magnetic resonance.

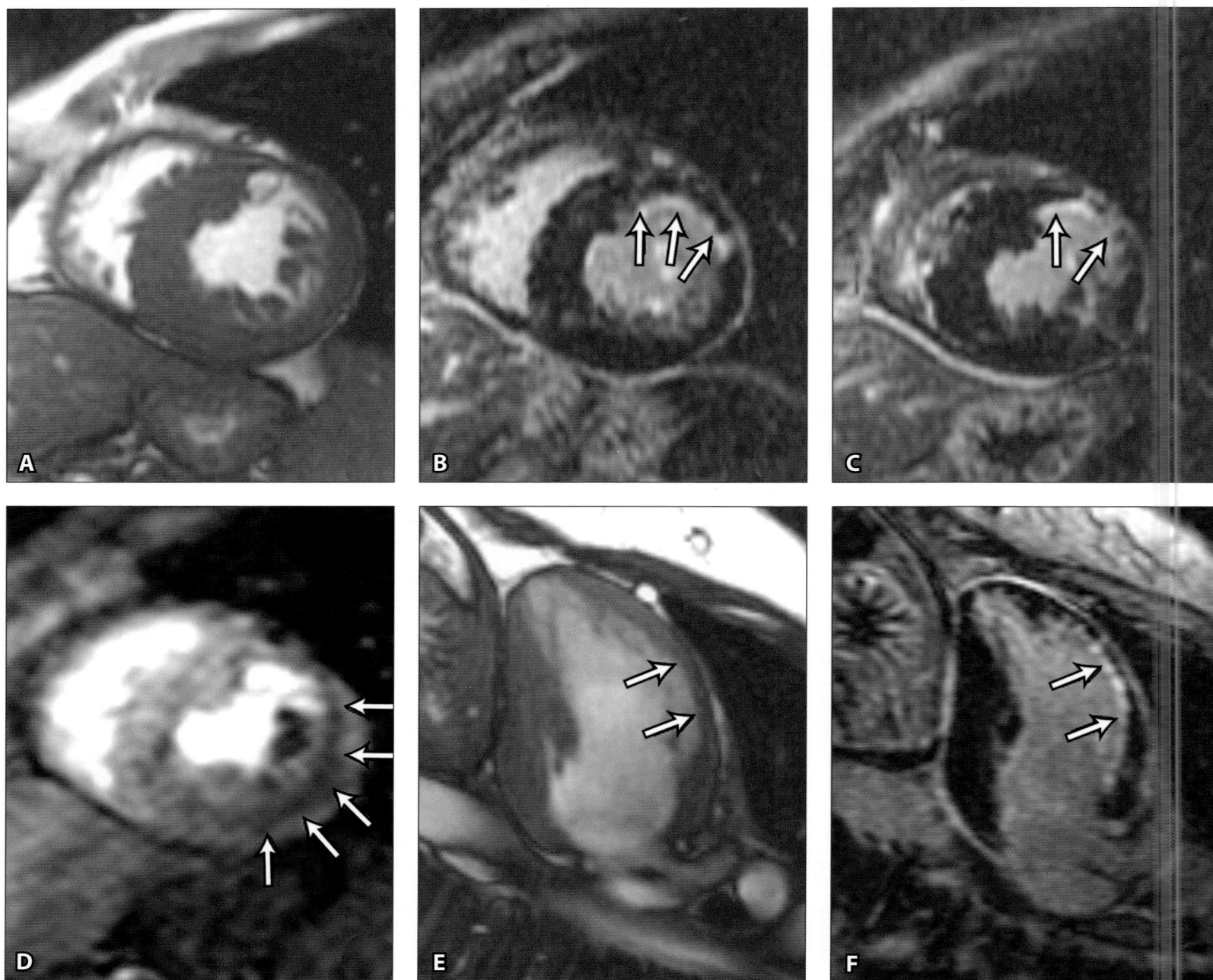

Figure 16-6. A 68-year-old women with diabetes was referred due to abnormal echocardiogram for preoperative assessment. Echocardiography detected anterior systolic wall motion abnormality. The systolic frame in **A** illustrates cardiac magnetic resonance (CMR) cine steady-state free precession imaging that confirmed the presence of an anterior and anterolateral region of hypokinesis. Late gadolinium enhancement imaging detected the presence of subendocardial infarction in the matching segments (**B**, **C**, and **D**). These findings were confirmed on the corresponding long axis views showing anterior wall thinning (**E**) and subendocardial infarction (**F**). During dobutamine stress infusion at a moderate dose of 30 mcg/kg/min, there is a large stress-induced perfusion defect involving the anterior, anterolateral, inferolateral, and inferior walls, indicating multivessel coronary artery disease. This patient was subsequently found to have severe three-vessel coronary stenosis and was treated with multivessel stenting.

Registration of Three-Dimensional Anatomic Cardiac Magnetic Resonance Data for Electrophysiologic Ablation

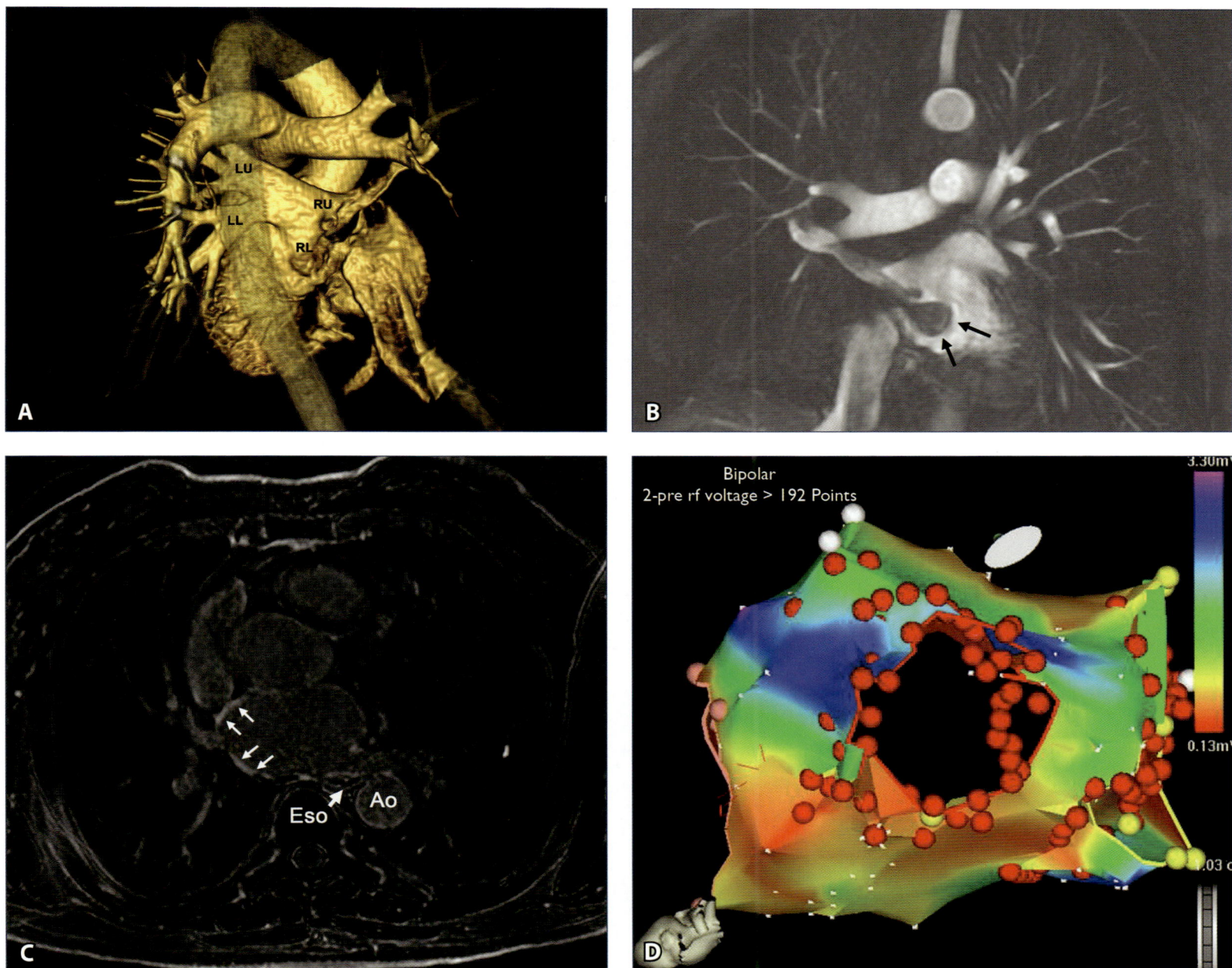

Figure 16-7. Registration of three-dimensional (3D) anatomic data from cardiac magnetic resonance (CMR) and electrophysiologic voltage mapping has been common practice in many tertiary care centers. 3D data from contrast-enhanced imaging of the left atrium (LA) and the locations of the pulmonary veins can be performed by acquiring a standard 3D magnetic resonance angiogram (MRA) at high spatial resolution while an intravenous bolus of gadolinium is injected. **A,** A coronal view of a 3D MRA of the LA, with the descending aorta translucent. The relative positions of the pulmonary veins and the presence of any accessory or anomalous pulmonary veins can be clearly depicted, which may ease the anatomic voltage mapping of the LA volume and contour. These coregistered data may ease radiofrequency ablation (RFA) of the LA to achieve electrical isolation of the pulmonary veins and retard the development of atrial fibrillation in some patients. In addition, adjacent structures including the esophagus and the descending aorta can be demonstrated relative to the LA volume; therefore, chance of procedural complication can be reduced. **B,** In the same patient as in **A,** the presence of a large left atrial thrombus (*arrows*) in a patient with atrial fibrillation, before the planned RFA. **C,** A novel technique demonstrating myocardial scar from RFA of the LA. Note late gadolinium enhancement (LGE) of the LA wall surrounding the right superior pulmonary vein (*arrows*). This is matched by the points of RFA recorded during the electrophysiology study (*red dots* on **D**). In a pilot study of 23 patients who underwent RFA of the LA for electrical isolation of the pulmonary veins, LGE detected LA scar from RFA at a high sensitivity and specificity [16,17]. The position of the esophagus (Eso) and the descending aorta (Ao) can also be readily identified (**C**).

Assessing the Anatomical Extent and Location of Radiofrequency Ablation in the Left Ventricle

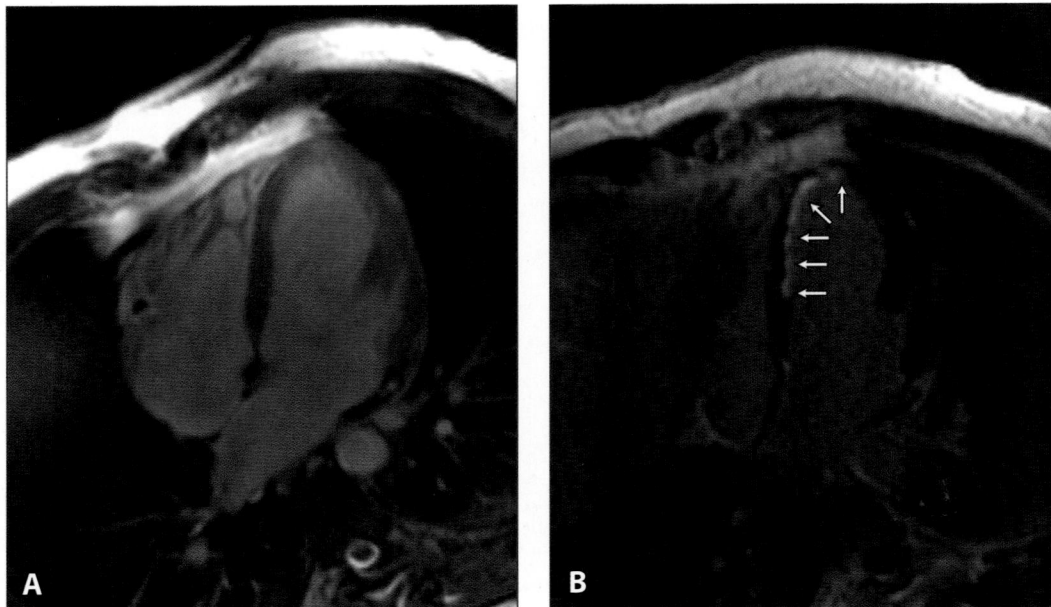

Figure 16-8. A 50-year-old physician experienced idiopathic nonsustained ventricular tachycardia. His symptoms were sufficiently debilitating to warrant radiofrequency ablation (RFA) treatment of the ectopic focus that was identified by voltage mapping to be in the left ventricle near the distal septum (**A**). **B,** After ablation, late gadolinium enhancement imaging provided accurate delineation of the segmental extent and transmural thickness of the myocardial damage caused by RFA (*arrows*).

Cardiac Magnetic Resonance Imaging of Cardiomyopathy of Unknown Etiology

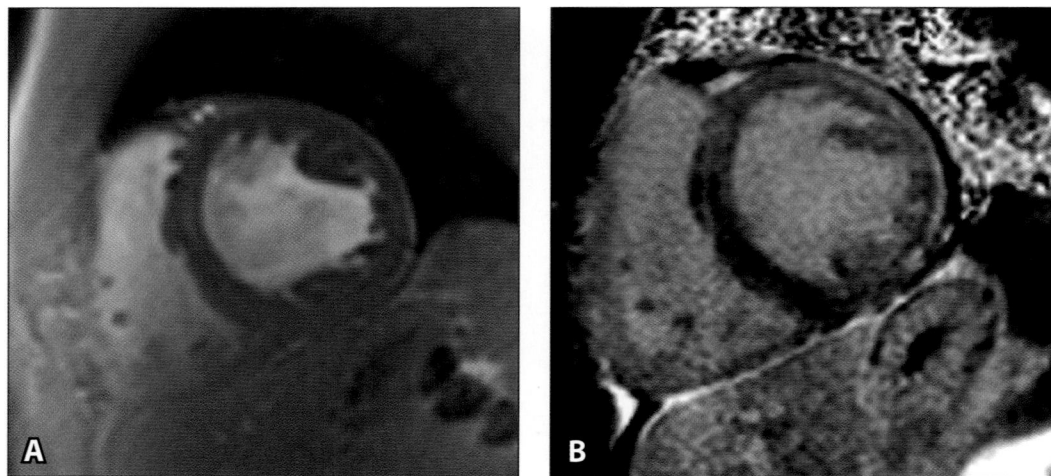

Figure 16-9. Acute myocarditis. A 20-year-old male student who was previously healthy developed an influenza-like illness while visiting Mexico. He developed worsened dyspnea and was found to have severe depression of left ventricular (LV) global systolic function and moderate LV dilatation. At hospital admission, he had frequent nonsustained ventricular tachycardia, physical findings consistent with cardiogenic shock, with an LV ejection fraction (LVEF) quantified by volumetric cine cardiac magnetic resonance (CMR) to be 25% (**A**). Serial blood and urine cultures revealed no bacterial pathogens. Endomyocardial biopsy revealed moderate interstitial fibrosis only. Contrast-enhanced late gadolinium enhancement (LGE) imaging demonstrated diffuse and patchy enhancement of the anterolateral and inferolateral wall (**B**). These CMR findings are consistent with diffuse acute myocardial inflammation and edema presumably from acute viral myocarditis. The patient fortunately followed a stable and then progressively improving clinical course in the months following initial presentation.

Diagnosing acute myocarditis is often challenged by nonspecific symptoms, echocardiography findings, and insensitivity of endomyocardial biopsy sampling. CMR LGE imaging provides two- or three-dimensional mapping of the extracellular accumulation of gadolinium diethylene triamine pentaacetic acid that corresponds to areas of active myocarditis. Mahrholdt *et al.* [18] studied 32 patients who were diagnosed with acute myocarditis by clinical criteria. It was reported that the lateral aspect of the left ventricle (LV) was often involved. Histopathologic analysis revealed active myocarditis in 90% when the biopsy samples were taken from areas with LGE guided by the CMR data, whereas only 10% had histopathologic evidence of active myocarditis when the samples were obtained in non–LGE-enhanced areas [18]. The same group of authors recently reported that parvovirus B19 often presents with epimyocardial involvement of the lateral wall and follows a more benign clinical course. However, viral type 6 of human herpesvirus 6 more often involved the interventricular septum and had a higher propensity to lead to chronic heart failure [19].

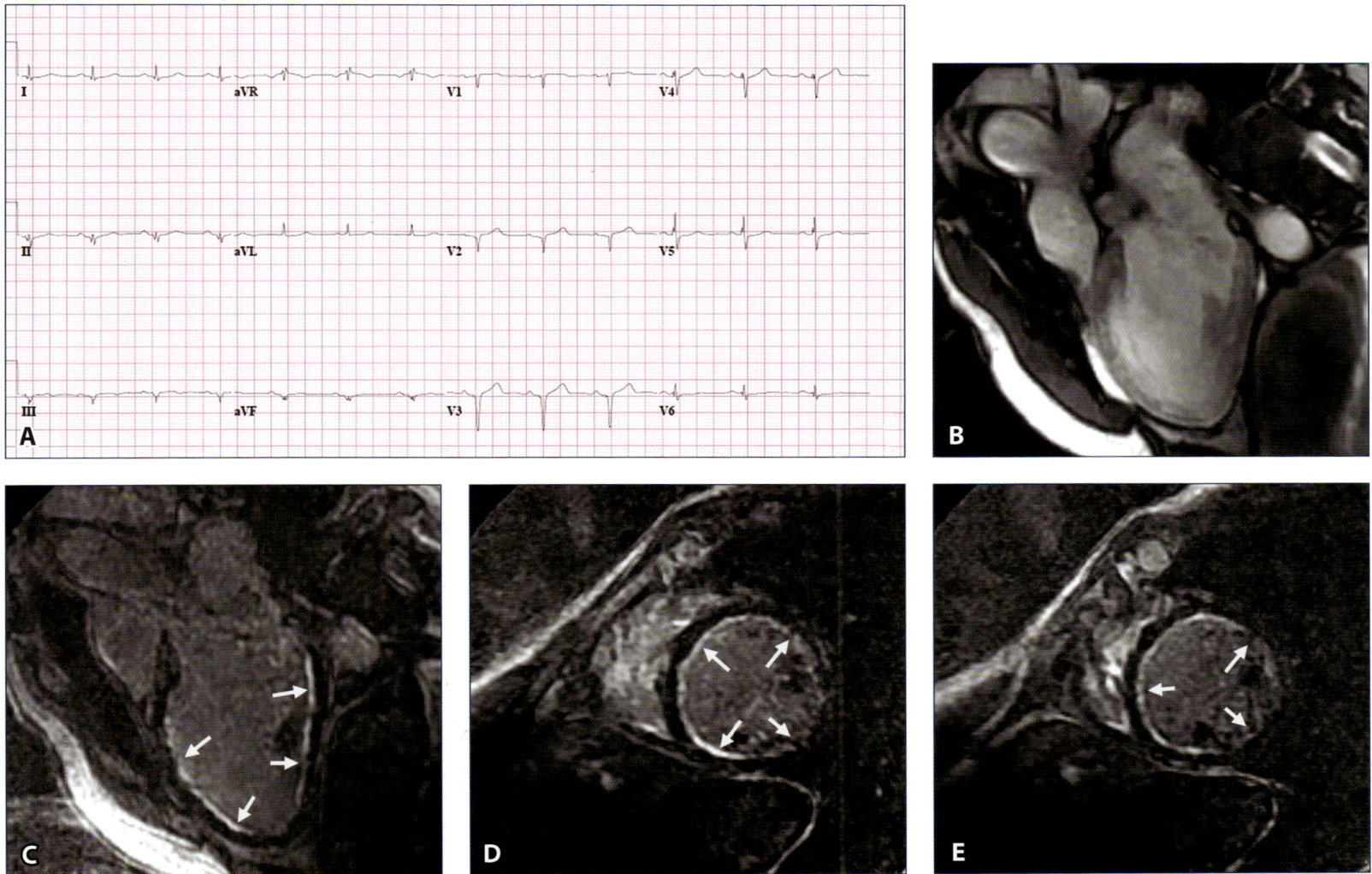

Figure 16-10. A 47-year-old male with a history of asthma, dyslipidemia, and distal polyneuropathy, developed increasing problems with sinusitis over several months and progressive dyspnea on exertion. **A,** Resting echocardiography (ECG) showed low voltage and formation of Q waves in both the precordial leads and the inferior leads. ECG revealed global hypokinesis with an estimated left ventricular ejection fraction (LVEF) of 45%, without regional wall motion abnormality.

Cardiac magnetic resonance (CMR) confirmed the presence of global hypokinesis at rest (LVEF, 41%) with moderate LV dilatation (**B**). There was no evidence of resting perfusion abnormality. Iron content quantified by T2-STAR gradient echo (T*) CMR technique was normal, excluding iron overloading condition as a cause of his cardiomyopathy. After gadolinium was administered intravenously, late gadolinium enhancement imaging demonstrated diffuse endomyocardial accumulation of gadolinium contrast that was not consistent with coronary artery distribution (**C, D,** and **E**). These findings in conjunction with the clinical setting in this case were consistent with a diagnosis of Churg Strauss systemic small-vessel vasculitis [20].

Effusive Constrictive Pericarditis

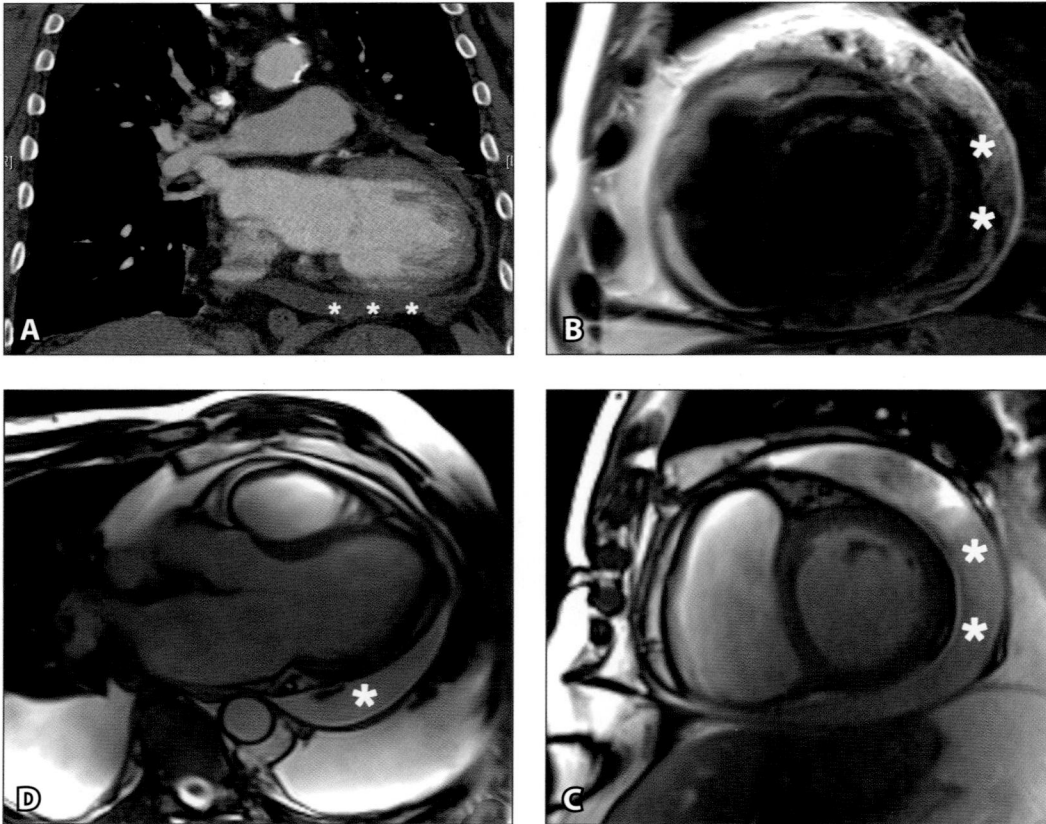

Figure 16-11. A 75-year-old male presented with a 5-month history of recurrent chest pain, progressive worsening of dyspnea, and bilateral edema of the lower extremities. Clinical examination was consistent with elevated venous pressure, raising a clinical suspicion of pericardial constriction. A moderate-sized pericardial effusion was seen in a CT scan (*asterisks* in **A**) but the pericardial thickness was reported to be normal (*asterisks* in **B**). Cardiac magnetic resonance (CMR) confirmed a large pericardial effusion that surrounds the left ventricle, estimating a total of more than 500 mL of pericardial fluid (*asterisks* in **C** and **D**). The pericardial fluid on T1 weighted imaging demonstrated intermediate-to-high signal intensity, which supported a diagnosis of an exudative content (**B**). Based on these findings, effusive constrictive pericarditis was diagnosed. Subsequent surgical exploration confirmed a bloody pericardial effusion with diffusely inflamed but normal thickness pericardium. No pathogen or malignancy was identified from any fluid culture in this case.

Pericardial Constriction

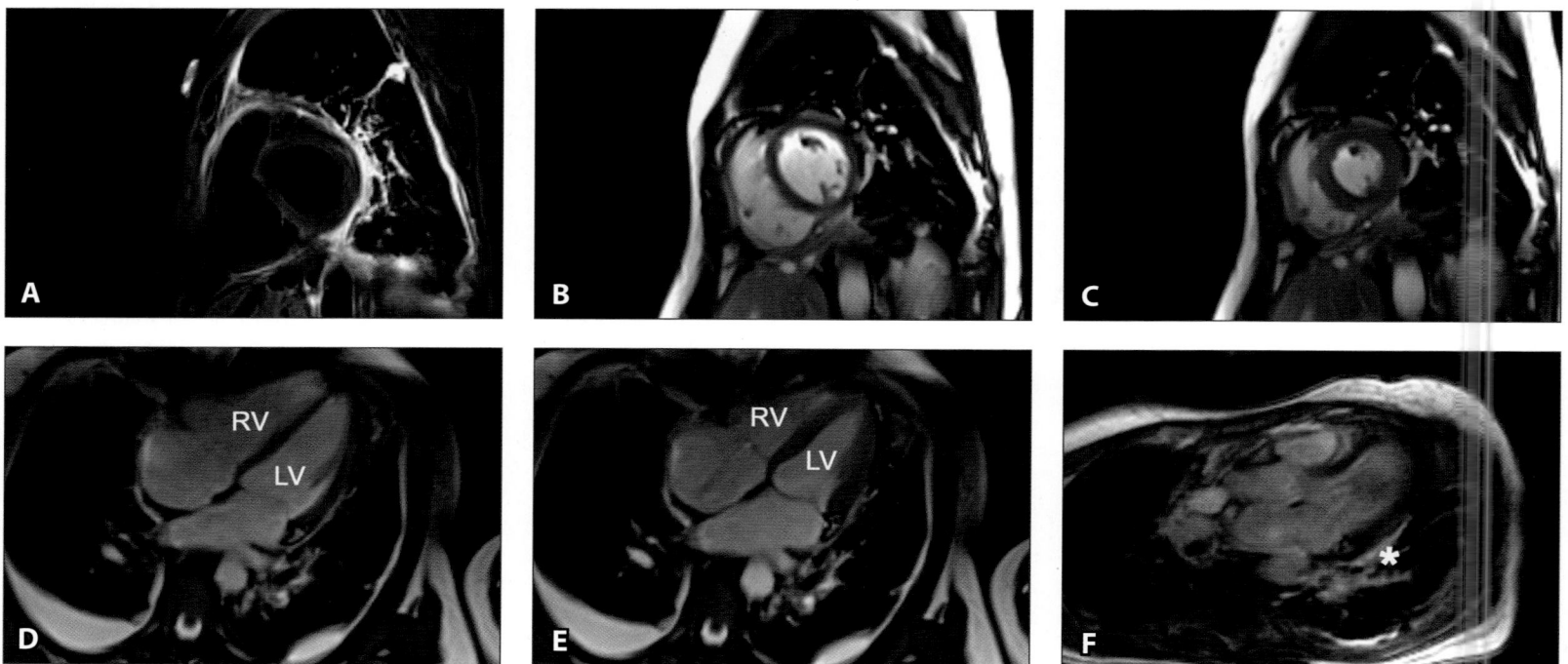

Figure 16-12. A 53-year-old woman presented with progressive dyspnea of 2-month duration. She had a history of Hodgkin's lymphoma treated with radiation, rheumatoid arthritis, and acute pericarditis, requiring pericardiectomy for cardiac tamponade, 10 years before this presentation. **A,** Marked adhesion of the pericardium to the adjacent pulmonary parenchyma. In **A, B, C, D,** and **E,** both ventricles were small in cavity size and there was marked bilateral atrial dilatation suggestive of abnormal diastolic filling. Marked concordant motion was noticed in the adjacent liver and lung tissues during systolic contraction. The right ventricle (RV) was tubular in shape during diastole, which was consistent with diastolic pericardial constriction (**D**). After contrast injection, late gadolinium enhancement imaging revealed marked fibrosis of the posterior aspects of the pericardial sac and adhesions formation with the adjacent pulmonary tissues (*asterisk* in **F**). There was bilateral pleural effusion (**D** and **E**).

Hypertrophic Cardiomyopathy

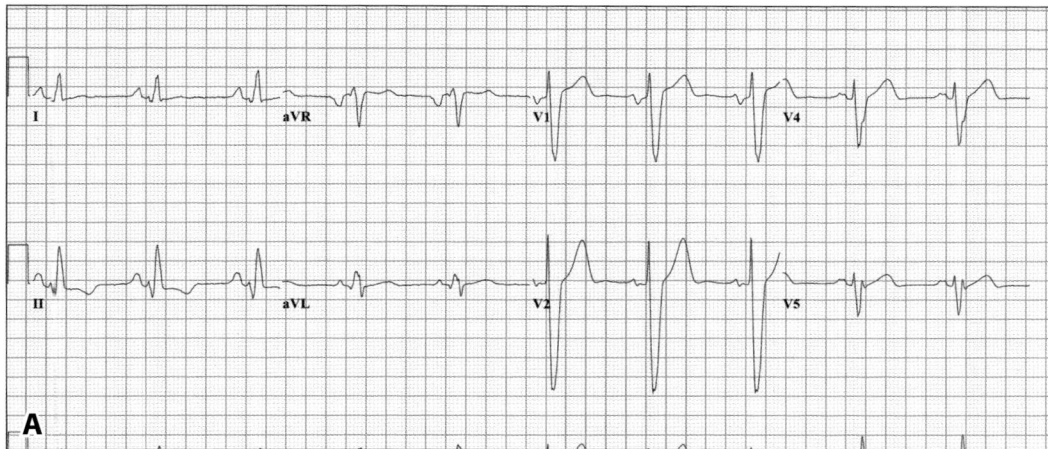

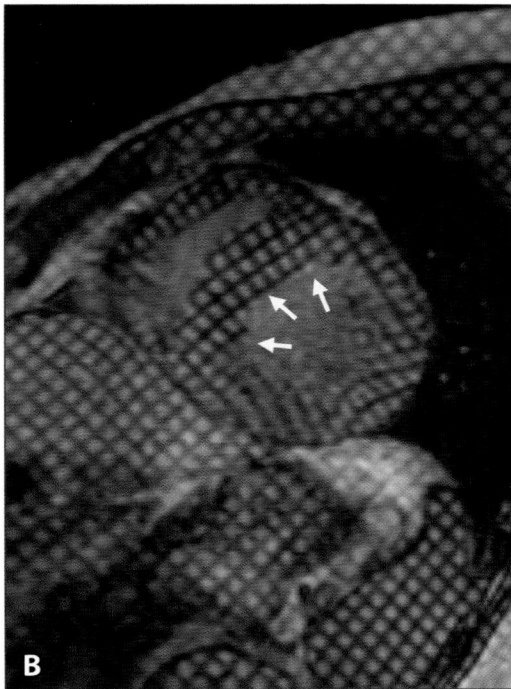

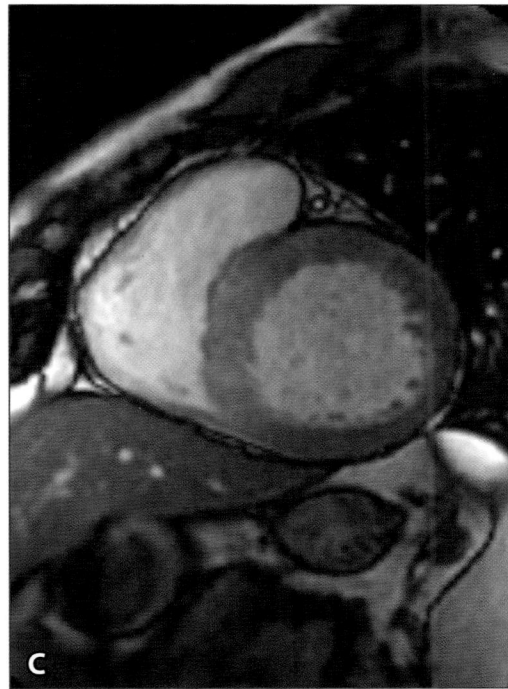

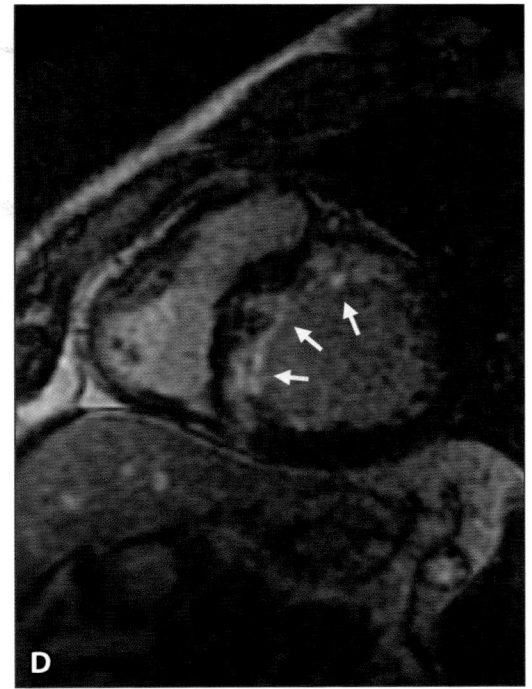

Figure 16-13. A 35-year-old lawyer with a strong family history of cardiac disease presented for assessment of an abnormal echocardiogram (ECG) and screening for hypertrophic cardiomyopathy (HCM). He had a strong family history of HCM in which his father, sister, and one of his paternal cousins died at a relatively young age. Genetic studies of other family members confirmed missense mutation of the β-myosin heavy chain disease, which was inherited in an autosomal dominant pattern. His resting ECG (**A**) demonstrated a left bundle branch block.

B and **C,** Cine short-axis functional imaging of the heart (tagged and cine steady-state free precession, respectively). In this myocardial tagging technique demonstrated in **B,** the grid lines represent tagged labeling of the myocardium at the beginning of systole. The tagging can be tracked throughout the rest of the cardiac cycle. **C** demonstrates a mildly dilated left ventricle (LV; 138 mL/m², normal < 112 mL/m²) with concentric hypertrophy of the LV but reduced left ventricular ejection fraction (LVEF) at 40%. LV mass was quantified to be 106 g/m² (normal < 83 g/m² for men). As demonstrated in **D,** in the segments with the most degree of segmental hypertrophy, there is extensive late gadolinium enhancement (LGE) with inhomogeneous signal intensity, which is consistent with myocardial fibrosis as a result of extensive myofibril disarray. **B,** A tagged image at end-systole. While there is no abnormality by systolic radial thickening seen on the cine steady-state free precession image on **C,** there is absence of systolic strain in the segments with extensive LGE, in contrast to the segments without LGE (*see* Ch. 6).

Apical Hypertrophic Cardiomyopathy

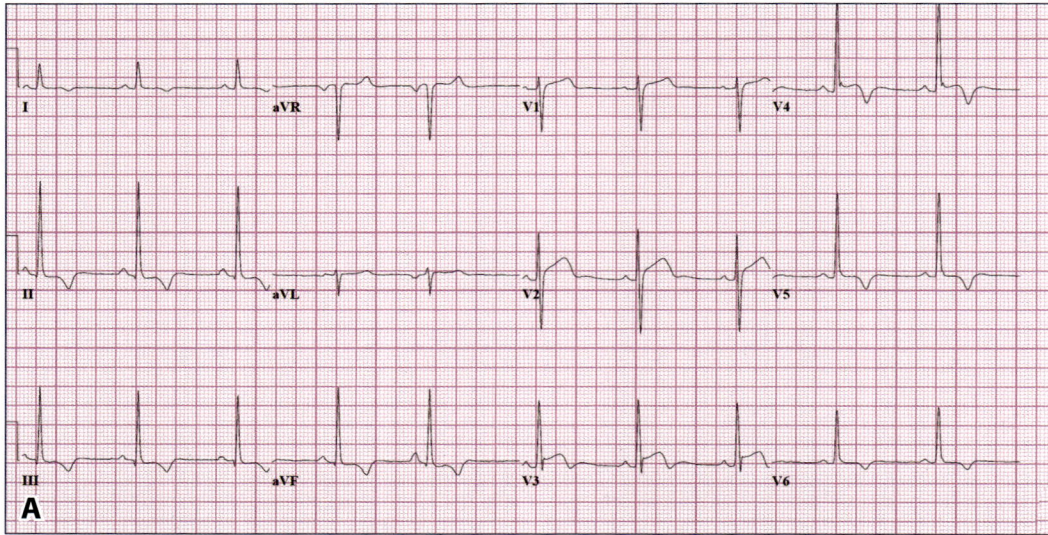

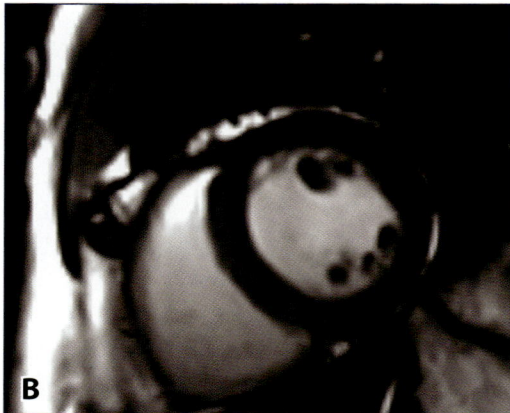

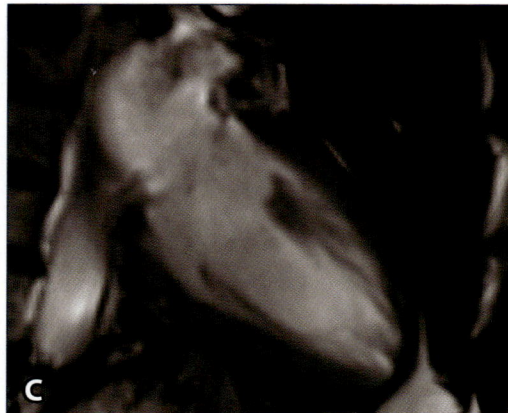

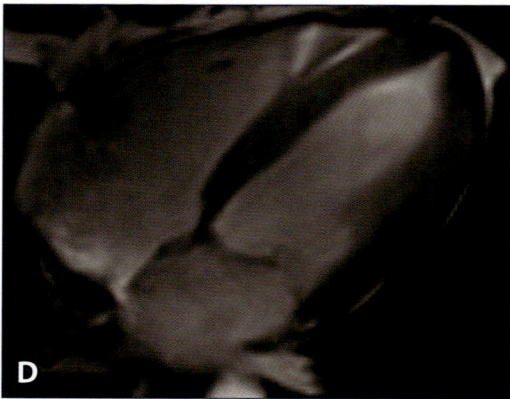

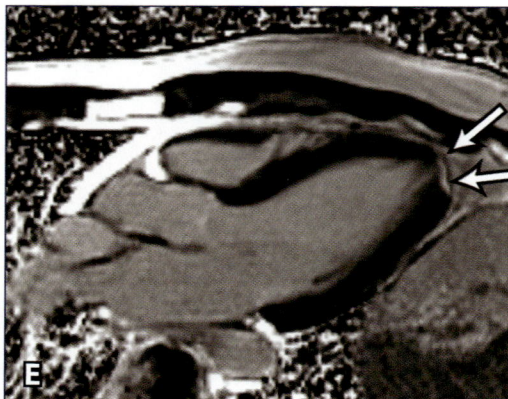

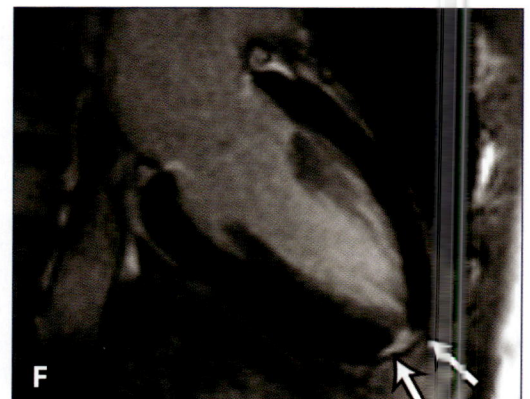

Figure 16-14. A 49-year-old male presented with recurrent dizziness during exertion for several years and a recent episode of syncope while playing tennis. On initial workup, he was found to have an abnormal echocardiogram with T-wave inversion of the anterolateral precordial leads and the inferior leads (**A**). These findings are suspicious for apical hypertrophic cardiomyopathy and cardiac magnetic resonance was referred. While the left ventricular (LV) mass is normal with normal systolic global function (**B** and **C**), the LV displays a spade-shape during systole, which is consistent with apical hypertrophy (**D**). After administration of gadolinium diethylene triamine pentaacetic acid contrast, there is late gadolinium enhancement of the LV apical cap, which suggests apical scar (**E** and **F**; *see* Ch. 6).

Left Ventricular Noncompaction

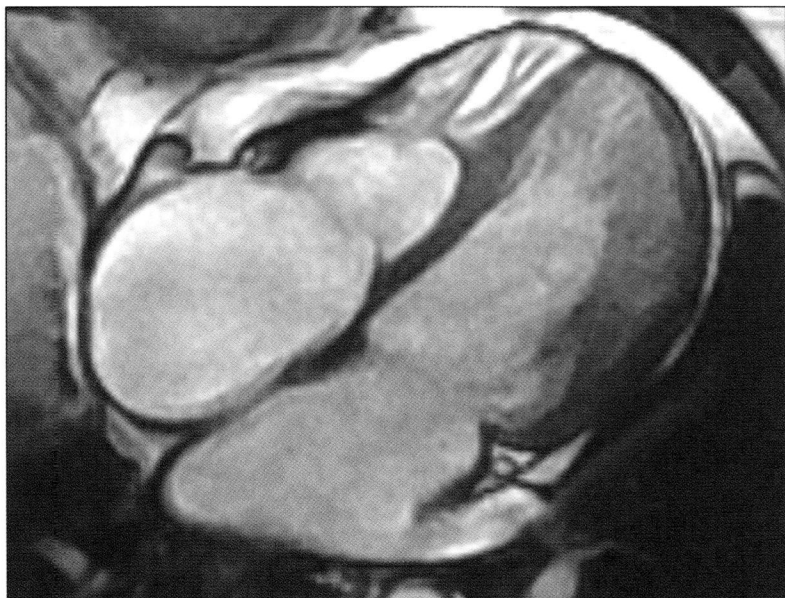

Figure 16-15. A 56-year-old male with a remote history of atrial septal defect repair and radiofrequency ablation of atrial flutter presented with new onset congestive heart failure. His left ventricular ejection fraction (LVEF) was quantified to be 25% with moderate LV dilatation. Cine cardiac magnetic resonance (CMR) demonstrated spongiform lateral wall of the LV. Current studies have suggested a noncompacted versus compacted (NC/C) ratio may differentiate pathological LV noncompaction from other causes of dilated cardiomyopathy. In a case-control cohort study, Petersen *et al.* [21] reported an NC/C ratio of more than 2:3 in diastole distinguished pathological noncompaction, with values for sensitivity, specificity, and positive and negative predictive values of 86%, 99%, 75%, and 99%, respectively.

Arrhythmogenic Right Ventricular Dysplasia

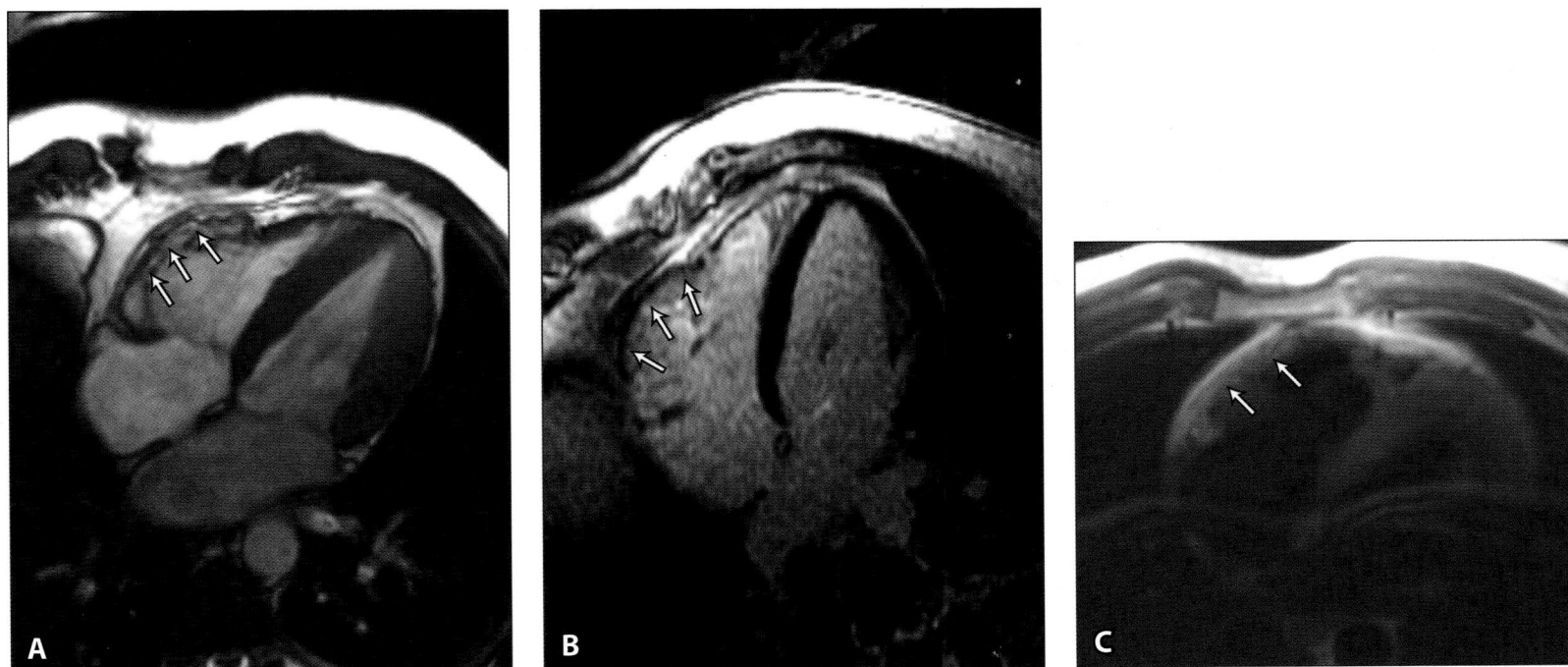

Figure 16-16. A 40-year-old man presented with recurrent near-syncope at rest. He reported a strong family history of sudden death in which his brother died suddenly at 35 years old. The patient has no cardiac risk factors and was referred to undergo cardiac magnetic resonance for assessment of arrhythmogenic right ventricular dysplasia (ARVD). **A,** Despite the RV global function being normal (RV ejection fraction, 47%), the basal RV was markedly thickened and was aneurysmal (systolic frame of a four-chamber cine view, note the hinge point at the mid-RV free wall). **B** and **C,** Late gadolinium enhancement imaging and double-inversion recovery fast-spin echo imaging of the matching four-chamber view. In addition to the aneurysmal morphology and dyskinesia of the right ventricular basal free wall, there is evidence of fibrosis (**B,** *arrows*) and fatty infiltration (**C,** *arrows*) in this corresponding RV segment (*see* Ch. 7).

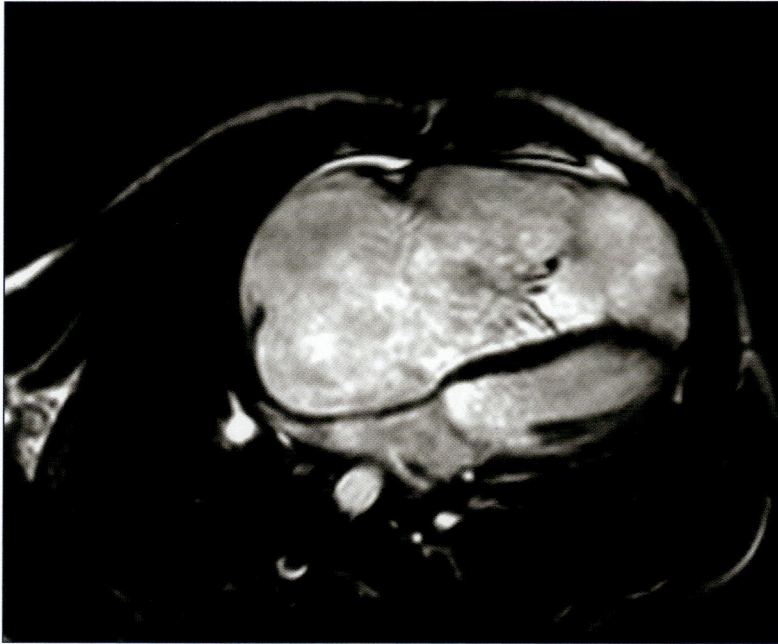

Figure 16-17. Case 1. An 18-year-old male with a history of congenital heart disease presents with recent worsening dyspnea on exertion and peripheral edema. This figure demonstrates the systolic frame of a cine steady-state free precession imaging of the four-chamber view. Note that there is severe anomaly of the tricuspid valve (TV) with resultant tricuspid regurgitation (TR). The septal leaflet of the TV is apically displaced 5 cm into the cavity of the right ventricle (RV). The right atrium (RA) is severely enlarged. These findings are diagnostic of Ebstein's anomaly.

By comparing the systolic flow volume across the pulmonary artery and the right ventricular stroke volume, the regurgitant fraction of the TV was 75%. Using quantitative methods, the RV was severely dilated at 285 mL/m² and the RV ejection fraction was moderately depressed at 33%. There is abnormal diastolic septal motion, which is consistent with markedly elevated right-sided volume overload. There is no evidence of atrial septal defect. By contrast-enhanced magnetic resonance angiography technique there is no coexisting anomaly of the pulmonary venous anatomy (*see* Ch. 10). (*Courtesy of* Dr. Tal Geva, Children's Hospital, Boston, MA).

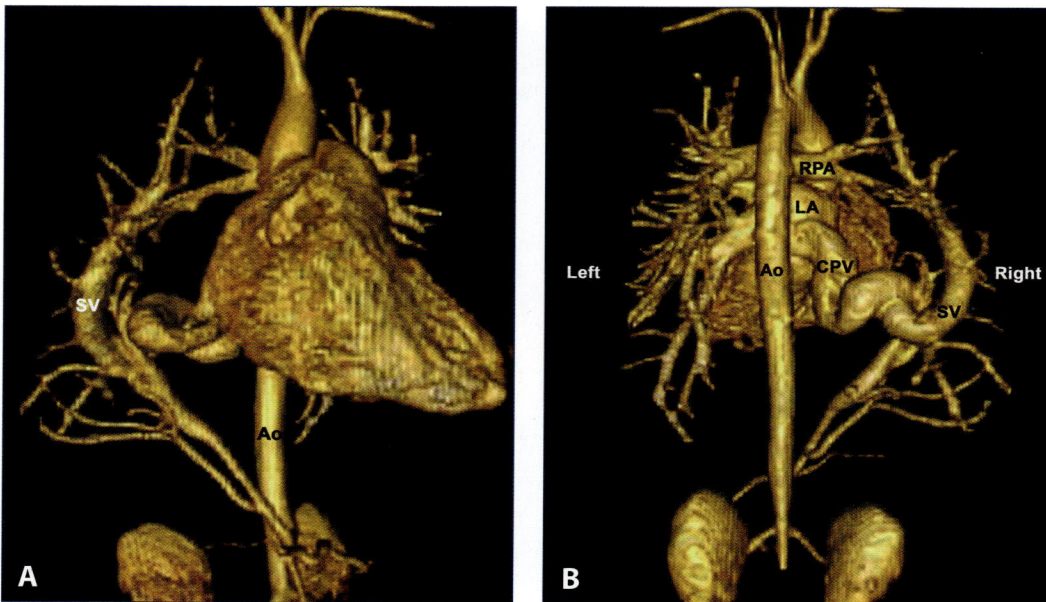

Figure 16-18. Case 2. A 17-year-old male with recurrent right lower-lobe pneumonia was referred for assessment of congenital heart disease. An antero-posterior coronal view of a three-dimensional (3D) magnetic resonance angiogram (MRA) (**A**) shows abnormal venous drainage of the right lung from both the right upper and middle lobes. These anomalous right-sided pulmonary veins joined together in forming a crescent-shaped pulmonary vein that assumes the shape of a scimitar and is thus termed *a scimitar vein* (SV). **B,** A postero-anterior coronal view of this 3D MRA. In this view, the SV was seen to join the pulmonary venous drainage from the right lower lobe and formed a single common pulmonary vein. The right lung is hypoplastic and the right pulmonary artery (RPA) could be seen in **B** to be hypoplastic. Most often in Scimitar syndrome, the anomalous right-sided pulmonary veins drain into the inferior vena cava causing a left-to-right shunt. In this case, the common pulmonary vein (CPV) drained into the left atrium (LA) directly and, by phase-contrast flow analysis, the pulmonary to asystemic flow ratio was therefore not elevated at 0.8 (*see* Ch. 00).

Acknowledgment

We are grateful for the expert assistance from Dr. Otavio Coelho in post-processing the images in the chapter.

References

1. Kellman P, Arai AE, McVeigh ER, Aletras AH: Phase-sensitive inversion recovery for detecting myocardial infarction using gadolinium-delayed hyperenhancement. *Magn Reson Med* 2002, 47:372–383.

2. Kellman P, Chung YC, Simonetti OP, *et al.*: Multi-contrast delayed enhancement provides improved contrast between myocardial infarction and blood pool. *J Magn Reson Imaging* 2005, 22:605–613.

3. Kim RJ, Fieno DS, Parrish TB, *et al.*: Relationship of MRI delayed contrast enhancement to irreversible injury, infarct age, and contractile function. *Circulation* 1999, 100:1992–2002.

4. Klem I, Heitner JF, Shah DJ, *et al.*: Improved detection of coronary artery disease by stress perfusion cardiovascular magnetic resonance with the use of delayed enhancement infarction imaging. *J Am Coll Cardiol* 2006, 47:1630–1638.

5. Ricciardi MJ, Wu E, Davidson CJ, *et al.*: Visualization of discrete microinfarction after percutaneous coronary intervention associated with mild creatine kinase-MB elevation. *Circulation* 2001, 103:2780–2783.

6. Wu E, Judd RM, Vargas JD, *et al.*: Visualisation of presence, location, and transmural extent of healed Q-wave and non-Q-wave myocardial infarction. *Lancet* 2001, 357:21–28.

7. Selvanayagam JB, Cheng AS, Jerosch-Herold M, *et al.*: Effect of distal embolization on myocardial perfusion reserve after percutaneous coronary intervention: a quantitative magnetic resonance perfusion study. *Circulation* 2007, 116:1458–1464.

8. Kwong RY, Chan AK, Brown KA, *et al.*: Impact of unrecognized myocardial scar detected by cardiac magnetic resonance imaging on event-free survival in patients presenting with signs or symptoms of coronary artery disease. *Circulation* 2006, 113:2733–2743.

9. Schwitter J, Nanz D, Kneifel S, *et al.*: Assessment of myocardial perfusion in coronary artery disease by magnetic resonance: a comparison with positron emission tomography and coronary angiography. *Circulation* 2001, 103:2230–2235.

10. Nagel E, Klein C, Paetsch I, *et al.*: Magnetic resonance perfusion measurements for the noninvasive detection of coronary artery disease. *Circulation* 2003, 108:432–437.

11. Schwitter J, Wacker CM, van Rossum AC, *et al.*: MR-IMPACT: comparison of perfusion-cardiac magnetic resonance with single-photon emission computed tomography for the detection of coronary artery disease in a multicentre, multivendor, randomized trial. *Eur Heart J* 2008, 29:480–489.

12. Kwong RY, Rekhraj S, Schussheim AE, *et al.*: Urgent assessment of emergency room chest pain patients with non-diagnostic electrocardiogram with adenosine stress magnetic resonance imaging. Presented at the American Heart Association Scientific Session. Anaheim, CA; November 14, 2001.

13. Ingkanisorn WP, Kwong RY, Bohme NS, *et al.*: Prognosis of negative adenosine stress magnetic resonance in patients presenting to an emergency department with chest pain. *J Am Coll Cardiol* 2006, 47:1427–1432.

14. Bodi V, Sanchis J, Lopez-Lereu MP, *et al.*: Prognostic value of dipyridamole stress cardiovascular magnetic resonance imaging in patients with known or suspected coronary artery disease. *J Am Coll Cardiol* 2007, 50:1174–1179.

15. Jahnke C, Nagel E, Gebker R, *et al.*: Prognostic value of cardiac magnetic resonance stress tests: adenosine stress perfusion and dobutamine stress wall motion imaging. *Circulation* 2007, 115:1769–1776.

16. Peters DC, Wylie JV, Hauser TH, *et al.*: Detection of pulmonary vein and left atrial scar after catheter ablation with three-dimensional navigator-gated delayed enhancement MR imaging: initial experience. *Radiology* 2007, 243:690–695.

17. Wylie JV Jr, Peters DC, Essebag V, *et al.*: Left atrial function and scar after catheter ablation of atrial fibrillation. *Heart Rhythm* 2008, 5:656–662.

18. Mahrholdt H, Goedecke C, Wagner A, *et al.*: Cardiovascular magnetic resonance assessment of human myocarditis: a comparison to histology and molecular pathology. *Circulation* 2004, 109:1250–1258.

19. Wagner A, Mahrholdt H, Thomson L, *et al.*: Effects of time, dose, and inversion time for acute myocardial infarct size measurements based on magnetic resonance imaging-delayed contrast enhancement. *J Am Coll Cardiol* 2006, 47:2027–2033.

20. Silva C, Moon JC, Elkington AG, *et al.*: Myocardial late gadolinium enhancement in specific cardiomyopathies by cardiovascular magnetic resonance: a preliminary experience. *J Cardiovasc Med (Hagerstown)* 2007, 8:1076–1079.

21. Petersen SE, Selvanayagam JB, Wiesmann F, *et al.*: Left ventricular non-compaction: insights from cardiovascular magnetic resonance imaging. *J Am Coll Cardiol* 2005, 46:101–105.

Index

Matrix metalloproteinase, 5
Mechanical assist devices, 119
Medina bifurcation lesion classification, 279
Medtronic Driver coronary stent, 273
Medtronic prosthetic aortic valve, 228
Metabolic syndrome, 16
Minimally invasive direct coronary artery bypass, 67
Mitral annular calcification, 346
Mitral leaflet systolic anterior motion, 124
Mitral prolapse, 299
Mitral regurgitation, 124, 221–225, 299
Mitral stenosis, 220–221
Mitral valve repair, 221, 224–225
Monocyte chemoattractant protein-1 deficiency, 2–3
Multidetector computed tomography, 347, 352, 354
Muscular dystrophy, 136–137
Myocardial fiber disarray, 124
Myocardial infarction
    cardiac magnetic resonance imaging in, 359–362
    definitions of, 26
    echocardiographic assessment of, 304
    implantable cardioverter-defibrillator after, 34
    management algorithms for, 36–37
    mechanical complications of, 33
    pharmacotherapy after, 31, 35–37
    radionuclide imaging in, 330–331, 337
    remodeling after, 30
    reperfusion after, 25, 27–30
    right ventricular, 32
    risk factors and, 12
    sequence of changes after, 24
    shock in, 32
    smoking cessation after, 13
    ST-segment elevation, 26–30
    transport options after, 28
Myocardial ischemia.
    See also Ischemic heart disease
    angina from, 41
    neuronal damage in, 337
    pathogenesis of, 331
Myocardial necrosis, 24–26
Myocardial oxygen requirement, 41
Myocardial perfusion
    positron emission tomography of, 329
    scintigraphy of, 325
    single photon emission computed tomography of, 328–330
Myocardial salvage
    reperfusion in, 25
Myocardial strain echocardiography, 311
Myocardial stunning, 332
Myocarditis, 138–143

diagnosis of, 139, 142–143, 368
    natural history and survival in, 140–142
    pathogenesis of, 138
    pathology of, 138–139, 141
Myocytes, 95, 333
Myofibers, 123

N

Natriuretic peptide, 97–98
Neuronal damage, 337
Nitrates, 58, 109, 112
Nuclear cardiology, 315–340.
    See also specific techniques
    computed tomography angiography versus, 351
    overview of, 315
Nutritional-hygienic therapy, 202

O

Obesity, 17
Off-pump coronary artery bypass grafting, 67

P

Pacing
    for cardiac resynchronization therapy, 185–187
    equipment and modes for, 184–185
    in heart failure, 114–115
Patent ductus arteriosus, 236
Percutaneous coronary intervention, 269–286
    after myocardial infarction, 27–30
    coronary artery bypass grafting versus, 65, 68
    hemodynamic support for, 284–286
    high-risk, 284–286
    history of, 29
    in-stent restenosis in, 275–276, 282
    invasive lesion assessment in, 270–272
    lesion subsets in, 278–283
    medical therapy versus, 64
    outcomes of, 29
    response to injury in, 269–270
    stent designs in, 272–275
    stent thrombosis in, 276–278
Percutaneous mitral valve repair, 221, 225
Perfusion-metabolism mismatch study, 334
Pericardial constriction, 370
Pericardial effusion, 146
Pericarditis, 144, 145–147
Peripheral artery disease, 71–75
Pheochromocytoma, 201–202
Physical activity in adolescents, 18
Physical inactivity, 17–18

Plaque
    atherosclerotic. See Atherosclerotic plaque
Platelet activation and aggregation, 34–35
Pleural effusion, 146
Port-access coronary artery bypass grafting, 66
Positron emission tomography
    after cardiac transplantation, 338
    in angina, 335
    in cardiomyopathy, 323, 334
    computed tomography angiography and, 340, 349
    in perfusion-metabolism mismatch, 334
    principles and imaging planes of, 315–319
    stress, 51, 329
Potassium, 191, 199–200
Potassium-sparing diuretics, 102
Pregnancy, 207
Preload-reducing drugs, 112
Primum atrial septal defect, 234
Proinflammatory pathways, 6
Prosthetic cardiac valves, 227–228
Pseudoaneurysms, 33
Pulmonary arterial hypertension
    idiopathic, 247, 263–265
    from pulmonary embolism, 258
    in sickle cell disease, 306
Pulmonary artery catheterization, 113
Pulmonary embolism, 252–255
    diagnosis of, 252–254, 308
    overview of, 247
    pathophysiology of, 250
    risk stratification in, 254–255
    therapy for, 256–261
Pulmonary stenosis, 237
Pulmonary thromboendarterectomy, 258
Pulmonic valve morphology, 303–304

Q

QRS complex, 161, 171

R

Radiation doses
    from computed tomography angiography, 350–351
Radiofrequency ablation of atrial fibrillation, 167, 368
Radionuclide-based imaging, 315–340.
    See also specific techniques
    in myocardial infarction, 330
Ramipril, 211
Reentry arrhythmias, 153–165
Relapsing idiopathic pericarditis, 145
Remodeling
    after myocardial infarction, 30
    in heart failure, 93–94, 107

W